MEDICAL RADIOLOGY
Radiation Oncology

Editors:
L.W. Brady, Philadelphia
H.-P. Heilmann, Hamburg
M. Molls, Munich
C. Nieder, Bodø

D1722041

J. J. Lu · L. W. Brady (Eds.)

Radiation Oncology
An Evidence-Based Approach

With Contributions by

A. A. Abitbol · R. R. Allison · B. Amendola · M. F. Back · J. J. Beitler · M. Biagioli · E. B. Butler
J. S. Butler · L. W. Brady · M. Chadha · A. Y. Chen · W-J. Chng · W. H. Choi · H. T. Chung
J. S. Cooper · B. R. Donahue · S. Fu · H. A. Gay · I. C. Gibbs · S. C. Han · L. B. Harrison
G. F. Hatoum · J. M. Herman · D. Hristov · K. Hu · B. J. Huth · A. J. Khan · F-M. Kong
L. Kong · K. LaFave · E. M. Landau · K. M. Lee · N. Lee · Y. Li · J. J. Lu · A. M. Markoe
V. K. Mehta · S. Mutyala · R. Ove · A. C. Paulino · T. M. Pawlik · J. A. Peñagarícano
C. L. Perkins · V. Ratanatharathorn · S. G. Soltys · M. M. Spierer · C. Takita · B. S. Teh
B-C. Wen · A. H. Wolfson · X. Wu · L. Xing · T. E. Yaeger · Q. Zhang · Z. Zhang

Foreword by

L. W. Brady · H.-P. Heilmann · M. Molls · C. Nieder

Introduction by J. J. Lu and L. W. Brady

With 150 Figures in 219 Separate Illustrations, 176 in Color and 147 Tables

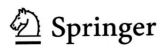 Springer

Jiade J. Lu, MD, MBA
Associate Professor and Consultant
Department of Radiation Oncology
National University Cancer Institute of Singapore
National University Health System
National University of Singapore
5 Lower Kent Ridge Road
Singapore 119074
Singapore
and
Distinguished Clinical Professor
Department of Radiation Oncology
Cancer Hospital of Fudan University
270 Dong An Road
Shanghai 200232
P. R. China

Luther W. Brady, MD
Hylda Cohn/American Cancer Society
Professor of Clinical Oncology, and
Professor, Department of Radiation Oncology
Distinguished University Professor
Drexel University, College of Medicine
Broad & Vine Sts., Mail Stop 200
Philadelphia, PA 19102-1192
USA

Medical Radiology · Diagnostic Imaging and Radiation Oncology
Series Editors:
A. L. Baert · L. W. Brady · H.-P. Heilmann · M. Knauth · M. Molls · C. Nieder

Continuation of Handbuch der medizinischen Radiologie
Encyclopedia of Medical Radiology

ISBN 978-3-642-09603-7   e-ISBN 978-3-540-77385-6

DOI 10.1007

Medical Radiology · Diagnostic Imaging and Radiation Oncology

© 2010, Springer-Verlag Berlin Heidelberg

Cover-Design and Layout: PublishingServices Teichmann, 69256 Mauer, Germany

Printed on acid-free paper – 21/3180xq
9 8 7 6 5 4 3 2 1

springer.com

Foreword

For the past ten years there have been significant scientific advances in biological sciences and healthcare. At the same time, there has been increased accountability and, in some instances, attempts to ration services as a mechanism to accomplish this. Although arbitrary clinical practice guidelines have been published, more rational bases to define optimal healthcare should be based on the identification of innovative approaches, outcome analysis in properly designed clinical trials, and careful assessment of current practice based on solid and creditable clinical research and evidence based decision making in medicine. The growth in basic and translational research data offers a guide to medical practice and is essential for the clinician to appraise and use published evidence for medical decisions. Evidence based medicine exemplifies the effect of teaching clinicians to evaluate research data by methodologic standards and to critically appraise published evidence from both a scientific and sociocultural perspective. Physicians are trained to maintain high standards of critical consciousness in methodologic domains, but not necessarily in the broader historic sociocultural domains surrounding them.

It is important for those practicing evidence based medicine to take full advantage of their encounters with patients, where the questions and answers that may arise can lead to providing the patient with the best available medical care. Appropriate and relevant clinical questions relate to the patient and the problem, to intervention, to a comparison intervention, and to outcome.

The present volume is specifically aimed at the utilization of evidence based medicine in outcome from radiation oncology. It stands as a significant and important standard by which all programs in management can be judged.

Philadelphia
Hamburg
Munich
Bodø

LUTHER W. BRADY
HANS-PETER HEILMANN
MICHAEL MOLLS
CARSTEN NIEDER

Introduction

JIADE J. LU and LUTHER W. BRADY

The practice of radiation oncology constantly involves decision making. Everyday, radiation oncologists are challenged with evaluating diagnostic and therapeutic options for cancer patients, and making decisions together with patients to ensure the best treatment of their disease. Historically, clinical experience and summarized expert knowledge served as important bases of medical practice. The rationales of medical decision making include those made in cancer management based largely on pathologic and physiologic rationales. The ability of physicians to provide effective medical care and rational decision making has long been assumed the valuable product of experience and expertise. When personal experience or understanding is lacking, clinicians usually turn to experts in the field for their opinions, or seek knowledge from textbooks.

While personal experience and expertise, as well as summarized knowledge, are valuable in providing references for daily practice in medicine, experience gained from physiologic/pathologic rationale-oriented practice faces several important pitfalls. One of the most concerning issues is the reliability of such practice, and decisions made according to the "obvious" situation according to our understanding of a disease (the perception of a physician) may not produce an effective outcome. Consistency of practice is another issue in empirical medicine, and close observation of the actual practices has demonstrated that even experienced physicians are likely to be unsystematic and inconsistent in medical decision making. Wide variations in patient care that are not related to differences in patients' preference, availability of treatment technology, or specific individual scenarios are often observed.

A recent example that illustrates the insufficiency of the pathologic/pathologic rationale in decision making is the concurrent use of erythropoietin with radiation therapy. It is well recognized that radiation is more effective against cancer cells with higher oxygen concentration. It has been demonstrated that the treatment outcome in patients with head and neck cancer or cervical cancer with high hemoglobin levels, for example, are superior to those with severe anemia during radiation therapy. While the efficacy of erythropoietin has been repeatedly demonstrated in patients with cancer or chemotherapy-induced anemia, it is reasonable to postulate that an increased hemoglobin level induced by erythropoietin may also improve outcome after radiation therapy. Based on this rationale, clinical trials were initiated to study whether correction of anemia during radiation therapy using certain drugs "should" improve the outcome. However, to the surprise of most researchers, although a reliable rise in hemoglobin concentration was observed with the use of medication, no benefit in local control, disease-free survival, and overall survival rates were observed when the medication was used concurrently with radiation therapy. In actual fact, treatment of anemia using erythropoietin during radiotherapy may impair tumor control, rather than improve the effectiveness of radiation (HENKE et al. 2003).

This example demonstrated the insufficiency of physiologic and pathologic reasoning to provide expected results, but also argued that experience and expertise were not reliable for preventing the mistreatment of patients. Since the detrimental effects of the medication on disease control was not always apparent immediately after the use of the medication, a cause–effect relationship could not be readily established. Accumulated experience in medical practice tends to be less systemic and may not be useful for recognizing cause–effect relationships typified above, especially when the time interval between the root cause and the effect is relatively protracted.

What Is Evidence-Based Medicine?

It is generally accepted that effective disease management and medical decision making rely on the best available scientific evidence, in combination with the clinician's experience and patients' preferences. The most common question posed upon hearing the term evidence-based medicine is: "Isn't that what we always do?" Many physicians, including radiation oncologists, may claim that clinical evidence is always incorporated in their practice. It is very true that much progress has been made in clinical research, and that medical decision making based on the results of scientific studies has increasingly prevailed; however, simply citing or using some research results is insufficient for effective clinical decision making and, alone, is far from evidence-based medical practice.

The Triad of Evidence-Based Medicine

Evidence-based medicine aims to utilize scientifically obtained evidence for medical practice and is defined as the conscientious, explicit, and judicious use of current best evidence in making decisions about the care of individual patients (SACKETT et al. 1996). It involves integrating the best available scientific evidence from systematic research on patients' condition, value, and expectations, as well as the attending physician's expertise in clinical decision making.

Although scientific evidence is one of the most important elements of evidence-based medicine (and effective medical practice requires routine application of the best evidence in patient care), a fundamental principle of evidence-based medicine is that evidence alone, even when obtained through systemic and exhaustive research, is not sufficient for effective clinical decision making. Systemically reviewed clinical evidence must be integrated with patients' expectations and value, together with clinical expertise. Effective decision making in medical practice requires the application of all three elements of evidence-based medicine (Fig. 1).

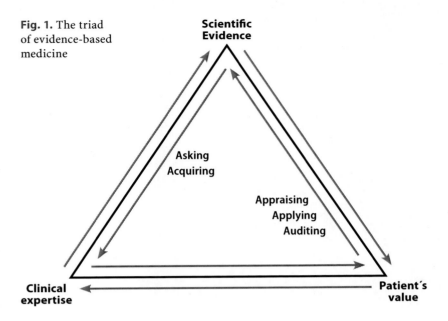

Fig. 1. The triad of evidence-based medicine

Hierarchy of Evidence

As scientific evidence plays a major role in the learning and practice of evidence-based medicine, it is necessary to briefly clarify the meaning of evidence in this context. The Cambridge dictionary defines "evidence" as anything that helps to prove that something is or is not true. This simple definition can be applied to clinical evidence of any specialty in medicine, including radiation oncology. Results obtained from basic science, animal, translational, as well as clinical research can all be used as medical evidence. Furthermore, observations made in the clinician's daily practice are also considered clinical evidence.

However, not all evidence in medicine is created equal, and not all evidence can be, or should be, used in decision making in patient care. The quality, i.e., the validity, relevance, and importance of clinical evidence differ significantly. Evidence-based medicine seeks to assess the quality of scientific evidence relevant to the risks and benefits of treatment (or in many cases, lack of treatment), with the purpose of improving the health of patients by means of decisions that will maximize patients' quality of life and life span. Merely applying study results without critical appraisal may not only be less useful, but potentially harmful or dangerous to patients.

Evidence used in any clinical decision making process can be categorized according to its quality based on the probability of freedom from error, and is usually classified by critical appraisal. The following four aspects are the most basic of critical appraisal: relevance, validity, consistency, and significance of the results. The quality of evidence can be differentiated according to those elements of quality.

In a simple sense, the quality of evidence, specifically its validity, can be differentiated according to the nature of the evidence. For a specific topic, when all other factors are equal, meta-analyses and systemic reviews based on randomized clinical trials, as well as well-designed and -powered randomized clinical trials, are usually of superior quality than retrospective series. Figure 2 is a simplified illustration of the quality of clinical evidence. However, it is important to remember that quality also depends on the relevance and importance of the evidence, and such factors depend largely on specific clinical scenarios.

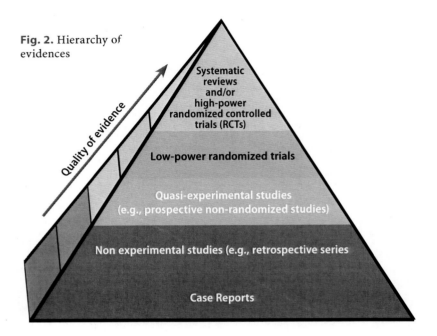

Fig. 2. Hierarchy of evidences

The "5As" Practice of Evidence-Based Medicine

Radiation oncology is an ever-changing field. With the development of new technology and treatment techniques, the management of cancer using ionizing or particle radiation is evolving on a monthly, if not daily, basis. Like any other forms of therapy, applying newly developed radiation techniques (such as imaging-guided radiation therapy and particle therapy) or treatment strategies (such as combined chemoradiotherapy) to a particular type of malignancy, or applying existing treatment techniques proven for one type of disease to a different type of cancer, requires vigorous testing and verification before it can be called standard. As a result, the field of radiation oncology is flooded with publications and literature.

While it is encouraging to observe the exponential growth in scientific research papers and literature published in this field, it is important to recognize that evaluating and understanding the scientific evidence in order that one can utilize it in decision making requires proficient skills and knowledge of evidence-based medicine, as well as sufficient time and effort.

Scientific evidence is one of the three integral parts of evidence-based medical practice; thus, understanding and being able to apply pertinent and best-available evidence for a particular clinical question is crucial in the practice of evidence-based medicine in radiation oncology. To achieve this purpose, the following five key steps (the "5As" cycle) should be considered sequentially (Fig. 3):

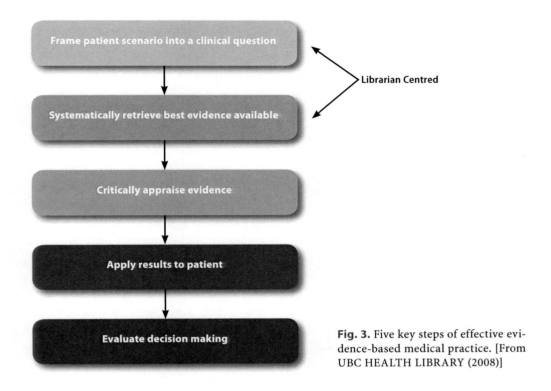

Fig. 3. Five key steps of effective evidence-based medical practice. [From UBC HEALTH LIBRARY (2008)]

1. Formulating a clinical question (Asking)
2. Acquiring relevant and complete information (Acquiring)
3. Critically appraising the quality (including validity and importance) of available evidence, or identifying the lack of evidence (Appraising)
4. Applying the knowledge in the clinical management of patients (Applying)
5. Evaluating the results of practice (Auditing)

A Strategy of Learning and Clinical Practice (Why Use Evidence-Based Medicine?)

Evidence-based medicine is probably more of a strategy of effective and efficient medical care than a scientific subject. The ultimate purpose of evidence-based medicine by practicing the "5As" cycle is to improve the quality of care for patients. However, clinical practice based on the essence of evidence-based medicine can also be used as a strategy of continuing medical education and professional development. Inevitably, physicians' knowledge deteriorates over time. The "5As" process of evidence-based medicine emphasizes a structural, systemic, and strategic search for and evaluation of evidence for questions encountered in daily clinical practice, to be used in decision making in patient management. Through such a process, clinicians and other health-care professionals continuously educate themselves and sharpen their knowledge.

Issues in the Practice of Evidence-Based Radiation Oncology

The basic principle of evidence-based medicine can largely be applied to any specialties in healthcare, including public health and policy making. However, specific issues encountered by clinicians in different specialties, including radiation oncologists, affect how they practice evidence-based medicine.

Formulating a Clinical Question in Oncology

Clinical questions encountered in the practice of radiation oncology are usually individualized based on the diagnoses, patients' medical conditions and preferences, as well as the availability of medical resources. However, as a disease category, cancer has been effectively categorized based on pathological diagnosis, differentiation, and staging. The value of the AJCC/UICC staging system on predicting outcome, thus facilitating the choice of treatment strategy for most types of cancers, has been repeatedly proven. In addition, with the development of molecular biology and genetics, other disease characteristics have been continuously discovered.

At the present time, a clinical question in cancer management can be formulated on the basis of pathologic diagnosis and cancer staging, combined with patients' characteristics and other disease-associated prognostic factors. For the purpose of knowledge development and learning, the clinical question of focus in the practice of evidence-based radiation oncology is usually "What is the most effective treatment of this malignancy at the current stage?"

Acquiring Relevant and Complete Information

Once the target question is formulated, the next step in the practice of evidence-based radiation oncology is to search for the relevant evidence. With the development of information technology and the Internet, obtaining an exhaustive amount of information through literature search using databases such as PubMed and ScienceDirect is no longer an issue. However, the problem that perturbs most practicing radiation oncologists is usually not insufficient, but rather excessive amounts of information of varying quality. While all professionals aim to keep abreast of developing research, differentiating the "relevant" and "complete" information from a flood of publications usually requires an enormous amount of time and effort, and is hardly achievable. It is usually not feasible for a clinician to find, read, and appraise all available evidence on his/her own. The time and effort needed to acquire and then crucially appraise information is currently an insurmountable obstacle standing between individual clinicians and the practice of evidence-based medicine, including radiation oncologists.

Evaluating the Quality of the Evidence

As mentioned previously, not all evidence is created equal. Much of the available evidence is not clinically relevant for decision making. The quality (i.e., validity and importance) of relevant and pertinent clinical evidence varies significantly. As the practice of evidence-based medicine involves the integration of the best available scientific evidence with expertise and patients' value in patient care, the critical appraisal of evidence obtained from systemically researched endeavor is crucial for identifying the best available and most relevant evidence.

To evaluate the quality of a piece of evidence, basic knowledge and skills in critical appraisal of medical publications are usually required. Often, formal training in literature research and review is necessary to attain proficiency in appraising scientific evidence. However, critical appraisal of scientific evidence is extremely time consuming and, as with the process of acquiring relevant and complete information, the time and effort required to critically appraise the literature comprises yet another insurmountable obstruction to the practice of evidence-based radiation oncology.

It is important for clinicians to understand that, in many instances, the only evidence available is of low quality. For example, the majority of available evidence used in guiding radiation therapy for rare tumors (such as cancer of the fallopian tube, cancer of urachus) are retrospective in nature. A lack of high-quality evidence does not preclude the feasibility of practicing evidence-based medicine in the treatment of these malignancies. One can always use the current best evidence after critical appraisal, bearing in mind that even the best is flawed.

Radiation Oncology: An Evidence-Based Approach

The traditional thoughts on evidence-based medicine described above emphasize searching the literature, appraising, and then summarizing search results with the focus on a particular clinical question. Although the basic understanding, required skills, and knowledge remain unchanged for the practice of evidence-based medicine, the process has gradually evolved with the increasing availability of sophisticated secondary information resources that differentiate and appraise high-quality evidence from the existing medical literature. The most direct product of an institutional exercise in evidence-based medicine is the development and utilization of protocolized diagnostic and treatment recommendations for a particular disease entity. In the field of clinical oncology, there is an increased use of guidelines or algorithms for disease management which have been developed by professional organizations. The Cancer Guidelines for Patients and Physicians developed by experts from the National Comprehensive Cancer Network (NCCN) is well known among clinical oncologists. In addition, the American Society of Clinical Oncology (ASCO) and the American Society of Therapeutic Radiology Oncology (ASTRO) also provide treatment recommendations for a number of malignancies or selected disease groups.

However, evidence-based medicine (including evidence-based radiation oncology) is a process of learning, developing, and practicing. The guidelines including the algorithms and pathways of diagnosis and treatment developed by NCCN, ASCO, or other professional organizations certainly provide crucial references to standardized and protocolized management of cancer. However, merely following the recommendations provided in the guidelines without knowing the underlying supporting evidence provides no benefit for acquiring new knowledge and expanding one's skill in cancer management. In other words, knowing "how" to practice does not equal knowing exactly "why" to practice in certain ways.

While the clinical question can be formulated on the basis of pathology, stage at diagnosis, as well as other prognostic factors of the disease and the patient, acquiring evidence in the field of radiation oncology is intricate, especially in an era when physicians are flooded with publications and information. Furthermore, the search for best evidence is especially difficult for clinicians in training due to insufficient search techniques and skills in critical appraisal of clinical evidence. Clinicians who are proficient in literature searches and appraisal may be impeded by the lack of time to update their knowledge and understanding of the new treatment techniques and strategies. In addition, healthcare professionals not trained in North America or Europe may experience both language and methodological difficulties.

Structured and Systemic Learning and Practice of Evidence-Based Radiation Oncology

The idea behind Radiation Oncology: An Evidence-Based Approach was formulated with the aim of facilitating the application of evidence-based medicine in radiation oncology and helping clinicians to utilize the best available medical evidence in their practice. The sole purpose of evidence-based radiation oncology is to improve the quality of cancer care through the utilization of the best available scientific evidence, in combination with clinicians' expertise and patients' value. The purpose of Radiation Oncology: An Evidence-Based Approach is to convey the knowledge gained in evidence-based radiation oncology, including the recommendations on cancer management and the supporting evidence in a simple, concise, efficient, and effective manner. It is not only a text for studying radiation oncology using an evidence-based approach, but also a practical reference for improving the quality of cancer care in daily practice.

Two of the most important tasks of this publication are: (1) to minimize the time and effort required of the reader to absorb and understand the pertinent knowledge, and (2) to maximize the opportunities to apply the knowledge in the daily practice of cancer care. As such, this publication was deliberately written and structured in a formulated fashion, and all entities were presented in a planned sequence: Recommendation and the grade of recommendation ("What" to do and the strength of recommendation) → Evidence and the level(s) of evidence ("Why" to do and the strength of the evidence) → Radiation therapy techniques ("How" to do and the detailed techniques). In addition, diagnosis and treatment algorithms were provided for the majority of commonly diagnosed malignancies.

Quality Control of a Quality-Improvement Endeavor

To ensure the quality of each topic included in Radiation Oncology: An Evidence-Based Approach, the project invited radiation oncologists with extensive experience in the field; many of the contributors have been responsible for developing the treatment standards in their subspecialties, including researchers of phase III randomized trials who have set the current management standard. Efforts were made to include scientific evidence of the highest quality. In addition, the results of clinical research from well-established multi-institutional study groups, such as RTOG, SWOG, ECOG, etc., were attributed the highest priority, and all evidence was critically appraised before its inclusion. Furthermore, personal opinions or institutional preferences were carefully avoided in the process of codification, and the grading of recommendations and evidence was reviewed by a second specialist, including one of the editors. For some entities provided in this publication where high-quality evidence is lacking (such as recommendations on follow-ups), recommendations were based on consensuses agreed upon by organizations such as the ASTRO expert panel, or other treatment guidelines such as NCCN.

The quality of clinical evidence and recommendations for treatment can be graded according to various grading systems. The non-unified grading systems advocated by different organizations have added yet another layer of obstruction to summarizing and codifying a reference like this. To assure that a "common language" is used between practitioners with different backgrounds, the grading systems for recommendations and levels of evidence endorsed and used by ASCO and the European Society of Medical Oncology (ESMO) were adopted (Table 1) (SMITH et al. 1997).

Table 1. Levels of evidence and grade of recommendations

Level	Type of Evidence
I	Evidence obtained form meta-analysis of multiple, well-designed, controlled studies. Randomized trials with low false-positive and low false-negative errors (high power).
II	Evidence obtained from at least one well-designed experimental study. Randomized trials with high false-positive and/or negative errors (low power).
III	Evidence obtained from well-designed, quasi-experimental studies such as nonrandomized, controlled, single group, pre-post, cohort, and time or matched case-control series.
IV	Evidence from well designed, nonexperimental studies such as comparative and correlational descriptive and case studies.
V	Evidence from case reports.

Grade	Grade of Recommendation
A	There is evidence of type I or consistent findings from multiple studies of type II, III, or IV.
B	There is evidence of type II, III, or IV and findings are generally consistent.
C	there is evidence of type II, III, or IV but findings are inconsistent.
D	There is little or no systemic empirical evidence

Evidence-Based Radiation Oncology: Practice with Caution

Although the application of evidence-based radiation oncology involves the use of currently available evidence of the highest quality, one cannot overemphasize the fact that scientific evidence alone is never sufficient for effective decision making in the practice of cancer care. The biggest challenge in evidence-based radiation oncology is to apply scientific evidence and standardized knowledge of cancer management generated from population studies to individual patients with unique clinical, psychological, and social circumstances. It is equally important to consider clinical expertise of radiation oncologists as well as patients' value and expectations in the decision-making process. In other words, the three elements presented in the "Triad of Evidence-Based Medicine" should be emphasized equal measure in daily practice.

The rapidly evolving field of radiation oncology also requires radiation oncologists to be vigilant with regard to updates in knowledge, since scientific evidence that may induce changes in the treatment standard of medical practice emerges continuously and constantly. While Radiation Oncology: An Evidence-Based Approach serves as a practical reference for clinicians wishing to utilize updated evidence for their practice and better understand the basis of those treatment strategies, it can never be updated enough and certainly contains gaps which constantly need to be filled in by the readers through the practice of the "5As" process of evidence-based medicine.

References

Henke M, Laszig R, Rübe C et al. (2003) Erythropoietin to treat head and neck cancer patients with anaemia undergoing radiotherapy: randomised, double-blind, placebo-controlled trial. Lancet 362(9392):1255–1260

Sackett DL, Rosenberg WM, Gray JA et al. (1996) Evidence based medicine: what it is and what it isn't. BMJ 312 (7023):71–72

Smith TJ, Somerfield MR (1997) The ASCO experience with evidence-based clinical practice guidelines. Oncology (Williston Park) 11:223–227

UBC Health Library wiki. Web 2.0. (2008) Five steps of EBM. Accessed on July 3rd, 2008 from http://hlwiki.slais.ubc.ca/index.php?title=Five_steps_of_EBM

Contents

Section XI: Metastatic Diseases

Section XII: Radiation Biology and Physics

Section I:
Head and Neck Cancers

Ocular and Orbital Tumors

Arnold M. Markoe

CONTENTS

Introduction and Objectives

Intraocular and orbital tumors are relatively rare disease entities. Approximately 2100 new cases of primary orbital or ocular tumors are diagnosed annually in the United States. While cancer metastases to the eye or the orbit comprise the majority of ocular and/or orbital tumors, the most common primary tumor of the eye in adults is intraocular melanoma.

The treatment of ocular and orbital tumors depends on the tumor types as well as the extent of the diseases. Radiation plays a major role in the treatment of ocular or orbital tumors. This chapter focuses on the management of the more commonly diagnosed primary tumors of the eye and orbit and examines:

● Recommendations for diagnoses and staging procedures of various diagnoses of intraocular and orbital tumors

● The staging systems and prognostic factors for malignancies of the eye and orbit

● Treatment recommendations for these tumors as well as their supporting scientific evidence

● Follow-up care and surveillance of survivors of ocular and orbital malignancies

Arnold M. Markoe, MD
Department of Radiation Oncology (D31),
Sylvester Comprehensive Cancer Center, University of
Miami/Miller School of Medicine, 1475 N.W. 12th Ave,
Miami, FL 33136, USA

1.1   Diagnosis, Staging, and Prognoses of Intraocular Melanoma

1.1.1   Diagnosis

Initial Evaluation

■ Intraocular melanoma is usually diagnosed on ophthalmologic examination. Patients may or may not present with symptoms at the time of diagnosis, depending on tumor size, location in the eye, and production of secondary retinal detachment.

■ Frequently, a patient is seen by an optometrist or ophthalmologist for an unrelated condition, then sent to a retinal specialist and ultimately to the ocular oncologist for an incidental finding. The overall delay for small tumors was up to 129 days as compared to 50 days for medium tumors and 34 days for large tumors (Level IV) (Damato 2001). The diagnosis is only made when seen by the ocular oncologist since almost 30% of patients referred to an ocular oncology service with a diagnosis of choroidal melanoma have an incorrect diagnosis (Level IV) (Khan and Damato 2007).

■ The essential diagnostic procedures include ocular examination, especially indirect ophthalmoscopy, fundus photograph, ultrasonography and fluorescein angiography.

■ With the exception of iris melanomas, which are amenable to biopsy, diagnosis is usually on a clinical basis and is in excess of 99% accurate (COMS, Level II) (Collaborative Ocular Melanoma Study Group 1990).

■ The disease incidence in men is $6.8/10^6$ and in women $5.3/10^6$ (McLaughlin et al. 2005) in the United States. In Europe, incidence rates increase from south to north from $< 2/10^6$ in Spain and southern Italy up to $> 8/10^6$ in Norway and Denmark (Virgili et al. 2007). This variation of incidence with altitude also holds for the United States (Yu et al. 2006) for internal ocular melanoma, but is the reverse for external ocular melanoma (eyelid and conjunctival melanoma).

Laboratory Tests

■ Initial blood tests should include a complete blood count with differential, basic blood chemistry, liver function tests, and renal function tests.

Imaging Studies

■ Intraocular melanoma is commonly a localized disease and imaging studies for distant metastasis is usually not indicated for asymptomatic patients, except for pre-treatment chest X-ray.

■ Ultrasound or CT scan of the abdomen is indicated to rule out hepatic metastasis in patients with abnormal liver function test or presenting with suggestive symptoms.

Pathology

■ Intraocular melanoma is commonly diagnosed clinically and biopsy of the intraocular lesion should be avoided.

■ Diagnosis is usually on a clinical basis and is in excess of 99% accurate (COMS, Level II) (Collaborative Ocular Melanoma Study Group 1990).

1.1.2   Staging

■ Intraocular melanoma is staged clinically by location of tumor in the eye and by tumor dimension and presence or absence of extrascleral extension.

■ The AJCC staging system (Table 1.1) gives the staging for uveal melanoma and melanoma of the ciliary body and choroid.

Table 1.1. Definition of TNM. These definitions apply to both clinical[*] and pathologic staging

Primary tumor (T)	
All uveal melanomas	
TX	Primary tumor cannot be assessed
T0	No evidence of primary tumor
Iris	
T1	Tumor limited to the iris
T1a	Tumor limited to the iris not more than 3 clock hours in size
T1b	Tumor limited to the iris more than 3 clock hours in size
T1c	Tumor limited to the iris with melanomalytic glaucoma
T2	Tumor confluent with or extending into the ciliary body and/or choroid
T2a	Tumor confluent with or extending into the ciliary body and/or choroid with melanomalytic glaucoma
T3	Tumor confluent with or extending into the ciliary body and/or choroid with scleral extension
T3a	Tumor confluent with or extending into the ciliary body with scleral extension and melanomalytic glaucoma
T4	Tumor with extraocular extension
Ciliary body and choroid	
T1[*]	Tumor 10 mm or less in greatest diameter and 2.5 mm or less in greatest height (thickness)
T1a	Tumor 10 mm or less in greatest diameter and 2.5 mm or less in greatest height (thickness) without microscopic extraocular extension
T1b	Tumor 10 mm or less in greatest diameter and 2.5 mm or less in greatest height (thickness) with microscopic extraocular extension
T1c	Tumor 10 mm or less in greatest diameter and 2.5 mm or less in greatest height (thickness) with macroscopic extraocular extension
T2[*]	Tumor greater than 10 mm but not more than 16 mm in greatest basal diameter and between 2.5 and 10 mm in maximum height (thickness)
T2a	Tumor 10 mm to 16 mm in greatest basal diameter and between 2.5 and 10 mm in maximum height (thickness) without microscopic extraocular extension
T2b	Tumor 10 mm to 16 mm in greatest basal diameter and between 2.5 and 10 mm in maximum height (thickness) with microscopic extraocular extension
T2c	Tumor 10 mm to 16 mm in greatest basal diameter and between 2.5 mm and 10 mm in maximum height (thickness) with macroscopic extraocular extension
T3[*]	Tumor more than 16 mm in greatest diameter and/or greater than 10 mm in maximum height (thickness) without extraocular extension
T4	Tumor more than 16 mm in greatest diameter and/or greater than 10 mm in maximum height (thickness) with extraocular extension
Regional lymph nodes (N)	
NX	Regional lymph nodes cannot be assessed
N0	No regional lymph node metastasis
N1	Regional lymph node metastasis
Distant metastasis (M)	
MX	Distant metastasis cannot be assessed
M0	No distant metastasis
M1	Distant metastasis

STAGE GROUPING	
I:	T1 N0 M0, T1a N0 M0, T1b N0 M0, T1c N0 M0
II:	T2 N0 M0, T2a N0 M0, T2b N0 M0, T2c N0 M0
III:	T3 N0 M0, T4 N0 M0
IV:	Any T N1 M0, Any T Any N M1

[*]**Note:** When basal dimension and apical height do not fit this classification, the largest tumor diameter should be used for classification. In clinical practice, the tumor base may be estimated in optic disc diameter (dd) (average: 1 dd = 1.5 mm). The height may be estimated in diopters (average: 3 diopters = 1 mm). Techniques such as ultrasonography, visualization, and photography are frequently used to provide more accurate measurements.

1.1.3 Prognostic Factors

- In general, prognosis of intraocular melanoma depends on tumor size and location in the eye. Treatment modality is not prognostically significant (Level II) (COLLABORATIVE OCULAR MELANOMA STUDY GROUP 2006).
- Patient survival has been related to age of the patient (older = poorer), but not gender or poverty level (BURR et al. 2007; COLLABORATIVE OCULAR MELANOMA STUDY GROUP 2006; ISAGER et al. 2006), as well as maximal basal tumor diameter (larger = poorer) (COMS 2006, Level II) (BERGMAN et al. 2005).
- Visual deterioration is related to the location of tumor relative to the foveola and optic nerve and to globe enucleation for either tumor recurrence or complications of treatment after radiation (Level IV) (BERGMAN et al. 2005). Obviously, if enucleation is the treatment, vision failure in the tumor containing eye is immediate and total.
- Tumor apical height, a history of diabetes, pretreatment visual acuity and tumor-associated retinal detachment and tumors that were not dome-shaped were also associated with poor visual outcome (MELIA et al. 2001).
- Tumors higher than 6 mm, tumors with low internal reflectivity, and tumors with an initial rate of height regression > 0.7 mm/month had a higher 5-year melanoma-related mortality. Response to brachytherapy is of prognostic significance. The initial height regression rate was 6.1% per month in patients who later developed metastases versus 4.3% per month in patients who did not (Level IV) (KAISERMAN et al. 2004).

1.2 Treatment of Intraocular Melanoma

1.2.1 Surgery

- Iris and conjunctival melanomas may be excised on a definitive basis. For other sites, surgery is usually reserved for tumors too large for radiation treatments or for patient reference.
- Enucleation is the surgical procedure of choice; however, if there is a large component of extras-

cleral extension, orbital exenteration may be preferable, followed by external beam irradiation.
- Transscleral local resection is not recommended as the standard surgical procedure for intraocular melanoma (Grade B). Although the procedure has been used in an effort to preserve the globe and vision, this technique has a local recurrence rate of 41% at 5 years compared with about 7% for brachytherapy (Level IV) (PUUSAARI et al. 2007).

1.2.2 Radiation Therapy

- Conventional external-beam radiation therapy is not recommended for the treatment of intraocular melanoma. External telecobalt treatment of the involved eye to 60 Gy has been attempted with poor results and, ultimately, visual or globe loss from complications.
- Proton beam and other hadron therapy can be recommended to treat intraocular melanoma (Grade B). It has been reported to have a 95% intraocular control rate (Level III) (DAMATO et al. 2005; DENDALE et al. 2006; DESJARDINS et al. 2003; GRAGOUDAS et al. 2002). Although initially varying among institutions, the tumor dose commonly used is currently approximately 60 cobalt Gy equivalent (CGE) delivered in four fractions.

  Since proton beam therapy requires accurate tumor localization, the patient usually requires surgery to implant markers to define the site for image-guided set-up. Even with fiducial guidance, about 50% of the local recurrences were at the tumor margin, possibly due to treatment planning errors and the majority of the rest were either extrascleral extension or uncontrolled tumor (Level III) (GRAGOUDAS et al. 2002).
- Stereotactic radiosurgery has been attempted using both the GammaKnife and the CyberKnife. These results are not mature enough for comparison with other techniques. However, from a pure physics viewpoint, proton beam delivers the lowest dose to the contralateral eye with the Gamma Knife delivering the highest dose. Scatter dosing into the pelvis of a phantom was nearly equivalent between the Gamma Knife and proton beam and was an order of magnitude smaller than the dose delivered by the CyberKnife (Level III) (ZYTKOVICZ et al. 2007).

Brachytherapy

- Brachytherapy is a mainstay radiation modality for the treatment of intraocular melanoma (Grade A). A variety of different isotopes and plaque designs have been employed for the purpose of brachytherapy of ocular melanoma. Results vary among institutions but are generally in the upper 80%–97% range for local intraocular control.
- Dose of brachytherapy is usually 85 Gy to the tumor apex plus 1 mm (to allow for scleral thickness) and usually allows for a 1- to 2-mm margin around the diameter of the tumor.
  For medium sized (T2) tumors, there does not appear to be any survival differences between ^{125}I plaque brachytherapy and enucleation in a randomized study of >1300 patients (Level II) (COLLABORATIVE OCULAR MELANOMA STUDY GROUP 2006).
  For small (T1) tumors, ^{125}I brachytherapy after observation until growth or until the tumor developed orange pigment is associated with a 5-year melanoma-specific mortality of about 4% and globe conservation in 97.8% of patients, according the results of a prospective series from the University of Miami (Level III) (SOBRIN et al. 2005).
  For large (T3) tumors local control rate was 91% at 5 years and 87% at 10 years. However, by 10 years, 34% of patients needed to be enucleated and 55% had developed metastatic disease (Level IV) (SHIELDS et al. 2002).
- Radiation complications will vary with size and location of tumor and choice of brachytherapy isotope. In the COMS study, cataracts occurred in 83% of study eyes by 5 years, but only 12% had undergone cataract surgery; when the lens dose was ≥24 Gy, 18% had cataract surgery but only 4% when the lens dose was < 12 Gy (Level II) (COLLABORATIVE OCULAR MELANOMA STUDY GROUP 2007).
  Risk factors for cataract development were age >65, male, and tumor diameter >10 mm (Level IV) (LUMBROSO-LE ROUIC et al. 2004). Cataract is the earliest complication to develop after brachytherapy and obviously occurs more frequently with anterior tumor than posterior tumors. Increasing tumor height correlates positively with cataracts, iris neovascularization, and persistent retinal detachment. As expected, maculopathy and optic neuropathy associate with

distance to the fovea and optic disk, respectively (Level IV) (PUUSAARI et al. 2004).
- Enucleation after brachytherapy can be recommended for local failure or for a blind painful eye despite other interventions to control complications. Treatment failure was the most common cause for enucleation within 3 years of treatment, whereas ocular pain was most common thereafter (COMS, Level II) (JAMPOL et al. 2002).
- The question of enucleation of non-seeing eyes or their preservation when no recurrence can be documented was addressed. Secondary enucleation for blind eyes with no evidence for recurrence did not appear to improve survival (Level IV) (AUGSBURGER et al. 2004).

1.2.3   Other Treatment Modalities

- An attempt to treat small choroidal melanomas by transpapillary thermotherapy alone indicated that the major side effect was retinal complications in over 75% of patients and that thermotherapy alone had an almost 30% local failure rate. Adjuvant thermotherapy after ^{125}I plaque brachytherapy for patients who were deemed radio-resistant led to no local failures with limited follow-up time (Level IV) (HARBOUR et al. 2003).

1.3   Follow-Ups and Surveillance

- Long-term follow-up after treatment of intraocular melanoma is recommended for early detection of recurrence and treatment complications, including secondary primary tumor induced by radiation therapy (Grade B).
- Long-term analysis of the COMS trials indicated that metastases from intraocular melanoma preferentially occur in liver, followed by lung, and then bone (Level II) (COLLABORATIVE OCULAR MELANOMA STUDY GROUP 2001; DIENER-WEST et al. 2005b).
- There would appear to be an association between ocular melanoma and the risk of developing second primary cancer with standardized incidence

ratios (SIR) from a high of 3.89 for liver cancer to 1.31 for prostate (Level IV) (SCELO et al. 2007). Conversely, there appears to be a significantly increased risk for ocular melanoma only after prostate cancer (SIR = 1.41). The increased risk of cutaneous melanoma after ocular melanoma (SIR = 2.38) may merely be related to greater skin cancer surveillance in ocular melanoma patients and may not be indicative of any common etiologic factors. In the COMS study, radiotherapy either by external beam for large tumors, pre-enucleation or brachytherapy with ^{125}I for medium tumors did not significantly increase the development of radiation-induced second primary cancers. Of the 222 patients who developed second primary cancers, there was a 5-year rate of 7.7% of second primary cancer, mostly of prostate (23% of 222) and breast (17%) (Level II) (DIENER-WEST 2005a).

Schedule and Work-Ups

- Patients could be followed up every 3–4 months in the first 2 years, every 6 months for an additional 3 years, and annually thereafter with their ophthalmologists and radiation oncologists (Grade D).
- Each follow-up should include a complete history and physical examination and a careful ophthalmological examination for non-surgically treated patients. As described above, after brachytherapy, tumors higher than 6 mm, tumor with low internal reflectivity and tumor with an initial rate of height regression > 0.7 mm/mo had a higher 5-year melanoma mortality. The initial height regression rate was 6.1% per month in patients who later developed metastases versus 4.3% per month in patients who did not (Level IV) (KAISERMAN et al. 2004).
- Laboratory and imaging studies are not routinely indicated in follow-up unless indicated by clinical symptoms (Grade D), except for CT scan of the chest to include the entire liver to be done annually for surveillance or if symptoms develop.

1.4 Diagnosis, Staging, and Prognoses of Primary Intraocular Lymphoma

1.4.1 Diagnosis

Initial Evaluation

- Primary intraocular lymphoma (PIOL) is a subset or a restricted form of primary central nervous system lymphoma (PCNSL) that involves the globe(s) in the absence of systemic or CNS lymphoma (LEVY-CLARKE et al. 2005; HORMIGO and DEANGELIS 2003; HORMIGO et al. 2004). PIOL often progresses to the brain and meninges.
- PIOL frequently presents as a chronic inflammatory state that resists corticosteroid therapy. Frequently, the disease presents in both eyes (ISOBE et al. 2006) with symptoms of blurred vision, decreased visual acuity, and floaters.

Laboratory Tests

- Initial laboratory tests should include a complete blood count, basic blood chemistry, liver and renal function tests, alkaline phosphatase, lactate dehydrogenase (LDH), and erythrocyte sedimentation rate (ESR) (GREENE et al. 2002).
- As in primary CNS lymphomas, CSF fluid should be tested for cell count, protein levels, cytology, flow cytometry and immunoglobin heavy chain gene rearrangement studies. Positive leptomeningeal involvement may change management and an elevated CSF protein is a poor prognostic factor (ABREY 2005).
- A bone marrow biopsy with aspirate is part of the recommended staging procedure.

Imaging Studies

- In addition to imaging studies utilized in the diagnosis and evaluation of other types of non-Hodgkin's lymphoma (NHL), a brain MRI is indicated in patients with primary intraocular lymphoma.

Pathology

- Pathologic diagnosis of PIOL is challenging. The procedure of choice for diagnosis is vitrectomy

(Grade B). In 83 patients retrospectively studied, 74 had diagnoses made by vitrectomy, six by choroid/retinal biopsy and three by ophthalmic examination only (Level IV) (GRIMM et al. 2007).

- The strategy for follow-up and surveillance after the completion of treatment of primary intraocular lymphoma resembles that of primary CNS lymphoma detailed in Chapter 31.

1.5 Treatment of Primary Intraocular Lymphoma

- Historically, primary intraocular lymphoma was considered to be associated with a risk for CNS involvement. Conversely, primary CNS lymphoma was considered to be associated with a risk for intraocular spread. Prior to effective systemic agents, this led to the en bloc irradiation of the globes, optic nerves, and brain.
- The current treatment of primary intraocular lymphoma includes chemotherapy regimens that are used for primary CNS lymphoma. The details of chemotherapy for primary CNS lymphoma are presented in Chapter 31.
- Radiation to the orbits to treat globes and optic nerves remain essential. Ocular radiation can be given with the induction chemotherapy if care is taken to exclude brain from the fields. Intravenous methotrexate (IV MTX) achieves micromolar levels in both aqueous and vitreous humors 4 h after infusion, but was much lower in the vitreous humor. In a series of nine patients with intraocular lymphoma treated with IV MTX, seven responded to the treatment at 8 gm/m² but three patients relapsed in the eye, requiring irradiation (Level IV) (BATCHELOR et al. 2003).
- In patients without other clinical manifestations, ocular irradiation and/or systemic chemotherapy fail to prevent CNS progression (Level IV) (HORMIGO et al. 2004).
- It is reasonable to treat patients with primary intraocular lymphoma who achieved complete response after chemotherapy to lower total dose of 30.6 Gy in conventional fractionation (Grade D). Such a strategy was studied in the treatment of primary CNS lymphoma. The use of the systemic regimen of Rituximab, MTX, procarbazine and vincristine (R-MVP) has allowed a decrease in the radiation to the brain in complete responders from 45 Gy to 30.6 and, most recently, to 23.4 Gy (Level III) (SHAH et al. 2007). Patients who had less than a complete response should be irradiated to 45 Gy.

1.6 Diagnosis, Staging, and Prognoses of Orbital Lymphoma

1.6.1 Diagnosis

Initial Evaluation

- The initial evaluation and diagnosis of orbital lymphoma resemble those performed in other types of NHL. Diagnosis and evaluation start with a complete history and physical examination (H&P). Attention should be paid to NHL-associated signs and symptoms: unexplained weight loss of more than 10% over 6 months prior to diagnosis, unexplained fever >38°C, and/or drenching night sweats that require change of bedclothes ("B" symptoms), shortness of breath, hemoptysis, pruritus, recent onset alcohol beverage intolerance and unusual fatigue.
  Orbital lymphoma is a rare manifestation of NHL that appears to have a higher incidence in Asian/Pacific Islanders, lower in whites and lower yet in blacks. Incidence increases with increasing age and has no gender preference (MOSLEHI et al. 2006). From 1975 to 2001, there appeared to be a rapid, steady increase in incidence among whites regardless of sex, varying between 6.0%–7.0% annually.
- Orbital lymphomas occur in conjunctival, lacrimal gland and sac locations. A thorough physical examination with special attention to these tissues, nodal sites in the head and neck area, oral cavity and oral pharynx, liver, and spleen.
- The majority of orbital lymphoma present as stage IAE, a small minority will have IIAE and higher staging (ESIK et al. 1996; HASEGAWA et al. 2003).

Laboratory Tests

- Initial laboratory tests should include a complete blood count, basic blood chemistry, liver and renal function tests, alkaline phosphatase, lactate dehydrogenase (LDH), and erythrocyte sedimentation rate (ESR) (GREENE et al. 2002).

- Bone marrow aspirate and biopsy should be considered, although the majority of orbital lymphoma present as stage IAE disease.

Imaging Studies

- CT scans of the head and neck, thorax, abdomen and pelvis are recommended to appropriately evaluate and stage NHL.
- Other imaging studies can be considered if indicated by the findings of H&P, laboratory tests, and CT scan.

Pathology

- Pathologic diagnosis of orbital lymphoma is mandatory prior to determining treatment. Diagnosis is by biopsy and PCR gene re-arrangement studies. Most cases of orbital lymphoma are of B-cell lineage. T-cell and NK/T cell diseases are rare. Orbital lymphomas are typically low-grade and largely of the extranodal marginal zone type (EMZL) of the mucosa-associated lymphoid tissue (MALT) lymphomas (Level IV) (RIGACCI et al. 2007).
- Historically, differentiation of orbital lymphoma from benign lymphoproliferative orbitopathy (orbital pseudotumor) on solely histopathologic grounds was difficult. With the advent of gene rearrangement reactions, monoclonality establishes the nature of the orbital lymphoma and absence of monoclonality favors the benign state.

1.6.2 Staging

- Orbital lymphoma is staged in an identical method to other types of NHL, and is staged clinically based on results of physical examination, laboratory tests, imaging studies, and bone marrow biopsy.
- The Ann Arbor Staging System is used for both Hodgkin's disease and NHL (Table 8.3) (GREENE et al. 2002)

1.6.3 Prognostic Factors

- The prognosis for stage IAE, low grade orbital lymphoma is excellent after definitive radiation therapy. The local control rate approaches 100%.

1.7 Treatment of Orbital Lymphoma

1.7.1 Radiation Therapy

- Radiation therapy is the mainstay treatment of orbital lymphoma (Grade A). Both surgery and chemotherapy have limited roles in the definitive treatment of Stage IAE orbital lymphoma. ESIK et al. (1996) examined various modes of treatment for primary orbital lymphoma. Of 37 patients, 17 were treated by radiotherapy, 13 by surgery alone and seven by chemotherapy. The 10-year local relapse free rate was 100%, 0%, and 42%, respectively (Level IV).
- Local control rates for the low grade orbital lymphoma range between 95% and 100% at 5 years, repeatedly confirmed in multiple single institution reports. The dose is generally 30 Gy–30.6 Gy, as used in various studies, depending on fraction size. Higher doses (40 Gy) are recommended for the intermediate grade orbital lymphoma. Dose to a total 45 Gy or more is indicated for the T and NK/T cell OL.

Radiation Technique

- The entire orbit needs to be encompassed in the irradiation field except for the very superficial conjunctival lymphomas (Grade B). When the entire orbit is not treated, recurrences tended to occur in initially uninvolved areas not treated in the initial target volume in 33% of cases (Level IV) (PFEFFER et al. 2004).
- Recurrences could be salvaged by repeat irradiation or surgery.

Radiation-Induced Side Effects and Complications

- Complications of irradiation are relatively unusual for low dose treatment of low grade orbital lymphoma. The main toxicity is, as expected, cataract formation in patients treated without a lens block (Level IV) (Zhou et al. 2005). Bhatia et al. (2002) report that only about 25% of patients develop cataracts, 2/3 grade 1 and 1/3 grade 3 (Level IV). Only male gender predicted for increased risk of cataract formation. Dose of treatment and treatment technique was not predictive except that if lens blocking was employed, no patient developed grade 3 lens toxicity or required surgical correction within the median 55-month follow-up range. There was a nearly 20% incidence of dry eye, all mild and only 1/47 patients developed neovascular glaucoma. No retinal or optic nerve injury was seen.

1.7.2 Chemotherapy and Immunotherapy

- Chemotherapy and/or immunotherapy may be efficacious for the treatment of low-grade orbital lymphoma; however, further investigation is needed before they can be recommended as the first line standard treatment.
  The utility of the anti-CD_{20} monoclonal antibody, Rituximab (Rituxan) in the treatment of orbital lymphomas has been recently examined in small case series with immature data. In one, eight patients were treated pre-operatively, and 5/8 had initial complete response, 2/8 had partial response and 1/8 had no response to Rituximab. Mean follow-up was 16.5 months and no comment on relapse was made (Level V) (Sullivan et al. 2004). The results of a second report revealed that 5/5 previously untreated patients had regression (extent not defined) and 0/3 patients treated with Retuximab after relapse responded. Of the five responders, four had early relapse of disease with a median time to progression of only 5 months (Level V) (Ferreri et al. 2005).
- Oral chlorambucil has been used as a single dose therapy for MALT orbital lymphoma. An average of four drug courses with a mean total dose of 600 mgm was given in 33 patients. Complete response was seen in 79% (26/33) but 4/26 had disease recurrence or relapse (Level IV) (Ben Simon et al. 2006).
- Chlorambucil and Rituximab have been combined to treat nine newly diagnosed orbital lymphoma patients (8/9 with EMZL) with a median

follow-up of 25 months; 8/9 (89%)) had complete response and 1/9 had partial response. All patients were alive without progression or late toxicities (Level IV) (Rigacci et al. 2007).

1.7.3 Potential Treatment Modalities

- Orbital lymphomas have been thought to possibly be antigen-driven disorders and since subsets of maltomas have been previously associated with infectious organisms (gastric NHL with *Helicobacter pylori* infection), it is not surprising that an association has been established between orbital lymphoma and *Chlamydia psittaci* (Cp). In Italy, 80% of the 40 orbital lymphoma samples examined carried Cp DNA (Level III) (Ferreri et al. 2004). However, in a series of 62 patients from the University of Miami, none of the specimens harbored Cp DNA (Level III) (Rosado et al. 2006). A similar finding was substantiated from the Northeastern United States (Level III) (Vargas et al. 2006). Interestingly, Korean results mirrored those in Italy (Yoo et al. 2007).
- Meta-analyses were performed, one examining the association of Cp and orbital lymphoma and the other focusing on the response of orbital lymphoma to antibiotic therapy. A collective of 458 orbital lymphoma cases were pooled from ten countries. Of these cases, 104 (23%) were positive for Cp and of the 346 cases that were maltomas, 25% (87 samples) were positive (Level I) (Husain et al. 2007). In all, 90% of the positive samples came from only three of the 11 pooled studies. This suggested a striking variability of Cp positively in orbital lymphoma across geographic regions and even within studies from the same region.
- With respect to the treatment of these orbital lymphoma with antibiotics, the Italian group in a prospective trial treated Cp positive (11) and negative (16) patients with 100 mgm Doxycycline twice daily for 3 weeks. Lymphoma regressed in 68% of positive patients and 38% of negative patients. The overall response rate (CR + PR) was 48% (Level III) (Ferreri et al. 2006). The meta-analysis identified three additional studies (overall 42 patients). This confirmed the overall response of 48% but objective response documentation was available for only 3/42 patients. Seven other patients experienced recurrence after ini-

tial response of disease stability with 6/7 of these recurrences occurring within the initial year of follow-up (Level IV) (Husain et al. 2007).

1.8 Follow-Ups and Surveillance

■ No follow-up schedule specific to orbital lymphoma can be recommended. Patients with orbital lymphoma can be followed-up in the same fashion as those with NHL.
Life-long follow-up after definitive treatment of NHL is recommended for detecting recurrence, secondary tumors or other long-term complications of radiation therapy or chemotherapy.

■ Follow-ups could be scheduled every 3 months for 2 years, then every 6 months for 3 additional years, then annually thereafter (Grade D).

■ Each follow-up should include a complete history and physical examination. Laboratory and imaging studies can be performed if clinically indicated.

1.9 Diagnosis of Benign Lymphoid Hyperplasia of the Orbit (Orbital Pseudotumor)

■ Presentations of benign lymphoid hyperplasia are similar to those observed in orbital lymphoma. Patients can present with a constellation of symptoms, none pathognomonic, which include orbital swelling, chemosis, proptosis, blepharoptosis, restricted eye motion, diplopia, and visual loss (Level IV) (Agir et al. 2007).

■ There is a high incidence of bilaterality at presentation for orbital pseudotumor (Level IV) (Austin-Seymour et al. 1985).

Pathology

■ Orbital pseudotumor is part of a spectrum of lymphocytic infiltrative orbital conditions that has orbital lymphoma at the most aggressive end.

■ Diagnosis tends to be one of exclusion. With the advent of gene rearrangement reactions, monoclonality establishes the nature of the orbital lymphoma and absence of monoclonality favors the benign state.

1.10 Treatment of Benign Lymphoid Hyperplasia of the Orbit (Orbital Pseudotumor)

■ Steroids are usually the first line of treatment for this disease.

Radiation Therapy

■ Many patients are sent for radiation after not responding to steroids, relapse after or during steroid taper, or when steroids are refused or medically contraindicated (Level IV) (Lanciano et al. 1990).

■ Radiation doses of 20 Gy with slight variation is recommended (Grade A). Excellent responses have been repeatedly reported in the literature. The local control rate is dependent on the presenting symptoms with complete response observed in 87% of orbits with soft tissue swelling, 82% with proptosis, 78% with restricted extraocular motility, and 75% with pain (Level IV) (Lanciano et al. 1990). Response may also depend on whether the patient has seen and failed steroids. Of naïve eyes irradiated, 100% cleared of symptoms but only 85% cleared when radiation was not the sole treatment (Level IV) (Barthold et al. 1986).

Immunotherapy

■ The use of Rituximab has been investigated for treating benign orbital pseudolymphomas; however, currently available evidence does not warrant routine use of Rituximab as a standard treatment. In a small series of 11 patients, intravenous Rituximab (375 mgm/m^2) weekly for 4 weeks were delivered and 10 patients (91%) responded. None of the responders has become refractory to the agent (Level III) (Witzig et al. 2007).

1.11 Diagnosis of Choroidal Hemangioma

- Choroidal hemangiomas are uncommon benign vascular tumors, and can be circumscribed or diffuse. The latter generally occur as part of the Sturge-Weber syndrome, and are usually evident at birth.
- The circumscribed tumors occur sporadically and are usually diagnosed when they cause visual disturbance due to development of exudative retinal detachment; retinal capillary hemangioma may occur as part of von Hippel-Lindau disease (VHL) (SINGH et al. 2005).

1.12 Treatment of Choroidal Hemangioma

- A variety of therapeutic modalities have been utilized to treat choroidal hemangiomas. The most common has been photocoagulation of the surface, which is a repetitive treatment that may require additional invasive management.
- Radiation therapy is indicated in patients with exudative retinal detachment including or threatening the fovea (Grade B). A total dose of 20 Gy of photon irradiation can be delivered, and approximately 64% of patients with circumscribed choroidal hemangiomas achieved complete resolution of subretinal fluid while the rest had residual serous retinal detachment distal to the fovea. Visual acuity was stabilized or improved in about 78% of patients (Level IV) (SCHILLING et al. 1997).
- In retinal capillary hemangiomas due to VHL disease, a small retrospective series of six eyes in five patients addressed the effect of radiation for salvaging standard therapy failure. Patients were given 21.6 Gy (1.8 Gy/fx) with improved visual acuity, stabilization of retinal detachment and reduced tumor volume in most eyes (Level IV) (RAJA et al. 2004).
- Radioactive eye-plaque brachytherapy has been used to treat circumscribed CH to 29 Gy (mean dose) at the apex. All five patients had complete resolution of subretinal fluid and reattachment

of the retina and all tumors decreased in height. A total of 60% of patients had improved visual acuity (Level IV) (AIZMAN et al. 2004). Cobalt application also produced retinal reattachment (Level IV) (ZOGRAFOS et al. 1998).

- Proton beam treatment to 20 CGE also produces retinal reattachment in circumscribed choroidal hemangiomas (Level IV) (FRAU et al. 2004; ZOGRAFOS et al. 1998). Treatment of diffuse choroidal hemangiomas is less effective with proton therapy. Proton and photon beam treatment appear equally effective (HOCHT et al. 2006).
- Complications secondary to low dose irradiation are usually mild. Maximum grade I optic neuropathy was seen in 41% of patients and retinopathy in 29.5% of cases (only one patient > grade II severity) has been reported.

References

Abrey LE (2005) Controversies in primary CNS lymphoma. Expert Rev Neurother 5:459–464

Agir H, Auburn N, Davis C et al. (2007) W(h)ither orbital pseudotumor? J Craniofac Surg 18:1148–1153

Aizman A, Finger PT, Shabto U et al. (2004) Palladium 103 (103Pd) plaque radiation therapy for circumscribed choroidal hemangioma with retinal detachment. Arch Ophthalmol 122:1652–1656

Augsburger JJ, Khouri L, Roumeliotis A et al. (2004) Enucleation versus preservation of blind eyes following plaque radiotherapy for choroidal melanoma. Can J Ophthalmol 39:372–379

Austin-Seymour MM, Donaldson SS, Egbert PR et al. (1985) Radiotherapy of lymphoid diseases of the orbit. Int J Radiat Oncol Biol Phys 11:371–379

Barthold HJ 2nd, Harvey A, Markoe AM et al. (1986) Treatment of orbital pseudotumors and lymphoma. Am J Clin Oncol 9:527–532

Batchelor TT, Kolak G, Ciordia R et al. (2003) High-dose methotrexate for intraocular lymphomas. Clin Cancer Res 9:711–715

Ben Simon GJ, Chung N, McKelvie P et al. (2006) Oral chlorambucil for extranodal, marginal zone, B-cell lymphoma of mucosa-associated lymphoid tissue of the orbit. Ophthalmology 113:1209–1213

Bergman L, Nilsson B, Lundell G et al. (2005) Ruthenium brachytherapy for uveal melanoma, 1979–2003: survival and functional outcomes in the Swedish population. Ophthalmology 112:834–840

Bhatia S, Paulino AC, Buatti JM et al. (2002) Curative radiotherapy for primary orbital lymphoma. Int J Radiat Oncol Biol Phys 54:818–823

Burr JM, Mitry E, Rachet B et al. (2007) Survival from uveal melanoma in England and Wales 1986 to 2001. Ophthalmic Epidemio 14:3–8

Collaborative Ocular Melanoma Study Group (COMS) (1990) Accuracy of diagnosis of choroidal melanomas in the Collaborative Ocular Melanoma Study: COMS report no. 1. Arch Ophthalmol 108:1268–1273

Collaborative Ocular Melanoma Study Group (COMS) (2001) Assessment of metastatic disease status at death in 435 patients with large choroidal melanoma in the Collaborative Ocular Melanoma study (COMS): COMS report no. 15. Arch Ophthalmol 119:670–676

Collaborative Ocular Melanoma Study Group (COMS) (2006) The COMS randomized trial of iodine 125 brachytherapy for choroidal melanoma: V. Twelve-year mortality rates and prognostic factors: COMS report no. 28. Arch Ophthalmol 125:1684–1693

Collaborative Ocular Melanoma Study Group (COMS) (2007) Incidence of cataract and outcomes after cataract surgery in the first 5 years after iodine 125 brachytherapy in the Collaborative Ocular Melanoma Study: COMS report no. 27. Ophthalmology 114:1363–1371

Damato B (2001) Time to treatment of uveal melanoma in the United Kingdom. Eye 15(pt 2):155–158

Damato B, Kacperek A, Chopra M et al. (2005) Proton beam radiotherapy of choroidal melanoma: the Liverpool-Clatterridge experience. Int J Radiat Oncol Phys 62:1405–1411

de Cremoux P, Subtil A, Ferreri AJ, Vincent-Salomon A et al. (2006) Re: Evidence for an association between Chlamydia psittaci and ocular adnexal lymphomas. J Natl Cancer Inst 98:365–366

Dendale R, Lumbroso-Le Rouic L, Noel G et al. (2006) Proton beam radiotherapy for uveal melanoma: results of Curie Institut-Orsay proton therapy center (ICPO). Int J Radiat Oncol Biol Phys 65:780–787

Desjardins L, Lumbroso L, Levy C et al. (2003) Treatment of uveal melanoma with iodine 125 plaques or proton beam therapy: indications and comparison of local recurrence rates. J Fr Ophthalmol 26:269–276

Diener-West M, Reynolds SM, Agugliaro DJ et al. (2005a) Second primary cancers after enrollment in the COMS trails for treatment of choroidal melanoma: COMS Report No. 25. Arch Ophthalmol 123:601–604

Diener-West M, Reynold SM, Agugliaro DJ et al. (2005b) Development of metastatic disease after enrollment in the COMS trails for treatment of choroidal melanoma: Collaborative Ocular Melanoma Study Group Report No. 26. Arch Ophthalmol 123:1639–1643

Esik O, Ikeda H, Mukai K et al. (1996) A retrospective analysis of different modalities for treatment of primary orbital non-Hodgkin's lymphomas. Radiother Oncol 38:13–18

Ferreri AJ, Guidoboni M, Ponzoni M et al. (2004) Evidence for an association between Chlamydia psittaci and ocular adnexal lymphomas. J Natl Cancer Inst 96:586–594

Ferreri AJ, Ponzoni M, Martinelli G et al. (2005) Bacteria-eradicating therapy with doxycycline in ocular adnexal MALT lymphoma: a multicenter prospective trial. J Natl Cancer Inst 98:1375–1382

Ferreri AJ, Ponzoni M, Guidoboni M et al. (2006) Rituximab in patients with mucosal-associated lymphoid tissue-type lymphoma of the ocular adnexa. Haematologica 90:1578–1579

Frau E, Rumen F, Noel G et al. (2004) Low-dose proton beam therapy for circumscribed choroidal hemangiomas. Arch Ophthalmol 122:1471–1475

Gragoudas ES, Lane AM, Munzenrider J et al. (2002) Long term risk of local failure after proton therapy for choroidal/ciliary body melanoma. Trans Am Ophthalmol Soc 100:43–48

Greene FL, Page DL, Fleming ID et al. (2002) American Joint Committee on Cancer, American Cancer Society. AJCC Cancer Staging Manual, 6th ed. Springer-Verlag, Berlin Heidelberg New York

Grimm SA, Pulido JS, Jahnke K et al. (2007) Primary intraocular lymphoma: an International Primary Central Nervous System Lymphoma Collaborative Group Report. Ann Oncol 18:1851–1855

Harbour JW, Meredith TA, Thompson PA et al. (2003) Trans-pupillary thermotherapy versus plaque radiotherapy for suspected choroidal melanomas. 110:2207–2214

Hasegawa M, Kojima M, Shioya M et al. (2003) Treatment results of radiotherapy for malignant lymphoma of the orbit and histopathologic review according to the WHO classification. Int J Radiat Oncol Biol Phys 57:172–176

Hocht S, Wachtlin J, Bechrakis NE et al. (2006) Proton or photon irradiation for hemangiomas of the choroid? A retrospective comparison. Int J Radiat Oncol Biol Phys 66:345–351

Hormigo A, DeAngelis LM (2003) Primary ocular lymphoma: clinical features, diagnosis and treatment. Clin Lymphoma 4:22–29

Hormigo A, Abrey L, Heineman MH et al. (2004) Ocular presentation of primary central nervous system lymphoma: diagnosis and treatment. Br J Haematol 126:202–208

Husain A, Roberts D, Pro B et al. (2007) Meta-analyses of the association between Chlamydia psittaci and ocular adnexal lymphoma and the response of ocular adnexal lymphoma to antibiotics. Cancer 110:809–815

Isager P, Engholm G, Overgaard J et al. (2006) Uveal and conjunctival malignant melanoma in Denmark 1943–97: observed and relative survival of patients followed through 2002. Ophthalmic Epidemio 13:85–96

Isobe K, Ejima Y, Tokumaru S et al. (2006) Treatment of primary intraocular lymphoma with radiation therapy: a multi-institutional survey in Japan. Leuk Lymphoma 47:1800–1805

Jampol LM, Moy CS, Murray TG et al. (2002) The COMS randomized trail of iodine 125 brachytherapy for choroidal melanoma: IV. Local treatment failure and enucleation in the first 5 years after brachytherapy. COMS report no. 19. Ophthalmology 109:2197–2206

Kaiserman I, Anteby I, Chowers I et al. (2004) Post-brachytherapy initial tumor regression rate correlates with metastatic spread in posterior uveal melanoma. Br J Ophthalmol 88:892–895

Khan J, Damato BE (2007) Accuracy of choroidal melanoma diagnosis by general ophthalmologists: a prospective study. Eye 21:595–597

Lanciano R, Fowble B, Sergott RC et al. (1990) The results of radiotherapy for orbital pseudotumor. Int J Radiat Oncol Biol Phys 18:407–411

Levy-Clarke GA, Chan CC, Nussenblatt RB (2005) Diagnosis and management of primary intraocular lymphoma 19:739–749, viii

Lumbroso-Le Rouic L, Charif Chefchaouni M, Levy C et al. (2004) 125I plaque brachytherapy for anterior uveal melanomas. Eye 18:911–916

McLaughlin CC, Wu XC, Jemal A et al. (2005) Incidence of noncutaneous melanomas in the US. Cancer 103:1000–1007

Melia BM, Abramson DH, Albert DM et al. (2001) Collaborative ocular melanoma study (COMS) randomized trial of I-125 brachytherapy for medium choroidal melanoma. I. Visual acuity after 3 years. COMS report no. 16. Ophthalmology 108:348–366

Moslehi R, Dvesa SS, Schairer C et al. (2006) Rapidly increasing incidence of ocular non-Hodgkin's lymphoma. J Natl Cancer Inst 98:936–939

Pfeffer MR, Rabin T, Tsvang L, Goffman J. et al. (2004) Orbital lymphoma: is it necessary to treat the entire orbit? Int J Radiat Oncol Biol Phys 60:527–530

Puusaari I, Heikkonen J, Kivela T (2004) Ocular complications after iodine brachytherapy for large uveal melanomas. Ophthalmology 111:1768–1777

Puusaari I, Damato B, Kivelä T (2007) Transscleral local resection versus iodine brachytherapy for uveal melanomas that are large because of tumor height. Graefes Arch Clin Exp Ophthalmol 245:522–533

Raja D, Benz MS, Murray TG et al. (2004) Salvage external beam radiotherapy of retinal capillary hemangiomas secondary to von Hippel-Lindau disease: visual and anatomic outcomes. Ophthalmology 111:150–153

Rigacci L, Nassi L, Puccioni M et al. (2007) Rituximab and chlorambucil as first-line treatment for low-grade ocular adnexal lymphomas. Ann Hematol 86:565–568

Rosado MF, Byrne GE Jr, Ding F et al. (2006) Ocular adnexal lymphoma: a clinicopathologic study of a large cohort of patients with no evidence for an association with Chlamydia psittaci. Blood 107:467–472

Scelo G, Boffetta P, Autier P et al. (2007) Associations between ocular melanoma and other primary cancers: an international population-based study. Int J Cancer 120:152–159

Schilling H, Sauerwein W, Lommatzsch et al. (1997) Long-term results after low dose ocular irradiation for choroidal haemangiomas. Br J Ophthalmol 81:267–273

Shah GD, Yahalom J, Correa DD et al. (2007) Combined immunochemotherapy with reduced whole-brain radiotherapy for newly diagnosed primary CNS lymphoma. J Clin Oncol 25:4730–4735

Shields CL, Naseripour M, Cater J et al. (2002) Plaque radiotherapy for large posterior uveal melanomas (> or = 8 mm thick) in 354 consecutive patients. Ophthalmology 109:1838–1849

Singh AD, Kaiser PK, Sears JE (2005) Choroidal hemangioma. Ophthalmol Clin North Am 18:151–161, ix

Sobrin L, Schiffman JC, Markoe AM et al. (2005) Outcomes of iodine 125 plaque radiotherapy after initial observation of suspected small choroidal melanomas: a pilot study. Ophthalmology 112:1777–1783

Sullivan TJ, Grimes D, Bunce I (2004). Monoclonal antibody treatment of orbital lymphoma. Ophthal Plast Reconstr Surg 20:103–106

Vargas RL, Fallone E, Feigar RE et al. (2006) Is there an association between ocular adnexal lymphoma and infection with Chlamydia psittaci? The University of Rochester experience. Leuk Res 30:547–551

Virgili G, Gatta G, Ciccolallo L et al. (2007) Incidence of uveal melanoma in Europe. Ophthalmology 114:2309–2315

Witzig TE, Inwards DJ, Habermann TM et al. (2007) Treatment of benign orbital pseudolymphomas with the monoclonal anti-CD20 antibody rituximab. Mayo Clin Proc 82:692–699

Yoo C, Ryu MH, Huh J et al. (2007) Chlamydia psittaci infection and clinicopathologic analysis of ocular adnexal lymphomas in Korea. Am J Hematol 82:821–823

Yu GP, Hu DN, McCormic SA (2006) Latitude and incidence of ocular melanoma. Photochem Photobiol 82:1621–1626

Zhou P, Ng AK, Silver B et al. (2005) Radiation therapy for orbital lymphoma. Int J Radiat Oncol Biol Phys 63:866–871

Zografos L, Egger E, Bercher L et al. (1998) Proton beam irradiation of choroidal hemangiomas. Am J Ophthalmol 126:261–268

Zytkovicz A, Daftari I, Phillips TL et al. (2007) Peripheral dose in ocular treatment with Cyberknife and Gamma Knife radiosurgery compared to proton radiotherapy. Phys Med Biol 52:5957–5971

Nasopharyngeal Cancer

2

NANCY LEE and LIN KONG

CONTENTS

N. LEE, MD
Department of Radiation Oncology, Memorial Sloan Kettering Cancer Center, 1275 York Avenue, Box 22, New York, NY 10021, USA
L. KONG, MD
Department of Radiation Oncology, Cancer Hospital of Fudan University, 270 Dong An Road, Shanghai 200032, P.R. China

Introduction and Objectives

Carcinoma of the nasopharynx is a relatively uncommon disease in Western countries, but is the most commonly diagnosed head and neck malignancy in Southeast Asia. Most nasopharyngeal cancers are of epithelial origin. The nonkeratinizing poorly or un-differentiated squamous cell carcinoma [i.e., World Health Organization (WHO) type II and III diseases] are the more commonly diagnosed pathologies in Asia and account for almost 95% of all cases; however, 75% of cases are WHO type I in North America. Radiation therapy is the primary treatment for nasopharyngeal cancer. As nasopharyngeal cancer tends to present with regional metastasis, and is sensitive to both chemotherapy and radiation therapy, multidisciplinary management is usually required for locally advanced disease. This chapter examines:

● Recommendations for diagnosis and staging procedures for nasopharyngeal cancer
● Staging systems and prognostic factors
● Management of nasopharyngeal cancer using radiation therapy (for early stage disease) and combined treatment based on radiation therapy and cytotoxic chemotherapy, as well as the supporting scientific evidence
● Techniques of radiation therapy including intensity-modulated radiation therapy
● Follow up care and surveillance of survivors

2.1 Diagnosis, Staging, and Prognoses

2.1.1 Diagnosis

Initial Evaluation

■ Diagnosis and evaluation of nasopharyngeal cancer initiates with a complete history and physical examination. Attention should be paid to disease-related signs and symptoms. The most common presenting symptom is a neck mass, while cervical lymph adenopathy occurs in nearly 90% of patients, and 50% of cases present with bilateral involvement (SKINNER et al. 1991; LINDGERB 1972; CHENG et al. 2001; CHOO and TANNOCK 1991. Other common presenting symptoms include epistaxis, nasal congestion (causing nasal twang in speech), hearing loss, otitis media, and headache.

■ A thorough physical examination including direct fiberoptic endoscopy of the nasopharynx, oropharynx, and hypopharynx is required to evaluate the extent of the disease. Characteristics of the metastatic lymph nodes including location, size, consistency, tenderness, and mobility should be carefully evaluated and recorded.

■ Patients with more advanced disease may present with cranial neuropathy. The most commonly involved cranial nerves (CN) include CN V and VI, but any cranial nerves may be involved in advanced nasopharyngeal cancer (WEI and SHAM 2005).

■ Although uncommon, approximately 3% of patients present with symptoms secondary to distant metastasis. The most common sites of distant spread include bone, lung, and liver (AHMAD and STEFANI 1986; CHOY et al. 1993).

■ Dental evaluation to assess and restore (when possible) or extract (when restoration impossible) decayed teeth is necessary in all patients who require radiation therapy at approximately 2 weeks prior to commencement of radiation therapy.

Laboratory Tests

■ Initial lab tests should include a complete blood count, basic blood chemistry, liver function tests, and renal function tests.

■ EBV-specific serologic tests including IgA antiviral capsule antigen (VCA) and Ig-G anti-early antigen (EA), which are usually positive in WHO type II and III nasopharyngeal cancers, are also recommended. Elevated results of both tumor markers are expected in more than 80% of nonkeratinized poorly or un-differentiated nasopharyngeal carcinoma (Level IV) (NEEL 1992).

Imaging Studies

■ Imaging studies with MRI and/or CT of the head and neck areas are mandatory to evaluate the extent of disease at the primary site, as well as in the regional lymph nodes. MRI is preferred over CT as it is more sensitive for detecting soft-tissue extension (such as parapharyngeal space) and bone involvement (Grade A). The sensitivity and specificity of MRI for detecting locoregional extension has been repeatedly demonstrated in both prospective and retrospective studies (Level III and IV) (POON et al. 2000; OLMI et al. 1995; SAKATA et al. 1999; SIEVERS et al. 2002).

CT scan is more sensitive to MRI in detecting early bone invasion; however, MRI is preferred for evaluating the extent of invasion of the base of the skull or cervical vertebrae (Level IV) (DILLON and HARNSBERGER 1991; SIEVERS et al. 2002).

■ Chest X-ray is indicated to rule out pulmonary metastasis, while CT with IV contrast of the thorax is required if the chest X-ray is equivocal.

■ Bone scan and liver ultrasound (or abdominal CT scan) should be considered in patients with more advanced disease, especially N3 diseases. However, routine use of bone scan and liver ultrasound is not recommended (Grade B). The incidence of distant metastases is associated with the extent of regional lymph node involvement. Results from a prospective trial revealed that the yield of bone scan, liver ultrasound, and chest X-ray combined was 0%, 1.8%, 4.8%, and 14.3% for N0, N1, N2, and N3 disease, respectively (Level III) (KUMAR et al. 2004). Similar results were reported in a retrospective study from Europe (Level IV) (CAGLAR et al. 2003).

■ FDG-PET is valuable for detecting local and regional disease as well as distant metastasis, and can be considered for initial evaluation and staging (Grade B). The sensitivity and specificity of FDG-PET have been demonstrated in several recently published reports:

Results from a retrospective study revealed that 18F FDG-PET is accurate in staging patients with nasopharyngeal cancer, especially in N3 diseases. However, the sensitivity and specificity over bone scan and/or abdominal CT or ultrasound for liver metastasis was not discussed (Level IV) (CHANG et al. 2005). In a prospective study, 18F FDG-PET was found to be more sensitive than bone scan for detecting bone metastasis in endemic nasopharyngeal carcinoma at initial staging. The sensitivity was 70% versus 36.7% (P = 0.006) in the patient-based analysis, and

55.6% versus 14.8% (P = 0.001) in the region-based analysis at the spine (Level III) (Liu et al. 2006). In a more recently published report by Liu et al. (2007), FDG-PET was found to be more sensitive than CT of the thorax and bone scan for detecting lung and bone metastasis, and was equally effective in detecting liver metastasis as compared to abdominal ultrasound (Level IV) (Table 2.1).

Pathology

- Histologic confirmation is mandatory for the diagnosis of nasopharyngeal cancer. Tissue for diagnosis can be obtained from the primary tumor site during endoscopic examination. Fine-needle aspiration (FNA) of an enlarged neck node can provide sufficient tissue for histological diagnosis, and can be used when primary tumor is not clinically detectable.

- Nearly all malignancies arising in the nasopharynx do so from the mucosa and consequently are squamous cell carcinomas. The World Health Organization (WHO) classifies NPC into three histopathologic types. WHO type I is a keratinizing squamous-cell carcinoma that is morphologically similar to other head and neck carcinomas, WHO type II is differentiated non-keratinizing carcinoma, and WHO type III is an undifferentiated carcinoma (Shanmugaratnam and Sobin 1991).

- Poorly differentiated nonkeratinizing (WHO type II) and undifferentiated carcinomas (WHO type III) have similar clinical behavior and account for approximately 95% of nasopharyngeal cancer in endemic regions (McGuire and Lee 1990). However, approximately 75% of nasopharyngeal cancer cases in North America are keratinized squamous cell carcinoma (WHO type I) (Marks et al. 1998).

2.1.2 Staging

- Nasopharyngeal cancer is usually staged clinically, as surgery has a limited role in the initial treatment of the disease. Clinical staging utilizes information from patient history and physical examinations, imaging studies, laboratory tests, and endoscopy.

- The American Joint Committee on Cancer (AJCC) Tumor Node Metastasis (TNM) staging system is the accepted standard for staging of nasopharyngeal cancer (Table 2.2) (Greene et al. 2002).

2.1.3 Prognostic Factors

- The stage at diagnosis is the most important prognostic factor for nasopharyngeal cancer.
  The value of the updated AJCC staging classification for nasopharyngeal cancer in predicting the prognosis has been repeatedly demonstrated. Reports from Asia, Europe, and North America have confirmed its value in defining the four prognostic categories (Level IV) (Chua et al. 2001; Cooper et al. 1998; Ma et al. 2001a,b; Ozyar et al. 1999).
  Based on the difference in failure patterns, patients with NPC can be divided into four different prognostic categories: (1) T1–2N0–1 (relatively good treatment outcome); (2) T3–4N0–1 (mainly local failure); (3) T1–2N2–3 (mainly regional and distant failure); and (4) T3–4N2–3 (local, regional, and distant failure) (Level IV) (Wei and Sham 2005).

- T classification of the AJCC staging system overall is of prognostic significance; however, T1 and T2a categories do not differentiate prognosis (Level IV) (Sham et al. 1992). Paranasopharyngeal extension (T2b) is an independent prognostic factor correlated with adverse local tumour

Table 2.1. Imaging and lab work-ups for diagnosis and staging of nasopharyngeal cancer

Imaging studies	Laboratory tests
MRI or CT scan of the head and neck area	Complete blood count
Chest X-ray	Serum chemistry
CT scan of the thorax (if equivocal chest X-ray)	Liver function tests
Bone scan (if clinically indicated)	Renal function tests
Liver scan or abdominal CT scan (if clinically indicated)	Alkaline phosphatase
FDG-PET (if clinically indicated)	EBV titers (Ig A anti-VCA and Ig G anti-EA)

Table 2.2. The AJCC Staging System for Nasopharyngeal Cancer [from Greene et al. (2002) with permission]

Primary tumor (T)	
TX	Primary tumor cannot be assessed
T0	No evidence of primary tumor
Tis	Carcinoma in situ
T1	Tumor confined to the nasopharynx
T2	Tumor extends to soft tissues
T2a	Tumor extends to the oropharynx and/or nasal cavity without parapharyngeal extension
T2b	Any tumor with parapharyngeal extension
T3	Tumor involves bony structures and/or paranasal sinuses
T4	Tumor with intracranial extension and/or involvement of cranial nerves, infratemporal fossa, hypopharynx, orbit, or masticator space
Regional lymph nodes (N)	
NX	Regional lymph nodes cannot be assessed
N0	No regional lymph node metastasis
N1	Unilateral metastasis in lymph node(s), 6 cm or less in greatest dimension, above the supraclavicular fossa
N2	Bilateral metastasis in lymph node(s), 6 cm or less in greatest dimension, above the supraclavicular fossa
N3	Metastasis in a lymph node(s) 6 cm and/or to supraclavicular fossa
N3a	Great than 6 cm in dimension
N3b	Extension to the supraclavicular fossa
Distant metastasis (M)	
MX	Distant metastasis cannot be assessed
M0	No distant metastasis
M1	Distant metastasis
STAGE GROUPING	
0:	Tis N0 M0
I:	T1 N0 M0
IIA:	T2a N0 M0
IIB:	T1 N1 M0, T2 N1 M0, T2a N1 M0, T2b N0 M0, T2b N1 M0
III:	T1 N2 M0, T2a N2 M0, T2b N2 M0, T3 N0 M0, T3 N1 M0, T3 N2 M0
IVA:	T4 N0 M0, T4 N1 M0, T4 N2 M0
IVB:	Any T N3 M0
IVC:	Any T Any N M1

control and increased distant spread (Sham and Choy 1991a,b; Cheng et al. 2001).

■ Patients with advanced N-category have higher risk of distant metastases. In a large retrospective study, risk factors for a poor outcome after radiation alone were evaluated. Advanced N-category and adenopathy in the lower neck were independent adverse prognostic factors for the development of distant metastases, while advanced T- and N-category were independent adverse prognostic factors for disease-specific survival (Level IV) (Geara et al. 1997).

Patients with adenopathy in the lower neck or supraclavicular area have significantly higher inci-

dence of distant metastases at presentation or after definitive treatment (Level IV) (Teo et al. 1991).

■ Primary tumor volume is an independent prognostic factor of local control and is more predictive with the AJCC/UICC staging system than with Ho's T stage classification. Validity of tumor volume has been confirmed in patients with T3 and T4 tumors (Chua et al. 1997; Chang et al. 2002; Shen et al. 2008; Sze et al. 2004). However, tumor volume is not an independent prognostic factor in early-stage nasopharyngeal carcinoma treated by radiotherapy alone (Chua et al. 2004a).

■ The WHO histopathologic classification is of prognostic significance, and WHO type III tumors have better prognosis: In a review of data from the Surveillance, Epidemiology, and End Results (SEER) database of the National Cancer Institute, 5-year overall survival rates for WHO grade I, II, and III tumors treated between 1990 and 1999 were 42%, 56%, and 69%, respectively (Level III) (LEE et al. 2005). The 5-year overall survival was 37% for WHO I, 55% for WHO II, and 60% for WHO III ($P < 0.001$) in the INT 0099 trial (Level IV) (AL-SARRAF et al. 2001).

■ Quantitative analysis of circulating EBV DNA in nasopharyngeal carcinoma has shown a positive correlation with disease stage and exhibiting prognostic importance (Level III and IV) (LIN et al. 2001, 2004; LE et al. 2005; CHAN et al. 2004). High posttreatment levels of EBV DNA may reflect microscopic residual tumor, and provide an even greater estimate of the chance of disease recurrence and death than pretreatment EBV DNA (Level III and IV) (LIN et al. 2004; LE et al. 2005; CHAN et al. 2004).

■ Anemia is an independent adverse effect for nasopharyngeal cancer treated with radiation therapy. CHUA et al. (2004b) investigated the impact of hemoglobin (Hb) levels on treatment outcome in patients with nasopharyngeal carcinoma treated in a randomized phase III trial aimed at comparing induction chemotherapy followed by radiotherapy or with radiotherapy alone. This study showed that Hb level during radiotherapy was an important prognostic factor with respect to local control and survival. Patients with Hb levels ≤ 11 g/dL during radiation had significantly poorer local control than patients with higher Hb levels (5-year local recurrence-free rate, 60% vs. 80%; $P = 0.0059$). The 5-year disease-specific survival for patients with Hb levels ≤ 11 g/dL and > 11 g/dL were 51% and 68%, respectively ($P = 0.001$) (Level IV) (CHUA et al. 2004b).

2.2 Treatment of Nasopharyngeal Cancer

2.2.1 General Principles

■ Radiation therapy is the standard treatment for nasopharyngeal cancer.
■ For early stage nasopharyngeal cancer (i.e., T1 and T2a, N0), radiation therapy alone is the treatment of choice (Grade A).

■ For locally advanced (i.e., T2b, T3, or T4 categories) or N+ diseases, concurrent chemotherapy and radiation is recommended and is currently the standard of care (Grade A).
■ Intensity-modulated radiation therapy (IMRT) should be considered for all patients for definitive treatment, if available (Grade B). IMRT provides significantly improved side-effect profile, as compared to conventional radiation or 3D conformal treatment.
■ Surgery has a limited role in the definitive treatment of nasopharyngeal carcinoma. However, neck dissection is indicated for patients with residual or recurrent neck adenopathy after definitive radiation therapy (Grade B).

2.2.2 Radiation Therapy for Early Stage Disease

■ Radiation therapy alone is recommended in the treatment of early stage nasopharyngeal cancer, and optimal outcome can be expected after radiotherapy (Grade A). The 10-year disease-specific survival, recurrence-free survival (RFS), local RFS, lymph node RFS, and distant metastasis-free survival rates for stage I NPC were 98%, 94%, 96%, 98%, and 98%, respectively after radiation therapy (Level IV) (CHUA et al. 2003a).
■ Higher dose of radiation is associated with improved disease control. Higher dose delivered by brachytherapy boost in addition to conventional external beam radiotherapy has been demonstrated to provided improved local control, and based on a literature review and the judgment of its panel of experts, the American Brachytherapy Society recommended 18 Gy in six fractions of high-dose-rate (HDR) brachytherapy over 3 days (two fractions per day, 6 h apart) 1–2 weeks after 60 Gy external beam radiation (Grade C) (NAG et al. 2001). This regimen was utilized in the series reported by LEVENDAG et al. (1998) and was found to be safe and effective (Level IV). Several retrospective series from Hong Kong also demonstrated comparable findings using similar dose schedules of HDR brachytherapy. CHANG et al. (1996) prescribed 5–16.5 Gy in between one and three fractions at a 1-week interval, while TEO et al. (2000a) used 18–24 Gy in three fractions over 15 days. Both of these techniques appeared effective and safe (Level IV).

Results of a more recently published prospective study revealed that the a 2-year local control rate of 94% at the primary site can be achieved with combined 3D conformal external-beam radiotherapy and high-dose-rate intracavitary brachytherapy (Level III) (Lu et al. 2004). However, the necessity of intracavitary brachytherapy for treating nasopharyngeal cancer in the era of IMRT becomes questionable. In a retrospective series from the University of California, San Francisco, local control at the primary site after combined external-beam radiation (including IMRT) with or without brachytherapy was > 90% at 5 years after treatment for T1, T2, and selected cases of more advanced disease (Level IV) (Lee et al. 2002a,b).

■ In the IMRT era, hyperfractionated radiation therapy is not routinely recommended for the treatment of early stage nasopharyngeal cancer (Grade B). The results of a prospective phase II trial showed that the 3-year local control and overall survival rates of stage II nasopharyngeal cancer treated to a total dose of 72 Gy in an accelerated concomitant boost (conformal radiotherapy) were 87.1% and 85.9%, respectively (Level III) (Lu et al. 2007). These rates were inferior to the local control and survival rates reported in patients treated with IMRT.

In addition, accelerated concomitant boost radiation using conventional technique without CT planning was associated with excess side effects and complications. A prospective randomized trial from Hong Kong aimed at studying the effect of accelerated concomitant boost radiation on locally advanced nasopharyngeal cancer was closed prematurely due to excessive toxicity, with no significant therapeutic benefits demonstrated (Level II) (Teo et al. 2000b).

■ Chemotherapy for early stage NPC has not been confirmed, and currently is not routinely recommended given the good treatment outcome after radiation therapy alone (Grade C). A survival benefit for chemoradiotherapy over RT alone was suggested in a retrospective study and a pooled analysis of two Phase III trials; however, it has not been addressed in any prospectively designed studies. Subgroup analysis showed the addition of chemotherapy benefited patients with T1-2, N0-1 NPC ($n = 208$ of the total 790 patients), the 5-year overall survival was 79% versus 67% ($p = 0.048$) (Chua et al. 2006). The benefit of chemoradiotherapy in early stage disease was also suggested

in a retrospective study of 32 patients with stage II NPC who received concomitant cisplatin and 5-FU with standard fraction RT, followed by 2-monthly post-RT chemotherapy cycles. With median follow-up of 44 months, locoregional control and DFS rates at 3 years were 100% and 97%, respectively (Cheng et al. 2000).

2.2.3 Combined Chemoradiation Therapy for Locoregionally Advanced NPC Concurrent Chemoradiation

■ Concurrent chemotherapy and radiation therapy followed by adjuvant chemotherapy is the current standard of care for patients with locally advanced nasopharyngeal cancer (T3, T4, or N+ diseases) (Grade A). The efficacy of chemotherapy delivered concurrently with radiotherapy has been demonstrated in a number of prospective randomized trials:

The landmark INT 0099 study randomly assigned 147 patients with locally advanced NPC to concurrent chemoradiotherapy (70 Gy) followed by adjuvant chemotherapy or the same dose of RT alone. Patients in the chemotherapy arm received cisplatin (100 mg/m^2) on days 1, 22, and 43 of standard RT followed by adjuvant cisplatin (80 mg/m^2 on day 1) and 5-FU (1000 mg/m^2 daily days 1 through 4), every 4 weeks for three cycles. The study was terminated early due to a highly significant 3-year survival advantage for chemoradiotherapy (76% versus 46%) (Level I) (Al-Sarraf et al. 1998).

A similar study from Singapore reported the outcome of 221 patients with NPC treated with RT alone (70 Gy over 7 weeks) or RT plus concurrent cisplatin (25 mg/m^2 days 1–4 during weeks 1, 4, and 7) followed by adjuvant cisplatin (20 mg/m^2 days 1–4) plus 5-FU (1000 mg/m^2 days 1–4), every 4 weeks for three cycles. The 3-year survival rate was significantly better with chemoradiotherapy (80% versus 65%), as was the 2-year cumulative incidence of distant metastases (13% versus 30%) (Level I) (Wee et al. 2005).

In contrast to these reports, a survival benefit for chemoradiotherapy was not shown in a preliminary report of a randomized trial designed identically to the INT 0099 regimen from Hong

Kong. Approximately 350 patients with T1-4N2-3M0 NPC were included. With a median follow-up of 2.3 years, the CRT arm had significantly better locoregional control (92% versus 82%) and 3-year failure-free survival (72% versus 62%), but similar rates of distant control, and overall survival. Longer follow-up is required to confirm these outcomes (Level II) (LEE et al. 2005).

■ Concurrent platinum-based chemoradiation therapy without adjuvant chemotherapy can also be recommended for definitive treatment for locally advanced nasopharyngeal cancer (Grade A). The benefit of concurrent chemoradiotherapy without additional adjuvant chemotherapy was addressed in three large trials: A study from Taiwan randomly assigned 284 patients with stage III or IV nasopharyngeal cancer radiation therapy alone or with cisplatin (20 mg/m^2 daily) plus 5-FU (400 mg/m^2 daily), both administered by continuous 96-h infusion on weeks 1 and 5 of RT. The 5-year overall survival (72% versus 54%), progression-free survival (72% versus 53%) and locoregional relapse rates (26% versus 46%) significantly favored chemoradiotherapy (Level I) (LIN et al. 2003).

A prospective randomized study from Hong Kong reported the outcome of 350 NPC patients treated with RT (66 Gy over 6.5 weeks) alone or RT with concurrent cisplatin (40 mg/m^2 weekly). Although the difference in 5-year progression-free survival with chemoradiotherapy was not statistically significant in the entire group, it was significant in the subgroup with T3/4 disease, after a follow-up of 5.5 years. In addition, the overall survival was significantly improved after combined treatment in patients with T3 or T4 tumors (Level I) (CHAN et al. 2005b).

A similar magnitude of benefit for chemoradiotherapy was seen in a Chinese trial that used weekly oxaliplatin (70 mg/m^2 over 2 h weekly) rather than cisplatin. However, the efficacy of oxaliplatin-based chemotherapy comparing to that of cisplatin needs further investigation (Level II) (ZHANG et al. 2005).

■ The effects of combined chemotherapy and radiation therapy on treatment outcome for locally advanced disease have been further confirmed by meta-analysis. LANGENDIJK and colleagues (2004) performed a meta-analysis of ten prospective randomized trials including 2450 patients aimed at determining the roles of neoadjuvant, concurrent, and adjuvant chemotherapy with de-

finitive radiation therapy. It was demonstrated that concurrent chemotherapy can provide a 20% survival benefits at 5 years after treatment [HR = 0.48, (95% CI, 0.32–0.72)]. However, neoadjuvant and adjuvant chemotherapy provided comparable results for locoregional recurrence and distant metastasis, but not on overall survival (Level I) (LANGENDIJK et al. 2004).

Two other meta-analyses, one with smaller sample size and another reported in abstract form, also confirmed concomitant chemotherapy in addition to radiation as probably being the most effective way to treat locally advanced NPC (Level I) (BAUJAT et al. 2006; THEPHAMONGKOL et al. 2004).

The Role of Neoadjuvant Chemotherapy

■ Neoadjuvant chemotherapy alone prior to radiation therapy (i.e., without concurrent chemotherapy) is not routinely indicated for definitive treatment of locally advanced nasopharyngeal carcinoma when followed by radiotherapy (Grade A). Neoadjuvant chemotherapy has not been demonstrated to improve overall survival if given before definitive radiotherapy in four randomized trials:

The preliminary results of a randomized trial reported by the International Nasopharynx Cancer Study Group showed that bleomycin, epirubicin, and cisplatin given prior to radiation significantly improved disease-free survival; however, local and distant control, as well as overall survival, were not statistically different in patients treated with radiation alone or combined therapy (VUMCA-I, Level II) (VUMCA 1996).

CHUA et al. (1998a) reported the results of the Asian-Oceanian Clinical Oncology Associations randomized trial comparing between two and three cycles of cisplatin-based (Cisplatin 60 mg/m^2 on day 1, epirubicin 110 mg/m^2 on day 1) induction chemotherapy followed by radiotherapy versus radiotherapy alone in the treatment of patients with locoregionally advanced nasopharyngeal carcinoma. Analysis of the 334 patients based on the intention to treat showed no significant difference in relapse free survival (48% vs. 42%, $P = 0.45$) or overall survival (78% vs. 71%, $P = 0.57$) between the two treatment arms (AOCOA trail, Level II) (CHUA et al. 1998a).

Another study conducted in China using a similar study design also failed to demonstrate sig-

nificant overall survival benefit (63% vs. 56%, $P = 0.11$) with the addition of neoadjuvant chemotherapy; however, neoadjuvant chemotherapy did associate with improved relapse-free survival rate (59% vs. 49%, $P = 0.05$) and local recurrence-free rate (82% vs. 74%, $P = 0.04$) (Level I) (MA et al. 2001).
A pooled data analysis of two previously reported Phase III studies totaling 784 patients revealed that the use of induction chemotherapy resulted in an absolute improvement of 8.2% in the recurrence-free survival rate ($P = 0.014$) and 5.4% in the disease-specific survival rate ($P = 0.029$) over 5 years. (Level III) (CHUA et al. 2005b).

■ Neoadjuvant chemotherapy prior to concurrent chemoradiation therapy can be considered in patients with locally advanced disease for improving local control (Grade B). Neoadjuvant chemotherapy is reasonable for reducing the tumor bulk of diseases with extensive intracranial extension or bulky neck adenopathy prior to concurrent chemoradiation therapy.
Despite lack of support from prospective randomized studies, several prospective phase II trails showed encouraging results: The overall survival rates for patients with locally advanced nasopharyngeal cancer treated with neoadjuvant chemotherapy plus concurrent chemoradiation therapy were in the range of 90% at 1–3 years post treatment (Level III) (AL-AMRO et al. 2005; CHAN et al. 2004; JOHNSON et al. 2004, 2005; RISCHIN et al. 2002).

The Role of Adjuvant Chemotherapy

■ Adjuvant chemotherapy is not routinely recommended for definitive treatment of locally advanced nasopharyngeal carcinoma (Grade A). Results of a randomized trial revealed that adjuvant chemotherapy after radiation therapy did not improve overall survival: ROSSI et al. (1988) randomized 229 patients with nonmetastatic NPC, including some early stage disease, to either radiation therapy or radiotherapy plus adjuvant chemotherapy (vincristine, doxorubicin, and cyclophosphamide) for 6 months. The overall and relapse-free survival rates in the two groups were nearly identical at about 60% and 55%, respectively (Level II) (ROSSI et al. 1988).

■ Whether adjuvant chemotherapy is necessary after concurrent chemoradiation therapy has not been tested in a prospective randomized fashion.

2.2.4 Radiation Therapy Techniques

Intensity-Modulated Radiation Therapy

■ IMRT is recommended for definitive treatment for all patients with nasopharyngeal cancer (Grade A). A number of retrospective reports comparing IMRT and 3D conformal radiation therapy revealed that IMRT has a much improved toxicity profile, especially in preserving parotid function. A landmark report from the University of California, San Francisco, demonstrated that the local progression-free, locoregional progression-free, and overall survival rates at 4 years reached 97%, 98%, and 88%, respectively. In addition, late grade 3 and 4 complications were seen in only eight of the group of 67 patients. And only one of 41 evaluable patients had Grade 2 xerostomia at 24 months, 32% had Grade 1, and 66% had Grade 0 or no xerostomia (Level IV) (LEE et al. 2002a,b). These results have been confirmed in other retrospective series (Level IV) (WOLDEN et al. 2006; SULTANEM et al. 2000; KAM et al. 2004; KWONG et al. 2004, 2006). Preliminary data from RTOG 0225, a prospective phase II trial, revealed that the 2-year local progression-free rate is 92% and locoregional progression-free rate is 90.5% after IMRT (Level III) (LEE et al. 2007). Furthermore, a small randomized trial compared the rates of delayed xerostomia between two-dimensional radiation therapy (2D-RT) and IMRT in 60 patients with early-stage (T1-T2b, N0-1, M0) nasopharyngeal carcinoma. The results revealed that at 1 year after treatment, patients treated with IMRT had lower incidence of severe xerostomia than those treated with 2D-RT (39.3% versus 82.1%; $p = 0.001$) (Level II) (KAM et al. 2007).

Treatment Technique of IMRT (Planning, Imaging, and Localization)

■ Treatment planning CT scans are required to define gross target volume(s), and clinical target volume(s). MRI scans (required unless medically contraindicated) aid in delineation of the treatment volume on planning CT scans. Image registration and fusion applications, if available, should be used to help in the delineation of target volumes.
All tissues to be irradiated must be included in the CT scan. CT scan thickness should be ≤ 0.3-cm slices through the region that contains the primary target volumes. The regions above and

below the target volume may be scanned with 0.5-cm slice thickness.

■ The treatment planning CT scan should be acquired with the patient in the same position and using the same immobilization device as for treatment. The immobilization device should include the head, neck, and shoulder area. When possible, the patient immobilization device should also be used for the MRI scan.

■ The gross tumor volume [GTV-P for primary and GTV-N for lymph node(s)] is defined as all known gross disease determined from CT, MRI, clinical information, and endoscopic findings. GTV-N is defined as any lymph nodes > 1 cm or nodes with a necrotic center.

High risk and low risk clinical target volume (CTV) should be defined. GTV (GTV-P and GTV-N) with a margin of ≥ 5 mm will be called the CTV70 (CTV70-P and CTV70-N).

The high risk CTV at the primary disease site (CTV 59.4-P) includes the entire nasopharynx, anterior 1/2 to 2/3 of the clivus (entire clivus, if involved), skull base (foramen ovale and rotundum bilaterally must be included for all cases), pterygoid fossae, parapharyngeal space, inferior sphenoid sinus (in T3-T4 disease, the entire sphenoid sinus) and posterior fourth to third of the nasal cavity and maxillary sinuses (to ensure pterygopalatine fossae coverage). The cavernous sinus should be included in high risk patients (T3, T4, bulky disease involving the roof of the nasopharynx). The outer most boundary of CTV 59.4-P should be at least 10 mm from the GTV-P.

The high risk lymph nodal regions (CTV 59.4-N) include upper deep jugular (junctional, parapharyngeal); subdigastric (jugulodigastric) (level II); midjugular (level III); posterior cervical (level V); retropharyngeal; submandibular (level I). If there are gross nodes in the low neck, low jugular and supraclavicular (level IV) lymph nodal regions should be considered high risk. IB lymph nodes can be spared if the patient is node-negative. In low risk node-positive patients presenting with isolated retropharyngeal nodes or isolated level IV nodes, level IB may also be spared or limited to the anterior border of the submandibular gland. The outer most boundary of the CTV 59.4-N should be at least 10 mm away from the GTV-N. The low risk CTV (CTV54) includes bilateral uninvolved lower neck nodal regions.

■ Neck node target volume delineation and typical IMRT plans are shown in Figures 2.1–2.3.

Dose Specifications

■ The recommended dose to the PTV 70 (i.e., CTV 70 with margin) is ~ 70 Gy in 33 fractions at 2.12 Gy per fraction.

■ The high risk PTV 59.4 (CTV 59.4 + margin) will receive 59.4 Gy in 33 fractions at 1.7–1.8 Gy per fraction.

■ The PTV54 (CTV54 + margin) will receive 54 Gy at 1.64 Gy per fraction. If the split beam technique is considered, the low neck or supraclavicular field may be treated with conventional AP or AP/PA fields for a total of 50 Gy at 2.0 Gy per fraction.

■ Treatment should be delivered once daily, five fractions per week. All targets should be treated simultaneously.

Critical Normal Structures Contour and Dose Limitations

■ Critical normal structures in the head and neck region, including the brainstem, spinal cord, optic nerves, chiasm, parotid glands, pituitary, temporomandibular (T-M) joints and middle and inner ears, skin (in the region of the target volumes), oral cavity, mandible, eyes, lens, temporal lobes, brachial plexus, esophagus (including postcricoid pharynx), and glottic larynx should be outlined.

■ If planning organ at risk volumes (PRVs) are used, the spinal cord PRV will be defined as a 3D margin at least 5 mm larger than the spinal cord to ensure that the PRV margin is at least 5 mm from any portion of the spinal cord. The brainstem PRV, chiasm PRV, and optic nerve PRV will be defined as at least 1 mm larger in all directions than the corresponding structure. Parotid glands: Mean dose < 26 Gy (should be achieved in at least one gland) or at least 20 cc of the combined volume of both parotid glands will receive < 20 Gy or at least 50% of one gland will receive < 30 Gy (should be achieved in at least one gland). Dose to the submandibular and sublingual glands and oral cavity should be kept at minimal if possible (Table 2.3).

Conventional Radiation Therapy

■ When IMRT is not available, 3D conformation radiation therapy can be utilized for the definitive treatment of nasopharyngeal cancer.

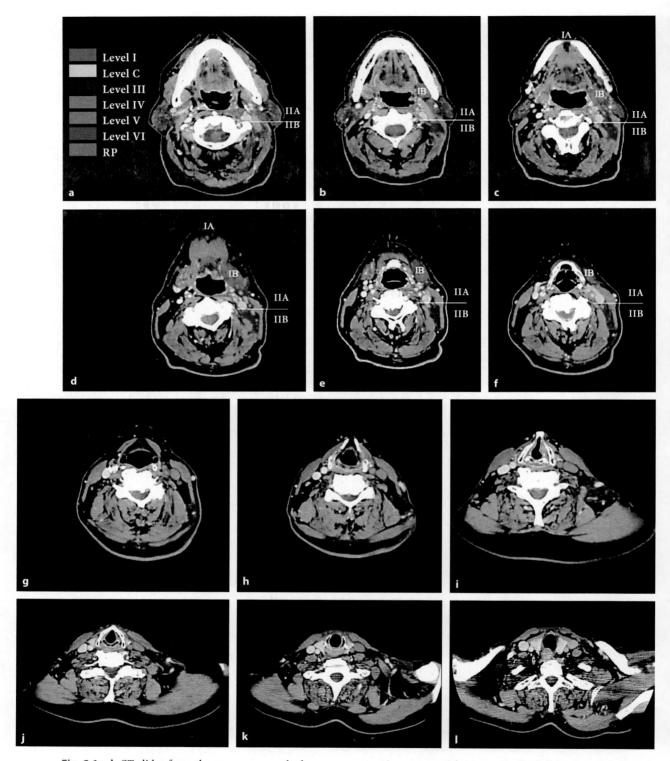

Fig. 2.1a–l. CT slides from the consensus reached among cooperative groups with respect to the delineation of the lymph node levels in the node-negative neck. These illustrations can be used as a reference for CTV delineation in nasopharyngeal cancer treatment

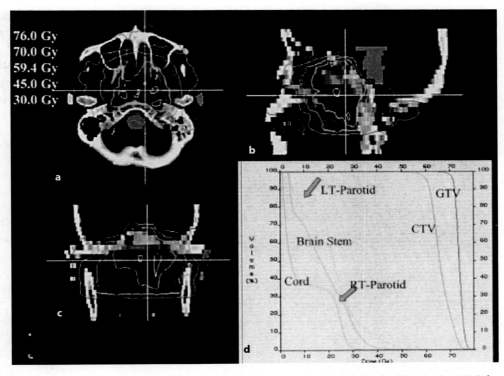

Fig. 2.2a–d. Isodose curves of an inverse IMRT plan delivered using multivane dynamic multi-leaf collimator (MIMiC) for a patient with T4N1 carcinoma of the nasopharynx displayed on the axial (**a**), coronal (**b**), and sagittal (**c**) planes through the centroid of the primary tumor and the dose volume histogram for the relevant structures (**d**). The gross tumor volume is shown in *red* and the clinical target volume is shown in *orange*. [From LEE et al. (2002b) with permission]

Table 2.3. Dose constraints of critical normal structures in IMRT for nasopharyngeal cancer treatment

Structure	True structure constraint	PRV constraint
Brainstem	54 Gy max dose	No more than 1% to exceed 60 Gy
Spinal cord	45 Gy max dose	No more than 1% to exceed 50 Gy
Optic nerves, chiasm	50 Gy max dose	54 Gy max dose
Mandible, TM joint	70 Gy, if not possible then no more than 1 cc to exceed 75 Gy	
Brachial plexus	66 Gy max dose	
Oral cavity (excluding PTVs)	Mean dose less than 40 Gy	
Each cochlea	No more than 5% receives 55 Gy or more	
Eyes	Max dose less than 50 Gy	
Lens	Max dose less than 25 Gy	
Glottic larynx	Mean dose less than 45 Gy	
Esophagus, postcricoid pharynx	Mean dose less than 45 Gy	

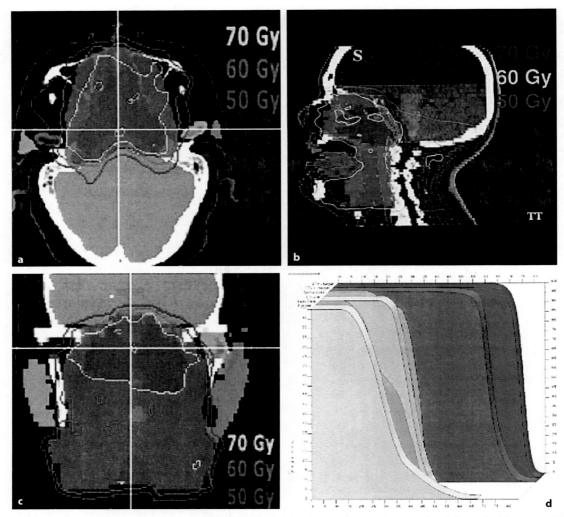

Fig. 2.3a–d. Isodose curves of an inverse IMRT plan using nine coplanar gantry angles delivered with conventional MLC for a patient with T3N0 carcinoma of the nasopharynx displayed on the axial (**a**), coronal (**b**), and sagittal (**c**) planes through the centroid of the primary tumor and the dose volume histogram for the relevant structures (**d**). The gross tumor volume is shown in *red* and the clinical target volume is shown in *magenta*. [From LEE et al. (2003) with permission]

Treatment Technique (Simulation and Field Arrangement)

■ The patient's head position should be hyperextended at the initial simulation so that there is adequate separation between the primary and retropharyngeal lymph nodes and the upper neck nodes. The head and neck, and in some cases the shoulders, are immobilized using a thermoplastic mask with the neck supported on a Timo (S-type, MED-TEC).

■ Tumor volumes including the involved neck adenopathy should be delineated on the planning CT scan.

■ The treatment can start with an opposed pair of large lateral opposing faciocervical fields that cover the primary tumor and the upper neck lymphatics in one volume, with matching lower anterior cervical field for lower neck lymphatics. The fields are designed as follows (Fig. 2.4):
Superiorly: the field border should be set at 2 cm superior to the tumor defined on the CT and/or MRI of the head and neck, and encompass the base of skull and sphenoid sinus.
Anteriorly: the field border should be set at 2 cm margin anterior to the tumor defined on CT and/or MRI, or to include posterior 1/3 of the maxillary sinus, whichever is more anterior.

Posteriorly: the posterior border should be set at 2 cm posterior to the mastoid process, or to include the involved cervical lymph node(s) with 1.5 cm margin, whichever is more posterior.

Inferiorly: the field border should be set at thyroid notch, preferably using a half-beam technique to allow matching with the lower neck field.

■ When the spinal cord dose reaches approximately 40 Gy, treatment can be continued to a total dose of 50 Gy with the lateral opposing faciocervical fields but with shrinkage of fields to avoid the spinal cord (off cord fields), and by treating the superior-posterior lymphatic with electron fields (Fig. 2.5).

■ The lower neck field is usually treated with anteroposterior and posteroanterior (AP/PA) fields with a midline block to spear larynx and spinal cord (Fig. 2.6).

■ Gross tumor (including primary and involved neck nodes) should be treated with additional 20 Gy to carry the total dose to approximately 70 Gy in conventional fractionations (Fig. 2.7).

Brachytherapy

■ Brachytherapy alone is not recommended for definitive treatment of nasopharyngeal carcinoma

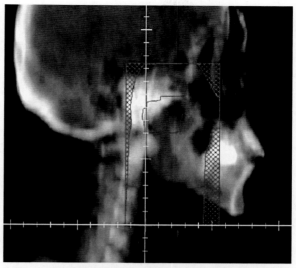

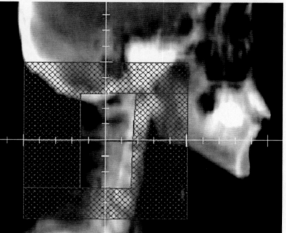

Fig. 2.5a,b. Off-cord fields (**a**) of the same patient after 40 Gy of conventional radiation delivered by the initial oppose lateral fields. The posterior neck fields (**b**) were treated using electron beam. The total dose to the off-cord fields were 10 Gy delivered in five daily fractions

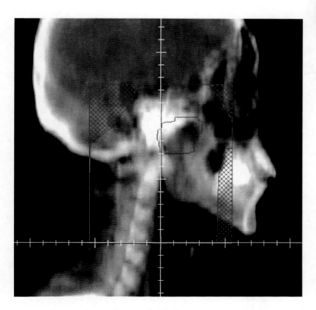

Fig. 2.4. Initial simulation field (lateral) using conventional radiotherapy for a patient with T2N0M0 undifferentiated carcinoma of the nasopharynx

due to the limitation of its effective treatment distance.

■ Brachytherapy as part of definitive treatment for nasopharyngeal carcinoma may be used as a boost treatment of T1 to T3 carcinoma of the nasopharynx after external beam irradiation or in the treatment of recurrent disease, either alone or in combination with external beam radiotherapy (Level III and IV) (Lee et al. 2002a,b; Lu et al. 2004).

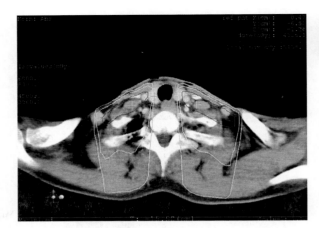

Fig. 2.6. Dose distribution of the lower neck area treated with AP/PA fields using conventional radiation

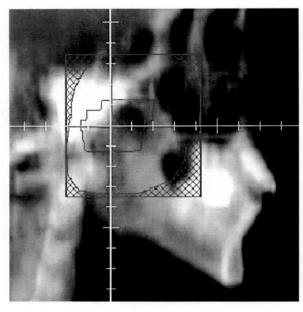

Fig. 2.7. Final boost fields to a total of 20 Gy delivered in ten daily fraction to bring the total dose to 70 Gy to the primary tumor

■ Various dose arrangements can be used for adjuvant brachytherapy. Total dose of 10 Gy given in two weekly fractions (i.e., 5 Gy in each session, 7 days apart), or 5–6 Gy in two daily fractions, 5–6 h apart, can be prescribed at the isodose curve that passes through the nasopharynx point as a boost treatment for T1 to T2 lesions after 65 Gy of external beam radiotherapy (Lee et al. 2002a,b; Lu et al. 2004). The dose for reirradiation of recurrent tumors depends on the previous dose of external beam radiotherapy

2.3 Treatment of Recurrent and Metastatic Nasopharyngeal Cancer

2.3.1 Treatment of Local Recurrence

■ Residual or recurrent disease in the nasopharynx can be managed with a second course of external radiotherapy. The second course of external radiotherapy with concurrent chemotherapy should be considered, although the risk of acute and late toxicities could be significant (Grade B). In a retrospective study reported by Poon et al. (2004), patients treated with a second course of radiation with chemotherapy achieved a 5-year actuarial overall survival rate of 26% (Level IV) (Poon et al. 2004). This result was supported by other retrospective series, with or without chemotherapy (Level IV) (Chua et al. 1998b; Leung et al. 2000).

■ Stereotactic radiotherapy or brachytherapy to the local recurrent focus can be considered for small local recurrence with a reduction in the incidence of complications from re-irradiation (Level IV) (Chua et al. 2003b; Xiao et al. 2001; Mitsuhashi et al. 1999; Choy et al. 1993; Kwong et al. 2001; Law et al. 2002). Kwong et al. (2001) reported the results of persistent and recurrent NPC treated with external radiotherapy followed by gold grain implants; the 5-year local tumor control rates were 87% and 63%, respectively, and the corresponding 5-year disease-free survival rates were 68% and 60% (Level IV) (Kwong et al. 2001).

■ The use of precision radiotherapy such as IMRT could improve the therapeutic ratio for local control (Chua et al. 2005a; Lu et al. 2004). Chua et al. (2005a) reported promising initial results of 31 locally recurrent NPC patients treated with reirradiation using IMRT. Preliminary results showed that good control of recurrent T1-3 NPC can be achieved using IMRT with a dose between 50 and 60 Gy, whereas the outcome for recurrent T4 tumor remained poor. Late toxicities were common but incidence of severe toxicities was relatively low (Level IV) (Chua et al. 2005a).

■ Nasopharyngectomy may be considered in a selected group of patients with local recurrence (Grade B). The efficacy of nasopharyngectomy has been demonstrated in several small series

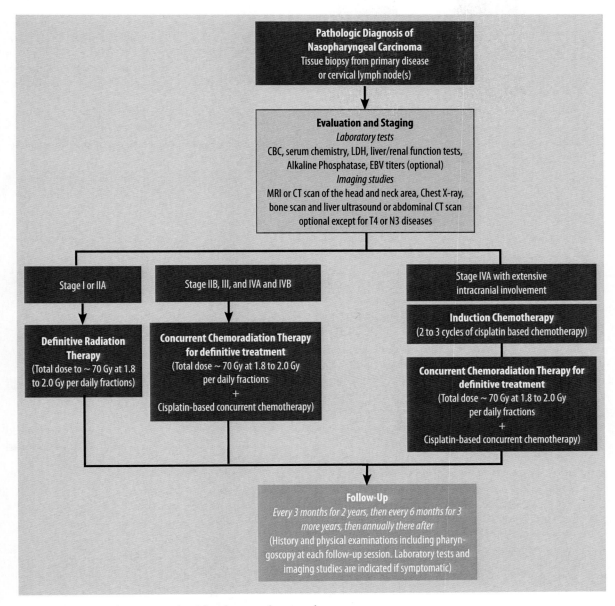

Fig. 2.8. A proposed treatment algorithm for nasopharyngeal cancer

from Asia: In one series of 60 recurrent NPC patients, the overall and relapse-free survival rates were 56% and 60%, and 30% and 40% at 2 and 5 years, respectively (Level IV) (Hsu et al. 2001). In another series of 37 patients with recurrent NPC treated with nasopharyngectomy, the 5-year overall survival and locoregional control rates were both in the range of 60% (Fee et al. 2002). A more recently reported prospective cohort of recurrent nasopharyngeal cancer from Taiwan revealed more optimal findings. The actuarial 3-year survival and local control

rate was 60% and 72.8%, respectively, for 38 patients with locally recurrent nasopharyngeal cancer after salvage surgery (Level IV) (Chang et al. 2004).

2.3.2 Treatment of Regional Recurrence

■ Isolated failure in the regional cervical lymph node(s) is usually rare, and occurs in less than

5% of cases after definitive radiation therapy for nasopharyngeal carcinoma (Level IV) (Huang et al. 1985).

- Radical neck dissection should be recommended for patients with isolated regional nodal failure (Grade B). Salvage surgery could achieve a 5-year tumor control rate of 66% in the neck, and a 5-year actuarial survival of 38% (Level IV) (Wei et al. 1990).
- Radiation can be reserved for patients with contraindication to surgery or who decline surgery (Grade B). However, the overall 5-year survival rate is around 20% for neck recurrence managed with a second course of external radiotherapy (Level IV) (Sham and Choy 1991b).

2.3.3 Treatment of Distant Metastasis (Stage IVC)

- Chemotherapy is the mainstay treatment for metastatic nasopharyngeal cancer (Grade A). An aggressive approach is recommended for metastatic NPC patients with good performance status, and response to chemotherapy can be expected in the majority of cases. Long-term survival has been reported; however, the reported median survival of patients with stage IV disease is usually less than 1 year, with active chemotherapy and palliative radiation (Level IV) (Choo and Tannock 1991; Fandi et al. 2000; Hui et al. 2004).
- Platinum-based chemotherapy regimens are among the most effective regimens for NPC and should be considered as first line chemotherapy for metastatic nasopharyngeal cancer.
- For patients with metastatic nasopharyngeal cancer who have developed resistance to platinum-based chemotherapy, newer agents including taxane, gemcitabine, and capecitabine can be considered (Grade B). Response rates ranging from 29% to 56% have been reported (Level III) (Chua et al. 2000; Ngan et al. 2002; Yeo et al. 1998).
- Molecular targeted therapy agents including cetuximab, sorafenib, and gefitinib have been tested in phase II studies in the treatment of stage IV nasopharyngeal cancer, but their routine use in treating this group of patients is not recommended (Grade B). Both agents were well tolerated in the treatment of stage IV nasopharyngeal cancer when used with platinum-based

chemotherapy, and were well tolerated. However, response to treatment is uncommon (partial response rate ranged from 0% to 12%) and no significant improvement in outcome is expected (Level III) (Chan et al. 2005a; Chua et al. 2008; Elser et al. 2007).

Table 2.4. Follow-up schedule after treatment for nasopharyngeal cancer

Interval	Frequency
First year	Every 1–3 months
Year 2	Every 2–4 months
Year 3–5	Every 4–6 months
Over 5 years	Annually

2.4 Follow-Ups

2.4.1 Post-Treatment Follow-Ups

- Life-long follow-up after definitive treatment of nasopharyngeal carcinoma is usually indicated for detection of recurrence or radiation-induced complications.

Schedule

- The intensity of follow-up is greatest in the first 2–3 years (the period of greatest risk for disease recurrence): every 1–3 months in the first year after treatment, every 2–4 months for the second year, every 4–6 months for year 3–5, then annually thereafter (Grade D) (NCCN 2008).

Work-Ups

- Each follow-up should include a complete history and physical examination and should include endoscopy (Chao et al. 2003).
- Biopsy of the primary area in the post-nasal space is not recommended, unless local disease progression is observed on endoscopy (Grade B). Serial biopsy results reported from Hong Kong showed that positive pathologic results could be expected in 6 weeks after the completion of radiation therapy, although most patients develop pathological remission in the primary site after

12 weeks (Level III) (KWONG et al. 1999). The yield of biopsy performed at 4 months after completion of definitive radiation therapy is less than 5% (Level III) (MA et al. 2006).

- CT scan for the head and neck area is not routinely indicated and should be performed for patients with persistent or newly onset symptoms (Grade B). CT results of "residual tumor" should not be used to determine salvage treatment unless disease progression is diagnosed.

  Residual tumor in the post nasal space may take up to 12 months to resolve, and there is a poor correlation between the findings on post-treatment CT and biopsy results (Level III) (MA et al. 2006).

- Chest X-ray and bone scan are not routinely indicated in asymptomatic patients in follow-up (Grade D) (NCCN 2008).

- Detection of the EBNA-1 and latent membrane protein-1 genes by RT-PCR has been suggested as a means of early detection of recurrent disease (Level III) (HAO et al. 2004). However, routine utilization for this testing cannot be recommended currently.

- Surveillance of TSH, speech and swallowing evaluation, as well as rehabilitation are suggested in patients with neck irradiation every 6–12 months (Grade D) (NCCN 2008).

References

Ahmad A, Stefani S (1986) Distant metastases of nasopharyngeal carcinoma: a study of 256 male patients. J Surg Oncol 33:194–197

Al-Amro A, Al-Rajhi N, Khafaga Y et al. (2005) Neoadjuvant chemotherapy followed by concurrent chemo-radiation therapy in locally advanced nasopharyngeal carcinoma. Int J Radiat Oncol Biol Phys 62:508–513

Al-Sarraf M, LeBlanc M, Giri PG et al. (1998) Chemoradiotherapy versus radiotherapy in patients with advanced nasopharyngeal cancer: phase III randomized Intergroup study 0099. J Clin Oncol 16:1310–1317

Al-Sarraf M, LeBlanc M, Giri P et al. (2001) Superiority of five year survival with chemo-radiotherapy vs. radiotherapy in patients with locally advanced nasopharyngeal cancer. Intergroup (0099) (SWOG 8892, RTOG 8817, ECOG 2388) Phase III study. Final Report. Proc Am Soc Clin Oncol 20:227a

Baujat B, Audry H, Bourhis J et al. (2006) Chemotherapy in locally advanced nasopharyngeal carcinoma: an individual patient data meta-analysis of eight randomized trials and 1753 patients. Int J Radiat Oncol Biol Phys 64:47–56

Caglar M, Ceylan E, Ozyar E (2003) Frequency of skeletal metastases in nasopharyngeal carcinoma after initiation of therapy: should bone scans be used for follow-up? Nucl Med Commun 24:1231–1236

Chan AT, Ma BB, Lo YM et al. (2004) Phase II study of neoadjuvant carboplatin and paclitaxel followed by radiotherapy and concurrent cisplatin in patients with locoregionally advanced nasopharyngeal carcinoma: therapeutic monitoring with plasma Epstein-Barr virus DNA. J Clin Oncol 22:3053–3060

Chan AT, Hsu MM, Goh BC et al. (2005a) Multicenter, phase II study of cetuximab in combination with carboplatin in patients with recurrent or metastatic nasopharyngeal carcinoma. J Clin Oncol 23:3568–3576

Chan AT, Leung SF, Ngan RK et al. (2005b) Overall survival after concurrent cisplatin-radiotherapy compared with radiotherapy alone in locoregionally advanced nasopharyngeal carcinoma. J Natl Cancer Inst 97:536–539

Chang CC, Chen MK, Liu MT et al. (2002) The effect of primary tumor volumes in advanced T-staged nasopharyngeal tumors. Head Neck 24:940–946

Chang KP, Hao SP, Tsang NM et al. (2004) Salvage surgery for locally recurrent nasopharyngeal carcinoma – a 10-year experience. Otolaryngol Head Neck Surg 131:497–502

Chang JT, Chan SC, Yen TC et al. (2005) Nasopharyngeal carcinoma staging by (18)F-fluorodeoxyglucose positron emission tomography. Int J Radiat Oncol Biol Phys 62:501–507

Chang JT, See LC, Tang SG et al. (1996) The role of brachytherapy in early-stage nasopharyngeal carcinoma. Int J Radiat Oncol Biol Phys 36:1019–1024

Chao SS, Loh KS, Tan LK et al. (2003) Modalities of surveillance in treated nasopharyngeal cancer. Otolaryngol Head Neck Surg 129:61–64

Cheng SH, Tsai,SYC, Yen KL et al. (2000) Concomitant radiotherapy and chemotherapy for early-stage nasopharyngeal carcinoma. J Clin Oncol 18:2040–2045

Cheng SH, Yen KL Jian JJ et al. (2001) Examining prognostic factors and patterns of failure in nasopharyngeal carcinoma following concomitant radiotherapy and chemotherapy: impact on future clinical trials. Int J Radiat Oncol Biol Phys 50:717–726

Choo R, Tannock I (1991) Chemotherapy for recurrent or metastatic carcinoma of the nasopharynx. A review of the Princess Margaret Hospital experience. Cancer 68:2120–2124

Choy D, Sham JS, Wei WI et al. (1993) Transpalatal insertion of radioactive gold grain for the treatment of persistent and recurrent nasopharyngeal carcinoma. Int J Radiat Oncol Biol Phys 25:505–512

Chua DT, Sham JS, Kwong DL et al. (1997) Volumetric analysis of tumor extent in nasopharyngeal carcinoma and correlation with treatment outcome. Int J Radiat Oncol Biol Phys 39:711–719

Chua DT, Sham JS, Choy D et al. (1998a) Preliminary report of the Asian-Oceanian Clinical Oncology Association randomized trial comparing cisplatin and epirubicin followed by radiotherapy versus radiotherapy alone in the treatment of patients with locoregionally advanced nasopharyngeal carcinoma. Cancer 83:2255–2258

Chua DT, Sham JS, Kwong DL et al. (1998b) Locally recurrent nasopharyngeal carcinoma: treatment results for patients with computed tomography assessment. Int J Radiat Oncol Biol Phys 41:379–386

Chua DT, Kwong DL, Sham JS et al. (2000) A phase II study of ifosfamide, 5-fluorouracil and leucovorin in patients with recurrent nasopharyngeal carcinoma previously treated with platinum chemotherapy. Eur J Cancer 36:736–741

Chua DT, Sham JS, Wei WI et al. (2001) The predictive value of the 1997 American Joint Committee on Cancer stage classification in determining failure patterns in nasopharyngeal carcinoma. Cancer 92:2845–2855

Chua DT, Sham JS, Kwong DL et al. (2003a) Treatment outcome after radiotherapy alone for patients with Stage I-II nasopharyngeal carcinoma. Cancer 98:74–80

Chua DT, Sham JS, Kwong PW et al. (2003b) Linear accelerator-based stereotactic radiosurgery for limited, locally persistent, and recurrent nasopharyngeal carcinoma: efficacy and complications. Int J Radiat Oncol Biol Phys 56:177–183

Chua DT, Sham JS, Leung LH et al. (2004a) Tumor volume is not an independent prognostic factor in early-stage nasopharyngeal carcinoma treated by radiotherapy alone. Int J Radiat Oncol Biol Phys 58:1437–1444

Chua DT, Sham JS, Choy DT (2004b) Prognostic impact of hemoglobin levels on treatment outcome in patients with nasopharyngeal carcinoma treated with sequential chemoradiotherapy or radiotherapy alone. Cancer 101:307–316

Chua DT, Sham JS, Leung LH et al. (2005a) Re-irradiation of nasopharyngeal carcinoma with intensity-modulated radiotherapy. Radiother Oncol 77:290–294

Chua DT, Ma J, Sham JS et al. (2005b) Long-term survival after cisplatin-based induction chemotherapy and radiotherapy for nasopharyngeal carcinoma: a pooled data analysis of two phase III trials. J Clin Oncol 23:1118–1124

Chua DT, Ma J, Sham JS et al. (2006) Improvement of survival after addition of induction chemotherapy to radiotherapy in patients with early-stage nasopharyngeal carcinoma: subgroup analysis of two Phase III trials. Int J Radiat Oncol Biol Phys 65:1300–1306

Chua DT, Wei WI, Wong MP et al. (2008) Phase II study of gefitinib for the treatment of recurrent and metastatic nasopharyngeal carcinoma. Head Neck [Epub ahead of print]

Cooper JS, Cohen R, Stevens RE (1998) A comparison of staging systems for nasopharyngeal carcinoma. Cancer 83:213–219

Dillon WP, Harnsberger HR (1991) The impact of radiologic imaging on staging of cancer of the head and neck. Semin Oncol 18:64–79

Elser C, Siu LL, Winquist E et al. (2007) Phase II trial of sorafenib in patients with recurrent or metastatic squamous cell carcinoma of the head and neck or nasopharyngeal carcinoma. J Clin Oncol 25:3766–3773

Fandi A, Bachouchi M, Azli N et al. (2000) Long-term disease-free survivors in metastatic undifferentiated carcinoma of nasopharyngeal type. J Clin Oncol 18:1324–1330

Fee WE Jr, Moir MS, Choi EC et al. (2002) Nasopharyngectomy for recurrent nasopharyngeal cancer: a 2- to 17-year follow-up. Arch Otolaryngol Head Neck Surg 128:280–284

Geara FB, Sanguineti G, Tucker SL et al. (1997) Carcinoma of the nasopharynx treated by radiotherapy alone: determinants of distant metastasis and survival. Radiother Oncol 43:53–61

Greene FL, Page DL, Fleming ID et al. (2002) American Joint Committee on Cancer, American Cancer Society. AJCC Cancer Staging Manual, 6th ed. Springer-Verlag, Berlin Heidelberg New York

Hao SP, Tsang NM, Chang KP (2004) Monitoring tumor recurrence with nasopharyngeal swab and latent membrane protein-1 and Epstein-Barr nuclear antigen-1 gene detection in treated patients with nasopharyngeal carcinoma. Laryngoscope 114:2027–2030

Hsu MM, Hong RL, Ting LL et al. (2001) Factors affecting the overall survival after salvage surgery in patients with recurrent nasopharyngeal carcinoma at the primary site: experience with 60 cases. Arch Otolaryngol Head Neck Surg 127:798–802

Huang SC, Lui LT, Lynn TC et al. (1985) Nasopharyngeal cancer: study III. A review of 1206 patients treated with combined modalities. Int J Radiat Oncol Biol Phys 11:1789–1793

Hui EP, Leung SF, Au JS et al. (2004) Lung metastasis alone in nasopharyngeal carcinoma: a relatively favorable prognostic factor. A study by the Hong Kong Nasopharyngeal Carcinoma Study Group. Cancer 101:300–306

Johnson FM, Garden A, Palmer JL et al. (2004) A Phase II study of docetaxel and carboplatin as neoadjuvant therapy for nasopharyngeal carcinoma with early T status and advanced N status. Cancer 100:991–998

Johnson FM, Garden AS, Palmer JL et al. (2005) A phase I/II study of neoadjuvant chemotherapy followed by radiation with boost chemotherapy for advanced T-stage nasopharyngeal carcinoma. Int J Radiat Oncol Biol Phys 63:717–724

Kam MK, Teo PM, Chau RM et al. (2004) Treatment of nasopharyngeal carcinoma with intensity-modulated radiotherapy: the Hong Kong experience. Int J Radiat Oncol Biol Phys 60:1440–1450

Kam MK, Leung SF, Zee B et al. (2007) Prospective randomized study of intensity-modulated radiotherapy on salivary gland function in early-stage nasopharyngeal carcinoma patients. J Clin Oncol 25:4873–4879

Kwong DL, Nicholls J, Wei WI et al. (1999) The time course of histologic remission after treatment of patients with nasopharyngeal carcinoma. Cancer 85:1446–1453

Kwong DL, Wei WI and Cheng AC et al. (2001) Long term results of radioactive gold grain implantation for the treatment of persistent and recurrent nasopharyngeal carcinoma. Cancer 91:1105–1113

Kwong DL, Sham JS, Leung LH et al. (2002) Preliminary results of radiation dose escalation for locally advanced nasopharyngeal carcinoma. Int J Radiat Oncol Biol Phys 64:374–381

Kwong DL, Pow EH, Sham JS et al. (2004) Intensity-modulated radiotherapy for early-stage nasopharyngeal carcinoma: a prospective study on disease control and preservation of salivary function. Cancer 101:1584–1593

Kumar MB, Lu JJ, Loh KS et al. (2004) Tailoring distant metastatic imaging for patients with clinically localized undifferentiated nasopharyngeal carcinoma. Int J Radiat Oncol Biol Phys 58:688–693

Langendijk JA, Leemans CR, Buter J et al. (2004) The additional value of chemotherapy to radiotherapy in locally advanced nasopharyngeal carcinoma: a meta-analysis of the published literature. J Clin Oncol 22:4604–4612

Law SC, Lam WK, Ng MF et al. (2002) Reirradiation of nasopharyngeal carcinoma with intracavitary mold brachytherapy: an effective means of local salvage. Int J Radiat Oncol Biol Phys 54:1095–1113

Le QT, Jones CD, Yau TK et al. (2005) A comparison study of different PCR assays in measuring circulating plasma Epstein-Barr virus DNA levels in patients with nasopharyngeal carcinoma. Clin Cancer Res 11:5700–5707

Lee AW, Lau WH, Tung SY et al. (2005) Preliminary results of a randomized study on therapeutic gain by concurrent chemotherapy for regionally-advanced nasopharyngeal carcinoma: NPC-9901 Trial by the Hong Kong Nasopharyngeal Cancer Study Group. J Clin Oncol 23:6966–6975

Lee JT, Ko CY (2005) Has survival improved for nasopharyngeal carcinoma in the United States? Otolaryngol Head Neck Surg 132:303–308

Lee N, Hoffman R, Phillips TL et al. (2002a) Managing nasopharyngeal carcinoma with intracavitary brachytherapy: one institution's 45-year experience. Brachytherapy 1:74–82

Lee N, Xia P, Quivey JM et al. (2002b) Intensity-modulated radiotherapy in the treatment of nasopharyngeal carcinoma: an update of the UCSF experience. Int J Radiat Oncol Biol Phys 53:12–22

Lee N, Xia P, Fischbein N et al (2003) Intensity-modulated radiotherapy for head and neck cancer: the UCSF experience focusing on target. Int J Radiat Oncol Biol Phys 57:49–60

Lee N, Harris J, Garden A et al. (2007) Phase II multi-institutional study of IMRT ± chemotherapy for nasopharyngeal carcinoma (RTOG 0225): preliminary results. Int J Radiat Oncol Biol Phys 69:S13–14

Leung TW, Tung SY, Sze WK et al. (2000) Salvage radiation therapy for locally recurrent nasopharyngeal carcinoma. Int J Radiat Oncol Biol Phys 48:1331–1338.

Levendag PC, Schmitz PI, Jansen PP et al. (1998) Fractionated high-dose-rate brachytherapy in primary carcinoma of the nasopharynx. J Clin Oncol 16:2213–2220

Lin JC, Chen KY, Wang WY et al. (2001) Detection of Epstein-Barr virus DNA the peripheral-blood cells of patients with nasopharyngeal carcinoma: relationship to distant metastasis and survival. J Clin Oncol 19:2607–2615

Lin JC, Jan JS, Hsu CY et al. (2003) Phase III study of concurrent chemoradiotherapy versus radiotherapy alone for advanced nasopharyngeal carcinoma: positive effect on overall and progression-free survival. J Clin Oncol 21:631–637

Lin JC, Wang WY, Chen KY et al. (2004) Quantification of plasma Epstein-Barr virus DNA in patients with advanced nasopharyngeal carcinoma. N Engl J Med 350:2461–2470

Lindberg R (1972) Distribution of cervical lymph node metastases from squamous cell carcinoma of the upper respiratory and digestive tracts. Cancer 29:1446–1449

Liu FY, Chang JT, Wang HM et al. (2006) [¹⁸F]fluorodeoxyglucose positron emission tomography is more sensitive than skeletal scintigraphy for detecting bone metastasis in endemic nasopharyngeal carcinoma at initial staging. J Clin Oncol 24:599–604

Liu FY, Lin CY, Chang JT et al. (2007) ¹⁸F-FDG PET can replace conventional work-up in primary M staging of nonkeratinizing nasopharyngeal carcinoma. J Nucl Med 48:1614–1619

Lu JJ, Shakespeare TP, Tan LK et al. (2004) Adjuvant fractionated high-dose-rate intracavitary brachytherapy after external beam radiotherapy in Tl and T2 nasopharyngeal carcinoma. Head Neck 26:389–395

Lu JJ, Kong L, Shakespeare TP et al. (2007) Prospective phase II trial of concomitant boost radiotherapy for stage II nasopharyngeal carcinoma. Oral Oncol [Epub ahead of print]

Lu TX, Mai WY, Teh BS et al. (2004) Initial experience using intensity-modulated radiotherapy for recurrent nasopharyngeal carcinoma. Int J Radiat Oncol Biol Phys 58:682–627

Ma J, Mai HQ, Hong MH et al. (2001a) Is the 1997 AJCC staging system for nasopharyngeal carcinoma prognostically useful for Chinese patient populations? Int J Radiat Oncol Biol Phys 50:1181–1189

Ma J, Mai HQ, Hong MH et al. (2001b) Results of a prospective randomized trial comparing neoadjuvant chemotherapy plus radiotherapy with radiotherapy alone in patients with locoregionally advanced nasopharyngeal carcinoma. J Clin Oncol 19:1350–1357

Ma X, Lu JJ, Loh KS et al. (2006) Role of computed tomography imaging in predicting response of nasopharyngeal carcinoma to definitive radiation therapy. Laryngoscope 116:2162–2165

Marks JE, Phillips JL, Menck HR (1998) The National Cancer Data Base report on the relationship of race and national origin to the histology of nasopharyngeal carcinoma. Cancer 83:582–588

McGuire LJ, Lee JC (1990) The histopathologic diagnosis of nasopharyngeal carcinoma. Ear Nose Throat J 69:229–236

Mitsuhashi N, Sakurai H, Katano S et al. (1999) Stereotactic radiotherapy for locally recurrent nasopharyngeal carcinoma. Laryngoscope 109:805–809

Nag S, Cano ER, Demanes DJ et al. (2001) The American Brachytherapy Society recommendations for high-dose-rate brachytherapy for head-and-neck carcinoma. Int J Radiat Oncol Biol Phys 50:1190–1198

Neel HB (1992) Nasopharyngeal carcinoma: diagnosis, staging, and management. Oncology 6:87–95; discussion 99–102

Ngan RK, Yiu HH, Lau WH et al. (2002) Combination gemcitabine and cisplatin chemotherapy for metastatic or recurrent nasopharyngeal carcinoma: report of a phase II study. Ann Oncol 13:1252–1258

Olmi P, Fallai C, Colagrande S et al. (1995) Staging and follow-up of nasopharyngeal carcinoma: magnetic resonance imaging versus computerized tomography. Int J Radiat Oncol Biol Phys 32:795–800

Ozyar E, Yildiz F, Akyol FH et al. (1999) Comparison of AJCC 1988 and 1997 classifications for nasopharyngeal carcinoma. American Joint Committee on Cancer. Int J Radiat Oncol Biol Phys 44:1079–1087

Poon PY, Tsang VH, Munk PL (2000) Tumour extent and T stage of nasopharyngeal carcinoma: a comparison of magnetic resonance imaging and computed tomographic findings. Can Assoc Radiol J 51:287–295

Poon D, Yap SP, Wong ZW et al. (2004) Concurrent chemoradiotherapy in locoregionally recurrent nasopharyngeal carcinoma. Int J Radiat Oncol Biol Phys 59:1312–1318

Rischin D, Corry J, Smith J et al. (2002) Excellent disease control and survival in patients with advanced nasopharyngeal cancer treated with chemoradiation. J Clin Oncol 20:1845–1852

Rossi A, Molinari R, Boracchi P et al. (1988) Adjuvant chemotherapy with vincristine, cyclophosphamide, and doxorubicin after radiotherapy in local-regional nasopharyngeal cancer: results of a 4-year multicenter randomized study. J Clin Oncol 6:1401–1410

Sakata K, Hareyama M, Tamakawa M et al. (1999) Prognostic factors of nasopharynx tumors investigated by MR imaging and the value of MR imaging in the newly published TNM staging. Int J Radiat Oncol Biol Phys 43:273–278

Sham JS, Choy D (1991a) Prognostic value of paranasopharyngeal extension of nasopharyngeal carcinoma on local control and short-term survival. Head Neck 13:298–310

Sham JS, Choy D (1991b) Nasopharyngeal carcinoma: treatment of neck node recurrence by radiotherapy. Australas Radiol 35:370–373

Sham JS, Wei WI, Nicholls J et al. (1992) Extent of nasopharyngeal carcinoma involvement inside the nasopharynx. Lack of prognostic value on local control. Cancer 69:854–859

Shanmugaratnam K, LH Sobin (1991) Histological typing of tumours of the upper respiratory tract and ear. In: Shanmugaratnam K, Sobin LH (eds) International histological classification of tumours: no 19. WHO, Geneva, pp 32–33

Shen C, Lu JJ, Gu Y et al. (2008) Prognostic impact of primary tumor volume in patients with nasopharyngeal carcinoma treated by definitive radiation therapy. Laryngoscope (in print)

Sievers KW, Greess H, Baum U et al. (2002) Paranasal sinuses and nasopharynx CT and MRI. Eur J Radiol 33:185–202

Skinner DW, Van Hasselt CA, Tsao SY (1991) Nasopharyngeal carcinoma: modes of presentation. Ann Otol Rhinol Laryngol 100:544–551

Sultanem K, Shu HK, Xia P et al. (2000) Three-dimensional intensity-modulated radiotherapy in the treatment of nasopharyngeal carcinoma: the University of California-San Francisco experience. Int J Radiat Oncol Biol Phys 48:711–722

Sze WM, Lee AW, Yau TK et al. (2004) Primary tumor volume of nasopharyngeal carcinoma: prognostic significance for local control. Int J Radiat Oncol Biol Phys 59:21–27

Teo PM, Leung SF, Yu P et al. (1991) A comparison of Ho's, International Union Against Cancer, and American Joint Committee stage classifications for nasopharyngeal carcinoma. Cancer 67:434–439

Teo PM, Leung SF, Lee WY et al. (2000a) Intracavitary brachytherapy significantly enhances local control of

early T-stage nasopharyngeal carcinoma: the existence of a dose-tumor-control relationship above conventional tumoricidal dose. Int J Radiat Oncol Biol Phys 46:445–458

Teo PM, Leung SF, Chan AT et al. (2000b) Final report of a randomized trial on altered-fractionated radiotherapy in nasopharyngeal carcinoma prematurely terminated by significant increase in neurologic complications. Int J Radiat Oncol Biol Phys 48:1311–1322

Thephamongkol, K, Zhou, J, Browman, G et al. (2004) Chemo-radiotherapy versus radiotherapy alone for nasopharyngeal carcinoma: a meta-analysis of 78 randomized controlled trials from English and non-English databases (abstract). Proc Am Soc Clin Oncol 23:491a

VUMCA (1996) Preliminary results of a randomized trial comparing neoadjuvant chemotherapy (cisplatin, epirubicin, bleomycin) plus radiotherapy vs. radiotherapy alone in stage IV (> or = N2, M0) undifferentiated nasopharyngeal carcinoma: a positive effect on progression-free survival. International Nasopharynx Cancer Study Group. VUMCA I trial. Int J Radiat Oncol Biol Phys 35:463–469

Wee J, Tan EH, Tai BC et al. (2005) Randomized trial of radiotherapy versus concurrent chemoradiotherapy followed by adjuvant chemotherapy in patients with American Joint Committee on Cancer/International Union against cancer stage III and IV nasopharyngeal cancer of the endemic variety. J Clin Oncol 23:6730–6738

Wei WI, Sham JS (2005) Nasopharyngeal carcinoma. Lancet 365:2041–2054

Wei WI, Lam KH, Ho CM et al. (1990) Efficacy of radical neck dissection for the control of cervical metastasis after radiotherapy for nasopharyngeal carcinoma. Am J Surg 160:439–442

Wolden SL, Chen WC, Pfister DG et al. (2006) Intensity-modulated radiation therapy (IMRT) for nasopharynx cancer: update of the Memorial Sloan-Kettering experience. Int J Radiat Oncol Biol Phys 64:57–62

Xiao J, Xu G, Miao Y (2001) Fractionated stereotactic radiosurgery for 50 patients with recurrent or residual nasopharyngeal carcinoma. Int J Radiat Oncol Biol Phys 51:164–170

Yeo W, Leung TW, Chan AT et al. (1998) A phase II study combination of paclitaxel and carboplatin in advanced nasopharyngeal carcinoma. Eur J Cancer 34:2027–2031

Zhang L, Zhao C, Peng PJ et al. (2005) Phase III study comparing standard radiotherapy with or without weekly oxaliplatin in treatment of locoregionally advanced nasopharyngeal carcinoma: preliminary results. J Clin Oncol 23:8461–8468

Cancer of the Oral Cavity and Oropharynx

Kenneth Hu and Louis B. Harrison

C O N T E N T S

Introduction and Objectives

Cancers of the oropharynx and oral cavity originate in central locations which can severely impact speech, mastication, taste, swallowing, and cosmesis and are curable with multiple treatment modalities. Disease control, quality of life, and organ function preservation represent important goals of treatment.

Oropharyngeal cancers are usually treated with organ preservation therapy compared to oral cavity lesions, for which radical resection is considered upfront because of excellent control with function preservation. For early stages of both diseases, single modality therapy is preferred whereas multidisciplinary treatment is needed for locoregionally advanced disease.

Important advances have been made with altered fractionation radiotherapy and incorporation of chemotherapy to improve disease control. More recent advances involve better targeting of tumor either through improved imaging, radiation delivery, or biologic therapies.

This chapter examines:

● Recommendations for diagnoses and staging work-up

● Staging systems and prognostic factors

● The role of brachytherapy in the treatment of oral cavity and oropharynx cancer

● Integration of chemotherapy in the definitive and adjuvant setting

● Intensity-modulated radiation therapy experience in the treatment of oropharynx cancer

● Altered fractionation in the definitive and postoperative setting

● Role of targeted therapy in the definitive management of oral cavity/oropharynx cancer

● Follow-up care and surveillance of survivors

K. Hu, MD
Department of Radiation Oncology, Beth Israel Medical Center, 10 Union Square East, Suite 4G, New York, NY 10003, USA
L. B. Harrison, MD
Department of Radiation Oncology, Beth Israel Medical Center, 10 Union Square East, Suite 4G, New York, NY 10003, USA

3.1 **Diagnosis, Staging, and Prognoses**

3.1.1   Diagnosis

Initial Evaluation

■ Diagnosis and evaluation of cancers of the head and neck begin with a complete history and physical examination. History of tobacco or alcohol use are the major risk factors for these tumors; tobacco use has the greatest impact and should be recorded (CRAWFORD et al. 1979). In addition, chewing areca or betel nuts, paan, and tobacco are risk factors for oral cancer, contributing to the high incidence found in Southern Asian countries (BALARAM et al. 2002; MERCHANT et al. 2000).

■ Cancer of the oral cavity can present as a non-healing ulcer, pain, bleeding, or ill-fitting denture. More advanced lesions may present with speech difficulties, dysphagia, otalgia, hypersalivation, and neck mass. These lesions may be preceded or associated with leukoplakia and erythroplakia which represent premalignant epithelial changes.

Oropharyngeal carcinomas present differently depending on their site of origin.

– Soft palate tumors often present in early stages due to ready visualization.

– Cancers of the base of the tongue are occult and often diagnosed in later stages due their remote location and because of the lack of pain fibers at the site. They commonly present with an asymptomatic neck node. However, symptoms may include foreign body sensation in the throat, otalgia due to referred pain from cranial nerve involvement, dysphagia, and changes in voice/articulation due to tongue fixation.

– Tonsillar lesions may present with pain, sore throat, dysphagia, trismus, and ipsilateral neck mass.

■ A thorough physical examination should be focused upon the head and neck area with special attention to tongue mobility, extension to adjacent sites including the nasopharynx, larynx or hypopharynx, and involvement of the primary echelon nodal drainage levels I and II for oral cavity and level II in oropharynx (Fig. 3.1).

– Level I: Submental and submandibular nodes

– Level II: Upper jugular nodes above the hyoid bone to skull base

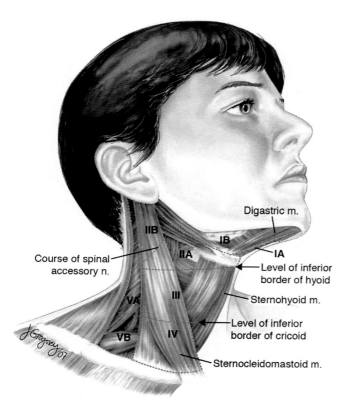

Fig. 3.1. Consensus nodal station as defined by American-Otolaryngology Head and Neck Society. Regional lymph nodes have been divided into levels I–V as follows: Level *I*, submental and submandibular nodes; level *II*, upper jugular nodes above the hyoid bone to skull base; level *III*, mid-jugular nodes between the hyoid and cricoid cartilages under the sternocleidomastoid muscle; level *IV*, lower jugular nodes; level *V*, posterior triangle nodes outlined by the trapezius muscle and posterior border of the sternocleidomastoid muscle (ROBBINS et al. 1991)

- Level III: Mid-jugular nodes between the hyoid and cricoid cartilages under the sternocleidomastoid muscle
- Level IV: Lower jugular nodes
- Level V: Posterior triangle nodes outlined by the trapezius muscle and posterior border of the sternocleidomastoid muscle (ROBBINS et al. 1991).

■ Whether in a clinically involved or negative neck, the spread of tumor into the nodal basins is orderly and predictable based on radical neck dissection data. The primary lymphatic drainage of the oropharynx are to the upper jugulodigastric node(s), as well as the retropharyngeal and parapharyngeal nodes, while oral cavity tumors drain primarily to submandibular nodes and upper jugular nodes (CANDELA et al. 1990; LINDBERG 1972; SHAH et al. 1990). In a clinically negative neck, nodal basins at greatest risk are levels II–IV in oropharynx cancer and I–III in oral cavity tumors (Table 3.1). Isolated skip nodal drainage to the lower level III–IV as well V is rare. In patients with clinical node-positive disease, comprehensive nodal coverage is required for both oral cavity and oropharynx cancers (Table 3.2) (Level IV) (SHAH et al. 1990).

■ Flexible endoscopy of the upper aerodigestive tract is crucial to evaluate the primary site in oropharyngeal cancer and to survey for metachronous lesions. Triple endoscopy including rigid endoscopy of the upper aerodigestive tract, esophagoscopy, and bronchoscopy should also be considered in oropharyngeal cancer.

Table 3.1. Percentage incidence and distribution of pathologically involved nodes in oral cavity and oropharyngeal cancers in clinical node-negative neck after elective radical neck dissection

Level of neck nodes	I	II	III	IV	V
Oropharynx (n=48)	2%	25%	19%	8%	2%
Oral Cavity (n=192)	20%	17%	9%	3%	0.5%

Table 3.2. Percentage incidence and distribution of pathologically involved nodes in oral cavity and oropharyngeal cancers in clinical node-positive neck after elective radical neck dissection

Level of neck nodes	I	II	III	IV	V
Oropharynx (n=165)	14%	71%	42%	28%	9%
Oral Cavity (n=324)	46%	43%	33%	15%	3%

■ Dental evaluation to assess and restore (when possible) or extract (when restoration impossible) decayed teeth is necessary for all patients requiring radiation therapy at approximately 2 weeks before radiation therapy begins.

Laboratory Tests

■ Initial laboratory tests should include a complete blood count, basic blood chemistry, liver, and renal function tests.

■ Testing for human papilloma virus in the biopsy specimen should be considered in oropharynx tumors, especially in patients without significant history of smoking (Grade B) (Level III) (WEINBERGER et al. 2006).

Imaging Studies

■ CT scans of the neck and chest are appropriate to evaluate and stage head and neck cancer. MRI may be useful to improve tumor delineation, especially the extent of soft tissue extension (such as depth of muscle invasion) in oral cancer patients with dental amalgam or in oropharyngeal cancer patients with trismus.

■ FDG-PET/CT scan is recommended for diagnosis and staging of head and neck cancer (Grade B). The results of a prospective study demonstrated that FDG-PET had higher sensitivities than CT or MRI for both primary tumor detection and cervical node detection, although the specificities were not different (Level III) (KIM MR et al. 2007). In addition, a retrospective study of 52 patients evaluated the relationship between the activity observed in the primary disease and the prognosis of the patients with oropharyngeal cancer, and showed that the median SUV was significantly higher in patients who failed treatment than that in the remaining controlled patients. Patients having tumors with a high SUV >6.0 had poorer local control (LC) and disease-free survival (DFS) ($p<0.05$) (Level IV) (KIM SY et al. 2007) (Table 3.3; Fig. 3.2).

3.1.2 Pathology

■ Histologic confirmation is critical to determine the histopathology and extent of disease spread to radiologically indeterminate nodes.

Table 3.3. Imaging and laboratory work-up for head and neck cancer

Imaging studies	Laboratory tests
– CT scan of neck and chest – MRI of head and neck if parapharyngeal/perineural spread is suspected, or to evaluate the primary site if there is severe artifact from dental amalgam – FDG-PET scan or PET/CT	– Complete blood count – Serum chemistry – Liver function tests – Renal function tests – HPV

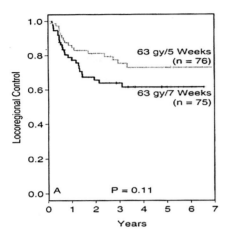
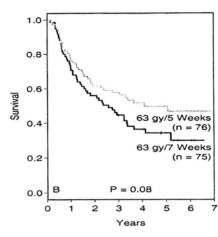

Fig. 3.2. Randomized trial of high-risk postoperative patients demonstrating need to keep the total treatment package time to <11 weeks either by starting treatment early or accelerating radiation delivery (KIM SY et al. 2007) (With permission from Society of Nuclear Medicine)

■ Tumor tissue can be obtained directly from the lesion(s) during examination or endoscopic examination. Typically fine-needle aspiration of a suspected lymph node or open biopsy of the primary site will yield sufficient cells for analysis (SHAHA and SHAH 1995).

■ More than 90% of all oral cavity and oropharyngeal cancers are squamous cell carcinomas (SCC); the remainders include minor salivary gland carcinomas, lymphoma, sarcoma, and melanoma (CRAWFORD et al. 1979).

3.1.3 Staging

■ Carcinomas of the oral cavity can be staged clinically and pathologically. Clinical staging utilizes information from examination of the oral cavity and the neck area, laboratory tests, endoscopy, as well as imaging studies (CT and/or MRI).

■ Clinical staging is usually used for squamous cell carcinomas of the oropharynx. Information from physical examination, direct or indirect endoscopy, and imaging studies. If surgery is employed in the treatment, information on the resected disease as well as nodal examination of pathology should be included for the pathological staging.

■ The American Joint Committee on Cancer (AJCC) Tumor Node Metastasis (TNM) staging system is the accepted standard for staging of both oral and oropharyngeal cancer (Table 3.4) (GREENE et al. 2002).

3.1.4 Prognostic Factors

■ The AJCC stage represents an important prognostic factor. Nodal involvement is the single most important prognostic factor which determines survival and upstages to advanced disease (GREENE et al. 2002)

■ In the postoperative setting, presence of extracapsular extension or positive margins are important predictors of locoregional recurrence and survival.

■ Other negative factors include poor performance status and male gender.

■ Human papilloma virus is implicated in the transformation of oropharynx with the subtype HPV-16 most associated with malignancy (DAHLSTRAND and DALIANIS 2005; WEINBERGER et al. 2006). HPV-positive oropharyngeal cancers have an improved prognosis related either to the biology of these tumors or the lack of associated

Table 3.4. The AJCC staging system for cancer of oral cavity and oropharynx [from GREENE et al. (2002) with permission]

Primary tumor (T): *oral cavity*	
TX	Primary tumor cannot be assessed
T0	No evidence of primary tumor
Tis	Carcinoma in situ
T1	Tumor 2 cm or less
T2	Tumor greater that 2 cm but up to 4 cm
T3	Tumor more than 4 cm in dimension
T4a	Tumor invades adjacent structures (cortical bone), into deep extrinsic muscle of tongue (genioglossus, hyoglossus, palatoglossus, and styloglossus), maxillary sinus, skin of face
T4b	Tumor invades masticator space, pterygoid plates, or skull base/encases internal carotid artery

Primary tumor (T): *oropharynx*	
T1	Tumor 2 cm or less in greatest dimension
T2	Tumor more than 2 cm but 4 cm or less in greatest dimension
T3	Tumor more than 4 cm in greatest dimension
T4a	Tumor invades the larynx, deep/extrinsic muscles of tongue, medial pterygoid, hard palate, mandible
T4b	Tumor invades lateral pterygoid muscle, pterygoid plates, lateral nasopharynx, skull base, or encases carotid artery

Regional lymph nodes (N)	
NX	Regional lymph nodes cannot be assessed
N0	No regional lymph nodes metastasis
N1	Metastasis in a single ipsilateral lymph node, 3 cm or less in greatest dimension
N2	Metastasis in a single ipsilateral lymph node, more than 3 cm but not more than 6 cm in greatest dimension, or in multiple ipsilateral lymph nodes, none more than 6 cm in greatest dimension, or in bilateral or contralateral lymph nodes, none more than 6 cm in greatest dimension
N2a	Metastasis in a single ipsilateral lymph node more than 3 cm but not more than 6 cm in greatest dimension
N2b	Metastasis in multiple ipsilateral lymph nodes, none more than 6 cm in greatest dimension
N2c	Metastasis in bilateral or contralateral lymph nodes, none more than 6 cm in greatest dimension
N3	Metastasis in lymph nodes more than 6 cm in greatest dimension

Distant metastasis (M)	
MX	Distant metastasis cannot be assessed
M0	No distant metastasis
M1	Distant metastasis

STAGE GROUPING	
0:	Tis N0 M0
I:	T1 N0 M0
II:	T2 N0 M0
III:	T3 N0 M0 or T1-3 N1 M0
IVA:	T4a N0-1M0 or T1-4a N2 M0
IVB:	Any T N3 M0 or T4b AnyN M0
IVC:	AnyT AnyN M1

smoking history in many of these patients (Level III) (WEINBERGER et al. 2006).

Management of Oral Cavity Cancer

3.2.1 General Principles

- In general, primary surgery is recommended for oral cavity cancer as single modality therapy in stage I and II with radical resection and selective neck dissection (Grade B). Surgical reconstruction to optimize functional outcomes including radial forearm free flap reconstruction should be considered (Grade B).
- For stage III/IV disease, radical resection with adjuvant radiation alone or with chemotherapy in high-risk patients should be considered (Grade B). High risk is defined by the presence of positive margins at the primary site or extracapsular nodal extension (Grade A). Other factors to be determined for risk stratification include lymphovascular, perineural invasion, level IV nodal involvement in an oropharynx/oral cavity primary, and presence of multiple nodes.
- For locoregionally advanced oral cavity tumors not candidates for resection, concurrent chemoradiation remains the standard (Grade A).

3.2.2 Treatment of Early-Stage Disease

Oral Tongue

- Traditional treatment for oral cavity tumors has been radical resection with or without adjuvant radiation as indicated by pathologic risk factors (Grade B). Reconstruction with free flaps most commonly from the radial forearm has yielded good functional/cosmetic outcomes. A surgical series from Memorial Sloan Kettering Cancer Center, New York, reported LC rates of 85%, 77%, and 50% for T1, T2, and T3 lesions, respectively (Level IV) (SPIRO et al. 1981).
- Radiation therapy alone serves as a reasonable alternative to surgery for early-stage squamous cell cancer of oral tongue (Grade B). The major

series documenting excellent locoregional control from definitive radiation therapy have been large single institution series integrating brachytherapy (Level IV) (Pernot et al. 1992, 1996; Gerbaulet et al. 1985; Mazeron et al. 1987, 1989, 1993; Goffinet et al. 1985; Puthawala et al. 1988; Harrison et al. 1992, 1996). A series from the Curie Institute in Paris of over 600 oral cavity tumors treated with brachytherapy reported LC for T1, T2, and T3 lesions of 86%, 80%, and 68%, respectively. Most of the T1 and T2 lesions were treated with brachytherapy alone (60–70 Gy over 6–9 days). Larger T2 and T3 tumors were treated with a combination of external-beam radiation therapy (EBRT) (50–55 Gy) and low-dose-rate (LDR) interstitial brachytherapy (20–30 Gy) (Level IV) (Pernot et al. 1992, 1996). High dose-rate techniques offer similar outcomes (Inoue et al. 1996; Yamazaki et al. 2003).

Floor of Mouth

- For early stage floor of mouth cancers, the combination of brachytherapy and EBRT or brachytherapy alone can be recommended (Grade B). These treatment strategies have shown excellent outcomes for early stage tumors. Pernot et al. (1996) reported the outcomes of 207 patients with floor of month cancers treated with definitive EBRT and brachytherapy or brachytherapy alone. The 5-year LC was 97%, 72%, and 51% for T1, T2, and T3, respectively (Level IV).

Buccal Mucosa

- Tumors of the buccal mucosa can invade a compartment at great risk for spread into the cheek and gingivobuccal sulcus, requiring generous treatment margins at the primary site and consideration of adjuvant radiation for close margins. If the lesion is accessible intraorally, surgery is generally preferred, followed by adjuvant radiation (Grade B). Results from surgical series show high incidence of locoregional failure after surgical resection alone, indicating the necessity for adjuvant therapy (Dixit et al. 1998). Diaz et al. (2003) reported on 119 patients of all stages with 71% of patients treated with surgery alone. There was 45% incidence of locoregional recurrences with 32% of failures involving the primary location (Level IV).

- Select lesions can be treated with radiation therapy, which may include interstitial brachytherapy, intra-oral cone, ipsilateral electrons or conformal EBRT with photons (Grade B). The European Group of Curietherapy reported on 748 buccal mucosa patients treated either with brachytherapy alone, brachytherapy with EBRT, or EBRT alone. LC rates were 81% for brachytherapy alone, 65% for combined treatment, and 66% for external radiation alone (Level IV) (Gerbaulet and Pernot 1985).

Lip

- Most lesions of the lips can be treated with either surgery or radiation alone. Surgery is preferred for small lesions without significant functional deficits. Lesions involving the lip commissure or which would result in microstomia after resection should be evaluated for radiation therapy.

- Radiation alone using brachytherapy or electron can be recommended in early-stage squamous cell carcinoma of the lip (Grade A). The European Group of Brachytherapy reported their results of over 1800 cases of lip cancer, which were treated with a radioactive implant (Level IV) (Mazeron et al. 1984). The LC was 98.4%, 96.6%, and 89.9% for T1, T2, and T3 lesions, respectively. Electron and orthovoltage beams have been reported in large retrospective series with LC from 94%–100% for T1–2 lesions (Level IV) (Petrovich et al. 1987; Sykes et al. 1996).

Postoperative Radiation Therapy for Early-Stage Oral Cavity Cancer

- Patients with positive close margins and perineural or lymphovascular invasion may be considered for adjuvant radiation therapy potentially with concurrent chemotherapy (Grade A). Analysis of patients studied in a phase III randomized trial revealed that early-stage lesions undergoing primary surgery may have pathologic factors associated with high risk of recurrence, including positive close margins and perineural or lymphovascular invasion (Level I) (Ang et al. 2001; Peters et al. 1993). Results from a recent prospective randomized trial demonstrated that patients with high-risk squamous cell carcinoma of the head and neck treated with radiation therapy (60–66 Gy in 30–33 daily fractions over 6–6.6 weeks) in combination with chemotherapy (CDDP 100 mg/m^2 in weeks 1, 4, and 7) achieved superior outcome in terms of DFS and LC rates as compared to those who received adjuvant radiation (66 Gy in 33 daily fractions over 6.6 weeks) alone. The results showed that the estimated 2-year locoregional rates were 82% and 72%, respectively, for both groups, in favor of combined chemoradiation therapy (RTOG 95-01, Level I) (COOPER et al. 2004). A similar study completed by the European Organization for Research and Treatment of Cancer (EORTC) showed similar findings for stage III and IV squamous cell carcinoma of the head and neck areas (EORTC 22931, Level I) (BERNIER et al. 2004). In both randomized trials, extracapsular extension (ECE) and positive margins were defined as high risk. In addition, the EORTC study included lymphovascular invasion (LVI), perineural invasion, and level IV and V lymph node involvement (for cancer of oral cavity) as additional high-risk factors, whereas the Radiation Therapy Oncology Group (RTOG) study included multiple lymph nodes as additional high-risk factors.

Tables 3.5 and 3.6 compare the study populations and outcomes of the RTOG 95-01 and EORTC 22931 trials.

- In patients receiving adjuvant radiation, the total treatment package time (day of surgery to the end of radiation therapy) should be limited to 11 weeks or less in high-risk patients (Grade B). In a prospective trial partly aimed at evaluating

Table 3.6. Comparison of outcomes from the RTOG 95-01 and EORTC 22931. Both groups showed the addition of concurrent chemotherapy improved locoregional control and disease-free survival

Postoperative CT/RT vs. RT results of EORTC/RTOG phase III trials	RTOG 95-01	EORTC 22931
Median follow-up	46 months	60 months
Loco-regional failure	Outcomes (CT/RT vs. RT) 3 years: 22% vs. 33% (p=0.01)	5 years: 18% vs. 31% (p=0.01)
Disease-free survival	3 years: 47% vs. 36% (p=0.04)	5 years: 47% vs. 36% (p=0.01)
Overall survival	3 years: 56% vs. 47% (p=0.09)	5 years: 53% vs. 40% (p=0.01)
Distant metastases	3 years: 20% vs. 23% (p=0.46)	5 years: 21% vs. 24% (p=0.01)
≥Grade 3 acute toxicity	22% vs 34% (p<0.0001)	44% vs 21% (p=0.001)
All late toxicity	21% vs 17% (p=0.29)	38% vs 41% (p=0.25)

Table 3.5. Comparison of study populations. In the RTOG study, a greater proportion of patients were oropharynx and had more advanced neck stage. In the EORTC study, more patients had positive margins/extracapsular extension (ECE) and received higher radiation doses

Post-operative chemoradiation vs. radiation: phase III trials	RTOG 95-01	EORTC 22931
No. of patients	459	334
OPX/OC/LX/HPX	42%/27%/21%/10%	30%/26%/22%/20%
T3–4	61%	66%
N2–3	94%	57%
With ECE and/or + margins	59%	70%
RT: receiving 66 Gy	13%	91%

the importance of the overall combined treatment duration on the treatment outcome, a trend toward higher LRC and survival rates was noted when PORT was delivered in 5 rather than 7 weeks for high-risk patients. The cumulative duration of combined surgery and radiation therapy had a significant impact on the locoregional control and overall survival rates (Level II) (ANG et al. 2001).

- If definitive radiation therapy is considered, integration of brachytherapy should be considered in combination with conventional external-beam radiation (Grade A). Excellent outcome have been repeatedly demonstrated using combined EBRT and brachytherapy in oral cavity tumors as well as oropharynx cancer. (Level IV) (PERNOT et al. 1992, 1996; GERBAULET et al. 1985; MAZERON et al. 1987, 1989, 1993; GOFFINET et al. 1985; PUTHAWALA et al. 1988; HARRISON et al. 1992, 1996).

- Selected oral tongue and floor of mouth cancers can be treated with adjuvant brachytherapy alone for positive margins with excellent LC (LAPEYERE et al. 2000; HU et al. 2004).

3.2.3 Treatment of Advanced Disease in Oral Cavity Cancer

■ For patients with advanced lesions for which primary resection offers the best chance of locoregional control, adjuvant radiation is usually required (Grade A). For high-risk patients, trials conducted by the RTOG and EORTC detailed above show a significant benefit for the addition of concurrent chemotherapy to conventional fractionated postoperative radiation (EORTC 22931 and RTOG 95-01, Level I) (BERNIER et al. 2004; COOPER et al. 2004). These two landmark trials (EORTC 22931 and RTOG 95-01) demonstrated a benefit with the use of postoperative concomitant chemotherapy with EBRT for high-risk head and neck squamous cell carcinomas including oral cavity cancers. Pooled analyses of the EORTC/RTOG trials confirm a locoregional control, disease-free and overall survival benefit for patients with ECE or positive margins. Patients with perineural invasion, lymphovascular invasion, presence of low level neck nodes in patients with oral cavity/oropharynx primaries trended towards a survival benefit (Level IV) (BERNIER et al. 2005).

■ For high risk cases in which patients are unable to tolerate chemotherapy, postoperative accelerated radiation by delayed concomitant boost (DCB) or conventional fractionated radiation starting within 4 weeks after surgery improves locoregional control and should be considered (ANG 1998; ANG et al. 2001).

■ A proposed algorithm for the treatment of oral cavity cancer is presented in Figure 3.3

3.3 Management of Oropharyngeal Cancer

3.3.1 Management of Early-Stage Disease

General Principles

■ Due to the central location of the oropharynx and its integral role in swallowing, speech, and phonation, management of oropharyngeal can-

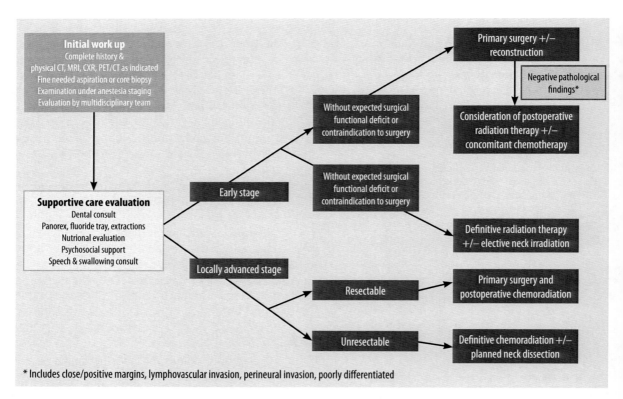

* Includes close/positive margins, lymphovascular invasion, perineural invasion, poorly differentiated

Fig. 3.3. A proposed algorithm for the management of oral cavity cancer

cer usually requires complex, multidisciplinary evaluation.

■ Treatment decisions depend both on the ability of a particular modality to control disease and its associated morbidity.

■ In contrast to oral cavity tumors, radiation therapy is chosen more often than surgery for either early or advanced lesions because of the significant likelihood of nodal spread and primary drainage into the retropharyngeal nodal basins which are not typically addressed surgically (Fig. 3.6).

■ For early-stage soft palate and pharyngeal wall cancers, many lesions are near midline leaving bilateral neck and retropharyngeal nodes at risk. In these patients, EBRT alone is often preferable for T1-2 lesions because of comprehensive nodal coverage with high rates of control (Grade B) (FEIN et al. 1993; AMDUR et al. 1987; MILLION et al. 1985; GWOZDZ et al. 1997). Also, functional deficits after surgery, such as uvulopalatal insufficiency, requiring prosthetic obturators to prevent reflux into the nasopharynx/nasal cavity may be avoided.

■ Special methods of delivering radiation such as brachytherapy or intensity-modulated radiation further improve upon treatment outcomes (Grade B) (EISBRUCH et al. 2001; DE ARRUDA et al. 2006; CHAO et al. 2000, 2004)

Surgery for Early Stage

■ Selected patients with small oropharyngeal lesions and a clinically negative neck can be managed with primary resection and elective neck dissection (Grade B). LACCOURREYE et al. (2005) recently reported a large experience using a mandibulotomy-sparing transoral approach for early-stage tonsillar lesions with excellent LC rates. However, a large percentage were treated with induction chemotherapy and postoperative radiation (Level IV).

External-Beam Radiation Therapy for Early-Stage Disease

■ Conventionally fractionated radiation therapy (CF) alone controls the majority of early-stage oropharyngeal lesions, especially of tonsil cancers, but may be suboptimal for T2 base of tongue and posterior pharyngeal wall cancers (Grade B). For tonsil cancers, several large single institutional series show excellent LC after CF alone (65–70 Gy delivered over 6.5–7 weeks at 1.8–2.0 Gy per daily fraction), approximating 80%–90% for T1 to T2 lesions and 63%–74% for T3 (Table 3.7) (Level IV). Table 3.8 illustrates the outcome of EBRT for base of tongue cancers (Level IV).

Table 3.7. Outcomes after definitive external-beam radiation for tonsil cancer from retrospective single institution series

Tonsillar carcinoma: local control and survival with external-beam radiation therapy													
Institution and study	No. of patients	Median follow-up (months)	T3–4 (%)	Local control (%)				Local control (%)				5-Year survival (%)	
				T1	T2	T3	T4	N0	N1	N2	N3	DFS	Overall
MDAC (REMMLER et al. 1985)	112	50	63	100	89	68	24	95	95	95	95	48	85
UFla (MENDENHALL et al. 2006)	503	24 (minimum)		94	79	59	50	NS	NS	NS	NS	–	–
Institut Curie (BATAINI et al. 1989)	698	60	72	89	84	63	43	NS	NS	NS	NS	NS	NS
Centre Alexis (PERNOT et al. 1992)[a]	277	36	36	89	86	69	–	NS	NS	NS	NS	62	NS
Henri Mondor (MAZERON et al. 1989)[a]	165	60	0	100	94	–	–	NS	NS	NS	NS	71	53

MDAC, MD Anderson Cancer Center; UFla, University of Florida; DFS, disease-free survival; NS, not significant. [a]With implant

Table 3.8. Outcomes after definitive external-beam radiation therapy alone for base of tongue cancer from retrospective single institution series

Institution and study	No. of patients	Median follow-up (years)	T3/T4 (%)	Local control (%)				Local control (%)				5-Year overall survival (%)			
				T1	T2	T3	T4	N0	N1	N2	N3	T1	T2	T3	T4
Institut Curie (Spanos et al. 1976)	166	5	58	96	57	45	23	86	79	58	61	49	29	23	16
MDAC (Jaulerry et al. 1991)	174	10[a]	54	91	71	78	52	NS	NS	NS	NS	100	58	38	20
U of Fla (Foote et al. 990)	84	8	54	89	88	77	36[b]	NS	NS	NS	NS	100	86	56	36[b]
Hospital Necker (Housset et al. 1987)	54	8	0	78	47	–	–	4	9	–	40	17	17	–	–

NS, not significant. [a] Extrapolated. [b]Average of stages IVa and IVb

Brachytherapy for Oropharynx Cancer

■ Brachytherapy has been a mainstay treatment for oropharyngeal cancers for decades and excellent results have been reported (Level IV) (Crook et al. 1988; Harrison et al. 1992, 1997; Housset et al. 1987; Goffinet et al. 1985; Puthawala et al. 1988).

■ Brachytherapy implantation of radioactive seeds directly into the target volume offers dose escalation to tumor and sparing of surrounding normal tissue by inverse square attenuation, producing excellent dose conformality with function preservation (Fig. 3.4). Normal tissue toxicity is further reduced because the dose of EBRT is re-

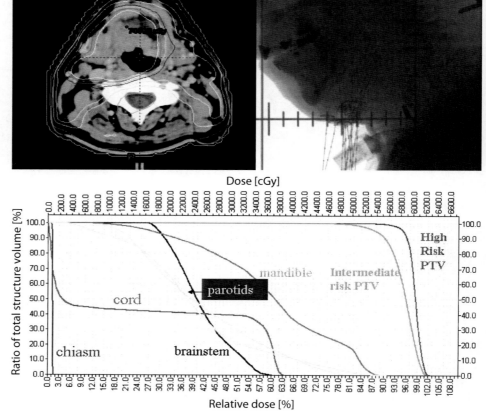

Fig. 3.4. Example of a 62-year-old male patient with a T2N2bM0 base of tongue carcinoma treated with combined external beam radiation and concurrent chemotherapy, brachytherapy implant and planned neck dissection. External beam radiation was delivered with intensity modulate radiation with a reduced dose of 59.4 Gy to the involved primary site and nodes followed by 20 Gy brachytherapy boost. Dose volume histogram demonstrating dose distribution from IMRT course only.

duced, especially in those receiving concurrent chemotherapy. Brachytherapy is typically used as a boost (20–30 Gy) after a reduced dose of conventional fractionated EBRT that treats the bilateral neck and primary site (50–54 Gy to the primary site, and 54–60 Gy to regional neck nodes) (Fig. 3.4).

■ Recent data indicate that a brachytherapy boost in combination with a reduced dose of external EBRT decreases the incidence of severe dysphagia compared to patients receiving a full course of external-beam treatment (Level IV) (LEVANDAG et al. 2007).

■ Base of tongue lesions are particularly ideal candidates for brachytherapy because LC is suboptimal

after conventional fractionated radiation, even for early-stage diseases. HARRISON et al. (1992, 1996) have reported long-term results of 68 patients treated with this strategy combined with planned neck dissension for patients presenting with involved neck nodes. At 5-year actuarial estimate, LC is as follows: T1 (n=17) 87%, T2 (n=32) 93%, T3 (n=17) 82%, regional control was 96%, and overall survival was 86% (Level IV). Near identical results using this approach for base of tongue lesions have been reported by PUTHAWALA et al. (1988) and GOFFINET et al. (1985). Equally excellent LC for early stage tonsil and soft palate cancers treated with combined EBRT and brachytherapy boost (Level IV) (GOFFINET et al. 1985).

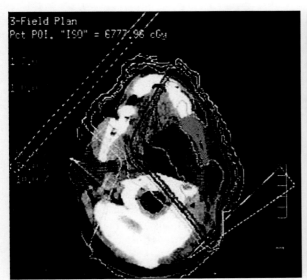

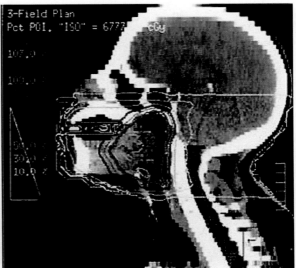

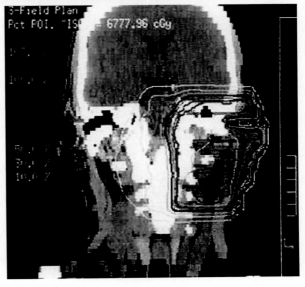

Fig. 3.5. Unilateral treatment of a lateralized early stage tonsil cancer. A patient treated with unilateral fields. This patient is a 50-year-old woman with a T2N0 squamous cell carcinoma of the left tonsil. Our plan is to treat this patient with definitive radiation therapy. This patient was treated with a three-field plan. This involves a wedged-pair plan, with a low-weighted right anterior oblique field, to help cover the tongue extension without overdosing the spinal cord. The planning tumor volume (PTV) is contoured. The primary site, extension along the soft palate, extension into the base of tongue, upper neck nodes, and retropharyngeal nodes are all included. An axial, sagittal, and coronal dose distribution shows that the PTV is well covered. The salivary gland tissue of the contralateral neck, especially the parotid gland, is well protected

Ipsilateral EBRT for Early-Stage Tonsil Cancer

- In general, most lateralized T1 to T2 lesions in patients with an N0 or N1 neck can be treated with ipsilateral radiation fields (Fig. 3.5) (Grade B). Such an approach minimizes irradiation to the contralateral salivary glands and reduces the incidence of xerostomia. Eisbruch et al. (2001) have demonstrated that patients treated unilaterally experience less xerostomia and better quality of life compared to those treated with intensity-modulated radiotherapy delivery of bilateral radiation with contralateral parotid sparing (Level III).
- Lesions that cross the midline, extensively involve the tongue base or soft palate, or associated with N2 or more advanced neck disease should receive comprehensive bilateral neck therapy (Grade B). A total of 228 patients with tonsillar carcinomas were treated with ipsilateral radiotherapy at Princess Margaret Hospital. Eligible patients typically had T1 or T2 tumors (191, T1–2; 30, T3; 7, T4) with N0 (133, N0; 35, N1; 27, N2-3) disease. Radiation was typically delivered with wedged pair Cobalt beams and ipsilateral low anterior neck field delivering 50 Gy in 4 weeks to the primary volume. At a median follow-up of 5.7 years, the 3-year LC rate was 77%, regional control 80%, and cause-specific survival 76%. Contralateral neck failure occurred in 3% (8/228). All patients with T1 lesions or N0 neck status had 100% contralateral neck control. Patients with a 10% or greater risk of contralateral neck failure included those with T3 lesions, lesions involving the medial 1/3 of the of the soft hemi palate, tumors invading the middle third of the ipsilateral base of tongue, and patients with N1 disease (Level IV) (O'Sullivan et al. 2001).

3.3.2 Management of Advanced-Stage Oropharyngeal Cancer

General Principles

- Locoregional failure is the primary pattern of failure after any treatment approach for advanced oropharyngeal cancer patients.
- Radiation alone provides suboptimal rates of LC in T3-4 lesions or patients with advanced N2/3 neck disease due to high rates of persistent disease after treatment compared to combined treatment, but may be considered in patients with intermediate stage cancers T1–2N1 or T2N0.
- For most patients with advanced oropharyngeal cancer, combined modality therapy with primary chemoradiation is recommended to maximize organ and function preservation (Grade A) (Fig. 3.6).
- In an effort to improve locoregional control, major strides have been made with the incorporation of altered fractionated radiation, chemotherapy, and biologic therapy.

Altered Fractionated Radiation

- Altered fractionated radiation therapy attempts to improve tumor control either by accelerating radiation treatment to overcome tumor repopulation or by dose escalation with hyperfractionation (HF) to utilize the radiation repair advantage of normal tissues over tumor (Ang et al. 1998).
- Radiation therapy can be successfully accelerated by DCB or a Danish regimen of six conventional treatments per week while dose escalation is best accomplished by HF (Grade A) (Level I) (Overgaard et al. 2003; Trotti et al. 2005). Altered fractionated radiation represents a reasonable treatment option for T2N0-1 base of tongue cancers or T3 tonsil lesions in patients who cannot tolerate chemotherapy (Grade A).
- Meta-analyses indicate a survival advantage of HF with dose escalation compared to CF, but no advantage is noted for accelerated radiation compared to CF (Level I) (Bourhis et al. 2006; Budach et al. 2006). A landmark trial conducted by the Radiation Therapy Oncology Group (RTOG 90-03) compared the leading US altered fractionated regimens [as described by Million et al. (1985), Gwozdz (1997), and Wang (1988)] for primarily stage III/IV head and neck cancers. A total of 1073 patients were randomized to: (1) CF 70 Gy/7 weeks, (2) split course accelerated fractionation (S-AF) with 1.6 Gy bid to 67.2 Gy over 6 weeks with an intentional 2-week break after 38.4 Gy, or (3) accelerated radiation by delayed concomitant boost (DCB) 72 Gy/6 weeks with bid last 12 days of treatment, and (4)) pure hyperfractionation (HF) with 1.2 Gy twice daily 81.6 Gy/7 weeks. At 8 years median follow-up, the DCB and HF arms had significantly better 8-year locoregional control compared to CF (48%

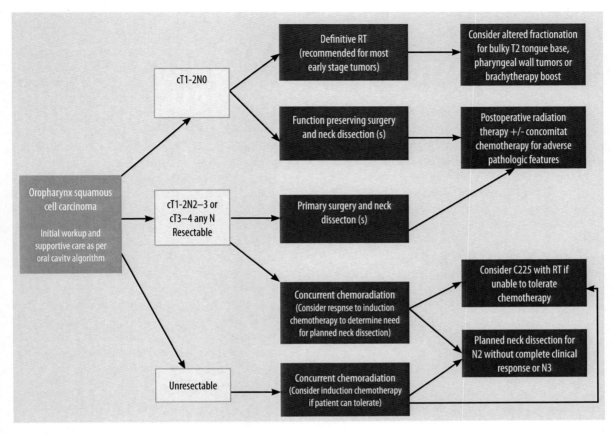

Fig. 3.6. A proposed algorithm for the management of cancer of oropharynx

vs. 49% vs. 41%, respectively) and improved DFS (30% vs. 31% vs. 21%, respectively) without significant difference in distant metastases (27% vs. 29% vs. 29%, respectively). Overall survival was 34% vs. 37% vs. 30%, respectively (Level I) (Fu et al. 2000).

■ Horiot et al. (1992) reported results of the EORTC 22791 randomized trial comparing an HF regimen of 1.15 cGy bid (4–6 h between fractions) to 80.5 Gy over 7 weeks versus conventional fractionation of 1.8–2.0 Gy to 70 Gy over 7–8 weeks in the treatment of 356 patients with T2-3N0-1 oropharyngeal cancers excluding the base of tongue. With a mean follow-up of about 4 years, HF improved 5-year actuarial local regional control compared to conventional fractionation (59% vs. 40%, respectively, $p=0.02$) with a trend toward improved survival (38% vs. 29%, respectively, $p=0.08$). T3 tumors benefited from HF but not T2 lesions (Level I) (Horiot et al. 1992).

Concurrent Radiation and Chemotherapy

■ Combined chemotherapy and radiation is the mainstay treatment of locally advanced oropharyngeal cancer (Grade A). Numerous overviews demonstrate the advantage of adding chemotherapy to radiation (Pignon et al. 2000; Monnerat et al. 2002; El-Sayed and Nelson 1996). A meta-analysis by Monnerat et al. (2002) concludes that concurrent chemotherapy offers an 8% survival benefit, induction chemotherapy 2% and adjuvant therapy a 1% benefit (Level I).

■ The French intergroup (GORTEC 94-01) phase III randomized trial established concurrent chemoradiation as the standard treatment for locoregionally advanced oropharynx cancer over conventional radiation alone. A total of 226 patients with stage III (32%) and IV (68%) were randomized to 70 Gy/7 weeks or 70 Gy with three cycles of concurrent carboplatin (70 mg/

$m^2/dx^4)/5$-fluorouracil (600 mg/m^2/dx^4) (weeks 1, 4, and 7). The initial report with a median follow-up of 35 months showed that patients in the combined modality arm had an approximately 20% improvement in 3-year locoregional control (66% vs. 42%, p=.03), DFS (42% vs. 20%, p=.04), and overall survival (51% vs. 31%, p=.02), but no difference in rate of distant metastases (11% vs. 11%, respectively). Long-term follow-up with a median follow-up of 5.5 years, confirms a 5-year overall survival (22.4% vs. 15.8%), DFS (26.6% vs. 14.6%), and locoregional control (47.6% vs. 24.7%) advantage with combined therapy (GORTEC 94-01, Level I) (CALAIS 1999; DENIS 2004).

Combining Chemotherapy with Altered Fractionated Radiation

- Efforts to further improve locoregional control and survival have explored combining concurrent chemotherapy with altered fractionated radiation as both approaches independently improve outcome for head and neck cancer patients.
- The present challenge is to find the optimal chemoradiation regimen(s), which offer high rates of locoregional control and organ function preservation with acceptable morbidity and the possibility of integration with new biologic agents or induction chemotherapy.
- The majority of phase III trials show a benefit of the addition of concurrent chemotherapy to altered fractionated radiation either with HF or DCB compared to the same radiation regimen alone. Two randomized trials included only patients with oropharynx or hypopharynx carcinoma in comparing the benefit of combining chemotherapy with altered fractionation versus the same altered fractionation alone: BENSADOUN et al. (2006) investigated the benefit of chemotherapy with HF for 163 unresectable oropharynx (n=123) or hypopharynx carcinoma (n=40) randomized to receive HF (1.2 bid to 80.4 Gy) with or without cisplatin (100 mg/m^2 days 1, 22, 43)/5-FU (750 mg/m^2/5 days on day 1, 430 mg/m^2/5 days on days 22, 43). Actuarial 2-year locoregional control, disease-free and overall survival were better in the patients receiving concurrent chemoradiation: 59% vs. 27.5% (p=0.0003), 48.2% vs. 25.2% (p=0.002) and 37.8% vs. 20.1% (p=0.038), respectively, (EORTC 22791, Level I) (BENSADOUN et al. 2006).

STARR et al. (2001) reported a benefit of the addition of chemotherapy to DCB in a German randomized trial of 246 stage III/IV oropharyngeal (n=178) and hypopharynx (n=62) carcinoma. In a 2×2 study, all patients were treated with DCB (69.6 Gy/5½ wks) randomized to receive carboplatin (70 mg/m^2)/5-FU (600 mg/m^2/d×5 days) on weeks 1 and 5 of RT and then randomized again to receive granulocyte colony stimulating factor (G-CSF) or not. At a median follow-up of 22 months, the 1- and 2-year rates of locoregional control were 69% and 51% after CT/RT compared to 58% and 45% after RT (p=0.14). Patients receiving G-CSF had reduced locoregional control (55 vs. 38%, p=.0072) and decreased mucositis (p=.06), raising the issue of possible tumor radioprotection with G-CSF. For both trials, the addition of chemotherapy sharply increased acute mucositis, hematologic toxicity, and feeding tube dependence (Level I). Table 3.9 lists the randomized phase III studies that compared the addition of concurrent chemotherapy to altered fractionated radiation therapy versus altered fractionated radiation alone.

Biologic Therapy

- Epidermal growth factor receptor (EGFR) is over-expressed in more than 90% of head and neck cancer cells and has a role in tumor proliferation, apoptosis, angiogenesis, and matrix metalloproteinase expression (HARARI et al. 2000). EGFR over-expression is considered a marker of radiation resistance (ANG et al. 2002).
- A pivotal phase III trial reported by BONNER et al. (2006) demonstrated the benefit of adding cetuximab (C225), the monoclonal antibody targeting EGFR, to radiation. A total of 424 patients with stage III/IV head and neck cancer (oropharynx comprised 64% of patients enrolled) were randomized to 7 weeks of C225 plus radiation (CF or altered fractionation) or radiation alone. No oral cavity patients were entered. At a median follow-up of 38 months, the C225/RT arm was superior to radiation therapy alone with respect to 3-year locoregional control (47% vss 34%, p<0.01), 3-year overall survival (55% vs. 45%, p=0.05) and median overall survival (54 months vs. 28 months, p = 0.02). With regard to toxicity, C225, unlike the addition of concurrent chemotherapy or the acceleration of radiation, did not significantly increase grade 3

or 4 mucositis (55% vs. 52%, respectively) but was associated with increased dermatitis 34% vs. 18%, $p=0.0003$) and infusion reaction (3%) (Level I).

■ The efficacy of C225 versus chemotherapy has not been compared directly in a randomized clinical trial.

Role of Induction Chemotherapy

■ Induction chemotherapy has been utilized to reduce tumor burden and predict successful treatment of tumors for organ preservation therapy (Grade A). With regard to survival benefit, multiple meta-analyses have shown a minor benefit of induction chemotherapy (Level I) (PIGNON et al. 2000; MONNERAT et al. 2002; EL-SAYED et al. 1996). Recent trials report that the addition of taxotere to cisplatin/5-fluorouracil (TPF) improves survival and organ preservation in patients treated with subsequent radiation or concurrent chemoradiation: An EORTC prospective trial randomized 358 locally advanced head and neck cancer patients to receive TPF (75 mg/ m^2 day 1, 750 mg/m^2 CI days 1–5, respectively) or 5-fluorouracil and cisplatin (PF) (100 mg/m^2 day 1, 1000 mg/m^2 CI days 1–5), respectively, followed by conventional or altered fractionated radiation. Patients in the TPF arm demonstrated superior response rate (68% vs. 54%, $p=0.007$), and had an increased 3-year overall survival (36.5% vs. 23.9%) at 51-month median follow-up. Patients who received TPF had less grade 3–4 toxicity and fewer toxic deaths (3.7% vs. 7.8%) compared to those receiving PF due to the reduced doses of platinum and 5-FU in the TPF regimen (EORTC 24971, Level I) (VERMORKEN et al. 2007). POSNER et al. (2007) reports a benefit of adding taxotere to PF followed by concurrent chemoradiation: 494 patients were randomized to three cycles of induction TPF (75 mg/m^2, 100 mg/m^2, 1000 mg/m^2) or three cycles of PF (100 mg/m^2, 1000 mg/m^2) followed by concurrent chemoradiation (70 Gy/7 weeks and weekly carboplatin AUC 1.5). At a median follow-up of 42 months, 3-year overall survival (62% vs. 48%, $p=0.0058$) and PFS were increased (49% vs. 37%, $p=0.004$) after TPF compared to PF (Level I).

3.4 Radiation Therapy Techniques for Cancer of the Oral Cavity and Oropharynx

3.4.1 Intensity-Modulated Radiation Therapy (IMRT)

■ Recent efforts to improve radiation dose conformality and reduce toxicity have been made with 3D and IMRT techniques to treat complex, irregularly shaped head and neck tumors. Cancers of the oropharynx are ideal sites for IMRT since the tumors often present in close proximity to sensitive normal tissues such as the parotid glands or involve the pharyngeal wall/retropharyngeal nodes close to the spinal cord. IMRT allows exquisite dose conformality with sparing of adjacent organs. Each radiation field is divided into a number of beamlets with the aid of an intensity modulator and inverse treatment planning. The different beamlets are added to form a cumulative dose distribution tailored to the shape of the tumor and respecting designated normal tissue tolerance constraints (Level III) (HUNT et al. 2001). IMRT also offers the possibility of differential dosing to the elective nodal basin, high-risk nodal areas and primary tumor sites with resultant modest accelerated radiation (Fig. 3.7) (DE ARRUDA et al. 2006; CHAO et al. 2000; BUTLER et al. 1999).

■ Early experience with IMRT shows encouraging locoregional control for oropharynx cancers, especially among the recently reported series in which LC over 90% is consistently reported (Table 3.10) (Levels III–IV) (DE ARRUDA et al. 2006; DAWSON et al. 2000; HUANG et al. 2003; LAWSON et al. 2008; CHAO et al. 2000).

■ IMRT regimens of 70 Gy in 33 or 37 fractions are well tolerated even with concurrent chemotherapy. A multi-institutional RTOG 0022 protocol has been completed and the results are pending.

■ To date, greatest benefit of IMRT compared to standard techniques has been to reduce the incidence of severe xerostomia, the primary quality-of-life complaint among long-term head and neck cancer survivors treated with radiation (Levels III–IV) (EISBRUCH et al. 2001; CHAO et al. 2001). It can prevent hearing loss and may

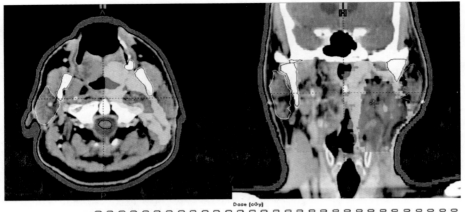

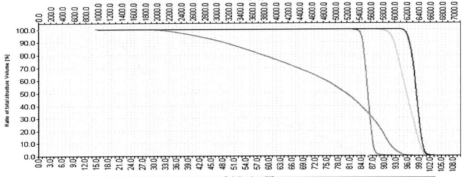

	Structure	Coverage [%] / [%]	Volume [cm³]	Min [cGy]	Max [cGy]	Mean [cGy]	Modal [cGy]	Median [cGy]
	L cochlea							
	L parotid	100.0 / 99.4	17.5	1809.3	6298.2	4815.4	5818.1	5170.4
	PTV 50.4	100.0 / 99.9	126.1	5095.7	5951.8	5551.5	5527.5	5550.1
	PTV 59.4	100.0 / 99.9	327.6	4445.5	6663.4	6199.6	6267.1	6199.6
	PTV 63	100.0 / 99.9	122.1	6014.8	6663.4	6361.3	6425.6	6363.9
	R cochlea							
	R parotid	100.0 / 99.7	30.8	832.7	5581.7	2776.2	1750.0	2142.8

Fig. 3.7. Example of a T2N1 base of tongue cancer treated with intensity-modulated radiation therapy

be useful to preserve swallowing function by decreasing dose to the cochlea and constrictor muscles (Level IV) (CHEN et al. 2006; EISBRUCH et al. 2004a).

Techniques of IMRT

- IMRT should be considered particularly for oropharyngeal tumors near the spinal cord such as those involving the posterior pharyngeal wall or nasopharynx, as well as for those where significant parotid sparing can be attained, such as those patients with negative contralateral neck nodes.
- The patient should be immobilized and the neck extended as described above. An isocenter should be selected to treat the primary and upper neck nodes for oropharyngeal cancers with a lower border matched to a low anterior neck field to treat the lower cervical and supraclavicular node.

Use of an extended mold to immobilize the shoulders is recommended. Need to decide whether placement of matchline at or below the arytenoids to attempt to spare the voice box.

- The nodal stations at risk and patterns of primary spread should be determined, as well as treatment to unilateral or bilateral neck. An extended field treating the primary and all regional nodes should be considered for patients with extensive lymphadenopathy involving multiple nodal levels.
- Treatment planning CT with contrast using 3-mm slice thickness should be performed over the primary and regional nodes. IV contrast is recommended. Fusion with PET and MRI should be considered.
- CTV encompassing gross tumor volume, microscopic disease, and potential for tumor spread should be outlined and stratified according to burden of disease – high risk: gross disease; inter-

mediate risk: areas with high likelihood of nodal disease or tumor spread; and low risk: elective nodal treatment. Expansion from CTV to PTV is typically 5–10 mm.

■ Care must be taken not to underdose regional nodes near the parotid as well as to evaluate dose at the matchline. If a patient has a clinically negative neck, the superior border of regional node delineation can end at the bottom of the C1 transverse process, sparing significant parotid tissue (Grégoire et al. 2000, 2003).

■ Consider treatment of skin in postoperative cases and in definitive cases with extensive nodal extracapsular extension or soft tissue extension at the primary site. If so, consider adding bolus.

Dose Fractionation

■ Simultaneous integrated boost technique to 70 Gy to high risk CTV, 59.4 Gy to intermediate risk, and 50–54 Gy to elective risk in 33 daily fractions can be used.

■ Alternatively, the RTOG studied 30 fractions to 66 Gy to high, 60 Gy to intermediate and 54 Gy to low risk regions without concurrent chemotherapy.

■ Prescription isodose should cover at least 95% of the PTV; no more than 20% shall receive >110% of prescribed dose; no more than 1% shall receive <93% of prescribed dose; and no more than 1% of normal tissues outside the PTV shall receive >110% the prescribed dose.

Dose Constraints to Normal Tissues

■ Dose to the temporal lobes should be limited to 60 Gy or less. Dose to the optic nerves and chiasm should be limited to 50 Gy or less, and no more than 1% (V1) should be treated to over 54 Gy.

■ Dose to the brainstem should be limited to 54 Gy or less, and no more than 1% (V1) should be treated over 60 Gy; dose to the spinal cord should be limited to 45 Gy, and no more than 1% (V1) should be treated to dose over 50 Gy.

■ Dose to the mandible should be limited to 70 Gy, and no more than 1% (V1) should be treated to doses over 75 Gy.

■ A total of 50% of the parotid bland should be treated to 26 Gy or less.

3.4.2 Conventional Radiation Therapy

Treatment Technique

■ Unilateral treatment of an early stage lateralized tonsil cancer using 3D conformal therapy.

Table 3.9. Randomized phase III studies evaluating the addition of concurrent chemotherapy to altered fractionated radiation compared to altered fractionation radiation alone

Study	No. of patients	2-Year overall survival difference	2-Year locoregional control difference
(Brizel et al. 1998) HF vs. HF+CDDP/5-FU	116	18%	26%
(Wendt et al. 1998) SC-AF vs. SC-AF+CDDP/5-FU	270	25%	19%
(Jeremic et al. 2000) HF vs. HF+ daily CDDP or CBCDA	130	22%	15%
(Starr et al. 2001) DCB vs DCB+ CBCDA/55FU	270	8%	6%
(Dobrowsky and Naude 2000) CHART vs. CHART+MMC	161	18%	16%
(Budach et al. 2005) HART vs. HART+MMC/5FU	384	7%	15%
(Bensadoun et al. 2006) HF vs. HF+5FU/CDDP	163	18%	31%

HF, hyperfractionation; SC-AF, split course accelerated fractionation; DCB, accelerated radiation by delayed concomitant boost; CHART, continuous hyperfractionated accelerated radiation therapy; HART, hyperfractionated accelerated radiation therapy; CDDP, cisplatin; 5FU, 5-fluorouracil; CBCDA, carboplatin; MMC:Mitomycin-C.

- Patients should be immobilized in an aquaplast mold with neck extension and shoulder board to separate the oropharynx site from the larynx.
- For tongue cancers, a bite block may be used to depress the tongue downward and away from the palate, allowing easier blocking of the palate and preventing a bolus effect from closure of the mouth.
- Palpable neck disease should be outlined with wire. The target volume of the parallel opposed fields should include the primary with margin plus draining lymph nodes of the upper neck with a high match above the arytenoids for oropharynx lesions and oral cavity lesions.
- Owing to the high probability of lymph node metastasis, these portals will also include the retropharyngeal lymph node groups up to the skull base.
- Fields are matched to a low anterior neck using a split isocenter technique with a spinal cord/vocal cord block in the LAN for oropharynx cancer or a lateral field cord block in patients with hypopharynx cancer (Fig. 3.8).
- Initial lateral fields are treated to 40–45 Gy followed by an off cord cone down to the primary and upper neck to a dose of 50–54 Gy and a final cone down to gross disease to a dose of 66–70 Gy for T3 and 70–80 Gy for a T4 lesion. Posterior necks are treated with electron strips using 6–9 MeV electrons to appropriate doses of 50–70 Gy.
- For lesions involving the posterior pharyngeal wall or retropharyngeal nodes, careful attention should be paid to the posterior border of the off cord block. Fein et al. (1993) showed that moving the posterior border from the middle to the posterior edge of the vertebral body improves LC.

Postoperative Radiation

- When postoperative radiation is administered, patients should be set up similarly to the description above. The match line should be above the arytenoids for oropharynx cancer and oral cavity lesions.
- A typical dose and fractionation schedule would be 63–66 Gy to high risk areas, 57.6–59.4 Gy to intermediate regions of the neck (in 1.8-Gy fractions), and 50–54 Gy to low-risk areas. The low anterior neck is treated to a dose of 50 Gy; the stoma (when present) is often boosted with electrons to 60 Gy.

3.4.3 Brachytherapy

- The dose with LDR Ir-192 interstitial brachytherapy ranges from 2000–3000 cGy at 40–60 cGy/h which is done approximately 3 weeks after the completion of EBRT. Mandibular lead lined shields can be used to decrease the incidence of osteoradionecrosis. Interstitial brachytherapy should not be ideally performed with lesions abutting/tethering mandible due to risk of osteoradionecrosis.

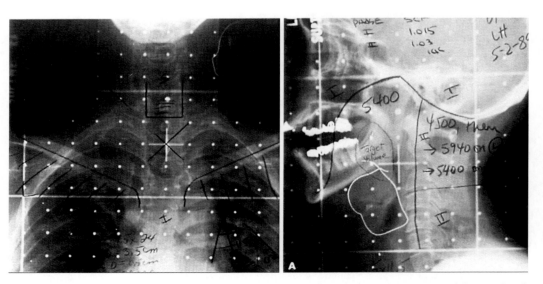

Fig. 3.8. Conventional technique used for definitive treatment of squamous cell carcinoma of the tonsil with neck node metastasis (wired)

3.5 Treatment-Induced Toxicities

■ The major sequelae of radiation therapy can be divided into acute and chronic side effects. These depend on total dose, fraction size, fractionation, prior or concomitant therapy (i.e., surgery or chemotherapy), and target volume.

3.5.1 Acute Toxicities

■ Acute toxicities during treatment which may persist up to 3 months after radiation treatment include: mucositis, pain, phlegm production, xerostomia, dysphagia, dysgeusia, dermatitis, weight loss, laryngeal edema, lhermitte's syndrome.

■ Mucositis is the major dose-limiting toxicity of radiation. Severe mucositis can result in treatment breaks, which can compromise locoregional control and cause infection in patients compromised by chemotherapy.

■ The addition of concurrent cisplatin toxicity doubles the grade 3 or 4 mucositis rates and adds a treatment mortality risk of 2% (Level I) (Bernier et al. 2004; Cooper et al. 2004). The addition of chemotherapy steeply increases mucositis, feeding tube dependence, dermatitis, hematologic suppression, and infection. The addition of C225 increases infusion reaction and dermatitis (Bonner et al. 2006).

Table 3.10. Single institution experience of intensity-modulated radiation therapy for the treatment of oropharynx cancer

Study	No. of patients (% OPX)	Median follow-up (months)	Locoregional control
(Chao et al. 2000)	52 (54%)	26	79%
(Eisbruch et al. 2004)	133 (60%)	32	84%
(Yao et al. 2004)	90 (71%)	29	Local control 96%
(de Arruda et al. 2006)	48 (100%)	18	Local control 98%
(Lawson et al. 2008)	34 (100% BOT)	20	Local control 90% 15% stricture

BOT, base of tongue.

3.5.2 Chronic Toxicities

■ Xerostomia, hypothyroidism, cervical fibrosis, dental decay, osteoradionecrosis, chondronecrosis, dysphagia/PEG dependence, cricopharyngeal stricture, fistula, epilation are potential toxicities, but their occurrence reduces with the use of IMRT.

■ With regard to chronic toxicity, the major issues after definitive radiation therapy are xerostomia which represents the main quality-of-life complaint, as well feeding tube dependence. The incidence of feeding tube dependence appears to be increased with concurrent chemoradiation, particularly after the addition of cisplatin chemotherapy to DCB.

■ In the Starr et al. (2001) trial, patients treated with chemoradiation treatment had more swallowing problems and continuous need for feeding tube (51% vs. 25%, p=.02) Other important side effects to consider include soft tissue and bone ulceration and necrosis, neck fibrosis, trismus, dental caries, epilation, and hypothyroidism.

■ Long-term complications after implant and EBRT include soft tissue ulcer, osteoradionecrosis, infection, and bleeding (Table 3.11).

Table 3.11. Complications secondary to chemoradiation therapy treatment for head and neck cancers. [Summarized from Brizel (2000), Trotti et al. (2003), and Zackrisson et al. (2003)]

Complications after chemoradiotherapy	Occurrence
Xerostomia	78%–95%
Mucositis/stomatitis	35%–75%
Chewing or eating difficulties	80%
Dysphagia	40%–65%
Anorexia/weight loss/malnutrition	55%–85%
Dysgeusia	90%
Infection	14%
Radiation necrosis	5%–15%

3.5 Follow-Up

3.5.1 Post-Treatment Follow-Up

■ Close follow-up of the patient is required especially during the first 2 years of treatment as locoregional failure is most likely to occur during this period.

- The risk of developing a secondary malignancy in the aerodigestive tract is 6%–8%/year and may be decreased by half if patients cease smoking or consuming alcohol (SPECTOR et al. 2001).
- Assessment of smoking cessation is recommended if applicable.

Schedule

- Follow-up every 1–3 months during the first year, every 2–4 months in the second year, every 4–6 months in years 3–5, then semiannually or annually after 5 years (Grade D) (NCCN 2008) (Table 3.12).

Table 3.12. Follow-up schedule after treatment for head and neck cancer

Interval	Frequency
First year	Every 1–3 months
Second year	Every 2–4 months
Year 3-5	Every 4–6 months
Over 5 years	Every 6–12 months

Work-Up

- Each follow-up should include a complete history and physical examination (especially the neck lymph node regions), as well as indirect laryngoscopic examination. Speech and swallowing evaluation and rehabilitation should be considered if clinically indicated.
- CT of the neck every 3 months during the first year and/or abdomen at 6, 12, and 24 months after completion of treatment can be considered (Grade D).
- PET/CT can be considered at 3 months in the definitively treated neck to rule out residual disease (Grade B). For follow-up after completion of treatment, PET/CT is best performed 3 months after the end of radiation therapy to monitor for persistent disease in the neck or primary site. High false-negative rates are noted in scans done earlier (Level III) (GREVEN et al. 2001; YAO et al. 2005, 2005; PORCEDDU et al. 2005).
- CT of the chest or chest X-ray should be performed if clinically indicated (Grade D) (NCCN 2008).
- Evaluation of thyroid function with thyroid-stimulating hormone (TSH) every 6–12 months if the neck is irradiated (Grade D) (NCCN 2008).
- Dental prophylaxis and speech/swallowing evaluation as needed.

References

Amdur RJ, Mendenhall WM, Parsons JT et al. (1987) Carcinoma of the soft palate treated with irradiation: analysis of results and complications. Radiother Oncol 9:185–194

Ang KK (1998) Altered fractionation in the management of head and neck cancer. Int J Radiat Biol 73:395–399

Ang KK, Trotti A, Brown BW et al. (2001) Randomized trial addressing risk features and time factors of surgery plus radiotherapy in advanced head-and-neck cancer. Int J Radiat Oncol Biol Phys 51:571–578

Ang KK, Berkey BA, Tu X et al.(2002) Impact of epidermal growth factor receptor expression on survival and pattern of relapse in patients with advanced head and neck carcinoma. Cancer Res 62:7350–7356

Balaram P, Sridhar H, Rajkumar T et al. (2002) Oral cancer in southern India: the influence of smoking, drinking, paan-chewing and oral hygiene. Int J Cancer 98:440–405

Bataini JP, Asselain B, Jaulerry C et al. (1989) A multivariate primary tumour control analysis in 465 patients treated by radical radiotherapy for cancer of the tonsillar region: clinical and treatment parameters as prognostic factors. Radiother Oncol 14:265–277

Bensadoun RJ, Benezery K, Dassonville O et al. (2006) French multicenter phase III randomized study testing concurrent twice-a-day radiotherapy and cisplatin/5-fluorouracil chemotherapy (BiRCF) in unresectable pharyngeal carcinoma: results at 2 years (FNCLCC-GORTEC). Int J Radiat Oncol Biol Phys 64:983–994

Bernier J, Domenge C, Ozsahin M et al. (2004) Postoperative irradiation with or without concomitant chemotherapy for locally advanced head and neck cancer. N Engl J Med 350:1945–1952

Bernier J, Cooper JS, Pajak TF et al. (2005) Defining risk levels in locally advanced head and neck cancers: a comparative analysis of concurrent postoperative radiation plus chemotherapy trials of the EORTC (#22931) and RTOG (# 9501). Head Neck 2005:843–850

Bonner J, Harari P, Giralt J et al. (2006) Radiotherapy plus cetuximab for squamous-cell carcinoma of the head and neck. N Engl J Med 354:567–578

Bourhis J, Overgaard J, Audry H et al. (2006) Hyperfractionated or accelerated radiotherapy in head and neck cancer: a meta-analysis. Lancet 368:843–854

Brizel DM, Albers ME, Fisher SR et al. (1998) Hyperfractionated irradiation with or without concurrent chemotherapy for locally advanced head and neck cancer. N Engl J Med 338:1798–1804

Brizel DM, Wasserman TH, Henke M et al. (2000) Phase III randomized trial of amifostine as a radioprotector in head and neck cancer. J Clin Oncol 18:3339–3345

Budach V, Stuschke M, Budach W et al. (2005) Hyperfractionated accelerated chemoradiation with concurrent fluorouracil-mitomycin is more effective than dose-escalated hyperfractionated accelerated radiation therapy alone in locally advanced head and neck cancer: final results of the radiotherapy cooperative clinical trials group of the German Cancer Society 95-06 Prospective Randomized Trial. J Clin Oncol 23:1125–1135

Budach W, Hehr T, Bucah V et al. (2006) A meta-analysis of hyperfractionated and accelerated radiotherapy and combined chemotherapy and radiotherapy regimens in unresected locally advanced squamous cell carcinoma of the head and neck. BMC Cancer 6:28

Butler EB, Teh BS, Grant WH 3rd et al. (1999) Smart (simultaneous modulated accelerated radiation therapy) boost: a new accelerated fractionation schedule for the treatment of head and neck cancer with intensity modulated radiotherapy. Int J Radiat Oncol Biol Phys 45:21–32

Calais G, Alfonsi M, Bardet E et al. (1999) Randomized trial of radiation therapy versus concomitant chemotherapy and radiation therapy for advanced-stage oropharynx carcinoma. J Natl Cancer Inst 91:2081–2016

Candela FC, Kothari K, Shah JP (1990) Patterns of cervical node metastases from squamous carcinoma of the oropharynx and hypopharynx. Head Neck 12:197–203

Chao KS, Low DA, Perez CA et al. (2000) Intensity-modulated radiation therapy in head and neck cancers: the Mallinckrodt experience. Int J Cancer 90:92–103

Chao KS, Deasy JO, Markman J et al. (2001) A prospective study of salivary function sparing in patients with head-and-neck cancers receiving intensity-modulated or three dimensional radiation therapy: initial results. Int J Radiat Oncol Biol Phys 49:907–916

Chao KS, Ozyigit G, Blanco AI et al. (2004) Intensity-modulated radiation therapy in the treatment of oropharyngeal cancer: impact of tumor volume. Int J. Radiat Oncol Biol Phys 59:43–50

Chen WC, Jackson A, Budnick AS et al. (2006) Sensorineural hearing loss in combined modality treatment of nasopharyngeal carcinoma. Cancer 106:820–829

Cooper JS, Pajak TF, Forastiere AA et al. (2004) Postoperative concurrent radiotherapy and chemotherapy for high-risk squamous-cell carcinoma of the head and neck. N Engl J Med 350:1937–1944

Crawford BE, Callihan MD, Corio RL et al. (1979) Oral pathology. Otolaryngol Clin North Am 12:29–43

Crook J, Mazeron JJ, Marinello G et al. (1988) Combined external irradiation and interstitial implantation for T1 and T2 epidermoid carcinomas of base of tongue: the Creteil experience (1971–1981). Int J Radiat Oncol Biol Phys 15:105–114

Dawson LA, Anzai Y, Marsh L et al. (2000) Patterns of local-regional recurrence following parotid-sparing conformal and segmental intensity-modulated radiotherapy for head and neck cancer. Int J Radiat Oncol Biol Phys 46:1117–1126

Dahlstrand HM, Dalianis T (2005) Presence and influence of human papillomaviruses (HPV) in tonsillar cancer. Adv Cancer Res 93:59–89

de Arruda FF, Puri DR, Zhung J et al. (2006) Intensity-modulated radiation therapy for the treatment of oropharyngeal carcinoma: the Memorial Sloan-Kettering Cancer Center experience. Int J Radiat Oncol Biol Phys 64:363–373

Denis F, Garaud P, Bardet E et al. (2004) Final results of the 94-01 French Head and Neck Oncology and Radiotherapy Group randomized trial comparing radiotherapy alone with concomitant radiochemotherapy in advanced-stage oropharynx carcinoma. J Clin Oncol 22:69–76

Diaz EM Jr, Holsinger FC, Zuniga ER et al. (2003) Squamous cell carcinoma of the buccal mucosa: one institution's experience with 119 previously untreated patients. Head Neck 25:267–273

Dixit S, Vyas RK, Toparani RB et al. (1998) Surgery versus surgery and postoperative radiotherapy in squamous cell carcinoma of the buccal mucosa: a comparative study. Ann Surg Oncol 5:502–510

Dobrowsky W, Naude J (2000) Continuous hyperfractionated accelerated radiotherapy with/without mitomycin C in head and neck cancers. Radiother Oncol 57:119–124

Dupont JB, Guillamondegui OM, Jesse RH (1978) Surgical treatment of advanced carcinomas of the base of tongue. Am J Surg 136:501–503

Eisbruch A, Kim HM, Terrell JE et al. (2001) Xerostomia and its predictors following parotid-sparing irradiation of head-and-neck cancer. Int J. Radiat Oncol Biol Phys 50:332–343

Eisbruch A, Schwartz M, Rasch C et al. (2004a) Dysphagia and aspiration after chemoradiotherapy for head-and-neck cancer: which anatomic structures are affected and can they be spared by IMRT? Int J Radiat Oncol Biol Phys 60:1425–1439

Eisbruch A, Marsh L, Dawson LA et al. (2004b) Recurrences near the base of skull following IMRT of head and neck cancer: implications for target delineation in the high neck and for parotid gland sparing. Int J Radiat Oncol Biol Phys 59:28–42

El-Sayed S, Nelson N (1996) Adjuvant and adjunctive chemotherapy in the management of squamous cell carcinoma of the head and neck region. A meta-analysis of prospective and randomized trials. J Clin Oncol 14:838–847

Fein DA, Mendenhall WM, Parsons JT et al. (1993) Pharyngeal wall carcinoma treated with radiotherapy: impact of treatment technique and fractionation. Int J Radiat Oncol Biol Phys 26:751–757

Foote RL, Parsons JT, Mendenhall WM et al. (1990) Is interstitial implantation essential for successful radiotherapeutic treatment of base of tongue carcinoma. Int J. Radiat Oncol Biol Phys 18:1293–1298

Fu KK, Pajak TF, Trotti A et al. (2000) A radiation therapy oncology group (RTOG) phase III randomized study to compare hyperfractionation and two variants of accelerated fractionation to standard fractionation radiotherapy for head and neck squamous cell carcinomas. First report of RTOG 9003. Int J Radiat Oncol Biol Phys 48:7–16

Gerbaulet A, Pernot A (1985) Cancer of the buccal mucosa – Proceedings of the 20th annual meeting of the European Curietherapy Group. J Eur Radiother 6:1–4

Goffinet DR, Fee WE Jr., Wells J et al. (1985) 192Ir pharyngoepiglottic fold interstitial implants. The key to successful treatment of base of tongue carcinoma by radiation therapy. Cancer 55:941–948

Greene F, Page D, Fleming I et al. (2002) AJCC Cancer Staging Manual, 6th edn. Springer-Verlag, Berlin Heidelberg New York

Grégoire V, Coche E, Cosnard G et al. (2000) Selection and delineation of lymph node target volumes in head and neck conformal radiotherapy. Proposal for standardizing terminology and procedure based on the surgical experience. Radiother Oncol 56:135–150

Grégoire,V, Levendag, P, Ang K et al. (2003) CT-based delineation of lymph node levels and related CTVs in the node-negative neck: DAHANCA, EORTC, GORTEC, NCIC, RTOG consensus guidelines. Radiother Oncol 69:227–236

Greven KM, Williams DW, Mcquirt WF et al. (2001) Serial positron emission tomography scans following radiation therapy of patients with head and neck cancer. Head Neck 23:942–946

Gwozdz JT, Morrison WH, Garden AS et al. (1997) Concomitant boost radiotherapy for squamous carcinoma of the tonsillar fossa. Int J. Radiat Oncol Biol Phys 39:127–135

Harari PM, Huang SM (2000) Modulation of molecular targets to enhance radiation. Clin Cancer Res 6:323–325

Harrison LB, Zelefsky MJ, Sessions RB et al. (1992) Base-of-tongue cancer treated with external beam irradiation plus brachytherapy: oncologic and functional outcome. Radiology 184:267–270

Harrison, LB, Lee H, Kraus DH et al. (1996) Long term results of primary radiation therapy for squamous cancer of the base of tongue. Radiother Oncol 39:S6

Harrison LB, Zelefsky MJ, Pfister D et al. (1997) Detailed quality of life assessment on long term survivors of primary radiation therapy for cancer of the base of tongue. Head Neck 19:169–175

Horiot JC, Le Fur R, N'Guyen T et al. (1992) Hyperfractionation versus conventional fractionation in oropharyngeal carcinoma: final analysis of a randomized trial of the EORTC cooperative group of radiotherapy. Radiother Oncol 25:231–241

Housset M, Baillet F, Dessarrd-Diana B et al. (1987) A retrospective study of three treatment techniques for T1-T2 base of tongue lesions: surgery plus postoperative radiation, external radiation plus interstitial implantation and external radiation alone. Int J Radiat Oncol Biol Phys 15:511–516

Hu KS, Sachdeva G, Harrison LB (2004) Adjuvant interstitial Iridium 192 brachytherapy for resected T1 and T2 cancers of the oral cavity with close or positive margins. Presented at 6th International Head and Neck conference, Washington DC, Aug 2004

Huang K, Lee N, Xia P et al. (2003) Intensity-modulated radiotherapy in the treatment of oropharyngeal carcinoma: a single institutional experience. Int J Radiat Oncol Biol Phys 57 S2:2303

Hunt MA, Zelefsky MJ, Wolden S et al. (2001) Treatment planning and delivery of intensity-modulated radiation therapy for primary nasopharynx cancer. Int J Radiat Oncol Biol Phys 49:623–632

Inoue T, Inoue T, Teshima T et al. (1996) Phase III trial of high and low dose rate interstitial radiotherapy for early oral tongue cancer. Int J Radiat Oncol Biol Phys 36:1201–1204

Jaulerry C, Rodriguez J, Brunin F et al. (1991) Results of radiation therapy in carcinoma of the base of the tongue. The Curie Institute experience with about 166 cases. Cancer 67:1532–1538

Jeremic B, Shibamoto Y, Milicic B et al. (2000) Hyperfractionated radiation therapy with or without concurrent low-dose daily cisplatin in locally advanced squamous cell carcinoma of the head and neck: a prospective randomized trial. J Clin Oncol 18:1458–1464

Kim MR, Roh JL, Kim JS et al. (2007) Utility of 18F-fluorodeoxyglucose positron emission tomography in the preoperative staging of squamous cell carcinoma of the oropharynx. Eur J Surg Oncol 33:633–638

Kim SY, Roh JL, Kim MR et al. (2007) Use of 18F-FDG PET for primary treatment strategy in patients with squamous cell carcinoma of the oropharynx. J Nucl Med 48:752–757

Laccourreye O, Hans S, Menard M et al. (2005) Transoral lateral oropharyngectomy for squamous cell carcinoma of the tonsillar region: II. An analysis of the incidence, related variables and consequences of local recurrence. Arch Otolaryngol Head Neck Surg 131:592–599

Lapeyre M, Hoffstetter S, Peiffert D et al. (2000) Postoperative brachytherapy alone for T1-2 N0 squamous cell carcinomas of the oral tongue and floor of mouth with close or positive margins. Int J Radiat Oncol Biol Phys 48:37–42

Lawson JD, Otto K, Chen A et al (2008) Concurrent platinum-based chemotherapy and simultaneous modulated accelerated radiation therapy for locally advanced squamous cell carcinoma of the tongue base. Head Neck 30:327–335

Levendag PC, Teguh DN, Voet P et al. (2007) Dysphagia disorders in patients with cancer of the oropharynx are significantly affected by the radiation therapy dose to the superior and middle constrictor muscle: a dose-effect relationship. Radiother Oncol 85:64–73

Lindberg R (1972) Distribution of cervical lymph node metastases from squamous cell carcinoma of the upper respiratory and digestive tracts. Cancer 29:1446–1449

Mazeron JJ, Richaud P (1984) Lip cancer. Report of the 18th annual meeting of the European Curietherapy Group. J Eur Radiother 5:50–56

Mazeron JJ, Marinello G, Crook J et al. (1987) Definitive radiation treatment for early stage carcinoma of the soft palate and uvula: the indications for iridium 192 implantation. Int J Radiat Oncol Biol Phys 13:1829–1837

Mazeron JJ, Crook J, Martin M et al. (1989) Iridium 192 implantation of squamous cell carcinomas of the oropharynx. Am J Otolaryngol 10:317–321

Mazeron JJ, Belkacemi Y, Simor JM et al. (1993) Place of iridium 192 implantation in definitive irradiation of faucial arch squamous cell carcinomas. Int J Radiat Oncol Biol Phys 27:251–257

Mendenhall WM, Morris CB, Amdur RJ et al. (2006) Definitive radiotherapy for tonsillar squamous cell carcinoma. Am J Clin Oncol 29:290–297

Merchant A, Husain SS, Hosain M et al. (2000) Paan without tobacco: an independent risk factor for oral cancer. Int J Cancer 86:128–131

Million RR, Parsons JT, Cassisi NJ (1985) Twice-a-day irradiation technique for squamous cell carcinomas of the head and neck. Cancer 55[suppl]:2096–2099

Monnerat C, Faivre S, Temam S et al. (2002) End points for new agents in induction chemotherapy for locally advanced head and neck cancers. Ann Oncol 13:995–1006

O'Sullivan B, Warde P, Grice B et al. (2001) The benefits and pitfalls of ipsilateral radiotherapy in carcinoma of the tonsillar region. Int J Radiat Oncol Biol Phys 51:332–343

Overgaard J, Hansen HS, Specht L et al. (2003) Five compared with six fractions per week of conventional radiotherapy of squamous-cell carcinoma of head and neck: DAHANCA 6 and 7 randomised controlled trial. Lancet 362:933–940

Pernot M, Malissard L, Taghian A et al. (1992) Velotonsillar squamous cell carcinoma: 277 cases treated by combined external irradiation and brachytherapy – results according to extension, localization, and dose rate. Int J Radiat Oncol Biol Phys 23:715–723

Pernot M, Hoffstetter S, Peiffert D et al. (1996) Role of interstitial brachytherapy in oral and oropharyngeal carcinoma: reflection of a series of 1344 patients treated at the time of initial presentation. Otolaryngol Head Neck Surg 115:519–526

Peters LJ, Goepfert H, Ang KK et al. (1993) Evaluation of the dose for postoperative radiation therapy of head and neck cancer: first report of a prospective randomized trial. Int J Radiat Oncol Biol Phys 26:3–11

Petrovich Z, Parker RG, Luxton G et al. (1987) Carcinoma of the lip and selected sites of head and neck skin. A clinical study of 896 patients. Radiother Oncol 8:11–17

Pignon JP, Bourhis J, Domenge C et al. (2000) Chemotherapy added to locoregional treatment for head and neck squamous-cell carcinomas: three meta-analyses of updated individual data. MACH-NC Collaborative Group. Meta-analysis of chemotherapy on head and neck cancer. Lancet 355:949–955

Posner MR, Hershock DM, Blajman CR (2007) Cisplatin and fluorouracil alone or with docetaxel in head and neck cancer. N Engl J Med 357:1705–1715

Porceddu SV, Jarmolowski E, Hicks RJ et al. (2005) Utility of positron emission tomography for the detection of disease in residual neck nodes after (chemo)radiotherapy in head and neck cancer. Head Neck 27:175–181

Puthawala AA, Syed AM, Eads DL et al. (1988) Limited external beam and interstitial 192iridium irradiation in the treatment of carcinoma of the base of the tongue: a ten year experience. Int J Radiat Oncol Biol Phys 14:839–848

Remmler D, Medina JE, Byers RM et al. (1985) Treatment of choice for squamous carcinoma of the tonsillar fossa. Head Neck Surg 7:206–211

Robbins KT, Medina JE, Wolfe GT et al. (1991) Standardizing neck dissection terminology. Official report of the Academy's Committee for Head and Neck Surgery and Oncology. Arch Otolaryngol Head Neck Surg 117:601–605

Shah JP, Candela FC, Poddar AK (1990) The patterns of cervical lymph node metastases from squamous carcinoma of the oral cavity. Cancer 66:109–113

Shaha AR, Shah JP (1995) Biopsy techniques in head and neck. Surg Oncol Clin North Am 4:15–28

Spanos WJ Jr. Shukovsky LJ, Fletcher GH (1976) Time, dose and tumour volume relationships in irradiation of squamous cell carcinomas of the base of the tongue. Cancer 37:2591–2599

Spector JG, Sessions DG, Haughey BH et al. (2001) Delayed regional metastases, distant metastases and second primary malignancies in squamous cell carcinomas of the larynx and hypopharynx. Laryngoscope 111:1079–1087

Spiro RH, Gerold FP, Strong EW (1981) Mandibular "swing" approach for oral and oropharyngeal tumors. Head Neck Surg 3:371–378

Starr S, Rudat V, Stuetzer H et al. (2001) Intensified hyperfractionated accelerated radiotherapy limits the additional benefit of simultaneous chemotherapy – results of a multicentric randomized German trial in advanced head-and-neck cancer. Int J Radiat Oncol Biol Phys 50:1161–1171

Sykes AJ, Allan E, Irwin C (1996) Squamous cell carcinoma of the lip: the role of electron treatment. Clin Oncol (R Coll Radiol) 8:384–386

Trotti A, Bellm LA, Epstein JB et al. (2003) Mucositis incidence, severity and associated outcomes in patients with head and neck cancer receiving radiotherapy with or without chemotherapy: a systematic literature review. Radiother Oncol 66:253–262

Trotti A, Fu K, Pajak T et al. (2005) Long term outcomes of RTOG 90-03: a comparison of hyperfractionation and two variants of accelerated fractionation to standard fractionation radiotherapy for head and neck squamous cell carcinoma. Int J Radiat Oncol Biol Phys 63:S70

Vermorken, Remenar E, Van Herpen, C et al. (2007) Cisplatin, fluorouracil, and docetaxel in unresectable head and neck cancer. N Engl J Med 357:1695–1704

Wang CC (1988) Local control of oropharyngeal carcinoma after two accelerated hyperfractination radiation therapy schemes. Int J Radiat Oncol Biol Phys 14:1143–1146

Weinberger PM, Yu Z, Haffty BG et al. (2006) Molecular classification identifies a subset of human papillomavirus-associated oropharyngeal cancers with favorable prognosis. J Clin Oncol 24:736–747

Wendt TG, Grabenbauer GG, Rodel CM et al. (1998) Simultaneous radiochemotherapy versus radiotherapy alone in advanced head and neck cancer: a randomized multicenter study. J Clin Oncol 16:1318–1324

Yamazaki H, Inoue T, Yoshida K et al. (2003) Brachytherapy for early oral tongue cancer: low dose rate to high dose rate. J Radiat Res (Tokyo) 44:37–40

Yao M, Graham MM, Hoffman HT et al. (2004) The role of post-radiation therapy FDG PET in prediction of necessity for post-radiation therapy neck dissection in locally advanced head-and-neck squamous cell carcinoma. Int J Radiat Oncol Biol Phys 59:1001–1010

Yao M, Smith RB, Graham MM et al. (2005) The role of FDG PET in management of neck metastasis from head-and-neck cancer after definitive radiation treatment. Int J Radiat Oncol Biol Phys 63:991–999

Yao M, Hoffman HT, Chang K et al. (2007) Is planned neck dissection necessary for head and neck cancer after intensity-modulated radiotherapy? Int J Radiat Oncol Biol Phys 68:707–713

Zackrisson B, Mercke C, Strander H et al. (2003 A systematic overview of radiation therapy effects in head and neck cancer. Acta Oncol 42:443–61

Major Salivary Gland Tumors

4

JONATHAN J. BEITLER, AMY Y. CHEN, and CHARLES L. PERKINS

CONTENTS

Introduction and Objectives

Malignancies of the parotid, submandibular, and sublingual glands account for approximately 4% of all head and neck cancers. A total of 80% of malignant major salivary gland tumors occur in the parotid gland. In adults, roughly a quarter of parotid tumors and one half of submandibular tumors are malignant.

Pathology of major salivary glands is complex and best arbitrated by the WHO classification. Fine-needle aspirations and even histological diagnoses can have surprisingly high rates of error. Histology does predict risk of lymphatic spread and perineural spread. Grade can predict the risk of local recurrence as well as regional spread. Surgery is the mainstay of treatment and adjuvant radiation is used liberally to optimize results.

This chapter examines:

● Recommendations for diagnosis and staging procedures for major salivary glands

● The staging systems, classification (pathology), and prognostic factors

● The management of salivary gland tumors using surgery, radiation therapy, or combined treatment and supporting scientific evidence

● Techniques of radiation therapy including intensity-modulated radiation therapy (IMRT)

● Follow-up care and surveillance of survivors

As the characteristics, natural history, presentation, and treatment strategy of the minor salivary glands differ significantly from those of the major salivary glands, the management of tumors of the minor salivary glands is not detailed in this chapter.

J. J. BEITLER, MD, MBA, FACR
Departments of Radiation Oncology and Otolaryngology, Emory University School of Medicine, 1365 Clifton Road NE, Atlanta, GA 30322–1013, USA

A. Y. CHEN, MD, MPH
C. L. PERKINS, MD, PhD
Emory University School of Medicine, 1365A Clifton Road NE, Atlanta, GA 30322–1013, USA

4.1 Diagnosis, Staging, and Prognoses

4.1.1 Diagnosis

Initial Evaluation

■ Diagnosis and evaluation of major salivary tumors start with a complete history and physical examination. Attention should be paid to disease-associated signs and symptoms, which are dependent on histologic types, grade, and primary origin. Salivary gland cancers can present as masses (mostly painless and fast growing), facial palsies, lymphatic disease, or even skin invasion. Tumors of the deep lobe may cause dysphagia, odynophagia, and referred ear pain.

■ The history should take careful note of possible risk factors. Prior ionizing radiation exposure to the head and neck is clearly associated with an increased risk of subsequent development of salivary gland cancer. This risk has been observed in atomic bomb survivors (Level IV) (LAND et al. 1996; SAKU et al. 1997), as well as patients treated with I-131 for thyroid cancer (Level IV) (HALL et al. 1991), or with external beam irradiation. The etiologic role of non-ionizing ultraviolet radiation has been controversial (Level IV) (SUN et al. 1999).

■ Clustering due to viral etiology – There is some evidence of a viral component to the development of salivary gland cancer. Human papilloma virus 16 and/or 18 have been detected in pathologic parotid lesions (Level III) (VAGELI et al. 2007) and polyomavirus injected into mice on the first day of life can induce salivary gland tumors (STANLEY et al. 1964) Furthermore, the increased incidence of salivary gland tumors in Alaskan Eskimos and Alaskan Indian women in the Arctic has been ascribed to a viral pattern of spread (Level IV) (LANIER et al. 1980).

■ The majority (> 80%) of parotid tumors are benign (pleomorphic adenoma) and 20% are malignant. Approximately 50% of submandibular tumors are benign while the other 50% are malignant; most tumors of the sublingual glands are malignant.

■ Though difficult to prove, generalizations about the pattern of malignancy within the parotid gland ring true (Level IV) (DAS et al. 2004). The malignant gradient increases from anterior to posterior and from superficial to deep (RUBIN and HANSEN 2008). The posterior mass is more likely to be malignant, as is the deep mass. The mass that causes facial nerve paralysis is likely malignant in nature. Masses of the submandibular gland and sublingual glands were more likely to be malignant compared to parotid gland. Malignancy is also more common with increasing age (Level IV) (MARTIN et al. 1989).

■ Early dental evaluation including imaging to assess and restore (when possible) or extract (when restoration is impossible or would cause an extensive delay) decayed teeth is required for all patients who need high-dose radiation therapy.

Laboratory Tests

■ Initial laboratory tests include a complete blood count and comprehensive metabolic panel, basic blood chemistry, liver and renal function tests, lactate dehydrogenase, and alkaline phosphatase are recommended for initial evaluation.

Imaging Studies

■ CT scan and/or MRI of the head and neck area are usually recommended for patients with tumor of the major salivary glands, except in small, discrete, and freely mobile tumors involving the superficial lobe of the parotid gland.

■ MRI is preferred over CT scan for deep-lobe tumors and tumors of submandibular and sublingual gland (Grade B). A carefully performed MRI can demonstrate soft tissue extension and document nerve involvement without the risks of ionizing radiation, and is particularly valuable in evaluating tumor of the deep parotid lobe (Level IV) (FEE and TRAN 2003).

■ FDG-PET or PET/CT can be considered for patients with high-grade malignancies (Grade B). Comparing PET/CT with CT alone in the evaluation of salivary gland malignancies, the extent of the tumor, regional spread to the nodes, and distant disease were all significantly more accurate for the PET/CT studies (Level III) (JEONG et al. 2007; ROH et al. 2007).

■ Imaging studies of the head and neck areas are important for detecting regional lymph adenopathy.

■ Appropriate imaging is important for ruling out distant disease. TERHAARD et al. (2004) found that distant metastases were found in the lung (43%), bones (21%), liver (5%), brain (1%), elsewhere (6%), and in multiple sites (24%) (Level IV).

■ Human immunodeficiency virus (HIV)-related parotid hypertrophy is commonly diagnosed by imaging, without a biopsy (Grade C) (BEITLER et al. 1999) (Table 4.1).

Table 4.1. Imaging and laboratory work-ups for diagnosis and staging of tumor of major salivary glands

Imaging studies	Laboratory tests
MRI and/or CT scan of the head and neck area Chest X-ray FDG-PET or PET/CT (optional)	Complete blood count Comprehensive metabolic panel

Pathology

■ Histological diagnosis is crucial to treatment decisions. Histological diagnosis may confirm or refute FNA-based diagnosis or grading and may exclude squamous cell cancers. The diagnosis of squamous cell carcinoma should prompt a vigorous search for a cutaneous primary tumor.

■ The procedure for definitive diagnosis of major salivary glands is tumor resection and pathologic study. Incisional or excisional biopsy should be avoided as they are associated with increased chances of recurrence and complications such as facial nerve damage.

■ Fine needle aspiration (FNA) is often the first diagnostic test and is particularly valuable for patients who are medically inoperable, decline surgery, or present with metastatic diseases. However, results from FNA can be unreliable. A negative or benign diagnosis does not exclude malignant disease (Grade B). The accuracy of FNA varies with the expertise of the pathologist. Tumor can be missed, and the relative scarcity of the tumor and the relative complexity of the WHO classification system further promote inaccuracy (Level III) (WESTRA 2007).

In a study of 712 patients undergoing FNA for a salivary mass, 73% had benign lesions and 20%

had neoplastic lesions. Sensitivity (the percentage of positive specimens that are true positives), specificity (the percentage of negative specimens that are true negative), and diagnostic accuracy (#true positive/#true negative) / (#true positive + #false positive + #false negative + #true negative) of FNA cytology for all neoplastic lesions of the salivary gland were 94.6%, 75.0%, and 91.1%, respectively (Level III) (DAS et al. 2004).

The vast majority of the studies performed to assess the accuracy of the FNA have been single institution studies where the FNA result was compared to the histological result. The potential for publication of only those results reflecting positively on the institution and the physicians is evident.

The College of the American Pathologists Interlaboratory Comparison Program in Nongynecologic Cytology took a prospective approach to evaluating the accuracy of FNA: Every quarter, five glass slides with accompanying clinical history were mailed to participating cytopathologists. The slides had been vetted by two Cytopathology Resource Committee cytopathologists who believed that the slides were representative, non-controversial, and of good technical quality. The reference cytopathologists had to agree on the general and specific diagnosis. Looking at the benign cases, there were 4642 responses and 4254 had the correct response, producing a specificity of 91%. Benign cases with high false-positive rates were monomorphic adenoma (53%) and intraparotid lymph nodes (36%). With respect to the malignant cases, there were 1607 responses, with 1096 being correct, giving a sensitivity of 68% and a false-negative rate of 32%. Malignant cases with high false-negative rates were lymphoma (57%), acinic cell carcinoma (49%), low-grade mucoepidermoid carcinoma (43%), and adenoid cystic carcinoma (33%). The overall diagnostic accuracy for making the correct specific reference diagnosis was a sobering 48% (Level II) (HUGHES et al. 2005).

CAJULIS et al. (1997) reported that while all 89% of the aspirations done by cytopathologists were diagnostic, only 77% of the 62 FNAs performed by the clinicians were diagnostic (Level III). One interpretation of these results is that clinicians need assistance in preparing the slide after aspiration. Sensitivity for detecting malignancy was 91% while the specificity for detecting a benign lesion was 96%.

■ The most common histologies for all salivary gland tumors are: Mucoepidermoid (21.7%), lymphoma (17.2%), squamous cell (16.1%), other adeno (12.8%) and acinar (10.3%) (DAVIES and WELCH 2006). For the parotid gland, mucoepidermoid is the most common malignancy; for the submandibular gland, adenoid cystic is the most common cancer (DAVIES and WELCH 2006).

In most cases the histology determines the tumor grade. Assignment of a specific grade is only applicable in mucoepidermoid carcinoma, adenocarcinoma not otherwise specified, or when either of those two histologies is identified as a carcinomatous element in a pleomorphic adenoma.

The histologic classification, as recommended by the second edition of the WHO (SEIFERT and SOBIN 1992) is shown in Table 4.2.

■ Just as cytologists face challenges to improve their diagnostic accuracy, the reproducibility of pathologic grading has been questioned. BRANDWEIN et al. (2001) reported on 20 slides from 20 cases of mucoepidermoid cancer circulated among five distinguished pathologists. Though the study used low, intermediate, and high grading (as compared to simply low versus high grade), interobserver agreement was poor (weighted kappa estimate, $\kappa = 0.49$). Comparing the five experts with an AFIP grading system, there were 46 discrepancies out of 100 pairs of grading events (Level III) (BRANDWEIN et al. 2001).

■ Histologic grade of mucoepidermoid carcinomas did not correlate with clinical behavior, according to a retrospective series of 391 patients with parotid tumor (Level IV) (CESINARO et al. 1994).

4.1.2 Staging

■ Primary tumors of the major salivary glands can be staged clinically or pathologically based on size of the primary tumor and tumor extension. Staging for neck nodes are identical to that of squamous cell carcinoma of other head and neck areas (see Chap. 6, Table 6.2).

■ The American Joint Committee on Cancer (AJCC) Tumor Node Metastasis (TNM) staging system is the accepted standard for staging of tumors of the major salivary glands (Table 4.3) (GREENE et al. 2002).

Table 4.2. WHO Classification, 2nd edition

Tumor type	
1	**Adenomas**
1.1	Pleomorphic adenoma
1.2	Myoepithelioma (myoepithelial adenoma)
1.3	Basal cell adenoma
1.4	Warthin tumor (adenolymphoma)
1.5	Oncocytoma (oncocytic adenoma)
1.6	Canalicular adenoma
1.7	Sebaceous adenoma
1.8	Ductal papilloma
1.8.1	Inverted ductal papilloma
1.8.2	Intraductal papilloma
1.8.3	Sialadenoma papilliferum
1.9	Cystadenoma
1.9.1	Papillary cystadenoma
1.9.2	Mucinous cystadenoma
2	**Carcinomas**
2.1	Acinic cell carcinoma
2.2	Mucoepidermoid carcinoma
2.3	Adenoid cystic carcinoma
2.4	Polymorphous low-grade adenocarcinoma (terminal duct adenocarcinoma)
2.5	Epithelial-myoepithelial carcinoma
2.6	Basal cell adenocarcinoma
2.7	Sebaceous carcinoma
2.8	Papillary cystadenocarcinoma
2.9	Mucinous adenocarcinoma
2.10	Oncocytic carcinoma
2.11	Salivary duct carcinoma
2.12	Adenocarcinoma
2.13	Malignant myoepithelioma (myoepithelial carcinoma)
2.14	Carcinoma in pleomorphic adenoma (malignant mixed tumor)
2.15	Squamous cell carcinoma
2.16	Small cell carcinoma
2.17	Undifferentiated carcinoma
2.18	Other carcinomas
3	**Nonepithelial tumors**
4	**Malignant lymphomas**
5	**Secondary tumors**
6	**Unclassified tumors**
7	**Tumor-like lesions**
7.1	Sialadenosis
7.2	Oncocytosis
7.3	Necrotizing sialometaplasia (salivary gland infarction)
7.4	Benign lymphoepithelial lesion
7.5	Salivary gland cysts
7.6	Chronic sclerosing sialadenitis of submandibular gland (Küttner tumor)
7.7	Cystic lymphoid hyperplasia in AIDS

Table 4.3. American Joint Committee on Cancer (AJCC) TNM Classification of Carcinoma cancer of Major Salivary Glands

Primary tumor (T)	
TX	Primary tumor cannot be assessed
T0	No evidence of primary tumor
T1	Tumor 2 cm or less in greatest dimension without extraparenchymal extension
T2	Tumor more than 2 cm but ont more than 4 cm in greatest dimension without extraparenchymal extension
T3	Tumor more than 4 cm and/or tumor having extraparenchymal extension
T4a	Tumor invades skin, mandible, ear canal, and/or facial nerve
T4b	Tumor invades skull base and/or pterygoid plates and/or encases carotid artery
Regional lymph nodes (N)	
NX	Regional lymph nodes cannot be assessed
N0	No regional lymph node metastasis
N1	Metastasis in a single ipsilateral lymph node, 3 cm or less in greatest dimension
N2	Metastasis in a single ipsilateral lymph node, more than 3 cm but not more than 6 cm greatest dimension, or in multiple ipsilateral lymph nodes, none more than 6 cm in greatest dimension, or in bilateral or contralateral lymph nodes, none more than 6 cm in greatest dimension
N2a	Metastasis in a single ipsilateral lymph node, more than 3 cm but not more than 6 cm in greatest dimension
N2b	Metastasis in multiple ipsilateral lymph nodes, none more than 6 cm in greatest dimension
N2c	Metastasis in bilateral or contralateral lymph nodes, none more than 6 cm in greatest dimension
N3	Metastasis in a lymph node, more than 6 cm in greatest dimension
Distant metastasis (M)	
MX	Distant metastasis cannot be assessed
M0	No distant metastasis
M1	Distant metastasis
STAGE GROUPING	
I:	T1 N0 M0
II:	T2 N0 M0
III:	T3 N0 M0, T1 N1 M0, T2 N1 M0, T3 N1 M0
IVA:	T4a N0 M0, T4a N1 M0, T1 N2 M0, T2 N2 M0, T3 N2 M0, T4a N2 M0
IVB:	T4b Any N M0, Any T N3 M0
IVC:	Any T Any N M1

4.1.3 Prognostic Factors

■ The Dutch Head and Neck Oncology Cooperative Group study found that the 10-year cumulative regional control for clinical +N/p+N, pN0, and clinical N0 patients was 75%, 94%, and 91%, respectively (Level IV) (TERHAARD et al. 2004). The 5-year relative survival rates from the American College of Surgeons National Cancer Data Base are presented in Table 4.4 (GREENE et al. 2002).

Table 4.4. The 5-year relative and observed survival rates from the American College of Surgeons National Cancer Data Base

Stage	5-Year relative survival rate	5-Year observed survival rate
I	86%	75%
II	66%	59%
III	53%	47%
IV	32%	28%

■ Histologic grade or cellular differentiation of the tumor is one of the most important prognostic factors affecting treatment outcome, including overall survival.

■ Histology can be predictive of predilection for lymphatic spread, perineural spread, as well as tendency to local recurrence. More than 30% of parotid cancers are mucoepidermoid carcinoma, which is usually slow growing and rarely metastasizes hematogenously. High-grade mucoepidermoid carcinoma is locally aggressive, may metastasize to regional lymph nodes in 40%–50% of cases and distantly in approximately 30% of cases.

Adenoid cystic carcinoma accounts for approximately 10% of parotid cancer, but is relatively more common in submandibular tumors, where it accounts for more than 40% of cases. Adenoid cystic carcinoma is associated with perineural invasion in more than 50% of cases. Disease growth or recurrence along the cranial nerves has been a distinct characteristic of adenoid cystic carcinoma, and extension of disease via nerve to skull base is probable. Regional nodal involvement by this entity is not common and occurs in less than 8% of cases at initial presentation; however, distant spread to lung occurs in approximately 50% of cases.

Approximately 10% of parotid cancers and 17% of submandibular cancers are acinic cancers. Malignant mixed tumors account for roughly 15% of parotid malignancy and 10% of submandibular cancers.

- Completeness of treatment is a significant prognostic factor for patients undergoing surgical resection. Multivariate analysis from the study reported by the Dutch Head and Neck Oncology Cooperative Group revealed that the status of the tumor margins ≥ 5 mm was associated with improved local control ($p = 0.07$) (Level IV) (Terhaard et al. 2004). For those patients undergoing a therapeutic neck dissection, margin status was an independent predictor of regional control (67% for positive margin, 83% for < 5-mm margin, and 91% regional control for a margin ≥ 5 mm, $p = 0.04$). Other authors have used 3-mm margins as the standard (Level IV) (Brandwein et al. 2001).
- Other significant independent prognostic features for regional control were complete facial paralysis (65% regional control for complete facial nerve paralysis versus 91% for no or partial paralysis), bone invasion, and the use of combined modality treatment (as detailed below).
- In Koul et al.'s (2007) review of 184 parotid malignancies, advanced age was also an independent prognostic feature correlating with poor local control (Level IV).
- The major pattern of failure for malignant tumors of the major salivary glands is development of distant metastases. In a population based review of 903 patients, Bhattacharyya and Fried (2005) found that increasing age, tumor size, grade, extraglandular extension, and nodal positivity negatively influenced survival (Level IV).

4.2 Treatment of Major Salivary Gland Cancers

4.2.1 General Principles

- For patients with malignant tumors of the major salivary glands being treated for cure, surgery is the gold standard (Grade B).
- For inoperable patients, radiation therapy is indicated for disease control (Grade B). Neutrons can

control 67% of tumors, compared to only 20%–25% for definitive treatment with high energy photons (Level IV) (Koh et al. 1989; Douglas et al. 2003; Mendenhall et al. 2005).

- Lymphomas of the major salivary glands and HIV-related benign parotid hypertrophy are treated non-surgically as discussed below (Grade B).
- Although response to chemotherapy has been well documented for metastatic salivary cancers, there is little persuasive literature to suggest that systemic therapy can effectively lower the rates of distant metastases.

4.2.2 Surgery

Carcinoma of the Parotid Gland

- A superficial parotidectomy is the surgery of choice for most parotid tumors. Excisional biopsy is not recommended as it may violate the surgical field and is associated with increased local recurrence.
- Approximately 90% of parotid tumors are located in the superficial lobe of the parotid gland. The superficial lobe can be resected using superficial parotidectomy or subtotal parotidectomy.
- The spinal accessory, facial, and greater auricular nerves are identified. The greater auricular nerve is usually sacrificed because of it's anatomic path through the SCM and parotid gland (Figs. 4.1–4.3).
- If a branch or the entire facial nerve is paralyzed prior to surgery, sacrifice of the nerve is usually necessary. However, if there is no facial nerve palsy preoperatively, surgeons try not to sacrifice any branch of the facial nerve. A transient facial nerve palsy may occur up to 40% of cases, especially if there are other concomitant medical comorbidities (Dulguerov et al. 1999; Guntinas-Lichius et al. 2006) (Level IV). A permanent facial nerve palsy is an unusual complication in the hands of experienced surgeons, occurring less than 5% of cases (Dulguerov et al. 1999; Guntinas-Lichius et al. 2006) (Level IV).
- For parotid tumors located in the deep lobe, total parotidectomy is the surgery of choice. The entire parotid gland with a margin of normal tissue is removed in the procedure.
- The goals of surgery are complete tumor resection with a ≥ 5-mm margin, as well as preservation of

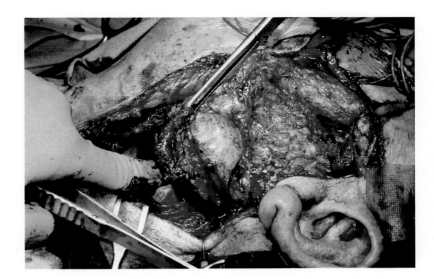

Fig. 4.1. Mass overlying facial nerve

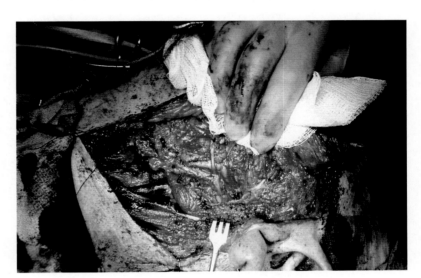

Fig. 4.2. Facial nerve main trunk and branches

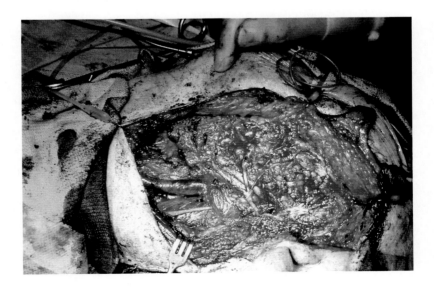

Fig. 4.3. Facial nerve main trunk and branches

as much function and anatomy as oncologically possible (Grade C). As mentioned above, the multivariate analysis from the Dutch Head and Neck Oncology Cooperative Group described above showed that the status of the tumor margins ≥5 mm was associated with improved local control ($p=0.07$) (Level IV) (TERHAARD et al. 2004). Other authors have used 3-mm margins as the standard (Level IV) (BRANDWEIN et al. 2001).

- Formal neck dissection is not necessarily indicated if the patient is clinically N0 and elective neck irradiation is planned (see Sect. 4.2.4) (Grade B). Level IIa nodes are best dissected along with the parotid for malignant lesions because of the proximity of these lymph nodes to the tail of the parotid and high rates of involvement (Level III) (CORLETTE et al. 2005). Lymph nodes along the external jugular vein also need to be dissected, particularly for metastatic parotid lesions from dermal primary (Grade B) (Level III) (ZBAREN et al. 2005; YING et al. 2006).

- For patients with clinically positive lymph nodes, a modified radical or selective neck dissection is indicated.

Carcinoma of the Submandibular Gland

- Resection of the submandibular gland can be performed for small tumor of the gland where the tumor is encased in normal tissue.
- More extensive surgery is required for lesions with extracapsular extension with involvement of adjacent tissues and cranial nerves.
- Neck dissection is not routinely indicated; however, elective neck dissection should be considered in large or high-grade tumors.

4.2.3 Adjuvant Radiation Therapy of the Primary

- Indications for post-operative radiation include positive or close margins, high-grade disease, perineural invasion, regional nodal involvement, lymphovascular invasion, or pathologic T3 or T4 disease, and recurrent disease (Grade B). The efficacy of adjuvant radiation therapy for this group of patients has been demonstrated in a number of retrospective studies including a case-control study. The reliance exclusively on grade to exclude the use of radiation should be performed with caution.

- The Dutch Head and Neck Oncology Cooperative Group studied 565 patients with salivary gland tumors and found surgery without post-operative radiation had a local failure relative risk of 9.7 (CI 4.4-21), which was the highest relative risk for any factor affecting local control (Level IV) (TERHAARD et al. 2004).

- KOUL et al.'s (2007) multivariate analysis found that the addition of adjuvant radiation decreased the hazard ratio of disease-specific death to 0.5 (CI 0.228–0.995) when compared to surgery alone and adjusted for tumor size (Level IV).

- Early experience from the Princess Margaret Hospital showed that patients with malignant tumor of parotid gland treated with surgery followed by adjuvant radiation therapy achieved superior recurrence-free survival at 10 years (62% versus 22%). An analysis for prognostic factors showed that the histology, tumor stage, regional metastases (N0 vs. N+), age, and damage to the facial nerve all influenced cause-specific survival (Level IV) (THERIAULT 1986).

A case-control study reported from Memorial Sloan-Kettering Cancer Center evaluated the efficacy of adjuvant radiotherapy and concluded that radiation is not routinely indicated for patients with low-grade stage I and II cancers of the major salivary glands. However, improved survival and local control were demonstrated in patients with locoregionally advanced diseases, i.e., stage III and IV or N+ cancers. In addition, a trend of improved outcome was found for high-grade diseases (Level IV) (ARMSTRONG 1990). In addition, results from a retrospective series of 178 patients treated at the M.D. Anderson Cancer Center revealed that patients with high-grade tumor of major salivary glands or tumor with perineural invasion benefited significantly from adjuvant radiation therapy. Patients who underwent combined surgery and radiation achieved 86% local control rate, versus 58% in those received surgery only (Level IV) (FRANKENTHALER 1991). The study also demonstrated that histological grade, perineural invasion, and presenting stage are the most significant prognostic factors.

4.2.4 Nodal Treatment Considerations

- In the era of IMRT, the addition of ipsilateral nodal irradiation to the primary site should have manageable late consequences.

In a study at UCSF, 131 patients with carcinoma of the salivary glands underwent elective neck irradiation with no subsequent neck failures. Conversely, out of 120 patients with salivary gland cancer who did not receive elective neck irradiation, 24 suffered neck failures at 10 years (nodal relapse rate of 0% versus 26%, $p = 0.0001$). The authors were unable to exclude any patient group from elective neck irradiation based on age, perineural invasion, T-stage, and primary site.

■ The low risk of lymphatic spread for acinic cell cancers and adenoid cystic cancers of the parotids is echoed throughout the literature, thus elective irradiation to the neck nodes is not indicated for these pathologies (Grade B). In the UCSF experience, there were no neck relapses for any of the patients who had adenoid cystic or acinic cell histology regardless of whether they received elective nodal irradiation (Level IV) (CHEN et al. 2007a).TERHAARD et al. (2004) found that the 10-year cumulative regional control for clinical +N/p+N, pN0 and clinical N0 patients was 75%, 94%, and 91% respectively. Independent prognostic features for regional control were complete facial paralysis (65% regional control for complete facial nerve paralysis versus 91% for no or partial paralysis, $p = 0.01$), and the use of combined modality treatment (67% for surgery alone versus 89% for surgery followed by post-operative radiation therapy, $p = 0.03$) (Level IV) (TERHAARD et al. 2004).

4.2.5 Radiation Therapy Techniques

Simulation and Field Arrangement

■ IMRT techniques are recommended for the treatment of parotid tumors (Grade B). A six-field plan is illustrated in Figure 4.4.

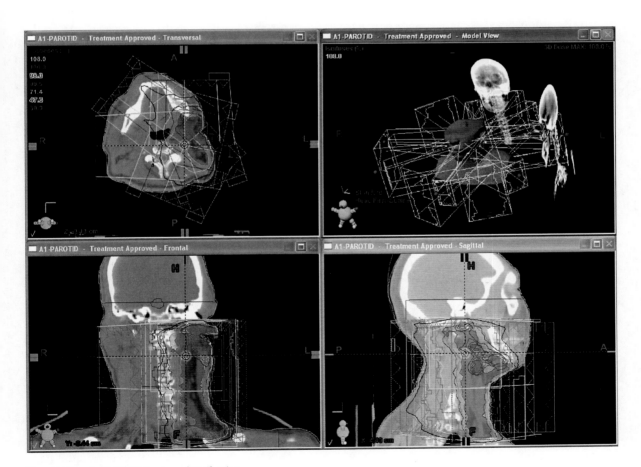

Fig. 4.4. Six-field IMRT isodose distribution

■ If IMRT technology is not available, ipsilateral wedge pair, the three-field, and the mixed electron-photon beam techniques are optimal techniques for providing relatively homogeneous dose distributions within the target area and for minimizing dose to the relevant normal structures (Level III) (YAPARPALVI et al. 1998).

■ Ideally, preoperative imaging should be fused with post-operative CT simulation to ensure an adequate plan to the primary site.

Dose and Fractionation

■ Doses to the primary tumor bed/resection area should be 60 Gy in once-daily fractions over 30 days, unless the surgical margins were unsatisfactory. Dose for elective neck irradiation is usually in the range of 50 Gy in 25 daily fractions.

■ When the en face mixed beam technique is used, the composition of the dose depends on the depth, size, and location of the tumor, and is determined by CT planning system. Approximately 80% electron and 20% photon can be commonly used.

■ Attention should be paid to the dose delivered to the adjacent normal organs and tissues including temporal lobes. Bolus can be used to avoid overdosing the temporal lobe. Cerrobend can be customized to block the intraoral structures.

4.2.6   Side Effects and Complications

■ Commonly observed acute side effects induced by external beam radiation therapy include dermatitis and mucositis; both are usually self-limited.

■ Severe long-term complications induced by radiation therapy are uncommon but can include partial xerostomia, decreased hearing and fibrosis.

■ Trismus can be a complication and should be addressed by speech pathology consultation.

4.3   Patterns of Failure

■ The major pattern of failure for malignant tumors of the major salivary glands is develop-

ment of distant metastases. In a population based review of 903 patients, BHATTACHARYYA and FRIED (2005) found that increasing age, tumor size, grade, extraglandular extension, and nodal positivity negatively influenced survival (Level IV).

■ There is little persuasive literature to suggest that systemic therapy can effectively lower the rates of distant metastases.

4.4   Treatment of Uncommon Major Salivary Gland Tumors

4.4.1   Treatment of Squamous Cell Carcinoma of Parotid

■ Because of the intraparotid drainage of cutaneous skin malignancies, most squamous cell cancers of the parotid gland are metastatic from the skin.

■ In patients with skin cancers metastatic to the parotid area, post-operative local radiation of 60 Gy or higher improved local control from 74% to 93%(10/13 vs 16/17 controlled) when compared to doses below 60 Gy (CHEN et al. 2007b). Post-operative irradiation to the parotid bed to a dose of at least 60 Gy is indicated (Grade B).

■ Ipsilateral neck irradiation for those patients with clinically N0 neck who had skin cancers which has spread to the parotid should also be performed (Grade B). Ipsilateral elective nodal irradiation from Levels IB to Level V for clinically N0 patients was effective in 15 patients, whereas there were seven neck failures in 14 patients with N0 necks who were observed. Their 5-year neck control rate was 45% (CHEN et al. 2007b).

4.4.2   Treatment of Benign Lymphoepithelial Cysts in HIV+ Patients

■ Immunocompromised patients can develop chronic cystic hyperplasia which results in a physical deformity that can be cosmetically devastating. The disease is usually bilateral and can persist despite anti-retroviral medication.

- As chronic cystic hyperplasia can recur after both aspiration and surgery, radiation therapy can be considered (Grade B). Doses of 24 Gy in 1.5-Gy daily fractions are well-tolerated and have long-term efficacy in 70% of patients (Level IV) (BEITLER et al. 1999).

4.5 Follow-Ups

4.5.1 Post-Treatment Follow-Ups

- Long-term follow-up after definitive treatment of malignant tumors of the major salivary glands is indicated, especially in high-grade tumors (Grade B). The probability of local and distant recurrence combined approaches 50%, as described in studies detailed above (Level IV).
- Local salvage is poor. TERHAARD et al. (2004) reported on 100 patients with local residual or recurrent disease. Salvage was attempted on 46 and only 17 of the original 100 were cured (Level IV).
- Regional salvage is poor. TERHAARD et al. (2004) reported on 61 patients with regional persistence or recurrence. Of the 61 patients, 15 were cured (Level IV).

4.5.2 Schedule

- Follow-ups could be scheduled every 3–4 months in the first 2 years, every 4–6 months over an additional 3 years and annually thereafter (Grade D) (Table 4.5).

Table 4.5. Proposed follow-up schedule after treatment for cancers of major salivary glands

Interval	Frequency
First 2 years	Every 3-4 months
Year 3–5	Every 4-6 months
Over 5 years	Annually

4.5.3 Work-Ups

- Each follow-up should include an interval history and physical examination.
- Annual chest X-ray can be considered for ruling out pulmonary metastasis: however, there is no evidence to support the use of any imaging studies in improving survival (Grade D). Bone scan and CT scan of the head and neck area are not routinely recommended in asymptomatic patients (Grade D).

References

Armstrong JG, Harrison LB, Spiro RH, Fass DE, Strong EW, Fuks ZY (1990) Malignant tumors of major salivary gland origin. A matched-pair analysis of the role of combined surgery and postoperative radiotherapy. Arch Otolaryngol Head Neck Surg 116:290–293

Beitler JJ, Smith RV, Brook A, Edelman M, Sharma A, Serrano M, Silver CE, Davis LW (1999) Benign parotid hypertrophy on +HIV patients: limited late failures after external radiation. Int J Radiat Oncol Biol Phys 45:451–455

Bhattacharyya N, Fried MP (2005) Determinants of survival in parotid gland carcinoma: a population-based study. Am J Otolaryngol 26:39–44

Brandwein MS, Ivanov K, Wallace DI, Hille JJ, Wang B, Fahmy A, Bodian C, Urken ML, Gnepp DR, Huvos A, Lumerman H, Mills SE (2001) Mucoepidermoid carcinoma: a clinicopathologic study of 80 patients with special reference to histological grading. Am J Surg Pathol 25:835–845

Cajulis RS, Gokaslan ST, Yu GH, Frias-Hidvegi D (1997) Fine needle aspiration biopsy of the salivary glands. A five-year experience with emphasis on diagnostic pitfalls. Acta Cytol 41:1412–1420

Cesinaro AM, Criscuolo M, Collina G, Galetti R, Migaldi M, Lo Bianco F (1994) Salivary gland tumors: revision of 391 cases according to the new WHO classification. Pathologica 86:602–605

Chen AM, Garcia J, Lee NY, Bucci MK, Eisele DW (2007a) Patterns of nodal relapse after surgery and postoperative radiation therapy for carcinomas of the major and minor salivary glands: what is the role of elective neck irradiation? Int J Radiat Oncol Biol Phys 67:988–994

Chen AM, Grekin RC, Garcia J, Bucci MK, Margolis LW (2007b) Radiation therapy for cutaneous squamous cell carcinoma involving the parotid area lymph nodes: dose and volume considerations. Int J Radiat Oncol Biol Phys 69:1377–1380

Corlette TH, Cole IE, Albsoul N, Ayyash M (2005) Neck dissection of level IIb: is it really necessary? Laryngoscope 115:1624–1626

Das DK, Petkar MA, Al-Mane NM, Sheikh ZA, Mallik MK, Anim JT (2004) Role of fine needle aspiration cytology in the diagnosis of swellings in the salivary gland regions: a study of 712 cases. Med Princ Pract 13:95–106

Davies L, Welch HG (2006) Epidemiology of head and neck cancer in the United States. Otolaryngol Head Neck Surg 135:451–457

Douglas JG, Koh WJ, Austin-Seymour M, Laramore GE (2003) Treatment of salivary gland neoplasms with fast neutron radiotherapy. Arch Otolaryngol Head Neck Surg 129:944–948

Dulguerov P, Marchal F, Lehmann W (1999) Postparotidectomy facial nerve paralysis: possible etiologic factors and results with routine facial nerve monitoring. Laryngoscope 109:754–762

Fee WE Jr, Tran LE (2003) Evaluation of a patient with a parotid tumor. Arch Otolaryngol Head Neck Surg 129:937–938

Frankenthaler RA, Luna MA, Lee SS, Ang KK, Byers RM, Guillamondegui OM, Wolf P, Goepfert H (1991) Prognostic variables in parotid gland cancer. Arch Otolaryngol Head Neck Surg 117: 1251–1256

Greene F, Page D, Fleming I et al. (2002) AJCC Cancer Staging Manual, 6th edn. Springer, Berlin Heidelberg New York

Guntinas-Lichius O, Klussmann JP, Wittekindt C, Stennert E (2006) Parotidectomy for benign parotid disease at a university teaching hospital: outcome of 963 operations. Laryngoscope 116:534–540

Hall P, Holm LE, Lundell G, Bjelkengren G, Larsson LG, Lindberg S, Tennvall J, Wicklund H, Boice JD Jr (1991) Cancer risks in thyroid cancer patients. Br J Cancer 64:159–163

Hughes JH, Volk EE, Wilbur DC (2005) Pitfalls in salivary gland fine-needle aspiration cytology: lessons from the College of American Pathologists Interlaboratory Comparison Program in Nongynecologic Cytology. Arch Pathol Lab Med 129:26–31

Jeong HS, Chung MK, Son YI, Choi JY, Kim HJ, Ko YH, Baek CH (2007) Role of 18F-FDG PET-CT in management of high-grade salivary gland malignancies. J Nucl Med 48:1237–1244

Koh WJ, Laramore G, Griffin T, Russell K, Griffin B, Parker R, Davis L, Pajak TF (1989) Fast neutron radiation for inoperable and recurrent salivary gland cancers. Am J Clin Oncol 12:316–319

Koul R, Dubey A, Butler J, Cooke AL, Abdoh A, Nason R (2007) Prognostic factors depicting disease-specific survival in parotid-gland tumors. Int J Radiat Oncol Biol Phys 68:714–718

Land CE, Saku T, Hayashi Y, Takahara O, Matsuura H, Tokuoka S, Tokunaga M, Mabuchi K (1996) Incidence of salivary gland tumors among atomic bomb survivors, 1950-1987. Evaluation of radiation-related risk. Radiat Res 146:28–36

Lanier AP, Blot WJ, Bender TR, Fraumeni JF Jr (1980) Cancer in Alaskan Indians, Eskimos, and Aleuts. J Natl Cancer Inst 65:1157–1159

Martin VT, Salmaso R, Onnis GL (1989) Tumors of salivary glands. Review of 479 cases with particular reference to histological types, site, age and sex distribution. Appl Pathol 7:154–160

Mendenhall WM, Morris CG, Amdur RJ, Werning JW, Villaret DB (2005) Radiotherapy alone or combined with surgery for salivary gland carcinoma. Cancer 103:2544–2550

Roh JL, Ryu CH, Choi SH, Kim JS, Lee JH, Cho KJ, Nam SY, Kim SY (2007) Clinical utility of 18F-FDG PET for patients with salivary gland malignancies. J Nucl Med 48:240–246

Rubin P, Hansen JT (2008) TNM staging atlas. Wolters Kluwer/Lippincott Williams & Wilkins, Philadelphia

Saku T, Hayashi Y, Takahara O, Matsuura H, Tokunaga M, Tokuoka S, Soda M, Mabuchi K, Land CE (1997) Salivary gland tumors among atomic bomb survivors, 1950–1987. Cancer 79:1465–1475

Seifert G, Sobin LH (1992) The World Health Organization's histological classification of salivary gland tumors. A commentary on the second edition. Cancer 70:379–385

Stanley HR, Dawe CJ, Law LW (1964) Oral tumors induced by polyoma virus in mice. Oral Surg Oral Med Oral Pathol 17:547–558

Sun EC, Curtis R, Melbye M, Goedert JJ (1999) Salivary gland cancer in the United States. Cancer Epidemiol Biomarkers Prev 8:1095–1100

Terhaard CH, Lubsen H, Van der Tweel I, Hilgers FJ, Eijkenboom WM, Marres HA, Tjho-Heslinga RE, de Jong JM, Roodenburg JL (2004) Salivary gland carcinoma: independent prognostic factors for locoregional control, distant metastases, and overall survival: results of the Dutch head and neck oncology cooperative group. Head Neck 26:681–692; discussion 692–683

Theriault C, Fitzpatrick PJ (1986) Malignant parotid tumors. Prognostic factors and optimum treatment. Am J Clin Oncol 9: 510–516

Vageli D, Sourvinos G, Ioannou M, Koukoulis GK, Spandidos DA (2007) High-risk human papillomavirus (HPV) in parotid lesions. Int J Biol Markers 22:239–244

Westra WH (2007) Diagnostic difficulties in the classification and grading of salivary gland tumors. Int J Radiat Oncol Biol Phys 69:S49–S51

Yaparpalvi R, Fontenla DP, Tyerech SK, Boselli LR, Beitler JJ (1998) Parotid gland tumors: a comparison of postoperative radiotherapy techniques using three dimensional (3D) dose distributions and dose-volume histograms (DVHS). Int J Radiat Oncol Biol Phys 40:43–49

Ying YL, Johnson JT, Myers EN (2006) Squamous cell carcinoma of the parotid gland. Head Neck 28:626–632

Zbaren P, Schupbach J, Nuyens M, Stauffer E (2005) Elective neck dissection versus observation in primary parotid carcinoma. Otolaryngol Head Neck Surg 132:387–391

Cancer of the Larynx and Hypopharynx

5

JAY S. COOPER

CONTENTS

J. S. COOPER, MD
Department of Radiation Oncology, Maimonides Cancer Center, 6300 Eighth Avenue, Brooklyn, NY 11220, USA

Introduction and Objectives

Carcinomas of the larynx and hypopharynx tend to present as local-regional disease that often requires multidisciplinary management. Preservation of function, as well as anatomy, can be paramount in the decision-making process. This tends to favor radiation therapy in the selection process. Treatment can, and should, be tailored to match the virulence of individual tumors and the impact of such therapy on individual patients.

This chapter examines:

- Recommendations for diagnosis and staging procedures for both laryngeal and hypopharyngeal cancer
- The staging systems and prognostic factors
- The management of laryngeal and hypopharyngeal cancers using unimodal and multimodal regimens based on surgery, radiation therapy, antibody therapy, and cytotoxic chemotherapy
- Techniques of radiation therapy
- Follow-up care

5.1 Diagnosis, Staging, and Prognosis

5.1.1 Diagnosis

Initial Evaluation

- Diagnosis and evaluation of laryngeal and hypopharyngeal cancer starts with a complete history and physical examination. Attention should be paid to disease-associated signs and symptoms and their chronology. Early onset hoarseness is more likely due to laryngeal lesion(s), while early onset difficulty swallowing is more likely from hypopharyngeal cancer.
- A thorough physical examination including direct fiberoptic endoscopy under local anesthesia and/or indirect mirror exam is required.

■ Dental evaluation to assess and restore (when possible) or extract (when restoration impossible) decayed teeth is necessary for all patients who require radiation therapy that includes a substantial volume of the parotid glands. The tooth socket generally requires approximately 2 weeks to heal before radiation therapy can begin.

Laboratory Tests

■ Initial laboratory tests should include a complete blood count, basic blood chemistry, liver function tests, and BUN/Creatinine.

Imaging Studies

■ Imaging studies with CT and/or MRI and/or PET/CT of the head and neck regions are required to evaluate the extent of the disease at the primary site, in regional lymph nodes, at distant sites, and to look for synchronous independent malignancies in the upper aerodigestive tract.
■ Three-dimensional imaging of the primary and regional neck nodes is routinely recommended. If radiation therapy is planned, scanning is ideally performed in radiation treatment position, using fixation devices such as thermoplastic facemasks and with the shoulders pulled or pushed down out of the path of lateral beams.
■ FDG-PET or PET/CT scans may be helpful in the evaluation of locally advanced laryngeal cancer or hypopharyngeal cancer (Grade B). A non-randomized prospective trial has demonstrated that the sensitivity, specificity, and accuracy approached 95%, superior to the results from CT scans (Level III) (GORDIN et al. 2006). In addition, high FDG uptake appears to be associated with poor survival in patients who have advanced laryngopharyngeal SCC (Level IV) (ROH et al. 2007; SCHWARTZ et al. 2004) (Table 5.1).

Table 5.1. Imaging and laboratory work-ups for cancer of the larynx or hypopharynx

Imaging studies	Laboratory tests
– CT scan or MRI of the head and neck area	– Complete blood count
– Chest X-ray or CT scan of chest	– Serum chemistry including BUN/creatinine
– FDG-PET or PET/CT (optional for locally advanced disease)	– Liver function tests

Pathology

■ Histologic diagnosis is mandatory for the diagnosis of cancer of the larynx and hypopharynx. Tissue for diagnosis can be obtained from the primary tumor site during endoscopic examination under anesthesia.
■ Nearly all malignancies arising in the larynx or hypopharynx do so from the mucosa and consequently are squamous cell carcinomas.
■ If regional adenopathy is present, sufficient tumor for diagnosis can often be obtained by fine-needle aspiration or core biopsy.

5.1.2   Staging

■ Carcinomas of the larynx and hypopharynx should always be assigned a clinical stage. Clinical staging utilizes information from history and physical examinations, imaging studies, laboratory tests, and endoscopy.
■ If surgery is performed, a pathologic stage should also be assigned. Pathologic staging is based on findings from clinical staging and examination of the resected specimen, including regional lymph nodes.
■ The American Joint Committee on Cancer (AJCC) Tumor Node Metastasis (TNM) staging system is the accepted standard for staging of both laryngeal and hypopharyngeal cancers (Table 5.2) (GREENE et al. 2002).

5.1.3   Prognostic Factors

■ Presenting stage is the most important prognostic factor for cancer of the larynx or hypopharynx.
■ Stage for stage, carcinomas of the larynx have a better prognosis than those arising in the hypopharynx.
■ Local control after radiation therapy is adversely influenced by increasing T category, prolonged overall treatment time, male gender, low pretreatment hemoglobin level, poor histologic differentiation, and/or failure to stop smoking (Level IV) (MENDENHALL et al. 2001; WARDE et al. 1998). Cause-specific survival rates at 5 years over 95% and 90% can be expected for T1 and T2 lesions, respectively.

Table 5.2. American Joint Committee on Cancer (AJCC) TNM classification of laryngeal and hypopharyngeal cancer [from GREENE et al. (2002) with permission]

	Primary tumor (T): glottis
TX	Primary tumor cannot be assessed
T0	No evidence of primary tumor
Tis	Carcinoma in situ
T1	Tumor limited to the vocal cord(s) with normal mobility
T2	Tumor extends to supraglottic and/or subglottis and/or with impaired cord mobility
T3	Tumor limited to the larynx with vocal cord fixation and/or invades paraglottic space and/or minor thyroid cartilage erosion
T4a	Tumor invades through the thyroid cartilage, and/or invades tissues beyond the larynx
T4b	Tumor invades prevertebral space, encases carotid artery, or invades mediastinal structures

	Primary tumor (T): supraglottis
TX	Primary tumor cannot be assessed
T0	No evidence of primary tumor
Tis	Carcinoma in situ
T1	Tumor limited to one subsite of supraglottis with normal vocal cord mobility
T2	Tumor invades mucosa of more than one adjacent subsite of supraglottis or glottis or region outside the supraglottis (e.g., mucosa of base of tongue, vallecula, medial wall of pyriform sinus) without fixation of the larynx
T3	Tumor limited to larynx with vocal cord fixation and/or invades any of the following: postcricoid area, pre-epiglottic tissues, paraglottic space, and/or minor thyroid cartilage erosion (e.g., inner cortex)
T4a	Tumor invades through the thyroid cartilage and/or invades tissues beyond the larynx(e.g., trachea, soft tissues of neck including deep extrinsic muscle of the tongue, strap muscles, thyroid or esophagus)
T4b	Tumor invades prevertebral space, encases carotid artery, or invades mediastinal structures

	Primary tumor (T): hypopharynx
TX	Primary tumor cannot be assessed
T0	No evidence of primary tumor
Tis	Carcinoma *in situ*
T1	Tumor limited to one subsite of hypopharynx, and 2cm or less in greatest dimension
T2	Tumor invades more than one subsite of hypopharynx or an adjacent site, or measures between 2 and 4 cm in greatest dimension, without fixation of hemilarynx
T3	Tumor measures greater than 4 cm or with fixation of hemilarynx
T4a	Tumor invades thyroid/cricoid cartilage, hyoid bone, thyroid gland, esophagus, or central compartment soft tissue
T4b	Tumor invades prevertebral fascia, encases carotid artery, or involves mediastinal structures

	Regional lymph nodes (N)
NX	Regional lymph nodes cannot be assessed
N0	No regional lymph node metastasis
N1	Metastasis in a single ipsilateral lymph node, 3 cm or less in greatest dimension
N2	Metastasis in a single ipsilateral lymph node, more than 3 cm but not more than 6 cm greatest dimension, or in multiple ipsilateral lymph nodes, none more than 6 cm in greatest dimension, or in bilateral or contralateral lymph nodes, none more than 6 cm in greatest dimension
N2a	Metastasis in a single ipsilateral lymph node, more than 3 cm but not more than 6 cm in greatest dimension
N2b	Metastasis in multiple ipsilateral lymph nodes, none more than 6 cm in greatest dimension
N2c	Metastasis in bilateral or contralateral lymph nodes, none more than 6 cm in greatest dimension Metastasis in a lymph
N3	node, more than 6 cm in greatest dimension

	Distant metastasis (M)
MX	Distant metastasis cannot be assessed
M0	No distant metastasis
M1	Distant metastasis

	STAGE GROUPING
0:	Tis N0 M0
I:	T1 N0 M0
II:	T2 N0 M0
III:	T3 N0 M0, T1 N1 M0, T2 N1 M0, T3 N1 M0
IVA:	T4a N0 M0, T4a N1 M0, T1 N2 M0, T2 N2 M0, T3 N2 M0, T4a N2 M0
IVB:	T4b Any N M0, Any T N3 M0
IVC:	Any T Any N M1

5.2 Definitive Treatment for Anatomic and Functional Organ Conservation

5.2.1 Lesions Incapable of Regional Metastasis

General Principles

- Limited extent squamous cell carcinoma of glottis (i.e., T1 or T2, N0) can be treated effectively by radiation therapy or, in select circumstances, by surgery (Grade A).
- Radiation therapy generally is the preferred option based on better subsequent voice quality. However, no high level evidence exists to select between treatment options, and numerous large retrospective studies have demonstrated similar control rates after surgery or radiation therapy.

Definitive Radiation Therapy

- Radiation therapy, by itself, is an effective treatment modality for the treatment of T1 or T2 squamous cell carcinoma of the glottic larynx (Grade A). The 5-year local control rates are approximately 85%–95% for T1 tumors and from 70% to 80% for T2 malignancies. The 5-year overall survival for stage I and II squamous cell carcinoma of glottic larynx is approximately 75% to 90% (more influenced by other factors than the tumor); the 5-year cause-specific survival is approximately 90%–100% (Level IV) (MENDENHALL et al. 2001, 2004; WARDE et al. 1998).

Techniques

- CT-based planning is recommended and the CT scan should be taken in the treatment position.
- A megavoltage accelerator (4 MV–6 MV energy photon beams) with a minimum source to isocenter distance of 100 cm is recommended. Care must be taken for patients who have far anterior disease that build up is considered. Some patients require thin bolus placed over the anterior skin.
- Carefully assess laryngeal motion upon swallowing to ensure that the target tumor remains in the treatment fields at all times during therapy. Small primary lesions of the glottic larynx do not pose a substantial risk of spreading to regional lymph nodes and treatment of the primary disease alone is sufficient.

- For practical purposes, bilateral field sizes as small as 5×5 cm, covering from the thyroid notch to the bottom of the cricoid cartilage and flashing skin to the anterior 1/3 of the vertebral body can be used (Grade A) (Figs. 5.1 and 5.2). The efficacy of this field arrangement has long been shown to be effective in retrospective studies (Level IV) (MENDENHALL et al. 2001, 2004). In addition, results from a small randomized study using 5×5 cm or 6×6 cm fields showed that the 5-year recurrence free survival approached 90% (Level II) (CHATANI et al. 1996).
- For anteriorly placed tumors without involvement of the posterior vocal cord, moving the posterior border anteriorly by 0.5 cm after a dose sufficient for subclinical disease (approximately 50 Gy for standard fractionation) is acceptable (Grade C). Such arrangement may reduce toxicity and does not appear to be associated with decreased tumor control. A smaller field size (5×5 cm vs. 6×6 cm) has been associated with less arytenoid edema in a prospective randomized trial (Level II) (CHATANI et al. 1996). However, the degree of edema has not been consistent across all studies (Level III) (ALLAL et al. 1997; AMDUR et al. 1995; ROVIROSA 1997).

Dose and Schedules

- T1 lesions of the glottic larynx need to be treated with at least 2 Gy per fraction per day [e.g., to a total dose of 66 Gy at 2 Gy per day (in 33 daily fractions)] (Grade A). Smaller daily fractions should

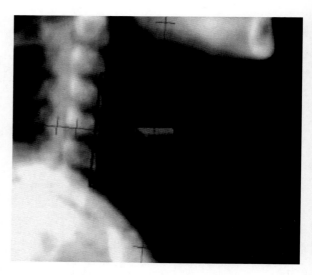

Fig. 5.1. Simulation film of a 6 × 6-cm field covering the glottis only for treatment of a T1N0M0 glottic tumor

Fig. 5.2. Dosimetry of parallel-opposed fields for T1N0M0 glottic cancer. Parallel-opposed, 6 × 6 fields were used with wedges and bolus

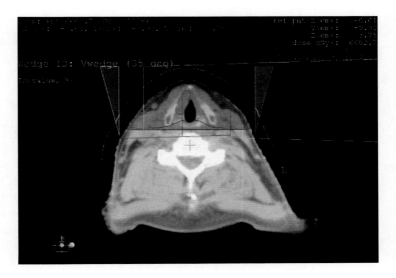

not be used as results from retrospective studies have suggested that they are associated with reduced local control rates (Level IV) (Schwaibold et al. 1998; Mendenhall et al. 1988; Kim et al. 1992; Rudoltz et al. 1993; Ricciardelli et al. 1994; Yu et al. 1997; Le et al. 1997). The small field size allows slight acceleration of dose. Some reports suggest that 2.25 Gy is more effective than 2 Gy per day for these lesions (i.e., 63 Gy at 2.25 Gy per fraction for 28 fractions) (Level II) (Le et al. 1997; Spector et al. 1999; Yamazaki et al. 2006).

■ T2 lesions of the glottic larynx can be treated to a total dose of 70 Gy at 2 Gy per day (in 35 daily fractions over 7 weeks).

■ Hyperfractionated radiation therapy [79.2 Gy in 66 fractions over 6.5 weeks (at 1.2 Gy per fractions, twice a day)] can be considered for better disease control (Grade B). While there is no compelling prospective evidence-based data to require it, there is suggestive data in support of this treatment strategy to improve local control (Level IV, II) (Garden et al. 2003; Trotti et al. 2006).

5.2.2   Small Lesions Capable of Regional Metastasis

General Principles

■ Small lesions (T1N0-small N1 and most T2N0) of the supraglottic larynx or (T1N0-1 and small T2N0)

of the hypopharynx can effectively be treated by radiation therapy or surgery (Grade A).

■ Radiation therapy is the preferred option when anatomic constraints would require total laryngectomy to close the surgical defect.

■ Chemotherapy is not indicated in the treatment of early stage squamous cell carcinoma of supraglottic larynx or hypopharynx capable of regional metastasis.

Definitive Radiation Therapy

■ Definitive radiation therapy provides effective treatment for small lesions (T1N0-1 and small T2N0) of the hypopharynx or (T1N0-small N1 and most T2N0) of the supraglottic larynx (Grade A). Results from a multi-institutional review of 115 patients with stage I and II squamous cell carcinoma showed that radiation therapy produced 5-year local control rates for hypopharyngeal tumors of approximately 85% and 65% for T1 and T2, respectively. The 5-year overall survival rate for hypopharyngeal tumors is approximately 65%; and the 5-year disease-specific survival is approximately 95% for T1, but only 70% for T2 lesions (Level IV) (Nakamura et al. 2006). The 5-year local control rates for supraglottic larynx tumors are close to 100% and 85% for T1 and T2, respectively. The 5-year overall survival rate for supraglottic larynx tumors is approximately 60% to 65% (more influenced by other factors than the tumor; 5-year disease-specific survival is approximately 90%–100%) (Level IV) (Hinerman et al. 2002).

Techniques

- Regional lymph nodes need to be included in the treatment volume even for N0 necks (Grade B) (Level III) (NCCN 2007).
- When conventional 3D planning is used for T1N0 supraglottic disease, 4–6 MV bilateral photon beams generally are used. These fields cover both the primary tumor and clinical/subclinical disease in the upper and mid anterior cervical nodal beds (levels 2 and 3 lymph node groups).
- For more extensive supraglottic disease the lateral fields are mated to a low anterior neck field and the volume of concern is extended to cover the low anterior cervical nodes (level 4 lymph node group).
- If macroscopic disease is evident in the anterior cervical lymph nodes, the volume of concern is extended to include the posterior cervical lymph nodes.
- Electron beams of 6–9 MeV generally are required to treat disease over the spinal cord for part of the treatment to protect the cord (Fig. 5.3).
- When conventional 3D planning is used for hypopharyngeal disease, 4–6 MV bilateral photon beams are mated to a low anterior neck field and the volume of concern includes the retropharyngeal lymph nodes up to the base of the skull, the upper, mid and low anterior cervical nodes and the posterior cervical nodes.
- Intensity-modulated radiation therapy (IMRT) techniques can be used to cover equivalent volumes of concern and are helpful when gross adenopathy that would overlie the spinal cord needs to be treated to doses required for macroscopic disease. However, to date, IMRT has not been as helpful in the management of tumors arising in the larynx or hypopharynx as it has been for nasopharyngeal and oropharyngeal disease.

Dose and Schedules

- Standard fractionation: 70 Gy in 35 fractions over 7 weeks to gross disease, 50 Gy to subclinical disease.
- Concomitant boost or hyperfractionated radiation therapy can be considered for patients with T2N0 hypopharyngeal cancer (Grade B). Patients who had T2N0 hypopharyngeal lesions were eligible for the RTOG 90-03 altered fractionation trial which, for the entire population enrolled, showed a local control benefit for altered fractionation (concomitant boost or hyperfractionated) therapy (RTOG 90-03, Level II) (Fu et al. 2000). (For an additional discussion of altered fractionation, see Section 5.2.3.)

5.2.3 Locally-Regionally Advanced Lesions

General Principles

- More advanced lesions than described previously (i.e., T2N1-3M0, T3-4N0-3M0 cancer of the larynx and hypopharynx) require more aggressive treatment than standard fractionation radiation therapy (Grade A), and are best treated by concurrent drug-enhanced radiation therapy (in relatively healthy patients) (Level I) or altered fractionation (in relatively unfit patients) (Level II, only supraglottic larynx and hypopharynx tumors were included in RTOG 9003).
- Results from prospective randomized trials support the superiority of concurrent targeted antibody (Level I) (Bonner et al. 2006) or chemotherapy- (Level I) (Adelstein et al. 2003; Forastiere et al. 2003) enhanced radiation therapy over radiation therapy alone for advanced disease.
- No prospective high level data exists to permit the head-to-head comparison of targeted antibody- vs. chemotherapy-enhanced treatment. However, considerably more data exists to support chemotherapy-enhanced radiation therapy.
- There are numerous drugs and combinations of drugs that appear to augment the effect of radiation therapy when given concurrently. However, the optimum regimen is not yet known (Grade B). It is not even clear how many drugs should be used concurrently with radiation therapy. Preliminary results from a randomized phase II trial revealed that concurrent radiation therapy and two-drug chemotherapy using either paclitaxel + cisplatin, 5-FU + cisplatin, or hydroxyurea + 5-FU was feasible (RTOG 97-03, Level II) (Garden et al. 2004).
- While de-escalation of the intensity of radiation therapy in combination with more intensive chemotherapy has been explored and reported (e.g., Merlano 2006), the preponderance of combined modality data (Grade A) has employed: (1) "full dose" standard fractionation therapy (Forastiere et al. 2003), (2) intensified altered fractionation radiation therapy (Adelstein et al. 2003; Brizel et al. 1998), or (3) intensified concomitant boost accelerated radiation therapy (Fu et al. 2000).
- Although the Department of Veterans Affairs Laryngeal Cancer Study initially created interest in sequential chemotherapy – radiation therapy regimens, they have since been supplanted by concurrent regimens (Grade A). The H&N meta-

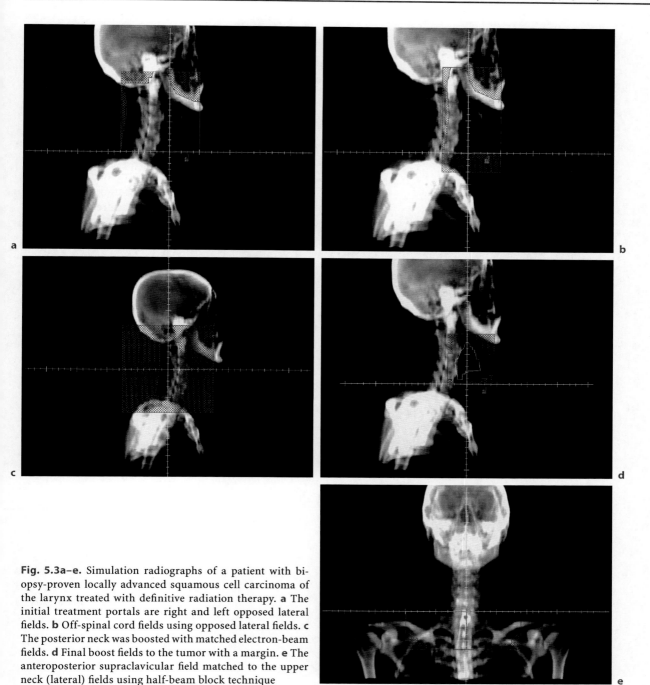

Fig. 5.3a–e. Simulation radiographs of a patient with biopsy-proven locally advanced squamous cell carcinoma of the larynx treated with definitive radiation therapy. **a** The initial treatment portals are right and left opposed lateral fields. **b** Off-spinal cord fields using opposed lateral fields. **c** The posterior neck was boosted with matched electron-beam fields. **d** Final boost fields to the tumor with a margin. **e** The anteroposterior supraclavicular field matched to the upper neck (lateral) fields using half-beam block technique

analysis reported by PIGNON et al. (2007) and results from the RTOG 9111 trial suggest that concurrent chemotherapy – radiation therapy regimens appear to be superior to sequential regimens in terms of organ preservation and survival (Level I) (FORASTIERE et al. 2003).

■ Intensified radiation therapy regimens in combination with chemotherapy currently are not routinely recommended (Grade B). Phase II trials suggest that intensified radiation regimens can be combined safely with drugs (Level III) (ANG et al. 2005). However, at least one prospective randomized trial suggested that the benefit of drug enhancement is somewhat abrogated by more intensive radiation therapy (Level II) (STAAR et al. 2001).

Definitive Radiation Therapy

■ Chemotherapy-enhanced radiation therapy is sufficiently potent that advanced lesions of the larynx or hypopharynx not associated with cartilage destruction can be offered larynx conserving therapy (rather than surgery and postoperative radiation therapy) without fear of significantly decreasing survival (Grade A) (Level I) (FORASTIERE et al. 2003; LEFEBVRE et al. 1996).

Techniques

■ The radiation therapy techniques for the treatment of locoregionally advanced squamous cell cancer of larynx and hypopharynx are similar to those described in Section 5.2.2.2.

Dose and Schedules

■ If standard fractionation is used, a total dose of 70 Gy at 2 Gy per daily fraction (in 35 fractions over 7 weeks) to gross disease is indicated. The prescribed dose to subclinical disease is 50 Gy at 2 Gy per daily fraction.

■ If concomitant boost radiotherapy therapy is used, a total dose of 72.0 Gy is given in 42 fractions over 6 weeks as 32.4 Gy in 18 fractions in 3½ weeks (1.8 Gy/fraction/day) to a relatively large field including subclinical disease followed by another 21.6 Gy in 12 fractions (1.8 Gy/fraction) to the same field, and a second daily fraction at least 6 h later consisting of 18.0 Gy in 12 fractions (1.5 Gy/fraction) to a small "boost field" for gross disease.

Chemotherapy and Targeted Therapy

■ Cisplatin-based chemotherapy delivered concurrently with radiation therapy (e.g., cisplatin 100 mg/m² IV days 1, 22, 43 of radiation therapy) is the "gold-standard" chemotherapy regimen for locoregionally advanced squamous cell carcinoma of the larynx or hypopharynx.

■ Cetuximab (Erbitux®) in an initial dose of 400 mg/m², followed by 250 mg/m² weekly for the duration of radiotherapy can be considered for patients with locoregionally advanced disease but unfit for standard chemotherapy (Grade A). Results of a (thus far single) multinational, prospective randomized study (described above) showed that treatment of locoregionally advanced head and neck cancer with concomitant radiotherapy plus cetuximab improves locoregional control

and reduces mortality without substantially increasing the common toxic effects associated with radiotherapy to the head and neck (Level I) (BONNER et al. 2006).

Outcome

■ Caution: The lesions included in this category are more heterogeneous than in other categories and the results of different treatments may reflect the differences in the patient populations treated more than treatment-related differences.

■ The 5-year local-regional control rates are approximately 35%–75% (FU et al. 2000; FORASTIERE et al. 2003; BONNER et al. 2006; ADELSTEIN et al. 2003; BRIZEL et al. 1998).

■ The 5-year overall survival rates are approximately 25%–55%.

■ The 5-year disease-free survival rates are approximately 25%–45%.

5.3 Beyond Organ Conservation

5.3.1 General Principles

■ Patients who have tumors that destroy cartilage (T4) have been excluded from trials testing organ conservation. At present, laryngectomy is the first step and mainstay of their treatment (Grade A). The 5-year local control is approximately 75% and the 5-year overall survival is approximately 40% for this group of patients after definitive treatment (Level I) (FORASTIERE et al. 2003; DEPARTMENT OF VETERANS AFFAIRS LARYNGEAL CANCER STUDY GROUP 1991).

5.3.2 Adjuvant Radiation Therapy

Treatment Techniques

■ Postoperative radiation therapy generally should be prescribed to the entire operative bed and draining nodes for risk features such as: T3–4 disease, N+ disease, extracapsular extension, microscopically involved margins of resection, perineural invasion (Grade A). Results from a multi-institutional prospective randomized trial revealed that patients with these risk factors had a significantly worse prognosis in terms of locoregional control and survival, as compared to those without such factors (Level I) (ANG et al. 2001).

■ Concurrent chemotherapy-enhanced postoperative radiation therapy should be considered for patients whose tumors demonstrate microscopic extension to a mucosal margin of the resected specimen and/or extracapsular extension of nodal disease (Grade A). Postoperative radiation therapy has been compared with combined chemotherapy-enhanced radiation therapy in two prospective randomized trials: In an RTOG study, 459 patients with high-risk squamous cell carcinoma were randomized to receive either radiotherapy alone or combined chemoradiation postoperatively. The total dose of radiation was 60–66 Gy in 30–33 fractions over 6–6.6 weeks. Intravenous cisplatin (100 mg/m^2 of body surface) on day 1, 22, and 43 was given in the combined regimen group. The results showed that the estimated 2-year locoregional rates were 82% and 72%, respectively, in favor of combined chemotherapy-enhanced radiation therapy; the disease-free survival was significantly longer in the combined-therapy group than in the radiotherapy group, although no significant difference in overall survival was detected. In addition, the incidence of acute adverse effects of grade 3 or greater was almost doubled in the combined-therapy group (77% versus 34%) (RTOG 95-01, Level I) (COOPER et al. 2004).

In a randomized trial completed by the European Organization for Research and Treatment of Cancer (EORTC), 334 patients with stage III or IV (non-metastatic) squamous cell carcinoma of the head and neck area received postoperative radiotherapy (66 Gy in 33 daily fractions) or combined chemoradiotherapy (essentially the same radiation and cisplatin-based chemotherapy regimen as in the RTOG trial detailed above). The results of the study largely mirrored those found in the RTOG trial. Locoregional control and progression-free survival were significantly improved with combined adjuvant treatment. In addition, overall survival rate was also significantly greater in the combined-therapy group than in the radiotherapy group (53% versus 40%). Severe (grade 3 or higher) adverse effects were doubled after combined therapy as compared to

radiation alone (41% versus 21%) (EORTC 22931, Level I) (BERNIER et al. 2004).

The data from both trials was subsequently pooled and in a previously unplanned retrospective analysis revealed that extracapsular extension (ECE) and/or microscopically involved surgical margins were the only risk factors for which the impact of chemotherapy-enhanced radiation therapy was significant in both trials. Patients who had two or more histopathologically involved lymph nodes, but without ECE and/or involved margins of resection did not appear to benefit from the addition of chemotherapy (Level IV) (BERNIER et al. 2005).

Doses and Schedules

■ Standard fractionation is recommended for adjuvant irradiation typically a total dose of 60–66 Gy at 2 Gy per fraction (in 30–33 fractions over 6–6½ weeks), as used in the RTOG randomized trial.

■ Cisplatin-based chemotherapy (100 mg/m^2 IV on days 1, 22, 43) with concurrent radiation therapy is the regimen best supported by the available literature.

5.4 Side Effects and Complications

■ Acute toxicity is related to the intensity of the treatment regimen; both the acceleration of radiation therapy and the addition of concomitant chemotherapy are associated with a greater incidence of grade 3–4 reactions (Level I) (TROTTI et al. 2006).

■ Limited extent, patchy mucositis is a common radiation-induced side effect and not an indication to "hold" treatment. Odynophagia is a common radiation-induced side effect that generally also does not constitute a reason for treatment interruption.

■ While there appears to be considerable variation in the onset of acute confluent grade 3 mucositis related to individual patients' inherent sensitivity to treatment, the shorter time to onset the longer the duration. More severe protracted mucositis is associated with a greater likelihood of late mucosal toxicity (Level IV) (DENHAM et al. 1999).

■ Xerostomia will occur if part of the parotid glands cannot be protected. Keeping the mean dose to the gland under 24–25 Gy is recommended (Grade B). It appears that limiting dose to this range helps to maintain clinically beneficial salivary flow (Level IV) (Eisbruch et al. 2001; Bussels et al. 2004; Blanco et al. 2005; Jellema et al. 2007).

■ Arytenoid edema is a well known consequence of irradiation. To what degree this effect is a function of dose delivered is unclear.

■ The cervical spinal cord may be more tolerant than the generally quoted acceptable risk at 45–50 Gy (Grade C); however, myelitis rarely does occur at this level and in light of the severity of this complication, keeping the dose under 50 Gy seems prudent in most circumstances (Level IV) (Marcus and Million 1990; Jeremic et al. 1991; Emami et al. 1991).

5.5   Follow-Up

5.5.1   Post-Treatment Follow-Up

■ Life-long follow-up is required for early detection of recurrence (initially) and detection of independent second malignancies (initially and long term) (Grade A).
Independent second malignancies of the upper aerodigestive tract are detected in approximately 3% of patients annually following successful treatment of a head and neck malignancy (Level I) (Cooper et al. 1989). There does not appear to be a time limitation for this risk.

Schedule

■ Follow-up should be scheduled every 1–3 months for the first year after treatment, every 2–4 months for the second year after treatment, every 4–6 months for the third through fifth years after treatment, and every 6–12 months thereafter (Grade D) (National Comprehensive Cancer Network 2007) (Table 5.3).

■ The majority of recurrences will occur within the first 2 years and nearly all within 3 years (Fu et al. 2000; Forastiere et al. 2003). Early stage glottic cancers can continue to recur up to 5 years after treatment (Mendenhall et al. 2001).

Work-Ups

■ Each follow-up examination should include an interval history and physical examination, including endoscopy or indirect mirror exam.

■ Imaging of the neck should be performed whenever patients develop new signs or symptoms suggestive of recurrence.

■ Imaging of the thorax looking primarily for new malignancies (not metastases) is recommended annually.

■ If a substantial portion of the thyroid has been irradiated, TSH levels should be monitored over the long term.

Table 5.3. Follow-up schedule after treatment of squamous cell carcinoma of the larynx or hypopharynx

Interval	Frequency
First year	Every 1–3 months
Second year	Every 2–4 months
Years 3–5	Every 4–6 months
Over 5 years	Every 6–12 months

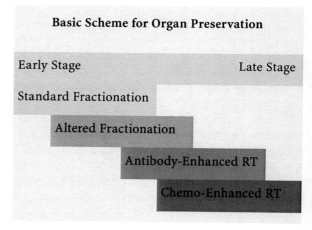

Fig. 5.4. A simplified treatment scheme for organ conservation therapy of cancers of the larynx and hypopharynx

References

Adelstein DJ, Li Y, Adams GL et al. (2003) An Intergroup phase III comparison of standard radiation therapy and two schedules of concurrent chemoradiotherapy in patients with unresectable squamous cell head and neck cancer. J Clin Oncol 21:92–98

Allal AS, Miralbell R, Lehmann W et al. (1997) Effect of arytenoid sparing during radiation therapy of early stage glottic carcinoma. Radiother Oncol 43:63–65

Amdur RJ, Conine FE, Harris RD et al. (1995) Arytenoid sparing during irradiation of early stage vocal cord cancer. Int J Radiat Oncol Biol Phys 32:801–808

Ang KK, Trotti A, Brown BW et al. (2001) Randomized trial addressing risk features and time factors of surgery plus radiotherapy in advanced head-and-neck cancer. Int J Radiat Oncol Biol Phys 51:571–578

Ang KK, Harris J, Garden AS et al. (2005) Concomitant boost radiation plus concurrent cisplatin for advanced head and neck carcinomas: radiation therapy oncology group phase II trial 99-14. J Clin Oncol 23:3008–3015

Bernier J, Domenge C, Ozsahin M et al. (2004) Postoperative irradiation with or without concomitant chemotherapy for locally advanced head and neck cancer. N Engl J Med 350:1945–1952

Bernier J, Cooper JS, Pajak TF et al. (2005) Defining risk levels in locally advanced head and neck cancers: a comparative analysis of concurrent postoperative radiation plus chemotherapy trials of the EORTC (# 22931) and RTOG (# 9501). Head Neck 2005:843–850

Blanco AI, Chao KS, El Naqa I et al. (2005) Dose-volume modeling of salivary function in patients with head-and-neck cancer receiving radiotherapy. Int J Radiat Oncol Biol Phys 62:1055–1069

Bonner JA, Harari PM, Giralt J et al. (2006) Radiotherapy plus cetuximab for squamous-cell carcinoma of the head and neck. N Engl J Med 354:567–578

Brizel DM, Albers ME, Fisher SR et al. (1998) Hyperfractionated irradiation with or without concurrent chemotherapy for locally advanced head and neck cancer. N Engl J Med 338:1798–1804

Bussels B, Maes A, Flamen P et al. (2004) Dose-response relationships within the parotid gland after radiotherapy for head and neck cancer. Radiother Oncol 73:297–306

Chatani M, Matayoshi Y, Masaki N et al. (1996) Radiation therapy for early glottic carcinoma (T1N0M0). The final results of prospective randomized study concerning radiation field. Strahlenther Onkol 172:169–172

Cooper JS, Pajak TF, Rubin P et al. (1989) Second malignancies in patients who have head and neck cancer: incidence, effect on survival and implications based on the RTOG experience. Int J Radiat Oncol Biol Phys 17:449–456

Cooper JS, Pajak TF, Forastiere AA et al. (2004) Postoperative concurrent radiotherapy and chemotherapy for high-risk squamous-cell carcinoma of the head and neck. N Engl J Med 350:1937–1944

Denham JW, Peters LJ, Johansen J et al. (1999) Do acute mucosal reactions lead to consequential late reactions in patients with head and neck cancer? Radiother Oncol 52:157–164

Department of Veterans Affairs Laryngeal Cancer Study Group (1991) Induction chemotherapy plus radiation compared with surgery plus radiation in patients with advanced laryngeal cancer. N Engl J Med 324:1685–1690

Eisbruch A, Kim HM, Terrell JE et al. (2001) Xerostomia and its predictors following parotid-sparing irradiation of head-and-neck cancer. Int J Radiat Oncol Biol Phys 50:695–704

Emami B, Lyman J, Brown A et al. (1991) Tolerance of normal tissue to therapeutic irradiation. Int J Radiat Oncol Biol Phys 21:109–122

Forastiere AA, Goepfert H, Maor M et al. (2003) Concurrent chemotherapy and radiotherapy for organ preservation in advanced laryngeal cancer. N Engl J Med 349:2091–2098

Fu KK, Pajak TF, Trotti A et al. (2000) A Radiation Therapy Oncology Group (RTOG) phase III randomized study to compare hyperfractionation and two variants of accelerated fractionation to standard fractionation radiotherapy for head and neck squamous cell carcinomas: first report of RTOG 9003. Int J Radiat Oncol Biol Phys 48:7–16

Garden AS, Forster K, Wong PF et al. (2003) Results of radiotherapy for T2N0 glottic carcinoma: does the "2" stand for twice-daily treatment? Int J Radiat Oncol Biol Phys 55:322–328

Garden AS, Harris J, Vokes EE et al. (2004) Preliminary results of Radiation Therapy Oncology Group 97-03: a randomized phase II trial of concurrent radiation and chemotherapy for advanced squamous cell carcinomas of the head and neck. J Clin Oncol 22:2856–2864

Gordin A, Daitzchman M, Doweck I et al. (2006) Fluorodeoxyglucose-positron emission tomography/computed tomography imaging in patients with carcinoma of the larynx: diagnostic accuracy and impact on clinical management. Laryngoscope 116:273–278

Greene F, Page D, Fleming I et al. (2002) AJCC Cancer Staging Manual, 6th edn. Springer, Berlin Heidelberg New York

Hinerman RW, Mendenhall WM, Amdur RJ et al. (2002) Carcinoma of the supraglottic larynx: treatment results with radiotherapy alone or with planned neck dissection. Head Neck 24:456–467

Jellema AP, Slotman BJ, Doornaert P et al. (2007) Unilateral versus bilateral irradiation in squamous cell head and neck cancer in relation to patient-rated xerostomia and sticky saliva. Radiother Oncol 85:83–89

Jeremic B, Djuric L, Mijatovic L (1991) Incidence of radiation myelitis of the cervical spinal cord at doses of 5500 cGy or greater. Cancer 68:2138–2141

Kim RY, Marks ME, Salter MM (1992) Early-stage glottic cancer: importance of dose fractionation in radiation therapy. Radiology 182:273–275

Le QT, Fu KK, Kroll S et al. (1997) Influence of fraction size, total dose, and overall time on local control of T1–T2 glottic carcinoma. Int J Radiat Oncol Biol Phys 39:115–126

Lefebvre JL, Chevalier D, Luboinski B et al. (1996) Larynx preservation in pyriform sinus cancer: preliminary results of a European Organization for Research and Treatment of Cancer phase III trial. EORTC Head and Neck Cancer Cooperative Group. J Natl Cancer Inst 88:890–899

Marcus RB Jr, Million RR (1990) The incidence of myelitis after irradiation of the cervical spinal cord. Int J Radiat Oncol Biol Phys 19:3–8

Mendenhall WM, Parsons JT, Million RR et al. (1988) T1–T2 squamous cell carcinoma of the glottic larynx treated with radiation therapy: relationship of dose-fractionation factors to local control and complications. Int J Radiat Oncol Biol Phys 15:1267–1273

Mendenhall WM, Amdur RJ, Morris CG et al. (2001) T1–T2 N0 squamous cell carcinoma of the glottic larynx treated with radiation therapy. J Clin Oncol 19:4029–4036

Mendenhall WM, Werning W, Hinerman RW et al. (2004) Management of T1–T2 glottic carcinomas. Cancer 100:1786–1792

Merlano M (2006) Alternating chemotherapy and radiotherapy in locally advanced head and neck cancer: an alternative? Oncologist 11:146–151

Nakamura K, Shioyama Y, Kawashima M et al. (2006) Multi-institutional analysis of early squamous cell carcinoma of the hypopharynx treated with radical radiotherapy. Int J Radiat Oncol Biol Phys 65:1045–1050

National Comprehensive Cancer Network (NCCN) Practice Guidelines in Oncology – v.1.2007: http://www.nccn.org/professionals/physician_gls/PDF/head-and-neck.pdf (Accessed on March 5, 2008)

Pignon JP, le Maître A, Bourhis J et al. (2007) MACH-NC Collaborative Group. Meta-Analyses of Chemotherapy in Head and Neck Cancer (MACH-NC): an update. Int J Radiat Oncol Biol Phys 69[2 Suppl]:S112–114

Ricciardelli EJ, Weymuller EA Jr, Koh WJ et al. (1994) Effect of radiation fraction size on local control rates for early glottic carcinoma. A model analysis for in vivo tumor growth and radio-response parameters. Arch Otolaryngol Head Neck Surg 120:737–742

Roh JL, Pae KH, Choi SH et al. (2007) 2-[^{18}F]-Fluoro-2-deoxy-D-glucose positron emission tomography as guidance for primary treatment in patients with advanced-stage resectable squamous cell carcinoma of the larynx and hypopharynx. Eur J Surg Oncol 33:790–795

Rovirosa A (1997) In relation to the arytenoid edema in the radiotherapy of the early vocal cord cancer: arytenoid shielding and small size of the field. Radiother Oncol 45:209–210

Rudoltz MS, Benammar A, Mohiuddin M (1993) Prognostic factors for local control and survival in T1 squamous cell carcinoma of the glottis. Int J Radiat Oncol Biol Phys 26:767–772

Schwaibold F, Scariato A, Nunno M et al. (1998) The effect of fraction size on control of early glottic cancer. Int J Radiat Oncol Biol Phys 14:451–454

Schwartz DL, Rajendran J, Yueh B et al. (2004) FDG-PET prediction of head and neck squamous cell cancer outcomes. Arch Otolaryngol Head Neck Surg 130:1361–1367

Spector JG, Sessions DG, Chao KS et al. (1999) Stage I (T1 N0 M0) squamous cell carcinoma of the laryngeal glottis: therapeutic results and voice preservation. Head Neck 21:707–717

Staar S, Rudat V, Stuetzer H et al. (2001) Intensified hyperfractionated accelerated radiotherapy limits the additional benefit of simultaneous chemotherapy – results of a multicentric randomized German trial in advanced head and neck cancer. Int J Radiat Oncol Biol Phys 50:1161–1171

Trotti A, Pajak T, Emami B et al. (2006) A randomized trial of hyperfractionation versus standard fractionation in T2 squamous cell carcinoma of the vocal cord. Int J Radiat Oncol Biol Phys 66:S15

Warde P, O'Sullivan B, Bristow RG et al. (1998) T1–T2 glottic cancer managed by external beam radiotherapy: the influence of pretreatment hemoglobin on local control. Int J Radiat Oncol Biol Phys 41:347–353

Yamazaki H, Nishiyama K, Tanaka E et al. (2006) Radiotherapy for early glottic carcinoma (T1N0M0): results of prospective randomized study of radiation fraction size and overall treatment time. Int J Radiat Oncol Biol Phys 64:77–82

Yu E, Shenouda G, Beaudet MP et al. (1997) Impact of radiation therapy fraction size on local control of early glottic carcinoma. Int J Radiat Oncol Biol Phys 37:587–591

Squamous Cell Carcinoma of Unknown Head and Neck Primary

Ling Kong and Ron R. Allison

CONTENTS

L. Kong, MD
Department of Radiation Oncology, Cancer Hospital of Fudan University, 270 Dong An Road, Shanghai 200032, P. R. China
R. R. Allison, MD
Department of Radiation Oncology, The Brody School of Medicine at ECU, 600 Moye Blvd., Greenville, NC 27834, USA

Introduction and Objectives

Squamous cell carcinoma adenopathy presenting above the clavicle from an unknown primary site is a rare and challenging diagnosis. In most cases, these are metastatic lesions arising from a head and neck origin. Advances in imaging have assisted in improving management of an unknown head and neck primary, as has better integration of surgery, radiation and, most recently, chemotherapy for this uncommon disease manifestation.

This chapter examines:

● Recommendations for diagnosis and staging procedures
● The staging system and prognostic factors
● Treatment recommendations for squamous cell carcinoma and poorly or un-differentiated carcinoma presenting as a cervical lymph node of unknown primary, as well as the supporting scientific evidence
● Radiation therapy, surgery, and chemotherapy treatment techniques
● Follow-up care and surveillance of survivors

A cervical lymph node with adenocarcinoma often originates from a non-head and neck site, although parotid, thyroid, and parathyroid primary should be ruled out. Squamous cell carcinoma of a parotid lymph node usually has a skin primary. These presentations are not addressed in this chapter.

6.1 Diagnosis, Staging, and Prognoses

6.1.1 Diagnosis

■ Diagnostic work-up aims to find the primary lesion (if possible) and define the extent of disease.
■ Diagnosis begins with a complete history including signs and symptoms attributable not only to a head and neck primary such as ear pain, but also a possible lung primary presenting with hoarseness or an esophageal primary with associated

dysphagia. Alcohol and tobacco use are pertinent aspects of the medical history.

- The initial physical exam should include a thorough head and neck examination including skin and scalp.
- Physical examination should detail the characteristic(s) of the nodal enlargement, particularly its location, dimensions, consistency, tenderness, and mobility.
- If suspicion is high or the node does not respond completely to antibiotics, biopsy for histology follows.

Initial Evaluation

- Fine-needle aspiration (FNA) offers diagnostic yield in most instances (Level II) (MUI et al. 1997).
- If a squamous cell or undifferentiated carcinoma is found on FNA, then panendoscopy under anesthesia enables direct visualization of the nasopharynx, oropharynx, hypopharynx, larynx, trachea, bronchial airway, and esophagus. This procedure permits multiple biopsies and may often locate the primary lesion, most commonly found in the nasopharynx, tonsil, and base of tongue (MENDENHALL et al. 2001). This procedure should be performed after imaging is completed.

Laboratory Tests

- Initial laboratory tests include a complete blood count, basic serum chemistries, liver function tests, and renal function tests.
- Should biopsy reveal a poorly or undifferentiated cancer, an Epstein-Barr virus (EBV) antibody level (i.e., IgA anti-VCA and IgA anti-EA) should be measured. High levels may indicate the possibility of the primary to be nasopharyngeal cancer, particularly in Asia (Level III) (LEE et al. 2000).

Imaging Studies

- Contrast CT of the head and neck assists in the detection of primary disease and helps define the extent of nodal involvement. Contrast MRI may be used in place of CT.
- PET/CT is recommended for detecting the primary disease and staging in unknown head and neck primary cancer (Grade A). PET/CT can de-

fine suspicious regions and lymph nodes to biopsy in the head and neck region, as well as identify metastases. The value of FDG-PET in the diagnosis and evaluation of unknown primary malignancies has been evaluated in numerous studies, and the results of a comprehensive review (meta-analysis) showed that FDG-PET is 88.3% sensitive, 74.9% specific, and 78.8% accurate in detecting the unknown primary. PET was also able to detect primary disease that went undetected by other modalities in 25% of cases. Furthermore, PET detected systemic metastatic disease in an additional 27% of cases missed by other modalities. However, FDG-PET has low specificity and a 40% false-positive rate in the tonsil (Level I) (RUSTHOVEN et al. 2004).

- PET/CT should be considered prior to panendoscopy or surgery as this imaging modality can assist and direct the surgeon to suspicious locations and also prevent unnecessary procedures in patients with widespread disease.
- FDG-PET scan may find primary disease below the clavicle and is therefore an important part of staging (Level III) (MILLER et al. 2005).
- Bone scan is unnecessary when FDG-PET (or PET/CT) is performed.

Table 6.1. Imaging and laboratory work-ups for cancer of unknown head and neck primary

Imaging studies	Laboratory tests
MRI and/or CT scan of the head and neck area	Complete blood count
	Serum chemistry
CT scan of thorax	Liver function tests
FDG-PET scan or PET/CT	Renal function tests
Bone scan (optional)	Serum EBV EA IgA and VCA IgA (for poorly or un-differentiated cancer, if EBV DNA by PCR is not performed)

Pathology

- FNA of the enlarged node permits histological diagnosis in 90% of cases (Grade B) (Level II) (MUI et al. 1997; PISHARODI 1997). FNA minimizes the risk of altering the accuracy of diagnostic imaging and is the preferred method for biopsy.
- Should FNA fail to yield diagnosis or if lymphoma is suspected, excisional biopsy should be undertaken.

■ Incisional biopsy is usually not recommended for tissue diagnosis of neck adenopathy (Grade B). Incisional biopsy is associated with increased risk of local failure and tumor seeding along the surgical site (Level III) (McGUIRT and McCABE 1978).

■ Squamous cell cancer or poorly differentiated carcinoma are the most common histologies associated with true unknown head and neck primaries and are the focus of this chapter.

■ Should histology prove to be adenocarcinoma, the primary is likely below the clavicle. Should these involved nodes be in the upper neck one must exclude salivary, thyroid, and parathyroid primaries, which is beyond the scope of this chapter. Similarly, Hodgkin's and non-Hodgkin's lymphoma may be diagnosed and management is found elsewhere in this book.

■ Evaluation of the nodal specimen for EBV genomic DNA using PCR may point to a nasopharynx primary (Level III) (LEE et al. 2000).

■ Detection of HPV-16 may point to an oropharynx primary (Level III) (BEGUM et al. 2007).

■ Panendoscopy under anesthesia with blind biopsy or biopsy assisted by imaging may detect the primary tumor in 40% of cases (Level III) (MENDENHALL et al. 2001).

■ Ipsilateral tonsillectomy is suggested for patients with submandibular, subdigastric and mid-jugular nodes as this may be the site of the primary disease in 25%–35% of patients (Level IV) (LAPEYRE et al. 1997; LEFEBVRE et al. 1990; MENDENHALL et al. 1998).

6.1.2 Staging

■ The extent of the nodal disease can be staged according to the N-category of the American Joint Committee on Cancer (AJCC) Tumor Node Metastasis (TNM) staging system for head and neck cancers. For suspicious nasopharyngeal primary (i.e., poorly or un-differentiated carcinoma with positive EBV DNA on PCR), the N classification of the AJCC staging system for nasopharyngeal cancer can be used (Table 6.2) (GREENE et al. 2002).

Table 6.2. The N classification of the AJCC staging system for squamous cell carcinoma of nasopharynx or other head and neck areas. [From GREENE et al. (2002) with permission]

	Nasopharyngeal cancer	Head and neck cancer other than nasopharyngeal cancer
NX	Regional lymph nodes cannot be assessed	Regional lymph nodes cannot be assessed
N0	No regional lymph node metastasis	No regional lymph node metastasis
N1	Unilateral metastasis in lymph node(s), 6 cm or less in greatest dimension, above the supraclavicular fossa	Metastasis in a single ipsilateral lymph node, 3 cm or less in greatest dimension
N2	Bilateral metastasis in lymph node(s), 6 cm or less in greatest dimension, above the supraclavicular fossa	Metastasis in a single ipsilateral lymph node, more than 3 cm but not more than 6 cm in greatest dimension, or in multiple ipsilateral lymph nodes, none more than 6 cm in greatest dimension, or in bilateral or contralateral lymph nodes, none more than 6 cm in greatest dimension
N2a		Metastasis in a single ipsilateral lymph node more than 3 cm but not more than 6 cm in greatest dimension
N2b		Metastasis in multiple ipsilateral lymph nodes, none more than 6 cm in greatest dimension
N2c		Metastasis in bilateral or contralateral lymph nodes, none more than 6 cm in greatest dimension
N3	Metastasis in (a) lymph node(s) > 6 cm and/or to supraclavicular fossa	Metastasis in a lymph node more than 6 cm in greatest dimension
N3a	Greater than 6 cm in dimension	
N3b	Extension to the supraclavicular fossa	

6.1.3   Prognostic Factors

■ Extent of nodal disease (presenting stage) is the key prognostic indicator for patients with an unknown primary head and neck cancer.

■ The location of the involved nodes is of critical significance. Low neck or supraclavicular nodes portend poor survival. Upper and mid cervical node metastasis, treated aggressively, have survival rates of 60% or greater at 5 years (KAMINSKY and BLOT 2006).

■ Advanced nodal staging, poor differentiation and extracapsular extension are negative prognostic indicators (NIEDER et al. 2001).

■ Treatment modality and technique are of prognostic significance: Combined modality treatment with surgery and radiation achieve higher local regional control rates, although survival outcomes may not be enhanced. In addition, wide field radiation which covers the major mucosal areas in the head and neck area was associated with a reduced manifestation of primary disease (Level IV) (DAVIDSON et al. 1994).

6.2   Treatment of Squamous Cell Carcinoma of Unknown Head and Neck Primary

6.2.1   General Principles

■ Treatment of squamous cell carcinoma of unknown head and neck primary requires a multidisciplinary team approach that may involve surgery, radiation, and chemotherapy. Treatment modality is defined by extent and location of adenopathy.

■ Limited N_1 disease, without extracapsular extension, of the mid-neck may be approached by neck dissection alone or ipsilateral neck radiation (Grade B).

■ N_1 disease found to have extracapsular spread or to be more extensive on neck dissection should have post-op radiation (Grade B).

■ Radiation is recommended in the treatment of N_2 category squamous cell carcinoma of unknown head and neck primary (Grade B). In general, both sides of the neck as well as mucosal sites at risk for harboring the primary tumor are included in the radiation portals.

■ N2 disease that is considered bulky or N3 disease undergo radiation with concomitant chemotherapy to improve local disease control (Grade B). If response is poor, clinically or radiographically, neck dissection may be added.

■ Supraclavicular adenopathy or patients found to have systemic disease may be offered a short course of radiation directed to the adenopathy for palliation.

6.2.2   Surgery

■ Surgery is rarely employed alone in the treatment of cancer of unknown head and neck primary. Surgery may be indicated as the sole treatment modality for the patient with limited N1 or N2A disease as long as no extracapsular extension is found and no incisional biopsy was undertaken (Grade A). These patients require close follow-up and must be reliable to undertake this limited treatment (Level IV) (NIEDER et al. 2001; IGANEJ et al. 2002; ERKAL et al. 2001; COSTER et al. 1992).

■ Modified neck dissection is generally undertaken to excise deep and superficial fascia including the nodal contents. As compared to radical neck dissection, the modified procedure may spare the sternocleidomastoid and digastric muscles, spinal accessory nerve, and the internal jugular vein. This allows for improved function and cosmesis without significantly higher local failure rates.

■ Bulky N_2 and N_3 nodes may not respond well to high dose radiotherapy or concomitant chemoradiotherapy. These patients may benefit from planned neck dissection 4–6 weeks after completion of external beam radiation (Grade B). Physical exam, CT, and FDG-PET may assist in the determination of residual disease and need for surgery (Level IV) (MENDENHALL et al. 1986).

■ Neck dissection is employed for salvage after local-regional recurrence following radiotherapy (Grade B) (Level IV) (GRAU et al. 2000).

6.2.3   Radiation Therapy

■ Radiation therapy plays a critical role for most patients diagnosed with an unknown primary of the head and neck.

- N1/N2A disease can be treated definitively with radiation therapy (Grade A). N1/N2A disease responds equally well to radiation and surgery in terms of local control and survival based on a large retrospective series from the University of Florida (100% local control and 70% cause-specific survival at 5 years) (Level IV) (MENDENHALL et al. 1998; MAULARD et al. 1992; COLLETIER et al. 1998).

- Patients with N2B, N2C, or N3 disease can be treated with definitive radiation therapy, or combined radiation and surgery (Grade A). N2B and N2C can be controlled in 80% of cases with radical radiation, neck dissection followed by radiation, or radiation followed by neck dissection. N3 disease can be controlled only 50% of the time with radical radiation or radiation combined with neck dissection (Level IV) (ERKAL et al. 2001; ARGIRIS et al. 2003; STROJAN and ANICIN 1998; WEIR et al. 1995).

- As combined chemoradiation therapy becomes the mainstay regimen for both definitive and adjuvant treatment of locally advanced squamous cell carcinoma of the head and neck area, patients with N2B, N2C, or N3 may also benefit from the addition of chemotherapy.

- Radiation is indicated for patients with a history of incisional biopsy or extracapsular spread for all N stages (Grade B) (Level IV) (ELLIS et al. 1991; MACK et al. 1993).

Radiation Technique

Field Arrangement

- The optimal volume and field arrangements are yet to be determined and remain a source of controversy.

- Nodal location assists in portal design: The oral cavity is generally excluded unless subdigastric lymphadenopathy is detected. The contralateral parotid gland can be spared in patients with ipsilateral nodal disease. As the hypopharynx and larynx rarely appear to be the source of disease these may be excluded from radiation portals to diminish morbidity (Level IV) (MILLION et al. 1994; BARKER et al. 2005).

- Appropriately designed smaller portals can be used in early stage (N1) disease (Grade A). Limited-field radiotherapy does not appear to diminish survival but may slightly increase risk of regional failure (Level IV) (GLYNNE-JONES et al. 1990; REDDY and MARKS 1997; WEIR et al. 1995; PAVLIDIS and FIZAZI 2005; SINNATHAMBY et al. 1997).

- N1 disease may be approached by a radiation portal directed to the ipsilateral neck through IMRT, direct photons and electrons, or a wedge pair (Level IV) (FRIESLAND et al. 2001; GLYNNE-JONES et al. 1990).

- Larger portals that encompass the bilateral upper and lower neck and also include the mucosal anatomy is recommended for patients with more extensive neck disease (Grade B). Such treatment arrangement has been associated with decreased risk of regional failure and development of a clinically detectable primary tumor at the cost of significantly higher permanent morbidity (Level IV) (ERKAL et al. 2001). The majority of patients, including those with N2 disease and above, undergo comprehensive radiation directed to (Fig. 6.1):

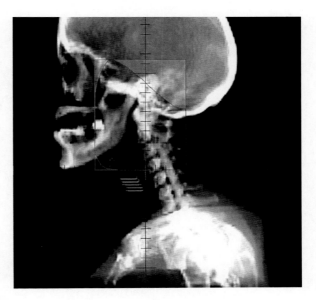

Fig. 6.1. A hypothetical upper portal. In this case, a half-beam arrangement is being used at the match line (Figs. 6.2 and 6.3 show different scenarios for the lower field)

Upper Neck Fields

- The upper neck fields should be designed to cover the nasopharynx, oropharynx, and the base of skull nodal basins using opposed lateral field arrangement or IMRT.

- Superiorly it should encompass the superior border of the nasopharynx with sufficient (1.5–2.0 cm) margin.

- The inferior border should be set at the thyroid notch. Half-beam technique can be used to ensure the match to the lower neck fields.

- Anteriorly to cover the base of tongue and tonsillar fossa with 2 cm margin to encompass the oropharynx and subdigastric nodes.
- Posterior border to be set at the level of the C2 spinous process to encompass the posterior cervical nodes. The spinal cord should be shielded at the tolerance dose, and the posterior neck area should be supplemented with electron fields.

Lower Neck Fields

- The lower neck fields [in anteroposterior and posteroanterior (AP/PA) arrangement] should include the mid and lower jugular nodes, as well as the ipsilateral if not bilateral supraclavicular region (Fig. 6.2).
- The superior border of the lower neck fields should match the inferior border of the upper neck fields, and half-beam technique can be used.
- The hypopharynx and larynx are rarely involved as sites of disease origin and may be excluded from the lower neck portal based on University of Florida data in which no failures at these sites were found (Level IV) (BARKER et al. 2005). The larynx block should cover only the medial part of the thyroid cartilage, and special attention should be paid to ensure the internal jugular vein lymph nodes which are situated along the lateral margin of the thyroid cartilage are not shielded.
- Coverage to the bilateral lateral supraclavicular area is usually not necessary for patients with N0 and N1 disease (Fig. 6.2). However, the lateral border of the lower neck field should be set to encompass the entire ipsilateral supraclavicular area for patients with lower neck disease or extensive adenopathy (Fig. 6.3).

Dose

- The definitive radiation dose to gross disease or the involved nodal area should achieve at least 70 Gy (if not higher) unless chemotherapy or surgery is planned.
- A dose of 64.8 Gy at 1.8 Gy or 66 Gy at 2-Gy fractions is suggested to all mucosal sites and the upper neck nodal basins.
- A dose of 50 Gy at 2-Gy per fraction is recommended for the low neck with additional dose to 70 Gy to clinically positive nodes in this portal.
- The total dose to the planned surgical sites in patients who will undergo planned neck dissection should be limited to a total dose of 60 Gy to minimize wound healing complications (Grade B) The results of a retrospective review from University of Florida showed that, although not statistically significant, higher total doses increased the complication rate, lower fraction sizes reduced the complication rate, and longer overall radiotherapy treatment times were associated with higher complication rates (Level IV) (TAYLOR et al. 1992).

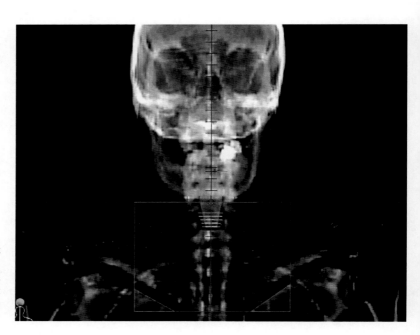

Fig. 6.2. Lower neck field with a larynx block and using a half-beam technique. For N0 or N1 disease, the lateral field borders may be narrower and do not necessarily need to include the entire supraclavicular field

Fig. 6.3. Lower neck field with larynx block and using a half-beam technique. The left supraclavicular field was extended in this case due to palpable left lower neck nodal disease

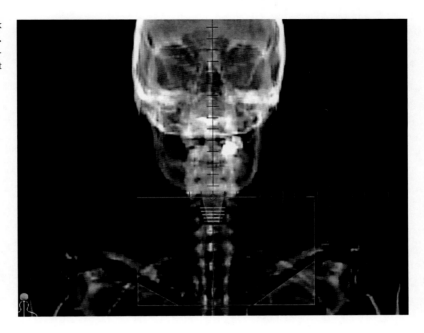

■ Patients with advanced disease treated for palliation may undergo a local field to the involved neck alone with 30 Gy in 10 daily fractions. This dose arrangement achieved a 60% palliation rate according to a retrospective study reported by ERKAL et al. (2001) (Level IV).

Radiation-Induced Side Effects

■ Commonly observed acute side effects include radiation-induced mucositis and dermatitis. Radiation-induced acute mucositis can be minimized by use of Carafate elixir and viscous lidocaine.

■ Xerostomia is a commonly observed long-term complication and intensive post-treatment dental care is critical for patients after conventional radiation treatment to the head and neck areas. IMRT to spare the contralateral parotid gland for patients with ipsilateral nodal disease may be possible. This is not suggested for patients with bilateral disease as it may underdose adenopathy.

■ High radiation doses in combination with chemotherapy may induce fibrotic changes.

■ Neck dissection following external beam radiation therapy has an increased risk of wound healing issues, particularly when doses of 60 Gy or greater were delivered to the operative bed (Level IV) (TAYLOR et al. 1992; MILLION et al. 1994; CARLSON et al. 1986).

8.2.4 Chemotherapy

■ The role of chemotherapy for unknown primary is evolving and platinum based chemotherapy has been increasingly used in patients with advanced neck adenopathy.

■ N3 disease is controlled poorly by radiation and surgery. Patients with N3 disease may particularly benefit from the addition of chemotherapy. The efficacy of combined chemoradiotherapy has been addressed in retrospective series: N2 and N3 patients have been treated with concurrent chemoradiation with excellent progression-free survival (87%) (Level IV) (ARGIRIS et al. 2003). Similarly, impressive local control of 95% following chemoradiation therapy after neck dissection was reported in a small retrospective series (Level IV) (SHEHADEH et al. 2006). However, substantial morbidity is to be expected with concomitant chemoradiotherapy.

■ Induction platinum-based chemotherapy for patients with advanced disease or poor performance status may also be an option for selected patients (Grade D) (ESMO 2007).

■ Targeted agents, such as cetuximab, have shown activity for head and neck cancer, particularly in elderly patients. Their use in the unknown primary is not documented, but may be beneficial as in locally advanced head and neck squamous cell carcinoma (PANIKKAR et al. 2008).

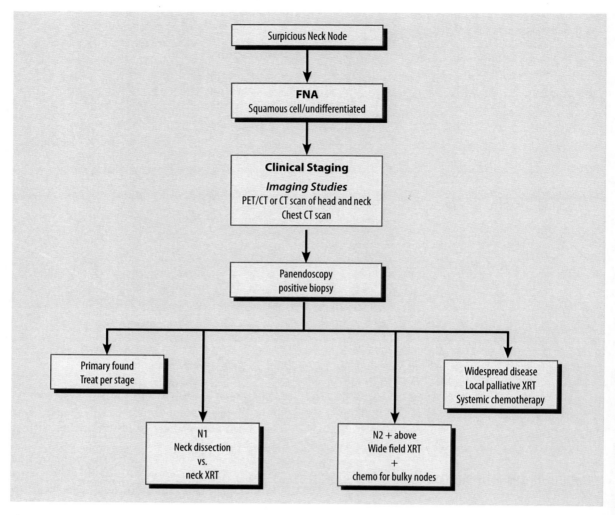

Fig. 6.4. A proposed treatment algorithm for head and neck squamous cell carcinoma of unknown primary

6.3 Follow-Ups

6.3.1 Post-Treatment Follow-Ups

▪ Follow-up after definitive treatment of squamous cell carcinoma of unknown head and neck primary is recommended for management of treatment-induced side effects, detection of disease recurrence, and emergence of primary disease. Diagnosis of the primary disease occurs in approximately 15% of patients with unknown head and neck primary within 5 years of treatment (Level IV) (ERKAL et al. 2001).

Schedule

▪ Follow-ups should be scheduled every 1–3 months for the first year, then every 4 months for the second year, every 6 months during years 3–5, and annually thereafter (Grade D).

Table 6.3. Follow-up schedule after treatment for unknown primary head and neck cancer

Interval	Frequency
Year 1	Every 1–3 months
Year 2	Every 4 months
Years 3–5	Every 6 months
> 5 Years	Annually

Work-Ups

- Each follow-up should include a complete history and physical examination, including endoscopic examination of the nasopharynx, oropharynx, larynx, and hypopharynx.
- Laboratory tests and imaging studies including CT scan of the head and neck area are not routinely indicated. There is no evidence to support the routine use of imaging work-ups for asymptomatic patients. Specific examinations should be performed if clinically indicated (ESMO 2007).

References

Argiris A, Smith SM, Stenson K et al. (2003) Concurrent chemoradiotherapy for N2 or N3 squamous cell carcinoma of the head and neck from an occult primary. Ann Oncol 14:1306–1311

Barker CA, Morris CG, Mendenhall WM (2005) Larynx-sparing radiotherapy for squamous cell carcinoma from an unknown head and neck primary site. Am J Clin Oncol 28:445–448

Begum S, Gillison ML, Nicol TL et al. (2007) Detection of human papillomavirus-16 in fine-needle aspirates to determine tumor origin in patients with metastatic squamous cell carcinoma of the head and neck. Clin Cancer Res 13:1186–1191

Carlson LS, Fletcher GH, Oswald MJ (1986) Guidelines for radiotherapeutic techniques for cervical metastases from an unknown primary. Int J Radiat Oncol Biol Phys 12:2101–2110

Colletier PJ, Garden AS, Morrison WH et al. (1998) Postoperative radiation for squamous cell carcinoma metastatic to cervical lymph nodes from an unknown primary site: outcomes and patterns of failure. Head Neck 20:674–681

Coster JR, Foote RL, Olsen KD et al. (1992) Cervical nodal metastasis of squamous cell carcinoma of unknown origin: indications for withholding radiation therapy. Int J Radiat Oncol Biol Phys 23:743–749

Davidson BJ, Spiro RH, Patel S et al. (1994) Cervical metastases of occult origin: the impact of combined modality therapy. Am J Surg 168:395–399

Ellis ER, Mendenhall WM, Rao PV et al. (1991) Incisional or excisional neck-node biopsy before definitive radiotherapy, alone or followed by neck dissection. Head Neck 13:177–183

Erkal HS, Mendenhall WM, Amdur RJ et al. (2001) Squamous cell carcinomas metastatic to cervical lymph nodes from an unknown head-and-neck mucosal site treated with radiation therapy alone or in combination with neck dissection. Int J Radiat Oncol Biol Phys 50:55–63

ESMO (2007) Clinical Recommendations for diagnosis, treatment and follow-up of cancers of unknown primary site. Ann Oncol 18 [Suppl 2]:ii81–ii82

Friesland S, Lind MG, Lundgren J et al. (2001) Outcome of ipsilateral treatment for patients with metastases to neck nodes of unknown origin. Acta Oncol 40:24–28

Glynne-Jones RG, Anand AK, Young TE et al. (1990) Metastatic carcinoma in the cervical lymph nodes from an occult primary: a conservative approach to the role of radiotherapy. Int J Radiat Oncol Biol Phys 18:289–294

Grau C, Johansen LV, Jakobsen J et al. (2000) Cervical lymph node metastases from unknown primary tumors. Results from a national survey by the Danish Society for Head and Neck Oncology. Radiother Oncol 55:121–129

Greene F, Page D, Fleming I et al. (2002) AJCC Cancer Staging Manual, 6th edn. Springer, Berlin Heidelberg New York

Iganej S, Kagan R, Anderson P et al. (2002) Metastatic squamous cell carcinoma of the neck from an unknown primary: management options and patterns of failure. Head Neck 24:236–246

Kaminsky MC, Blot E (2006) Squamous cell carcinoma of a unknown primary tumor located in the cervical lymph nodes. In Fizazi K (ed) Carcinoma of an unknown primary site, 1st edn. Taylor & Francis Books LLC, New York

Lapeyre M, Malissard L, Peiffert D et al. (1997) Cervical lymph node metastasis from an unknown primary: is a tonsillectomy necessary? Int J Radiat Oncol Biol Phys 39:291–296

Lee WY, Hsiao JR, Jin YT et al. (2000) Epstein-Barr virus detection in neck metastases by in-situ hybridization in fine-needle aspiration cytologic studies: an aid for differentiating the primary site. Head Neck 22:336–340

Lefebvre JL, Coche-Dequeant B, Van JT et al. (1990) Cervical lymph nodes from an unknown primary tumor in 190 patients. Am J Surg 160:443–446

Mack Y, Parsons JT, Mendenhall WM et al. (1993) Squamous cell carcinoma of the head-and-neck: management after excisional biopsy of a solitary metastatic neck node. Int Int J Radiat Oncol Biol Phys 25:619–622

Maulard C, Housset M, Brunel P et al. (1992) Postoperative radiation therapy for cervical lymph node metastases from an occult squamous cell carcinoma. Laryngoscope 102:884–890

McGuirt WF, McCabe BF (1978) Significance of node biopsy before definitive treatment of cervical metastatic carcinoma. Laryngoscope 88:594–597

Mendenhall WM, Million RR, Cassisi NJ (1986) Squamous cell carcinoma of the head and neck treated with radiation therapy: the role of neck dissection for clinically positive neck nodes. Int J Radiat Oncol Biol Phys 12:733–740

Mendenhall WM, Mancuso AA, Parsons JT et al. (1998) Diagnostic evaluation of squamous cell carcinoma metastatic to cervical lymph nodes from an unknown head and neck primary site. Head Neck 20:739–744

Mendenhall WM, Mancuso AA, Amdur RJ et al. (2001) Squamous cell carcinoma metastatic to the neck from an unknown head and neck primary site. Am J Otolaryngol 22:261–267

Miller FR, Hussey D, Beeram M et al. (2005) Positron emission tomography in the management of unknown primary head and neck carcinoma. Arch Otolaryngol 131:626–629

Million RR, Cassisi NJ, Mancuso AA (1994) The unknown primary. In: Million RR, Cassisi NJ (eds) Management of head and cancer: a multidisciplinary approach, 2nd edn. JB Lippincott, Philadelphia, pp 311–320

Mui S, Li T, Rasgon BM et al. (1997) Efficacy and cost-effectiveness of multihole fine-needle aspiration of head and neck masses. Laryngoscope 107:759–764

Nieder C, Gregoire V, Ang KK (2001) Cervical lymph node metastases from occult squamous cell carcinoma: cut down a tree to get apple. Int J Radiat Oncol Biol Phys 50:727–733

Panikkar RP, Astsaturov I, Langer CJ (2008) The emerging role of cetuximab in head and neck cancer: a 2007 perspective. Cancer Invest 26:96–103

Pavlidis N, Fizazi K (2005) Cancer of unknown primary (CUP). Crit Rev Oncol Hematol 54:243–250

Pisharodi LR (1997) False-negative diagnosis in fine-needle aspiration of squamous-cell carcinoma of head and neck. Diagn Cytopathol 17:70–73

Reddy SP, Marks JE (1997) Metastatic carcinoma in the cervical lymph nodes from an unknown primary site: results of bilateral neck plus mucosal irradiation vs. ipsilateral neck irradiation. Int J Radiat Oncol Biol Phys 37:797–802

Rusthoven KE, Koshy M, Paulino AC (2004) The role of fluorodeoxyglucose positron emission tomography in cervical lymph node metastases from an unknown primary tumor. Cancer 101:2641–2649

Shehadeh NJ, Ensley JF, Kucuk O et al. (2006) Benefit of postoperative chemoradiotherapy for patients with unknown primary squamous cell carcinoma of the head and neck. Head Neck 28:1090–1098

Sinnathamby K, Peters LJ, Laidlaw C et al. (1997) The occult head and neck primary: to treat or not to treat? Clin Oncol (R Coll Radiol) 9:322–329

Strojan P, Anicin A (1998) Combined surgery and postoperative radiotherapy for cervical lymph node metastases from an unknown primary tumor. Radiother Oncol 49:33–40

Taylor JM, Mendenhall WM, Parsons JT et al. (1992) The influence of dose and time on wound complications following post-radiation neck dissection. Int J Radiat Oncol Biol Phys 23:41–46

Weir L, Keane T, Cummings B et al. (1995) Radiation treatment of cervical lymph node metastases from an unknown primary: an analysis of outcome by treatment volume and other prognostic factors. Radiother Oncol 35:206–2011

Thyroid Cancer

Roger Ove and Ron R. Allison

CONTENTS

R. Ove, MD, PhD
Department of Radiation Oncology, Leo Jenkins Cancer Center, The Brody School of Medicine at ECU, 600 Moye Blvd., Greenville, NC 27834, USA
R. R. Allison, MD
Department of Radiation Oncology, The Brody School of Medicine at ECU, 600 Moye Blvd., Greenville, NC 27834, USA

Introduction and Objectives

Thyroid cancer is a relatively rare malignancy, occurring in less than 1% of the population. However, benign thyroid nodules are quite prevalent, found in 50% of the population (Ezzat et al. 1994). Benign nodules are up to three times more common in women than in men, and there is a similar increased incidence of malignancy. Yet, the mortality rates remain higher for men, perhaps due to the age of diagnosis, with thyroid cancer occurring more often in older males than females.

Three main histological variants of thyroid cancer are recognized: differentiated, medullary, and anaplastic. The differentiated types include papillary, follicular, and Hürthle cell. The majority of patients tend to present with differentiated carcinoma, 80% having papillary carcinoma, 11% follicular, 3% Hürthle cell, and medullary carcinoma occurring in 4%. Only 2% of patients present with anaplastic thyroid carcinoma (Hundahl et al. 1998).

This chapter examines:

● Diagnosis, staging, and assessing risk

● Histological subtypes

● Treatment recommendations for differentiated thyroid cancer, with supporting evidence

● Treatment recommendations for medullary thyroid cancer, with supporting evidence and discussion of familial syndromes

● Treatment recommendations for anaplastic thyroid cancer, with supporting evidence

● The roles of ^{131}I and external beam radiotherapy, their respective supporting evidence, and a discussion of radiotherapy technique.

The management of lymphoma of the thyroid gland is not discussed, as its management is equivalent to lymphoma diagnosed elsewhere in the neck, a topic discussed in other chapters.

7.1 Diagnosis, Staging, and Prognosis

7.1.1 Diagnosis

Initial Evaluation

- Diagnosis and evaluation of thyroid cancer initiates with a complete history and physical examination (H&P), and attention should be paid to disease-associated signs and symptoms. Benign thyroid nodules are common. The selection of patients for observation versus biopsy is based on an estimate of risk. The majority of lesions found incidentally are asymptomatic, usually detected during routine physical exam or scans performed for other reasons. For these incidentally found nodules, biopsy is of low yield if the lesions are smaller than 1 cm (Level IV) (Tan and Gharib 1997).
- If a nodule is greater than 4 cm, there is a higher risk of malignancy and fine needle aspiration (FNA) is recommended. Symptoms also increase the likelihood that a biopsy will be positive. Nodules that are fixed to adjacent structures or associated with regional lymphadenopathy, or give rise to other symptoms such as vocal cord paralysis or dysphagia, yield a higher risk of a thyroid cancer diagnosis. Other factors that increase the likelihood of a positive biopsy are age less than 15 years or greater than 60 years, a history of exposure to ionizing radiation, family history of thyroid carcinoma, the presence of familial syndromes associated with thyroid carcinoma, or the presence of suspicious findings by ultrasound examination, such as central hypervascularity, an irregular border, or microcalcifications (Level IV) (Frates et al. 2005).
- Many patients present with a palpable thyroid nodule or a nodule seen on routine imaging. FNA of the nodule is the primary means of diagnosis.
- Serum thyrotropin (thyroid-stimulating hormone, or TSH) should ideally be measured prior to the FNA.
- Serum calcitonin can also be measured and this is advised by some, but is not universally recommended (Level IV) (Singer et al. 1996).
- Papillary and medullary carcinoma can be accurately diagnosed by FNA. Anaplastic carcinoma can sometimes be difficult to distinguish from undifferentiated variants of a more favorable histology by FNA alone. It is particularly difficult to distinguish follicular carcinoma from benign adenomas. Additional tissue is required to determine if there is vascular invasion or capsular penetration for this histology, and therefore a surgical biopsy is typically necessary.

Laboratory Tests

- T3, T4, TSH, and thyroglobulin (Tg) should be measured.
- Calcitonin should be measured if there is concern that the carcinoma may be medullary. If medullary carcinoma is diagnosed, CEA and calcium along with urine and serum catecholamines should also be measured, in addition to calcitonin.
- A diagnosis of medullary thyroid cancer warrants an evaluation for familial cancer syndromes, including familial medullary thyroid cancer (FMTC) and MEN 2. These syndromes are associated with mutations in the RET proto-oncogene on chromosome 10, and specific mutations will dictate prophylactic surgery in family members.

Imaging Studies

- Ultrasound is the imaging modality of choice, and can be used to more extensively examine the neck as well as the primary site. CT with contrast should be avoided, as it would make it difficult to treat with ^{131}I. MRI can be useful to evaluate adenopathy in the neck.
- In cases where an FNA is nondiagnostic, checking a serum TSH and a thyroid ^{123}I or technetium-99m scan can identify patients with a hot nodule, which are almost invariably benign follicular adenomas. A low TSH with a hotspot on such scanning indicates an autonomously functioning nodule, requiring therapy for thyrotoxicosis. Repeating a nondiagnostic biopsy can often yield a diagnostic result. Patients with a cold nodule and a biopsy suspicious for carcinoma should proceed to surgery.
- Following surgery, ^{131}I or ^{123}I scans are useful in assessing residual disease, activity in the surgical bed, or a residual thyroid remnant. ^{123}I is more expensive, but has the advantage of decreased interference with possible subsequent ^{131}I therapy (Level III) (Hilditch et al. 2002).

Pathology

- The prognosis of thyroid cancer is largely dependent on the histological variant. Typically, papillary differentiation carries a good prognosis, but there are certain histological subsets for which the risk of recurrence is substantially higher. These include anaplastic transformation, tall cell papillary variants, and columnar variants. Mixed follicular papillary types, which are characterized by papillary cytology and follicular morphology, do not carry a worse prognosis (Level IV) (Mazzaferri 1993; Tielens et al. 1994).

- Follicular carcinoma can be more aggressive than papillary carcinoma. It tends to occur as a solitary encapsulated tumor and there may be capsular invasion and/or blood vessel invasion. Without evidence of vascular invasion or capsular penetration, it is not possible to distinguish follicular carcinoma from adenoma, and hence a more generous biopsy than FNA is required. Rarely a follicular carcinoma will invade surrounding tissues, and this characteristic is associated with a higher chance of metastases.

- Hürthle cell carcinoma (oncocytic carcinoma) is diagnosed when he majority of the tumor mass consists of Hürthle cells. The term oncocyte refers to a cell that has become abnormally swollen, due to the accumulation of mitochondria. They can occur in a variety of malignancies and may also be benign. While Hürthle cell tumors are morphologically similar to follicular tumors, cytologically they appear to be more closely related to papillary then follicular carcinomas. It can be difficult to distinguish benign collections of Hürthle cells from malignant Hürthle cells based on FNA or frozen section alone. Larger tumors are more likely to be malignant and can be more aggressive, and their clinical course can be more difficult to predict. The 10-year survival rate is roughly 10 percentage points worse than for follicular carcinoma. The incidence of distant metastases is twice that of follicular carcinoma.

- Anaplastic thyroid cancer is an undifferentiated carcinoma. It is often found in association with better differentiated types of thyroid cancer, most commonly papillary. FNA is accurate in 90% of cases, but it can be difficult to distinguish anaplastic carcinoma from less well differentiated variants of favorable histologies, such as tall cell and columnar papillary types. There is evidence that differentiated types can transform into anaplastic carcinoma, and this often involves loss of p53 function. Spindle cell, giant cell, and squamoid types have been described, but these distinctions have no impact on prognosis. Grossly, the tumor is a rapidly enlarging unencapsulated mass that infiltrates surrounding tissue.

7.1.2 Staging

- Multiple staging systems to stratify the risk of thyroid carcinoma have been developed. The most widely used is the AJCC 6th edition, which like several other staging systems in use for thyroid carcinoma, includes age as an important factor for the well differentiated histologies (Greene et al. 2002). Other factors that have played a role in defining staging systems include tumor size, nodal metastases, extent, invasion, patient age, and completion of dissection. None of these systems is entirely satisfactory, and many clinicians do not incorporate age into their clinical decision-making, although it is clearly the most important prognostic factor.

- Table 7.1 presents the AJCC 6th edition TNM classification system (Greene et al. 2002), while Table 7.2 presents the stage grouping. Note that all anaplastic carcinomas are by definition stage IV.

Table 7.1. American Joint Committee on Cancer (AJCC) 6th edition (Greene et al. 2002) staging for thyroid cancer. This does not apply to lymphoma

Primary tumor (T)	
TX	Primary tumor cannot be assessed
T0	No evidence of primary tumor
T1	2 cm or less, limited to the thyroid
T2	More than 2 cm, less than or equal to 4 cm, limited to thyroid
T3	More than 4 cm or minimal extrathyroid extension
T4a	Invasion of larynx, trachea, esophagus, recurrent laryngeal nerve, or subcutaneous soft tissues. Anaplastic carcinoma contained by thyroid capsule
T4b	Invasion of prevertebral fascia, encasement of carotid or mediastinal vessels. Anaplastic carcinoma with extrathyroidal extension
Regional lymph nodes (N)	
NX	Regional nodes cannot be assessed
N0	No regional node metastases
N1	Regional node metastases
N1a	Level VI
N1b	Other regional nodes
Distant metastases (M)	
MX	Distant metastases cannot be assessed
M0	No distant metastases
M1	Distant metastases

Regional nodes: central compartment, lateral cervical, upper mediastinal. For multiple tumors, the largest determines the classification. All anaplastic carcinoma is T4 and group stage IV

Table 7.2. American Joint Committee on Cancer (AJCC) 6th edition (GREENE et al. 2002) stage grouping for thyroid cancer. Hürthle cell carcinoma is considered a follicular carcinoma with regard to staging

STAGE GROUPING	
Papillary or follicular, under 45 years of age	
Stage I	Any T Any N M0,
Stage II	Any T Any N M1
Papillary or follicular, 45 years and older	
Stage I	T1 N0 M0
Stage II	T2 N0 M0
Stage III	T3 N0 M0, T1-3 N1a M0
Stage IVA	T4a Any N M0, T1-3 N1b M0
Stage IVB	T4b Any N M0
Stage IVC	Any T Any N M1
Medullary carcinoma	
Stage I	T1 N0 M0
Stage II	T2 N0 M0
Stage III	T3 N0 M0, T1-3 N1a M0
Stage IVA	T4a Any N M0, T1-3 N1b M0
Stage IVB	T4b Any N M0
Stage IVC	Any T Any N M1
Anaplastic carcinoma	
Stage IVA	T4a Any N M0
Stage IVB	T4b Any N M0
Stage IVC	Any T Any N M1

- Other risk classification systems include MACIS (metastases, age, completeness of resection, invasion, size), AMES (age, metastases, extent, size), and AGES (age, grade, extent, size). Each of these systems yields a numerical score that is correlated with survival (CADY and ROSSI 1988; HAY et al. 1993; SHERMAN et al. 1998).

7.1.3 Prognosis

- Prognosis is highly dependent upon histology.
- Low-risk patients with follicular or papillary carcinomas have a roughly 99% 20-year survival rate.

- Patients with anaplastic thyroid carcinoma are incurable and have a dismal prognosis, typically surviving less than 1 year after diagnosis.
- Other factors that can influence survival and the risk of recurrence include primary tumor size, lymph node metastases, degree of local invasion or capsular penetration, and distant metastases.
- Patients under 45 years of age with papillary or follicular carcinoma can have a surprisingly good outcome despite having systemic metastases. Nonetheless, metastases still portend a poor prognosis, and 50% of patients die within 5 years in the setting of pulmonary metastases, even with favorable histology.
- The ability to concentrate ^{131}I is a major prognostic factor in determining how patients with metastatic disease will do. Patients with medullary carcinoma or anaplastic thyroid cancer tend to have tumors which do not concentrate iodine, and hence do not have the option of that modality.

7.2 Treatment of Papillary and Follicular Thyroid Cancer

7.2.1 Surgical Management

- Surgery is the mainstay of treatment for differentiated papillary and follicular thyroid cancer.
- The degree of resection required remains controversial, but at present the majority of experts believe that a total thyroidectomy is required (Grade C) (WITT 2008). For some low-risk carcinomas, there are advocates of ipsilateral lobectomy, but this can complicate the follow-up and is not widely supported. In addition, should a recurrence or second primary be found in the residual gland, surgery is technically more difficult and morbidity is increased (DEGROOT and KAPLAN 1991).
- The question of ipsilateral resection versus more complete resection was addressed by the Mayo Clinic, with findings of no difference in survival between the two groups but a higher incidence of local recurrence with limited surgery (Level IV) (HAY et al. 1998). Other series have reported a local recurrence rate approaching 30% after partial resection, and also an increase in subse-

quent pulmonary metastases (MAZZAFERRI and JHIANG 1994).

■ Lobectomy can be considered for a solitary differentiated lesion less than 1 cm in size, with no evidence of vascular invasion, capsule involvement, or other adverse features that might warrant subsequent adjuvant therapy (Level III) (MAZZAFERRI and JHIANG 1994). However, some patients with higher risk disease continue to undergo such partial resections, and there may be socioeconomic factors influencing medical practice (BILIMORIA et al. 2007).

■ The motivation for limited or ipsilateral surgery is reduced surgical morbidity. The long-term complications of most concern after thyroidectomy are injury to the recurrent laryngeal nerve and hypoparathyroidism. Surgical morbidity is correlated with the experience of the surgeon. In the hands of surgeons with an adequate case load (> 100 cases per year), these complications occur at a rate of 2%–5% (SOSA et al. 1998). Subtotal thyroidectomy reduces the incidence of nerve injury roughly by half, and reduces the risk of hypoparathyroidism by an order of magnitude (UDELSMAN et al. 1996; UDELSMAN 2008).

■ Contraindications to lobectomy include age less than 15 years, age greater than 45 years, history of prior radiation exposure, distant metastases, cervical lymph node metastases, extrathyroidal extension, tumor size greater than 4 cm, or a more aggressive histology such as tall cell or columnar variants. Should a patient proceed to lobectomy and be found to have more aggressive histology, multifocal disease, positive margins, positive cervical nodes, or extrathyroidal extension, completion of the thyroidectomy is indicated.

■ Surgical neck dissection is indicated if preoperative imaging or physical examination indicates adenopathy. Neck dissection typically involves a central neck dissection (level VI), and functional lateral neck dissection including levels II through V, sparing the spinal accessory nerve, internal jugular vein, and sternocleidomastoid muscle.

■ Radionuclide imaging preoperatively with ^{131}I or ^{123}I is useful to verify that a differentiated tumor is in fact iodine avid. Iodine uptake is not universal in differentiated thyroid cancer, especially the Hürthle cell variant where only 10%–30% of cases are avid. Lack of iodine avidity in the setting of locally extensive disease is an indication for postoperative radiotherapy.

■ Thyroid hormone replacement with Synthroid is indicated after total thyroidectomy. In the setting of iodine avid thyroid cancer, thyroid replacement therapy is dosed to a level sufficient to suppress TSH below the lower limit of normal.

7.2.2 Radioactive Iodine (^{131}I)

■ Radioactive iodine can be used both as adjuvant therapy to treat residual microscopic disease, as well as to ablate the residual thyroid remnant after partial resection. Adjuvant radioactive iodine is typically delivered to patients with high-risk features or those with positive iodine imaging after completion of resection. A thyroid scan is usually done 1–12 weeks after thyroidectomy, and prior to this scan thyroid replacement is withdrawn or recombinant TSH is given to raise the level of TSH, to improve the sensitivity of the scan. The presence of an elevated thyroglobulin above 1 ng/ml is also an indication of residual carcinoma, and in addition adverse pathological findings may lead clinicians to recommend adjuvant ^{131}I despite a negative scan.

■ Patients with a significant risk for recurrence should also undergo iodine therapy for the purpose of ablating the remnant, to facilitate follow-up.

■ The typical dose of ^{131}I is 100–200 mCi (Grade B). Such treatment typically delivers 80 Gy to the surgical bed or residual disease. For remnant ablation, 50 mCi is sufficient, which delivers approximately 30 Gy to the remnant (BAL et al. 1996). ^{131}I is a beta emitter with a half life of 8 days, and delivers little systemic dose.

■ A large retrospective series from Princess Margaret Hospital showed no benefit to radioiodine therapy for low risk differentiated patients (less than 45 years of age with T1 tumors) (Level IV) (BRIERLEY et al. 2005).

■ Following delivery of radioiodine, a post-treatment scan is typically performed to verify efficacy. Patients with T4 disease and older than 40–45 years of age should be considered at this point for adjuvant external beam radiotherapy.

■ Radioiodine ablation is not recommended to ablate the residual thyroid for patients undergoing partial thyroidectomy. Such limited resections should be restricted to patients with very low risk disease, for which therapeutic ^{131}I and diagnostic iodine scans are not indicated. If pathological findings from a partial thyroidectomy are adverse and adjuvant therapy is being considered, completion thyroidectomy should be completed first.

■ Hürthle cell thyroid cancer can be viewed as a variant of follicular thyroid cancer, although less often iodine avid than the more common differentiated histologies. However, Hürthle cell cancers are iodine avid frequently enough that iodine imaging should be performed, in which case therapeutic iodine is effective (Level IV) (Besic et al. 2003).

■ Treatment with ^{131}I requires that Synthroid (T4) be withheld for 6 weeks prior to treatment, and the patient is placed on a low iodine diet. Cytomel (T3) is given for the first 3 of these weeks, and then also stopped. Prior to treatment, a diagnostic iodine scan is done to help determine the therapeutic dose, and treatment is given within 5 days of the scan. Some clinicians do not perform the diagnostic scan due to concern over inhibiting uptake of iodine during therapy (referred to as stunning). This can be mitigated by using ^{123}I, which can also inhibit therapeutic uptake but to a lesser degree than [131]I (Level III) (Hilditch et al. 2002). A scan is again performed 1 week to 10 days after therapy, and this scan may show additional foci of disease not detected on the diagnostic scan, due to the higher dose used. Another diagnostic scan is repeated 4–6 months later, and the process continues until a negative scan is obtained.

■ The lifetime limit for total activity of ^{131}I administration is generally quoted as 1000 mCi, although this is not based on reliable data (Grade D). Each administration of therapeutic iodine delivers a dose to blood and bone marrow of roughly 2 Gy. The bone marrow recovers from this dose well, and as treatments are typically 6 months apart, pancytopenia generally is not a problem. The cumulative dose limit is instead based on the theoretical risk of radiation-induced malignancies, and the possibility of pulmonary injury for patients with diffuse pulmonary metastases.

7.2.3   Systemic Chemotherapy

■ There is little evidence suggesting a benefit to systemic chemotherapy for differentiated thyroid carcinoma (Grade C). Doxorubicin has shown some promise for anaplastic thyroid cancer, in

particular with radiotherapy, and this drug has been more widely studied than others.

■ A randomized cooperative group study (ECOG) compared doxorubicin alone versus doxorubicin and cisplatin for advanced stage thyroid cancer, including differentiated, medullary, and anaplastic (Level II) (Shimaoka et al. 1985). Response rates were relatively low (23%), and there was no significant difference between the arms. However, the complete responses (CR) did differ between the arms, with five CRs seen in the combination arm and none in the single agent arm (p = 0.03), and several patients remained disease free for a substantial period.

7.2.4   Radiation Therapy

■ No prospective randomized trials have been performed to evaluate the role of external beam radiotherapy.

■ Indications for external beam radiotherapy for differentiated thyroid cancer in the setting of poor iodine uptake include incomplete resection, invasion of adjacent structures in the neck, extracapsular extension of nodal disease, and involvement of mediastinal nodes (Level IV) (Simpson and Carruthers 1978; Tubiana et al. 1985; Simpson et al. 1988; Farahati et al. 1996). External beam radiotherapy is also recommended after resection of local or regional recurrences.

■ For iodine avid tumors, ^{131}I radioiodine treatment typically delivers radiotherapy more conformally and to a higher dose than can be achieved with external beam equipment. Another advantage of ^{131}I is that it also treats undetected systemic metastases.

■ For completely resected papillary carcinomas with high risk features, there is compelling evidence to support the use of external beam radiotherapy (Grade B). There have been no prospective trials, and an attempt at a large randomized trial failed to accrue patients and was abandoned (Level IV) (Biermann et al. 2003). However, a retrospective review evaluated external beam radiotherapy for both follicular and papillary thyroid cancer with T4 disease. Subgroup analysis indicated that radiotherapy provided a significant benefit for patients older than 40 years with invasive papillary thyroid cancer with lymph node involvement, in comparison to those treated with surgery and iodine therapy alone (Level IV) (Farahati et al. 1996). This study showed no benefit to adjuvant radiotherapy for follicular carcinoma with these risk factors (completely resected node positive T4). Similarly, a series of 382 differentiated thyroid cancer patients from Princess Margaret Hospital showed a benefit to RT only for patients with papillary histology and microscopic residual disease (Level IV) (Tsang et al. 1998). Others have also recommended the addition of external beam radiotherapy for papillary patients with T4 disease, N1b (lateral cervical nodes), or bulky nodes (> 2 cm) (Level IV) (Chow et al. 2002, 2006; Lee and Tuttle 2006).

■ The case for adjuvant external beam radiotherapy for completely resected but locally advanced follicular carcinoma is less well supported than for the papillary variant, in view of the subset analyses in the above studies (Grade C). However, this lack of benefit for follicular histology is not uniformly reported, with a large retrospective review showing that 10-year cause-specific survival was improved with the addition of external beam radiotherapy, for older patients with completely resected T4 disease, improving from 65% to 81% (Level IV) (Brierley et al. 2005). This study included well differentiated thyroid carcinoma of both papillary and follicular types. Local control was also improved for these high-risk completely resected patients. Follicular carcinoma is more likely than papillary to present with locally advanced disease (Level IV) (Sherman et al. 1998).

■ Hürthle cell thyroid cancer is frequently not iodine avid, and external radiotherapy should be considered postoperatively in high-risk cases. Radiotherapy has been shown to be effective in the adjuvant setting for high-risk cases, for salvaging recurrences, and for palliation of metastases (Level IV) (Foote et al. 2003).

■ In the case of gross residual disease, retrospective data more clearly supports a role for radiotherapy (Grade B). Royal Marsden Hospital reported on a series of 49 patient with gross residual disease, all of whom received radioiodine therapy and external beam radiotherapy to substantial dose of 60–75 Gy (Level IV) (O'Connell et al. 1994). Complete responses were seen in 37.5%, with a similar number of nonresponders, and the remaining 25% saw a partial benefit. Survival was on 27%, much worse than for those with only microscopic residual, and clearly every attempt must be made to surgically eradicate gross disease. A similar series of patients with gross residual treated with or without external beam radiotherapy, yielded a 50% reduction in local failure (Level IV) (Tubiana et al. 1985). However, Princess Margaret Hospital reported a 62% local recurrence rate (Level IV) (Tsang et al. 1998). In some of these series the dosing was inadequate by modern standards, and it is possible that dose escalation with intensity modulation techniques will improve on these results.

7.3 Treatment of Medullary Thyroid Cancer

■ Medullary thyroid cancer is derived from the neuroendocrine C cells of the thyroid, cells that are commonly located in the upper portion of the thyroid lobes. These cells produce calcitonin. The majority of cases (80%) are sporadic, the remaining associated with familial syndromes such as multiple endocrine neoplasia (MEN 2A and 2B). Both MEN 2A and 2B are associated with medullary carcinoma and pheochromocytoma, and the MEN 2A variant is also associated with parathyroid tumors. Familial tumors tend to arise at earlier ages.

■ The high incidence of familial syndromes in patients with this diagnosis warrants genetic testing. Specific mutations of RET proto-oncogene on chromosome 10 are associated with MEN 2 and FMTC. This proto-oncogene codes for a membrane associated tyrosine kinase receptor expressed in neuroendocrine cells. The possibility of MEN 2 syndrome necessitates exclusion of pheochromocytoma (MEN 2A and 2B) and hyperparathyroidism (MEN 2A) prior to surgery, and these should be excluded even if MEN 2 is not suspected.

7.3.1 Surgical Management

■ Surgery is the primary treatment for medullary thyroid cancer, due to the lack of evidence that radiotherapy can eradicate macroscopic disease and the relative inefficacy of systemic therapy (Grade B).

■ Medullary carcinoma is not iodine avid.

■ Total thyroidectomy is recommended for all patients, and the degree of neck dissection depends on preoperative imaging, degree of invasion, presence of involved nodes, and the need for parathyroid resection in some cases (SAAD et al. 1984).

■ A central neck dissection (the level VI nodal station) is generally recommended (Grade B). If this level is involved, or the primary tumor is greater than 1 cm, levels II through V are also dissected. There is a lower threshold for more extensive neck dissection in patients with MEN 2B. Functional neck dissections are preferred, and radical dissection is not recommended unless there is evidence of involvement of the adjacent structures. In the case of hyperparathyroidism, care should be taken to leave adequate parathyroid tissue, and cryopreserve parathyroid tissue for possible later implantation.

■ Calcitonin should be measured a few months postoperatively, and if elevated additional imaging is warranted. The serum half life of calcitonin is 12 min. In the absence of distant metastases, comprehensive neck dissection can normalize calcitonin in roughly a third of patients. In some series, the mediastinum was also dissected, but it is unclear if this is necessary or beneficial.

■ Thyroid replacement therapy is given after thyroidectomy for medullary carcinoma, but it unnecessary to administer doses sufficient to suppress TSH.

7.3.2 Systemic Therapy

■ Chemotherapy for medullary thyroid cancer has not established efficacy for recurrent disease or in the setting of distant metastases, and such treatment should be performed on a clinical trial if possible. Dacarbazine-based regimens have been utilized, with modest response rates (Level III) (ORLANDI et al. 1994; WU et al. 1994). Clinical trials are currently exploring the use of tyrosine kinase inhibitors. Radio-immunotherapy utilizing radioisotopes bound to anti-CEA antibodies has shown some promise in early clinical trials (Level IV) (CHATAL et al. 2006).

7.3.3 Radiation Therapy

■ Adjuvant external beam radiotherapy should be considered for high-risk medullary thyroid can-

cer (Grade B). Historically, this histology has a reputation for being unresponsive to radiation (QUAYLE and MOLEY 2005; VEZZOSI et al. 2007). While the results of surgical resection for subcentimeter primary lesions is quite good, exceeding 90% disease-free survival, this drops to under 50% for tumors greater than 1 cm. Medullary thyroid tends to progress more slowly than other thyroid cancer variants, but nonetheless is more difficult to control. This slow growth may have contributed to its reputation for being radioresistant.

■ Radiotherapy is unlikely to be effective in eradicating gross disease, and surgical resection of gross disease should be performed if possible. In the postoperative setting, radiotherapy can provide some benefit. In a small series of locally advanced cases from M. D. Anderson cancer center, locoregional control was 87% at 5 years. All of the patients had stage IV disease, half had mediastinal involvement, and a third had positive margins (Level IV) (SCHWARTZ et al. 2008).

■ Due to the long natural history of the disease, and the lack of effective alternative therapies, postoperative radiotherapy should be considered for high-risk patients even in the setting of metastatic disease.

■ Radiotherapy was used at the Royal Marsden Hospital in the setting of elevated calcitonin postoperatively (Level IV) (FERSHT et al. 2001). While calcitonin was typically not normalized after radiotherapy, local control was improved from 41% to 71%. The failure to normalize calcitonin likely reflects metastatic disease, and indeed, recent studies have shown a high incidence of bone marrow involvement for locally advanced cases (Level III) (MIRALLIE et al. 2005).

7.4 Treatment of Anaplastic Thyroid Cancer

■ Anaplastic thyroid cancer carries a dismal prognosis, with a median survival of approximately 6 months. Aggressive locoregional therapy with chemoradiation can improve survival, but the disease remains universally fatal. Other histologies, such as lymphoma and poorly differentiated follicular carcinoma, can be misinterpreted as anaplastic carcinoma. An adequate biopsy specimen must be obtained to distinguish it from diagnoses with a more favorable outcome and different management.

7.4.1 Surgical Management

■ Except in cases of small tumors confined within the thyroid capsule, surgical resection does not improve survival (Grade B) (VENKATESH et al. 1990). However, aggressive local and regional management is warranted in view of the high likelihood of dying from airway compromise. In addition, rare cases of prolonged survival are almost invariably those that have been resected at diagnosis. If technically resectable, a total thyroidectomy should be performed along with selective dissection of the involved node bearing regions of the neck. If unresectable, surgery with the intent of protecting the airway is appropriate. Most cases are diagnosed via FNA, and some cases undergo total thyroidectomy due to the difficulty in distinguishing the pathology from other thyroid malignancies.

7.4.2 Systemic Therapy

■ Systemic agents have not been shown to improve survival. Chemotherapy, typically doxorubicin-based, is often used in radiosensitizing doses concurrently with hyperfractionated radiotherapy. Palliative systemic chemotherapy may be indicated in patients with good performance status, preferably in the setting of a clinical trial. No survival benefit has been demonstrated, although taxanes have some activity.

■ Combretastatin A4 phosphate (CA4P), a biologic agent that targets tumor vasculature, has shown efficacy in vitro and in tumor xenograft models, and led to one prolonged tumor remission in an early clinical trial (YEUNG et al. 2007). A clinical trial is currently underway using this agent with carboplatin and paclitaxel.

■ Trials are also underway exploring the use of tyrosine kinase inhibitors, such as the multiple target inhibitor sorafenib, in conjunction with conventional chemotherapy for anaplastic thyroid cancer.

7.4.3 Radiation Therapy

■ Hyperfractionated radiotherapy with concurrent doxorubicin chemotherapy, though toxic, has demonstrated the best results (Grade B) (Level III) (KIM and LEEPER 1983; TALLROTH et al. 1987; DE CREVOISIER et al. 2004). This improves the median survival to 1 year, although the disease remains incurable. The primary benefit that justifies this toxicity is a change in the pattern of failure from one of airway compromise to distant metastases (Level III) (KIM and LEEPER 1987).

■ Radiotherapy is typically delivered at 1.6 Gy bid to a total of 57.6 Gy, with weekly low-dose doxorubicin (10 mg/m^2), based on Sloan Kettering experience (Level III) (KIM and LEEPER 1987). Doxorubicin is a potent radiosensitizer, and the regional morbidity of this regimen is considerable. Rapid proliferation of anaplastic thyroid cancer motivated treatment with hyperfractionated regimens, to keep pace with tumor repopulation.

■ In view of the tendency to repopulate rapidly, and the consequences of local failure, potential benefits of IMRT should be weighed against the time required to plan such therapy. IMRT can be useful as a boost to conventional therapy, allowing radiotherapy to start without unnecessary delay.

7.5 Radiation Therapy Techniques

■ Radiotherapy dosing and field recommendations vary little based on histology, and large randomized trials have not been done to optimize these factors, due to the relative rarity of the disease. In general, the nodal regions treated include levels II–VI of the neck, and the superior mediastinum. Fields tend to extend from the angle of the mandible to the carina.

■ See Figure 7.1 for a typical beam arrangement. This region is usually treated in an AP/PA fashion, often with low energy photons from the anterior beam and high energy from the posterior, and the dose is taken to 40–44 Gy. The surgical bed and dissected neck is then boosted to 60 Gy, delivered in an off-cord manner, usually with a set of oblique fields. This dose is appropriate for microscopic disease in the postoperative (hypoxic)

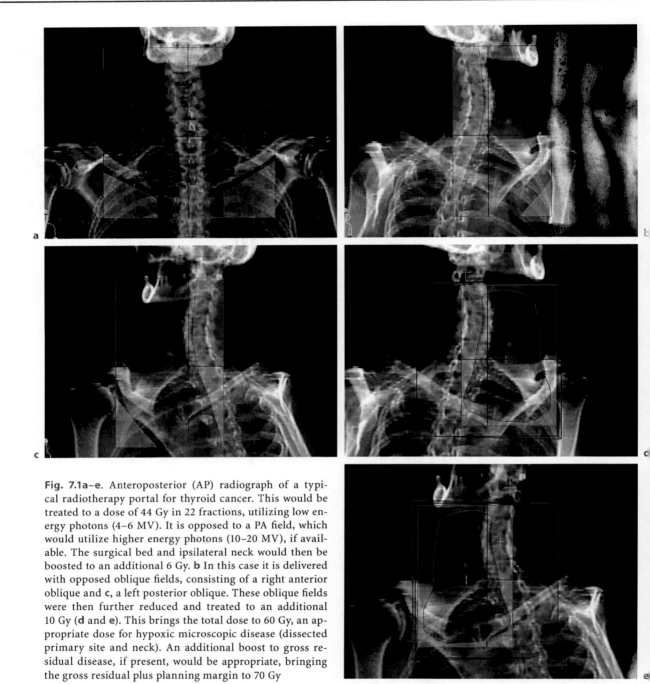

Fig. 7.1a–e. Anteroposterior (AP) radiograph of a typical radiotherapy portal for thyroid cancer. This would be treated to a dose of 44 Gy in 22 fractions, utilizing low energy photons (4–6 MV). It is opposed to a PA field, which would utilize higher energy photons (10–20 MV), if available. The surgical bed and ipsilateral neck would then be boosted to an additional 6 Gy. **b** In this case it is delivered with opposed oblique fields, consisting of a right anterior oblique and **c**, a left posterior oblique. These oblique fields were then further reduced and treated to an additional 10 Gy (**d** and **e**). This brings the total dose to 60 Gy, an appropriate dose for hypoxic microscopic disease (dissected primary site and neck). An additional boost to gross residual disease, if present, would be appropriate, bringing the gross residual plus planning margin to 70 Gy

setting, and is based more on general head and neck cancer recommendations than specifics of thyroid cancer. In this example there is an intermediate off-cord boost to 50 Gy, before reducing fields further. Gross residual disease should be boosted to approximately 70 Gy.

■ Dose recommendations have varied widely in the literature, due a lack of radiobiological and clinical data (Grade C). Recommendations have ranged from 40 Gy to approximately 70 Gy (SIMPSON and CARRUTHERS 1978; FORD et al. 2003). One study suggested improved outcomes for both local control and survival at higher doses, but patient numbers were small (FORD et al. 2003).

■ In the case of anaplastic carcinoma, the maximum dose is approximately 60 Gy delivered in a hyperfractionated fashion with concurrent radiosensitizing chemotherapy. Boosting beyond this level is not advised, as the regimen is toxic enough at 60 Gy, and pattern of failure is primarily systemic after that dose.

■ Treating thyroid carcinoma with radiotherapy can be technically difficult due to the geometry of the neck and upper mediastinum. This is due to the varying thicknesses of portions of the body, and made more complex because of the length of spinal cord adjacent to the treatment volume. Reproducible and accurate patient immobilization is essential. Obtaining acceptable dosimetry in this region often requires multiple beam segments, and other techniques including lateral fields and electrons have been reported (TUBIANA et al. 1985; TSANG et al. 1998).

■ Intensity modulated radiotherapy (IMRT) has been found to be useful in improving dosimetric target coverage and in lowering the spinal cord dose (Grade C) (Level IV) (POSNER et al. 2000; NUTTING et al. 2001). As the standard radiotherapy fields cover the inferior portions of the parotid glands, IMRT should be able to reduce xerostomia, as has been shown with other head and neck malignancies. Esophageal and pharyngeal toxicity should be reduced with IMRT. Figure 7.2 illustrates a comparison of dose distributions for the upper neck and mediastinum for IMRT and the conventional field arrangement described in Figure 7.1.

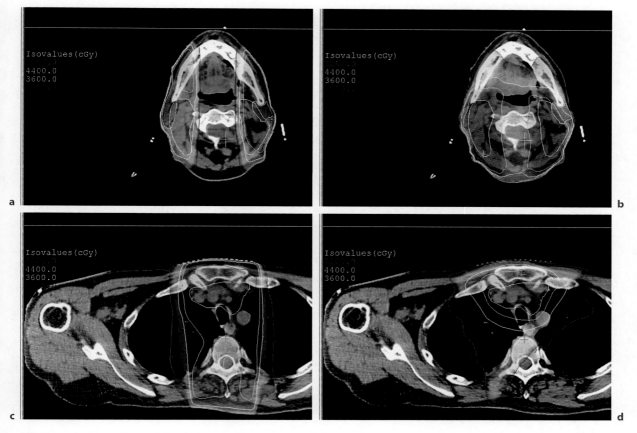

Fig. 7.2a–d. Comparison of the dosimetry for conventional therapy (see Fig. 7.1) and intensity modulated radiotherapy (IMRT). IMRT is useful for thyroid cancer as it allows better sparing of the spinal cord, better conformation of dose over portions of the body of different thickness (neck and chest), and in some cases sparing of the parotid glands. IMRT was delivered with seven nonopposed coaxial beams, each composed of 6 MV photons and modulated with a multi-leaf collimator. **a** Depicts the dosimetry at the level of upper level II for conventional therapy, compared with **b** IMRT. With conventional therapy the hotspots overlap the parotid glands, while with IMRT these are spared somewhat. With IMRT target coverage is improved, at the expense of large volumes of the head and neck that now receive a low dose, regions that may receive no dose with conventional therapy. **c** A similar comparison in the superior mediastinum for conventional therapy, compared with **d**, IMRT. Note the improved conformality of the high dose region. A primary benefit of IMRT for thyroid cancer is that the high dose region is further from the spinal cord, reducing the risk of cord complications due to patient positioning errors

7.6   Follow-Up

- Follow-up is dependent on histology (due to iodine avidity of the majority of differentiated cases).
- Physical examination remains important for all types.
- Laboratory studies commonly used for differentiated histology include thyroid function tests, including thyroglobulin, TSH, free T3, and thyrotropin. Imaging for these cases is typically done with ultrasound, although MRI of the neck is also an option.
- Radioiodine imaging is often performed, and is of added utility in that the degree of uptake can influence salvage treatment recommendations. However, this test requires withdrawal of thyroid supplements. A modern alternative to thyroxine withdrawal is the use of recombinant TSH.
- For medullary and anaplastic thyroid carcinoma, thyroid labs and radioiodine imaging are of no utility. Contrast CT can be used for these cases. Serum calcitonin is useful for following medullary thyroid cancer.
- For patients with MEN 2 syndrome, annual screening for hyperparathyroidism and pheochromocytoma are necessary.

References

Bal C, Padhy AK, Jana S et al. (1996) Prospective randomized clinical trial to evaluate the optimal dose of ^{131}I for remnant ablation in patients with differentiated thyroid carcinoma. Cancer 77:2574–2580

Besic N, Vidergar-Kralj B, Frkovic-Grazio S et al. (2003) The role of radioactive iodine in the treatment of Hürthle cell carcinoma of the thyroid. Thyroid 13:577–584

Biermann M, Pixberg MK, Schuck A et al. (2003) Multicenter study differentiated thyroid carcinoma (MSDS). Diminished acceptance of adjuvant external beam radiotherapy. Nuklearmedizin 42:244–250

Bilimoria KY, Bentrem DJ, Linn JG et al. (2007) Utilization of total thyroidectomy for papillary thyroid cancer in the United States. Surgery 142:906–913; discussion 913 e1–2

Brierley J, Tsang R, Panzarella T et al. (2005) Prognostic factors and the effect of treatment with radioactive iodine and external beam radiation on patients with differentiated thyroid cancer seen at a single institution over 40 years. Clin Endocrinol (Oxf) 63:418–427

Cady B, Rossi R (1988) An expanded view of risk-group definition in differentiated thyroid carcinoma. Surgery 104:947–953

Chatal JF, Campion L, Kraeber-Bodere F et al. (2006) Survival improvement in patients with medullary thyroid carcinoma who undergo pretargeted anti-carcinoembryonic-antigen radioimmunotherapy: a collaborative study with the French Endocrine Tumor Group. J Clin Oncol 24:1705–1711

Chow SM, Law SC, Mendenhall WM et al. (2002) Papillary thyroid carcinoma: prognostic factors and the role of radioiodine and external radiotherapy. Int J Radiat Oncol Biol Phys 52:784–795

Chow SM, Yau S, Kwan CK et al. (2006) Local and regional control in patients with papillary thyroid carcinoma: specific indications of external radiotherapy and radioactive iodine according to T and N categories in AJCC 6th edition. Endocr Relat Cancer 13:1159–1172

De Crevoisier R, Baudin E, Bachelot A et al. (2004) Combined treatment of anaplastic thyroid carcinoma with surgery, chemotherapy, and hyperfractionated accelerated external radiotherapy. Int J Radiat Oncol Biol Phys 60:1137–1143

DeGroot LJ, Kaplan EL (1991) Second operations for "completion" of thyroidectomy in treatment of differentiated thyroid cancer. Surgery 110:936–939; discussion 939–940

Ezzat S, Sarti DA, Cain DR et al. (1994) Thyroid incidentalomas. Prevalence by palpation and ultrasonography. Arch Intern Med 154:1838–1840

Farahati J, Reiners C, Stuschke M et al. (1996) Differentiated thyroid cancer. Impact of adjuvant external radiotherapy in patients with perithyroidal tumor infiltration (stage pT4). Cancer 77:172–180

Fersht N, Vini L, A'Hern R et al. (2001) The role of radiotherapy in the management of elevated calcitonin after surgery for medullary thyroid cancer. Thyroid 11:1161–1168

Foote RL, Brown PD, Garces YI et al. (2003) Is there a role for radiation therapy in the management of Hürthle cell carcinoma? Int J Radiat Oncol Biol Phys 56:1067–1072

Ford D, Giridharan S, McConkey C et al. (2003) External beam radiotherapy in the management of differentiated thyroid cancer. Clin Oncol (R Coll Radiol) 15(6):337–341

Frates MC, Benson CB, Charboneau JW et al. (2005) Management of thyroid nodules detected at US: Society of Radiologists in Ultrasound consensus conference statement. Radiology 237:794–800

Greene FL, Page DL, Fleming ID et al. (2002) American Joint Committee on Cancer, American Cancer Society. AJCC Cancer Staging Manual, 6th edn. Springer-Verlag, Berlin Heidelberg New York

Hay ID, Bergstralh EJ, Goellner JR et al. (1993) Predicting outcome in papillary thyroid carcinoma: development of a reliable prognostic scoring system in a cohort of 1779 patients surgically treated at one institution during 1940 through 1989. Surgery 114:1050–1057; discussion 1057–1058

Hay ID, Grant CS, Bergstralh EJ et al. (1998) Unilateral total lobectomy: is it sufficient surgical treatment for patients with AMES low-risk papillary thyroid carcinoma? Surgery 124:958–964; discussion 964–966

Hilditch TE, Dempsey MF, Bolster AA et al. (2002) Selfstunning in thyroid ablation: evidence from comparative studies of diagnostic ^{131}I and ^{123}I. Eur J Nucl Med Mol Imaging 29:783–788

Hundahl SA, Fleming ID, Fremgen AM et al. (1998) A National Cancer Data Base report on 53,856 cases of thyroid carcinoma treated in the US, 1985–1995. Cancer 83:2638–2648

Kim JH, Leeper RD (1983) Treatment of anaplastic giant and spindle cell carcinoma of the thyroid gland with combination Adriamycin and radiation therapy. A new approach. Cancer 52:954–957

Kim JH, Leeper RD (1987) Treatment of locally advanced thyroid carcinoma with combination doxorubicin and radiation therapy. Cancer 60:2372–2375

Lee N, Tuttle M (2006) The role of external beam radiotherapy in the treatment of papillary thyroid cancer. Endocr Relat Cancer 13:971–977

Mazzaferri EL (1993) Management of a solitary thyroid nodule. N Engl J Med 328:553–559

Mazzaferri EL, Jhiang SM (1994) Long-term impact of initial surgical and medical therapy on papillary and follicular thyroid cancer. Am J Med 97:418–428

Mirallie E, Vuillez JP, Bardet S et al. (2005) High frequency of bone/bone marrow involvement in advanced medullary thyroid cancer. J Clin Endocrinol Metab 90:779–788

Nutting CM, Convery DJ, Cosgrove VP et al. (2001) Improvements in target coverage and reduced spinal cord irradiation using intensity-modulated radiotherapy (IMRT) in patients with carcinoma of the thyroid gland. Radiother Oncol 60:173–180

O'Connell ME, A'Hern RP, Harmer CL (1994) Results of external beam radiotherapy in differentiated thyroid carcinoma: a retrospective study from the Royal Marsden Hospital. Eur J Cancer 30A:733–739

Orlandi F, Caraci P, Berruti A et al. (1994) Chemotherapy with dacarbazine and 5-fluorouracil in advanced medullary thyroid cancer. Ann Oncol 5:763–765

Posner MD, Quivey JM, Akazawa PF et al. (2000) Dose optimization for the treatment of anaplastic thyroid carcinoma: a comparison of treatment planning techniques. Int J Radiat Oncol Biol Phys 48:475–483

Quayle FJ, Moley JF (2005) Medullary thyroid carcinoma: including MEN 2A and MEN 2B syndromes. J Surg Oncol 89:122–129

Saad MF, Ordonez NG, Rashid RK et al. (1984) Medullary carcinoma of the thyroid. A study of the clinical features and prognostic factors in 161 patients. Medicine (Baltimore) 63:319–342

Schwartz DL, Rana V, Shaw S et al. (2008) Postoperative radiotherapy for advanced medullary thyroid cancer – local disease control in the modern era. Head Neck 30:883–888

Sherman SI, Brierley JD, Sperling M et al. (1998) Prospective multicenter study of thyrois carcinoma treatment: initial analysis of staging and outcome. National Thyroid Cancer Treatment Cooperative Study Registry Group. Cancer 83:1012–21

Shimaoka K, Schoenfeld DA, DeWys WD et al. (1985) A randomized trial of doxorubicin versus doxorubicin plus cisplatin in patients with advanced thyroid carcinoma. Cancer 56:2155–2160

Simpson WJ, Carruthers JS (1978) The role of external radiation in the management of papillary and follicular thyroid cancer. Am J Surg 136:457–460

Simpson WJ, Panzarella T, Carruthers JS et al. (1988) Papillary and follicular thyroid cancer: impact of treatment in 1578 patients. Int J Radiat Oncol Biol Phys 14:1063–1075

Singer PA, Cooper DS, Daniels GH et al. (1996) Treatment guidelines for patients with thyroid nodules and well-differentiated thyroid cancer. American Thyroid Association. Arch Intern Med 156:2165–2172

Sosa JA, Bowman HM, Tielsch JM et al. (1998) The importance of surgeon experience for clinical and economic outcomes from thyroidectomy. Ann Surg 228:320–330

Tallroth E, Wallin G, Lundell G et al. (1987) Multimodality treatment in anaplastic giant cell thyroid carcinoma. Cancer 60:1428–1431

Tan GH, Gharib H (1997) Thyroid incidentalomas: management approaches to nonpalpable nodules discovered incidentally on thyroid imaging. Ann Intern Med 126:226–231

Tielens ET, Sherman SI, Hruban RH et al. (1994) Follicular variant of papillary thyroid carcinoma. A clinicopathologic study. Cancer 73:424–431

Tsang RW, Brierley JD, Simpson WJ et al. (1998) The effects of surgery, radioiodine, and external radiation therapy on the clinical outcome of patients with differentiated thyroid carcinoma. Cancer 82:375–388

Tubiana M, Haddad E, Schlumberger M et al. (1985) External radiotherapy in thyroid cancers. Cancer 55[9 Suppl]:2062–2071

Udelsman R (2008) Is total thyroidectomy the procedure of choice for papillary thyroid cancer? Nat Clin Pract Oncol 5:184–185

Udelsman R, Lakatos E, Ladenson P (1996) Optimal surgery for papillary thyroid carcinoma. World J Surg 20:88–93

Venkatesh YS, Ordonez NG, Schultz PN et al. (1990) Anaplastic carcinoma of the thyroid. A clinicopathologic study of 121 cases. Cancer 66:321–330

Vezzosi D, Bennet A, Caron P (2007) Recent advances in treatment of medullary thyroid carcinoma. Ann Endocrinol (Paris) 68:147–153

Witt RL (2008) Initial surgical management of thyroid cancer. Surg Oncol Clin N Am 17:71–91, viii

Wu LT, Averbuch SD, Ball DW et al. (1994) Treatment of advanced medullary thyroid carcinoma with a combination of cyclophosphamide, vincristine, and dacarbazine. Cancer 73:432–436

Yeung SC, She M, Yang H et al. (2007) Combination chemotherapy including combretastatin A4 phosphate and paclitaxel is effective against anaplastic thyroid cancer in a nude mouse xenograft model. J Clin Endocrinol Metab 92:2902–2909

Section II:
Breast Cancer

Breast Cancer

Manjeet Chadha

CONTENTS

M. Chadha, MD
Department of Radiation Oncology, Beth Israel Medical Center, 10 Union Square East, Suite 4G, New York, NY 10003, USA

Introduction and Objectives

Worldwide breast cancer incidence accounts for approximately 25% of all cancers diagnosed in women and almost 15% of all cancer deaths. It is one of the most common malignancies in the Western world and has the highest incidence in North America. The breast cancer risk varies within age groups; for example, the risk from birth to 39 years is one in 229 (0.44%), from age 40–59 years one in 24 (4.14%), from age 60–70 years one in 13 (7.53%), and from birth to death the probability of developing breast cancer is one in seven (13.4%) (Jemal et al. 2007).

The evolution in the management of breast cancer often serves as a model for conservative therapy in cancer care allowing organ preservation. Further managing breast cancer also illustrates the importance of multidisciplinary care and the need to have a team of specialists to achieve better clinical outcomes.

In most instances, the local and regional extent of disease is treated by surgery and/or radiation therapy (RT). The distant disease risk is treated by systemic therapy including chemotherapy, endocrine therapy, biologic therapy, or any combination of these agents. A discussion that provides an opportunity for shared-decision-making with the patient is an important step towards arriving at the best treatment approach for any given patient. To achieve this goal, ▷

patient awareness and education of treatment options and clinical outcomes is very important. In many States in the US the physicians are required by law to discuss treatment options of breast-conserving surgery plus RT and modified radical mastectomy with eligible patients.

This chapter examines the recommendations for:

● Breast cancer diagnosis and staging
● Treatment of:
  – Stage 0 (DCIS, LCIS)
  – Stage I through Stage IIB (T1-2, N0-1)
  – Stage IIB (T3N0) and Stage III
● Radiation treatment delivery
● Follow-up and screening guidelines

8.1 Diagnosis, Staging, Risk Factors, and Prognostic Factors

8.1.1 Diagnosis

Initial Evaluation

■ Initial evaluation requires a complete medical history and physical examination. The medical history will include a detailed history pertaining of the breast cancer and associated risk factors. A complete physical examination with special attention to the breast exam and draining lymph nodes must be performed. The breast exam should be completed both in sitting and supine positions.

■ Most patients who present with early-stage breast cancer are asymptomatic and the cancer is detected by screening mammography. In other instances, patients may present with a palpable breast lump, and rarely report bloody nipple discharge as the only presenting symptom. Inflammatory breast cancer, which is an aggressive sub-type, presents with a cluster of clinical symptoms including erythema and an inflammatory type of reaction with skin edema (peau d'orange). Paget's disease presents with an eczematoid change involving the nipple areola and associated mass or bloody nipple discharge.

Laboratory Tests

■ Initial laboratory tests should include a complete blood count, basic blood chemistry, liver function tests, and BUN/creatinine.

Imaging Studies

■ Mammography and ultrasonography are the most commonly used diagnostic imaging techniques. With ongoing studies and accumulating clinical experience, there is an emerging role for breast MRI in selected cases (Level I) (Lord et al. 2007).

■ Breast imaging reporting data system (BI-RAD) is a radiographic classification of mammographic lesions and is the established standard for reporting findings on mammogram (Table 8.1).

■ Breast MRI requires a special coil to obtain high-resolution high-contrast images. Due to its high sensitivity and low specificity, MRI screening is used in selected high-risk patient populations which include young women with previous diagnosis of breast cancer, patients with known genetic mutations, known LCIS, history of lymphoma with prior RT, occult breast cancer with a biopsy-proven axillary lymph node, and patients with augmentation or reconstruction using implants (Kriege et al. 2004; Lehman et al. 2007).

■ Body CT scan is indicated in patients presenting with locally advanced disease. When available, FDG-PET scans or PET/CT can be ordered for staging and documenting metastatic disease.

Table 8.1. The breast imaging reporting and data system (BI-RADS). [From American College of Radiology (2003) with permission]

Category	Assessment	Recommendation
0	Incomplete study	Need additional imaging and/or prior mammograms for comparison
1	Negative	Routine screening
2	Benign findings	Routine screening
3	Probably benign findings	Initial short-interval follow-up to establish stability
4	Suspicious abnormality	Biopsy should be considered
5	Highly suggestive of malignancy	Appropriate action should be taken
6	Known, suggestive of malignancy	Appropriate action should be taken

■ Bone scan is an optional study and only performed when there are symptoms related to the skeletal system or in patients with advanced stage of disease. Liver scans are optional studies that are obtained when there is questionable abnormality detected on CT scan or on liver chemistry.

Pathology

■ Prior to initiating any treatment, a pathologic diagnosis of cancer must be confirmed. This is usually obtained by performing a fine-needle aspirate or core-needle biopsy. The palpable or sonographically identified lesions are subjected to ultrasound guided biopsies; a stereotactic-guided biopsy is performed for non-palpable lesions and MRI-directed biopsies for lesions detected on MRI alone.

■ A thorough pathology evaluation and standardized reporting is an essential component of treating breast cancer. The College of American Pathologists' (CAP) protocols for reporting the pathology of all breast specimens is recommended to ensure standardized reporting of pathology findings. The reference for the CAP template is available through the CAP website (*www.cap.org*).

■ Request for biomarkers that include estrogen receptors (ER), progesterone receptors (PR), and HER-2 status should be stated at the time of pathology review.

■ The multifocal or multicentric nature of the disease described in the pathology report is an important factor in deciding optimal local treatment. A lesion is defined to be 'multifocal' when multiple foci of cancer are identified within the same quadrant. 'Multicentric' disease is defined when foci of cancer are noted in multiple quadrants of the breast.

8.1.2 Staging

■ The American Joint Committee on Cancer (AJCC) revised the breast cancer staging in 2002. The sixth edition of the Cancer Staging Manual includes the most current TNM staging system used for breast cancer (GREENE et al. 2002).

■ The goals of the revised staging were to categorize patients within uniform cohorts for better assessment of prognosis and treatment (Table 8.2).

8.1.3 Risk Factors

■ The exact etiology of breast cancer is unknown; however, there are a number of genetic and acquired risk factors that have been associated with a higher incidence of the disease.

■ *Gender:* The female gender is at risk. The female:male ratio is 100:1 (JEMAL et al. 2007).

■ *Age:* The incidence of breast cancer increases with advancing years. However, the patients of younger age have a worse prognosis.

■ *Race:* There is a five-fold difference in the incidence of breast cancer in Western countries compared to Japan, Thailand, and India where the incidence tends to be very low. Breast cancer survival rates in African American and Hispanic populations is lower than in Caucasian women. Young age, advanced stage, and poor pathology risk factors are more often seen in African American women (MOORMEIER 1996).

■ *Hormonal milieu:* Early menarche, late menopause, nulliparity, late primi, and exogenous unopposed estrogens in premenopausal women are some of the factors associated with a higher risk of developing breast cancer.

■ The use of oral contraceptives and the risk of breast cancer has been studied in a large meta-analysis trial (COLLABORATIVE GROUP ON HORMONAL FACTORS IN BREAST CANCER 1996) The analysis of 54 studies including 53,297 women with breast cancer and 100,239 women without breast cancer noted the following results:
  – A modest increase in the risk of breast cancer was observed with oral contraceptive use.
  – The risk of breast cancer decreased to background levels after 10 years of discontinuation of contraception use.
  – The limitations of the study were that it was based on clinical data on oral contraceptive pills with the hormone dose that is no longer recommended. It is believed that the more recent use of lower dose oral contraceptive pills may not be associated with this increased risk.

■ The risk from hormone replacement therapy (HRT) was studied in the 16,608 postmenopausal women who participated in the Women's Health Initiative Study Group (WRITING GROUP FOR THE WOMEN'S HEALTH INITIATIVE INVESTIGATORS 2002). The study randomization was between HRT and placebo. At a mean follow-up of 5.2 years they observed a 26% increased risk of developing

Table 8.2. American Joint Committee on Cancer (AJCC) TNM classification of carcinoma cancer of breast. [From GREENE et al. (2002)]

Primary tumor (T)	
TX	Primary tumor cannot be assessed
T0	No evidence of primary tumor
Tis	Carcinoma in situ
Tis (DCIS)	Ductal carcinoma in situ
Tis (LCIS)	Lobular carcinoma in situ
Tis (Paget's)	Paget's disease of the nipple with no tumor
T1	Tumor 2 cm or less in greatest dimension
T1mic	Microinvasion 0.1 cm or less in greatest dimension
T1a	Tumor more than 0.1 cm but not more than 0.5 cm in greatest dimension
T1b	Tumor more than 0.5 cm but not more than 1 cm in greatest dimension
T1c	Tumor more than 1 cm but not more than 2 cm in greatest dimension
T2	Tumor more than 2 cm but not more than 5 cm, in greatest dimension
T3	Tumor more than 5 cm in greatest dimension
T4	Tumor of any size with direct extension to (a) chest wall or (b) skin, only as described below
T4a	Extension to chest wall, not including pectoralis muscle
T4b	Edema (including peau d'orange) or ulceration of the skin of the breast, or satellite skin nodules confined to the same breast
T4c	Both T4a and T4b
T4d	Inflammatory carcinoma
Regional lymph nodes (N)	
NX	Regional lymph nodes cannot be assessed (e.g., previously removed)
N0	No regional lymph node metastasis
N1	Metastasis to movable ipsilateral axillary lymph node(s)
N2	Metastases in ipsilateral axillary lymph nodes fixed or matted, or in clinically apparent ipsilateral internal mammary nodes in the absence of clinically evident axillary lymph node metastasis
N2a	Metastasis in ipsilateral axillary lymph nodes fixed to one another (matted) or to other structures
N2b	Metastasis only in clinically apparent ipsilateral internal mammary nodes and in the absence of clinically evident axillary lymph node metastasis
N3	Metastasis in ipsilateral infraclavicular lymph node(s) with or without axillary lymph node involvement, or in clinically apparent ipsilateral internal mammary lymph node(s) and in the presence of clinically evident axillary lymph node metastasis; or metastasis in ipsilateral supraclavicular lymph node(s) with or without axillary or internal mammary lymph node involvement
N3a	Metastasis in ipsilateral infraclavicular lymph node(s)
N3b	Metastasis in ipsilateral internal mammary lymph node(s) and axillary lymph node(s)
N3c	Metastasis in ipsilateral supraclavicular lymph node(s)
Distant metastasis (M)	
MX	Distant metastasis cannot be assessed
M0	No distant metastasis
M1	Distant metastasis
STAGE GROUPING	
0:	Tis N0 M0
I:	T1* N0 M0
IIA:	T0 N1 M0, T1* N1 M0, T2 N0 M0
IIB:	T2 N1 M0, T3 N0 M0
IIIA:	T0 N2 M0, T1* N2 M0, T2 N2 M0, T3 N1 M0, T3 N2 M0
IIIB:	T4 N0 M0, T4 N1 M0, T4 N2 M0
IIIC:	Any T N3 M0
IV:	Any T Any N M1

* includes T1 mic

breast cancer among the women receiving HRT compared with placebo. When prescribing HRT, an individualized evaluation of the risk:benefit ratio should be carefully evaluated.

- *Previous history of breast cancer:* Results in approximately a five-fold increase in the risk of developing another cancer.
- *Radiation exposure:* Previous radiation exposure is known to increase the risk of breast cancer with a latency period of 15–20 years (BHATIA et al. 1996; YAHALOM et al. 1992).
- *Family history:* There is a two- to three-fold increased incidence of breast cancer when there is a history of a first-degree relative having breast cancer. This incidence rises to ten-fold among women where the mother and sister was affected with breast cancer.
- *Genetic mutations:* Hereditary mutations account for approximately 10% of all breast cancers diagnosed, while in the other 85%–90% of patients the breast cancer is a sporadic event (GARBER and OFFIT 2005; MARTIN and WEBER 2000). BRCA1/BRCA2 carriers are at high risk of developing breast cancer at a younger age. The lifetime breast cancer risk among BRCA carriers may range from 50%–85%. Further studies evaluating the impact of genetic mutations among the general breast cancer population still need to be pursued.
- *Diet and obesity:* It is suggested that the incidence of breast cancer may be related to environmental and dietary factors that are rich in animal fat (CHLEBOWSKI et al. 2006).
- *History of proliferative breast disease/benign disease:* Women who have a history of hyperplasia and lobular carcinoma in situ are at an increased risk of developing breast cancer. Lobular carcinoma in situ is markedly known to increase the risk of subsequent invasive breast cancer (8- to 11-fold).

Table 8.3. 5-Year survival by stage of disease. [From BALCH et al. (2002) with permission]

Stage	5-Year survival
0	100%
I	98%
IIA	88%
IIB	76%
IIIA	56%
IIIB, IIIC	49%
IV	16%

8.1.4 Prognostic Factors

- The individualized treatment plan for any given patient should be based on prognostic factors.
- The stage at diagnosis is the most important prognostic factor (Table 8.3).
- Axillary lymph node status remains an independent predictor of patient outcome.
- Histology and grade of the primary tumor has prognostic significance. The prognosis of invasive lobular is similar to invasive ductal, whereas subtypes including tubular, medullary, and mucinous have a more favorable prognosis.
- Tumor hormone receptor and HER-2 status are prognostic factors that also influence treatment.
- Patient age and menopausal status also influence outcome.
- Cancer genomic analysis evaluating the contribution of 16 cancer related genes in the patients own tumor appears to have prognostic and predictive value.

8.2 Management of Stage 0 Disease

- Stage 0 breast cancer includes ductal carcinoma in situ and lobular carcinoma in situ (HARRIS 2004; SILVERSTEIN 1997; SILVERSTEIN and LAGIOS 2006). The diagnosis of in-situ cancer is generally made on mammography. With the widespread use of screening mammography there is an increase in the overall incidence of in-situ lesions. Approximately 20% of all breast cancers diagnosed are in situ.

8.2.1 Lobular Carcinoma In Situ (LCIS)

- The biologic behavior of LCIS illustrates that this lesion is associated with an increased risk for bilateral breast cancer. The incidence of subsequent breast cancer among women with LCIS is 20%–25% when followed over a duration of 15 years (HAAGENSEN et al. 1981).
- Pleomorphic LCIS has been recognized as an aggressive variant that has a greater potential for progressing to invasive cancer (ANDERSON et al. 2006). In the future, a better understanding of the natural history supported by clinical evidence from outcome data on histologic variants of LCIS might influence our treatment recommendations.

Therapy Recommendations for LCIS

■ With a diagnosis of LCIS preventive interventions for risk reduction of subsequent cancer events is recommended (Grade A); the diagnosis is also an indication for following screening guidelines in high-risk patients (Grade A).

■ Risk reduction may be achieved by either of the following:
  – Chemoprevention strategy using tamoxifen or raloxifene (Grade A).
  – No local treatment for the breast per se is indicated, however, the option of bilateral mastectomy through individualized risk assessment under special circumstances like BRCA1/2 mutations or strong family history (Grade B) may be performed.

■ The benefit of chemoprevention was evaluated in the NSABP-P1 tamoxifen trial (NSABP-P1, Level I) (FISHER et al. 2005), which randomized healthy patients at high risk of breast cancer to receive placebo vs. tamoxifen for 5 years. Among all patients receiving tamoxifen the relative risk of invasive and non-invasive breast cancer was reduced by 49% and 50%, respectively. Among the 13,388 women enrolled in the study, 826 had LCIS. At a follow up of 69 months, a 56% reduction in the incidence of invasive cancer in the LCIS patient group was observed. Results from the STAR trial conducted by the NSABP randomized patients between tamoxifen and raloxifene (NSABP-P2; Level I) (VOGEL et al. 2006). They observed both agents to be effective in reducing second cancer events. Based on these results, tamoxifen in the premenopausal patient and raloxifene in the postmenopausal patient is an effective therapeutic intervention for risk reduction in women with LCIS.

8.2.2   Ductal Carcinoma In Situ (DCIS)

■ DCIS arises from the ductal epithelium. This histologic pattern includes comedo and non-comedo subtypes. The non-comedo subtypes described are micropapillary, papillary, cribriform, and solid.

■ With a diagnosis of DCIS, the subsequent risk of infiltrating duct cell cancer is increased by eight to ten-fold. This risk is higher with comedo histology (Level IV) (WARD et al. 1992).

■ Van Nuys classification of DCIS is based on nuclear grade and presence of comedo necrosis (Grade C). Group 1 is non-high grade without necrosis; Group 2, non-high grade with necrosis; and Group 3, high grade. Risk of recurrence is lowest in Group 1 and highest in Group 3 (Level IV) (SILVERSTEIN 2003).

■ Unlike LCIS, DCIS tends to be more unilateral than bilateral.

■ The poor prognostic variables for DCIS include young age, positive or close margins of resection, high nuclear grade, necrosis, and size of the lesion.

Therapy Recommendations for DCIS

General

■ Patients with a diagnosis of DCIS who have mammographically-detected calcifications should have a post-lumpectomy, pre-RT mammogram to establish the new baseline, and also to document whether there is any radiographic evidence of residual calcifications.

■ *Local treatment* options in the management of DCIS include:
  – Lumpectomy with adjuvant RT (Grade A). The goal of lumpectomy is to remove the tumor with associated microcalcifications in its entirety and achieve negative surgical margins.
  – Lumpectomy alone (Grade B).
  – Total mastectomy with/without sentinel lymph node biopsy with/without reconstruction (Grade B).

Role of RT

■ NSABP B-17 is a phase III study that randomized patients between lumpectomy and lumpectomy plus 50 Gy RT. A total of 391 patients were treated by lumpectomy alone, while 399 patients received RT following lumpectomy. Patients with all subtypes of DCIS benefited from RT with an overall recurrence rate of 16% at 12-years follow-up compared to 32% among the observation group. Approximately 50% of the recurrence had in-situ histology and the other 50% had invasive recurrences (NSAPB B-17, Level I) (FISHER et al. 1998b).

■ The limitations of the NSAPB B-17 study are that the margin width was not reported and data on post-lumpectomy mammograms documenting removal of all radiographic microcalcifications was not routinely performed.

- A prospective phase III clinical trial completed by the European Organization of Research and Treatment of Cancer (EORTC) randomized 1010 patients with DCIS with documented negative margins on lumpectomy to receive 50 Gy RT vs. observation (BIJKER et al. 2006). At 4-year follow-up they reported benefit of RT with a lower recurrence rate of 9% among the irradiated patients compared with 16% in the observation group (EORTC 108-53, Level I) (BIJKER et al. 2006).

Role of Observation After Lumpectomy

- Observation after lumpectomy has been studied in a recent multi-institutional ECOG 5194 single-arm prospective study. In this study, patients with low risk DCIS were treated with lumpectomy alone. The results identified a favorable subset as patients with low- to intermediate-grade DCIS with median tumor size of 6 mm and a clear margin width of 5–10 mm. At 5 years, the local recurrence rate for this group was 6.8% compared to 13.7% among those with small high-grade DCIS. The results suggest that there may be a select group of patients with DCIS who may be observed following lumpectomy (ECOG 5194, Level II) (HUGHES et al. 2006).
- Retrospective studies evaluating patients with DCIS treated by excision alone suggests that there is an incremental improvement in local control by achieving large, clear margins on excision. It may be possible to select subgroups of DCIS who are at low risk for recurrence and may not benefit from the administration of RT at initial diagnosis (Level IV) (MACDONALD et al. 2005). However, a recent study completed by WONG et al. (2006) noted otherwise. Among a favorable group of patients with grade 1 or 2 DCIS $\leq$2.5 cm on mammogram and with negative resection margins >1 cm a relatively high local failure rate of 12% at 5 years was observed (Level IV).

Role of Tamoxifen

- The NSABP B-24 trial aimed to study the effect of tamoxifen in the prevention of tumor recurrence or secondary breast cancer in patients treated for DCIS (FISHER et al. 1999). RT was used for post-operative adjuvant treatment. In this trial, 1804 women with the diagnosis of DCIS were treated with lumpectomy and RT. This was followed by randomization to placebo vs. tamoxifen at a dose of 20 mg daily for 5-years. A total of 902 women received tamoxifen and 902 women were observed. The margins of resection were positive in 16% of the patients enrolled in this study. At 7-year follow-up, they reported an overall reduction in cancer events when tamoxifen was used. In the ipsilateral breast the recurrence rate decreased from 11% to 8% and in the contralateral breast the reduction in cancer events reduced from 4.9% to 2.3% (NSABP B-24, Level I) (FISHER et al. 1999).

- In a subsequent publication, the response to tamoxifen with respect to the ER status was evaluated. In ER-positive patients, tamoxifen resulted in a 59% reduction of all breast cancer events, whereas in ER-negative patients, only a 20% reduction was observed (Level I) (ALLRED et al. 2002).

- The UK COORDINATING COMMITTEE ON CANCER RESEARCH (2003) completed a four-arm randomized trial. Patients were randomized after lumpectomy with negative margins to observation vs. RT alone vs. tamoxifen alone vs. tamoxifen and RT. The study enrolled 1701 patients and reported failure rates observed at a median follow-up of 53 months The results on reported local relapse rates were 22%, 18%, 8%, and 6% for patients enrolled to no treatment, tamoxifen alone, RT alone, and both RT and tamoxifen, respectively. Patients receiving any RT had a 6% relapse rate compared to 14% relapse for patients receiving no RT (UKCCCR, Level I).

8.2.3 Radiation Therapy Dose Fraction Schedule

- All the level I data evaluating the efficacy of RT in the management of DCIS used whole breast RT fields.
- The recommended RT is conventionally delivered in opposed tangential fields to the ipsilateral breast.
- Irradiation of the regional nodal areas is not required because the risk of nodal metastasis is low.
- The dose of RT to whole breast is 45–50 Gy in 1.8–2.0 Gy fractions. An additional 10–16 Gy dose is delivered to the boost. Generally, the boost volume includes the surgical bed with a 1.5–2-cm margin.
- Field arrangements, simulation, and dosimetric considerations are detailed in Section 8.5.

8.3 Management of Stage I Through Stage IIB Diseases

8.3.1 General Therapy Principles

- The standard of care in breast-conserving therapy (BCT) includes adjuvant radiation after lumpectomy (Grade A). The efficacy of postoperative RT after lumpectomy has been repeatedly demonstrated through various prospective randomized trials (Table 8.4). A number of Phase III randomized trials have shown that lumpectomy and axillary dissection, followed by RT is equivalent to modified radical mastectomy. BCT is the preferred treatment option for the majority of patients with early-stage invasive breast cancer and allows for organ preservation (Grade A).
- The value of RT following lumpectomy in the elderly population has been studied in Phase III trials completed in North America. In the early results, RT does not appear to improve overall survival, but its use is noted to significantly improve local control (Grade A).
- The logistical problems associated with conventional ERT include a protracted time commitment from the patient, commuting issues for those women who live at great distances from the hospital/centers has led investigators to study alternative accelerated dose fraction schedules. Partial breast irradiation is delivered to the lumpectomy volume only by using either brachytherapy or conformal external beam RT (ERT) therapy technique (Grade B). Early results suggest the safety and efficacy of using partial breast irradiation in carefully selected patients.
- Accelerated whole breast RT using varied dose fraction schedules has been investigated in Canada and Europe. Early outcome data suggest that a large fraction size is well tolerated by the breast and may be safely used to administer an accelerated schedule resulting in an overall shorter course of treatment (Grade B).

8.3.2 Treatment Recommendations for Stage I Through Stage IIB

Breast-Conserving Therapy vs. Mastectomy

- As noted in Table 8.4 (VERONESI et al. 2002; FISCHER et al. 2002b; BLICHERT-TOFT et al. 1992; ARRIAGADA et al. 1996; JACOBSON et al. 1995;

Table 8.4. Lumpectomy and whole breast RT vs. mastectomy

Institution	Years	Patients (n)	Overall survival (%)	Follow-up years
Milan	1973–1980	349 (M)	Same	@ 20 years
		352 (Q + XRT)		
NSABP-B06	1976–1984	590 (M)	Same	@ 20 years
		629 (L + XRT)		
Danish Breast Cancer	1983–1987	429 (M)	82%	@ 6 years
Cooperative Group		430 (L + XRT)	79%	
Institut Gustave-Roussy	1972–1979	91 (M)	65%	@ 15 years
Breast Cancer Group		88 (L + XRT)	73%	
NCI	1980–1986	116 (M)	75%	@ 10 years
		121 (L + XRT)	77%	
EORTC 10801	1980–1986	426 (M)	63%	@ 8 Years
		456 (L + XRT)	58%	

Q, Quadrantectomy; M, mastectomy; L, lumpectomy; XRT, whole breast external beam RT.

van Dongen et al. 2000) and the meta-analysis by the Early Breast Cancer Trialists' Collaborative Group (1995), there is established level I evidence that notes that BCT is equivalent to mastectomy. However, mastectomy is performed when BCT is clinically contraindicated or when mastectomy is the patient's preference. The clinical contraindications to BCT include multicentricity, unfavorable ratio of tumor size to breast, advanced-stage disease, pregnancy, and collagen vascular disease. Even though we have robust supporting evidence on the use of BCT for early stage disease, a significant number of patients still undergo a modified radical mastectomy. This is primarily attributed to lack of patient education and awareness of treatment options, as well as management influenced by surgeon bias (Morrow et al. 2001; American College of Surgeons Report).

Administering a Boost After Whole Breast RT

■ Most radiation oncologists administer a boost with electrons and, on occasion, with photons to administer a higher dose to the lumpectomy site with the objective of improving local control (Bartelink et al. 2001; Antonini et al. 2007; Romestaing et al. 1997). Boost irradiation to the tumor bed is recommended after whole breast RT (Grade A).

■ The EORTC conducted a randomized trial to evaluate the impact of additional RT dose to the lumpectomy site. The study enrolled 5569 patients with stage I and II disease. All patients underwent a lumpectomy with negative margins and were randomized to receive 50 Gy ERT to breast vs. 50 Gy ERT to breast and 16 Gy boost. The boost treatment was associated with a lower recurrence rate of 4.3% vs. 7.3% among patients receiving no boost. The maximum benefit of boost dose was observed in the younger women aged ≤40 years (EORTC 22881–10882, Level I) (Bartelink et al. 2001; Antonini et al. 2007). Another randomized boost vs. no boost trial was conducted in Lyon. In this study, patients received 50 Gy whole breast RT followed by randomization to receive 10 Gy boost vs. no boost. A total of 1024 patients with tumors less than 3 cm were enrolled. At a median follow-up of 3 years the local relapse rate in the boost arm was 3.6% compared to 4.5% in the non-boost arm. No difference in the cosmesis was observed

between the two groups (Level I) (Romestaing et al. 1997).

Patient Selection for Safely Eliminating RT

■ Adjuvant RT is currently recommended in all patients after lumpectomy, regardless of the size of the primary disease, age of patient, and hormonal receptor (Grade A). A number of studies have focused on whether we can identify subsets of patients in whom RT may be safely eliminated.

■ NSABP B21 evaluated the potential for eliminating post-lumpectomy ERT for very small invasive tumors and ER-positive patients receiving antiestrogen therapy. The study enrolled 1009 patients with tumor size ≤ 1 cm. The randomization following lumpectomy was tamoxifen vs. placebo and RT vs. tamoxifen and RT. At 8-years median follow-up, the study results reported RT and tamoxifen to have the lowest relapse rate at 2.8%; the RT and placebo had a local relapse rate of 9.3% and tamoxifen alone had a local relapse rate of 16.5% (NSABP –B21, Level I) (Fisher et al. 2002a).

In a study limited to post-menopausal patients, women over the age of 50 years, with stage I/II disease irrespective of ER status, were randomized following lumpectomy to receive tamoxifen and RT vs. tamoxifen alone. The study enrolled 769 patients. The 5-year local failure rate was much lower when treating with RT and tamoxifen as compared to tamoxifen alone, 0.6% vs. 7.7% ($p<0.001$). The findings of the study illustrate a high local failure rate with a short follow-up establishing RT as the recommended treatment after lumpectomy (Level I) (Fyles et al. 2004).

■ The objective of the CALGB C9343/INT trial was to evaluate the role of post-lumpectomy RT in the elderly. The study enrolled 636 patients over the age of 70 years with ER-positive stage T1N0 disease. Following lumpectomy, patients were randomized to tamoxifen alone vs. tamoxifen and RT. At 5-year follow-up they observed statistically significant differences with a lower recurrence rate when both tamoxifen and RT were used, 1% vs. 4% ($p< 0.001$). However, no difference in survival was observed between the two groups. When treating the very elderly, one could consider individualizing the risk benefits of adjuvant treatment with regards to the patient's overall health and co-morbidities (CALGB C9343, Level I) (Hughes et al. 2004).

Accelerated Partial Breast Irradiation

■ Although RT to the whole breast is considered the standard treatment course, administering partial breast irradiation may be an effective treatment (Grade B) (McCormick 2005). Accelerated partial breast irradiation (APBI) can significantly reduce the overall treatment time of adjuvant RT, and its efficacy has been shown in non-randomized trials.

■ A Phase II trial that included 199 patients with early stage cancer treated all patients with partial breast brachytherapy. Using either high-dose-rate (HDR) or low-dose-rate (LDR) brachytherapy. Matched-pair analysis with women treated with whole breast RT was performed. At a median follow-up of 65 months, the local failure rate was 1% and the results observed were comparable to those achieved with whole breast RT (Level III) (Vicini et al. 2003).

■ The RTOG completed a Phase II trial of brachytherapy alone following lumpectomy for stage I/II breast cancer. Following lumpectomy and axillary dissection, patients either received a dose of 34 Gy in ten fractions over 5 days through HDR brachytherapy treatments or 45 Gy over 3.5–5 days using LDR brachytherapy. They reported an overall actuarial survival of 93% and less than 1% local failure per year (Level III) (Arthur et al. 2006).

■ There is an ongoing phase III randomized prospective trial, i.e., RTOG 0413/NSABP B39 (Radiation Therapy Oncology Group 2004). The eligible patients include stage 0–II breast cancer, all histologic subtypes are eligible. Patients with up to three positive nodes are allowed to enroll. The randomization is between whole breast RT 45–50 Gy followed by a boost delivering 60–66 Gy to the lumpectomy site and partial breast irradiation with either brachytherapy technique delivering 34 Gy in ten fractions or 3D external beam partial breast treatment delivering 3.85 Gy in ten fractions. The study is projected to enroll in excess of 3000 patients.

Accelerated Whole Breast Radiation Therapy

■ One of the limitations of the accepted ERT treatment is that it requires patients to receive at least a 6-week course of RT on a daily schedule from Monday through Friday. Published Phase III reports suggest that a large fraction size is well tolerated by the breast and may be safely used to administer an accelerated schedule resulting in an overall shorter course of treatment (Grade B) (Whelan et al. 2002; Dewar et al. 2007). However, longer follow-up and more clinical data need to be acquired. Whelan et al. (2002) randomly assigned 1234 women to receive either the "long" arm (*n* = 612) delivering 50 Gy in 25 fractions over 35 days, or the "short" arm (*n* = 622) delivering 42.5 Gy in 16 fractions over 22 days (2.65 Gy per day). At a median follow-up of 69 months, the 5-year local recurrence-free survival was 97.2% in the short RT arm and 96.8% in the long RT arm. The local breast recurrence rates reported at 5 years were 2.87% and 2.9% (*p* = 0.83), respectively. Overall and disease-free survival was also equivalent (Level I).

Radiation Therapy Dose Fraction Schedule

■ All the level I data evaluating the efficacy of RT in the management of early-stage invasive breast cancer used whole breast RT fields.

■ The recommended RT is conventionally delivered in opposed tangential fields to the ipsilateral breast.

■ Irradiation of the regional nodal areas is indicated when there is significant burden of metastatic disease in the lymph nodes.

■ The dose of RT to whole breast is 45–50 Gy in 1.8–2.0-Gy fractions. Boost volume is generally defined as the lumpectomy cavity plus a 1.5–2-cm margin. Another 10- 16 Gy boost is prescribed for a total dose of 60–66 Gy at the lumpectomy site. The dose to the regional nodes, when indicated, is in the range of 50 Gy.

Alternative dose fraction schedules are used for patients participating in protocols.

■ Field arrangements, simulation, and dosimetric considerations are detailed in Section 8.5.

8.4   Radiation Therapy Techniques for the Intact Breast

Treatment Technique and Field Arrangements

■ *Breast irradiation:* Radiation therapy is conventionally delivered using opposed tangential fields to the ipsilateral breast. A volume-based dosimetric plan should be evaluated in all cases. Therefore, CT simulation is recommended (Grade A). This would assure adequate coverage of target and maximize sparing and limiting the dose to lung and heart. A recent phase III study has very nicely illustrated the benefit of minimizing hot spots within the target volume (Level I) (DONOVAN et al. 2007; PIGNOL 2006). Achieving homogenous dose distribution may require using wedges or intensity-modulated RT with forward planning or inverse planning technique.

■ *Boost:* The lumpectomy boost volume includes the lumpectomy cavity with a 1.5- to 2-cm margin. The most commonly used beam for boost is the electrons, on occasion, when treating deep-seated cavity photons may be used. There is limited experience using brachytherapy for boost.

■ *Regional nodes:* In a negative axilla or an adequately dissected axilla with low residual tumor burden (1–3 positive nodes) may not require the addition of an RT field that targets the lymph node bearing area. This added radiation field is associated with increased morbidity and lack of clear evidence of therapeutic benefit. On the other hand, if a patient has 1–3 positive nodes and the axillary dissection is inadequate, i.e., only a limited number of nodes (6 or less) are removed, or following a positive sentinel lymph node, a formal axillary dissection is not performed. The plan should include RT to the regional lymph node. Also, when more than 4 nodes are positive RT to regional lymph nodes should be planned.

Dose Fraction Schedule

■ The most commonly used fraction schedule to the whole breast is 45–50 Gy in 1.8–2.0 Gy per fraction. This is followed by boost treatment. Generally, a dose of another 10–16 Gy boost is prescribed for a total dose of 60–66 Gy to the lumpectomy site. When indicated, the lymph node stations are treated using a supraclavicular field with or without a posterior axilla boost field. The prescribed dose to the regional nodes is in the range of 50 Gy in 1.8–2.0 Gy fractions.

8.5 Management of Locally Advanced (Stage IIB and III) Diseases

8.5.1 General Therapy Principles

■ For locally advanced disease the optimal treatment of local, regional, and systemic risk of breast cancer, requires a multimodality approach.
■ Among operable patients, generally the surgical procedure for the primary tumor and draining lymph nodes is performed upfront, followed by adjuvant chemotherapy, hormone therapy, and RT based on individualized risk.
■ Among patients with large tumors neoadjuvant chemotherapy may facilitate operability.

8.5.2 Surgery

■ Patients presenting with large tumors undergo modified radical mastectomy with a level I/II axillary dissection. In this category, only patients presenting with unifocal breast cancer and favorable tumor-to-breast ratio may be candidates for a breast-conserving operation that includes a lumpectomy and axillary dissection.

8.5.3 Adjuvant Radiation Therapy After Mastectomy

■ Following mastectomy, patients with locally advanced-stage disease are at a substantial risk for local and regional recurrence when left untreated (TAGHIAN et al. 2004; KATZ et al. 2000; NIELSEN et al. 2006). Locoregional relapse is a challenging problem for the patient and clinician alike. On average, the probability of controlling a localized relapse is 50%.
■ Postmastectomy RT (PMRT) has consistently been shown to improve local regional control of disease (Grade A). The EARLY BREAST CANCER TRIALISTS' COLLABORATIVE GROUP (2005b) completed a meta-analysis of 78 randomized trials that included over 42,000 women. In all these studies one of the treatment arms included postoperative RT. The results noted an improvement in local control when RT was used and reported

a 17%–19% benefit from RT at 5-years. The added absolute benefit of RT was also noted among patients receiving chemotherapy. The 15-year overall survival noted an absolute benefit of RT in the order of 5.3% after BCT and 4.4% after mastectomy and axillary dissection. These benefits were noted among all age groups, tumor grade, nodal status, and receptor status (EBCTCG RT, Level I).

■ PMRT is routinely indicated for patients presenting with stage T3/4 tumor, more than four axillary lymph nodes with evidence of metastases, or when the lymph node metastasis has extracapsular extension and positive margins on mastectomy (Grade A). HARRIS et al. (1999), RECHT et al. (2001), and TAGHIAN et al. (2004) systemically reviewed clinical data on 5758 lymph node-positive breast cancers that were treated with mastectomy and had enrolled in one of the five listed NSABP trials (B15, B16, B18, B22, B25). The majority of isolated failures involved either the chest wall or the supraclavicular nodes. The significant clinical factors associated with a risk of local recurrence in the range of 25% were ≥ four positive nodes, tumors greater than 5 cm, young age (below 40 years), and suboptimal axillary dissection < six nodes retrieved (Level I).

■ At least three randomized studies have also shown a survival advantage in addition to the benefit in locoregional control, although others do not illustrate that conclusion:
The Danish Breast Cooperative Group reported on the impact of PMRT on 1708 premenopausal patients with stage II and III breast cancer. At 10-year follow-up, the addition of PMRT to chemotherapy had a local failure rate of 9% compared with 32% without PMRT. They also reported a significant improvement in disease-free survival and overall survival at 34% and 45% compared to 48% and 54%, respectively (Level I) (OVERGAARD et al. 1997). In the postmenopausal population, a similar magnitude of benefit of RT over tamoxifen alone on local control disease-free survival, and overall survival was reported in 1375 women with stage II and III disease. The common critique of these results is focused on the low median number of lymph nodes reported in the axillary dissection (Level I) (OVERGAARD et al. 1999).
A similar experience reported by the British Columbia Trial (RAGAZ et al. 2005) limited to premenopausal patients reported the benefit of PMRT administered to the chest wall and regional nodes. At a median follow-up of 14.5 years, significant improvements in local control, disease-free survival, and overall survival were observed in favor of RT with chemotherapy over chemotherapy alone. The most significant benefit was seen in the 1–3 lymph node-positive group with extracapsular spread (Level I).

8.5.4 Radiation Therapy Technique for Postmastectomy RT

Treatment Technique and Field Arrangements

■ *Chest wall irradiation:* RT is commonly delivered using opposed tangential fields to encompass the ipsilateral chest wall. A volume-based dosimetric plan should be evaluated in all cases. Therefore, CT simulation is recommended. This would assure adequate coverage of target while limiting the dose to lung and heart.
Achieving homogenous dose distribution may require using wedges or intensity-modulated RT with forward planning or inverse planning technique.

■ *Boost:* There is no consensus on whether the mastectomy scar should receive a boost. Most contemporary techniques do not use scar boost.

■ *Regional nodes:* If the axilla is adequately dissected and there is no extracapsular extension, the residual tumor burden from metastatic disease in the axilla may not justify the addition of an RT field to include the axilla. RT field overlapping an adequately dissected axilla is associated with increased morbidity and with little supplemental therapeutic benefit. On the other hand, if the patient has had an inadequate axillary dissection, or there is evidence of extracapsular extension, the lateral border of the supraclavicular field includes the axilla with intent to treat. The lymph node stations are treated using an anterior supraclavicular field with or without a posterior axilla boost field. The internal mammary nodes (IMN) can be encompassed by using deep tangential beam with blocks or a separate matched IMN field may be used.

Dose Fraction Schedule

- The most commonly used dose fraction schedule to the chestwall and regional node is 50 Gy in 1.8–2.0 Gy per fraction.
- For patients treated with BCT, a dose of another 10–16 Gy boost is prescribed for a total dose of 60–66 Gy to the lumpectomy site.

8.6 Chemotherapy

Adjuvant Chemotherapy

- For high-risk disease, chemotherapy is associated with improved overall survival, disease-free survival, and local control. This has been repeatedly demonstrated for this group of patients by prospective randomized trials (Grade A) (HARRIS 2004; EARLY BREAST CANCER TRIALISTS' COLLABORATIVE GROUP 2005a). Detailed discussions of these trials are beyond the scope of this chapter.
- For early stage the clinical data shows that, although systemic therapy improves local control, it does not obviate the role of RT in patients with early-stage invasive ductal carcinoma (Grade A). In a randomized trial from Europe which enrolled 585 patients with stage I/II breast cancer, T size < 4 cm, and negative margins of resection, patients were randomized to lumpectomy vs. lumpectomy and RT. All patients were then prescribed systemic therapy. ER-negative patients received CMF (cyclophosphamide, methotrexate, fluorouracil 5FU) chemotherapy and ER-positive patients received tamoxifen. The patients that received lumpectomy and adjuvant systemic therapy alone had a local failure rate of 24.5% vs. 5.8% among the patients who also received RT ($p<0.01$) (Scottish Trial, Level I) (FORREST et al. 1996).
- The EBCTCG completed a meta-analysis on chemo-/hormone therapy (EARLY BREAST CANCER TRIALISTS' COLLABORATIVE GROUP 2005a). This meta-analysis included 194 randomized trials. The results reported a benefit to using anthracycline-based chemotherapy and hormone therapy in the ER-positive patients. Patients who received an anthracycline-containing chemotherapy regimen for at least 6 months experienced a reduction in breast cancer mortality by 38% and 20% among the premenopausal and postmenopausal women, respectively. Tamoxifen of 5 years' duration is more effective than the shorter 1- to 2-year course. The absolute benefits at 5 years without chemotherapy were 12% and with chemotherapy 11% (EBCTCG chemo/HT; Level I).

- NSABP B-31 included high-risk HER-2 positive breast cancer patients who were randomized and received either adriamycin, cyclophosphamide and paclitaxel, or the same chemotherapy plus trastuzumab. Results on 3351 patients reported that the trastuzumab arm had a better 3-year disease-free survival and overall survival at 87% and 94% compared to 75% and 92% for the patients who received chemotherapy alone However, trastuzumab was associated with a higher cardiac toxicity (NSABP B-31 & NCCTG N9831, Level I) (ROMOND et al. 2005).

Sequencing of Chemotherapy and Radiation Therapy

- When patients are advised RT, the scheduled RT generally begins 3–4 weeks after the last chemotherapy cycle. Further, for patients receiving herceptin, radiotherapy course can be administered concomitantly.
- The sequencing of chemotherapy and RT may impact the first site of failure but is not known to influence overall outcome (Grade A). In patients with close or positive surgical margins, if re-excision is not feasible, RT should be considered prior to chemotherapy. In a prospective randomized trial which enrolled 244 patients with stage I/II disease, patients were randomized to receive either four cycles of anthracycline-based chemotherapy followed by RT, or initial RT followed by the same the chemotherapy regimens. At 11-year follow-up, no difference in the overall survival, distant metastases, between the two arms was observed. Patients with clinical close margins seemed to benefit from receiving the RT first. The local recurrence with RT first was 4% compared to 32% with chemotherapy first. Patients with positive margins experienced similar local failure rates of 20%–23% (Level I) (RECHT et al. 2004).

Sequencing of Chemotherapy and Surgery

■ Although chemotherapy is usually delivered following surgery, no difference was observed in outcome between pre- vs. postoperative chemotherapy. The NSABP B-18 trial enrolled 1523 patients and randomized all cases to four cycles of pre- or postoperative chemotherapy using four cycles of doxorubicin and cyclophosphamide (AC regimen). The results of this prospective randomized trial showed that no difference can be found in overall survival and disease-free survival between patients treated in either sequence at 9 years. However, those treated with preoperative AC chemotherapy achieved a higher rate of BCT when the size of the primary tumor at presentation was > 5 cm (NSABP B-18, Level I) (FISHER et al. 1998).

Neoadjuvant Chemotherapy

■ Neoadjuvant chemotherapy is often used to address the systemic risk upfront, as well as to assess response to the chemotherapy regimen prescribed. Effective cytoreduction might obviate the need for a modified radical mastectomy (Grade A). Neoadjuvant chemotherapy converts mastectomy to BCT in 20%–30% of cases; CR and PR rates on neoadjuvant therapy range between 20%–40% and 10%–20%, respectively. BCT may be appropriate among patients achieving a good response to neoadjuvant chemotherapy. In the NSABP-B 18 trial, the women randomized to the neoadjuvant arm had 12% more lumpectomies resulting in BCT (NSABP B-18, Level I) (FISHER et al. 1998).

■ Multiple retrospective reviews have reported the feasibility of BCT for advanced stage disease. CHEN et al. (2004) completed a retrospective review on 340 patients who received neoadjuvant chemotherapy followed by BCT. With appropriate selection, this sequencing can offer breast conservation with acceptable local failure rates of 5% at 5 years (Level IV). KUERER et al. (1999) also reported on 372 patients diagnosed as having locally advanced disease. All patients received four cycles of neoadjuvant AC. They reported a better outcome for patients who had experienced at least a partial response to chemotherapy. The 5-year overall survival was 89% among the responders compared to 64% among non-responders (Level IV).

8.7 Post-Therapy Follow-Up Guidelines

■ Follow-up after treatment of breast cancer is recommended for all patients (Grade D). Ideally, follow-up of patients should be performed by a multidisciplinary team.

■ The recommended follow-up schedule is as follows: every 3–6 months for years 1–3; every 6 months for years 4 and 5, and annually thereafter.

■ Each follow-up visit requires an interval history and a physical examination that includes a breast exam. Follow-up mammograms are obtained 6 months after completion of therapy is performed. Subsequent mammograms are obtained annually. A short follow-up mammogram may be obtained on a case-by-case basis and is at the discretion of the radiologist. Dedicated MRI breast follow-up may be used in selected situations, i.e., when the patient is identified as being at high risk, has dense breast on mammogram, or is a carrier of BRCA mutations.

■ Other imaging studies are obtained only if clinical history and physical findings warrant this.

References

Allred D, Bryant J, Land S et al. (2002) Estrogen receptor expression as a predictive marker of effectiveness of tamoxifen in the treatment of DCIS: findings from the NSABP Protocol B-24. Breast Cancer Res Treat 76:S36, (abstract 30)

American College of Radiology (2003) Breast imaging reporting and data system (BI-RADs), 4th edn. American College of Radiology, Reston, VA

Anderson BO, Calhoun KE, Rosen EL et al. (2006) Evolving concepts in the management of lobular hyperplasia. J Natl Compr Canc Netw 4:511–522

Antonini N, Jones H, Horiot J et al. (2007) Effect of age and radiation dose on local control after breast conserving treatment. EORTC trial 22881–10882. Radiother Oncol 82:265–271

Arriagada R, Le MG, Rochard F et al. (1996) Conservative treatment versus mastectomy in early breast cancer: patterns of failure with 15 years of follow up data. Institut Gustave-Roussy Breast Cancer Group. JCO 14:1558–1564

Arthur DW, Winter K, Kuske RR et al. (2006) A phase II trial of brachytherapy alone following lumpectomy for select breast cancer: tumor control and survival outcomes of RTOG 95–17. Int J Radiat Oncol Biol Phys 66:S29–30 [suppl] (abstract 51)

Balch CM et al. (2002) Breast cancer. In: Greene FL, Page DL, Fleming ID et al. (eds) AJCC Cancer staging manual, 6th edn. Springer, Berlin Heidelberg New York, pp 209–220

Bartelink H, Horiot JC, Poortsmans P et al. (2001) Recurrence rates after treatment of breast cancer with standard radiotherapy with or without additional radiation. N Engl J Med 245:1378–1387

Bhatia S, Robison LL, Oberlin O et al. (1996) Breast cancer and other second neoplasms after childhood Hodgkin's disease. N Engl J Med 334:745–751

Bijker N, Meijnen P, Peterse JL et al. (2006) Breast-conserving treatment with or without radiotherapy in ductal carcinoma-in-situ: ten-year results of European Organization for Research and Treatment of Cancer randomized phase III trial 10853 – a study by the EORTC Breast Cancer Cooperative Group and EORTC Radiotherapy Group. J Clin Oncol 24:3381–3387

Blichert-Toft M, Rose C, Andersen JA et al. (1992) Danish randomized trial comparing breast conservation therapy with mastectomy: six years of life-table analysis. Danish Breast Cancer Cooperative Group. J Natl Cancer Inst Monogr 11:19–25

Chen AM, Meric-Bernstam F, Hunt KK et al. (2004) Breast conservation after neoadjuvant chemotherapy: the MD Anderson experience. J Clin Oncol 22:2303–2312

Chlebowski RT, Blackburn GL, Thomson CA et al. (2006) Dietary fat reduction and breast cancer outcome: interim efficacy results from the Women's Intervention Nutrition Study. J Natl Cancer Inst 98:1767–1776

Collaborative Group on Hormonal Factors in Breast Cancer (1996) Breast Cancer and hormonal contraceptives: collaborative reanalysis of individual data on 53,297 women with breast cancer and 100,239 women without breast cancer from 54 epidemiological studies. Lancet 347:1713–1727

Dewar JA, Haviland JS, Agrawal RK et al. (2007) Hypofractionation for early breast cancer: first results of the UK standardization of breast radiotherapy (START) trials [Abstract]. J Clin Oncol ASCO annual meeting Proceedings Part I; 25(18s) (June 20 Supplement):LBA518

Donovan E, Bleakley N, Denholm E et al. (2007) Randomised trial of standard 2D radiotherapy (RT) versus intensity modulated radiotherapy (IMRT) in patients prescribed breast radiotherapy. Radiother Oncol 82:254–264

Early Breast Cancer Trialists' Collaborative Group (1995) Effects of radiotherapy and surgery in early breast cancer. An overview of the randomized trials. N Engl J Med 333:1444–1455

Early Breast Cancer Trialists' Collaborative Group (2005a) Effects of chemotherapy and hormonal therapy for early breast cancer on recurrence and 15-year survival: an overview of the randomized trials. Lancet 365:1687–1717

Early Breast Cancer Trialists' Collaborative Group (2005b) Effects of radiotherapy and of differences in the extent of surgery for early breast cancer on local recurrence and 15-year survival: an overview of the randomized trials. Lancet 366:2087–2106

Fisher B, Bryant J, Wolmark N, Mamounas E, Brown A, Fisher ER, Wickerham DL, Begovic M, DeCillis A, Robidoux A, Margolese RG, Cruz AB Jr, Hoehn JL, Lees AW, Dimitrov NV, Bear HD (1998a) Effect of preoperative chemotherapy on the outcome of women with operable breast cancer. J Clin Oncol 16:2672–2685

Fisher B, Dignam JJ, Wolmark N et al. (1998b) Lumpectomy and radiation therapy for the treatment of intraductal breast cancer: findings from the National Surgical Adjuvant Breast and Bowel Project B-17. J Clin Oncol 16:441–452

Fisher B, Dignam JJ, Wolmark N et al. (1999) Tamoxifen in treatment of intraductal breast cancer: National Surgical Adjuvant Breast and Bowel Project B-24 randomized control trial. Lancet 353:1993–2000

Fisher B, Bryant J, Dignam JL et al. (2002a) Tamoxifen, radiation therapy, or both for prevention of ipsilateral breast tumor recurrence after lumpectomy in women with invasive breast cancers of one centimeter or less. N Engl J Med 20:4141–4149

Fisher B, Anderson S, Bryant J et al. (2002b) Twenty year follow up of a randomized trial comparing total mastectomy, lumpectomy, and lumpectomy plus irradiation for the treatment of invasive breast cancer. N Engl J Med 347:1233–1241

Fisher B, Costantino JP, Wickerman DL et al. (2005) Tamoxifen for prevention of breast cancer: report of the National Surgical Adjuvant Breast and Bowel Project P-1 Study. J Natl Cancer Inst 97:1652–1662

Forrest AP, Stewart HJ, Everington D et al. (1996) Randomized controlled trial of conservation therapy for breast cancer: 6 year analysis of the Scottish trial. Lancet 348:708–713

Fyles AW, McCready DR, Manchul LA et al. (2004) Tamoxifen with or without breast irradiation in women 50 years of age or older with early breast cancer. N Engl J Med 351:963–970

Garber JE, Offit K (2005) Hereditary cancer predisposition syndromes. J Clin Oncol 23:276–292

Greene F, Page D, Fleming I et al. (2002) AJCC Cancer Staging Manual, 6th edn. Springer, Berlin Heidelberg New York

Haagensen CD, Bodian C, Haagensen DE Jr. (1981) Breast carcinoma. Risk and detection. W. B. Saunders, Philadelphia, PA

Harris JR (2004) Diseases of the breast. Lippincott Williams and Wilkins, Philadelphia

Harris JR, Halpin-Murphy P, Neese MM et al. (1999) Consensus statement on post mastectomy radiation therapy. Int J Radiat Oncol Biol Phys 44:989–990

Hughes KS, Schnaper LA, Berry D et al. (2004) Lumpectomy plus tamoxifen with or without irradiation in women 70 years of age or older with early stage breast cancer. N Engl J Med 351:971–977

Hughes L, Wong M, Page D et al. (2006) Five year results of an intergroup study E 5194: local excision alone (without radiation treatment) for selected patients with ductal carcinoma in situ. San Antonio Breast Cancer Symposium, abstract 29

Jacobson JA, Danforth DN, Cowan KH et al. (1995) Ten-year

results of a comparison of conservation with mastectomy in the treatment of stage I and II breast cancer. N Engl J Med 332:907–911

Jemal A, Siegel R, Ward E (2007) Cancer statistics, 2007. CA Cancer J Clin 57:43–66

Katz A, Strom EA, Buchholz TA et al. (2000) Locoregional recurrence patterns after mastectomy and doxorubicin-based chemotherapy: implications for postoperative irradiation. J Clin Oncol 18:2817–2827

Kriege M, Brekelmans C, Boetes C et al. (2004) Efficacy of MRI and mammography for breast cancer screening in women with a familial or genetic predisposition N Engl J Med 351:427

Kuerer HM, Newman LA, Smith TL et al. (1999) Clinical course of breast cancer patients with complete pathological primary tumor and axillary lymph nodes response to doxorubicin-based neoadjuvant chemotherapy. J Clin Oncol 14:460–469

Lehman C, Gatsonis C, Kuhl CK et al. (2007) MRI evaluation of the contralateral breast in women with recently diagnosed breast cancer. N Engl J Med 356:1295–1303

Lord SJ, Lei W, Craft P et al. (2007) A systematic review of the effectiveness of magnetic resonance imaging (MRI) as an addition to mammography and ultrasound in screening young women at high risk of breast cancer. Eur J Cancer 43:1905–1917

MacDonald HR, Silverstein MJ, Mabry H et al. (2005) Local control in ductal carcinoma in situ treated by excision alone: incremental benefit of larger margins. Am J Surg 190:521–525

Martin AM, Weber BL (**2000**) Genetic and hormonal risk factors in breast cancer. J Natl Cancer Inst 92:1126–1135

McCormick B (2005) Partial breast radiation for early stage breast cancers: hypothesis, existing data, and a planned phase III trial. J Natl Compr Canc Netw 3:301–307

Moormeier J (1996) Breast cancer in black women. Ann Intern Med 124:897–905

Morrow M, White J, Moughan J et al. (2001) Factors predicting the use of breast-conserving therapy in stage I and II breast carcinoma. J Clin Oncol 19:2254–2262

Nielsen HM, Overgaard M, Grau C et al. (2006) Study of failure pattern among high-risk breast cancer patients with or without postmastectomy radiotherapy in addition to adjuvant systemic therapy: long term results from the Danish breast Cancer Cooperative Group DBCG 82b and c randomized studies. J Clin Oncol 24:2268–2275

Overgaard M, Hansen PS, Overgaard J et al. (1997) Postoperative radiotherapy in high-risk premenopausal women with breast cancer who receive adjuvant chemotherapy. Danish Breast cancer Cooperative Group DBCG 82b Trial. N Engl J Med 337:949–955

Overgaard M, Jensen MB, Overgaard J et al. (1999) Postoperative radiotherapy in high risk postmenopausal breast cancer patients given adjuvant tamoxifen: Danish Breast cancer Cooperative Group DBCG 82c randomized trial. Lancet 353:1641–1648

Pignol J-P, Olivotto E, Rakovitch WE et al. (2006) Phase III randomized study of intensity modulated radiation therapy vs. standard wedging adjuvant breast radiotherapy. Int J Rad Oncol Bio Phys 66:S1

Radiation Therapy Oncology Group (2007) National Surgical Adjuvant Breast and Bowel Project B-39/Radiation Therapy Oncology Group 0413 Protocol. A randomized phase III study of conventional whole breast irradiation (WBI) versus partial breast irradiation (PBI) for women with stage 0, I, or II breast Cancer. http://www.rtog.org/members/protocols/0413/0413.pdf

Ragaz J, Olivotto I, Spinelli J et al. (2005) Locoregional radiation therapy in patients with high-risk breast cancer receiving adjuvant chemotherapy: 20 year results of the British Columbia randomized trial. J Natl Cancer Inst 97:116–126

Recht A, Edge SB, Solin LJ et al. (2001) Postmastectomy radiotherapy: guidelines of the American society of Clinical Oncology. J Clin Oncol 19:1539–1569

Recht A, Gome SE, Henderson IC et al. (2004) Impact on outcome of delay in starting radiotherapy. J Clin Oncol 22:1341–1342

Romestaing P, Lehingue Y, Carrie C et al (1997) Role of 10 Gy boost in the conservative treatment of early stage breast cancer: results of a randomized trial. J Clin Oncol 15:963–968

Romond EH, Perez EA, Bryant J et al. (2005) Trastuzumab plus adjuvant chemotherapy for operable HER2-positive breast cancer. N Engl J Med 353:1673–1684

Silverstein MJ (ed) (1997) Ductal carcinoma in situ of the breast. Williams & Wilkins, Baltimore

Silverstein MJ (2003) The University of Southern California/Van Nuys prognostic index for ductal carcinoma in situ of the breast. Am J Surg 186:337–343

Silverstein MJ, Lagios M (**2006**) Should all patients undergoing breast conserving therapy for DCIS receive radiation therapy? J Surg Oncol **95:605–609**

Taghian A, Jeong JH, Mamounas E et al. (2004) Patterns of locoregional failure in patients with operable breast cancer treated by mastectomy and adjuvant chemotherapy with or without tamoxifen and without radiotherapy: results from five National Surgical Adjuvant Breast and Bowel Project randomized clinical trials. J Clin Oncol 22:4247–4254

UK Coordinating Committee on Cancer Research (2003) Radiotherapy and tamoxifen in women with completely excised ductal carcinoma in situ of the breast in UK, Australia, and New Zealand: randomized controlled trial. Lancet 362:95–102

van Dongen JA, Voogd AC, Fentiman IS et al. (2000) Long-term results of a randomized trial comparing breast-conserving therapy with mastectomy: European organization for research and treatment of cancer 10801 trial. J Natl Cancer Inst 92:1143–1150

Veronesi U, Cascinelli N, Mariani L et al. (2002) Twenty year follow up of a randomized study comparing breast-conserving surgery with radical mastectomy for early breast cancer. N Engl J Med 347:1227–1232

Vicini FA, Kestin L, Chen P et al. (2003) Limited-field radiation therapy in the management of early stage breast cancer. J Natl Cancer Inst 95:1205–1211

Vogel VG, Costantino JP, Wickerman DL et al. (2006) Effects of tamoxifen vs raloxifene on risk of developing invasive breast cancer and other disease outcomes: the NSABP study of Tamoxifen and Raloxifene (STAR) P-2 trial. JAMA 295:2727–2741

Ward BA, McKhann CF, Ravikumar TS. et al. (1992) Ten-year follow-up of breast carcinoma in situ in Connecti-cut. Arch Surg 127:1392–1395

Whelan T, MacKenzie R, Julian J et al. (2002) Randomized trial of breast irradiation schedules after lumpectomy for women with lymph node-negative breast cancer. J Natl Cancer Inst 94:1143–50

Wong JS, Kaelin CM, Troyan SL et al. (2006) Prospective study of wide excision alone for DCIS of the breast. J Clin Oncol 24:1031–1036

Writing group for the Women's Health Initiative Investiga-tors (2002) Risk and benefits of estrogen plus progestin in healthy postmenopausal women; principal results from the women's Health initiative randomized control trial. JAMA 288:321–333

Yahalom J, Petrek JA, Biddinger PW et al. (1992) Breast can-cer in patients irradiated for Hodgkin's disease: a clini-cal and pathologic analysis of 45 events in 37 patients. J Clin Oncol 10:1674–1681

Section III:
Tumors of the Thorax

Non-Small Cell Lung Cancer

Jiade J. Lu and Ron R. Allison

CONTENTS

Introduction and Objectives

Non-small-cell lung cancer (NSCLC), unless in its earliest stage, is a systemic disease that requires multidisciplinary management. Accurate staging is crucial to determine resectability as resection is currently the best means to prolong survival. The gold standard for resectable disease remains surgery, though equivalent outcomes appear possible for selected T1N0/T2N0 lesions treated by radiosurgery. Patients with stage IB disease and beyond benefit from adjuvant chemotherapy. Those with stage III disease require concurrent chemoradiation. In addition, innovative interventions are needed for these individuals as outcomes remain poor in this subgroup.

This chapter examines:

- Recommendations for diagnosis and staging procedures

- The staging system and prognostic factors

- Treatment recommendations as well as the supporting scientific evidence for definitive and adjuvant treatment for early stage resectable NSCLC

- The use of combined chemotherapy and radiotherapy for definitive treatment of locally advanced disease

- Systemic chemotherapy and palliative radiation for metastatic disease

- Follow-up care and surveillance of survivors

J. J. Lu, MD, MBA
Department of Radiation Oncology, National University Cancer Institute of Singapore, National University Health System, National University of Singapore, 5 Lower Kent Ridge Road, Singapore 119074, Singapore
R. R. Allison, MD
Department of Radiation Oncology, The Brody School of Medicine at ECU, 600 Moye Blvd., Greenville NC, 27834, USA

9.1 Diagnosis, Staging, and Prognosis

9.1.1 Diagnosis

Initial Evaluation

- Diagnosis and evaluation of NSCLC starts with a complete history and physical examination (H&P). Presenting signs and symptoms depend on the location and extent of the tumor.
- Attention should be paid to tobacco use, exposure to environmental carcinogens, weight loss, bone pain, neurologic signs, and NSCLC-associated paraneoplastic syndromes. Although paraneoplastic syndromes are comparatively uncommon in NSCLC, squamous cell carcinoma of the lung may present with hypercalcemia due to parathyroid-like hormone production. Adenocarcinoma of the lung may be associated with clubbing and hypertrophic pulmonary osteoarthropathy and the Trousseau syndrome of hypercoagulability.
- Thorough physical examination should be performed to exclude atelectasis, pleural effusion, airway obstruction, hepatomegaly, supraclavicular and neck lymphadenopathy, and in particular, neurologic symptoms.

Laboratory Tests

- Initial laboratory tests should include a complete blood count, basic serum chemistry, liver function tests, renal function tests, alkaline phosphatase, and lactate dehydrogenase (LDH). Serum LDH is prognostically important in NSCLC.
- Adequate pulmonary function is required when lobectomy, pneumonectomy, or definitive dose

Table 9.1. Imaging and laboratory work-ups for NSCLC

Imaging studies	Laboratory tests
– PET/CT or FDG-PET scan – MRI or CT of brain with contrast (optional for stage I and II) – Chest X-ray – CT of chest/upper abdomen – Bone scan (optional)	– Complete blood count – Serum chemistry – Liver function tests – Renal function tests – Alkaline phosphatase – LDH – Pulmonary function tests

radiation therapy is attempted. However, tumor obstruction may provide a falsely low FEV_1. In these cases curative radiation/chemoradiation is still possible and recommended (BECKLES et al. 2003).

Imaging Studies

- A PET/CT scan is recommended (Grade A). Diagnostic imaging studies are required to evaluate the extent of the disease in the thorax as well as distant metastasis. Contrast CT of the brain, neck, thorax, and abdomen with bone scan may be used as substituted, but is inferior to PET/CT.
- Mediastinoscopy and biopsy is indicated for lymph nodes greater than 1.0 cm in shortest transverse axis or positive on FDG-PET (Grade B). CT alone is not adequate for detecting mediastinal lymphadenopathy. Prospective evaluation of CT and mediastinoscopy in mediastinal lymph node staging revealed the sensitivity, specificity, and accuracy of CT was 63%, 57%, and 59%, respectively; therefore, CT alone is not adequate for mediastinal staging (Level III) (GDEEDO et al. 1997). A lymph node is considered normal if its short axis is < 1 cm on CT. Results from a large retrospective study showed metastasis was found in 20% of mediastinal lymph nodes < 1.5 cm in shortest diameter (Level IV) (DE LEYN et al. 1997).
- FDG-PET/CT scan is optimal for staging as it is more specific and sensitive than CT alone for detecting distant metastasis and mediastinal lymphadenopathy (Grade A). Results from a prospective study for the impact of FDG-PET on preoperative staging of NSCLC showed the sensitivity and specificity of PET for the detection of both mediastinal and distant metastatic disease was 95% and 83%, respectively, significantly higher than those from CT alone (Level III) (PIETERMAN et al. 2000). In addition, results from a prospective randomized study revealed the addition of FDG-PET scan significantly reduced the number of unnecessary thoracotomies (PLUS multicentre trial, Level I) (VAN TINTEREN et al. 2002).
- Brain CT or MRI is not routinely indicated for stage I and II NSCLC, but should be used when signs and symptoms of brain metastases are present. When definitive surgery or chemoradiation is indicated for stage III disease, brain CT or MRI should be considered (Grade B). Asymptomatic

brain metastases occur in approximately 30% of stage II and III patients within 2 years after diagnosis. When compared to CT, MRI did not show a higher preoperative detection rate in patients without neurologic symptoms. The detection rate for patients with stage I or II NSCLC was 4%, and that for stage III disease was 11.4% (Level III) (YOKOI et al. 1999).

■ A bone scan is unnecessary for staging when FDG-PET is performed (Grade B). The accuracy in detecting bone metastasis by FDG-PET was 96% versus 66% by bone scan in a retrospective series (Level IV) (BURY et al. 1998). Furthermore, results from a small prospective nonrandomized trial which included 53 patients with small-cell lung cancer or advanced stage NSCLC showed that FDG-PET is the most accurate method for detecting bone metastasis compared to bone scan and SPECT (Level III) (SCHIRRMEISTER et al. 2001).

■ Isolated adrenal or liver mass on CT, abdominal ultrasound, or PET/CT may require biopsy for pathologic confirmation of metastasis for patients otherwise considered curable due to the risk of false positive results (Grade B) (PORTE et al. 1999).

■ Table 9.1 lists the recommended laboratory and imaging tests for the evaluation and staging of NSCLC.

Pathology

■ Pathologic confirmation of NSCLC is imperative prior to the initiation of any treatment. Tissue for pathologic diagnosis can be obtained via fine-needle biopsy of the primary tumor, sputum cytology, or from a metastasis including a pleural effusion.

Approximately 80% of centrally located tumors can be diagnosed with sputum cytology (with three samples), but the yield is only 20% for small peripheral lesions.

■ Bronchoscopy or CT-guided biopsies are generally successful to gain histologic diagnosis in virtually all patients. Mediastinoscopy is suggested to avoid futile surgeries for unresectable patients.

A Chamberlain procedure may be used to stage AP window nodes.

■ When a pleural effusion is observed, a thoracentesis is indicated to rule out malignant pleural effusion.

9.1.2 Staging

■ NSCLC can be staged clinically and pathologically. Clinical staging utilizes information from H&P, imaging studies, and laboratory tests; pathologic staging is based on findings from clinical staging and procedures such as mediastinoscopy, thoracentesis, thoracoscopy, and examination of the resected specimen.

■ The 2007 American Joint Committee on Cancer Tumor Node Metastasis (TNM) staging system is presented in Table 9.2 (GREENE et al. 2002).

9.1.3 Prognostic Factors

■ The prognosis of patients with NSCLC is directly associated with presenting characteristics. Advanced pretreatment stage, poor performance status, and weight loss of 10% or more within 6 months prior to the diagnosis are the most important adverse prognostic factors in NSCLC (GREENE et al. 2002; STANLEY 1980).

■ The pathologic subtype of NSCLC (i.e., squamous cell carcinoma, adenocarcinoma, and large cell undifferentiated carcinoma) is not prognostically important, especially in locally advanced disease. Nevertheless, adenocarcinoma has a higher propensity to metastasize to the brain.

■ For stage I and II diseases, the size of the primary tumor is prognostically important (GROOME et al. 2007).

■ Malignant pleural or pericardial effusion is associated with poor prognosis. Although staged as T4 disease in the current TNM staging system, the prognoses of patients with malignant pleural or pericardial effusion is similar to those with distant metastases, and definitive surgery or radiation therapy is usually not indicated (GROOME et al. 2007).

■ Sites of distant metastases may be important prognostically. Metastasis to liver and bone are associated with shorter survival compared to metastasis to other organs such as adrenal glands (STANLEY 1980).

■ Currently no biologic markers are routinely utilized for determination of prognosis of lung cancer.

Table 9.2. American Joint Committee on Cancer (AJCC) TNM classification of non-small-cell lung cancer [from GREENE et al. (2002) with permission]

Primary tumor (T)	
TX	Primary tumor cannot be assessed, or tumor proven by the presence of malignant cells in sputum or bronchial washings but not visualized by imaging or bronchoscopy
T0	No evidence of primary tumor
Tis	Carcinoma in situ
T1	Tumor 3 cm or less in greatest dimension, surrounded by lung or visceral pleura, without bronchoscopic evidence of invasion more proximal than the lobar bronchus (i.e., not in the main bronchus)
T2	Tumor with any of the following features of size or extent: – More than 3 cm in greatest dimension – Involves main bronchus, 2 cm or more distal to the carina – Invades the visceral pleura – Associated with atelectasis or obstructive pneumonitis that extends to the hilar region but does not involve the entire lung
T3	Tumor of any size that directly invades any of the following: chest wall (including superior sulcus tumors), diaphragm, mediastinal pleura, parietal pericardium; or tumor in the main bronchus less than 2 cm distal to the carina but without involvement of the carina; or associated atelectasis or obstructive pneumonitis of the entire lung
T4	Tumor of any size that invades any of the following: mediastinum, heart, great vessels, trachea, esophagus, vertebral body, carina; or separate tumor nodules in the same lobe; or tumor with malignant pleural effusion
Regional lymph nodes (N)	
NX	Regional lympy node (s) cannot be assessed
N0	No regional lympy node metastasis
N1	Metastasis to ipsilateral peribronchial and/or ipsilateral hilar lymph nodes, and intrapulmonary nodes including involvement by direct extension of the primary tumor
N2	Metastasis to ipsilateral mediastinal and/or subcardinal lymph nodes(s)
N3	Metastasis to contralateral mediastinal, contralateral hilar, ipsilateral or contralateral scalene, or supraclavicular lymph nodes(s)
Distant metastasis (M)	
MX	Distant metastasis cannot be assessed
M0	No distant metastasis
M1	Distant metastasis present (includes separate tumor nodules (s) in a different lobe (ipsilateral or contralateral)
STAGE GROUPING	
Occult Carcinoma: TX N0 M0	
0:	Tis N0 M0
IA:	T1 N0 M0
IB:	T2 N0 M0
IIA:	T1 N1 M0
IIB:	T2 N1 M0, T3 N0 M0
IIIA:	T1 N1 M0, T2 N2 M0, T3 N1 M0, T3 N2 M0
IIIB:	Any T N3 M0, T4 Any N M0
IV:	Any T Any N M1

9.2   Treatment of Resectable NSCLC

9.2.1   General Principles

■ Complete surgical resection is the standard treatment for stage I, II, and resectable IIIA NSCLC. External beam radiation is the definitive treatment of choice for medically inoperable patients or patients who decline surgery.

■ Radiosurgery has become an alternative choice to resection for stage I/II patients who are medically inoperable or those who decline surgery (Grade B).

■ For stage IA NSCLC, adjuvant radiation therapy or chemotherapy has no role after complete resection (Grade A).

■ For stage IB, IIA, and IIB lesions, adjuvant radiation therapy after complete resection is not indicated; however, cisplatin-based chemotherapy has been shown to improve treatment outcome in adjuvant settings and is usually recommended (Grade A).

■ For resectable IIIA NSCLC, adjuvant chemotherapy has been shown to improve treatment outcome and should be recommended (Grade A). However, routine use of postoperative radiation directed to the mediastinum in patients with completely resected stage IIIA NSCLC is controversial. Adjuvant radiation therapy is indicated if microscopic (positive margin) or macroscopic residual disease is suspected after surgical resection in early stage NSCLC.

■ Preoperative radiation therapy is usually not indicated for resectable NSCLC (Grade A). The role of neoadjuvant chemotherapy in resectable NSCLC is controversial.

9.2.2 Surgery

■ Lobectomy is the standard surgery for resectable NSCLC (Grade A). Results from a randomized trial reported by the Lung Cancer Study Group revealed that local recurrence after wedge resection for stage T1N0M0 diseases was approximately 18% versus 6% after lobectomy (LCSG 821, Level I) (GINSBERG and RUBINSTEIN 1995). In addition, results from lobectomy were equal to those of pneumonectomy, if complete tumor resection could be achieved (CHURCHILL et al. 1950). Mortality associated with lobectomy is less than 3% in modern series (BOFFA et al. 2008).

■ Complete mediastinal lymphadenectomy enables accurate pathologic staging and information for patient selection for adjuvant radiotherapy (N2 disease).

■ The 5-year overall survival for patients with pathological stage I after complete surgical resection is approximately 70%, while that for pathological stage II is approximately 50% (MOUNTAIN 2000).

■ Most treatment failures for early stage NSCLC after complete surgical resection are due to metastatic recurrences rather than locoregional failure (Level IV) (FELD et al. 1984; PAIROLERO et al. 1984; THOMAS and RUBINSTEIN 1990).

9.2.3 Adjuvant Chemotherapy

■ Chemotherapy is not indicated in the treatment of stage IA NSCLC after surgical resection and may be detrimental.

■ Adjuvant chemotherapy is usually recommended in stage IB, IIA, IIB, and IIIA NSCLC after complete resection (Grade A). Numerous randomized studies have confirmed that adjuvant chemotherapy can improve outcome when used after complete resection (IALT, ANITA, LACE meta-analysis, Level I) (ARRIAGADA et al. 2004; DOUILLARD et al. 2006; PIGNON et al. 2006). Adjuvant chemotherapy may improve outcome for patients whose primary lesions are larger than 4 cm in diameter. A significant survival benefit of 12% at 4 years was seen with the addition of chemotherapy (CALGB 9633, Level II) (STRAUSS et al. 2004).

■ The role of neoadjuvant chemotherapy in resectable NSCLC is controversial and should not be routinely considered for resectable NSCLC (Grade C). Survival benefits were observed in two randomized trials in stage IIIA NSCLC in which patients received cisplatin-based induction chemotherapy and surgery versus surgery alone (Level I) (ROSELL et al. 1999; ROTH et al. 1998). However, overall survival improvement was not observed in a randomized trial that enrolled 355 patients with resectable stage IB–IIIA NSCLC, although the median disease-free survival was extended from 13 to 27 months after induction chemotherapy (Level I) (DEPIERRE et al. 2002).

Regimens

■ Cisplatin-based chemotherapy regimens (e.g., cisplatin 50 mg/m^2 on days 1 and 8 every 4 weeks for four cycles, and vinorelbine 25 mg/m^2 weekly for 16 weeks for four cycles) should be considered in the adjuvant setting (Grade A). The majority of published randomized trials mentioned above utilized cisplatin-based multiagent chemotherapy regimens (Level I).

■ Alkylating agents are not recommended due to their association with shorter survival (Grade A). Results from the NSCLC Collaborative Group individual-patient meta-analysis (17 trials) revealed a significant survival disadvantage associated with the use of adjuvant alkylating agents (Level I) (NON-SMALL CELL LUNG CANCER COLLABORATIVE GROUP 1995).

9.2.4 Radiation Therapy

Adjuvant Radiation

- Postoperative radiation therapy (PORT) is indicated when microscopic or macroscopic residual disease is suspected after surgical resection.
- For stage I and II NSCLC, post-operative radiation therapy is not recommended after complete resection (Grade A). The PORT meta-analysis of nine trials (2128 patients) found a significant detrimental effect of adjuvant thoracic irradiation on overall survival of patients with stage I and II NSCLC (i.e., lower nodal status) (PORT Meta-analysis, Level I) (PORT 1998). This finding was confirmed by the results of a more recently published randomized European trial in which patients with stage I–IIIA NSCLC were randomized to surgery alone or surgery followed by 60 Gy of thoracic irradiation. The 5-year overall survival rate was 43% for the control group and 30% for the radiotherapy group. The detrimental effect of PORT was specific to patients with stage II disease (Level I) (DAUTZENBERG et al. 1999).
- For stage IIIA NSCLC, PORT can be considered in N2 disease for locoregional control, but its routine use after complete resection is controversial (Grade B). According to a large retrospective study that included 7465 patients with NSCLC, survival was improved with adjuvant radiation in patients with N2 disease, but PORT reduced survival in patients with N0 disease (SEER, Level IV) (LALLY et al. 2006). In randomized trials or meta-analysis, although locoregional recurrence was found to be reduced by PORT, no benefit or detrimental effects on survival has been observed after complete resection followed by mediastinal radiation (STEPHENS et al. 1996; LUNG CANCER STUDY GROUP 1986). Furthermore, addition of concurrent cisplatin-based chemotherapy to PORT did not improve locoregional control or survival, as compared with radiation alone (INT 0115/ECOG E3590, Level I) (KELLER et al. 2000).
- Preoperative radiation therapy alone is not recommended for resectable NSCLC (Grade A). Results from two randomized clinical trials revealed that preoperative radiation therapy followed by surgery in both operable and marginally inoperable NSCLC provided no advantage over surgery alone (NCI and VAMC, Level I) (WARRAM 1975).
- Preoperative concurrent chemoradiation may be of benefit to patients with stage IIIA disease, who have biopsy proven N2 nodes. Combination cisplatinum and etoposide concurrent with radiation offer a 3-year survival rate of 27%. Patients who achieved a pathologic complete response had a tripling of medial survival (SWOG 8805, Level III) (ALBAIN et al. 1995).

Radiation Technique – Adjuvant Setting

- The gross tumor volume (GTV) and clinical target volume (CTV) in the adjuvant setting encompass suspected residual gross and microscopic disease as indicated by both preoperative imaging studies and postoperative surgical clips, surgical and pathology reports, as well as postoperative imaging studies.
- The GTV and CTV are expanded to take into account motion, generating internal target volumes (ITVs) for each, which are then expanded to the planning target volume (PTV) which takes into account setup error.
- Elective nodal radiation can be omitted in the adjuvant setting for Stage I/II NSCLC as nodal failure rates are below 10% (Level IV) (ROSENZWEIG et al. 2001). Adjuvant radiation for stage IIIA (N2 disease) only includes involved lymph node stations (SENAN et al. 2002).
- Dose to microscopic disease (positive margin) is 60 Gy with conventional fractionation. With gross residual disease, the addition of concurrent chemotherapy should be considered, as should radiation dose escalation (Level II) (PEREZ et al. 1980). Simulation, beam energy, and delivery are similar to those described and utilized in definitive radiation for unresectable disease (see below).

Definitive Radiation

- Fractionated radiation therapy remains the standard treatment for patients with early stage but medically inoperable NSCLC, and for patients who decline surgery. Local failure rates remain high even when dose excalation is attempted by conventional fractionation. Doses of 70–90 Gy in 2-Gy treatment offered local control to only 50%–70% of patients (Level IV) (BRADLEY 2005).
- The efficacy of chemotherapy in patients with stage I or II NSCLC after definitive radiation therapy is unknown at this time and requires further study.
- Radiosurgery (stereotactic lung radiosurgery) is the emerging optimal treatment technique for T1/

T2 N0 M0 NSCLC. For selected patients, outcomes appear equivalent to surgery. Local control rates were of greater than 90% at 2-year follow-up, with only 3% serious morbidity. The 5-year survival for medically operable patients who refused surgery was 88% (Level IV) (ONISHI et al. 2004, 2007).

- For medically inoperable stage IIIA NSCLC, combined chemotherapy and radiation therapy should be considered in patients with good performance status (ECOG 0, 1, or possibly 2). The treatment regimen and techniques are identical to unresectable stage IIIA/IIIB disease.

Radiosurgery Technique

- Radiosurgery enables the delivery of a small number of large fractions to minimize tumor repopulation. Figure 9.1 illustrates a typical radiosurgery isodose plan.
- The biological equivalent dose (BED_{10}) of 100 Gy is required to offer local control of lesions ≤ 4 cm (Grade B). By delivering the BED_{10} of 100 Gy to the PTV, high local control rates with low complications are possible. In a retrospective multi-institutional review, delivering a BED < 100 resulted in a 27% local failure rate compared to 8% local failure with a BED > 100 Gy. Survival with doses less than 100 BED was 70% versus 88% with BED > 100 ($p < 0.05$) (Level IV) (ONISHI et al. 2004).

- BED_{10} of 100 Gy can be delivered safely via several different regimens including 12 Gy $\times$ 4 or 10 Gy $\times$ 5. Doses of 20 Gy $\times$ 3 can be toxic especially when treating central lesions (Level III) (TIMMERMAN et al. 2006).
- Optimal radiosurgery requires careful treatment planning to define the PTV, generally by measuring motion on CT Scan. Radiosurgery treatment delivery also requires precise targeting, often assisted by image-guided radiation therapy (IGRT) and limiting of respiratory motion by stereotacticradiosurgerybody frame or via gated radiation delivery (CHANG et al. 2006).
- Immobilization via a Vac-Loc bag and Tbar minimizes motion to 7 mm or less, > 95% of the time.

Radiosurgery Morbidity

- Normal tissue tolerance is not yet clearly defined for hypofractionated irradiation to the intrathoracic tissues, bone, and soft-tissue.
- Acute morbidity induced by radiosurgery is rare. Late complications may occur one year or more after surgery, and may include fistula, bleeding, fibrosis, pneumonitis, pneumonia, brachial plexopathy for apical lesions and liver toxicity for basal lesions (Level IV) (ONISHI et al. 2007). Rib fracture and soft tissue fibrosis are also possible with stereotactic radiosurgery.

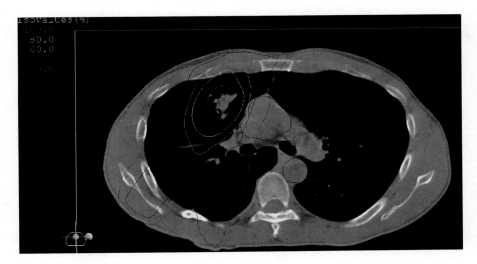

Fig. 9.1. Hypofractionated curative radiosurgery, 10 Gy $\times$ 5 fractions every other day. Note the GTV is encompassed by the 100% isodose, and the 80% isodose encompasses microscopic tumor extension. Vascular structures are limited below the 60% isodose line. (Image courtesy of Hiram Gay, MD)

9.3   Treatment of Surgically Unresectable Stage III NSCLC

9.3.1   General Principles

- For unresectable or medically inoperable stage IIIA and IIIB NSCLC, combined radiation and chemotherapy is the treatment of choice for patients with good performance status (ECOG 0, 1, or possibly 2) (Grade A).
- Radiation therapy and chemotherapy should be utilized concurrently (Grade A). The role of induction chemotherapy before and consolidation chemotherapy after concurrent chemoradiation are not yet proven and should not be routinely utilized.
- Stage IIIB NSCLC with malignant pleural effusion, malignant pericardial effusion, and/or pleural dissemination are usually treated as metastatic cases.

9.3.2   Systemic Chemotherapy

- Combined chemotherapy and radiation therapy should be considered as the definitive treatment of choice for stage IIIA and IIIB NSCLC (Grade A). The efficacy of induction chemotherapy (cisplatin + vinblastine) followed by radiation therapy (60 Gy given in 30 fractions) was compared with radiation therapy alone in the treatment of stage III NSCLC in a CALGB randomized trial. Results from the 7-year follow-up revealed that patients receiving 5 weeks of induction chemotherapy had a 4.1-month increase of median survival, compared to those treated with radiation alone (CALGB 8433, Level I) (DILLMAN et al. 1996). These results were confirmed in a three-arm randomized trial from RTOG in which 490 patients with unresectable stage II–IIIB NSCLC were randomized to induction chemotherapy followed by radiation (same regimen as in the CALGB 8433 trial) or one of two radiation alone arms (twice daily radiation at 1.2 Gy/fraction to a total of 69.6 Gy versus conventional radiation to a total of 60 Gy). The median survival of patients who received induction chemotherapy followed by radiation was 13.2 months, significantly better than patients treated with radiation alone (12 months

and 11.4 months for twice daily and conventional radiation, respectively) (RTOG 8088, Level I) (SAUSE et al. 2000). This benefit was seen only for patients with good performance status and minimal weight loss.

- Chemotherapy is usually delivered concurrently with radiation therapy (Grade A). Results from a number of phase III randomized trials have suggested improvements in locoregional control and survival when chemotherapy is used in this fashion with radiation therapy. A phase III randomized trial from Japan treated 320 patients with unresectable stage III NSCLC with concurrent chemotherapy (cisplatin, vindesine, and mitomycin) and radiation (two courses of 28-Gy treatment, with 10 days break in between) or sequential chemotherapy (same regimen) followed by radiation (56 Gy in 28 daily fractions). The medial survival durations were 16.5 months versus 13.3 months, significantly superior in the concurrently treated group. The 5-year overall survival was 15.8% and 8.9%, respectively, favoring concurrent chemoradiation (West Japan Lung Cancer Group Study, Level I) (FURUSE et al. 1999). The sequencing of chemotherapy and radiation was also studied in a RTOG phase III trial. Patients with medically inoperable or unresectable stage II and III NSCLC were randomized to receive concurrent chemotherapy (cisplatin + vinblastine) and radiation (1.8 Gy daily to a total of 63 Gy), sequential chemoradiation (same chemotherapy and radiation regimens), and concurrent chemotherapy (cisplatin + etoposide) and hyperfractionated radiotherapy (1.2 Gy twice daily to a total of 69.6 Gy). The results were reported in abstract form, which revealed that concurrent chemotherapy and daily radiation improved median survival (17.1 months) as compared to the other two treatment strategies (15.2 months and 14.6 months, respectively, for concurrent chemotherapy + twice daily radiation and sequential chemoradiation) (RTOG 9410, Level I) (CURRAN et al. 2003). A French randomized trial treated 205 patients with unresectable stage III NSCLC with either cisplatin- and vinorelbine-based chemotherapy followed by 66 Gy radiation therapy (given in 33 daily fractions), or concurrent radiation (same dose regimen) and chemotherapy (cisplatin + etoposide) followed by consolidation chemotherapy consisting of cisplatin and vinorelbine. Concurrent chemoradiotherapy improved the median survival duration to 16.3 months compared to 14.5 months from the sequential treatment, although the difference did not reach statistical significance (GLOT NPC 95-01, Level I) (FOURNEL et al. 2005).

■ No evidence supports the use of induction chemotherapy (carboplatin-based) prior to concurrent chemoradiation therapy (Grade A). Results from a randomized trial where 366 patients were randomized to concurrent radiation (66 Gy given in 33 daily fractions) and chemotherapy (weekly carboplatin + paclitaxel) or the same chemoradiation regimen preceded by two cycles of induction chemotherapy revealed no significant difference in 1-year overall survival rates (48% vs. 54%) or medial survival time (11.4 months vs. 14 months) (CALGB 39801, Level I) (VOKES et al. 2002).

Regimens

■ Various platinum-based chemotherapy regimens have been utilized in combination with radiation therapy. Cisplatin-based chemotherapy regimens such as cisplatin + etoposide are commonly used. Other regimens including carboplatin + paclitaxel, cisplatin+ paclitaxel, and cisplatin + vinorelbine have also been studied.

■ Between two and four cycles of chemotherapy can be used in combination with radiation for unresectable stage III NSCLC (Grade D). The optimal duration of cisplatin-based chemotherapy used as induction, concurrent, and/or adjuvant treatment with radiation or unresectable NSCLC is debatable, and the role of consolidation chemotherapy is unknown.

9.3.3 Radiation Therapy

Treatment Technique

Simulation

■ CT-based planning is recommended, and CT scan should be taken in the treatment position with arms raised above head (treatment position) with 3-mm-thick slices.

■ Intravenous contrast is not recommended for planning CT as it may compromise the treatment planning calculation. Fusion of a CT with contrast may be needed if IV contrast is necessary for tumor delineation.

■ Pulmonary lesions should be delineated with the "lung window" setting; lymph nodes should be outlined using a "mediastinal window" setting.

Target Delineation (see Fig. 9.2)

■ GTV is visible tumor on imaging including all nodes on CT ≥ 1 cm, though PET/CT is far more accurate to delineate nodal spread.

■ CTV is the region of microscopic disease spread. It expands the GTV by 6 mm for squamous lesions and 8 mm for adenocarcinomas.

■ PTV is the CTV with margin for motion and setup error. About 85% of lesions move less than 1 cm. Lesions near the diaphragm often move more than 1 cm.

■ ITV is the CTV with explicit measurement of motion usually via CT scan. Delineation of motion is critical when highly conformal, IMRT, or stereotacticradiosurgery fields are employed as the risk of geographic miss is increased.

■ Motion can be minimized by Vac-Loc bags and stereotactic body frames with diaphragm compression; motion can be accounted for by gated delivery of therapy, breath-hold techniques, or active tracking devices.

Beam Energy and Dose Calculation

■ Megavoltage accelerator with a minimum source to isocenter distance of 100 cm is recommended.

■ Only 6-MV to 10-MV energy photon beams are to be used for any field arrangement, including oblique or other fields.

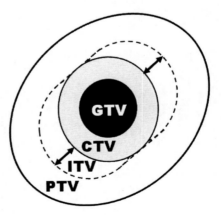

Fig. 9.2. Important terminology in lung radiotherapy: *GTV*, gross tumor volume; *CTV*, clinical tumor volume; *ITV*, internal target volume; *PTV*, planning target volume

- Doses are to be calculated with heterogeneity correction; i.e., correction is to be made for density differences between air spaces, lung, water-density, or bony tissue for 3D planning.
- IMRT may be advantageous as it better limits dose to normal lung as compared to conventional delivery.

Field Arrangement

Involved-Field Radiation (See Fig. 9.3)

- Involved-field radiation is a new paradigm to minimize normal tissue toxicity, particularly pneumonitis risk.
- Radiation port defined exclusively on abnormal or hot spots on PET/CT, with no attempt to include radiologically uninvolved nodal basins, as approximately 10% nodal failure rate is found with this technique (Level IV) (Rosenzweig et al. 2001).
- From a practical viewpoint, involved field radiation is still a relatively large field (as compared to stereotactic radiosurgery) so many nodal basins are still encompassed

Large-Field Thoracic Radiation

- Large-Field thoracic radiation is a classis approach encompassing gross and microscopic regions of spread, which includes all abnormal regions on radiology as well as mediastinum, hilum, and ipsilateral supraclavicular fossa (except for lower lobe lesions)
- The large field size limits therapeutic outcomes due to risk of pneumonitis and significant acute esophagitis

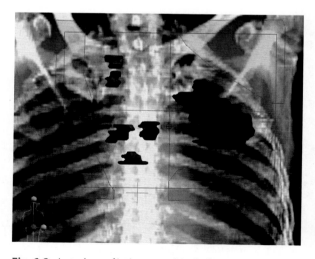

Fig. 9.3. Anterior radiation portal including GTV (*red*) and PET positive lymph nodes (*blue*)

Dose and Fractionation

- Thoracic irradiation to a total dose of 60 Gy administered in conventional fractionation (1.8 Gy or 2.0 Gy per fraction) should be used for definitive treatment of NSCLC (Grade A). However, high local failure rates, up to 40%, are reported with this dose (Level I) (Perez et al. 1980).
- Several studies have examined dose escalation with conventional fractionation and concomitant chemotherapy. It appears that 74 Gy in 2 Gy per fraction with concurrent chemotherapy improves both local control and extends survival to 22 months (Level IV) (Bradley 2005). These results need to be confirmed in randomized trials.
- Hyperfractionated radiation therapy has not been shown to be more efficacious than conventional radiation in definitive treatment of NSCLC. The RTOG compared hyperfractionation of 1.2 Gy bid from 60–77 Gy. Optimal outcome was seen at 69.6 Gy with a 3-year 20% survival rate. When 69.6 Gy bid was later compared to sequential chemotherapy with 60 Gy conventional fractionation in a randomized trial, outcomes were statistically superior with conventional therapy (RTOG 8808, Level I). The RTOG 9410 then compared the total dose of 69.6 Gy given at 1.2 Gy twice daily with concurrent chemotherapy, conventional fractionation with concurrent chemotherapy, and sequential chemoradiation. Conventional radiotherapy with concurrent chemotherapy offered the best survival outcome (RTOG 9410, Level I) (Curran et al. 2003).
- Continuous hyperfractionated accelerated radiation therapy (CHART) delivers 54 Gy in at 1.5 Gy per fraction three times a day (TID), 7 days a week. Hyperfractionated accelerated radiation therapy (HART) delivers 57 Gy in 1.5 Gy per fraction TID, 5 days a week. The CHART and HART offered only 20% local control at 2 years and similar 12-month survival (Level II) (Mehta et al. 1998; Saunders et al. 1999).
- Split course of radiation should not be used in the treatment of NSCLC for curative treatment (Grade A). This is associated with poorer outcome but may be a means for palliative therapy with minimal morbidity (Perez et al. 1980).
- The combination of involved field radiation with stereotactic radiosurgery boost to the primary tumor could be considered as a means to improve local control and survival in lung cancer.

Side Effects and Complications

Radiation-Induced Side Effects and Complications

- Esophagitis is the most common radiation-induced side effect during treatment. It may be severe with concomitant chemotherapy. Carafate elixir and lidocaine elixir may be palliative.
- Radiation-induced myocarditis or transverse myelitis rarely occurs at doses lower than 50 Gy.
- Radiation-induced pneumonitis is a diagnosis of exclusion and occurs in ~ 10% of patients 4–6 weeks after treatment. It is associated with the amount of normal lung treated above 20 Gy (V20), as well as the mean lung dose. Radiographic evidence of radiation change and subsequent fibrosis of the lung will occur within lung volume receiving 40 Gy (Level III) (BRADLEY and MOVSAS 2006).
- Other side effects include bone marrow toxicity, skin pigmentation, brachial plexopathy, and epilation depending on the site and dose of irradiation.

Dose Limiting Structures

- Dose of radiation to the spinal cord should be limited to 45 Gy (1.8–2.0 Gy daily) (Level IV) (EMAMI et al. 1991).
- Dose to the esophagus should be limited to 60 Gy for 1/3 of the esophagus, or 55 Gy for the entire esophagus.
- V40 of the heart should be limited to 50% or less.
- V20 of bilateral lung should be limited to ≤30% as probability of pneumonitis increases rapidly when more than V20 >30% (Level III) (BRADLEY and MOVSAS 2006).
- Delivering a V20 <20 Gy offers minimal pneumonitis risk (BRADLEY and MOVSAS 2006).

9.4 Treatment of Superior Sulcus Tumor and "Marginally Unresectable" NSCLC

9.4.1 General Principles

- Preoperative chemoradiation therapy followed by surgery is recommended for the treatment of "Pancoast" tumor (superior sulcus tumor) (Grade B).
- The concept of "marginally unresectable" NSCLC has not been uniformly defined.
- For stage I/II marginally unresectable patients, pre-op chemotherapy followed by post-operative chemotherapy is recommended. Focal post-op radiation therapy should be used if residual disease is present (Grade B).
- For stage IIIA marginally unresectable patients, preoperative chemotherapy may downstage for surgery, followed by postoperative chemotherapy. Postoperative radiation is included for N2 nodes or residual disease (ROTH et al. 1998; DEPIERRE et al. 2002) (Grade B).

9.4.2 Induction Treatment

- Preoperative radiation therapy followed by surgery has been the treatment of choice for patients with "Pancoast" tumor (superior sulcus tumor). Long-term survival can reach 40%–50% if complete resection is achievable after induction chemoradiation.
- Surgery is contraindicated for superior sulcus tumors with extensive brachial plexus involvement, mediastinal involvement of nodes, and subclavian artery extension. MRI, PET/CT, and mediastinoscopy can determine resectability (EMAMI et al. 1991).
- Concurrent chemotherapy and radiation therapy (45 Gy given in 25 daily fractions) should be considered for patients with superior sulcus tumor followed by evaluation for resection (Grade B). Although randomized study comparing the efficacy of induction radiation and chemoradiation has never been performed, results from a SWOG phase II study revealed that pathologic complete or near-complete response reached 65% after concurrent cis-platinum and etoposide induction chemotherapy and 45 Gy of radiation therapy (Level III) (RUSCH et al. 2007).
- Evaluation of resectability should be performed after induction chemoradiotherapy. If resection is not feasible, continuation of chemotherapy and radiation to a definitive dose should be offered.
- Due to critical surrounding normal structures and minimal motion of these lesions, IMRT should be favored.

9.4.3 Treatment of Marginally Unresectable Disease

■ Marginally unresectable disease can be down-staged to resection in many instances by preoperative chemotherapy and, if successful, postoperative chemotherapy is continued. Patients with residual disease or N2 nodes can be offered involved field radiation (French Thoracic Cooperative Group, Level I) (Depierre et al. 2002).

■ In stage IIIA disease, concurrent chemoradiotherapy (45 Gy) may be employed to downstage. If resectable, postoperative chemotherapy is delivered. If unresectable, concurrent chemoradiation to definitive doses are offered (INT 0139, Level I) (Albain et al. 2005).

■ There is no evidence to support the routine use of surgery after combined chemoradiation for definitive treatment in patients with "marginally unresectable" NSCLC.

9.5 Treatment of Metastatic NSCLC

9.5.1 General Principles

■ Systemic chemotherapy is indicated for stage IIIB (pleural and/or pericardial effusion) and stage IV NSCLC patients with good performance statues (ECOG 0, 1, or possibly 2) (Grade A).

■ Palliative thoracic irradiation is commonly used to treat hemoptysis, excessive cough, dyspnea, and other symptoms caused by locally advanced pulmonary lesions.

9.5.2 Systemic Chemotherapy

■ Cisplatin in combination with one of the newer agents (such as vinorelbine, paclitaxel, docetaxel, and gemcitabine) should be considered as first line treatment in most patients with good performance status (ECOG 0 or 1) (Grade A). Results from numerous randomized trials have confirmed that platinum-based two-drug chemotherapy regimens using newer agents improves survival in advanced stage NSCLC compared to cisplatin alone, or used with first generation

agents (such as etoposide). A phase III randomized trial compared the efficacy of cisplatin plus paclitaxel, gemcitabine, or docetaxel, or carboplatin plus paclitaxel and showed no difference in these combinations (Level I) (Schiller et al. 2002).

■ For elderly patients or patients with poor performance status (ECOG 2), single-drug chemotherapy can be considered (Grade A) (Level I) (Jatoi and Aranguren 2007).

■ First-line chemotherapy should be discontinued after 4 cycles if clinical response is not achieved (Grade D). There is no evidence that supports the use of maintenance chemotherapy after 4–6 cycles.

9.5.3 Palliative Radiotherapy

■ Palliative thoracic irradiation is commonly used for relieving symptoms caused by advanced pulmonary disease or distant metastases.

■ Radiation is indicated when symptoms occur and prophylactic irradiation to the chest is usually not indicated (Grade A). A multicenter randomized controlled trial investigating the effects of immediate palliative radiation (17 Gy given in two fractions 1 week apart or 10 Gy single-fraction) to chest versus delayed treatment until the onset of symptoms on symptom control, quality of life, and survival in 230 patients with NSCLC who were not candidates for curative treatment, found no difference between the two groups of patients (Level I) (Falk et al. 2002).

■ Various total dose and fraction arrangements can be considered for controlling thoracic symptoms: 30–39 Gy administered in 10–13 fractions, 5 days per week, or 20 Gy over five fractions are commonly used.

■ Higher dose radiation regimens for palliation are preferred over lower dose (hypofractionated) regimens (Grade A). Higher dose regimens may be associated with modest survival benefits in which patients with incurable NSCLC. An MRC randomized study compared the efficacy of 17 Gy of chest radiation given in two fractions 1 week apart and 39 Gy of radiation delivered in 13 fractions, 5 days per week, found that although more hypofractionated irradiation led to rapid symptom palliation and less toxicity (dysphagia), patients in the higher dose arm had significantly longer survival (9 months vs. 7 months) (MRC Lung Cancer

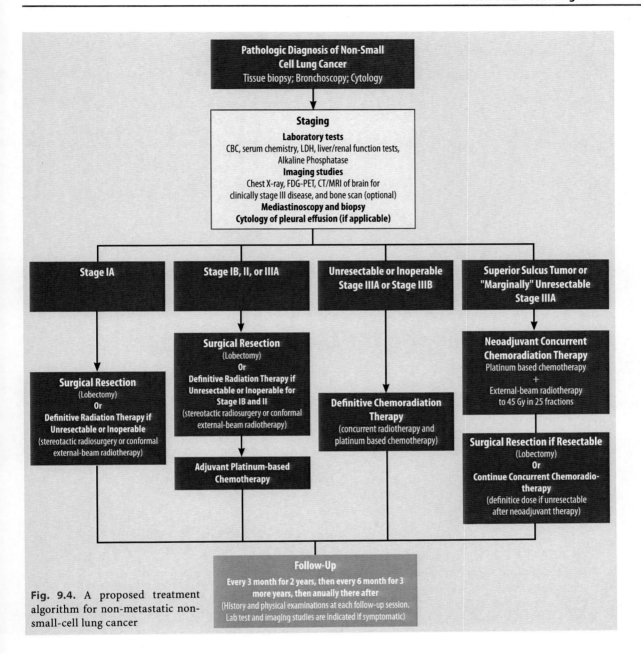

Fig. 9.4. A proposed treatment algorithm for non-metastatic non-small-cell lung cancer

Working Party, Level I). (MACBETH et al. 1996). Results from a similarly designed phase III randomized study from Canada revealed similar findings. Patients with uncurable NSCLC who received 20 Gy of chest radiation over five fractions had better symptom relief and 2 months longer median survival time compared to patients treated with 10 Gy thoracic irradiation in one fraction (NCIC CTG SC.15, Level I) (BEZJAK et al. 2002).

■ Whole brain radiation therapy with or without stereotactic radiosurgery (for between one and four brain metastases) or surgical resection (for solitary brain metastasis) is usually indicated for stage IV NSCLC with intracranial metastases (Grade A). Brain metastases occur in approximately 30% of patients with NSCLC, and palliative treatment for brain metastasis in patients with NSCLC usually follows the common strategy for CNS metastasis.

■ Palliative radiation for bone pain and prevention of fracture in weight-bearing bone in patients with bone metastasis is commonly used, and usually follows the common strategy of radiation for bone metastases.

9.6 Follow-Ups

9.6.1 Post-Treatment Follow-Ups

■ Life-long follow-up is required for all patients with NSCLC treated with curative intent.

Schedule

■ Follow-ups could be scheduled every 3 months initially in the first 2 years after treatment, then every 6 months thereafter through year 5. Annual follow-up is recommended for long-term survivors after 5 years (Table 9.3) (Grade D) (PFISTER et al. 2004).

Table 9.3. Follow-up schedule

Interval	Frequency
First 2 years	Every 3 months
Year 3–5	Every 6 months
Over 5 years	Annually

Work-Ups

■ Each follow-up examination should include a complete history and physical examination.
■ There is no clear role for routine imaging studies for asymptomatic patients. Imaging studies (including chest X-ray, CT scan of the chest and/or abdomen, CT or MRI of the brain, bone scan, and PET/CT) and blood tests (including complete blood count, serum chemistry, renal and liver function tests) should not be performed routinely in asymptomatic patients during follow-up (Grade B). Results from multiple large retrospective reviews indicated that aggressive surveillance after curative treatment did not improve overall outcome and was not cost effective (Level IV) (WALSH et al. 1995; YOUNES et al. 1999).
■ Screening for secondary primary lung cancer with chest X-ray or CT scan in long-term survivors of NSCLC is investigational and is not routinely recommended, although risk of secondary primary lung cancer ranges at 1%–2% per year.

Acknowledgments

Our thanks go to Jim Naves and Kevin Sahadeo, medical dosimetrists, for their expert assistance with the radiotherapy treatment figures.

References

Albain KS, Rusch VW, Crowley JJ et al. (1995) Concurrent cisplatin/etoposide plus chest radiotherapy followed by surgery for stages IIIA (N2) and IIIB non-small-cell lung cancer: mature results of Southwest Oncology Group phase II study 8805. J Clin Oncol 13:1880–1892

Albain KS, Swann RS, Rusch VR et al. (2005) Phase III study of concurrent chemotherapy and radiotherapy (CT/RT) vs CT/RT followed by surgical resection for stage IIIA(pN2) non-small cell lung cancer (NSCLC): outcomes update of North American Intergroup 0139 (RTOG 9309). J Clin Oncol 23:16S

Arriagada R, Bergman B, Dunant A, Le Chevalier T, Pignon JP, Vansteenkiste J (2004) Cisplatin-based adjuvant chemotherapy in patients with completely resected non-small-cell lung cancer. N Engl J Med 350:351–360

Beckles MA, Spiro SG, Colice GL, Rudd RM (2003) The physiologic evaluation of patients with lung cancer being considered for resectional surgery. Chest 123[1 Suppl]:105S–114S

Bezjak A, Dixon P, Brundage M et al. (2002) Randomized phase III trial of single versus fractionated thoracic radiation in the palliation of patients with lung cancer (NCIC CTG SC.15). Int J Radiat Oncol Biol Phys 54:719–728

Boffa DJ, Allen MS, Grab JD et al. (2008) Data from The Society of Thoracic Surgeons General Thoracic Surgery database: the surgical management of primary lung tumors. J Thorac Cardiovasc Surg 135:247–225

Bradley J (2005) A review of radiation dose escalation trials for non-small cell lung cancer within the Radiation Therapy Oncology Group. Semin Oncol 32[2 Suppl 3]:S111–113

Bradley J, Movsas B (2006) Radiation pneumonitis and esophagitis in thoracic irradiation. Cancer Treat Res 128:43–64

Bury T, Barreto A, Daenen F, Barthelemy N, Ghaye B, Rigo P (1998) Fluorine-18 deoxyglucose positron emission tomography for the detection of bone metastases in patients with non-small cell lung cancer. Eur J Nucl Med 25:1244–1247

Chang J, Balter P, Liao Z et al. (2006) Preliminary report of image-guided hypofractionated stereotactic body radiotherapy to treat patients with medically inoperable stage I or isolated peripheral lung recurrent non-small cell lung cancer. Int J Radiat Oncol Biol Phys 66:5480

Non-small Cell Lung Cancer Collaborative Group (1995) Chemotherapy in non-small cell lung cancer: a meta-analysis using updated data on individual patients from 52 randomised clinical trials. Non-small Cell Lung Cancer Collaborative Group. BMJ 311:899–909

Churchill ED, Sweet RH, Soutter L, Scannell JG (1950) The surgical management of carcinoma of the lung; a study of the cases treated at the Massachusetts General Hospital from 1930 to 1950. J Thorac Surg 20:349–365

Curran W, Scott C, Langer C et al. (2003) Long-term benefit is observed in a Phase III comparison of sequential vs concurrent chemo-radiation for patients with unresected Stage III NSCLC: RTOG 94-10. Am Soc Clin Oncol 22:633

Dautzenberg B, Arriagada R, Chammard AB et al. (1999) A controlled study of postoperative radiotherapy for patients with completely resected nonsmall cell lung carcinoma. Groupe d'Etude et de Traitement des Cancers Bronchiques. Cancer 86:265–273

De Leyn P, Vansteenkiste J, Cuypers P et al. (1997) Role of cervical mediastinoscopy in staging of non-small cell lung cancer without enlarged mediastinal lymph nodes on CT scan. Eur J Cardiothorac Surg 12:706–712

Depierre A, Milleron B, Moro-Sibilot D et al. (2002) Preoperative chemotherapy followed by surgery compared with primary surgery in resectable stage I (except T1N0), II, and IIIa non-small-cell lung cancer. J Clin Oncol 20:247–253

Dillman RO, Herndon J, Seagren SL, Eaton WL, Jr., Green MR (1996) Improved survival in stage III non-small-cell lung cancer: seven-year follow-up of cancer and leukemia group B (CALGB) 8433 trial. J Natl Cancer Inst 88:1210–1215

Douillard JY, Rosell R, De Lena M et al. (2006) Adjuvant vinorelbine plus cisplatin versus observation in patients with completely resected stage IB–IIIA non-small-cell lung cancer [Adjuvant Navelbine International Trialist Association (ANITA)]: a randomised controlled trial. Lancet Oncol 7:719–727

Lung Cancer Study Group (1986) Effects of postoperative mediastinal radiation on completely resected stage II and stage III epidermoid cancer of the lung. The Lung Cancer Study Group. N Engl J Med 315:1377–1381

Emami A, Schwartz JH, Borkan SC (1991)Transient ischemia or heat stress induces a cytoprotectant protein in rat kidney. Am J Physiol 260[4 Pt 2]:F479–485

Falk SJ, Girling DJ, White RJ et al. (2002) Immediate versus delayed palliative thoracic radiotherapy in patients with unresectable locally advanced non-small cell lung cancer and minimal thoracic symptoms: randomised controlled trial. BMJ 325(7362):465

Feld R, Rubinstein LV, Weisenberger TH (1984) Sites of recurrence in resected stage I non-small-cell lung cancer: a guide for future studies. J Clin Oncol 2:1352–1358

Fournel P, Robinet G, Thomas P et al. (2005) Randomized phase III trial of sequential chemoradiotherapy compared with concurrent chemoradiotherapy in locally advanced non-small-cell lung cancer: Groupe Lyon-Saint-Etienne d'Oncologie Thoracique-Groupe Francais de Pneumo-Cancerologie NPC 95-01 Study. J Clin Oncol 23:5910–5917

Furuse K, Fukuoka M, Kawahara M et al. (1999) Phase III study of concurrent versus sequential thoracic radiotherapy in combination with mitomycin, vindesine, and cisplatin in unresectable stage III non-small-cell lung cancer. J Clin Oncol 17:2692–2699

Gdeedo A, Van Schil P, Corthouts B, Van Mieghem F, Van Meerbeeck J, Van Marck E (1997) Prospective evaluation of computed tomography and mediastinoscopy in mediastinal lymph node staging. Eur Respir J 10:1547–1551

Ginsberg RJ, Rubinstein LV (1995) Randomized trial of lobectomy versus limited resection for T1 N0 non-small cell lung cancer. Lung Cancer Study Group. Ann Thorac Surg 60:615–22; discussion 22–23

Greene FL, Page DL, Fleming ID et al. (2002) American Joint Committee on Cancer, American Cancer Society. AJCC Cancer Staging Manual, 6th edn. Springer-Verlag, Berlin Heidelberg New York

Groome PA, Bolejack V, Crowley JJ et al. (2007) The IASLC Lung Cancer Staging Project: validation of the proposals for revision of the T, N, and M descriptors and consequent stage groupings in the forthcoming (seventh) edition of the TNM classification of malignant tumours. J Thorac Oncol 2:694–705

Jatoi A, Aranguren D (2007) A critical look at the role of chemotherapy in older patients with non-small cell lung cancer. J Thorac Oncol 2:83–90

Keller SM, Adak S, Wagner H et al. (2000) A randomized trial of postoperative adjuvant therapy in patients with completely resected stage II or IIIA non-small-cell lung cancer. Eastern Cooperative Oncology Group. N Engl J Med 343:1217–1222

Lally BE, Zelterman D, Colasanto JM, Haffty BG, Detterbeck FC, Wilson LD (2006) Postoperative radiotherapy for stage II or III non-small-cell lung cancer using the surveillance, epidemiology, and end results database. J Clin Oncol 24:2998–3006

Macbeth FR, Bolger JJ, Hopwood P et al. (1996) Randomized trial of palliative two-fraction versus more intensive 13-fraction radiotherapy for patients with inoperable non-small cell lung cancer and good performance status. Medical Research Council Lung Cancer Working Party. Clin Oncol (R Coll Radiol) 8:167–175

Mehta MP, Tannehill SP, Adak S et al. (1998) Phase II trial of hyperfractionated accelerated radiation therapy for nonresectable non-small-cell lung cancer: results of Eastern Cooperative Oncology Group 4593. J Clin Oncol 16:3518–3523

Mountain CF (2000) The international system for staging lung cancer. Semin Surg Oncol 18:106–15

Onishi H, Araki T, Shirato H et al. (2004) Stereotactic hypofractionated high-dose irradiation for stage I nonsmall cell lung carcinoma: clinical outcomes in 245 subjects in a Japanese multi-institutional study. Cancer 101:1623–1631

Onishi H, Shirato H, Nagata Y et al. (2007) Hypofractionated stereotactic radiotherapy (HypoFXSRT) for stage I non-small cell lung cancer: updated results of 257 patients in a Japanese multi-institutional study. J Thorac Oncol 2[7 Suppl 3]:S94–100

Pairolero PC, Williams DE, Bergstralh EJ, Piehler JM, Bernatz PE, Payne WS (1984) Postsurgical stage I bronchogenic carcinoma: morbid implications of recurrent disease. Ann Thorac Surg 38:331–338

Perez CA, Stanley K, Rubin P et al. (1980) Patterns of tumor recurrence after definitive irradiation for inoperable non-oat cell carcinoma of the lung. Int J Radiat Oncol Biol Phys 6:987–994

Pfister DG, Johnson DH, Azzoli CG et al. (2004) American Society of Clinical Oncology treatment of unresectable non-small-cell lung cancer guideline: update 2003. J Clin Oncol 22:330–353

Pieterman RM, van Putten JW, Meuzelaar JJ et al. (2000) Preoperative staging of non-small-cell lung cancer with positron-emission tomography. N Engl J Med 343:254–261

Pignon JP, Tribodet H, Scagliotti GV et al. (2006) Lung Adjuvant Cisplatin Evaluation (LACE): a pooled analysis of five randomized clinical trials including 4,584 patients. J Clin Oncol 24[Suppl 18]:366S (abstract 7008)

Porte HL, Ernst OJ, Delebecq T et al. (1999) Is computed tomography guided biopsy still necessary for the diagnosis of adrenal masses in patients with resectable non-small-cell lung cancer? Eur J Cardiothorac Surg 15:597–601

PORT (1998) Postoperative radiotherapy in non-small-cell lung cancer: systematic review and meta-analysis of individual patient data from nine randomised controlled trials. PORT Meta-analysis Trialists Group. Lancet 352:257–263

Rosell R, Gomez-Codina J, Camps C et al. (1999) Preresectional chemotherapy in stage IIIA non-small-cell lung cancer: a 7-year assessment of a randomized controlled trial. Lung Cancer 26:7–14

Rosenzweig KE, Sim SE, Mychalczak B, Braban LE, Schindelheim R, Leibel SA (2001) Elective nodal irradiation in the treatment of non-small-cell lung cancer with three-dimensional conformal radiation therapy. Int J Radiat Oncol Biol Phys 50:681–685

Roth JA, Atkinson EN, Fossella F et al. (1998) Long-term follow-up of patients enrolled in a randomized trial comparing perioperative chemotherapy and surgery with surgery alone in resectable stage IIIA non-small-cell lung cancer. Lung Cancer 21:1–6

Rusch VW, Giroux DJ, Kraut MJ et al. (2007) Induction chemoradiation and surgical resection for superior sulcus non-small-cell lung carcinomas: long-term results of Southwest Oncology Group Trial 9416 (Intergroup Trial 0160). J Clin Oncol 25:313–318

Saunders M, Dische S, Barrett A, Harvey A, Griffiths G, Palmar M (1999) Continuous, hyperfractionated, accelerated radiotherapy (CHART) versus conventional radiotherapy in non-small cell lung cancer: mature data from the randomised multicentre trial. CHART Steering committee. Radiother Oncol 52:137–148

Sause W, Kolesar P, Taylor SI et al. (2000) Final results of phase III trial in regionally advanced unresectable non-small cell lung cancer: Radiation Therapy Oncology Group, Eastern Cooperative Oncology Group, and Southwest Oncology Group. Chest 117:358–364

Schiller JH, Harrington D, Belani CP et al. (2002) Comparison of four chemotherapy regimens for advanced non-small-cell lung cancer. N Engl J Med 346:92–98

Schirrmeister H, Glatting G, Hetzel J et al. (2001) Prospective evaluation of the clinical value of planar bone scans, SPECT, and (^{18})F-labeled NaF PET in newly diagnosed lung cancer. J Nucl Med 42:1800–1804

Senan S, Burgers S, Samson MJ et al. (2002) Can elective nodal irradiation be omitted in stage III non-small-cell lung cancer? Analysis of recurrences in a phase II study of induction chemotherapy and involved-field radiotherapy. Int J Radiat Oncol Biol Phys 54:999–1006

Stanley KE (1980) Prognostic factors for survival in patients with inoperable lung cancer. J Natl Cancer Inst 65:25–32

Stephens RJ, Girling DJ, Bleehen NM, Moghissi K, Yosef HM, Machin D (1996) The role of post-operative radiotherapy in non-small-cell lung cancer: a multicentre randomised trial in patients with pathologically staged T1–2, N1–2, M0 disease. Medical Research Council Lung Cancer Working Party. Br J Cancer 74:632–639

Strauss GM, Herndon J, Maddaus MA et al. (2004) Randomized clinical trial of adjuvant chemotherapy with paclitaxel and carboplatin following resection in Stage IB Non-Small Cell Lung Cancer (NSCLC): Report of Cancer and Leukemia Group B (CALGB) Protocol 9633. In: 2004 ASCO Annual Meeting Proceedings, p 7019

Thomas P, Rubinstein L (1990) Cancer recurrence after resection: T1 N0 non-small cell lung cancer. Lung Cancer Study Group. Ann Thorac Surg 49:242–246; discussion 246–247

Timmerman R, McGarry R, Yiannoutsos C et al. (2006) Excessive toxicity when treating central tumors in a phase II study of stereotactic body radiation therapy for medically inoperable early-stage lung cancer. J Clin Oncol 24:4833–4839

van Tinteren H, Hoekstra OS, Smit EF et al. (2002) Effectiveness of positron emission tomography in the preoperative assessment of patients with suspected non-small-cell lung cancer: the PLUS multicentre randomised trial. Lancet 359:1388–1393

Vokes EE, Herndon JE II, Crawford J et al. (2002) Randomized phase II study of cisplatin with gemcitabine or paclitaxel or vinorelbine as induction chemotherapy followed by concomitant chemoradiotherapy for stage IIIB non-small-cell lung cancer: cancer and leukemia group B study 9431. J Clin Oncol 20:4191–4198

Walsh GL, O'Connor M, Willis KM et al. (1995) Is follow-up of lung cancer patients after resection medically indicated and cost-effective? Ann Thorac Surg 60:1563–1570; discussion 1570–1572

Warram J (1975) Preoperative irradiation of cancer of the lung: final report of a therapeutic trial. A collaborative study. Cancer 36:914–925

Yokoi K, Kamiya N, Matsuguma H et al. (1999) Detection of brain metastasis in potentially operable non-small cell lung cancer: a comparison of CT and MRI. Chest 115:714–719

Younes RN, Gross JL, Deheinzelin D (1999) Follow-up in lung cancer: how often and for what purpose? Chest 115:1494–1499

Small Cell Lung Cancer

JIADE J. LU

CONTENTS

J. J. LU, MD, MBA
Department of Radiation Oncology, National University Cancer Institute of Singapore, National University Health System, National University of Singapore, 5 Lower Kent Ridge Road, Singapore 119074, Singapore

Introduction and Objectives

Small-cell lung cancer (SCLC) accounts for 15%–20% of all lung cancer cases. It is a systemic disease that requires multidisciplinary management. Both chemotherapy and radiation therapy are important treatment modalities in curative and palliative treatment of SCLC.

This chapter examines:

● Recommendations for diagnosis and staging procedures
● The staging systems and prognostic factors
● Treatment recommendations for both limited- and extensive-stage SCLC, as well as the supporting scientific evidence
● The use of prophylactic cranial irradiation (PCI) in both limited- and extensive-stage SCLC
● Techniques of thoracic irradiation and PCI
● Follow-up care and surveillance of survivors

10.1 Diagnosis, Staging, and Prognoses

10.1.1 Diagnosis

Initial Evaluation

■ Diagnosis and evaluation of small-cell lung cancer (SCLC) starts with a complete history and physical examination. Attention should be paid to history, signs and symptoms specific to SCLC, including its paraneoplastic syndromes.
■ The most common endocrinologic syndrome is the syndrome associated with inappropriate secretion of antidiuretic hormone (SIADH) (LIST et al. 1986).
■ Atrial natriuretic peptide (ANP) syndrome can produce hypotension, natriuresis, and hypona-

tremia; physical findings of myasthenia gravis-like symptoms may indicate Eaton-Lambert syndrome; ectopic adrenocorticotropic hormone (ACTH) production syndrome results in cushingoid symptoms, and usually indicates poor prognosis (DIMOPOULOS et al. 1984).

■ Most SCLC associated paraneoplastic syndromes respond to therapy.

Laboratory Tests

■ Initial laboratory tests should include a complete blood count, basic serum, liver function tests, renal function tests, alkaline phosphatase, and lactate dehydrogenase (LDH). Serum LDH is prognostically important.

■ Adequate pulmonary function is required when thoracic radiotherapy is indicated. However, tumor obstruction may provide a falsely poor result of pulmonary function. In such cases, definitive chemoradiation is still possible and recommended.

Imaging Studies

■ Diagnostic imaging studies are required to evaluate the extent of the disease in the thorax as well as distant metastasis.

■ Imaging studies utilized for SCLC are similar to those of non-small cell lung cancer (NSCLC). CT scan of the thorax and upper abdomen is required to evaluate the extent of disease.

■ MRI or CT scan of brain and radionuclide bone scan are indicated in all cases to rule out brain or bone metastasis when SCLC is considered. The most common sites of distant metastases include liver (62%), adrenals (42%), brain (40%), and bone (37%) (LINE and DEELEY 1971).

■ Any evidence of distant metastasis on imaging study should preclude further investigations of other metastatic disease(s) unless local treatment is indicated by symptoms (Grade D).

■ Although SCLC is avid to fluorodeoxyglucose (FDG), currently FDG-PET scan is not routinely recommended for staging of small-cell lung cancer (Grade B). Although FDG-PET was found to be more sensitive and specific than CT scans for non-brain distant metastases in a retrospective series, upstaging or downstaging of patients with SCLC was observed in less than 10% of cases when FDG-PET is used (Level III) (BRADLEY et al. 2004; BRINK et al. 2004).

Table 10.1. Imaging and laboratory work-ups for SCLC

Imaging studies	Laboratory tests
– Chest X-ray	– Complete blood count
– CT of chest/abdomen	– Serum chemistry
– CT or MRI of brain	– Liver function tests
– Bone scan	– Renal function tests
– PET/CT (optional)	– Alkaline phosphatase
	– LDH
	– Pulmonary function test

Pathology

■ Tissue (specimen) for pathology diagnosis can be obtained via fine needle biopsy of the primary tumor, sputum cytology, or from metastatic area including pleural effusion.

■ As the treatment strategy for SCLC differs significantly from NSCLC, pathologic confirmation of SCLC is imperative prior to the initiation of any treatment.

■ Invasive mediastinal staging is not necessary once a diagnosis of SCLC is established, as surgery has a limited role in the treatment of SCLC.

■ When pleural effusion is observed on chest X-ray, thoracentesis is indicated to rule out malignant pleural effusion.

■ In cases where no sign of extensive disease is observed, bone marrow aspirate and/or biopsy should be performed in patients with equivocal bone scan or elevated alkaline phosphatase or LDH.

10.1.2 Staging

■ SCLC is usually staged clinically. The more commonly used Veterans' Administration (VA) Lung Study Group criteria for SCLC staging include limited- and extensive-stage (STAHEL et al. 1989).

■ Recent cooperative group trials in North America require staging of all SCLC patients with the AJCC TNM system to avoid variable interpretations of the VA criteria. The 2002 American Joint Committee on Cancer Tumor Node Metastasis (TNM) staging system for lung cancer is presented in Table 9.2 (see Chap. 9).

Limited Stage

■ Limited-stage SCLC is confined to one hemithorax and regional lymph nodes, and can be encompassed in a single radiation port. Involvement of ipsilateral supraclavicular lymph nodes is generally considered as limited-stage.

■ Approximately 40% of SCLC cases are categorized as limited-stage at diagnosis (GOVINDAN et al. 2006).

■ The corresponding AJCC stages for limited-stage SCLC include stages I–IIIB (except for pleural effusion).

Extensive Stage

■ Extensive-stage SCLC refers to diseases that cannot be included in a single radiation port, and usually has metastatic disease outside the ipsilateral thorax.

■ Common sites of distant metastasis include the brain, bone, liver, and bone marrow.

■ Contralateral supraclavicular lymph nodes and/or pleural effusion denote extensive stage, although both conditions are not explicitly defined in the staging criteria.

■ The corresponding AJCC stages for extensive stage SCLC include IIIB (pleural and/or pericardial effusion) and IV.

■ Approximately two thirds of SCLC cases are extensive at presentation.

10.1.3 Prognosis

■ The prognosis of patients with SCLC is directly associated with the presenting characteristics.

Main Prognostic Factors

■ Extensive stage, poor performance status, and weight loss (more than 5% within 6 months prior to diagnosis) are the most important adverse prognostic factors for SCLC (PAESMANS et al. 2000).

■ For limited-stage disease, the median survival is 18–20 months with concurrent chemoradiation. The 2- and 5-year survival rates are approximately 40% and 15%–25%, respectively (TURRISI et al. 1999).

■ For extensive-stage disease, the median survival after treatment is in the range of 8–10 months with 2-year survival of 10% or less.

Other Prognostic Factors

■ When other factors are equal, male gender, advanced age, high serum LDH level, higher number of organs involved in metastases (in extensive disease), metastases to the liver, central nervous system, and bone marrow, as well as more advanced disease (> stage I by TNM criteria) within limited-stage are associated with poor prognoses (BYHARDT et al. 1986; CERNY et al. 1987; ALBAIN et al. 1991).

10.2 Treatment of Limited-Stage SCLC

10.2.1 General Principles

■ SCLC is usually a systemic disease at diagnosis, and chemotherapy is the mainstay treatment for limited-stage (Grade A).

■ Thoracic radiation therapy to the involved field delivered concurrently with chemotherapy is usually recommended and can significantly improve the treatment outcome (Grade A).

■ The utilization of surgical resection should be limited to diagnosis or early-stage (T1-2N0M0 confirmed by PET CT) SCLC, followed by systemic chemotherapy (Grade B).

10.2.2 Systemic Chemotherapy

■ Chemotherapy is the mainstay treatment for limited-stage SCLC (Grade A) (LOEHRER et al. 1988).

■ Approximately 80%–90% of cases of limited-stage SCLC achieve partial or complete response to chemotherapy; however, response is usually short-lived (Level IV) (CHUTE et al. 1997).

Regimens

■ Concurrent cisplatin and etoposide (EP regimen) is the preferred chemotherapy regimen for limited-stage SCLC used with concurrent radiotherapy (Grade A). A phase III study from Europe randomly assigned 436 patients with SCLC to EP regimen or CAV (cyclophosphamide, epirubicin, and vincristine)-based chemotherapy. Of all patients, 214 with limited-stage disease were treated with concurrent radiation started at cycle 3 of their chemotherapy. The median survival for limited-stage patients treated with the EP regimen was 14.5 months, as compared to 9.7 months in those who received CAV regimen chemotherapy (Level I) (SUNDSTRØM et al. 2002).

- Carboplatin-based chemotherapy can also be used with radiation therapy for the treatment of limited-stage SCLC (Grade B). A randomized trial from Greece compared the efficacy of etoposide-cisplatin or etoposide-carboplatin in SCLC (limited- and extensive-stage). Patients who achieved response to chemotherapy were treated with thoracic irradiation. The results revealed that overall response and complete response rates, as well as median survival, did not differ significantly in the two groups (Hellenic Co-operative Oncology Group, Level II) (SKARLOS et al. 1994).

Dose

- Between four and six 3-weekly courses of cisplatin and etoposide are usually prescribed [e.g., Etoposide 100–120 mg/m^2 intravenously (IV) on days 1–3, and cisplatin 60–90 mg/m^2 IV on day 1] (Grade A). No evidence supports the use of more than six cycles of chemotherapy (i.e., maintenance chemotherapy), and treatment-induced side effects increase with prolonged use of chemotherapy (Level I, II) (BYRNE et al. 1989; GIACCONE et al. 1993; SCULIER et al. 1996).

10.2.3 Thoracic Radiation Therapy

- Thoracic irradiation in combination with concurrent chemotherapy is recommended for definitive treatment of limited-stage SCLC (Grade A). The addition of thoracic irradiation to chemotherapy significantly reduced the risk of locoregional failure by 25% and significantly improved the overall survival in limited-stage SCLC, as demonstrated in two meta-analyses. In a meta-analysis by PIGNON et al. (1992), 13 randomized trials including more than 2400 patients with limited-stage SCLC were analyzed. The addition of thoracic irradiation to chemotherapy

provided an absolute benefit overall survival of 5.4% at 3 years. The relative risk of death in the combined treatment group compared with chemotherapy alone was 0.86 (95% CI, 0.78 to 0.94; p=0.001) (Level I).
The results of a second meta-analysis by WARDE and PAYNE (1992) that included 11 randomized trials revealed that the absolute difference in 2-year survival was 5.4% with the addition of thoracic irradiation to chemotherapy (Level I).

Treatment Technique

Simulation

- CT-based planning is recommended, and CT scan should be taken in the treatment position with arms raised above head (treatment position).
- Intravenous contrast is not recommended for planning CT as it may compromise the treatment planning calculation. Fusion of a CT with contrast may be needed if IV contrast is necessary for tumor and lymph node delineation.
- Pulmonary lesions should be delineated with the "lung window" setting; lymph nodes should be outlined using a "mediastinal window" setting.

Beam Energy and Dose Calculation

- Megavoltage accelerator with a minimum source to isocenter distance of 100 cm is recommended.
- Only 6 MV–10 MV energy photon beams are to be used for any field arrangement, including oblique or other fields.

Field Arrangement

Involved Field Radiation

- Gross tumor volume (GTV) that includes primary tumor and involved lymph nodes (defined as PET scan or pathologic positive, or > 1.5 cm in largest dimension on thoracic CT) plus 1.5- to 2-cm margin (Fig. 10.1) (CURRAN 2001).
- Elective lymph node irradiation is usually not recommended. Ipsilateral hilum/mediastinum should be treated to 36 Gy (1.5 Gy twice daily) or 40–45 Gy (1.8–2.0 Gy daily) in rare cases without lymph node involvement (Fig. 10.2).
- The involved field arrangement is adopted by various collaborative research groups including RTOG as the field arrangement of choice (Grade D) (RADIATION THERAPY ONCOLOGY GROUP 2007).

Fig. 10.1. Anteroposterior field of involved field radiation therapy for limited-stage small-cell lung cancer. Planning tumor volume encompassed the involved area with a margin of 2 cm

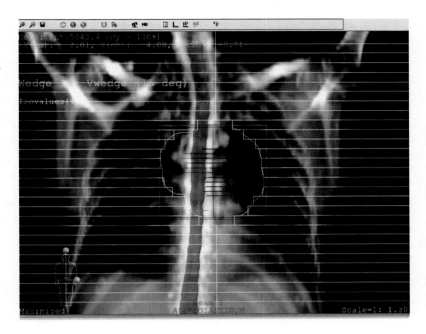

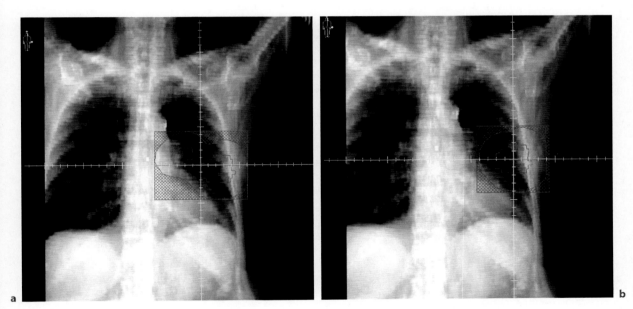

Fig. 10.2a,b. The anterior radiation field of a peripheral small-cell lung cancer case without lymph node involvement. **a** Irradiation to the primary tumor with elective ipsilateral hilar lymph node treatment to 36 Gy (1.5 Gy twice daily). **b** The boost field for the primary tumor was treated to an additional 9 Gy

■ In cases where chemotherapy was initiated prior to the start of thoracic radiation, post-chemotherapy tumor volume should be used as GTV (Grade B). A subgroup of patients (191 cases) with limited-stage SCLC in a SWOG initiated randomized trial who had partial response or stable disease after induction chemotherapy were randomized to receive radiation using a pre- or post-induction tumor volume, with treatment portals designed according to tumor extent before or after induction chemotherapy, respectively. No difference in survival was detected with either radiation field arrangement (Level II) (KIES et al. 1987).

LIENGSWANGWONG et al. (1994) reported the results of a retrospective study intended to determine the appropriate volume that should be encompassed by thoracic radiation treatments for patients with limited-stage SCLC who have responded to initial chemotherapy. The use of radiation fields that encompass post-chemotherapy tumor volumes does not increase the risk of intrathoracic failures including marginal failures (Level IV) (LIENGSWANGWONG et al. 1994).

Large-Field Thoracic Radiation

- Uninvolved ipsilateral hilum and bilateral mediastinum from thoracic inlet to 5 cm below carina can be considered as clinical tumor volume (CTV) for thoracic irradiation.
- Uninvolved contralateral hilum and contralateral supraclavicular area should not be involved in the treatment field. Unilateral supraclavicular area could be included in upper lobe disease only.
- There is no evidence to support that irradiating subclinical disease using the large-field technique can improve outcome when concurrent chemoradiation is used for limited-stage SCLC.

Dose and Fractionation

Accelerated Hyperfractionation

- External beam radiation therapy to a total dose of 45 Gy delivered twice daily (i.e., 1.5 Gy bid) is currently the dose of choice for limited-stage SCLC radiation (Grade A). Results from a randomized study showed that the 5-year overall survival of patients treated with 45 Gy radiation therapy over 15 days (1.5 Gy twice daily) and concurrent EP chemotherapy reached 26%, versus 16% in patients who received the same chemotherapy regimen with 45 Gy of thoracic radiation over 25 fractions at 1.8 Gy per daily fraction (ECOG/RTOG, Level I) (TURRISI et al. 1999).
- Twice-daily radiation given in split course does not improve outcome compared with once-daily radiation, thus should not be considered in routine practice (Grade A). No difference was observed in treatment outcome in terms of overall survival and local progression rates in a phase III trial aimed to compare twice-daily radiotherapy (two courses of 24 Gy in 16 fractions, twice a day, spaced by 2.5 weeks) versus continuous once-daily radiotherapy (50.4 Gy in 28 fractions over 5.5 weeks). Radiotherapy was initiated with the

4th cycle of chemotherapy in the trial, and all patients received six cycles of identical EP chemotherapy regimen (NCCTG, Level I) (BONNER et al. 1999).

Conventional Fractionation

- When twice-daily radiotherapy is not feasible, once-daily thoracic radiation at conventional fractionation (i.e., 1.8–2.0 Gy/day) to a total dose of 54 Gy or higher can be considered (Grade B). A phase I study reported that 56–70 Gy delivered at 2 Gy per daily fraction is well tolerated when given with concurrent EP chemotherapy (radiation started at the 4th cycle of chemotherapy) (Level III) (CHOI et al. 1998).

  Results from a phase II trial that used conventional radiation to a total dose of 70 Gy with concurrent chemotherapy revealed such a regimen was feasible. The median survival was 19.8 months for the entire group (CALGB, Level III) (BOGART et al. 2002).

Side Effects and Complications

Radiation-Induced Side Effects and Dose Limiting Structures

- Dose of radiation to the spinal cord should be limited to ≤ 36 Gy (1.5 Gy twice daily) or 45 Gy (1.8–2.0 Gy daily) (Grade C) (EMAMI et al. 1991).
- Dose to the esophagus should be limited to 60 Gy for 1/3 of the esophagus, or 55 Gy for the entire esophagus (Grade C) (EMAMI et al. 1991). Esophagitis is a common radiation-induced side effect during treatment, and usually does not constitute a reason for treatment interruption.
- V_{20} of bilateral lung should be limited to $\leq 30\%$ as probability of pneumonitis increases rapidly when more than $V_{20} > 30\%$ (Level II) (BYHARDT et al. 1993).

  Radiation-induced pneumonitis is a diagnosis of exclusion and occurs in ~10% of patients 4–6 weeks after treatment. It is associated with the amount of normal lung treated above 20 Gy (V_{20}), as well as the mean lung dose; radiographic evidence of radiation change and subsequent fibrosis of the lung will occur within lung volume receiving 40 Gy (Level III) (MOVSAS et al. 1997; CLAUDE et al. 2004; BYHARDT et al. 1993).
- V_{40} of the heart should be limited to 50% or less. Radiation-induced myocarditis rarely occurs at doses lower than 50 Gy.

- Other side effects include bone marrow toxicity, skin pigmentation, brachial plexopathy, and hair loss (in chest), depending on the site of irradiation.

10.2.4 Timing of Thoracic Radiation

- Thoracic radiation should be initiated early in the chemotherapy course starting at the first or second cycle of chemotherapy (Grade A). A randomized trial completed by the NCI of Canada compared thoracic radiation (40 Gy in 15 fractions over 3 weeks) initiated early during chemotherapy (cyclophosphamide, doxorubicin, and vincristine [CAV] alternating with etoposide and cisplatin [EP] every 3 weeks for a total of six cycles) in week 3 to radiation initiated concurrent with the last cycle of chemotherapy in week 15. The results showed progression-free survival and overall survival rates were significantly superior in the early radiation arm. Additionally, patients treated in the late radiation arm had a significantly higher risk of brain metastases (NCIC, Level I) (MURRAY et al. 1993).
Similar results were seen when accelerated hyperfractionated radiation was utilized. Thoracic radiation given during weeks 1–4 provided improved survival compared to same radiation regimen delivered in weeks 6–9 of chemotherapy. The median survival time was 34 months and 26 months, in early and late radiation groups, respectively. The estimated 5-year survival rates were 30% and 15%, respectively, favoring early initiation of irradiation (Level II) (JEREMIC et al. 1997).

10.2.5 Prophylactic Cranial Irradiation

- Prophylactic cranial irradiation (PCI) is part of the standard treatment for SCLC with complete response after chemotherapy or chemoradiation (Grade A). Results from the PCI Overview Collaborative Group meta-analysis showed that patients who achieved complete response after chemotherapy or combined chemoradiation had improved overall survival after PCI. The 3-year survival rates were 20.7% versus 15.3% for patients receiving PCI and control group patients ,

respectively (PCI Overview Collaborative Group, Level I) (AUPERIN et al. 1999).
- PCI should also be recommended for SCLC with partial response after chemotherapy or chemoradiation (Grade B). Results from a randomized study from Europe revealed that PCI can improve survival in patients with extensive-stage SCLC who developed response to chemotherapy. Although limited-stage SCLC was not included in the study, it is reasonable to infer that a similar benefit from PCI can be expected if partial response is achieved in limited-stage disease after chemoradiation (EORTC 22993-08993, Level II) (SLOTMAN et al. 2007).

Timing of PCI

- PCI should be initiated once complete response is achieved after chemoradiation (Grade B). Results from a retrospective study revealed late start of PCI may adversely affect the prognosis of patients (Level IV) (SUWINSKI et al. 1998).

Dose and Fractionation

- Different radiation doses and fractionation have been utilized in various studies. A dose of 25 Gy delivered in 10 daily fractions (2.5 Gy/day) to 36 Gy delivered in 18 daily fractions (2 Gy/day) can be used (Grade B) (KOTALIK et al. 2001).
- Total equivalent dose less than 24 Gy (calculated in 2 Gy per daily fraction) should not be used for PCI (Grade A). A randomized study from the UK has shown that a dose of 24 Gy in 12 daily fractions (2 Gy/day) or equivalent total dose lower than that does not improve patients' prognosis compare to control (UK02 of UKCCCR/EORTC, Level I) (GREGOR et al. 1997).
- Fraction dose of less than 3 Gy per daily fraction is recommended (Grade B). Cognitive and neurologic function may be impaired when higher fraction dose is used, as suggested in two retrospective studies (Level IV) (KOMAKI et al. 1995; JOHNSON et al. 1990).

10.2.6 Surgery

- Surgery after definitive chemotherapy can be considered in stage I SCLC (Grade B). The results of a prospective nonrandomized trial from

Canada showed that adjuvant surgery (thoracotomy) significantly improved median survival of patients with stage I SCLC, as compared to patients treated with chemotherapy only. Improvement in survival was not seen in patients with more advanced disease (Level III) (SHEPHERD et al. 1989).

■ There is no evidence to support the routine use of surgery after chemotherapy as a replacement strategy of combined chemoradiation therapy for early stage SCLC, including stage I disease.

10.3 Treatment of Extensive-Stage SCLC

10.3.1 Systemic Chemotherapy

■ Chemotherapy is the mainstay treatment for extensive stage SCLC. Approximately 70% of cases of extensive stage SCLC achieve partial or complete response to chemotherapy; however, response to chemotherapy is usually limited to 6–8 months only (CHUTE et al. 1997; LOEHRER et al. 1988).

Chemotherapy Regimen

■ Between four and six 3-weekly courses of cisplatin-based chemotherapy is usually recommended [e.g., Etoposide 100–120 mg/m^2 intravenously (IV) on days 1–3, and cisplatin 60–90 mg/m^2 IV on day 1] (Grade A). Maintenance chemo-therapy after six cycles does not improve outcome, but treatment-induced side effects increase with prolonged chemotherapy (Level I) (GIACCONE et al. 1993; SCULIER et al. 1996; BEITH et al. 1996).

10.3.2 Radiation Therapy

■ Thoracic radiation should not be included in the initial treatment of the definitive therapy for extensive stage SCLC, and is usually reserved for palliation of symptomatic metastases or intrathoracic lesions.

Consolidation Radiotherapy

■ In patients who achieved partial response to chemotherapy, the efficacy of post-chemotherapy thoracic irradiation for consolidation treatment to residual disease is not proven.

Prophylactic Cranial Irradiation

■ PCI should be considered in all SCLC patients who achieve response to chemotherapy (Grade A). Results from a randomized study revealed that patients with extensive-stage SCLC who received PCI had lower risk of symptomatic brain metastases. PCI was associated with an increase in median disease-free survival from 12.0 weeks to 14.7 weeks and in median overall survival from 5.4 months to 6.7 months. The 1-year survival rates were 27.1% versus 13.3% for patients who received PCI and patients in the control group, respectively, (EORTC, Level I) (SLOTMAN et al. 2007).

■ The radiation field arrangement, dose, and fractionation are identical to those used in PCI in limited-stage disease.

Palliation

■ Radiotherapy is commonly utilized to palliate symptoms from metastatic diseases such as bone and brain metastasis, or extensive and symptomatic local disease in patients with extensive SCLC.

■ Figure 10.3 presents a proposed treatment algorithm for SCLC.

Table 10.2. Follow-up schedule

Interval	Frequency
First year	Every 2–3 months
Year 2–3	Every 3–4 months
Year 4–5	Every 4–6 months
Over 5 years	Annually

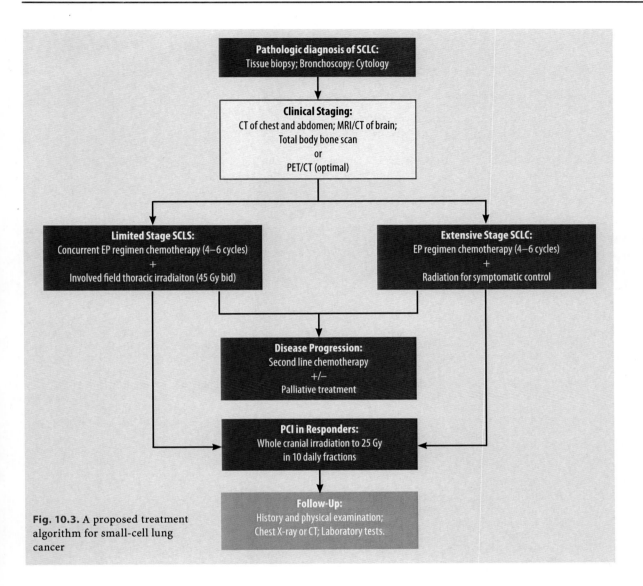

Fig. 10.3. A proposed treatment algorithm for small-cell lung cancer

10.4.1 Post-Treatment Follow-Ups

■ Life-long follow-up is recommended for all patients treated for SCLC for early detection of recurrence as well as second primary lung cancer (Grade D).

Schedule

■ Follow-ups could be scheduled every 2–3 months initially in the first year after treatment, then every 3–4 months in year 2–3, then every 4–6 months in year 4–5. Annual follow-up is recommended for long-term survivors after 5 years (Grade D) (National Comprehensive Cancer Network 2008).

Work-Ups

■ Each follow-up examination should include a complete history and physical examination.
■ Imaging and laboratory tests including chest X-ray or CT scan, complete blood count, and basic serum chemistry can be ordered if clinically indicated; CT or MRI of the brain is indicated when neurologic symptoms occur; total body bone scan or PET/CT can be ordered if signs and symptoms indicate bone or distant metastasis.

References

Albain KS, Crowley JJ, Livingston RB (1991) Long-term survival and toxicity in small-cell lung cancer. Expended Southwest Oncology Group experience. Chest 99: 1425–1432

Auperin A, Arriagada R, Pignon JP et al. (1999) Prophylactic cranial irradiation for patients with small-cell lung cancer in complete remission. Prophylactic Cranial Irradiation Overview Collaborative Group. N Engl J Med 341: 476–484

Beith JM, Clarke SJ, Woods RL et al. (1996) Long-term follow-up of a randomised trial of combined chemoradiotherapy induction treatment, with and without maintenance chemotherapy in patients with small cell carcinoma of the lung. Eur J Cancer 32A: 438–443

Bogart J, Herndon J, Lyss AP et al. (2002) 70 Gy thoracic radiotherapy is feasible concurrent with chemotherapy for limited stage small cell lung cancer: preliminary analysis of a CALGB phase II trial. Int J Radiat Oncol Biol Phys 54[2 suppl]:103

Bonner JA, Sloan JA, Shanahan TG et al. (1999) Phase III comparison of twice-daily split-course irradiation versus once-daily irradiation for patients with limited stage small cell lung carcinoma. J Clin Oncol 17: 2681–2691

Bradley JD, Dehdashti F, Mintun MA et al. (2004) Positron emission tomography in limited-stage small-cell lung cancer: a prospective study. J Clin Oncol 22:3248–3254

Brink I, Schumacher T, Mix M et al. (2004) Impact of [18F] FDG-PET on the primary staging of small-cell lung cancer. Eur J Nucl Med Mol Imaging 31:1614–1620

Byhardt RW, Hartz A, Libnoch JA et al. (1986) Prognostic influence of TNM staging and LDH levels in small cell carcinoma of the lung (SCLC). Int J Radiat Oncol Biol Physs 12:771–777

Byhardt RW, Martin L, Pajak TF et al. (1993) The influence of field size and other treatment factors on pulmonary toxicity following hyperfractionated irradiation for inoperable non-small cell lung cancer – analysis of a Radiation Therapy Oncology Group protocol. Int J Radiat Oncol Biol Phys 27:537–544

Byrne MJ, van Hazel G, Trotter J et al. (1989) Maintenance chemotherapy in limited small-cell lung cancer: a randomized controlled clinical trial. Br J Cancer 60:413–418

Cerny T, Blair V, Anderson H, et al. (1987) Pretreatment prognostic factors and scoring system in 407 small cell lung cancer patients. Int J Cancer 39:146–149

Choi NC, Herndon JE 2nd, Rosenman J et al. (1998) Phase I study to determine the maximum-tolerated dose of radiation in standard daily and hyperfractionated-accelerated twice-daily radiation schedules with concurrent chemotherapy for limited-stage small-cell lung cancer. J Clin Oncol 16:3528–3536

Chute JP, Venzon DJ, Hankins L et al. (1997) Outcome of patients with small-cell lung cancer during 20 years of clinical research at the US National Cancer Institute. Mayo Clin Proc 72:901–912

Claude L, Pérol D, Ginestet C et al. (2004) A prospective study on radiation pneumonitis following conformal radiation therapy in non-small-cell lung cancer: clinical and dosimetric factors analysis. Radiother Oncol 71:175–181

Curran WJ Jr. (2001) Combined-modality therapy for limited-stage small cell lung cancer. Semin Oncol 28[2 Suppl 4]:14–22

Dimopoulos MA, Fernandez JF, Samaan NA et al. (1984) Paraneoplastic Cushing's syndrome as an adverse prognostic factor in patients who die early with small cell carcinoma of the lung. Am J Med 77:851–857

Emami B, Lyman J, Brown A et al. (1991) Tolerance of normal tissue to therapeutic irradiation. Int J Radiat Oncol Biol Phys 21:109–122

Giaccone G, Dalesio O, McVie GJ et al. (1993) Maintenance chemotherapy in small-cell lung cancer: long-term results of a randomized trial. European Organization for Research and Treatment of Cancer Lung Cancer Cooperative Group. J Clin Oncol 11:1230–1240

Govindan R, Page N, Morgensztern D et al. (2006) Changing epidemiology of small-cell lung cancer in the United States over the last 30 years: analysis of the surveillance, epidemiologic, and end results database. J Clin Oncol 24:4539–4544

Gregor A, Cull A, Stephens RJ et al. (1997) Prophylactic cranial irradiation is indicated following complete response to induction therapy in small cell lung cancer: results of a multicentre randomized trial. United Kingdom Coordinating Committee for Cancer Research (UKCCCR) and the European Organization for Research and Treatment of Cancer (EORTC). Eur J Cancer 33:1752–1758

Jeremic B, Shibamoto Y, Acimovic L et al. (1997) Initial versus delayed accelerated hyperfractionated radiation therapy and concurrent chemotherapy in limited small-cell lung cancer: a randomized study. J Clin Oncol 15:893–900

Johnson BE, Patronas N, Hayes W et al. (1990) Neurologic, computed cranial tomographic, and magnetic resonance imaging abnormalities in patients with small-cell lung cancer: further follow-up of 6- to 13-year survivors. J Clin Oncol 8:48–56

Kies MS, Mira JG, Crowley JJ et al. (1987) Multimodal therapy for limited small cell lung cancer: a randomized study of induction combination chemotherapy with or without thoracic radiation in complete responders; and with wide-field versus reduced-field radiation in partial responders; a Southwest Oncology Group study. J Clin Oncol 5:592–600

Komaki R, Meyers CA, Shin DM et al. (1995) Evaluation of cognitive function in patients with limited small-cell lung cancer prior to and shortly following prophylactic cranial irradiation. Int J Radiat Oncol Biol Phys 33:179–182

Kotalik J, Yu E, Markman BR et al. (2001) Practice guideline on prophylactic cranial irradiation in small-cell lung cancer. Int J Radiat Oncol Biol Phys 50:309–316

Liengswangwong V, Bonner JA, Shaw EG et al. (1994) Limited stage small-cell lung cancer: patterns of intrathoracic recurrence and the implications for thoracic radiotherapy. J Clin Oncol 12:496–502

Line DH, Deeley TJ (1971) The necropsy findings in carcinoma of the bronchus. Br J Dis Chest 65:238–242

List AF, Hainsworth JD, Davis BW et al. (1986) The syndrome of inappropriate secretion of antidiuretic hormone (SIADH) in small cell lung cancer. J Clin Oncol 4:1191–1198

Loehrer PJ Sr, Einhorn LH, Greco FA (1988) Cisplatin plus etoposide in small cell lung cancer. Semin Oncol 15[3 Suppl 3]:2–8

Movsas B, Raffin TA, Epstein AH et al. (1997) Pulmonary radiation injury. Chest 111:1061–1076

Murray N, Coy P, Pater JL et al. (1993) Importance of timing for thoracic irradiation in the combined modality treatment of limited-stage small-cell lung cancer. The National Cancer Institute of Canada Clinical Trials Group. J Clin Oncol 11:336–344

National Comprehensive Cancer Network (2008) Clinical practice guidelines in oncology: small-cell lung cancer. Available at http://www.nccn.org/ Accessed on March 30, 2008

Paesmans M, Sculier JP, Lecomte J et al. (2000) Prognostic factors for patients with small cell lung carcinoma: analysis of a series of 763 patients included in 4 consecutive prospective trials with a minimum follow-up of 5 years. Cancer 89:523–533

Pignon JP, Arriagada R, Ihde DC et al. (1992) A meta-analysis of thoracic radiotherapy for small-cell lung cancer. N Engl J Med 327:1618–1624

Radiation Therapy Oncology Group (2007) Active lung cancer protocols. Available at http://www.rtog.org/members/active.html#lung. Accessed on October 23, 2007

Sculier JP, Paesmans M, Bureau G et al. (1996) Randomized trial comparing induction chemotherapy versus induction chemotherapy followed by maintenance chemotherapy in small-cell lung cancer. European Lung Cancer Working Party. J Clin Oncol 14:2337–2344

Shepherd FA, Ginsberg RJ, Patterson GA et al. (1989) A prospective study of adjuvant surgical resection after chemotherapy for limited small cell lung cancer. A University of Toronto Lung Oncology Group study. J Thorac Cardiovasc Surg 97:177–186

Skarlos DV, Samantas E, Kosmidis P et al. (1994) Randomized comparison of etoposide-cisplatin vs. etoposide-carboplatin and irradiation in small-cell lung cancer. A Hellenic Co-operative Oncology Group study. Ann Oncol 5:601–607

Stahel RA, Ginsberg R, Havermann K et al (1989) Staging and prognostic factors in small cell lung cancer: a consensus. Lung Cancer 5:119–126

Sundstrøm S, Bremnes RM, Kaasa S et al. (2002) Cisplatin and etoposide regimen is superior to cyclophosphamide, epirubicin, and vincristine regimen in small-cell lung cancer: results from a randomized phase III trial with 5 years' follow-up. J Clin Oncol 20:4665–4672

Slotman B, Faivre-Finn C, Kramer G et al. (2007) Prophylactic cranial irradiation in extensive small-cell lung cancer. N Engl J Med 357:664–672

Suwinski R, Lee SP Withers HR (1998) Dose-response relationship for prophylactic cranial irradiation in small-cell lung cancer. Int J Radiat Oncol Biol Phys 40:797–806

Turrisi AT 3rd, Kim K, Blum R et al. (1999) Twice-daily compared with once-daily thoracic radiotherapy in limited small-cell lung cancer treated concurrently with cisplatin and etoposide. N Engl J Med 340:265–271

Warde P, Payne D (1992) Does thoracic irradiation improve survival and local control in limited-stage small-cell carcinoma of the lung? A meta-analysis. J Clin Oncol 10:890–895

Thymoma

11

Feng-Ming (Spring) Kong and Jiade J. Lu

CONTENTS

F.-M. (Spring) Kong, MD, PhD, MPH
Radiation Oncology, Veteran Administration Health Center and University Hospital Department of Radiation Oncology, University of Michigan, 1500 E Medical Center Drive, Ann Arbor, MI 48109, USA
J. J. Lu, MD, MBA
Department of Radiation Oncology, National University Cancer Institute of Singapore, National University Health System, National University of Singapore, 5 Lower Kent Ridge Road, Singapore 119074, Singapore

Introduction and Objectives

Thymoma is a tumor originating from the epithelial cells of the thymus. Thymic tumors are the most commonly diagnosed tumors in the anterior mediastinum in adults, accounting for approximately 50% of anterior mediastinal tumors. Thymoma is usually an indolent disease with a potential of local invasion.

This chapter examines:

- Recommendations for diagnosis and staging procedures
- Staging systems and prognostic factors
- Treatment recommendations for both resectable and unresectable diseases
- The use of chemotherapy in both resectable and unresectable disease and the role of radiation therapy
- Techniques of radiation therapy
- Follow-up care and surveillance of survivors

11.1 Diagnosis, Staging, and Prognoses

11.1.1 Diagnosis

Initial Evaluation

- Approximately one-third of patients with thymoma are diagnosed incidentally on chest X-ray.
- Diagnosis and evaluation of thymoma starts with a complete history and physical examination (H&P). Attention should be paid to thymoma-specific history, signs, and symptoms including cough, chest pain, dysphagia, superior vena cava syndrome, and thymoma-associated paraneoplastic syndromes including myasthenia gravis.
- Lymph node metastases are rare in thymomas, but are present in 40% of thymic carcinomas.

- Myasthenia gravis occurs in approximately 30%–45% of cases of thymoma, and 10%–15% of patients with myasthenia gravis will develop thymoma during their course of disease. Myasthenia gravis is an uncommon manifestation of thymic carcinoma (LÓPEZ-CANO et al. 2003).
- Other commonly seen paraneoplastic syndromes associated with thymoma include pure red cell aplasia, hypogammaglobulinemia, and various types of autoimmune disorders and vasculitides. Paraneoplastic syndromes are rare in thymic carcinoma.

Laboratory Tests

- Initial lab tests should include a complete blood count, basic blood chemistry, liver and renal function tests, and other studies directed by the presenting syndromes. Serum α-fetoprotein and β-HCG in male patients should be performed to rule out germ cell tumor.

Imaging Studies

- CT scan of the thorax is the most important imaging study for mediastinal tumors and is usually required to evaluate the characteristics and extent of the disease.
- MRI can be considered for distinguishing anterior mediastinal tumors (Grade B). While CT is superior to MRI of the chest in the diagnosis of anterior mediastinal tumors, MRI is more valuable for evaluating thymic cyst such as thymic cyst with hemorrhage or inflammation which mimic solid tumor despite low enhancement (Level III) (TOMIYAMA et al. 2007).
- Octreotide scanning for diagnosis and staging of thymoma or thymic carcinoma should not be routinely considered. Octreotide scanning was reported to be accurate for diagnosing thymoma in a small prospective series of 18 cases (Level III) (LASTORIA et al. 1998). However, whether octreotide scanning provides additive value over its value over traditional diagnostic process is unknown.
- The use of FDG-PET scans for diagnosis and staging of thymoma is currently under investigation and should not be routinely utilized.

Pathology

- Clinical diagnosis of a thymoma is usually sufficient for small tumors, especially in cases associated with paraneoplastic syndromes. Biopsy

of the tumor is usually necessary for large and locally invasive tumor for pathological diagnosis, or when lymphoma or germ cell tumors are considered (Grade C). The results from a retrospective series from Johns Hopkins Hospital revealed improved survival in patients who underwent biopsy before tumor resection (Level IV) (WILKINS et al. 1999). However, case reports raised concerns of tumor spillage into the pleura space when the capsule was breached during biopsy (Level V) (MORAN et al. 1992).

- Biopsy can be performed using CT-guided core needle biopsy, anterior mediastinoscopy. Video-assisted thoracoscopy or open surgical biopsy by limited anterior mediastinotomy may be necessary if fine-needle aspiration or core biopsy is insufficient to establish the diagnosis.
- Tumor spillage into pleural space or seeding along needle track secondary to biopsy procedures has not been confirmed.
- Approximately 50% of thymomas are localized within a capsule without infiltration at diagnosis, and the vast majority (90%–95%) are localized and resectable. Small and encapsulated disease should be excised for diagnosis and treatment.
- Thymoma can be classified histologically into six subtypes according to the WHO classification (Table 11.1) (ROSAI 1999). Thymic carcinoma (type C) represents less than 1% of the thymic malignancies. The WHO classification of thymoma is of prognostic significance.

Table 11.1. World Health Organization pathologic classification of thymoma

Type	Histologic description	5-/10-Year survival
– A	– Medullary thymoma	– 100/95%
– AB	– Mixed thymoma	– 93/90%
– B1	– Predominately cortical thymoma	– 89/85%
– B2	– Cortical thymoma	– 82/71%
– B3	– Thymic carcinoma	– 71/40%
– C	– Well-differentiated thymic carcinoma	– 23%
	– Thymic carcinoma	

11.1.2 Staging

- Two pathological staging systems exist for the staging of thymoma.
- The staging system proposed by MASAOKA et al. (1981) is based on the histological finding of lo-

cal invasion and has been widely adopted for the staging of thymoma (Table 11.2).

■ The staging system proposed by the Groupe d'Etudes des Tumerus Thymiques (GETT) is based on the extent of surgical resection (Table 11.3) (GAMONDÈS et al. 1991).

11.1.3 Prognostic Factors

■ The most important determinants of long-term survival in thymoma include stage, completeness of resection, and histologic classification of the disease.

■ The stage (i.e., invasiveness) of the tumor is the main prognostic factor of thymoma. The 10-year overall survival ranges between 90% to 100% for Masaoka stage I and II, 50%–60% for stage III, and 0%–10% for stage IV diseases (Level IV) (MAGGI et al. 1986; QUINTANILLA-MARTINEZ et al. 1994; BLUMBERG et al. 1995).

■ Completeness of resection and the use of post-operative adjuvant radiation therapy for incompletely resected cases are significant prognostic factors (Level IV) (MYOJIN et al. 2000; RENA et al. 2005).

■ The WHO classification is an independent prognostic factor of thymoma. The significance of the WHO classification in predicting long-term outcome of thymoma has been confirmed by a number of studies. The 10-year disease-free survival of type A and AB disease approaches 95%–100%. That of type B1, B2, and B3 diseases approximates 85%, 70%, and 40%, respectively (Level IV) (CHEN et al. 2002; KONDO et al. 2004; RENA et al. 2005; OKUMURA et al. 2002). The median survival of patients with thymic carcinoma is approximately 2 years, and the 10-year overall survival average 33% (ENG 2004). The presence of myasthenia gravis at diagnosis is not an independent predictor of overall survival after definitive treatment, but may indicate favorable prognosis in advanced diseases (Level IV) (CHEN et al. 2002; KONDO and MONDEN 2005; LUCCHI 2005).

■ Age, gender, and disease-free interval are not independent predictors of overall survival (Level IV) (PESCARMONA et al. 1990; QUINTANILLA-MARTINEZ et al. 1994; BLUMBERG et al. 1995).

Table 11.2. Masaoka staging system of thymomas

Stage	Description	5-Year survival
I	Macroscopically completely encapsulated and microscopically no capsular invasion	94%–100%
II	Microscopically invasion into capsule (A); or macroscopically invasion into surrounding fatty tissue or mediastinal pleura (B)	86%–95%
III	Macroscopically invasion into neighboring organs (i.e., pericardium, great vessels, or lung). (A) Without invasion of great vessels and (B) with invasion of great vessels	56%–69%
IV	Pleural or pericardial dissemination (A) Lymphogenous or hematogenous metastases (B)	11%–50%

Table 11.3. GETT staging system of thymomas

Stage	Description	5-Year survival
Ia	Encapsulated tumor, totally resected	100%
Ib	Macroscopically encapsulated tumor, totally resected, but the surgeon suspects mediastinal adhesions and potential capsular invasion	60%–87%
II	Invasive tumor, totally resected	85%
IIIa	Invasive tumor, subtotally resected	65%
IIIb	Invasive tumor, biopsy	40%
IVA	Supraclavicular metastasis or distant pleural implant	
IVB	Distant metastases	

11.2 Treatment of Resectable Thymoma

11.2.1 General Principles

■ Surgery is the mainstay treatment for potentially resectable thymoma (Grade A).
■ Adjuvant treatment of any type is usually not justified for stage I disease after complete resection.
■ Postoperative radiation therapy may be recommended for stage II and stage III thymoma after complete resection for local control (Grade C).
■ Postoperative radiation therapy is recommended for incompletely resected stage III and IVA thymoma (Grade B).
■ Currently there is no evidence to support the use of adjuvant chemotherapy in the treatment of thymoma after surgical resection.

11.2.2 Surgery

■ Complete resection is the treatment of choice for surgically resectable thymoma (Grade A). Completeness of surgical resection is of prognostic significance. Incomplete resection leads to poor results even with postoperative radiotherapy or chemoradiotherapy for locally advanced disease (Level IV) (Myojin et al. 2000; Rena et al. 2005).
■ Median sternotomy is the standard procedure for most cases of thymoma. Other surgical techniques such as cervical approaches or video-assisted thoracic surgery have been reported, but their efficacy in comparison with median sternotomy approach needs to be confirmed.
■ Preoperative preparation (including plasmapheresis) for patients with myasthenia gravis may be necessary to avoid respiratory complications in the perioperative period.
■ Perioperative mortality is less than 1% in modern series.

11.2.3 Adjuvant Radiation Therapy

■ For encapsulated thymoma (Masaoka stage I), adjuvant treatment after complete resection is not justified (Grade A). The disease-specific survival of patients with encapsulated thymoma approaches 100%, and locoregional recurrence rate is less than 5% after surgery alone (Level IV) (Curran et al. 1988; Maggi 1991).
■ For stage II disease, adjuvant radiation therapy may be recommended after resection (Grade C). Although close to 100% of stage II thymoma can be completely resected, results from retrospective series showed that the local recurrent rate approached 30% after complete resection of stage II thymoma, as compared to less than 10% for those receiving postoperative radiation therapy (Level IV) (Curran et al. 1988; Haniuda et al. 1996; Ogawa et al. 2002). However, results from other retrospective studies did not confirm such findings (Level IV) (Mangi et al. 2002; Kondo and Monden 2003).
■ For stage III thymoma, adjuvant radiation therapy after surgery may be recommended after resection, especially in type B2 and B3 diseases (Grade C). Complete resection is possible in approximately 60% of stage III thymoma. Results from a number of retrospective series have indicated that adjuvant radiation therapy after complete resection is beneficial for local control in stage II and III thymoma (Level IV) (Curran et al. 1988; Gripp et al. 1998; Ogawa et al. 2002). In a recently published large retrospective review of 228 resected thymoma cases, adjuvant radiation therapy was given to 42 patients. No patients receiving adjuvant radiation after complete resection had recurrence, as compared to 33% local recurrence rate among those receiving complete resection only (Level IV) (Ströbel et al. 2004).
   However, results from a small series from Japan revealed that the recurrence rates for stage III patients with or without adjuvant radiation were 23% and 26%, respectively, after complete resection (Level IV) (Kondo and Monden 2003).
■ Complete resection is usually not feasible for stage IVA thymoma. For incompletely resected stage III and stage IVA cases, adjuvant radiation therapy is recommended (Grade B). Results from numerous retrospective studies have confirmed that adjuvant radiotherapy can improve local control and overall survival rates.
   Radiation to the entire mediastinum was found to improve local control in stage III and IVA thymoma after surgery. In a retrospective study from Italy which included 77 patients with stage

III and IVA diseases, complete resection was achieved in 56% of stage III cases and in no patients with stage IVA diseases. Intrathoracic relapses occurred in 15.2% of patients in stage III and in 50% of patients in stage IVA disease, but only seven relapses (9.1%) were within the limits of the radiation field (Level IV) (URGESI et al. 1990).

In the above-mentioned study by STRÖBEL et al. (2004), 75 patients with B2 and B3, stage III, or higher thymomas had incomplete resection of their primary diseases. The recurrence rate of patients who received adjuvant chemoradiation therapy was 34%, as compared to 78% in patients without adjuvant treatment (Level IV) (STRÖBEL et al. 2004).

11.2.4 Chemotherapy

■ Currently, chemotherapy cannot be recommended for routine use after complete or partial resection of thymoma (Grade C). Thymoma is relatively sensitive to chemotherapy; however, chemotherapy is usually used for induction treatment for unresectable thymomas. In a French multicenter retrospective review of 90 cases with stage III and IVA thymomas, a subgroup (59) of patients received postoperative chemotherapy, with or without radiation. The results showed that chemotherapy was not a significant prognostic factor after partial resection or biopsy (Level IV) (MORNEX et al. 1995).

11.3 Treatment of Unresectable Thymoma

11.3.1 General Principles

■ A combined multimodality approach including induction chemotherapy, radiation therapy, and/or surgery should be considered for unresectable thymoma (Grade A).
■ The use of radiotherapy as induction therapy for unresectable thymoma is justified if chemotherapy is contraindicated (Grade C).

11.3.2 Induction Chemotherapy

■ Induction chemotherapy followed by radiation therapy or surgery (with or without radiation) is usually indicated for unresectable thymoma (Grade A). Thymoma is relatively sensitive to chemotherapy, and response rates to induction chemotherapy ranges from 60%–77%.

An Intergroup phase II trial treated 26 patients with limited-stage unresectable thymoma with four cycles of induction cisplatin-doxorubicin-cyclophosphamide chemotherapy, followed by external beam radiation (54 Gy in conventional fractionation) to the primary disease and regional lymph nodes. Complete or partial response were seen in 16 of 26 cases, and the progression-free and overall survival rates at 5 years were 54% and 52%, respectively (Level III) (LOEHRER et al. 1997).

A phase II trial from the M. D. Anderson Cancer Center treated 22 patients with invasive and unresectable disease with induction chemotherapy (cyclophosphamide, doxorubicin, cisplatin, and prednisone) followed by surgical resection, followed by adjuvant radiation therapy and consolidated chemotherapy. Response was observed in 77% of patients, and 21 patients underwent complete resection (16 patients) or incomplete resection (five patients). The overall survival rate was 95% and 79% at 5 and 7 years, respectively (Level III) (KIM et al. 2004).

11.3.3 Induction Chemoradiation

■ Induction chemoradiation followed by surgery can also be used in unresectable thymoma (Grade C). WRIGHT et al. (2008) treated 10 patients with cisplatin and etoposide along with 45 Gy of radiation over the past 10 years with acceptable toxicity and no treatment-related mortality. There were seven stage II (post-treatment) and three stage IVA patients – the 5-year survival was 60% in all patients and 85% in the stage III patients (Level IV) (WRIGHT et al. 2008).

11.3.4 Adjuvant and Neoadjuvant Radiation Therapy

■ Radiation therapy is usually recommended after induction chemotherapy followed by surgical resection for unresectable cases. Adjuvant radiation seems most appropriate in the setting of incomplete resections or close margins.

- Adjuvant chemoradiation can also be used following neoadjuvant chemotherapy and surgery (Grade B). In a prospective series of 45 cases of unresectable stage III thymic tumors, induction and adjuvant chemotherapy was found to be effective and safe. The 10-year survival rates after induction chemotherapy, surgery, followed by adjuvant chemotherapy for patients with thymoma or well-differentiated thymic carcinoma were 90% and 85%, respectively. The 8-year survival for patients with thymic carcinoma was 56% (Level III) (VENUTA et al. 2003).

- Preoperative radiation therapy can be used for unresectable thymoma if induction chemotherapy is contraindicated (Grade C). A small retrospective series from Japan of 12 patients with unresectable thymoma was treated with preoperative radiation therapy followed by surgery. Complete resection was possible by concomitant resection of the surrounding tissues, mainly pericardium and/or brachiocephalic vein in nine of the 12 patients (Level IV) (AKAOGI et al. 1996). The use of preoperative radiation therapy was also reported by other studies and results have shown that preoperative treatment to increase the complete resection rate could improve the overall survival of these patients (Level IV) (BRETTI et al. 2004; OHARA et al. 1990).

- A dose of 40–50 Gy can be considered in 1.8- to 2.0-Gy daily fractions for preoperative radiation therapy (Grade D).

- For surgically unresectable or medically inoperable cases after induction chemotherapy, radiation therapy can be used for local treatment (Grade B). As in cases with gross residual after surgery, a total dose of 60–70 Gy may be needed for patients with unresectable disease (Grade D). Lower radiation dose may be associated with higher chances of disease progression or recurrence.
  The progression-free and overall survival rates at 5 years were 54% and 52%, respectively, after induction chemotherapy followed by radiation to a total dose of 54 Gy, as reported in the above mentioned Intergroup phase II trial (Level III) (LOEHRER et al. 1997).

11.4 Radiation Therapy Techniques

11.4.1 Simulation, Target Volumes, and Field Arrangement

- CT-based planning is highly recommended. CT scan should be taken in the treatment position with arms raised above the head (treatment position). Simulations of considering target motion are encouraged whenever possible. CT scan can be performed at the end of natural inhale, exhale, and under free breathing, when more sophisticated techniques like 4D CT or gated CT, active breathing control (ABC) are not available.

- The gross tumor volume (GTV) should include any grossly visible tumor. Surgical clips indicative of gross residual tumor should be included for postoperative cases.

- The clinical tumor volume (CTV) for postoperative radiation therapy should encompass the potential site with residual disease, the entire thymus (for partial resection cases), and any potential sites with residual diseases. The treatment field should include CTV plus 1.5- to 2-cm margin for motion and set-up errors.

- Extensive elective nodal irradiation (entire mediastinum and bilateral supraclavicular nodal regions) is not recommended (Grade B). Thymomas do not commonly metastasize to regional lymph nodes, thus elective nodal irradiation is often substantially morbid without any evidence of clinical benefit (Level IV) (RUFFINI et al. 1997).

- The planning target volume (PTV) should consider the target motion and daily set-up error. The PTV margin should be based on individual patient's motion, the simulation techniques used (with and without inclusion motion) and reproducibility of daily set-up of each clinic.

- Radiation beam arrangements depend on the shape of PTV aiming to confine the prescribed high dose to the target and minimize dose to adjacent critical structures. Anterior-posterior and posterior-anterior (AP/PA) ports weighting more anteriorly (Fig. 11.1), or wedge pair technique (Fig. 11.2) may be considered.

- Three-dimensional conformal plan (Fig. 11.3) and intensity-modulated radiation therapy (IMRT) (Fig. 11.4) may further improve the dose distribution and decrease dose to normal tissue.

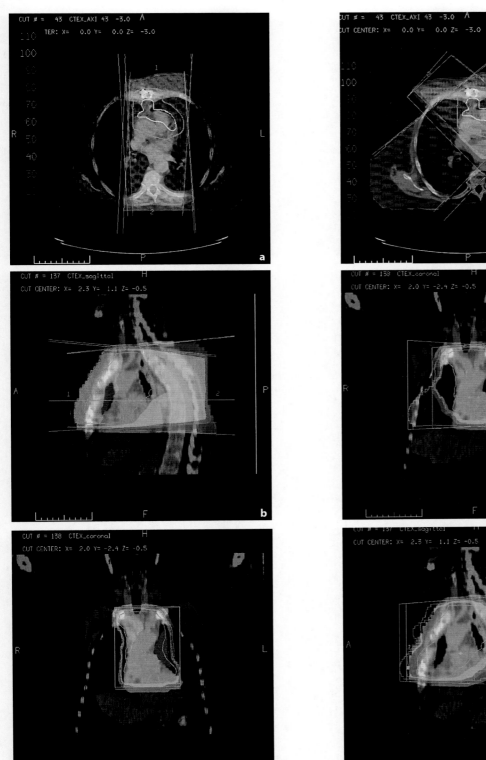

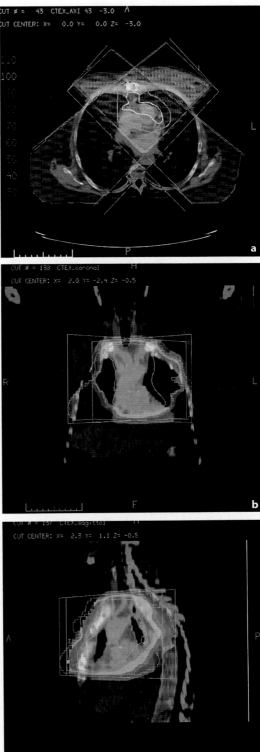

Fig. 11.1a–c. Isodose distribution of an AP/PA traditional field arrangement in a postoperative case (prescription dose=54 Gy to the ICRU reference point)

Fig. 11.2a–c. Isodose distribution of a wedge paired field arrangement in a postoperative case (prescription dose = 54 Gy to the ICRU reference point)

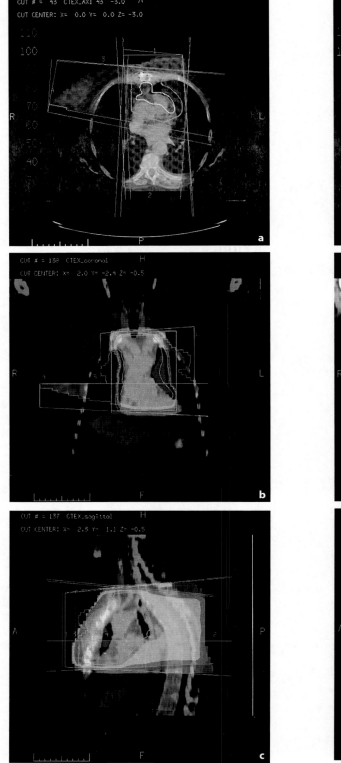

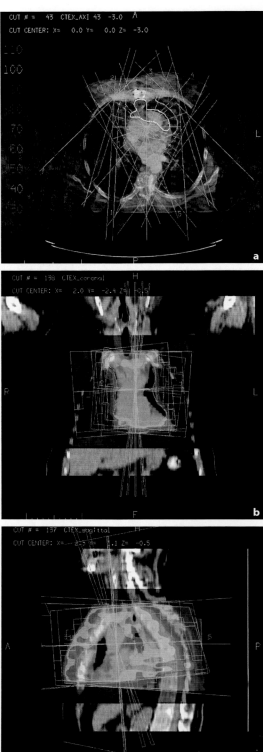

Fig. 11.3a–c. Isodose distribution of a 3 D conformal radiation therapy in a postoperative case (prescription dose = 54 Gy to the ICRU reference point)

Fig. 11.4a–c. Isodose distribution of an intensity modulated radiation therapy (IMRT) in a postoperative case (prescription dose = 54 Gy to the planning target volume)

■ These techniques, though commonly used during traditional 2D era, can generate excessive dose to normal tissue (Figs. 11.5 and 11.6).

11.4.2 Dose and Fractionation

■ The dose and fractionation schemes of radiation therapy depend on the completeness of surgical resection.

■ For adjuvant treatment, the radiation dose consists of 45–50 Gy for clear/close margins, 54 Gy for microscopically positive resection margins, and 60 Gy for grossly positive margins, if conventional fractionation (1.8–2.0 Gy per daily fraction) is recommended (Grade D).

■ A total dose of 60–70 Gy may be needed for patients with gross residual disease after surgery, although there is no clear evidence of a dose-response relationship for thymoma due to the rarity of the disease (Grade D) (Level IV) (MORNEX et al. 1995).

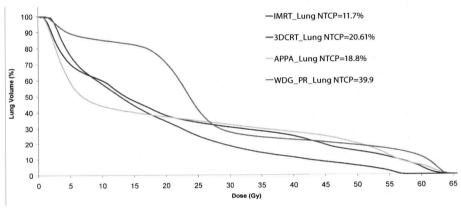

Fig. 11.5. Comparison of lung dose volume histograms (DVH) treated with various techniques. NTCP = normal tissue complication probability

Technique	Radiation Therapy (RT)	Mean Lung Dose
IMRT	Intensity Modulated RT	17.2 Gy
3DCRT	3-D Conformal RT	21.4 Gy
APPA	Anterior/Posterior 2DRT	20.6 Gy
WDG	Wedge Paired 2DRT	27.8 Gy

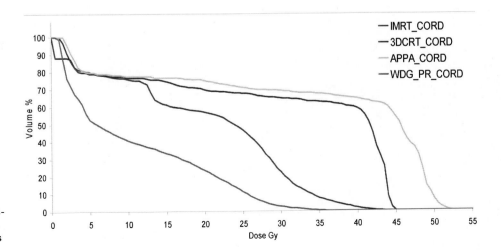

Fig. 11.6. Comparison of cord dose volume histograms (DVH) treated with various techniques

11.5 Side Effects and Complications

11.5.1 Radiation-Induced Side Effects and Complications

- Commonly seen acute side effects secondary to radiation treatment for thymoma include fatigue, skin erythema, odynophagia, dysphagia, cough, or mild dyspnea.
- Late complications include radiation-induced lung toxicities (such as pneumonitis, fibrosis), radiation-induced cardiac diseases (such as pericarditis or myocarditis), and myelopathy (rarely).
- To avoid late toxicities to lung, the mean lung dose should be limited to 20 Gy, and V_{20} of total lung with exclusion of gross tumor volume should be limited to $\leq 30\%$ (Grade B). Radiation-induced lung toxicity is associated with many lung dosimetric factors such as volume receiving ≥ 20 Gy (V_{20}) and the mean lung dose. The risk for developing radiation-induced lung toxicity increases substantially if mean lung dose is >20 Gy (Level III) (Kong et al. 2006; Wang et al. 2006).
- To avoid radiation-induced heart disease, V_{40} of the heart should be limited to 50% or less (Grade B). Radiation-induced myocarditis rarely

occurs at doses lower than 50 Gy. Dose of radiation to the spinal cord should be limited to 45 Gy (1.8–2.0 Gy daily) (Grade C) (Level IV) (Emami 1991).

11.6 Follow-Ups

11.6.1 Post-Treatment Follow-Ups

- Life-long follow-up is required for thymoma patients after definitive treatment (Grade B). Late recurrences up to 12% occurring 10–20 years after surgery has been reported (Level IV) (Wilkins 1999).
- Follow-ups could be scheduled every 4–6 months initially in the first 2 years after treatment, then annually thereafter (Grade D) (NCCN 2008).
- Each follow-up examination should include a complete history and physical examination. Annual thoracic CT scan is recommended by the National Comprehensive Cancer Network clinical practice guidelines (Grade D) (NCCN 2008). Other imaging studies and lab studies should be ordered according to clinical findings on follow-up examinations.

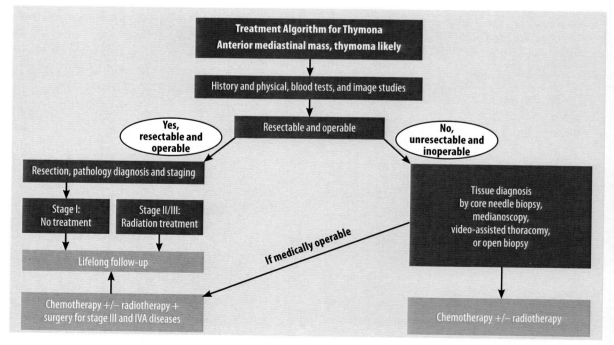

Fig. 11.7. A proposed treatment algorithm for thymoma

Acknowledgments

We are in debt to Daniel Tatro, CMD and Randall Ten Haken, PhD from the University of Michigan, USA for the treatment plan figures.

References

Akaogi E, Ohara K, Mitsui K et al. (1996) Preoperative radiotherapy and surgery for advanced thymoma with invasion to the great vessels. J Surg Oncol 63:17–22

Blumberg D, Port JL, Weksler B et al. (1995) Thymoma: a multivariate analysis of factors predicting survival. Ann Thorac Surg 60:908–913

Bretti S, Berruti A, Loddo C et al. (2004) Piemonte Oncology Network. Multimodal management of stages III–IVa malignant thymoma. Lung Cancer 44:69–77

Chen G, Marx A, Wen-Hu C et al. (2002) New WHO histologic classification predicts prognosis of thymic epithelial tumors: a clinicopathologic study of 200 thymoma cases from China. Cancer 95:420–429

Curran WJ Jr, Kornstein MJ, Brooks JJ et al. (1988) Invasive thymoma: the role of mediastinal irradiation following complete or incomplete surgical resection. J Clin Oncol 6:1722–1727

Emami B, Lyman J, Brown A et al. (1991) Tolerance of normal tissue to therapeutic irradiation. Int J Radiat Oncol Biol Phys 21:109–122

Eng TY, Fuller CD, Jagirdar J et al. (2004) Thymic carcinoma: state of the art review. Int J Radiat Oncol Biol Phys 59:654–664

Gamondès JP, Balawi A, Greenland T et al. (1991) Seventeen years of surgical treatment of thymoma: factors influencing survival. Eur J Cardiothorac Surg 5:124–131

Gripp S, Hilgers K, Wurm R et al. (1998) Thymoma: prognostic factors and treatment outcomes. Cancer 83:1495–1503

Haniuda M, Miyazawa M, Yoshida K et al. (1996) Is postoperative radiotherapy for thymoma effective? Ann Surg 224:219–224

Kim ES, Putnam JB, Komaki R et al. (2004) Phase II study of a multidisciplinary approach with induction chemotherapy, followed by surgical resection, radiation therapy, and consolidation chemotherapy for unresectable malignant thymomas: final report. Lung Cancer 44:369–379

Kondo K, Monden Y (2005) Thymoma and myasthenia gravis: a clinical study of 1,089 patients from Japan. Ann Thorac Surg 79:219–224

Kondo K, Monden Y (2003) Therapy for thymic epithelial tumors: a clinical study of 1,320 patients from Japan. Ann Thorac Surg 76:878–884

Kondo K, Yoshizawa K, Tsuyuguchi M et al. (2004) WHO histologic classification is a prognostic indicator in thymoma. Ann Thorac Surg 77:1183–1188

Kong FM, Hayman JA, Griffith KA et al. (2006) Final toxicity results of a radiation-dose escalation study in patients with non-small-cell lung cancer (NSCLC): predictors for radiation pneumonitis and fibrosis. Int J Radiat Oncol Biol Phys 65:1075–1086

Lastoria S, Vergara E, Palmieri G et al. (1998) In vivo detection of malignant thymic masses by indium-111--DTPA-D-Phe1-octreotide scintigraphy. J Nucl Med 39:634–639

Loehrer PJ Sr, Chen M, Kim K et al. (1997) Cisplatin, doxorubicin, and cyclophosphamide plus thoracic radiation therapy for limited-stage unresectable thymoma: an intergroup trial. J Clin Oncol 15:3093–3099

López-Cano M, Ponseti-Bosch JM, Espin-Basany E et al. (2003) Clinical and pathologic predictors of outcome in thymoma-associated myasthenia gravis. Ann Thorac Surg 76:1643–1649

Lucchi M, Ambrogi MC, Duranti L et al. (2005) Advanced stage thymomas and thymic carcinomas: results of multimodality treatments. Ann Thorac Surg 79:1840–1844

Maggi G, Giaccone G, Donadio M et al. (1986) Thymomas. A review of 169 cases, with particular reference to results of surgical treatment. Cancer 58:765–776

Maggi G, Casadio C, Cavallo A et al. (1991) Thymoma: results of 241 operated cases. Ann Thorac Surg 51:152–156

Mangi AA, Wright CD, Allan JS et al. (2002) Adjuvant radiation therapy for stage II thymoma. Ann Thorac Surg 74:1033–1037

Masaoka A, Monden Y, Nakahara K, Tanioka T (1981) Follow-up study of thymomas with special reference to their clinical stages. Cancer 48:2485–2492

Moran CA, Travis WD, Rosado-de-Christenson M et al. (1992) Thymomas presenting as pleural tumors. Report of eight cases. Am J Surg Pathol 16:138–144

Mornex F, Resbeut M, Richaud P et al. (1995) Radiotherapy and chemotherapy for invasive thymomas: a multicentric retrospective review of 90 cases. The FNCLCC trialists. Fédération Nationale des Centres de Lutte Contre le Cancer. Int J Radiat Oncol Biol Phys 32:651–659

Myojin M, Choi NC, Wright CD et al. (2000) Stage III thymoma: pattern of failure after surgery and postoperative radiotherapy and its implication for future study. Int J Radiat Oncol Biol Phys 46:927–933

National Comprehensive Cancer Network (2008) Clinical practice guidelines in oncology: non-small-cell lung cancer. Available at http://www.nccn.org/professionals/physician_gls/PDF/nscl.pdf . Accessed on March 8, 2007

Ogawa K, Uno T, Toita T, Onishi H et al. (2002) Postoperative radiotherapy for patients with completely resected thymoma: a multi-institutional, retrospective review of 103 patients. Cancer 94:1405–1413

Ohara K, Okumura T, Sugahara S et al. (1990) The role of preoperative radiotherapy for invasive thymoma. Acta Oncol 29:425–429

Okumura M, Ohta M, Tateyama H et al. (2002) The World Health Organization histologic classification system reflects the oncologic behavior of thymoma: a clinical study of 273 patients. Cancer 94:624–632

Pescarmona E, Rendina EA, Venuta F et al. (1990) Analysis of prognostic factors and clinicopathological staging of thymoma. Ann Thorac Surg 50:534–538

Quintanilla-Martinez L, Wilkins EW Jr, Choi N et al. (1994) Thymoma. Histologic subclassification is an independent prognostic factor. Cancer 74:606–617

Rena O, Papalia E, Maggi G et al. (2005) World Health Organization histologic classification: an independent prognostic factor in resected thymomas. Lung Cancer 50:59–66

Rosai J (1999) Histological typing of tumors of the thymus, 2nd edn. Springer-Verlag, Berlin Heidelberg New York

Ruffini E, Mancuso M, Oliaro A et al. (1997) Recurrence of thymoma: analysis of clinicopathologic features, treatment, and outcome. J Thorac Cardiovasc Surg 113:55–63

Ströbel P, Bauer A, Puppe B et al. (2004) Tumor recurrence and survival in patients treated for thymomas and thymic squamous cell carcinomas: a retrospective analysis. J Clin Oncol 22:1501–1509

Tomiyama N, Honda O, Tsubamoto M et al. (2007) Anterior mediastinal tumors: diagnostic accuracy of CT and MRI. Eur J Radiol 2007 Nov 17; [Epub ahead of print]

Urgesi A, Monetti U, Rossi G et al. (1990) Role of radiation therapy in locally advanced thymoma. Radiother Oncol 19:273–280

Venuta F, Rendina EA, Longo F et al. (2003) Long-term outcome after multimodality treatment for stage III thymic tumors. Ann Thorac Surg 76:1866–1872

Wang SL, Liao Z, Vaporciyan AA et al. (2006) Investigation of clinical and dosimetric factors associated with postoperative pulmonary complications in esophageal cancer patients treated with concurrent chemoradiotherapy followed by surgery. Int J Radiat Oncol Biol Phys 64:692–699

Wilkins KB, Sheikh E, Green R et al. (1999) Clinical and pathologic predictors of survival in patients with thymoma. Ann Surg 230:562–572

Wright CD, Choi NC, John C. Wain JC et al. (2008) Induction chemoradiotherapy followed by resection for locally advanced Masaoka stage III and IVA thymic tumors. Ann Thorac Surg 85:385–389

Esophageal Cancer

12

JIADE J. LU

CONTENTS

J. J. Lu, MD, MBA
Department of Radiation Oncology, National University Cancer Institute of Singapore, National University Health System, National University of Singapore, 5 Lower Kent Ridge Road, Singapore 119074, Singapore

Introduction and Objectives

Esophageal cancer is a highly malignant disease with a cure rate of less than 20%. Less than 40% of patients present with localized and resectable disease. Both surgery and combined chemoradiation therapy are important therapeutic modalities in curative treatment for esophageal cancer. Radiation therapy plays an important role in palliation of symptoms caused by advanced local or metastatic disease.

This chapter examines:

● Recommendations for diagnosis and staging procedures

● The staging systems and prognostic factors

● Treatment recommendations as well as the supporting scientific evidence for esophagectomy and neoadjuvant and adjuvant treatment for resectable esophageal cancer

● The use of concurrent chemotherapy and radiotherapy for definitive treatment of locally advanced esophageal cancer

● Palliative radiation (external beam radiation therapy and brachytherapy) for symptomatic control in advanced diseases

● Follow-up care and surveillance of survivors

12.1 Diagnosis, Staging, and Prognoses

12.1.1 Diagnosis

Initial Evaluation

■ Diagnosis and evaluation of esophageal cancer starts with a complete history and physical examination (H&P). Attention should be paid to esophageal cancer-specific history, signs, and symptoms including tobacco and alcohol use, dietary history, obesity, weight loss, gastroesophageal reflux disease (GERD), dysphagia, odynophagia, cough, hoarseness, hematemesis, and hemoptysis.

■ Thorough physical examination should be performed with attention to aerodigestive track as well as cervical and/or supraclavicular lymphadenopathy.

■ Panendoscopy (triple endoscopy) examines the trachea, larynx, pharynx, and esophagus. Panendoscopy allows direct visualization of characterization, measurement of tumor extent, as well as biopsy for pathologic diagnosis.

Laboratory Tests

■ Initial laboratory tests should include a complete blood count, basic serum chemistry, liver function tests, renal function tests, and alkaline phosphatase.

Imaging Studies

■ CT scans of chest and abdomen are required to evaluate local extension, regional lymph nodes, and to rule out distant metastasis.

■ Endoscopic ultrasonography (EUS) should be performed to evaluate the depth of invasion from the primary disease, as well as periesophageal and regional nodal involvement (Grade B). The accuracy of EUS for evaluating T and N classifications approaches 90% and 80%, respectively, as compared to 70% and less than 60%, respectively, for CT of thorax (Level III) (KELLEY et al. 2001; PICUS et al. 1983; SALONEN et al. 1987).

■ Barium esophagram can be used to detect tracheoesophageal (TE) fistula and delineate the proximal and distal tumor margins. TE fistula is a relative contraindication of radiation therapy, and usually requires stent placement prior to treatment.

■ FDG-PET is highly encouraged for initial evaluation and staging (Grade B). The sensitivity and specificity of PET over CT scan alone have been repeatedly recognized in prospective studies (Level III) (KATO et al. 2005; KATSOULIS et al. 2007; FLAMEN et al. 2000; RANKIN et al. 1998). In addition, response of esophageal cancer in terms of reduction in metabolic activity on FDG-PET after definitive chemoradiation is of prognostic

value (Level III) (OTT et al. 2006; WIEDER et al. 2004).

■ Bone scan is indicated for patients with elevated alkaline phosphatase or if bone pain is reported. Bone scan is optional if FDG-PET is performed.

■ Imaging and laboratory work-ups required for the diagnosis and staging of esophageal cancer are listed in Table 12.1.

Table 12.1. Imaging and laboratory work-ups for esophageal cancer

Imaging studies	Laboratory tests
– Barium esophagram	– Complete blood count
– Endoscopic ultrasonography (EUS)	
– CT of chest and abdomen	– Serum chemistry
– FDG-PET scan or PET/CT	– Liver function tests
	– Renal function tests
– Bone scan (optional)	– Alkaline phosphatase

Pathology

■ Tissue for pathology diagnosis can be obtained during initial examination using endoscopy.

■ Pathologic confirmation of esophageal cancer is imperative prior to the initiation of any treatment. Treatment and prognosis of the more commonly diagnosed adenocarcinoma and squamous cell carcinoma (comprising 95% of all esophageal cancer cases combined) are substantially different from those of the more rarely diagnosed malignancies such as leiomyosarcoma, lymphoma, and malignant melanoma.

12.1.2 Staging

■ Esophageal cancer can be staged clinically and pathologically: Clinical staging utilizes information from H&P, imaging studies, endoscopy, and laboratory tests; Pathologic staging is based on findings from clinical staging and procedures such as esophagectomy and examination of the resected specimen.

■ The 2002 American Joint Committee on Cancer Tumor Node Metastasis (TNM) staging system is presented in Table 12.2.

Table 12.2. American Joint Committee on Cancer (AJCC) TNM classification of carcinoma of esophagus [from GREENE et al. (2002) with permission]

Primary tumor (T)	
TX	Primary tumor cannot be assessed
T0	No evidence of primary tumor
Tis	Carcinoma in situ
T1	Tumor invades lamina propria or submucosa
T2	Tumor invades muscularis propria
T3	Tumor invades adventitia
T4	Tumor invades adjacent structures
Regional lymph nodes (N)	
NX	Regional lymph node metastasis cannot be assessed
N0	No regional lymph node metastasis
N1	Regional lymph node metastasis
Distant metastasis (M)	
MX	Distant metastasis cannot be assessed
M0	No distant metastasis
M1	Distant metastasis present
Tumors of the lower thoracic esophagus:	
M1a	Metastasis in celiac lymph nodes
M1b	Other distant metastasis
Tumors of the midthoracic esophagus:	
M1a	Not applicable
M1b	Nonregional lymph node and/or other distant metastasis
Tumors of the upper thoracic esophagus:	
M1a	Metastasis in cervical lymph nodes
M1b	Other distant metastasis
STAGE GROUPING	
0:	Tis N0 M0
I:	T1 N0 M0
IIA:	T2 N0 M0, T3 N0 M0
IIB:	T1 N1 M0, T2 N1 M0
III:	T3 N1 M0, T4 Any N M0
IVA:	Any T Any N M1a
IVB:	Any T Any N M1b

* Used with permission of the American Joint Committee on Cancer (AJCC), Chicago, Illinois. The original and primary source for this information is the AJCC Cancer Staging Manual, 6th Edition (2002) published by Springer-Verlag New York.

12.1.3 Prognostic Factors

■ The prognosis of patients with esophageal cancer is directly associated with the presenting characteristics.

■ Stage is the most important prognostic factor in predicting patients' outcome.

■ The significance of pathologic subtypes of esophageal cancer (squamous cell carcinoma vs. adenocarcinoma) on prognosis has not been confirmed. For resectable cases, results from a large single-center series showed that the 5-year overall survival is better in adenocarcinoma than in squamous cell carcinoma (47% vs. 37%), as the probability of regional nodal metastasis is higher in the latter (Level IV) (SIEWERT et al. 2001). However, difference in survival was not observed in locally advanced esophageal cancer treated with chemoradiation between the two subtypes (Level II) (AL-SARRAF et al. 1997).

■ The size of the primary tumor and depth of tumor invasion are prognostically significant (CREHANGE et al. 2007; GREENE et al. 2002). However, anatomic location does not appear to be a significant prognostic factor (GREENE et al. 2002).

■ Male gender, advanced age (65 years of age or above), weight loss, and poor performance status have been associated with poor prognosis in esophageal cancer (Level III/IV) (CREHANGE et al. 2007; HUSSEY et al. 1980; PEARSON 1977).

■ Currently no biologic markers can be routinely recommended for determination of prognosis of esophageal cancer.

12.2 Treatment of Resectable Esophageal Cancer

12.2.1 General Principles

■ Stages I–III and selective IVA esophageal cancer are potentially resectable for cure, and approximately 30%–40% of patients with esophageal cancer present with potentially resectable disease.

■ Esophagectomy is the standard treatment for resectable cancer of thoracic esophagus. Cancer of the cervical esophagus (beginning at the level of the lower border of the cricoid cartilage and ending at the thoracic inlet at the level of suprasternal notch) is usually treated with radiation therapy or combined chemoradiotherapy for locally advanced disease without surgery.

- For stage T1-2 N0 M0 thoracic esophageal cancer, neoadjuvant or adjuvant treatment is not indicated, unless microscopic or macroscopic residual (including positive margins) is suspected after resection.
- For surgically resectable stage IIA (T3 N0 M0), IIB-IVA cancer of thoracic esophagus, induction chemoradiotherapy may further improve the treatment outcome and should be considered (Grade A). However, if esophagectomy is performed without induction therapy, chemoradiotherapy can be considered for adjuvant treatment (Grade B).
- Preoperative or postoperative radiotherapy (or chemotherapy) alone is usually not recommended for esophageal cancer before or after complete resection (Grade A).
- For patients with medically inoperable esophageal cancer or who decline surgery, external beam radiation is the definitive treatment of choice for stage T1-2 N0 M0 disease. Concurrent chemoradiotherapy should be considered for locally advanced lesions.

12.2.2 Surgical Resection

- Surgery is considered as the primary treatment for resectable esophageal cancer, with the exception of cancer of the cervical esophagus.
- Surgery alone is usually indicated for stage I and IIA thoracic esophageal cancer; however, surgery as a monotherapy for resectable but more advanced disease is questionable. The 5-year survival rates of less than 40% only after surgery alone for locally advanced esophageal cancer in contemporary surgical series suggested adjuvant treatment is necessary (HULSCHER et al. 2002; KELSEN et al. 1998).
- Esophagectomy can be accomplished by a transhiatal or transthoracic approach. The optimal surgical approach for esophageal cancer is debatable. Results of a randomized trial comparing transhiatal versus transthoracic approach in patients with adenocarcinoma of esophagus revealed no significant differences in 5-year

overall and disease-free survival rates, although transhiatal esophagectomy was associated with lower morbidity (Level I) (HULSCHER et al. 2002).

12.2.3 Preoperative (Neoadjuvant) Treatment

Preoperative Radiation Therapy

- Radiation therapy alone given preoperatively is not recommended in the treatment of resectable esophageal cancer (Grade A). Results from numerous randomized trials of various sizes comparing esophagectomy with or without preoperative radiotherapy revealed no improvement in respectability or overall survival rates from the addition of preoperative radiation (Level I or II) (ARNOTT et al. 1992; GIGNOUX et al. 1987; LAUNOIS et al. 1981; WANG et al. 1989). In addition, results from a meta-analysis including samples from five randomized studies showed no significance between patients treated with preoperative radiotherapy followed by surgery as compared to surgery alone, although a trend of reduction of risk of death (11% at 5 years) was noticed (Oesophageal Cancer Collaborative Group meta-analysis, Level I) (ARNOTT et al. 2005).

Pre- or Peri-operative Chemotherapy

- Chemotherapy alone given preoperatively is not routinely recommended in potentially resectable esophageal cancer (Grade A). The rate of pathologic complete response (CR) after neoadjuvant chemotherapy is low, and improvement of curative resection has not been demonstrated.

An Intergroup randomized trial reported the outcome of 440 patients with local and operable esophageal cancer (squamous cell carcinoma or adenocarcinoma) treated with surgery only or surgery with three cycles of pre- and two cycles of postoperative chemotherapy (cisplatin + 5 FU). The rate of CR after neoadjuvant chemotherapy was merely 2.5%, and there is no difference in the 2-year local control (32% vs. 31%) or overall survival rates (23% vs. 26%). Results from long-term follow-ups were also negative. In addition, there were no differences in survival between patients with squamous cell carcinoma or adenocarcinoma (INT0113/RTOG 89-11, Level I) (KELSEN et al. 1998, 2007).

A similar study from the Medical Research Council Oesophageal Cancer Working Group randomly assigned 802 patients with resectable esophageal cancer of any cell type to either two cycles of chemotherapy (cisplatin + 5-FU) followed by surgery or surgery alone. The results indicated that patients receiving neoadjuvant chemotherapy had a statistically improved 2-year survival rate (43% versus 34%). However, the benefit of neoadjuvant chemotherapy on survival was questionable because clinicians could choose to give preoperative radiotherapy to patients irrespective of randomization. In addition, preoperative CT scan was not required for staging (Level II) (MRC OESOPHAGEAL CANCER WORKING GROUP 2002).

GEBSKI et al. (2007) performed a meta-analysis of eight randomized controlled trials comparing neoadjuvant chemotherapy with surgery versus surgery alone, comprising more than 1700 patients with local and operable esophageal cancer. The results revealed that neoadjuvant chemotherapy did not have a survival benefit [hazard ratio for mortality 0.88 (0.75–1.03)] for squamous cell carcinoma, but may be beneficial for adenocarcinoma, although only one of the eight trials reported treatment effects of neoadjuvant chemotherapy (Level I) (GEBSKI et al. 2007).

Preoperative Chemoradiotherapy

- Preoperative chemotherapy given concurrently with radiation should be considered in potentially resectable locally advanced [stage IIA (T3 N0 M0) to IVA] cancer of the thoracic esophagus (Grade A). Radiation therapy techniques including simulation, field arrangement, and dose/fractionation are similar to those used in definitive treatment for unresectable esophageal cancer. Chemotherapy regimens consisting of cisplatin and 5-FU [e.g., two cycles of cisplatin (100 mg/m^2, day 1) and 5-FU (1000 mg/m^2/d, 4 days) spaced 4 weeks apart, as used in the CALGB9781 trial] with current external-beam radiation therapy to 50.4 Gy can be considered. (TEPPER et al. 2006).

Neoadjuvant concurrent radiation and cisplatin and 5-FU-based chemotherapy can produce a pathological complete response (pCR) rate of approximately 25%, and patients who achieved pCR had improved treatment outcome (Level I) (STAHL et al. 2005; WALSH et al. 1996).

In a randomized trial from Ireland, WALSH et al. (1996) randomly assigned 113 patients with adenocarcinoma of the esophagus to surgery alone or neoadjuvant chemotherapy (cisplatin + 5-FU) and radiation therapy (40 Gy in 15 fractions over 3 weeks) followed by surgery. The results revealed that approximately 25% of patients achieved pCR after concurrent chemoradiation. A significantly improved 3-year overall survival rate after preoperative chemoradiation plus surgery was demonstrated, as compared to surgery alone (32% versus 6%); however, these results were criticized because of the lower than expected survival of patients treated with surgery alone (Level I) (WALSH et al. 1996).

BOSSET et al. (1997) randomly assigned 282 patients with squamous cell carcinoma of the esophagus to surgery alone or concurrent cisplatin-based chemotherapy and radiation therapy (split course) followed by surgery. Although median survival after either treatment regimen showed no difference (18.6 months for both groups), patients receiving neoadjuvant chemoradiotherapy had a significantly higher rate of curative resection, local control and disease-free survival. However, the postoperative mortality in the combined treatment arm was significantly higher as compared to surgery alone (12% vs. 4%) (Level I) (BOSSET et al. 1997).

In the recently reported meta-analysis by GEBSKI et al. (2007), ten randomized controlled trials comparing neoadjuvant chemoradiotherapy plus surgery versus surgery alone, comprising more than 1200 patients with local and operable esophageal cancer, were included. The results revealed that neoadjuvant combined chemoradiation significantly improved 2-year overall survival [hazard ratio for mortality 0.81 (0.70–0.93, $p=0.002$)]. The benefit of neoadjuvant chemoradiation was found in both squamous cell carcinoma or adenocarcinoma. In addition, no benefit was demonstrated in patients who received sequential preoperative chemotherapy and radiotherapy (Level I) (GEBSKI et al. 2007). The advantage of neoadjuvant chemoradiation was also reported in an earlier meta-analysis of nine randomized trials comprising more than 1100 patients (Level I) (URSHEL and VASAN 2003).

12.2.4 Postoperative (Adjuvant) Treatment

Postoperative Radiation Therapy

- Postoperative radiation therapy is not routinely indicated in the treatment of esophageal cancer after complete resection (Grade A). Radiation given after complete resection does not improve survival, but may reduce locoregional recurrence in locally advanced diseases. Results from three randomized trials comparing esophagectomy alone or esophagectomy followed by radiation therapy reported no survival advantage with the addition of adjuvant radiotherapy (Level I) (FOK et al. 1993; TÉNIÈRE et al. 1991; ZIEREN et al. 1995). A recently published randomized trial from China reported the outcome of 549 patients with thoracic squamous cell carcinoma treated with surgery or surgery plus adjuvant radiation therapy, and confirmed that postoperative radiation has no effect on overall survival. However, a retrospective review of all cases according to the extent of metastasis revealed that the 5-year survival of patients with involved lymph nodes treated with surgery followed by radiation therapy was 34.1%, as compared to 17.6% in patients who received surgery alone (Level IV) (XIAO et al. 2005).

Postoperative Chemotherapy

- Chemotherapy alone given postoperatively is not routinely indicated after complete resection of esophageal cancer (Grade B). Results from prospective randomized trials have not demonstrated a survival benefit from the addition of chemotherapy after surgery. A Japanese Esophageal Oncology Group trial randomly assigned patients with resectable squamous cell carcinoma of esophagus to surgery alone or surgery followed by adjuvant cisplatin and vindesine. The results showed no benefit in 5-year overall survival from the addition of postoperative chemotherapy (JAPANESE ESOPHAGEAL ONCOLOGY GROUP, Level I) (JAPANESE ESOPHAGEAL ONCOLOGY GROUP 1993). In a study reported by the Japanese Clinical Oncology Group, 242 patients with esophageal squamous cell carcinoma were randomly assigned to receive surgery alone or surgery followed by cisplatin and 5-FU. Although the 5-year disease-free survival (primary end point) was significantly improved with adjuvant chemotherapy in patients with nodal involvement, the study failed to demonstrate an overall survival benefit (JCOG9204, Level I) (ANDO et al. 2003). However, it is important to note that newer chemotherapy agents may be more efficacious for adjuvant treatment of esophageal cancer. In a collaborative phase II study, 59 patients with stage T2 N+ and T3-4 adenocarcinoma of the distal esophagus, gastroesophageal (GE) junction, and gastric cardia were treated with adjuvant chemotherapy (cisplatin + paclitaxel) followed by surgery. The 2-year overall survival was 60%, significantly improved from 38% of the historic control (ECOG/E8296, Level III) (ARMANIOS et al. 2004).

Postoperative Chemoradiotherapy

- For locally advanced disease, if esophagectomy is performed without induction therapy, chemoradiotherapy may be considered for adjuvant treatment (Grade B). The effects of postoperative chemoradiotherapy have not been thoroughly examined for locally advanced squamous cell carcinoma; however, adjuvant chemoradiation may improve treatment outcome in patients with adenocarcinoma of the esophagus. Approximately 20% of patients treated in the Intergroup 0116 trial had primary adenocarcinoma of the GE junction or proximal stomach with involvement of the GE junction. The subgroup analysis of patients with gastroesophageal disease of the trial revealed a significant survival advantage in the adjuvantly treated group (INT0116, Level II) (MACDONALD et al. 2001).

12.2.5 Treatment of Medically Inoperable Esophageal Cancer

- Radiation therapy is the mainstay treatment for medically inoperable but potentially resectable esophageal cancer.
- For stage T1-2 N0 M0 diseases, external beam radiation therapy alone to a total dose of approximately 60 Gy in conventional fractionation should be considered for definitive treatment (Grade D).
- For stage IIA (T3 N0 M0) to IVA diseases, concurrent chemoradiotherapy with curative intent is the treatment of choice if the patient is medically fit for combined treatment.

12.3 Treatment of Locally Advanced Unresectable Esophageal Cancer

12.3.1 General Principles

■ Current chemotherapy and radiation therapy is the standard treatment for locally advanced and surgically unresectable esophageal cancer (Grade A).
■ External beam radiation therapy alone can be considered for definitive treatment when chemotherapy is contraindicated.
■ The role of surgery after definitive chemotherapy has not been proven and should not be routinely recommended (Grade A).

12.3.2 Concurrent Chemoradiotherapy

■ Combined chemotherapy and radiation therapy is the definitive treatment of choice for unresectable or medically inoperable locally advanced esophageal cancer (Grade A). The RTOG 8501 trial randomly assigned patients to either radiation (64 Gy in 32 fractions over 6.4 weeks) alone, or concurrent chemotherapy [two cycles of cisplatin (75 mg/m^2 day 1) and FU (1000 mg/m^2/d by continuous infusion for 4 days)] and radiotherapy (50 Gy in 25 fractions over 5 weeks). Patients in the chemoradiation arm received two more cycles of cisplatin and FU after radiation. The results of the RTOG 8501 trial showed that overall survival was significantly improved in the combined treatment arm. The 2-year overall survival and local recurrence rates were 38% versus 10%, and 16% versus 24%, respectively, both in favor of the chemoradiation arm (RTOG 85-01, Level I) (HERSKOVIC et al. 1992). Updated trial results from COOPER et al. (1999) revealed that at 5 years of follow-up, survival rates were 26% and 0% for patients who received chemoradiotherapy or radiation therapy alone, respectively (Level I).

12.3.3 Surgery After Definitive Chemoradiotherapy

■ Surgery after definitive chemoradiotherapy is not routinely recommended (Grade A). "Adjuvant" surgery may improve local control after definitive chemoradiation, but its effect on survival has not been demonstrated.

In a randomized trial from Germany, 172 patients with locally advanced but potentially resectable squamous cell carcinoma (SCC) of esophagus were treated with three cycles of induction chemotherapy (cisplatin, etoposide, 5-FU, leucovorin) followed by concurrent chemotherapy (cisplatin + etoposide) and external beam radiotherapy (40 Gy). Patients were then randomized to receive either further concurrent chemoradiation (to 60–65 Gy) or surgery. No survival benefit was observed with the addition of surgery to combined chemoradiation: The median survival and 3-year overall survival rates were 16 months versus 15 months and 31% versus 24%, respectively, without significant difference. However, 2-year progression-free survival was 64.3% versus 40.7%, significantly improved with the addition of surgery ($p=0.003$). It is interesting to note that the subgroup of patients who achieved pathologic CR after chemoradiation had an improved survival rate (50% at 5 years after treatment) (Level I) (STAHL et al. 2005).

A recently published French randomized trial treated 444 patients with T3 N0-1 M0 potentially resectable thoracic esophageal cancer with concurrent chemotherapy (cisplatin + 5-FU) and radiation therapy (two split courses of 15 Gy given at 3 Gy per fraction, 2 weeks apart, or 46 Gy given in 23 fractions). A total of 259 patients with clinical partial or CR were subsequently randomized to receive further combined chemoradiation or surgery. The median survival and overall survival rates were 19.3 months versus 17.7 month and 40% versus 34%, respectively, for the two groups, without significant differences. However, the 3-month mortality rates were 9.3% and 0.8%, respectively, significantly worse in patients who received surgery after chemoradiation. Surgery after chemoradiotherapy offered no improvement in outcome in locally advanced esophageal cancer, at least in responders to chemoradiation (FFCD9102, Level I) (BEDENNE et al. 2007).

12.3.4 Radiation Therapy Techniques

Dose and Fractionation

■ External beam radiation therapy to a total dose of 50.4 Gy at 1.8 Gy/fraction, in combination with concurrent cisplatin + 5-FU chemotherapy is currently the standard regimen for definitive treatment (Grade A). The Intergroup 0123 trial randomly assigned 236 patients with locally advanced esophageal cancer (T1-4, N0/1) to radiation to a total dose of 50.4 Gy or 64.8 Gy at 1.8 Gy/fraction. Concurrent chemotherapy (cisplatin + 5-FU) was used in both groups. The results revealed no differences in locoregional failure rates (56% versus 52%) and 2-year overall survival rates (31% versus 40%), as well as in median survival (13 months versus 18 months) (INT 0123, Level I) (Minsky et al. 2002).

- Continuous-course radiation therapy is preferred over split-course radiation (Grade A). A randomized phase III trial from France compared standard versus split-course irradiation with concurrent chemotherapy for definitive treatment for squamous cell carcinoma of esophagus. Its results showed standard course irradiation was associated with improved local control rates (57% versus 29%) as well as 2-year survival rates (37% versus 23%), as compared to split course radiation (FFCD9305, Level I) (Jacob et al. 1999).

An ancillary study of the above mentioned French FFCD9102 phase III randomized trial compared protracted chemoradiation with split-course chemoradiation for T3 N0-1 M0 tumor of the thoracic esophagus. Two radiation schemes (46 Gy in 23 fractions over 4.5 weeks, or split-course radiation with two 1-week courses of 15 Gy spaced 2 weeks apart) were allowed in the FFCD9102 trial. Responders to chemoradiation were randomized to either surgery or further chemoradiotherapy (continuous-course radiation to 20 Gy in 10 fractions, or 15 Gy in 1 week in the split-course arm). The 2-year local relapse-free survival rate was 76.7% versus 56.8%, respectively, for protracted and split-course radiation (p=0.002), although no statically significant difference was found in overall survival. In addition, the 2-year local recurrence-free survival rate was higher with continuous-course radiation whether patients were resected or not (FFCD9102, Level II) (Crehange et al. 2007).

Simulation and Planning

- CT-based treatment planning is highly recommended for defining gross tumor volume (GTV) and planning target volume (PTV). An individualized immobilization device (e.g., Alpha cradle,

Smithers Medical Products, Inc. North Canton, OH) should be used during planning and treatment.
- CT scan should be taken in the treatment position with arms placed overhead (supine for proximal and distal diseases, and prone for mid-esophageal primaries are recommended) with 3- to 5-mm-thick slices from the level of cricoid cartilage to upper abdomen. Oral and IV contrast should be administered to better define the esophagus and the disease.
- The tumor volume should be defined by CT, EUS, or esophagram, whichever is larger. PET/CT scan is recommended for planning purposes, but should be utilized with other diagnostic tests (Grade B). GTV adjustment was required in more than 50% of cases with the utilization of FDG-PET and CT fusion in a small prospective trial (Level III) (Moureau-Zabotto et al. 2005).
- The clinical tumor volume (CTV) is defined to include GTV with 4-cm proximal and distal margins, and 1-cm radial margins. The planning tumor volume (PTV) is defined as CTV plus 1–2 cm expansion for set-up errors and organ movement.
- Peri-esophageal nodes are usually included in the treatment field arranged as described above. Elective radiation therapy to other clinically uninvolved lymph nodes is usually not performed in thoracic esophageal cancer.
- Normal tissues to be delineated include, but are not limited to, both lungs, skin, heart, spinal cord, esophagus, and liver for organ identification, lung correction, and dose-volume histograms. For disease located in distal esophagus, contour of intestine, liver, stomach, and/or kidneys may be needed.

Field Arrangement

- Radiation treatment of esophageal cancer can be delivered in a number of ways: A three-field (two anterior oblique and one posterior) technique (single-phase treatment, Fig. 12.1), or a two-phase arrangement using an AP/PA field (to approximately 36 Gy) followed by boost treatment with opposed lateral, oblique, or AP plus two posterior oblique fields (to the total dose of 50.4 Gy) can be planned (Fig. 12.2).

Attention should be paid to limit the radiation dose to dose-limiting organs including spinal cord, lungs, heart, liver, and kidneys. In addition,

Fig. 12.1. Field arrangement using a PA and two anterior oblique fields for a patient with squamous cell carcinoma of the mid-lower esophagus

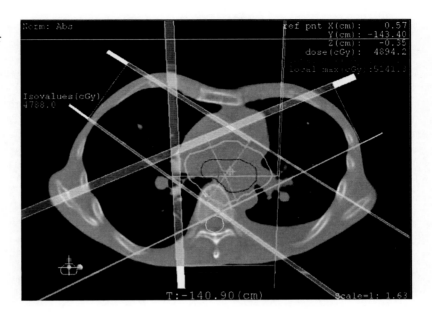

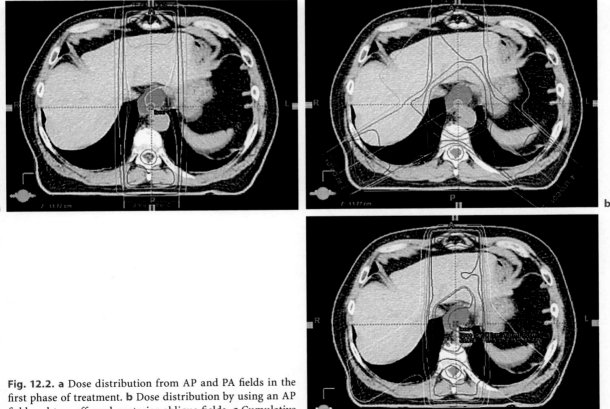

Fig. 12.2. a Dose distribution from AP and PA fields in the first phase of treatment. **b** Dose distribution by using an AP field and two off-cord posterior oblique fields. **c** Cumulative dose distribution [from HONG et al. (2006) with permission)

dose inhomogeneity should be limited to 5% or less (HONG et al. 2006).

- Bilateral supraclavicular nodes should be included for diseases located above the carina including cervical primaries: A pair of AP/PA fields should be used for the initial 39.6 Gy followed by oblique fields to 10.8 Gy to exclude the spinal cord. The supraclavicular field, which is excluded from the oblique fields, can be supplemented with electrons to bring the total dose up to 50.4 Gy calculated 3 cm from the skin surface. For distal esophageal cancers, celiac lymph nodes (located at T12 level) should be included in the treatment fields (Fig. 13.1, see Chap. 13).

- Intensity-modulated radiation therapy (IMRT) can be recommended for cervical esophageal cancer treatment (Grade D). The benefit of IMRT in the treatment of thoracic esophagus has not been demonstrated in clinical trials; however, results from a dosimetric study suggested its advantage over three-dimensional conformal radiation (WU et al. 2004).

Brachytherapy

- Brachytherapy alone is not recommended for definitive treatment of esophageal cancer due to the limitation of its effective treatment distance.

- Brachytherapy as part of definitive treatment for esophageal cancer is usually not recommended after definitive dose of external beam radiation (Grade B). Esophageal brachytherapy has not been shown to be efficacious for definitive treatment as an adjuvant to external beam radiotherapy but is related to increased adverse effects.
  Results from an RTOG phase I/II prospective study showed the median survival time for patients who received concurrent cisplatin-/5-FU-based chemotherapy and external beam radiation (50 Gy in 25 fractions over 5 weeks) followed by adjuvant brachytherapy after 2 weeks [15 Gy in three weekly fractions for high-dose-rate (HDR), or 20 Gy for low-dose-rate (LDR) during week 8] was 11 months; however, the incidence of fistula after such treatment reached 12% (RTOG 9207, Level III) (GASPER et al. 2000).

- American Brachytherapy Society (ABS) consensus guidelines suggested that brachytherapy should be performed with caution if used after definitive chemoradiation for esophageal cancer. Patients with unifocal cancer of the thoracic esophagus, primary tumor ≤ 10 cm in length confined to esophageal wall, and no regional lymph node or systemic metastases are good candidates for adjuvant brachytherapy. The recommended dose of brachytherapy was 10 Gy in two weekly fractions (5 Gy each) for HDR or 20 Gy in a single course at 0.4–1 Gy/h for LDR, and should not be used with concurrent chemotherapy (Grade D) (GASPAR et al. 1997).

Radiation-Induced Side Effects and Dose Limiting Structures

- Radiation-induced side effects and complications depend on the location of the primary tumor and the treatment fields. The critical normal structures commonly located within treatment fields include spinal cord, lungs, and heart. Attention should be paid to the radiation dose to intestine, stomach, liver, and kidney for diseases of the lower thoracic esophagus and GE junction.

- Commonly observed adverse effects associated with radiation include esophagitis (dysphagia and odynophagia) and pneumonitis.

- Dose of radiation to the spinal cord should be limited to 45 Gy (1.8–2.0 Gy daily) (Grade C) (Emami et al. 1991). V_{20} of bilateral lung should be limited to ≤ 30% as probability of pneumonitis increases rapidly when more than $V_{20} > 30\%$ (Level III) (BYHARDT et al. 1993). V_{40} of the heart should be limited to 50% or less, and the dose to the entire heart should be limited to 30 Gy.

- Incidence of death related to chemoradiation therapy was approximately 2% as reported in the RTOG8501 and INT0123 trials (HERSKOVIC et al. 1992; MINSKY et al. 2002).

12.4 Palliative Treatment of Esophageal Cancer

12.4.1 General Principles

- Radiation (external beam radiation therapy or intraluminal brachytherapy) is frequently utilized to palliate symptoms caused by the primary disease (e.g., dysphagia) or metastases.

- Chemotherapy given concurrently with radiation can further improve the palliative results, and is recommended in medially fit patients with metastatic esophageal cancer (Grade B).
- Systemic chemotherapy is usually indicated for symptomatic palliation of metastatic esophageal cancer (Grade C). Distant metastasis occurs in 25%–30% of cases at diagnosis, and is a major cause of treatment failure. The most common sites of distant metastasis include lung, liver, bone, kidney, and pleura. However, randomized trials have failed to consistently demonstrate a survival advantage with the use of chemotherapy (van Meerten and van der Gaast 2005).
- Other useful treatment modalities for palliation include photodynamic therapy (PDT), balloon dilatation, alcohol or chemotherapeutic injection, placement of plastic or expandable metal prosthesis.

12.4.2 Palliative Radiation Therapy

External Beam Radiation Therapy

- External beam radiation therapy, with or without chemotherapy, is indicated for palliative treatment of dysphagia, a common presenting symptom of advanced esophageal cancer (Grade B). The efficacy of radiation for palliation of esophageal cancer has been demonstrated in numerous retrospective trials. External beam radiation therapy either used alone or in combination with chemotherapy offers symptomatic relief in more than 70% of cases.
  The results of a retrospective analysis of 120 patients with esophageal cancer treated with concurrent chemoradiotherapy revealed that 45% and 83% of patients had symptomatic relief within 2 weeks and 6 weeks of treatment initiation, respectively (Level IV) (Coia et al. 1993).
  A phase I/II trial from Canada prospectively treated 22 patients with dysphagia from advanced incurable esophageal cancer with palliative radiation (30 Gy in 10 fractions) with a concurrent single course of chemotherapy (5-FU, 1000 mg/m^2, days 1–4 and mitomycin-C 10 mg/

m^2, day 1). The results showed that the combined regimen was well tolerated, and close to 70% patients achieved a CR (i.e., no difficulty on swallowing) with a median time to normalization of swallowing of 5 weeks (Level III) (Hayter et al. 2000).
- A range of dose and fractionation of external beam radiation can be considered for symptomatic palliation: 30 Gy administered in 10 fractions to the primary tumor with 2 cm margins in AP-PA arrangement, to dose/fractionation in the range of definitive treatment, i.e., 50.4 Gy at 1.8 Gy/fraction has been used.

Brachytherapy

- Brachytherapy can be utilized for rapid symptomatic (dysphagia) palliation in selected groups of patients (Grade A). A Danish randomized trial randomly assigned 209 patients with dysphagia from inoperable carcinoma of the esophagus or GE junction to either single-dose brachytherapy (12 Gy) or stent placement. Its results showed that dysphagia improved more rapidly after stent placement, but long-term relief of dysphagia was better after brachytherapy. Additionally, stent placement had significantly more complications than brachytherapy (33% versus 21%) (Level I) (Homs et al. 2004).
- The efficacy of external beam radiation therapy and brachytherapy in dysphagia palliation has not been compared. However, due to the short effective range of treatment, the utilization of intraluminal brachytherapy is usually limited.
- American Brachytherapy Society (ABS) consensus guidelines recommended brachytherapy alone without external beam radiation, dosed at 10–14 Gy in one to two weekly fractions for HDR or 25–40 Gy in one or two fractions at 0.4–1.0 Gy/h for LDR to be used for palliative treatment for recurrent esophageal cancer after external beam radiation or patients with short life expectancy. In previously un-irradiated patients, the addition of external beam radiation before brachytherapy may prolong the duration of palliation (Grade C) (Gaspar et al. 1997) (Fig. 12.3).

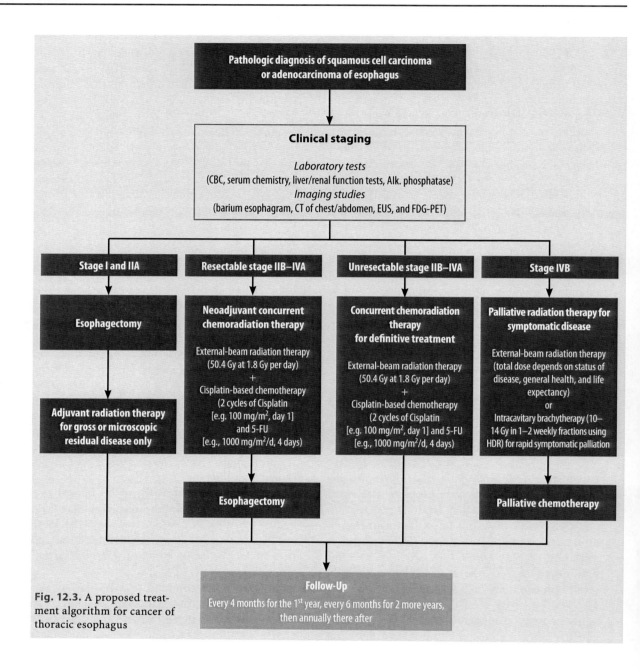

Fig. 12.3. A proposed treatment algorithm for cancer of thoracic esophagus

12.5   Follow-Ups

12.5.1   Post-Treatment Follow-Ups

■ Life-long follow-up after definitive treatment of esophageal cancer is usually indicated for detection of local or distant failures.

■ Local failure is a major cause of treatment failure and the rates of locoregional failure range from 30%

to 50% after surgery or definitive concurrent chemoradiotherapy (HERSKOVIC et al. 1992; HULSCHER et al. 2002; KELSEN et al. 1998; MINSKY et al. 2002).

Schedule

■ Follow-ups could be scheduled every 4 months for 1 year, then every 6 months for 2 more years, then annually thereafter (Table 12.3) (Grade D) (NATIONAL COMPREHENSIVE CANCER NETWORK 2008).

Table 12.3. Follow-up schedule after treatment for esophageal cancer

Interval	Frequency
First year	Every 4 months
Year 2–3	Every 6 months
Over 3 years	Annually

Work-Ups

■ Each follow-up should include a complete history and physical examination. Laboratory tests include complete blood count and serum chemistry, endoscopy, chest X-ray, and CT of the chest are required when clinically indicated (Grade D) (NATIONAL COMPREHENSIVE CANCER NETWORK 2008).

■ Although changes of metabolic activity on FDG-PET after neoadjuvant treatment may be of prognostic importance, currently FDG-PET cannot be recommended routinely for follow-up (Grade D). The value of PET-guided therapy for residual disease has not been confirmed.

Results from a prospective nonrandomized trial from Japan found that metabolic response after neoadjuvant chemotherapy was a significant predictor for recurrence after chemotherapy followed by surgery for esophageal cancer. The 3-year overall survival rates for patients with or without metabolic response were 70% versus 35%, respectively (p=0.01) (Level III) (OTT et al. 2006).

Change of metabolic activity measured by FDG-PET after neoadjuvant chemoradiation is a strong predictor of median survival time for squamous cell carcinoma of esophagus: 16–23 months for responders versus 6–7 months for non-responders (Level III) (WIEDER et al. 2004). Results of a retrospective study also showed that the post-treatment standardized uptake value (SUV) on PET/CT predicted for disease-free survival after definitive chemoradiotherapy for esophageal cancer (Level III) (KONSKI et al. 2007).

References

Al-Sarraf M, Martz K, Herskovic A et al. (1997) Progress report of combined chemoradiotherapy versus radiotherapy alone in patients with esophageal cancer: an intergroup study. J Clin Oncol 15:277–284

Ando N, Iizuka T, Ide H et al. (2003) Surgery plus chemotherapy compared with surgery alone for localized squamous cell carcinoma of the thoracic esophagus: a Japan Clinical Oncology Group Study – JCOG9204. J Clin Oncol 21:4592–4596

Armanios M, Xu R, Forastiere AA et al. (2004) Adjuvant chemotherapy for resected adenocarcinoma of the esophagus, gastro-esophageal junction, and cardia: phase II trial (E8296) of the Eastern Cooperative Oncology Group. J Clin Oncol 22:4495–4499

Arnott SJ, Duncan W, Kerr GR et al. (1992) Low dose preoperative radiotherapy for carcinoma of the oesophagus: results of a randomized clinical trial. Radiother Oncol 24:108–113

Arnott SJ, Duncan W, Gignoux M et al. (2005) Preoperative radiotherapy for esophageal carcinoma. Cochrane Database Syst Rev (4):CD001799

Bedenne L, Michel P, Bouché O et al. (2007) Chemoradiation followed by surgery compared with chemoradiation alone in squamous cancer of the esophagus: FFCD 9102. J Clin Oncol 25:1160–1168

Bosset J, Gignoux M, Triboulet J et al. (1997) Chemoradiotherapy followed by surgery compared with surgery alone in squamous-cell cancer of the esophagus. N Engl J Med 337: 161–167

Byhardt RW, Martin L, Pajak TF et al. (1993) The influence of field size and other treatment factors on pulmonary toxicity following hyperfractionated irradiation for inoperable non-small cell lung cancer – analysis of a Radiation Therapy Oncology Group protocol. Int J Radiat Oncol Biol Phys 27:537–544

Coia LR, Soffen EM, Schultheiss TE et al. (1993) Swallowing function in patients with esophageal cancer treated with concurrent radiation and chemotherapy. Cancer 71:281–286

Cooper JS, Guo MD, Herskovic A et al. (1999) Chemoradiotherapy of locally advanced esophageal cancer: long-term follow-up of a prospective randomized trial (RTOG 85-01). Radiation Therapy Oncology Group. JAMA 281:1623–1627

Crehange G, Maingon P, Peignaux K et al. (2007) Phase III trial of protracted compared with split-course chemoradiation for esophageal carcinoma: Federation Francophone de Cancerologie Digestive 9102. J Clin Oncol 25:4895–4901

Emami B, Lyman J, Brown A et al. (1991) Tolerance of normal tissue to therapeutic irradiation. Int J Radiat Oncol Biol Phys 21:109–122

Flamen P, Lerut A, Van Cutsem E et al. (2000) Utility of positron emission tomography for the staging of patients with potentially operable esophageal carcinoma. J Clin Oncol 18:3202–3210

Fok M, Sham JS, Choy D et al. (1993) Postoperative radiotherapy for carcinoma of the esophagus: a prospective, randomized controlled study. Surgery 113:138–147

Gaspar LE, Nag S, Herskovic A et al. (1997) American Brachytherapy Society (ABS) consensus guidelines for brachytherapy of esophageal cancer. Int J Radiat Oncol Biol Phys 38:127–132

Gaspar LE, Winter K, Kocha WI et al. (2000) A phase I/II study of external beam radiation, brachytherapy, and concurrent chemotherapy for patients with localized carcinoma of the esophagus (Radiation Therapy Oncology Group Study 9207): final report. Cancer 88:988–995

Gebski V, Burmeister B, Smithers BM et al. (2007) Survival benefits from neoadjuvant chemoradiotherapy or chemotherapy in oesophageal carcinoma: a meta-analysis. Lancet Oncol 8:226–234

Gignoux M, Roussel A, Paillot B et al. (1987) The value of preoperative radiotherapy in esophageal cancer: results of a study of the E.O.R.T.C. World J Surg 11:426–432

Greene FL, Page DL, Fleming ID et al. (2002) American Joint Committee on Cancer, American Cancer Society. AJCC Cancer Staging Manual, 6th edn. Springer-Verlag, Berlin Heidelberg New York

Hayter CR, Huff-Winters C, Paszat L et al. (2000) A prospective trial of short-course radiotherapy plus chemotherapy for palliation of dysphagia from advanced esophageal cancer. Radiother Oncol 56:329–333

Herskovic A, Martz K, al-Sarraf M et al. (1992) Combined chemotherapy and radiotherapy compared with radiotherapy alone in patients with cancer of the esophagus. N Engl J Med 326:1593–1598

Homs MY, Steyerberg EW, Eijkenboom WM et al. (2004) Single-dose brachytherapy versus metal stent placement for the palliation of dysphagia from oesophageal cancer: multicentre randomised trial. Lancet 364:1497–1504

Hong TS, Crowley EM, Killoran J et al. (2006) Considerations in treatment planning for esophageal cancer. Semin Radiat Oncol 17:53–61

Hulscher JB, van Sandick JW, de Boer AG et al. (2002) Extended transthoracic resection compared with limited transhiatal resection for adenocarcinoma of the esophagus. N Engl J Med 347:1662–1669

Hussey D, Barakley T, Bloedorn F (1980) Carcinoma of the esophagus, 3rd edn. Lea & Febiger, Philadelphia

Jacob J, Seitz JF, Langlois C et al. (1999) Definitive concurrent chemo-radiation therapy in squamous cell carcinoma of the esophagus: preliminary results of a French randomized trial comparing standard versus split-course irradiation (FN- CLCC-FFCD9305). Proc Am Soc Clin Oncol 18:1035a

Japanese Esophageal Oncology Group (1993) A comparison of chemotherapy and radiotherapy as adjuvant treatment to surgery for esophageal carcinoma. Chest 104:203–207

Kato H, Miyazaki T, Nakajima M et al. (2005) The incremental effect of positron emission tomography on diagnostic accuracy in the initial staging of esophageal carcinoma. Cancer 103:148–156

Katsoulis IE, Wong WL, Mattheou AK et al. (2007) Fluorine-18 fluorodeoxyglucose positron emission tomography in the preoperative staging of thoracic oesophageal and gastro-oesophageal junction cancer: a prospective study. Int J Surg 5:399–403

Kelly S, Harris KM, Berry E et al. (2001) A systematic review of the staging performance of endoscopic ultrasound in gastro-oesophageal carcinoma. Gut 49:534–539

Kelsen DP, Ginsberg R, Pajak TF et al. (1998) Chemotherapy followed by surgery compared with surgery alone for localized esophageal cancer. N Engl J Med 339:1979–1984

Kelsen DP, Winter KA, Gunderson LL et al. (2007) Long-term results of RTOG trial 8911 (USA Intergroup 113): a random assignment trial comparison of chemotherapy followed by surgery compared with surgery alone for esophageal cancer. J Clin Oncol 25:3719–3725

Konski AA, Cheng JD, Goldberg M et al. (2007) Correlation of molecular response as measured by 18-FDG positron emission tomography with outcome after chemoradiotherapy in patients with esophageal carcinoma. Int J Radiat Oncol Biol Phys 69:358–363

Launois B, Delarue D, Campion JP et al. (1981) Preoperative radiotherapy for carcinoma of the esophagus. Surg Gynecol Obstet 153:690–692

Macdonald JS, Smalley SR, Benedetti J et al. (2001) Chemoradiotherapy after surgery compared with surgery alone for adenocarcinoma of the stomach or gastroesophageal junction. N Engl J Med 345:725–730

Minsky BD, Pajak TF, Ginsberg RJ et al. (2002) INT 0123 (Radiation Therapy Oncology Group 94-05) Phase III trial of combined modality therapy for esophageal cancer: high-dose versus standard-dose radiation therapy. J Clin Oncol 20:1167–1174

Moureau-Zabotto L, Touboul E, Lerouge D et al. (2005) Impact of CT and 18F-deoxyglucose positron emission tomography image fusion for conformal radiotherapy in esophageal carcinoma. Int J Radiat Oncol Biol Phys 63:340–345

MRC (Medical Research Council) Oesophageal Cancer Working Group (2002) Surgical resection with or without preoperative chemotherapy in esophageal cancer: a randomized controlled trial. Lancet 359:1727–1733

National Comprehensive Cancer Network (2008) Clinical practice guidelines in oncology: esophageal Cancer. Version 1.2008. Available at http://www.nccn.org/professionals/physician_gls/PDF/esophageal.pdf. Accessed on May 22, 2008

Ott K, Weber WA, Lordick F et al. (2006) Metabolic imaging predicts response, survival, and recurrence in adenocarcinomas of the esophagogastric junction. J Clin Oncol 24:4692–4698

Pearson JG (1977) The present status and future potential of radiotherapy in the management of esophageal cancer. Cancer 39[2 Suppl]: 882–890

Picus D, Balfe DM, Koehler RE et al. (1983) Computed tomography in the staging of esophageal carcinoma. Radiology 146:433–438

Rankin SC, Taylor H, Cook GJ et al. (1998) Computed tomography and positron emission tomography in the preoperative staging of oesophageal carcinoma. Clin Radiol 53:659–665

Salonen O, Kivisaari L, Standertskjöld-Nordenstam CG et al. (1987) Computed tomography in staging of oesophageal carcinoma. Scand J Gastroenterol 22:65–68

Siewert JR, Stein HJ, Feith M et al. (2001) Histologic tumor type is an independent prognostic parameter in esophageal cancer: lessons from more than 1,000 consecutive resections at a single center in the Western world. Ann Surg 234:360-367; discussion 368–369

Stahl M, Stuschke M, Lehmann N et al. (2005) Chemoradiation with and without surgery in patients with locally advanced squamous cell carcinoma of the esophagus. J Clin Oncol 23:2310–2317

Ténière P, Hay JM, Fingerhut A et al. (1991) Postoperative radiation therapy does not increase survival after curative resection for squamous cell carcinoma of the middle and lower esophagus as shown by a multicenter controlled trial. French University Association for Surgical Research. Surg Gynecol Obstet 173:123–130

Tepper J, Krasna M, Niedzwiecki D et al. (2006) Superiority of tri-modality therapy to surgery alone in esophageal caner: results of CALGB 9781. J Clin Oncol 24[suppl 18S]:4012

Urschel JD, Vasan H (2003) A meta-analysis of randomized controlled trials that compared neoadjuvant chemoradiation and surgery to surgery alone for resectable esophageal cancer. Am J Surg 185:538–543

van Meerten E, van der Gaast A (2005) Systemic treatment for oesophageal cancer. Eur J Cancer 41:664–672

Walsh TN, Noonan N, Hollywood D et al (1996) A comparison of multimodel therapy and surgery for esophageal adenocarcinoma. N Engl J Med 335:462–467

Wang M, Gu XZ, Yin WB et al. (1989) Randomized clinical trial on the combination of preoperative irradiation and surgery in the treatment of esophageal carcinoma: report on 206 patients. Int J Radiat Oncol Biol Phys 16:325–327

Wieder HA, Brucher BL, Zimmermann F et al. (2004) Time course of tumor metabolic activity during chemoradiotherapy of esophageal squamous cell carcinoma and response to treatment. J Clin Oncol 22:900–908

Wu VW, Sham JS, Kwong DL (2004) Inverse planning in three-dimensional conformal and intensity-modulated radiotherapy of mid-thoracic oesophageal cancer. Br J Radiol 77:568–572

Xiao ZF, Yang ZY, Miao YJ et al. (2005) Influence of number of metastatic lymph nodes on survival of curative resected thoracic esophageal cancer patients and value of radiotherapy: report of 549 cases. Int J Radiat Oncol Biol Phys 62:82–90

Zieren HU, Müller JM, Jacobi CA et al. (1995) Adjuvant postoperative radiation therapy after curative resection of squamous cell carcinoma of the thoracic esophagus: a prospective randomized study. World J Surg 19:444–449

Section IV:
Cancers of the Gastrointestinal Tract

Gastric Cancer

ZHEN ZHANG

CONTENTS

Introduction and Objectives

Gastric cancer is the second leading cause of cancer-related death worldwide. Surgery is the primary treatment modality for resectable gastric cancer. An estimated 50% of the disease is resectable. However, the cure rate after surgery alone for locally advanced cancer is low, while the overall survival rate after completed D2 is around 30% in most parts of the world other than Japan, where the rate approaches 60%. Adjuvant treatment, which include perioperative chemotherapy and postoperative chemoradiotherapy has been demonstrated to improve survival for locally advanced gastric cancer.

This chapter examines:

- Recommendations for diagnosis and staging procedures for adenocarcinoma of the stomach
- The staging systems and prognostic factors
- Treatment recommendations as well as the supporting scientific evidence for surgery and adjuvant treatment for resectable gastric cancer
- Surgery in combination with neoadjuvant chemotherapy or adjuvant chemoradiation for locally advanced gastric cancer
- Systemic chemotherapy and palliative radiation for metastatic diseases
- Follow-up care and surveillance of survivors

The management of other types of gastric cancer, including gastric lymphoma, carcinoid tumors, and sarcoma, is detailed in other chapters.

Z. ZHANG, MD
Department of Radiation Oncology, Cancer Hospital of Fudan University, 270 Dong An Road, Shanghai 200232, P. R. China

13.1 Diagnosis, Staging, and Prognoses

13.1.1 Diagnosis

Initial Evaluation

- Diagnosis and evaluation of gastric cancer starts with a complete history and physical examination (H&P). Attention should be paid to gastric cancer-specific history, signs, and symptoms including *Helicobacter pylori* infection, weight loss and persistent abdominal discomfort, dysphagia, melena, nausea and vomiting, and early satiety.
- Thorough physical examination should be performed with attention to an abdominal mass and Blumer's rectal shelf (for drop metastases into the peritoneal reflection in the prerectal and postvesical space), as well as left supraclavicular lymphadenopathy.
- Upper gastrointestinal endoscopy allows direct visualization and measurement of the characterization and extent of tumor, while biopsy enables pathologic diagnosis.
- Staging laparoscopy can be used to rule out peritoneal spread when neoadjuvant therapy or surgery with curative intent is planned. Peritoneal metastases are found in 20%–30% of endoscopic ultrasonography (EUS)-staged cases beyond T1, as well as CT-negative patients (FEUSSNER et al. 1999; WATT et al. 1989).

Laboratory Tests

- Initial laboratory tests should include a complete blood count, basic blood chemistry, liver function tests, and renal function tests.
- Serologic marker tests (including CEA, CA125, CA19-9 and CA72-4) are not routinely indicated (Grade B). The serum levels of these marks may be elevated in about 44% of gastric cancer patients; however, the sensitivity and specificity are low and wide ranging, from 6% to 31%, which limit their routine use as diagnostic tests (Level III) (CARPELAN-HOLMSTROM et al. 2002; LAI et al. 2002).

Imaging Studies

- CT scan of abdomen and pelvis are required to evaluate local extension, regional and distant lymph nodes, ascites, and to rule out distant metastasis (Grade B). CT scan can accurately assess the T-category of the primary lesion in 43%–70% patients (Level III) (DAVIES et al. 1997; MINAMI et al. 1992; DUX et al. 1999). The sensitivity and specificity rates of CT regional adenopathy detection range from 65% to 97%, and 49% to 90%, respectively (Level III) (D'ELIA et al. 2000; KIENLE et al. 2002).
- Endoscopic ultrasonography (EUS) is required to evaluate the depth of invasion of primary gastric cancer, especially in early lesions, as well as regional nodal involvement (Grade B). The accuracy of EUS for differentiation tumor stage (T1–T4) ranges from 77% to 93% (WILLIS et al. 2000; KELLY et al. 2001). Nodal staging accuracy ranges from 65% to 90%, slightly greater as compared to CT (Level III) (WILLIS et al. 2000; TSENDSUREN et al. 2006).
- Barium study can be used to detect patients with linitis plastica in relatively normal endoscopic appearance for the decreased distensibility of the stiff, 'leather-flask' stomach.
- Chest X-ray is recommended to rule out pulmonary metastasis. CT scan of the chest is indicated for proximal gastric cancer to evaluate disease extension to the esophagus and regional lymph nodes, as well as thoracic metastasis.
- FDG-PET can be used for preoperative staging to screen for distant metastases; however, its value in evaluating the extent of primary disease and peritoneal spread has not been supported by clinical evidence. Up to one third of patients with gastric cancer have disease that was not FDG-avid. It may be a useful tool in some gastric cancer patients but is not routinely indicated for all gastric patients due to its limitation. PET scan will not identify most peritoneal disease (Level II) (SHAH 2007); (Level III) (CHEN et al. 2005) (Table 13.1).

Table 13.1. Imaging and laboratory work-ups for esophageal cancer

Imaging studies	Laboratory tests
– CT of abdomen and pelvis	– Complete blood counts
– Chest X-ray or CT of thorax	
– Endoscopic ultrasonography	– Serum chemistry
– Barium study (optional)	– Liver function tests
– FDG-PET scan or PET/CT (optional)	– Renal function tests
	– Alkaline phosphatase

Pathology

- Pathologic confirmation of gastric cancer is imperative prior to the initiation of any treatment. Adenocarcinomas comprise 90%–95% of all gastric malignancies. Treatment and prognosis are different from those more rarely occurring malignancies such as lymphoma, leiomyosarcoma, carcinoid tumors, adenoacanthomas, and squamous cell carcinomas.
- Adequate tissue sampling for pathologic diagnosis can usually be obtained during initial examination using upper gastrointestinal endoscopy.
- Numerous pathologic classifications for gastric adenocarcinoma exist. The WHO classification based on light microscopy is the most commonly used: adenocarcinomas are graded into well, moderately, or poorly differentiated patterns of gastric adenocarcinoma. Other than the degree of differentiation, subtyping of adenocarcinomas may also take into account traditional histopathological characteristics such as intestinal or diffuse subtype, based on growth patterns (FENOGLIO-PREISER et al. 2000).

  Other less commonly used classifications of gastric cancer include the Borrmann classification which consists of four categories based on the gross morphology. The Lauren classification divides gastric cancer into two groups based on epidemiologic studies.

13.1.2 Staging

- Gastric cancer can be staged clinically and pathologically: Clinical staging utilizes information from H&P, imaging studies, endoscopy, and laboratory tests; pathologic staging is based on findings from clinical staging and procedures such as laparoscopy, gastrectomy, and examination of the resected specimen.
- Depending on the depth of invasion into the gastric wall and regional lymph node status, localized gastric carcinomas are divided into early and locoregionally advanced stages.
- Two staging systems are currently in use for gastric cancer. The 2002 American Joint Committee on Cancer staging system based on tumor/node/metastasis (TNM) (Table 13.2) (GREENE et al. 2002). The Japanese staging system for gastric cancer is based on refined anatomic involvement (especially that of the elaborate lymph node stations) and is not widely utilized in non-Asian countries (Table 13.3).

Table 13.2. American Joint Committee on Cancer (AJCC) TNM classification of gastric cancer [from GREENE et al. (2002) with permission]

Primary tumor (T)	
TX	Primary tumor cannot be assessed
T0	No evidence of primary tumor
Tis	Carcinoma in situ: intraepithelial tumor without invasion of the lamina propria
T1	Tumor invades lamina propria or submucosa
T2	Tumor invades muscularis propria or submucosa
T2a	Tumor invades muscularis propria
T2b	Tumor invades submucosa
T3	Tumor penetrates scrosa (visceral peritoneum) without invasion of adjacent structures
T4	Tumor invades adjacent structures

Regional lymph nodes (N)	
NX	Regional lymph node(s) cannot be assessed
N0	No regional lymph node metastasis
N1	Metastasis in 1–6 regional lymph nodes
N2	Metastasis in 7–15 regional lymph nodes
N3	Metastasis in more than 15 regional lymph nodes

Distant metastasis (M)	
MX	Distant metastasis cannot be assessed
M0	No distant metastasis
M1	Distant metastasis

STAGE GROUPING	
0:	Tis N0 M0
IA:	T1 N0 M0
IB:	T1 N1 M0, T2a/b N1 M0
II:	T1 N2 M0, T2a/b N1 M0, T3 N0 M0
IIIA:	T2a/b N2 M0, T3 N1 M0, T4 N0 M0
IIIB:	T3 N2 M0
IV:	T4 N1-3 M0, T1-3 N3 M0, Any T Any N M1

Table 13.3. Japanese surgical staging system for gastric cancer

Definitions	
S0	No serosal invasion
S1	Suspected serosal invasion
S2	Definite serosal invasion
S3	Adjacent organ involvement
N1	Perigastric lymph nodes
N2	Lymph nodes around the left gastric artery, common hepatic artery, splenic artery, and celiac axis
N3	Lymph nodes in the hepatoduodenal ligament, posterior aspect of pancreas, and root of mesentery
N4	Periaortic and middle colic lymph nodes
P0	No peritoneal metastases
P1	Adjacent peritoneal involvement
P2	A few scattered metastases to distant peritoneum
P3	Many distant peritoneal metastases
H0	No liver metastases
H1	Metastases limited to one lobe
H2	A few bilateral metastases
H3	Numerous bilateral metastases

STAGE GROUPING	
Stage I	S0, N0, P0, H0
Stage II	S1, N0-1, P0, H0
Stage III	S2, N0-2, P0, H0
Stage IV	S3, N3-4, P1-3, H1-3

13.1.3 Prognostic Factors

- The prognosis of patients with gastric cancer is directly associated with the presenting characteristics. Advanced stage, poor performance status, weight loss, and abdominal pain at diagnosis are associated with adverse outcomes in gastric cancer.

- Stage is the most important prognostic factor in predicting patients' outcome. Gastric cancer with a limited depth of invasion has a much more favorable prognosis and survival rates from 85%–95% have been reported for early stage disease (T1 category without nodal involvement) (Level IV) (Everett and Axon 1997; Craanen et al. 1991; Eckardt et al. 1990). Survival decreases with more tumor invasive depth into the stomach wall. The 5-year survival rates of T3 to T4 lesions decrease significantly, from 30% to 5% in Japa-

nese studies and 47% to 15% in Western studies, respectively (Noguchi et al. 1989; Bonenkamp et al. 1995; Meyers et al. 1987). Cure of diseases with distant metastasis or peritoneal seeding is dismally low.

- Regional nodal involvement adversely affects the prognosis. The number and locations of the affected lymph nodes are both significant factors for prognosis. Classification of the nodal groups advocated by The Japanese Research Society for Gastric Cancer are as follows: N1 nodes, perigastric lymph nodes; N2 nodes, nodes around the left gastric artery, common hepatic artery, splenic artery and celiac axis; N3 nodes, nodes in the hepatoduodenal ligament, posterior aspect of pancreas, and root of mesentery; N4 nodes, periaortic and middle colic lymph nodes (Nishi et al. 1986).

  The prognosis of the level of lymph node metastases is significant. From level I to III lymph nodes according to the Japanese Classification of gastric cancer, numbers of positive level II nodes have more influence on the prognosis in patients with node-positive gastric cancer. Early stage gastric cancer has a favorable 5-year survival of over 80%; however, the survival rate decreases in relation to the lymph node metastasis with approximate 77% for N1 and 60% for N2. Involvement of more than three or four nodes was an independent poor prognostic determinant (Level IV) (Folli et al. 2001; Saito et al. 2007; Adachi et al. 2000; Shimada et al. 2001; Ichikura et al. 1993; Kodera et al. 1998).

- Tumor location of the primary tumor has been suggested to be prognostically significant. The prognosis of proximal cancers is less favorable than that of distal lesions (Levels IV) (Fein et al. 1985; Heberer et al. 1988).

- Pathologic features including gross and microscopic appearance, tumor grade are not independent prognostic factors relative to tumor stage. These features provide some prognostic information. Diffuse type pathology cases are associated with worse treatment results compared with intestinal type (Level II) (Macdonald et al. 2004). Borrmann's type I and II tumors have relatively favorable 5-year survival rates compared with type IV carcinomas (Level IV) (Dent et al. 1979; Tsukiyama et al. 1988).

- Currently, no biologic markers can be routinely utilized for determining prognosis of gastric cancer.

13.2 Treatment of Resectable Gastric Cancer

13.2.1 General Principles

- Surgery is the primary treatment of resectable gastric cancer. Total gastrectomy or subtotal gastrectomy has been the main surgical procedure for resectable gastric cancer depending on the extent and location of the tumor: A subtotal gastrectomy can be utilized for diseases located in the body or distal stomach.

  The optimal standard surgical principles have not reached consensus. The most controversial aspect of surgery for gastric cancer is the extent of lymph node dissection required.

- For resectable clinical stage T2 or higher or node-positive tumors, neoadjuvant or adjuvant treatment may further improve the treatment outcome and is recommended (Grade A). Recent evidence also supports the use of surgery with neoadjuvant and adjuvant (perioperative) chemotherapy, or surgery with adjuvant chemoradiation therapy for locoregionally advanced gastric cancer (Grade A).

- For patients with locally advanced unresectable gastric cancer, treatment options including concurrent chemoradiation, preoperative chemotherapy with or without radiation, or maximal resection with intraoperative radiation therapy (IORT) can be considered (Grade B).

- For patients who have distant metastasis, peritoneal seeding, or are medically inoperable, concurrent chemoradiation or chemotherapy alone can be considered for palliation.

13.2.2 Surgical Resection

- Surgical resection of the stomach and regional lymph nodes is the primary therapy of curable gastric cancer (Grade A). Following surgical resection of early stage gastric cancer 5-year survival rates of 80% or higher can be achieved ,while the same rate is 30% or less for patients with extensive lymph node involvement (Everett and Axon 1997; Agboola 1994).

- For tumors limited to the mucosa or submucosa (T1 classification or less), surgical resection alone is sufficient in most cases. Modalities including endoscopic mucosal resection and minimal access surgery have been applied to selected early

gastric cancer patients. For low-risk patients, adjuvant therapy is usually not recommended. Node-negative T1 tumors are associated with a favorable 5-year survival of more than 90% (Kooby et al. 2003).

- Subtotal gastrectomy is the procedure of choice if a 5-cm margin can be achieved (Grade B). Total gastrectomy is not necessary if a sufficient margin can be obtained.

  The choice of surgical procedure is based on tumor location. The preferred treatment for body or antrum lesions of stomach is a radical subtotal resection (Level I) (Bozzetti et al. 1999). Proximal or extensive gastric cancers usually require a total gastrectomy to achieve adequate margins.

- The extent of lymph node dissection has not been determined; however, it is accepted that extended lymphadenectomies are not necessary (Grade C). Results of two randomized trials has demonstrated that extended dissection of regional nodes were not associated with improved survival: A large multicenter randomized trial from the Netherlands (the Dutch trial) and a randomized trial reported by the Medical Research Council compared D1 versus D2 dissection in patients with gastric cancer. The results from both trials showed no significant differences in 5-year survival among the patients who received either nodal dissection, but higher postoperative mortality and morbidity rates were observed in the patients undergoing D2 dissection (Bonenkamp et al. 1999; Hartgrink et al. 2004; Cuschieri et al. 1999).

  However, the debate on nodal dissection is not solved (Mansfield 2004). The Japanese Research Society for Gastric Cancer (JRSGC) has provided guidelines for the standardization of surgical treatment and pathological evaluation, and considered surgery without D2 dissection inadequate (Kajitani 1981). The results from a randomized trial from Taipei revealed that the overall 5-year survival was significantly improved in patients who received D3 surgery than those who received D1 dissection (59.5% versus 53.6%, respectively). More importantly, a low mortality rate was observed from the study (Level II) (Wu et al. 2006) These finding were confirmed by the results from a randomized trial from Japan, which reported a hospital mortality rate of 0.8% (JCOG 95-01, Level I) (Sasako et al. 2006; Sano et al. 2004). An Italian study also showed similar results on postoperative mortality (Level II) (Degiuli et al. 2004).

Results from a number of retrospective trials suggested that D2 gastrectomy with pancreas- and spleen-sparing procedure may be safe when performed in high-volume centers and that may confer a survival benefit in selected patients (Grade B). Nonrandomized gastric cancer studies from Germany, England, Norway, and the United States reported mortality between 4% and 5%, morbidity between 22% and 30.6% postoperatively, and 5-year survival between 26.3% and 55% for patients who underwent D2 dissections. These results indicated D2 dissections appear to improve survival.

Splenectomy is not routinely recommended for the purpose of adequate removal of station 10 and 11 lymph nodes in D2 dissection but spleen- and pancreas-preserving lymphadenectomies are becoming more popular (Fenoglio-Preiser et al. 1996).

Endoscopic mucosal dissection (EMR) has been increasingly used in selected patients with early-stage gastric cancer. Indications for EMR include tumor size < 3 cm, absence of ulceration, well-differentiated histology, absence of lymph node metastasis, and no evidence of invasive findings (Ono et al. 2001; Hiki et al. 1995; Noda et al. 1997). There is no defined standard for managing incomplete resection after EMR. Gastrectomy has generally been recommended. Close endoscopic follow-up with or without further resection may be appropriate for some cases. Chemoradiation may be another alternative modality for endoscopically treated early gastric cancer.

13.2.3 Postoperative Treatment

The suboptimal outcome after surgery alone for gastric cancer indicated the necessity of adjuvant treatment for locally or locoregionally advanced adenocarcinoma of the stomach. Adjuvant treatment for gastric cancer could involve radiation therapy, chemotherapy, or combined chemoradiotherapy.

Postoperative Radiation Therapy

Postoperative radiation therapy alone is not indicated for gastric cancer after complete surgical resection (Grade B). A prospective randomized trial reported by the British Stomach Cancer Group (BSCG) compared surgery alone versus surgery followed by postoperative chemotherapy or postoperative radiation. The results showed postoperative radiation therapy improved local-regional control but provided no survival benefit for patients, suggesting combined with chemotherapy may be helpful to improve survival rates (Level II) (Allum et al. 1989; Hallissey et al. 1994).

Postoperative Chemotherapy

The role of postoperative chemotherapy alone in patients after complete resection of gastric cancer has not been fully confirmed. As the efficacy of peri-operative chemotherapy and adjuvant chemoradiotherapy have been confirmed in the treatment of resectable locally advanced gastric cancer, adjuvant chemotherapy alone is not routinely recommended for locally advanced gastric cancer (Grade C). Results of randomized clinical trials of adjuvant chemotherapy have not demonstrated a consistent improvement on survival benefit when compared with surgery alone in gastric cancer:
The International collaborative cancer groups (ICCG) and an Italian study evaluated FAM-based chemotherapy (fluorouracil, adriamycin, and mitomycin) regimen in resected high-risk gastric cancer. However, neither overall survival nor relapse rates were affected by the addition of the chemotherapy (Level II) (Coombes et al. 1990; DeVita et al. 2006).
The European Organization for Research and Treatment of Cancer (EORTC) and ICCG conducted two randomized phase III trials independently to compare adjuvant chemotherapy (FAMTX or FEMTX) following surgery to surgery alone. Both studies failed to demonstrate a significant difference with the addition of postoperative chemotherapy. In addition, the pooled analysis of these two studies did not demonstrate any significant change on overall survival with chemotherapy, and the 5-year survival was 52% and 51% in patients treated with surgery plus FAMTX chemotherapy or surgery alone, respectively, or 33% and 36% in patients treated with surgery plus FEMTX chemotherapy or surgery alone (Level II) (Nitti et al. 2006).

The results of a recently published randomized trial from Japan reported a significant improvement in overall survival with a single oral chemotherapeutic agent, S-1, given postoperatively (80 mg/m^2, daily, for 4 weeks and 2 weeks' break).

S-1 is a compound drug consisting of the oral fluoropyrimidine prodrug tegafur and the enzyme inhibitors gimeracil and oteracil. It reduces the toxic effects associated with fluorouracil by inhibiting orotate phosphoribosyltransferase. There was a significant survival benefit of adjuvant therapy comparing surgery alone with 3-year survival from 70% to 80% and with a low incidence of toxicity (Level II) (Sakuramoto et al. 2007). Two other randomized trials in Japan involving patients with advanced gastric cancer have shown the non-inferiority of S-1 to the continuous infusion of 5-FU and the activity of S-1 in combination with cisplatin (Level II) (Boku et al. 2007; Narahara et al. 2007). However, these results should be evaluated and verified in Western populations prior to any change in practice.

- The effects of postoperative chemotherapy in gastric cancer have been evaluated by a number of meta-analyses. Many of the individual randomized trials included in meta-analyses had small numbers of patients, using chemotherapy regimens of limited efficacy. Overall, there is a trend with an odds ratio from 0.8–0.94 of advantage of adjuvant chemotherapy; however, the low quality of many of these studies weaken the impact to conclude a definitive result regarding the value of postoperative chemotherapy of gastric cancer (Level I) (Hermans et al. 1993; Earle and Maroun 1999; Hu et al. 2002).

In a comprehensive review and meta-analysis recently reported by Liu et al. (2008), a total of 4919 gastric cancer patients treated with surgery and adjuvant chemotherapy in 23 randomized trials were analyzed. Trials utilizing peri-operative or preoperative chemotherapy were excluded. The analysis reported a benefit of adjuvant chemotherapy and a pooled relative risk of death was 0.85 (95% CI: 0.80–0.90) was observed (Level I). An up to 18% reduction of death risk benefit of adjuvant chemotherapy compared with surgery alone was reported in two additional analyses. However, adequately powered randomized trials and individual patient data analyses were recommended by the authors (Level I) (Panzini et al. 2002; Mari et al. 2000; Janunger et al. 2001).

Postoperative Chemoradiation Therapy

- Postoperative concurrent chemoradiation is indicated for resected high-risk stage II–III B gastric cancer patients (Grade A). The efficacy of combined chemoradiation therapy has been demonstrated in randomized trials of various sizes:

The Mayo clinic performed the first trial to evaluate postoperative chemoradiotherapy versus surgery alone, and 62 patients were enrolled. Local control was achieved in 61% of patients treated with adjuvant chemoradiation and 45% in the surgery-alone group. The 5-year survival also favored the adjuvant therapy group (20% versus 4%) (Level II) (Moertel 1984).

The randomized phase III trial Intergroup 0116 compared postoperative chemoradiation with observation. This study demonstrated an overall survival benefit in combined adjuvant therapy. Patients who received postoperative therapy had a significant improvement in median survival (26 months versus 35 months at 7-year follow up, $p = 0.006$), and 3-year overall survival (50% versus 41%, $p = 0.005$). Local and regional failure decreased in the chemoradiation group (19% versus 29% and 65% versus 72%). However, only 10% of patients received planned surgical resection (i.e., D2 dissection) (INT 01-16, Level II) (Macdonald et al. 2001).

- Adjuvant chemoradiation therapy is recommended after D2 resection for patients with locally or locoregionally advanced gastric cancer (Grade B); however, randomized trial data is lacking. A large retrospective adjuvant chemoradiation analysis from Korea indicated an overall survival benefit for postoperative therapy as compared to surgery alone: the 5-year survival rates were 57% versus 51%, respectively, in favor of postoperative treatment ($p=0.005$). Local control was significantly improved with postoperative chemoradiation therapy (15% versus 22%, $p=0.005$); however, no difference in distant metastasis (38%) was observed (Level IV) (Kim et al. 2005).

13.2.4 Pre- or Peri-operative Treatment

Peri-operative Chemotherapy

- Peri-operative chemotherapy can be recommended as one of the standard treatment regimens for patients with locally or locoregionally advanced but resectable gastric cancer (Grade A). The results of a randomized phase III trial from Britain demonstrated that the addition of three cycles of peri- and post-operative chemotherapy using an ECF regimen (epirubicin 50 mg/m² day 1, cisplatin

60 mg/m^2 d1 and 5-FU 200 mg m^2 for 21 days) to surgery significantly improved survival in patients with potentially curable gastric cancer: The 5-year overall survival rates were 36% versus 23% for patients treated with or without peri-operative chemotherapy. In addition, it was observed that chemotherapy produced significant tumor downstaging and increased resectability (MAGIC Study, Level I) (CUNNINGHAM et al. 2006).

Preoperative Chemoradiotherapy

■ Preoperative chemoradiation therapy cannot be routinely offered for resectable gastric cancer at this stage, as the efficacy of such strategy has not been confirmed by phase III randomized trials. Research on neoadjuvant chemoradiation for patients with gastric cancer is limited to phase II trials: The RTOG 99-04 trial included 49 patients treated with two cycles of induction 5-FU, leucovorin, and cisplatin followed by irradiation (45 Gy) with concurrent continuous 5-FU and weekly paclitaxel preoperatively. The results revealed 27% pathological CR and 77% R0 resection rates (RTOG 99-04, Level III) (OKAWARA et al. 2005; AJANI et al. 2006).

Two phase II studies from the M. D Anderson Cancer Center also indicated the possible effect of neoadjuvant chemoradiation therapy. One enrolled 33 patients treated with induction chemotherapy of 5-FU, leucovorin, and cisplatin followed by chemoradiation of 45 Gy in 25 fractions concurrently with 5-FU. The pathological complete and partial response was observed in 64% patients (Level III) (AJANI et al. 2004). The second study included 41 resectable gastric cancer patients treated with two cycles of induction chemotherapy of 5-FU, paclitaxel, and cisplatin followed by 45 Gy irradiation with concurrent 5-FU and paclitaxel. The 25% pathological CR and 78% R0 resection rate was achieved (Level III) (AJANI et al. 2005). These data form the basis for future evaluation of pre- versus postoperative chemoradiotherapy strategies for localized resectable gastric cancer.

■ Although there are no published phase III trials aimed at studying the effect of preoperative chemoradiation on gastric cancer, two randomized trials of esophagus cancer included either gastric cardia or GE junction lesions: The randomized trial by WALSH et al. (1996) assigned 113 patients with lesions of esophagus and gastric cardia comparing immediate surgery to preoperative 5-FU/cisplatin-based chemotherapy and radiation therapy (to a total dose of 40 Gy in 15 daily fractions) followed by surgical resection. A significant survival improvement was demonstrated with combined therapy in 3-year survival of 32% versus 6% of the surgery-alone arm (Level III). The prospective randomized CALGB 9871 was a phase III trial of preoperative chemoradiation (5-FU/cisplatin and 50.4 Gy in 28 fractions) versus surgery alone for treatment of esophageal carcinoma. Patients with GE junction lesions were included in the trial. It was closed due to poor accrual of 56 patients for a targeted patient enrollment of 500. Although accrual was well below that planned, the observed 5-year survival of 39% in the preoperative therapy arm versus 16% in the surgery alone arm suggests that combined modality is an appropriate treatment for this disease (CALGB 98-71, Level III) (KRASNA et al. 2006). It is important to note that the numbers of patients with gastric cardia lesions are limited in both studies, and the results of the trials cannot be directly applied to gastric cancer treatment.

Preoperative Radiation Therapy

■ Radiation therapy is not routinely indicated in the treatment of resectable gastric cancer (Grade C). As the effects of adjuvant chemotherapy and radiation therapy, as well as perioperative chemotherapy, have been confirmed by well designed multi-institutional randomized trials, preoperative radiation is not recommended as a standard practice for potentially resectable gastric cancer. Prospective randomized trials from Russia and one from China have demonstrated the effect of preoperative radiotherapy in the treatment of resectable gastric cancer; however, regimens including dose and fractionation used in the studies were not standardized. Further investigations with randomized trials are needed to confirm the efficacy of neoadjuvant radiation therapy before it can be recommended as part of standard treatment.

■ Three prospective randomized Russian trials have evaluated radiotherapy alone (20 Gy in four fractions in the first two trials and 32 Gy in the third trial) in potentially resectable gastric cancer. Although survival advantage was observed in these trials with preoperative therapy, there were some methodological uncertainties and their applicability to gastric cancer in other countries is not clear (Level II) (Kossé 1990; Skoropad et al. 2000; Talaev et al. 1990).

■ A well designed randomized trial from China compared preoperative radiation (40 Gy in 20 fractions) with surgery alone in patients with clinically resectable gastric cardia disease. A significant improvement in survival and local regional disease control were observed with the preoperative-radiation arm to the surgery-only arm. The 5-year survival rate was 30% versus 20%, $p=0.0094$, with local relapse rates of 39% versus 52%, $p<0.025$. However, only patients with adenocarcinoma of gastric cardia were included in this single institutional randomized trial (Level I) (Zhang et al. 1998).

■ A randomized trial from Georgetown University 293 patients with gastric cancer (resectable and unresectable) to preoperative radiation therapy, preoperative radiation with postoperative hyperthermia, or gastrectomy alone. The results of this trial showed that preoperative radiation therapy of 20 Gy delivered in four fractions (5 Gy per fraction) did not improve overall survival as compared to surgery alone. However, patients with unresectable gastric cancer benefited significantly from preoperative radiotherapy with or without hyperthermia (Level II) (Shchepotin et al. 1994).

13.3 Treatment of Locally Advanced Unresectable Gastric Cancer

13.3.1 General Principles

■ Neoadjuvant chemoradiation therapy followed by surgery and adjuvant chemotherapy, or neoadjuvant chemotherapy followed by surgery and adjuvant chemoradiation can be considered for patients with unresectable gastric cancer or residual tumor after resection.

■ Radical subtotal or total gastrectomy may be indicated in some patients to achieve symptomatic palliation.

13.3.2 Surgery

■ Limited gastric resection is recommended for symptomatic control and may alleviate symptoms such as hemorrhage, symptomatic obstruction, perforation, and pain by ulceration (Grade B). Resection may be associated with benefit of prolongation of survival but is not confirmed in randomized trials. However, palliative surgery has been shown to improve quality of life for patients with bulky or proximal tumors (Level III) (Haugstvedt et al. 1989; Monson et al. 1991).

13.3.3 Radiation and Chemotherapy

■ Combined radiation and chemotherapy may be considered for patients of unresectable gastric cancer, or for patients with residual tumor after surgical resection (Grade C). Data from randomized studies of postoperative combined chemoradiation in patients with locally unresectable gastric cancer were inconsistent.

In an early randomized study reported by the Mayo Clinic, combined therapy of radiotherapy (35–37.5 Gy over 4–5 weeks) and chemotherapy (5-FU) were given to patients with unresectable gastric cancer after surgery, as compared to surgery alone. Mean and overall survival rates were significantly improved in the combined modality group (13 versus 5.9 months and 12% versus 0% for 5-year survival) (Level II) (Moertel et al. 1969).

■ Two randomized trials conducted by GITSG compared the effect of combined chemoradiotherapy and chemotherapy in patients with locally advanced unresectable gastric cancer. The first trial compared chemotherapy (5-FU and MeCCNU) and split-course radiation (50 Gy delivered in split courses spaced 2 weeks apart) with chemotherapy alone in patients with locally unresectable gastric cancer. Approximately 25% of patients who received chemoradiation died or deteriorated earlier within the first 10 weeks of treatment. However, further follow-up revealed that a significant improvement in 4-year survival was observed in the combined modality group (18% versus 6%) (Level II) (Schein et al. 1982).

In the second study from GITSG, radiation was delivered in continuous course, and doxorubicin was added to the chemotherapy regimen and chemotherapy was delivered before combined modality therapy. However, close to 50% of the patients in the combined treatment group did not receive planned therapy, and the outcome of the combined therapy group did not show improvement of survival (Level II) (GASTROINTESTINAL TUMOR STUDY GROUP 1982).

■ A retrospective analysis of 60 patients with unresectable, incompletely resected, or recurrent gastric or gastroesophageal junction adenocarcinoma was reported by the Mayo Clinic. The results indicated that in patients with recurrent disease, the number of sites involved and the use of external-beam radiation and IORT to a total dose of more than 54 Gy were of borderline significance in regard to survival (Level IV) (HENNING et al. 2000). The median survival time for the entire group of patients was 11.6 months, similar to those reported in the randomized trials.

13.3.4 Neoadjuvant Chemotherapy and Radiotherapy

■ Neoadjuvant chemotherapy in patients with resectable gastric cancer to improve survival has been confirmed in the MAGIC trial. The resectability may be improved. The role of neoadjuvant chemotherapy to increase resectability or improve survival in patients with locally advanced unresectable gastric cancer has not yet been demonstrated.

■ KANG et al. (1996) performed a small randomized trial of 107 patients with locally advanced gastric cancer to receive between two and three cycles of chemotherapy followed by surgery versus surgery alone. Pathological complete response of 7% was observed. No significant improvement in survival (55% versus 55% of 2 years) but borderline increased resectable rate was observed with neoadjuvant chemotherapy (71% versus 61%) (Level II).

■ Radiation should be considered incorporated into the study design for initially unresectable tumor due to high incidence of local regional relapse after neoadjuvant chemotherapy. As detailed above, the survival benefit reported by WALSH et al. (1996) in a trial of chemoradiation followed by surgery versus surgery alone in patients with esophagus and gastric cardia tumors can be references for future trial design (Level III).

13.3.5 Treatment of Medically Inoperable Gastric Cancer

■ For patients with inoperable gastric cancer due to their medical conditions, definitive treatment with external beam radiation to a total dose of 45–50.5 Gy in 25–28 fractions with concurrent 5-FU-based chemotherapy can be considered (Grade D).

■ If combined treatment is not feasible, single modality management with radiation therapy or chemotherapy can be considered for palliation (Grade D).

13.4 Radiation Therapy Techniques

13.4.1 Dose and Fractionation

■ External beam radiation therapy to a total dose of 45 Gy at 1.8 Gy/fraction combined with current 5-FU-based chemotherapy is the standard regimen for adjuvant treatment (Grade A). In the above mentioned Intergroup 0116 study, patients in the treatment arm received adjuvant chemoradiation to a total dose of 45 Gy at 1.8 Gy/fraction and concurrent chemotherapy (5-FU and leucovorin) (Level II) (MACDONALD et al. 2001).

■ For patients with gross residual disease, a field reduction technique is recommended for boost to 50–55 Gy.

13.4.2 Simulation and Planning

■ The optimal target of adjuvant radiation treatment for gastric cancer is yet to be determined. A field that encompasses tumor bed, major lymph node regions, as well as any residual disease is reasonable, due to the high likelihood of local and regional recurrence in these areas (Grade D) (TEPPER and GUNDERSON 2002).

■ CT-based treatment planning is highly recommended for defining clinical target volume (CTV) and planning target volume (PTV). An individualized immobilization device (e.g., Alpha cradle, Smithers Medical Products, Inc. North Canton, OH) should be used for simulation and treatment. CT scan with a slice thickness of 3–5 mm should be performed with the patient in a supine treatment position with arms placed overhead, preferably 2–3 h after a meal.

■ The treatment target should be defined by CT (pre- and postoperative) and surgical findings, and depends on both the location and depth of invasion of the primary tumor (T category), as well as the location and extent of known nodal involvement (N category). When the invasion of primary tumor is deeper than subserosa (T2b or above), the tumor bed should be irradiated.

The lymph node chain should be included in the radiation field if there is nodal involvement (N+). Major lymph nodes at risk include the lesser and greater curvature, celiac axis, pancreaticoduodenal, splenic, suprapancreatic, porta hepatis and para-aortics. For resected tumor with positive or closer (less than 5 cm) margins, the residual stomach should be included (TEPPER and GUNDERSON 2002).

- The margin should be added to CTV to generate planning target volume (PTV) to account for individual's organ motion and daily setup uncertainties. For postoperative radiation, a preoperative CT is preferred as a reference.

- Normal tissues to be delineated include spinal cord, liver, distal esophagus, and kidneys for organ identification and dose-volume histograms. For tumor at GE junction, heart and mediastinum may need to be contoured.

13.4.3 Field Arrangement

- Although AP/PA with or without lateral fields (three- or four-field arrangement) are practical, multiple fields with 3D conformal techniques should be considered for sparing more normal tissue if possible (SMALLEY et al. (2002).

- Currently, no recommendation can be given for standard volume delineation. In a prospective study reported by CHUNG et al. (2004), tumor volume delineation between radiation oncologists differed significantly, in both clinical tumor volume (measured as total volume in cm^3) on 3D planning, as well as area of treatment field (measured as total volume in cm^2) on 2D planning, for adjuvant radiotherapy for gastric cancer using the treatment regimen indicated in the Intergroup 0116 trial (Level III).

- The suggested field of treatment depends on the location of the primary disease and the status of lymph node involvement: For proximal gastric tumor at the GE junction and cardia, the propensity to lymph node spread to the gastric antrum, periduodenal, and porta hepatic nodes is lower. These regions can be excluded to spare as much liver and right kidney as possible.

For distal gastric tumor, periduodenal, peripancreatic, and porta hepatic nodes should be included in the treatment fields, whereas periesophageal, pericardia, and splenic hilar nodes can be excluded for their lower likelihood of involvement. For tumors in the body of the stomach, all above-mentioned major lymph nodes should be included in the treatment field.

Figure 13.1 depicts nodal stations in the abdomen. Table 13.4 summarizes the draining lymph node groups of various gastrointestinal structures.

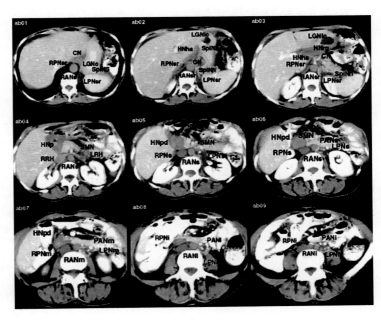

Fig. 13.1. CT images depict nodal stations in the abdomen

Table 13.4. Gastrointestinal lymphatic system [from MARTINEZ-MONGE et al. (1999) with permission]

Anatomic site	First echelon nodal group	Subgroup	Category	Abbreviation
Gastric cardia	Left gastric nodes	Juxtacardiac	Main	LGNc
Gastric lesser curvature	Left gastric nodes	Gastropancreatic	Main	LGNlc
		Lesser curvature	Main	LGNlc
Gastric antrum and pylorus	Hepatic nodes	Right gastroepiploic	Main	HNrg
		Infrapyloric	Main	HNp
		Suprapyloric	Main	HNp
Greater omentum	Hepatic nodes	Right gastroepiploic	Main	HNrg
		Infrapyloric	Main	HNp
		Supropyloric	Main	HNp
Gastric greater curvature	Splenic nodes	Suprapancreatic	Main	SpINs
Duodenum	Hepatic nodes	Infrapyloric	Main	HNP
		Retropyloric	Main	HNp
		Pancreaticoduodenal	Main	HNpd
	Superior mesenteric nodes	Postpancreaticoduodenal	Main	SMN
Pancreas	Hepatic nodes	Infrapyloric, suprapyloric	Main	HNp
		Pancreaticoduodenal	Main	HNpd
		Hepatic artery	Main	HNha
	Splenic nodes	Suprapancreatic	Main	SpINs
		Splenic hilum	Main	SpINh
	Left gastric nodes	Gastropancreatic	Main	LGNIc
	Superior mesenteric nodes	Root of mesentery	Main	SMN
		Middle colic	Main	SMN
		Postpancreaticoduodenal	Main	SMN
	Right paraaortic nodes	Superior	Main	RPNs
	Left paraaortic nodes	Superior	Main	LPNs
Spleen	Splenic nodes	Splenic hilum	Main	SpINh
Liver	Hepatic nodes	Gallbladder, hepatic artery	Main	HNha
	Celiac axis nodes		Main	CN
	Left gastric nodes	Lesser curvature	Main	LGNIc
	Diaphragmatic nodes	Anterior, lateral	Main	DNa, lat
	Paraesophageal nodes	Inferior	Main	PENi
	Renal hilum nodes		Main	RRH, LRH
Gallbladder and cystic duct	Hepatic nodes	Gallbladder	Main	HNha
		Foramen of Winslow	Main	HNha
Hepatic duct	Hepatic nodes	Foramen of Winslow	Main	HNha
Common bile duct	Hepatic nodes	Foramen of Winslow	Main	HNha
		Postpancreaticoduodenal	Main	HNhaHNpd

- 3D conformal treatment with mono-isocentric split-field technique or intensity-modulated radiation therapy (IMRT) can be considered for gastric cancer treatment. It is desired to deliver highly conformal dose to the target while reducing the dose to the surrounding critical structures. The benefit of IMRT over 3D conformal radiation has been suggested by many publications; however it needs to be further confirmed by the clinical outcome (Level III) (WIELAND et al. 2004).
- Figure 13.2 depicts a postoperative radiation fields for a ptient with T3N1 gastric cancer of the antral primary

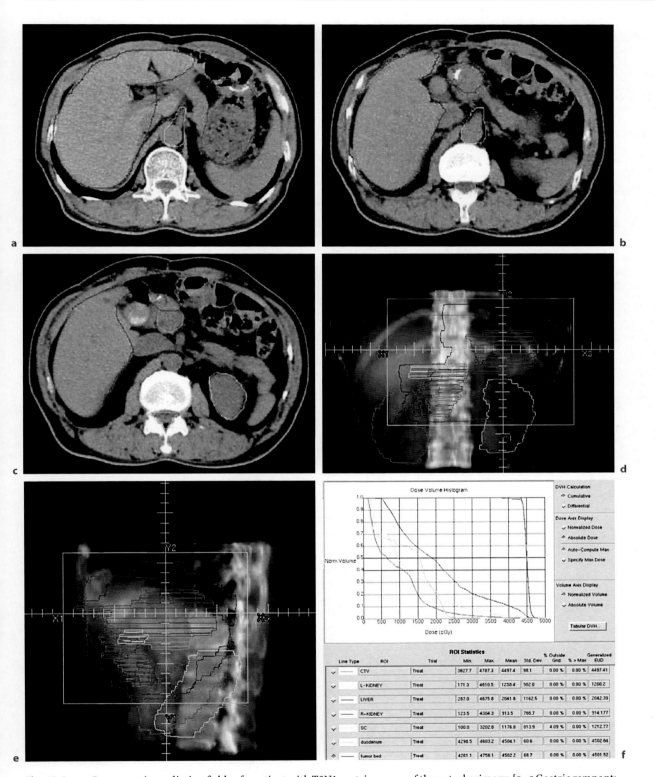

Fig. 13.2. a–c Postoperative radiation fields of a patient with T3N1 gastric cancer of the antral primary. [**a–c** Gastric remnant; tumor bed (*red*); celiac artery (*light orange*); porta hepatis (*light blue*); right kidney (*light orange*); pancreatic head (*orange*)]. **d–f** DRR and DVH of 3D conformal plan

13.4.4 Intraoperative Radiation

■ IORT alone or with external beam radiation may be considered for the treatment of locally advanced gastric cancer (Grade C). Randomized trials have examined the efficacy of IORT in combination with surgery for patients with gastric carcinoma. The limited data suggested that IORT may improve locoregional control in selected patients with gastric cancer; however, most trials failed to demonstrate a benefit in overall survival.

■ ABE et al. (1988) performed a randomized trial of 211 patients with gastric cancer comparing surgery only with surgery and IORT (28–35 Gy). Advantage of combined therapy was observed in patients with locally advanced gastric cancer. For stage IV disease, 15% patients who received IORT were alive at 5 years compared to no survivors in the surgery alone group (Level II). In a prospective randomized trial reported by SINDELAR et al. (1993), surgical resection alone was compared to surgery and IORT (20 Gy) followed by external beam radiation (50 Gy in 25 fractions) in locally advanced gastric cancer. The results revealed no significant difference in patients who received surgery or combined treatment; however, locoregional disease failures occurred in 44% patients treated with IORT and in 92% of patients who received surgery only ($p < 0.001$). Complication rates were similar between IORT and control patients (Level II).
A more recently published study compared surgery followed by chemoradiation and surgery plus IORT followed by chemoradiation. A group of 94 patients with locally advanced gastric cancer were treated with surgery followed by chemoradiation, with or without IORT. The results revealed that the 3-year locoregional control rates were 77% versus 63%, respectively, in favor of IORT-treated patients. However, no difference in overall survival was observed (Level IV) (FU et al. 2008).

13.4.5 Side Effects and Complications

Radiation-Induced Side Effects and Complications

■ Toxicities and complications of radiation depend on the location of the target and treatment fields. The critical normal structures for gastric treat-ment located within treatment fields include liver, kidneys, spinal cord, and heart.

■ Gastritis is a common radiation-induced side effect during treatment and does not constitute a reason for treatment interruption.

■ Radiation-induced kidney dysfunction is dose- and volume-dependent and associated with incidence of renovascular hypertension. A dose of approximately 20 Gy, given over 3–5 weeks, is considered the radiation tolerance dose. A progressive decrease in relative left kidney function of approximately 11% at 6 months and 52% at 18 months in AP/PA parallel opposed field technique was observed (Level III) (JANSEN et al. 2007).

■ Other side effects may include fatigue, skin reaction, bone marrow toxicity, and/or diarrhea depending on the site and volume of irradiation.

13.4.6 Dose Limiting Structures

■ V20 of one functional kidney should not exceed 75%.

■ Radiation dose to the spinal cord should be less than 45 Gy (1.8–2.0 Gy/day); V40 of the heart should be limited to 50% or less; V30 of the liver should be limited to 60% or less (Level IV) (EMAMI et al. 1991).

13.5 Palliative Treatment of Gastric Cancer

13.5.1 General Principles

■ Limited gastric resection can be used for relief of symptoms such as obstruction, hemorrhage, and ulceration or gastric perforation (Grade B).

■ Radiation therapy is frequently recommended to palliate symptoms such as pain, dysphagia, obstruction, and bleeding (Grade B).

■ Chemotherapy concurrently combined with radiation can be considered in palliation treatment of advanced gastric cancer (Grade B).

■ Systemic chemotherapy can be considered for metastatic gastric cancer; however, the effect of chemotherapy on prolonging survival has not been confirmed.

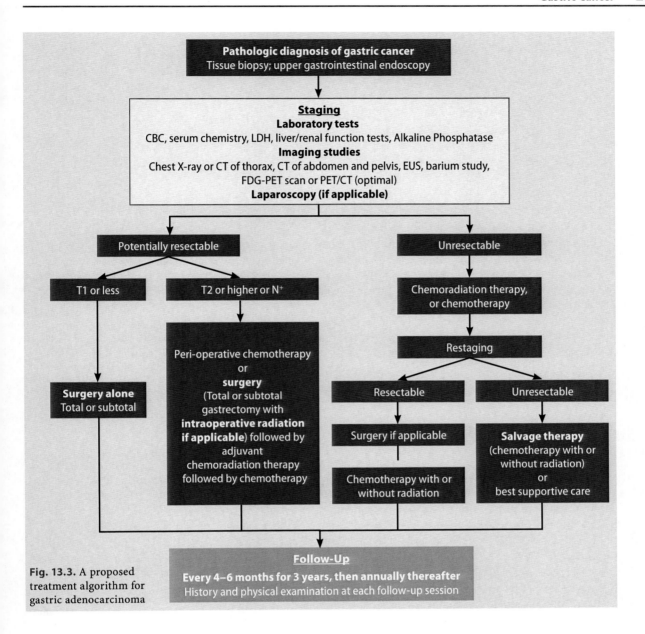

Fig. 13.3. A proposed treatment algorithm for gastric adenocarcinoma

13.5.2 Palliative Radiation Therapy

■ Dysphagia/obstruction, hemorrhage, and pain are the more common presenting symptoms of advanced gastric cancer. Radiation alone or in combination with chemotherapy is recommended in symptomatic palliation of advanced gastric cancer (Grade B). Radiation offers relief of symptoms in approximately 70% of patients. The outcomes of retrospective analyses of patients with gastric cancer treated with palliative radiation or concurrent chemoradiation revealed 70%–81% symptom control rates (Level IV) (Kim et al. 2007). Some reports showed radiation alone had symptom control in 54% patients with bleeding and 25% patients with obstruction of gastric cancer (Level IV) (Tey et al. 2007).

■ Relationship between dose response and clinical effects in palliative radiation is not consistent. Various doses to the primary tumor range from 30 Gy in 10 fractions to the dose fractionation for definitive treatment, i.e., 50.4 Gy at 1.8 Gy/ fraction have been used. A retrospective study showed bleeding can be palliated with 30 Gy in

10 daily fractions and no obvious dose response was evident (Level IV) (Tey et al. 2007). The role of higher biologically effective dose of radiation remains to be established in prospective randomized studies.

13.5.3 Combined Chemoradiation Therapy

■ Chemotherapy concurrently combined with radiation can be considered in palliative treatment of advanced gastric cancer (Grade B). In a prospective trial aimed to study the effects of combined radiation therapy and chemotherapy (razoxane, used as a radiosensitizer), partial response was achieved in 89% patients and local control in 64%. The median time to an in-field recurrence was 7 months. Rapid pain relief was achieved in 96% of patients (Level III) (Rhomberg et al. 1996).

13.6   Follow-Ups

13.6.1 Post-Treatment Follow-Ups

■ Life-long follow-up after definitive treatment of gastric cancer is usually indicated.

Schedule

■ Each follow-up should include a complete history and physical examination. Laboratory tests include complete blood count and multichannel serum chemistry; radiologic imaging or endoscopy are required when clinically indicated (Grade D) (NCCN 2008).
■ Follow-ups could be scheduled every 4–6 months initially in the first 3 years after treatment and annually thereafter (Grade D) (NCCN 2008) (Table 13.5).

Table 13.5. Follow-up schedule

Interval	Frequency
First 3 years	Every 4–6 months
Over 3 years	Annually

Work-Ups

■ Each follow-up examination should include a complete history and physical examination. There is no clear role for routine imaging studies for asymptomatic patients.

References

Abe M, Takahashi M, Ono K et al. (1988) Japan gastric trials in intraoperative radiation therapy. Int J Radiat Oncol Biol Phys 15:1431–1433

Adachi Y, Shiraishi N, Suematsu T et al. (2000) Most important lymph node information in gastric cancer: multivariate prognostic study. Ann Surg Oncol 7:503–507

Agboola O (1994) Adjuvant treatment in gastric cancer. Cancer Treat Rev 20:217–240

Ajani JA, Mansfield PF, Janjan N et al. (2004) Multi-institutional trial of preoperative chemoradiotherapy in patients with potentially resectable gastric carcinoma. J Clin Oncol 22:2774–2780

Ajani JA, Mansfield PF, Crane CH et al. (2005) Paclitaxel-based chemoradiotherapy in localized gastric carcinoma: degree of pathologic response and not clinical parameters dictated patient outcome. J Clin Oncol 23:1237–1244

Ajani JA, Winter K, Okawara GS et al. (2006) Phase II trial of preoperative chemoradiation in patients with localized gastric adenocarcinoma (RTOG 9904): quality of combined modality therapy and pathologic response. J Clin Oncol 24:3953–3958

Allum WH, Hallissey MT, Ward LC et al. (1989) A controlled, prospective, randomised trial of adjuvant chemotherapy or radiotherapy in resectable gastric cancer: interim report. British Stomach Cancer Group. Br J Cancer 60:739–744

Boku N, Yamanoto S, Shirao K et al. (2007) Randomized phase III study of 5-fluorouracil (5-FU) alone versus combination of irinotecan and cisplatin (CP) versus S-1 alone in advanced gastric cancer (JCOG 9912). J Clin Oncol 25:200s

Bonenkamp JJ, Songum I, Hermans J et al. (1995) Randomized comparison of morbidity after D1 and D2 dissection for gastric cancer in 996 Dutch patients. Lancet 345:745–748

Bonenkamp JJ, Hermans J, Sasako M (1999) Extended lymph-node dissection for gastric cancer. Dutch Gastric Cancer Group. N Engl J Med 340:908–914

Bozzetti F, Marubini E, Bonfanti G et al. (1999) Subtotal versus total gastrectomy for gastric cancer: five-year survival rates in a multicenter randomized Italian trial. Italian Gastrointestinal Tumor Study Group. Ann Surg 230:170–178

Carpelan-Holmstrom M, Louhimo J, Stenman UH et al. (2002) CEA, CA 19-9 and CA 72-4 improve the diagnostic accuracy in gastrointestinal cancers. Anticancer Res 22:2311

Chen J, Cheong JH, Yun MJ et al. (2005) Improvement in preoperative staging of gastric adenocarcinoma with position emission tomography. Cancer 103:2383–2390

Chung HT, Shakespeare TP, Wynne CJ et al. (2004) Evaluation of a radiotherapy protocol based on INT0116 for completely resected gastric adenocarcinoma. Int J Radiat Oncol Biol Phys 59:1446–1453

Coombes RC, Schein PS, Chilvers CE et al. (1990)A randomized trial comparing adjuvant fluorouracil, doxorubicin, and mitomycin with no treatment in operable gastric cancer. J Clin Oncol 8:1362–1369

Craanen ME, Dekker W, Ferwerda J et al. (1991) Early gastric cancer: a clinicopathologic study. J Clin Gastroenterol 13:274–283

Cunningham D, Allum WH, Stenning SP et al. (2006) Perioperative chemotherapy versus surgery alone for resectable gastroesophageal cancer. N Engl J Med 355:11–20

Cuschieri A, Weeden S, Fielding J et al. (1999) Patient survival after D1 and D2 resection for gastric cancer: longterm results of the MRC randomized surgical trial. Surgical Cooperative Group. Br J Cancer 79:1522–1530

Davies J, Chalmers AG, Sue-Ling HM et al. (1997) Spiral computed tomography and operative staging of gastric carcinoma: a comparison with histopathological staging. Gut 41:314–319

Degiuli M, Sasako M, Calgaro M et al. (2004) Morbidity and mortality after D1 and D2 gastrectomy for cancer; interim analysis of the Italian Gastric Cancer Study Group (IGCSG) randomized surgical trial. Eur J Surg Oncol 30:3030–308

D'Elia F, Zingarelli A, Palli D et al. (2000) Hydro-dynamic CT preoperative staging of gastric cancer: correlation with pathological findings. A prospective study of 107 cases. Eur Radiol 10:1877–1885

Dent DM, Werner ID, Novis B et al. (1979) Prospective randomized trial of combined oncological therapy for gastric carcinoma. Cancer 44:385–391

DeVita F, Giuliani F, Gebbia V et al. (2006) Surgery plus ELFE (epirubicin-leucovorin-fluorouracil-etoposide) versus surgery alone in radically resected gastric cancer. J Clin Oncol 24:182

Dux M, Richter GM, Hansmann J et al. (1999) Helical hydro-CT for diagnosis and staging of gastric carcinoma. J Comput Assist Tomogr 23:913–922

Earle CC, Maroun JA (1999) Adjuvant chemotherapy after curative resection for gastric cancer in non-Asian patients: revisiting a meta-analysis of randomised trials. Eur J Cancer 35:1059–1064

Eckardt V, Giebler W, Kanzler G et al. (1990) Clinical and morphological characteristics of early gastric cancer. A case-control study. Gastroenterology 98:708–714

Emami B, Lyman J, Brown A et al. (1991) Tolerance of normal tissue to therapeutic irradiation. Int J Radiat Oncol Biol Phys 21:109–122

Everett SM, Axon AT (1997) Early gastric cancer in Europe. Gut 41:142–150

Fein R, Kelsen DP, Geller N et al. (1985) Adenocarcinoma of the esophagus and gastroesophageal junction: prognostic factors and results of therapy. Cancer 56:2512–2518

Fenoglio-Preiser CM, Noffsinger AE, Belli J et al. (1996) Pathologic and phenotypic features of gastric cancer. Semin Oncol 23:292–306

Fenoglio-Preiser CM, Carneiro F, Correa P et al. (2000) Gastric cancer. In: Hamilton SR, Aaltonen LA (ed) World Health Organization classification of tumours. Pathology & genetics. IARC Press, Lyon, France, pp 39–52

Feussner H, Omote K, Fink U et al. (1999) Pretherapeutic laparoscopic staging in advanced gastric carcinoma. Endoscopy 31:342–347

Folli S, Morgagni P, Roviello F et al. (2001) Risk factors for lymph node metastases and their prognostic significance in early gastric cancer (EGC) for the Italian Research Group for Gastric Cancer (IRGGC). Jpn J Clin Oncol Oct 31:495–499

Fu S, Lu JJ, Zhang Q et al. (2008) Intraoperative radiotherapy combined with adjuvant chemoradiotherapy for locally advanced gastric adenocarcinoma. Int J Radiat Oncol Biol Phys 2008 (Epub ahead of print)

Gastrointestinal Tumor Study Group (1982) A comparison of combination chemotherapy and combined modality therapy for locally advanced gastric carcinoma. Cancer 49:1771–1777

Greene F, Page D, Fleming I et al. (2002) AJCC Cancer Staging Manual, 6th edn. Springer-Verlag, Berlin Heidelberg New York

Hallissey MT, Dunn JA, Ward LC et al. (1994) The second British Stomach Cancer Group trial of adjuvant radiotherapy or chemotherapy in resectable gastric cancer: five-year follow-up. Lancet 343:1309–1312

Hartgrink HH, van de Velde CJ, Putter H et al. (2004) Extended lymph node dissection for gastric cancer: who may benefit? Final results of the randomized Dutch gastric cancer group trial. J Clin Oncol 22:2069–2077

Haugstvedt T, Viste A, Eide GE et al. (1989) The survival benefit of resection in patients with advanced stomach cancer: the Norwegian multicenter experience. Norwegian Stomach Cancer Trial. World J Surg 13:617–621

Heberer G, Teichmann RK, Kramling HJ et al. (1988) Results of gastric resection for carcinoma of the stomach: the European experience. World J Surg 12:374–381

Henning GT, Schild SE, Stafford SL et al. (2000) Results of irradiation or chemoirradiation for primary unresectable, locally recurrent or grossly incomplete resection of gastric adenocarcinomas. Int J Radiat Oncol Biol Phys 46:109–118

Hermans J, Bonenkamp JJ, Boon MC et al. (1993) Adjuvant therapy after curative resection for gastric cancer: meta-analysis of randomized trials. J Clin Oncol 11:1441–1447

Hiki Y, Shimao H, Mieno H et al. (1995) Modified treatment of early gastric cancer: evaluation of endoscopic treatment of early gastric cancers with respect to treatment indication groups. World J Surg 19:517–522

Hu JK, Chen ZX, Zhou ZG et al. (2002) Intravenous chemotherapy for resected gastric cancer: meta-analysis of randomized controlled trials. World J Gastroenterol 8:1023–1028

Ichikura T, Tomimatsu, Okusa Y et al. (1993) Comparison of the prognostic significance between the number of metastatic lymph nodes and nodal stage base on their location in patients with gastric cancer. J Clin Oncol 11:1894–1900

Jansen EP, Saunders MP, Boot H et al. (2007) Prospective study on late renal toxicity following postoperative chemoradiotherapy in gastric cancer. Int J Radiat Oncol Biol Phys 67:781–785

Janunger KG, Hafstrom L, Nygren P et al. (2001) A systematic overview of chemotherapy effects in gastric cancer. Acta Oncol 40:309–326

Kajitani T (1981) The general rules for the gastric cancer study in surgery and pathology. Part I. Clinical classification. Jpn J Surg 11:127–139

Kang YK, Choi DW, Im YH et al. (1996) Phase III randomized comparison of neoadjuvant chemotherapy followed by surgery versus surgery for locally advanced stomach cancer. Proc Am Soc Clin Oncol 15:215 (abstract 503)

Kelly S, Harris KM, Berry E et al. (2001) A systematic review of the staging performance of endoscopic ultrasound in gastro-oesophageal carcinoma. Gut 49:534–539

Kienle P, Buhl K, Kuntz C et al. (2002) Prospective comparison of endoscopy, endosonography and computed tomography for staging of tumours of the oesophagus and gastric cardia. Digestion 66:230–236

Kim MM, Rana V, Janjan NA et al. (2007) Clinical benefit of palliative radiation therapy in advanced gastric cancer. Acta Oncol 26:1–7

Kim SH, Lim DH, Lee J et al. (2005) An observation study suggesting clinical benefit for adjuvant postoperative chemoradiation in a population of over 500 cases after gastric resection with D2 nodal dissection for adenocarcinoma of the stomach. Int J Radiat Oncol Biol Phys 63:1279–1285

Kodera Y, Yamamura Y, Shimizu Y et al. (1998) The number of metastatic lymph nodes: a promising prognosis determinant for gastric carcinoma in the latest edition of the TNM classification. J Am Coll Surg 187:597–603

Kooby DA, Suriawinata A, Klimstra DS et al. (2003) Biologic predictors of survival in node-negative gastric cancer. Ann Surg 237:828–835

Kossé VA (1990) Combined treatment of gastric cancer using hypoxic radiotherapy. Vopr Onkol 36:1349–1353

Krasna M, Tepper JE, Niedzwiecki D et al. (2006) Trimodality therapy is superior to surgery alone in esophageal cancer: results of CALGB 9871. Gastrointestinal Cancer Symposium, abstract 4

Lai IR, Lee WJ, Huang MT et al. (2002) Comparison of serum CA72-4, CEA, TPA, CA19-9 and CA125 levels in gastric cancer patients and correlation with recurrence. Hepatogastroenterology 49:1157–1160

Liu TS, Wang Y, Chen SY et al. (2008) An updated meta-analysis of adjuvant chemotherapy after curative resection for gastric cancer. Eur J Surg Oncol (in press)

Macdonald JS, Smalley S, Benedetti J et al. (2001) Chemoradiotherapy after surgery compared with surgery alone for adenocarcinoma of the stomach or gastroesophageal junction. N Engl J Med 345:725–730

Macdonald JS, Smalley S, Benedetti N et al. (2004) Postoperative combined radiation and chemotherapy improves disease-free survival overall survival (OS) in resected adenocarcinoma of the stomach and gastroesophageal junction: update of the result of Intergroup Study INT-0116 (SWOG 9008) GI cancer symposium, abstract 6

Mansfield PF (2004) Lymphadenectomy for gastric cancer. J Clin Oncol 22:2759–2761

Mari E, Floriani I, Tinazzi A et al. (2000) Efficacy of adjuvant chemotherapy after curative resection for gastric cancer: a meta-analysis of published randomised trials. A study of the GISCAD (Gruppo Italiano per lo Studio dei Carcinome dell'Apparato Digerente). Ann Oncol 11:837–843

Martinez-Monge R, Fernandes PS, Gupta N et al. (1999) Cross-sectional nodal atlas: a tool for the definition of clinical target volumes in three-dimensional radiation therapy planning. Radiology 211:815–828

Meyers WC, Damiano RJ Jr, Rotolo FS et al. (1987) Adenocarcinoma of the stomach: changing patterns over the last four decades. Ann Surg 205:1–8

Minami M, Kawauchi N, Itai Y et al. (1992) Gastric tumors: radiologic-pathologic correlation and accuracy of T staging with dynamic CT. Radiology 185:173–178

Moertel CG, Childs DS, Jr, Reitemeier RJ et al. (1969) Combined 5-fluorouracil and supervoltage radiation therapy of locally unresectable gastrointestinal cancer. Lancet 2:865–867

Moertel CG, Childs DS, O'Fallon JR et al. (1984) Combined 5-fluorouracil and radiation therapy as a surgical adjuvant for poor prognosis gastric carcinoma. J Clin Oncol 2:1249–1254

Monson JR, Donohue JH, McIlrath DC et al. (1991) Total gastrectomy for advanced cancer. A worthwhile palliative procedure. Cancer 68:1863–1868

Narahara H, Koizumi W, Hara T et al. (2007) Randomized phase III study of S-1 + cisplatin in the treatment for advanced gastric cancer (The SPIRITS trial) SPIRITS: S-1 plus cisplatin vs S-1 in RCT in the treatment for stomach cancer. J Clin Oncol 25:201s

Nishi M, Nakajima T, Kajitani T (1986) The Japanese Research Society for Gastric Cancer: the general rules for the gastric cancer study and an analysis of treatment results based on the rules. Cancer of the stomach. Grune & Stratton, New York, p 107

Nitti D, Wils J, Dos Santos JG et al. (2006) Randomized phase III trials of adjuvant FAMTX or FEMTX compared with surgery alone in resected gastric cancer. A combined analysis of the EORTC GI Group and the ICCG. Ann Oncol 17:262–269

Noda M, Kodama T, Atsumi M et al. (1997) Possibilities and limitations of endoscopic resection for early gastric cancer. Endoscopy 29:361–365

Noguchi Y, Imada T, Matsumoto A et al. (1989) Radical surgery for gastric cancer: a review of the Japanese experience. Cancer 64:2053–2062

Okawara GS, Winter K, Donohue JH et al. (2005) A phase II trial of preoperative chemotherapy and chemoradiotherapy for potentially resectable adenocarcinoma of the stomach (RTOG 99-04). Proc Am Soc Clin Oncol 22:312s

Ono H, Kondo H, Gotoda T et al. (2001) Endoscopic mucosal resection for treatment of early gastric cancer. Gut 48:225–229

Panzini I, Gianni L, Fattori PP et al. (2002) Adjuvant chemotherapy in gastric cancer: a meta-analysis of randomized trials and a comparison with previous meta-analyses. Tumori 88:21–27

Rhomberg W, Bohler F, Eiter H (1996) Radiotherapy and razoxane in the palliative treatment of gastric cancer. Radiat Oncol Invest 4:27–32

Saito H, Fukumoto Y, Osaki T et al. (2007) Prognostic significance of level and number of lymph node metastases in patients with gastric cancer. Ann Surg Oncol 14:1688–1693

Sakuramoto S, Sasako M, Yamaguchi T et al. (2007) Adjuvant chemotherapy for gastric cancer with S-1, an oral fluoropyrimidine. N Engl J Med 357:1810–1820

Sano T, Sasako M, Yamamoto S et al. (2004) Gastric cancer surgery: morbidity and mortality results from a prospective randomized controlled trial comparing D2 and extended para-aortic lymphadenectomy – JCOG 9501. J Clin Oncol 22:2767–2773

Sasako M, Sano T, Yamamoto S et al. (2006) Randomized phase III trial of standard D2 versus D2 + para-aortic lymph node (PAN) dissection (D) for clinically M0 advanced gastric cancer: JCOG 9501. J Clin Oncol 24(part I):18s

Schein PS, Smith FP, Woolley PV et al. (1982) Current management of advanced and locally unresectable gastric carcinoma. Cancer 50[11 suppl]:2590–2596

Shah MA, Yeung H, Trocola R, et al. 2007) The characteristics and utility of FDG-PET/CT scans in patients with localized gastric cancer (GC). GI symposium, abstract 2

Shchepotin IB, Evans SR, Chorny V et al. (1994) Intensive preoperative radiotherapy with local hyperthermia for the treatment of gastric carcinoma. Surg Oncol 3:37–44

Shimada S, Yagi Y, Honmyo U et al. (2001) Involvement of three or more lymph nodes predicts poor prognosis in submucosal gastric carcinoma. Gastric Cancer 4:54–59

Sindelar WF, Kinsella TJ, Tepper JE et al. (1993) Randomized trial of intraoperative radiotherapy in carcinoma of the stomach. Am J Surg 165:178–186

Skoropad VY, Berdov BA, Mardynski YS et al. (2000) A prospective, randomized trial of pre-operative and intraoperative radiotherapy versus surgery alone in resectable gastric cancer. Eur J Surg Oncol 26:773–779

Smalley SR, Gunderson L, Tepper JE et al. (2002) Gastric surgical adjuvant radiotherapy consensus report-rationale and treatment implementation. Int J Radiat Oncol Biol Phys 52:283–293

Talaev MI, Starinskii VV, Kovalev BN et al. (1990) Results of combined treatment of cancer of the gastric antrum and gastric body. Vopr Onkol 36:1485–1488

Tepper JE, Gunderson LL (2002) Radiation treatment parameters in the adjuvant postoperative therapy of gastric cancer. Semin Radiat Oncol 12:187–195

Tey J, Back MF, Shakespeare TP et al. (2007) The role of palliative radiation therapy in symptomatic locally advanced gastric cancer. Int J Radiat Oncol Biol Phys 67:385–388

Tsendsuren T, Jun SM, Mian XH. (2006) Usefulness of endoscopic ultrasonography in preoperative TNM staging of gastric cancer. World J Gastroenterol 12:43–47

Tsukiyama I, Akine Y, Kajiura Y et al. (1988) Radiation therapy for advanced gastric cancer. Int J Radiat Oncol Biol Phys 15:123–127

Walsh TN, Noonau N, Hollywood D et al. (1996) A comparison of multimodal therapy and surgery to esophageal adenocarcinoma. N Engl J Med 335:462–467

Watt I, Stewart I, Anderson D et al. (1989) Laparoscopy, ultrasound and computed tomography in cancer of the oesophagus and gastric cardia: a prospective comparison for detecting intra-abdominal metastases. Br J Surg 76:1036–1039

Wieland P, Dobler B, Mai S et al. (2004) IMRT for postoperative treatment of gastric cancer: covering large target volumes in the upper abdomen: a comparison of a step-and-shoot and an arc therapy approach. Int J Radiat Oncol Biol Phys 59:1236–1244

Willis S, Truong S, Gribnitz S et al. (2000) Endoscopic ultrasonography in the preoperative staging of gastric cancer: accuracy and impact on surgical therapy. Surg Endosc 14:951–954

Wu CW, Hsiung CA, Lo SS et al. (2006) Nodal dissection for patients with gastric cancer: a randomized controlled trial. Lancet Oncol 7:309–315

Zhang ZX, Gu XZ, Yin WB et al. (1998) Randomized clinical trial on the combination of preoperative irradiation and surgery in the treatment of adenocarcinoma of gastric cardia (AGC) – report on 370 patients. Int J Radiat Oncol Biol Phys 42:929–934

Pancreatic Cancer

14

VIVEK K. MEHTA

CONTENTS

V. K. MEHTA, MD
Swedish Cancer Institute, 1221 Madison Street, Seattle, WA 98104, USA

Introduction and Objectives

Pancreatic cancer is a challenging disease to treat.

This chapter examines:
- Recommendations for diagnosis and staging procedures
- The staging systems and prognostic factors
- Treatment recommendations as well as the supporting scientific evidence for definitive and adjuvant treatment for early stage resectable pancreatic cancer
- The use of combined chemotherapy and radiotherapy for definitive treatment of locally advanced disease
- Systemic chemotherapy and palliative radiation for metastatic diseases
- Follow-up care and surveillance of survivors

14.1 Diagnosis, Staging, and Prognoses

14.1.1 Diagnosis

Initial Evaluation

- Diagnosis and evaluation of pancreatic cancer starts with a complete history and physical examination (H&P). Presenting signs and symptoms depend on the location and extent of the tumor. Possible signs of pancreatic cancer include jaundice, pain, and weight loss.
- The physical examination rarely confirms the diagnosis of localized pancreatic cancer. In advanced disease, palpable lymph nodes, hepatomegaly (from metastases), splenomegaly from portal vein obstruction, gallbladder (i.e., Courvoisier sign), ascites, or an abdominal mass might be appreciated.

■ Possible risk factors for pancreatic cancer that should be obtained in the history include smoking, long-standing diabetes, and chronic pancreatitis. Hereditary conditions such as hereditary pancreatitis, multiple endocrine neoplasia type-1 syndrome, hereditary nonpolyposis colon cancer (HNPCC: Lynch syndrome), von Hippel-Lindau syndrome, ataxia telangiectasia, and the familial atypical multiple mole melanoma syndrome may be predisposing conditions.

Laboratory Tests

■ Initial laboratory tests should include a complete blood count, basic blood chemistry, liver function tests, renal function tests, alkaline phosphatase, and lactate dehydrogenase (LDH). Patients with jaundice may show elevations in bilirubin.
■ CA 19-9 (serum carbohydrate antigenic determinant) is a tumor marker that is often elevated in patients with pancreatic cancer and is usually tested (Grade B). The reference range of CA 19-9 is less than 33–37 U/mL. It is more reliable in patients with more advanced disease. In one large study, CA 19-9 had a sensitivity of 92%, a specificity of 73%, and a total accuracy of 82% (Level IV) (SAFI et al. 1987).
■ Positive cytology from washings obtained at laparoscopy or laparotomy is equivalent to M1 disease.

Imaging Studies

■ A CT scan of the thorax, abdomen, and pelvis should be obtained for diagnosis and evaluation of the extent of disease (Grade A). The CT of the abdomen should be performed according to a defined pancreas protocol such as triphasic cross-sectional imaging and thin slices. The reported sensitivity is high, ranging between 89%–97% (Level III) (MIURA et al. 2006; SCHIMA et al. 2002).
■ Endoscopic ultrasound is useful in evaluating small lesions of the pancreas, determining local vascular invasion and obtaining tissue diagnosis (Grade B). It is an accurate tool for detecting pancreatic cancer, particularly when the lesion is small (in this situation, it is superior to CT) (Level III) (MERTZ et al. 2000). Endoscopic ultrasound can also localize lymph node metastases.
■ Endoscopic retrograde cholangiopancreatography is very sensitive for detecting pancreatic cancer. It is an invasive procedure, thus there is a real but small risk of complications.

■ PET and PET/CT may be helpful in differentiating between benign and malignant lesions (Grade B). FDG-PET has a sensitivity of 71%–100% and a specificity of 64%–90%. Results from prospective imaging studies revealed that FDG-PET had higher sensitivity and specificity compared to CT in diagnosing pancreatic carcinoma (92% and 85% versus 65% and 62%). Overall, PET suggested potential alterations in clinical management in 43% of patients suspected with primary pancreatic cancer (Level III) (ROSE et al. 1999). Results from another prospective study also demonstrated that FDG-PET is more sensitive than helical CT for detecting pancreatic cancer: The sensitivity for the detection of pancreatic cancer was higher for endoscopic ultrasound (EUS) (93%) and FDG-PET (87%) than for CT (53%). In addition, FDG-PET is useful for identifying metastatic disease (Level III) (MERTZ et al. 2000). However, it is important to note that FDG-PET does not replace, but is complementary to, CT imaging (MIURA et al. 2006) (Table 14.1).

Pathology

■ The necessity of obtaining a cytologic or tissue diagnosis of pancreatic cancer prior to surgery is controversial. On the one hand, needle aspiration is associated with a small risk of contaminating the peritoneum with cancer cells. Others argue that the operation has significant morbidity and should be only undertaken in patients with a known diagnosis. Finally, a pathologic diagnosis is generally preferred prior to initiation of chemotherapy, radiation therapy, or non-operative palliation.
■ EUS-directed fine-needle aspiration (FNA) is theoretically preferable to a CT-guided FNA in patients with resectable disease because of the much lower risk of peritoneal seeding.

Table 14.1. Imaging and laboratory work-ups for pancreatic cancer

Imaging studies	Laboratory tests
– CT of chest/abdomen/pelvis	– Complete blood count
– EUS	– Serum chemistry
– FDG-PET scan or PET/CT	– Liver function tests
– ERCP	– Renal function tests
	– Alkaline phosphatase
	– LDH
	– CA 19-9, CEA

14.1.2 Staging

■ Pancreatic cancer can be staged clinically and pathologically: Clinical staging utilizes information from H&P, imaging studies, and laboratory tests; pathologic staging is based on findings from clinical staging and procedures such as laparoscopy, exploratory laparotomy, EUS, and endoscopic retrograde cholangiopancreatography (ERCP).

■ Diagnostic staging laparoscopy is advocated by some experts to rule out sub-radiologic metastases (especially for body and tail lesions or for patients with high clinical suspicion of metastatic disease) (Grade D).

■ The 2007 American Joint Committee on Cancer Tumor Node Metastasis (TNM) staging system is presented in Table 14.2 (GREENE et al. 2002).

14.2 Treatment of Resectable Pancreatic Cancer

14.2.1 General Principles

■ Complete surgical resection is the mainstay treatment for respectable pancreatic cancer, although only a few patients are cured with surgery alone (Grade A). Subtotal resection or debulking surgery has no proven benefit.

■ Radiation therapy, chemotherapy, or combined chemoradiation is not routinely recommended preoperatively. Preoperative or neoadjuvant therapy has not been studied in large prospective studies. After a complete resection (R0 resection), adjuvant radiotherapy with 5-FU (Grade C)

Table 14.2. American Joint Committee on Cancer (AJCC) TNM classification of carcinoma cancer of exocrine pancreas [from GREENE et al. (2002) with permission]

Primary tumor (T)	
TX	Primary tumor cannot be assessed
T0	No evidence of primary tumor
Tis	Carcinoma in situ
T1	Tumor limited to the pancreas, 2 cm or less in greatest dimension
T2	Tumor limited to the pancreas, more than 2 cm in greatest dimension
T3	Tumor extends beyond the pancreas but without involvement of the celiac axis or the superior mesenteric artery
T4	Tumor involves the celiac axis or the superior mesenteric artery (unresectable primary tumor)
Regional lymph nodes (N)	
NX	Regional lymph nodes cannot be assessed
N0	No regional lymph node metastasis
N1	Regional lymph node metastasi
Distant metastasis (M)	
MX	Distant metastasis cannot be assessed
M0	No distant metastasis
M1	Distant metastasis
STAGE GROUPING	
0:	Tis N0 M0
IA:	T1 N0 M0
IB:	T2 N0 M0
IIA:	T3 N0 M0
IIB:	T1 N1 M0, T2 N1 M0, T3 N1 M0
III:	T4 Any N M0
IV	Any T Any N M1

or gemcitabine alone (Grade B) can be recommended.

■ After a subtotal resection (R1 resection), adjuvant chemotherapy (5-FU-based) and radiation therapy is indicated (Grade A).

14.2.2 Surgical Resection

■ Surgical resection is the only curative treatment modality for pancreatic cancer, and should be considered in all operable and resectable patients (Grade A). Resectable pancreatic tumors of the head, body, or tail are tumors without any evidence of distant metastases, a clear fat plane around celiac and superior mesenteric arteries (SMA), superior mesenteric vein and portal vein (NATIONAL COMPREHENSIVE CANCER NETWORK 2008).

■ The 5-year disease free survival for resected pancreatic cancer without additional therapy is generally 10% or less. In the Charite Onkologie (CONKO)-001 trial, the median disease free interval was 6.9 months and 5-year overall survival of 5.5% for the observation arm (OETTLE et al. 2007).

■ An R1 resection (residual microscopic disease) experiences similar overall survival to those with de novo presentation of locally advanced disease (i.e., 9–12 months median survival, and a 5-year survival rate of close to 0%) (PISTERS et al. 2003). Unfortunately, incomplete resections are common and the incidences of positive margins were reported to be as high as 51% (Level IV) (WILLET et al. 1993; MOUTARDIER et al. 2004).

■ Some practice guidelines suggest that resections should be done at institutions that perform at least 20 pancreatic resections annually (Grade B) (NATIONAL COMPREHENSIVE CANCER NETWORK 2008). There is an inverse relationship between surgical morbidity/mortality and surgical volume for pancreaticoduodenectomy (Level IV) (BIRKMEYER et al. 2002).

14.2.3 Adjuvant Chemotherapy

■ Chemotherapy is indicated for adjuvant treatment of pancreatic cancer after completed resection (Grade B). The efficacy of chemotherapy on pancreatic cancer using single agent or a combination of medications has been reported.

Single Agent Adjuvant Chemotherapy

■ The efficacy of gemcitabine-based chemotherapy was recently demonskated. The CONKO-001 trial randomized patients with resected pancreatic cancer to adjuvant gemcitabine versus observation. Adjuvant gemcitabine improved disease free survival (13.4 versus 6.9 months) but overall survival was not improved. In a "qualified" analysis meant to exclude patients in the treatment arm that did not receive at least one cycle of chemotherapy and those patients in the observation arm that received adjuvant chemotherapy or radiotherapy, there was a small but statistically significant survival improvement of 24.2 versus 20.5 months ($p=0.02$) (Level II) (OETTLE et al. 2007).

■ A randomized trial (ESPAC-3 trial) intended to compare the effect of adjuvant 5-FU to adjuvant gemcitabine-based chemotherapy has completed the accrual of patients; however, the results are still pending.

Combination Chemotherapy

■ A European study compared AMF (doxorubicin, mitomycin, and 5-FU) for six cycles after surgery to an observation group. The AMF group had improved median survival (23 months versus 11 months, $p=0.02$) and 2-year survival rate (43% versus 32%, $p=0.04$), but no survival advantage was seen at 3 years (Level II) (BAKKEVOLD et al. 1993).

■ The Virginia Mason Cancer Center single institution trial consisted of 43 patients treated with radiation, continuous infusion 5-FU, cisplatin, and interferon alpha, followed by 4 months of infusional 5-FU. The 2- and 5-year survival rates of 64% and 55% are promising. (Level IV) (PICOZZI et al. 2003).
The Virginia Mason regimen is being tested in an American College of Surgeons Oncology Group (ACOSOG) multi-institutional trial (Z05031). The accrual has been completed but the results are pending.

■ Pooled analysis of two randomized trials (GERCOR/GISCAD: Gemcitabine/Oxaliplatin versus Gemcitabine; German multi-center trial: gemcitabine plus cisplatin versus gemcitabine) was presented at the ASCO 2006. The conclusion was that high performance patients may achieve a greater benefit in progression-free survival (5.8

versus 3.5 months, $p<0.001$) and overall survival (10.6 versus 6.4 months, $p<0.001$) from treatment with a gemcitabine/platinum doublet (Level II) (Louvet et al. 2006).

14.2.4 Radiation Therapy

Adjuvant Radiation

■ Radiation therapy, in combination with chemotherapy, is recommended as the local treatment modality for adjuvant treatment of pancreatic cancer (Grade C). The high rate of local failure after surgical resection provides a strong rationale for the role of radiation after surgery. In the CONKO-001 trial, local recurrence was 34% in the gemcitabine-treated patients and 41% in the observation arm. Recurrence rates in patients with R1 resections are typically even higher, in excess of 60%.
The effects of postoperative radiation therapy on pancreatic cancer have been studied in a number of randomized trials. However, the results from these trials varied, largely due to small sample size or poor study design.

■ The first randomized trial providing evidence in favor of adjuvant therapy was conducted by the Gastrointestinal Tumor Study Group (GITSG). In this trial, Kalser and Ellenberg (1985) compared observation to bolus fluorouracil (5-FU) plus split-course radiation followed by 2 years of 5-FU. A total of 43 patients were evaluable and an improvement in median survival of 20 versus 11 months ($p=0.35$), and in 2-year survival of 42% versus 15% was shown in favor of the adjuvant chemoradiation group (GITSG, Level II). This study was stopped early because the adjuvant radiation therapy arm was doing so much better. Similar results were obtained when additional patients were treated with the same adjuvant chemoradiotherapy regimen (the experimental arm). This study was recently updated and the survival advantage persisted to 10 years.

■ The RTOG 9704 trial randomized patients with resected pancreatic cancer to either pre- and post-chemoradiation 5-FU or pre- and post-chemoradiation gemcitabine, with both groups receiving concurrent chemoradiation using infusional 5-FU. For the group with tumors of the head of the pancreas, a 3-year survival improvement was seen in the arm that received gemcitabine compared to the arm that received 5-FU (32% versus 21%) ($p=0.33$), with a hazard ratio of 0.76 (CI = 0.61–0.97). When the analysis included pancreatic body and tail tumors, no significant improvement in survival was revealed. More than 85% of patients completed therapy in both arms (RTOG, Level I) (Regine et al. 2006).

■ The EORTC 40891 trial compared observation to adjuvant infusional 5-FU and split-course radiation. Only 114 of the 127 patients included had tumor of the head of the pancreas. Among all patients, the 2-year survival between the treatment and control groups was 51% versus 41%, but this was not statistically significant. In a subgroup analysis of head of pancreas patients, 2-year survival was 37% versus 23% for the control arm (Level II) (Klinkenbijl et al. 1999). This study is often criticized because of the inclusion of patients with positive margins after resection, patients with ampullary tumors, the lack of maintenance chemotherapy, the split-course radiotherapy regimen, and the lack of radiation quality assurance.

■ The ESPAC-1 was a study designed to test whether patients would benefit from adjuvant chemotherapy alone (5-FU/Leucovorin), chemoradiotherapy (40 Gy split-course with 5-FU) or observation. Not all the patients were randomized and the study was a 2 × 2 design. The authors concluded that adjuvant chemotherapy was beneficial and that adjuvant chemoradiotherapy was detrimental because the 5-year survival was 20% in the two chemotherapy arms, and 10% in the two RT arms. There are a number of criticisms of this study including the "non-randomized" component, the lack of quality assurance, the fact that only 90 patients received the prescribed RT dose, and the split dose of RT (40 Gy). Also, this seldom mentioned but a 2 × 2 factorial design is only valid if there is not thought to be any interaction between the two treatment arms. Because 5-FU is a known radiosensitizing agent, there is an interaction between the two treatment arms which may invalidate the conclusions (Level II) (Neoptolemos 2001, 2004).

■ EORTC 40013-22012 is a randomized phase II trial that is designed to evaluate adjuvant gemcitabine versus adjuvant gemcitabine followed by chemoradiation. This study is closed to accrual.

Definitive Radiation

- Combined chemoradiation therapy is indicated for unresectable or inoperable pancreatic cancer. As described below, most studies reported have suggested that chemoradiotherapy is superior to radiotherapy alone as adjuvant therapy following surgery.
- In patients who are not candidates for chemotherapy, discussion about the role of radiotherapy alone should be performed in a thoughtful and careful manner.

14.3 Treatment of Unresectable Pancreatic Cancer

14.3.1 General Principles

- Definitive chemoradiation therapy should be offered to patients with unresectable or inoperable pancreatic cancer without evidence of distant metastasis (Grade B).
- Gemcitabine or gemcitabine-based combination therapy without radiation therapy may be considered as an alternative to 5-FU-based chemoradiotherapy in patients with locally advanced, unresectable disease (Grade B). Although the efficacy of gemcitabine-based chemotherapy has been demonstrated, chemotherapy alone has not been compared to combined chemoradiation therapy in phase III randomized trials.
- When definitive treatment is not feasible due to poor medical condition or patients' preference, palliative chemotherapy and/or radiation therapy is often used for symptomatic control.

14.3.2 Concurrent Chemoradiotherapy

- Patients with unresectable but non-metastatic pancreatic cancer should be offered definitive chemoradiotherapy (Grade B). 5-FU-based chemotherapy can be considered for combined chemoradiotherapy.
  In a randomized trial reported by GITSG, 194 patients with unresectable adenocarcinoma of the pancreas were randomly assigned to high-dose (60 Gy) radiation therapy alone, high-dose radiation plus 5-FU, or moderate-dose (40 Gy) radiation plus 5-FU. Median survival with radiation alone was only 5.5 months. Both 5-FU-containing treatment regimens produced a highly significant survival improvement when compared with radiation alone, with an overall median survival of 10 months. The 1-year overall survival rates were 40% versus 10% for patients treated with or without chemotherapy, respectively. However, survival differences between high or moderate doses of radiation were not observed (Level II) (MOERTEL et al. 1981).
  The FFCD-SFRO was a phase III trial comparing chemoradiotherapy (cisplatin and 5-FU) followed by gemcitabine versus gemcitabine alone in patients with locally advanced non-resectable pancreatic cancer. The study was stopped before the planned inclusion due to lower survival with combined chemoradiation, as compared to gemcitabine treatment alone. Gemcitabine alone had less toxicity and improved median survival (14.3 versus 8.4 months, $p=0.014$) (Level II) (CHAUFFERT et al. 2006).

Chemotherapy Regimen

- Gemcitabine or gemcitabine-based combination therapy without radiation therapy may be considered as an alternative to 5-FU-based chemoradiotherapy in patients with locally advanced, unresectable disease (Grade A).
  Gemcitabine has been demonstrated to improve the disease-related symptoms associated with unresectable or metastatic pancreatic cancer. Patients with advanced and symptomatic pancreas cancer were randomized to receive either gemcitabine 1,000 mg/m² weekly for seven cycles followed by 1 week of rest, then weekly for three cycles every 4 weeks thereafter or to 5-FU 600 mg/m² once weekly. The clinical benefit response (a composite measure of pain, performance status, and weight) was measured to be 23.8% in patients treated with gemcitabine and only 4.8% in patients treated with 5-FU. The median survival durations were 5.6 months for gemcitabine-treated patients and 4.4 months for 5-FU-treated patients. The survival rate at 12 months was 18% for gemcitabine patients and 2% for 5-FU patients (Level I) (BURRIS et al. 1997).
  Results from a randomized phase II study revealed that patients with locally advanced or metastatic adenocarcinoma of the pancreas were

randomized to 2200 mg/m^2 gemcitabine over 30 min or 1500 mg/m^2 over 150 min on days 1, 8, and 15 of a 4-week cycle. Slow infusion resulted in increased median survival (5 months versus 8 months, $p = 0.063$) and decreased toxicity (Level II) (TEMPERO et al. 2003).

14.4 Treatment of "Marginally Unresectable" Pancreatic Cancer

14.4.1 General Principles

- The National Comprehensive Cancer Network (NCCN) defines patients that are borderline resectable as tumors that are going to have a high likelihood of an incomplete (R1 or R2) resection (NATIONAL COMPREHENSIVE CANCER NETWORK 2008). For tumors in the head and body, criteria for borderline resectable patients include severe unilateral SMV/portal impingement, tumor abutment on SMA, gastroduodenal artery encasement up to origin at the hepatic artery, tumors with limited involvement of the IVC, SMV occlusion, or colon/mesocolon invasion.
- Decisions about resectability should be made after multidisciplinary consultation with reference to appropriate radiographic studies.

14.4.2 Induction Therapy and Surgery

- Neoadjuvant treatment has theoretical benefits but has not been that well studied. The neoadjuvant treatment studies often include small numbers of patients, and have used a variety of criteria to define resectability or marginally resectable disease.
- Most of the studies have used either bolus or infusional 5-FU and a wide range of radiation doses (30–50 Gy) The ability to downstage resectable tumors or to convert "unresectable" to resectable tumors has been reported in some small studies and not in others.
- For tumors where there is a higher likelihood of an incomplete (R1 or R2) resection, the NCCN guidelines suggest neoadjuvant chemoradiotherapy be given prior to surgery.

14.5 Treatment of Metastatic Pancreatic Cancer or Recurrent Cancer

14.5.1 General Principles

- Systemic chemotherapy can be administered to patients with metastatic disease at diagnosis or when patients become symptomatic from their disease.

14.5.2 Chemotherapy

- Gemcitabine at 1000 mg/m^2 over 30 min, weekly for 3 weeks every 28 days, is considered standard front-line therapy. Fixed dose rate gemcitabine (10 mg/m^2/min) may substitute standard infusion of gemcitabine over 30 min
- Gemcitabine combinations (gemcitabine + erlotinib, gemcitabine + cisplatin, gemcitabine + fluoropyrimidine) have shown a small improvement in response rate or time to progression, but definitive evidence of a survival benefit remains elusive.
- Second-line therapy may consist of gemcitabine or gemcitabine combinations.

14.5.3 Palliative Radiotherapy

- Palliative pancreatic irradiation is commonly used for relieving pain symptoms caused by advanced abdominal disease or distant metastases.

14.6 Radiation Therapy Treatment Technique

- ABRAMS and colleagues (2007) reviewed the radiotherapy delivered in RTOG 97-04 and demonstrated that suboptimal delivery of radiation therapy can be a more significant prognostic factor than the identity of the adjuvant chemoradiotherapeutic agent (Level IV).

Simulation and Treatment Planning

- CT simulation and 3D treatment planning is considered a standard and is highly recommended. Simulation is performed with the patient supine, arms above the head, while oral contrast is used to visualize the small bowel and IV contrast is used to delineate vessels and the kidneys.

- The tumor and nodal groups at risk should be delineated using preoperative and postoperative imaging studies, as well as the findings at surgery. 3D planning is necessary to optimize dose distributions while maintaining dose to liver, kidneys, small bowel, and spinal cord.

- In general, treatment volumes should encompass primary tumor as well as regional lymph nodes. For cancer in the pancreatic head, the pancreaticoduodenal, suprapancreatic, celiac nodes, and porta hepatic should be included in the treatment fields. The entire duodenal loop should be included.

  For lesions in the body/tail, the pancreaticoduodenal, porta hepatic, lateral suprapancreatic, and splenic hilum nodes should be covered. Usually, the porta hepatic and duodenal bed do not need to be covered.

  Lymph nodal stations to be encompassed in the treatment of pancreatic cancer were described and depicted in Table 13.4 and Figure 13.1 (see Chap. 13).

- Fluoroscopy at the time of simulation or verification to evaluate organ movement during respiration, or 4D treatment planning to account for organ movement should be considered if those technologies are available.

Conventional Field Arrangement

- Conventional treatment plans will often use a three- or four-field technique. The following field arrangement was utilized in the RTOG 9704 trial (Figs. 14.1–14.4):

  In the anteroposterior/posteroanterior (AP/PA) fields, the upper border of the fields will be the mid-T11 vertebral body and lower border of L3 vertebral body.

  Right lateral 2- to 3-cm margins to the preoperative tumor extent should be maintained. In tumors of the body or tail region, the right edge may be moved to a minimum of 2 cm from the right edge of the vertebral bodies, as long as a margin of 2–3 cm is maintained on preoperative primary tumor extent, to allow sparing of the right kidney while covering nodal areas at high risk.

  Left lateral margin of 2–3 cm from the preoperative primary tumor extent or 2 cm from the left edge of the vertebral bodies, whichever is most lateral.

  In the lateral fields, the posterior border should split the anterior vertebral bodies in half. The anterior border should be set at 1.5–2 cm anterior to the anterior aspect of the primary tumor as defined on preoperative CT scan and at least 3.5–4 cm anterior to the anterior edge of the vertebral bodies, whichever is most anterior.

  Shaped blocks are useful in limiting radiation to these organs. There might be field reductions as the dose is increased above normal tissue tolerances.

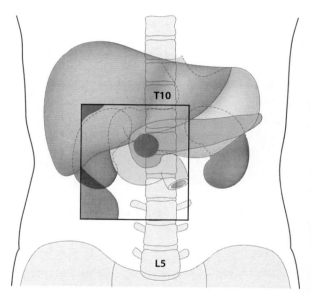

Fig. 14.1. AP field, with blocking, for pancreatic head lesion

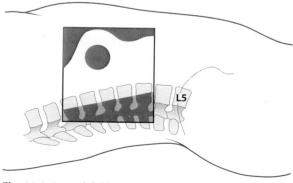

Fig. 14.2. Lateral field, with blocking

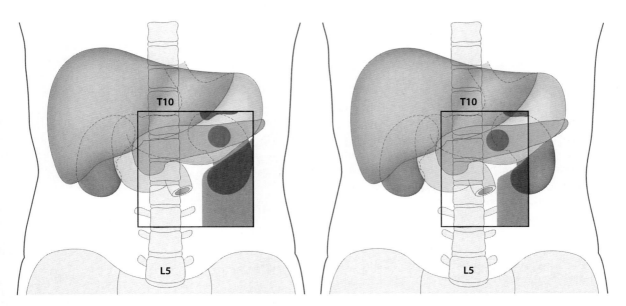

Fig. 14.3. AP field, with blocking, for pancreatic body lesion

Fig. 14.4. AP field, with blocking, for pancreatic tail lesion

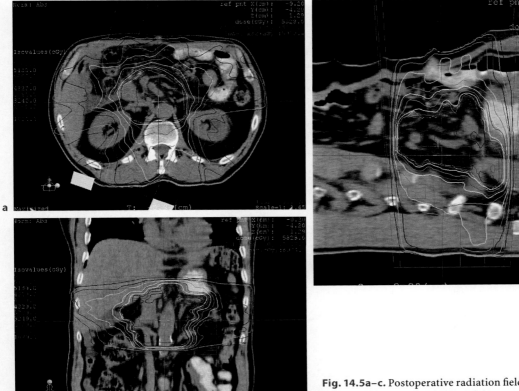

Fig. 14.5a–c. Postoperative radiation fields using IMRT of a patient with adenocarcinoma of the pancreatic head. Doses to small bowel, kidneys, and liver were limited as compared to four-field arrangement for conventional radiation

IMRT Treatment Planning

- Intensity-modulated radiation therapy (IMRT) is increasingly being used in the planning of patients with pancreatic cancer. The advantages to IMRT include improved coverage of the target tissues and reduced dose to the nearby normal tissues (Fig. 14.5). Results from a number of dosimetric studies have indicated that IMRT has the potential to significantly improve radiation therapy of pancreatic cancers by reducing normal tissue (particularly small bowel and kidney) dose, and simultaneously allow escalation of dose to further enhance locoregional control (Level III) (Brown et al. 2006; Landry et al. 2002). Preliminary results from clinical studies have demonstrated that combined IMRT and chemotherapy were well tolerated and efficacious for both resectable and unresectable pancreatic cancers (Level IV) (Ben-Josef et al. 2004; Milano et al. 2004). Because of the steep dose gradients and improved dose conformity, image-guided radiotherapy techniques are also increasingly being employed (Xing et al. 2006).

Beam Energy and Dose Calculation

- Most centers will treat with higher energy beams if available.
- 6 MV can be used for IMRT.

Dose and Fractionation

- Adjuvant or resected pancreatic cancer
- Standard fractionation consists of 1.8–2.0 Gy per daily fraction to a total dose of 45–50.4 Gy in 25–28 fractions.
- 5-FU-based chemotherapy is administered concurrently.
- Unresectable pancreatic cancer
- Standard fractionation consists of 1.8–2.0 Gy per daily fraction to a total dose of 54–60 Gy.
- 5-FU-based chemotherapy is administered concurrently.

Normal Tissue Tolerances

- Particularly for pancreatic cancer irradiation, the equivalent of one kidney is limited to less than 20 Gy. The whole liver is limited to less than 20 Gy, and 60% of the liver is limited to less than 30 Gy. Efforts should be made to exclude the small bowel

and liver as much as possible by utilizing megavoltage beams and multiple shaped ports.
- The spinal cord dose should be limited to < 45 Gy.

 14.7 Follow-Ups

14.7.1 Post-Treatment Follow-Ups

- Life-long follow-up is required for all patients with pancreatic cancer treated with curative intent.

Schedule

- Follow-ups could be scheduled every 3–6 months for 2 years, then annually thereafter (Grade D) (National Comprehensive Cancer Network 2008).

Work-Ups

- Each follow-up examination should include a complete history and physical examination. Laboratory tests (including CA 19-9) and abdominal CT can be considered at each follow-up (Grade D) (NCCN 2008).

References

Abrams RA, Winter KA, Regine WF et al. (2007) Correlation of RTOG 9704 (adjuvant therapy of pancreatic adenocarcinoma radiation therapy quality assurance scores with survival. J Clin Oncol 25[18S]:4523

Bakkevold KE, Arnesjø B, Dahl O et al. (1993) Adjuvant combination chemotherapy (AMF) following radical resection of carcinoma of the pancreas and papilla of Vater – results of a controlled, prospective, randomised multicentre study. Eur J Cancer 29A:698–703

Ben-Josef E, Shields AF, Vaishampayan U et al. (2004) Intensity-modulated radiotherapy (IMRT) and concurrent capecitabine for pancreatic cancer. Int J Radiat Oncol Biol Phys 59:454–459

Birkmeyer JD, Siewers AE, Finlayson EV et al. (2002) Hospital volume and surgical mortality in the United States. N Engl J Med 346:1128–1137

Brown MW, Ning H, Arora B et al. (2006) A dosimetric analysis of dose escalation using two intensity-modulated radiation therapy techniques in locally advanced pancreatic carcinoma. Int J Radiat Oncol Biol Phys 65:274–283

Burris HA 3rd, Moore MJ, Andersen J et al. (1997) Improvements in survival and clinical benefit with gemcitabine as first-line therapy for patients with advanced pancreas cancer: a randomized trial. J Clin Oncol 15:2403–2413

Chauffert B, Mornex F, Bonnetain F et al. (2006) Phase III trial comparing initial chemoradiotherapy (intermittent cisplatin and infusional 5-FU) followed by gemcitabine vs. gemcitabine alone in patients with locally advanced non metastatic pancreatic cancer: A FFCD-SFRO study. J Clin Oncol 24[18S, Part I]:4008

Greene F, Page D, Fleming I et al. (2002) AJCC Cancer Staging Manual, 6th edn. Springer-Verlag, Berlin Heidelberg New York

Kalser MH, Ellenberg SS (1985) Pancreatic cancer. Adjuvant combined radiation and chemotherapy following curative resection. Arch Surg 120:899–903

Klinkenbijl JH, Jeekel J, Sahmoud T et al. (1999) Adjuvant radiotherapy and 5-fluorouracil after curative resection of cancer of the pancreas and periampullary region: phase III trial of the EORTC gastrointestinal tract cancer cooperative group. Ann Surg 230:776–784

Landry JC, Yang GY, Ting JY et al. (2002) Treatment of pancreatic cancer tumors with intensity-modulated radiation therapy (IMRT) using the volume at risk approach (VARA): employing dose-volume histogram (DVH) and normal tissue complication probability (NTCP) to evaluate small bowel toxicity. Med Dosim 27:121–129

Louvet C, Hincke A, Labianca R et al. (2006) Increased survival using platinum analog combined with gemcitabine as compared to gemcitabine single agent in advanced pancreatic cancer (APC): pooled analysis of two randomised trials, the GERCOR/GISCAD Intergroup Study and a German Multicenter Study. J Clin Oncol 24[18S, Part I]:4003

Mertz HR, Sechopoulos P, Delbeke D et al. (2000) EUS, PET, and CT scanning for evaluation of pancreatic adenocarcinoma. Gastrointest Endosc 52:367–371

Milano MT, Chmura SJ, Garofalo MC et al. (2004) Intensity-modulated radiotherapy in treatment of pancreatic and bile duct malignancies: toxicity and clinical outcome. Int J Radiat Oncol Biol Phys 59:445–53

Miura F, Takada T, Amano H et al. (2006) Diagnosis of pancreatic cancer. HPB (Oxford) 8:337–342

Moertel CG, Frytak S, Hahn RG et al. (1981) Therapy of locally unresectable pancreatic carcinoma: a randomized comparison of high dose (6000 rads) radiation alone, moderate dose radiation (4000 rads + 5-fluorouracil), and high dose radiation + 5-fluorouracil: The Gastrointestinal Tumor Study Group. Cancer 48:1705–1710

Moutardier V, Turrini O, Huiart L et al. (2004) A reappraisal of preoperative chemoradiation for localized pancreatic

head ductal adenocarcinoma in a 5-year single-institution experience. J Gastrointest Surg 8:502–510

National Comprehensive Cancer Network (2008) Clinical practice guidelines in oncology: pancreatic adenocarcinoma. Version I.2008. Available at http://nccn.org/professionals/physician_gls/PDF/rectal.pdf. Accessed on March 26, 2008

Neoptolemos JP, Dunn JA, Stocken DD et al. (2001) Adjuvant chemoradiotherapy and chemotherapy in resectable pancreatic cancer: a randomised controlled trial. Lancet 358:1576–1585

Neoptolemos JP, Stocken DD, Friess H et al. (2004) A randomized trial of chemoradiotherapy and chemotherapy after resection of pancreatic cancer. N Engl J Med 350:1200–1210

Oettle H, Post S, Neuhaus P et al. (2007) Adjuvant chemotherapy with gemcitabine vs observation in patients undergoing curative-intent resection of pancreatic cancer: a randomized controlled trial. JAMA 297:267–277

Picozzi VJ, Kozarek RA, Traverso LW (2003) Interferon-based adjuvant chemoradiation therapy after pancreaticoduodenectomy for pancreatic adenocarcinoma. Am J Surg 285:476–480

Regine WF, Winter KW, Abrams R et al. (2006) RTOG 9704 a phase III study of adjuvant pre and post chemoradiation (CRT) 5-FU vs. gemcitabine (G) for resected pancreatic adenocarcinoma. J Clin Oncol 24[18S, Part I]:4007

Rose DM, Delbeke D, Beauchamp RD et al. (1999) 18Fluorodeoxyglucose-positron emission tomography in the management of patients with suspected pancreatic cancer. Ann Surg 229:729–738

Safi F, Roscher R, Bittner R et al. (1987) High sensitivity and specificity of CA 19-9 for pancreatic carcinoma in comparison to chronic pancreatitis. Serological and immunohistochemical findings. Pancreas 2:398–403

Schima W, Függer R, Schober E et al. (2002) Diagnosis and staging of pancreatic cancer: comparison of mangafodipir trisodium-enhanced MR imaging and contrast-enhanced helical hydro-CT. AJR Am J Roentgenol 179:717–724

Tempero M, Plunkett W, Ruiz Van Haperen V et al. (2003) Randomized phase II comparison of dose-intense gemcitabine: thirty-minute infusion and fixed dose rate infusion in patients with pancreatic adenocarcinoma. J Clin Oncol 21:3402–3408

Willett CG, Lewandrowski K, Warshaw AL et al. (1993) Resection margins in carcinoma of the head of the pancreas. Implications for radiation therapy. Ann Surg 217:144–148

Xing L, Thorndyke B, Schreibmann E et al. (2006) Overview of image-guided radiation therapy. Med Dosim 31:91–112

Hepatocellular Carcinoma, Gallbladder Cancer, and Cholangiocarcinoma

Joseph M. Herman and Timothy M. Pawlik

CONTENTS

J. M. Herman, MD, MSc
Department of Radiation Oncology and Molecular Radiation Sciences, Sidney Kimmel Comprehensive Cancer Center at Johns Hopkins, 401 N. Broadway Suite Suite 1440, Baltimore, MD 21231-2410, USA
T. M. Pawlik, MD, MPH
Division of Surgical Oncology at Johns Hopkins, 600 N Wolfe Street, Halsted 614, Baltimore, MD 21287, USA

Introduction and Objectives

Hepatobiliary carcinomas represent tumors that originate either from the gallbladder, the liver parenchyma, or bile ducts (cholangiocarcinoma). Hepatocellular cancer is the seventh most common cancer in the world and most common in men aged 50–60 years. The strongest risk factor for hepatocellular cancer is cirrhosis (risk of hepatocellular cancer is at 1%–2% per year) (Fattovich et al. 1995). Cirrhosis can be caused by viral infections including hepatitis B or C. Alcohol and hemochromatosis are other causes of cirrhosis. Aflatoxins and hepatitis itself (independent of underlying cirrhosis) are also strong risk factors for hepatocellular cancer. >>>

Gallbladder cancer is the most common biliary tract tumor and is most common in women aged 70–75 years. Gallbladder cancer is associated with gall stones, chronic cholecystitis, calcified gallbladder (porcelain gallbladder), polyps, and carcinogens (nitrosamines).

Extrahepatic cholangiocarcinoma occurs more frequently than intrahepatic cholangiocarcinoma and is seen equally in men and woman aged 60–70 years. The incidence of intrahepatic cholangiocarcinoma, however, has been rising faster than its extrahepatic counterpart. Cholangiocarcinoma is correlated with choledochal cysts, thorotrast, sclerosing cholangitis, liver flukes, hepatolithiasis, and ulcerative colitis.

In 2007, an estimated 19,160 people will develop hepatocellular or intrahepatic bile duct cancer (male/female 13,650/5,510) and 16,780 will die of their disease (JEMAL et al. 2007). A total of 9,250 patients will develop gallbladder or extrahepatic bile duct cancer, resulting in 3,250 deaths. While surgery remains the primary treatment for hepatobiliary carcinomas, many tumors are found to be unresectable at diagnosis. Several technologies have emerged as definitive or bridge therapy to resection and/or transplantation. Both chemotherapy and radiation remain an integral part of the treatment of hepatobiliary carcinomas.

This chapter examines:

- Overview of hepatocellular cancer, gallbladder cancer, and cholangiocarcinoma (intrahepatic/extrahepatic)
- Staging systems and prognostic factors
- Treatment recommendations for hepatocellular cancer, gallbladder cancer, and cholangiocarcinoma
- Summary of available literature documenting outcomes with chemotherapy and radiation
- Emerging technologies such as stereotactic radiation therapy and radioembolization
- Novel chemotherapeutic and targeted therapies available for the treatment of hepatobiliary carcinomas

15.1 Diagnosis, Staging, and Prognoses

15.1.1 Diagnosis

Initial Evaluation (Presentation)

- Patients with intrahepatic cholangiocarcinoma or hepatocellular carcinoma may present with dull pain in the upper abdominal or epigastric area. Weight loss and fatigue are also common and can be more prominent in patients with cir-

rhosis. Paraneoplastic symptoms include hypercholesterolemia, erythrocytosis, hypercalcemia, and hypoglycemia. Many patients may have no symptoms relating to the underlying tumor, but may have symptoms relating to their underlying liver insufficiency.

- Patients with advanced gallbladder cancer commonly complain of pain and jaundice and may have weight loss, anorexia, and fatigue. The majority of gallbladder cancers (70%), however, are diagnosed incidentally following cholecystectomy.
- Patients with distal or hilar cholangiocarcinoma often present with jaundice. Abdominal pain, weight loss, anorexia, fatigue, fever, and night sweats are common.

Laboratory Tests

- Required laboratory tests for hepatocellular carcinoma include Alpha-fetoprotein (AFP) which is elevated in 60%–90% of patients. Physicians should also collect creatinine, alkaline phosphatase, albumin, PT/PTT (INR), bilirubin, and test for Hepatitis B/C. C-reactive protein, PIV-KA-II, and standard laboratory tests (complete blood counts, serum chemistry, etc.) should also be obtained.
- There are no specific tumor markers for gallbladder cancer. Carbohydrate antigen 19-9 (CA 19-9) can sometimes be elevated.
- CC (both intra- and extrahepatic) may be associated with elevations in CA 19-9; however, biliary obstruction can also lead to an elevated CA 19-9 which decreases after stenting.

Imaging/Diagnostic Studies

- Standard tests of hepatocellular carcinoma and gallbladder cancer include a liver ultrasound, abdominal/chest CT, and/or MRI (Table 15.1) (Grade A) (MILLER et al. 2007). Patients with chronic liver disease who are at risk for hepatocellular carcinoma should undergo periodic liver screening for focal liver tumor detection, usually with ultrasonography (US) with MRI being used when US is equivocal (Grade B) (OLIVA and SAINI 2004).
- The utility of FDG-PET in hepatocellular carcinoma in the evaluation and staging of hepatobiliary tumors is still unclear, and should be ordered when there is suspicion of extrahepatic disease

Table 15.1. Imaging and laboratory work-up for hepatobiliary cancers

Imaging studies	Laboratory tests
– Liver MRI/MRCP	– Complete blood count
– Abdominal ultrasonography	– Serum chemistry, including liver function tests
– CT of chest and abdomen	– Coagulation studies (PT, PTT)
– Bone scan (optional, hepatocellular carcinoma)	– Serum CA 19-9 and CEA (cholangiocarcinoma)
– Transhepatic or endoscopic cholangiography (cholangiocarcinoma)	– AFP (hepatocellular carcinoma)
	– Hepatitis tests (HBsAg, HBsAb, HBcAb, anti-HCV)

AFP, Alpha-fetoprotein; anti-HCV, antibody to hepatitis C virus; CEA, carcinoembryonic antigen; CT, computed tomography; HBcAb, hepatitis B core antibody; HBsAb, hepatitis B surface antibody; HBsAg, hepatitis B surface antigen; MRCP, magnetic resonance cholangiopancreatography; MRI, magnetic resonance imaging; PT, prothrombin time; PTT, partial thromboplastin time

by other methods (Grade C). Yoon et al. (2007) compared CT, MRI, and FDG-PET on 87 patients with newly diagnosed hepatocellular carcinoma. Extrahepatic metastases were identified in 24 of 87 (33%) patients. The location and frequency of metastases were: lung, 12; lymph nodes, 19; and bone, 11. All extrahepatic metastases were detected by FDG-PET. In addition, FDG-PET identified four lymph node metastases and six bone metastases that were not found using conventional methods. The initial TNM stage based on the conventional staging work-up was changed in four cases after FDG-PET. Extrahepatic metastasis was significantly more frequent in patients with intrahepatic tumors > 5 cm in size ($p = 0.045$) (Level III). Overall, the sensitivity of FDG-PET for detection of hepatocellular carcinoma is reported to be around 50%–70%. Some investigators have reported that 11C-Acetate PET imaging may have a higher sensitivity and specificity as a radiotracer compared with FDG-PET for the evaluation of hepatocellular carcinoma lesions/metastatic disease (Level III) (Ho et al. 2003).

- Endoscopic retrograde cholangiopancreatography/magnetic resonance cholangiopancreatography (ERCP/MRCP) and endoscopic ultrasound (EUS) can help in the diagnosis of gallbladder cancer and cholangiocarcinoma (Grade A). These studies are also critical in assisting the surgeon to determine resectability. Biliary brushing at the

time of cholangiography may assist in diagnosis; however, it must be kept in mind that brushings have a high false-negative rate.

- Although PET/CT may help select which patients who are better candidates for surgical resection for cholangiocarcinoma, obtaining a PET/CT is currently not standard practice in patients with disease that is deemed resectable by standard imaging (Grade C). Kim et al. (2008) evaluated the utility of PET/CT scans in 123 patients with suspected resectable cholangiocarcinoma. The sensitivity, specificity, positive predictive value (PPV), negative predictive value (NPV), and accuracy of PET/CT in primary tumor detection were 84.0%, 79.3%, 92.9%, 60.5%, and 82.9%, respectively (Level III). PET/CT was able to significantly predict the presence of regional lymph nodes metastases (75.9% vs. 60.9%, $p = 0.004$) and distant metastases (88.3% vs. 78.7%, $p = 0.004$) when compared to CT scans. However, for patients with resectable disease, the value of FDG-PET or PET/CT is not confirmed. In addition, interpretation of PET/CT findings may be limited in those cholangiocarcinoma patients with pre-existing biliary stents.

Pathology

- With potentially resectable hepatocellular carcinoma, a biopsy may be performed if: (1) AFP < 400 ng/ml and is negative for hepatitis B surface antigen or (2) AFP < 4000 ng/ml with positive hepatitis B antigen (Grade C). However, the role of biopsy in hepatocellular carcinoma is controversial (National Comprehensive Cancer Network 2008).
  There are various histologic types of hepatocellular carcinoma and fibrolamellar is associated with a better prognosis.

- Most gallbladder carcinomas and cholangiocarcinomas are adenocarcinomas; however, small cell carcinoma and other rare histologies have also been reported. Gallbladder cancer is classified as papillary, nodular, or tubular.

- CC is typically divided on the basis of location: intrahepatic, extrahepatic, or hilar (Klatskin's tumor). Grossly, they are sclerotic, with a diffuse firm thickening of the duct. Almost all are mucin-producing adenocarcinoma. Intrahepatic cholangiocarcinoma can be further subdivided into three major macroscopic subtypes: mass forming, periductal infiltrating, and intraductal growth.

15.1.2 Staging

■ The AJCC/UICC (6th edition) staging of hepatocellular carcinoma, gallbladder cancer, and cholangiocarcinoma is presented in Table 15.2.

Other hepatocellular carcinoma staging systems include the CLIP (Cancer of the Liver Italian Program), the Okuda, and the BCLC (Barcelona Clinic Liver Cancer) scoring systems. All staging systems are based on a combination of clinical

Table 15.2. American Joint Committee on Cancer (AJCC) TNM classification for hepatobiliary cancers. [From GREENE et al. (2002) with permission]

Primary tumor (T): liver and intrahepatic cholangiocarcinoma	
TX	Primary tumor cannot be assessed
T0	No evidence of primary tumor
Tis	Carcinoma in situ
T1	Solitary tumor without vascular invasion
T2	Solitary tumor with vascular invasion, or multiple tumors, none more than 5 cm
T3	Multiple tumors more than 5 cm or tumor involving a major branch of the portal or hepatic veins
T4	Tumors with direct invasion of adjacent organs other than the gallbladder or with perforation of the visceral peritoneum
Primary tumor (T): gallbladder	
TX	Primary tumor cannot be assessed
T0	No evidence of primary tumor
Tis	Carcinoma in situ
T1	Tumor invades lamina propria or muscle layer
T1a	Tumor invades lamina propria
T1b	Tumor invades muscle layer
T2	Tumor invades perimuscular connective tissue; no extension beyond serosa or into the liver
T3	Tumor perforates the serosa (visceral peritoneum) and/or directly invades the liver and/or one other adjacent organ or structure, such as the stomach, duodenum, colon, or pancreas, omentum, or extrahepatic bile ducts
T4	Tumor invades main portal vein or hepatic artery or invades multiple extrahepatic organs or structures
Primary tumor (T): extrahepatic cholangiocarinoma	
TX	Primary tumor cannot be assessed
T0	No evidence of primary tumor
Tis	Carcinoma in situ
T1	Tumor confined to the bile duct histologically
T2	Tumor invades beyond the wall of the bile duct
T3	Tumor invades the liver, gallbladder, pancreas, and/or unilateral branches of the portal vein (right or left) or hepatic artery (right or left)
T4	Tumor invades any of the following: main portal vein or its branches bilaterally, common hepatic artery, or other adjacent structures such as the colon, stomach, duodenum, or abdominal wall
Regional lymph nodes (N)	
NX	Regional lymph node metastasis cannot be assessed
N0	No regional lymph node metastasis
N1	Regional lymph node metastasis
Distant metastasis (M)	
MX	Distant metastasis cannot be assessed
M0	No distant metastasis
M1	Distant metastasis present

and radiographic factors used to predict prognosis in patients with hepatocellular carcinoma. In general, the AJCC staging system is utilized for patients undergoing resection or transplantation, while the CLIP staging system has been advocated for patients undergoing non-surgical therapies.

- For cholangiocarcinoma, Bismuth-Corlette classification determines the extent of bile duct involved with tumor. The Jarnagin staging system predicts for resectability.

15.1.3 Prognostic Factors

Hepatocellular Carcinoma

- For hepatocellular carcinoma, primary prognostic factors include resectability, Child-Pugh Class (A-C), MELD (model for end-stage liver disease) score, fibrosis, size of future liver remnant, vascular invasion, tumor grade, size > 5 cm, > 3 tumors, poor performance status, and extrahepatic disease.
- The prognosis of patients with hepatocellular carcinoma is often correlated with the extent of fibrosis/cirrhosis and overall liver function based on the Child-Pugh classification (Table 15.3). The number, size, and location of lesions have also been shown to be prognostic (Level IV) (Pawlik et al. 2005). Tumor grade and the presence of vascular invasion (major > microscopic) are also strong predictors of survival.
- The 5-year survival rate after liver transplantation in patients with hepatocellular carcinoma has increased (25% for 1987–1991, compared to 47% for 1992–1996, and 61% for 1997–2001) (Level IV) (Yoo et al. 2003). This is in comparison to the 5-year survival in patients undergoing surgical resection alone (44.3%) (Level IV) (Poon et al. 2000).

Gallbladder Cancer

- For gallbladder cancer, favorable prognostic factors include early T-stage, no lymph node metastasis, a successful en bloc R0 resection with lymphadenectomy, adjuvant therapy, and no evidence of metastatic disease.
- The probability of metastasis is relatively high for gallbladder cancer (primarily peritoneal and/or intrahepatic metastasis). Patients with early-stage and resectable gallbladder cancer,

papillary pathology, and well-differentiated disease with associated metaplasia have a better prognosis.

- After curative resection alone, the prognosis is poor for all gallbladder cancer stages, with a pooled overall 5-year survival rate of approximately 5% (range, 3%–65%). The overall 5-year survival rate reported by Piehler and Crichlow (1978) for a surgical series of 6222 cases was 4.1% (Level IV).
- Kayahara and Nagakawa (2007) evaluated the predictive value of stage in determining survival in 4,774 patients with gallbladder cancer between 1988 and 1997. Stage correlated well with 5-year survival rates: 77% for stage I disease, 60% for stage II disease, 29% for stage III disease, 12% for stage IVA disease, and 3% for stage IVB disease (Level IV).
- Lymph node involvement is an important prognostic factor in gallbladder cancer, being closely associated with extent of the primary malignancy. The lymph node metastasis rate increases in frequency with increasing pathologic T-stage. Shimada et al. (1997) reported the overall lymph node metastasis rate in gallbladder cancer to be 63.4%. Those rates for T1, T2, and T3–4 disease were 0%, 61.9%, and 81.3%, respectively (Level IV). Pawlik et al. (2007) similarly demonstrated that the overall rate of lymph node metastasis increased with T-stage: T1b, 13%, T2, 31%, and T3, 46% (Level IV). In another study of 73 patients who underwent curative resection, Shimada et al. (2000) found 5-year survival rates to be 77.0% in pN0 cases and 27.3% in pN1 cases ($p < 0.01$) (Level IV).

Cholangiocarcinoma

- Patients who underwent complete resection with negative margins and without nodal involvement have the most favorable prognosis. Frequently, a concomitant liver resection is required to achieve an R0 margin in patients with hilar cholangiocarcinoma.
- Patients with margin and node-negative cholangiocarcinomas have the most favorable prognosis. Unfortunately, 30%–50% of all cholangiocarcinoma patients have node-positive or metastatic disease at presentation.

15.2 Treatment of Hepatocellular Carcinoma

15.2.1 General Principles

- Hepatocellular carcinoma is an aggressive tumor which typically occurs in patients with pre-existing cirrhosis or chronic liver disease.
- Curative options for hepatocellular carcinoma include partial hepatectomy or total hepatectomy with liver transplantation (Grade A). Unfortunately, most (70%–80%) patients are diagnosed in late stage, thus precluding them from surgical consideration.
- Many patients are unable to undergo curative resection because of advanced underlying liver disease which is typically classified based on the Child-Pugh classification (Table 15.3). In addition, many hepatocellular carcinoma patients are not candidates for transplantation due to

Table 15.3. Child-Pugh classification of severity of liver disease. Modified Child-Pugh classification of severity of liver disease according to the degree of ascites, the plasma concentrations of bilirubin and albumin, the prothrombin time, and the degree of encephalopathy

Parameter	Points assigned		
	1	2	3
Ascites	Absent	Slight	Moderate
Bilirubin, mg/dl	≤ 2	2–3	> 3
Albumin, g/dl	> 3.5	2.8–3.5	< 2.8
Prothrombin time Seconds over control or INR	1–3 < 1.8	4–6 1.8–2.3	> 6 > 2.3
Encephalopathy	None	Grade 1–2	Grade 3–4

A total score of 5–6 is considered grade A (well-compensated disease); 7–9 is grade B (significant functional compromise); and 10–15 is grade C (decompensated disease). These grades correlate with 1- and 2-year patient survival.

Grade	Points	1-Year patient survival (%)	2-Year patient survival (%)
A: well-compensated disease	5–6	100	85
B: significant functional compromise	7–9	80	60
C: decompensated disease	10–15	45	35

advanced malignancy that is outside the Milan criteria (e.g., solitary tumor ≤ 5 cm or up to three tumors all ≤ 3 cm) on presentation.

15.2.2 Curative Surgical Resection

- The proposed algorithm for the treatment of hepatocellular carcinoma is illustrated in Fig. 15.1. Surgical resection of hepatocellular carcinoma may be appropriate in the setting where there is no major vascular invasion and the patient has well-compensated liver function (Child-Pugh A) (Grade A). The size, number, and location of lesions can also dictate surgical resectability (Level IV) (Pawlik et al. 2005).
- It is imperative to determine the hepatic reserve prior to resection. The Cancer of the Liver Italian program (CLIP) staging classification takes into account the tumor stage as well as hepatic function to predict survival (Cancer of the Liver Italian Program 2000). Specifically, one should ensure an adequate future liver remnant (FLR) of at least 40%–50% based on pre-operative CT volumetry. In cases where the FLR is inadequate, portal vein embolization to induce hypertrophy of the FLR may be considered (Level III) (Seo et al. 2007).
- Modern surgery can lead to operative mortality rates of up to 3% with 5-year survival rates approaching 50%–90% (Bruix and Llovet 2002). Recurrence rates following surgical resection alone can be as high as 70%.

15.2.3 Transplant

- In the setting of hepatocellular carcinoma, a total hepatectomy and orthotopic liver transplantation (OLT) removes both the underlying diseased cirrhotic liver as well as the malignant macroscopic/microscopic disease. However, patients need to be carefully selected (Grade A). Recently, 11 studies were reviewed to determine the incidence of hepatocellular carcinoma recurrence following OLT to identify prognostic variables of recurrence (Level I) (Zimmerman et al. 2008). Recurrence was seen in approximately 20% of OLT patients and was likely the result of microscopic extrahepatic disease. These findings underscore the importance of accurate clinical staging and patient selection prior to transplantation.

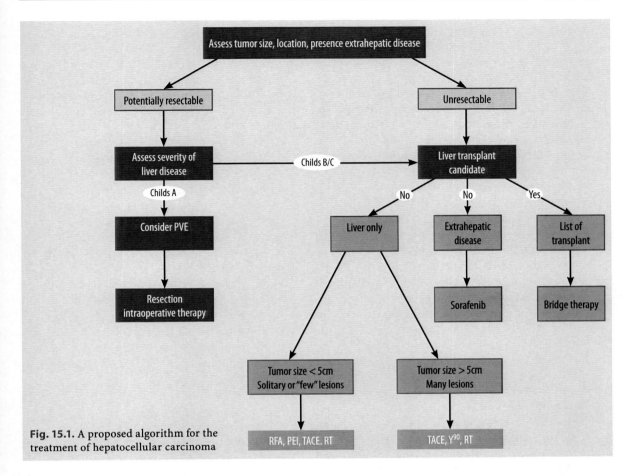

Fig. 15.1. A proposed algorithm for the treatment of hepatocellular carcinoma

■ Currently, the Milano/Mazzaferro criteria determines which hepatocellular carcinoma patients are eligible for liver transplantation (tumor ≤ 5 cm or up to three tumors all ≤ 3 cm) (Grade A). Liver transplantation has been reported to result in a 5-year survival of 70%–90% in well selected patients (Level IV) (Jonas et al. 2001; Yao et al. 2001). In these cases, OLT for hepatocellular carcinoma is slightly worse than survival rates in patients undergoing OLT for non-malignant causes.

■ Allocation of donor livers is determined by the model for end stage liver disease (MELD), a model which predicts survival in patients with cirrhosis.

■ While a patient is waiting for a transplant, bridging therapy with transarterial chemoembolization (TACE), radiofrequency ablation (RFA), or partial hepatectomy may be considered, although this data is limited (Grade D). Bridge therapy is probably most appropriate for those patients with anticipated long (> 6 months) wait times.

■ Because of the limited availability of organs, living-donor liver transplantation (LDLT) is an increasingly popular alternative (Grade C). LDLT enables recipients to avoid a long pre-transplantation waiting time. Subsequent ablative techniques (described below) can reduce tumor growth to ensure that patients continue to fulfill the Milan criteria for transplantation (Kassahun et al. 2006).

■ For smaller (< 3- to 4-cm) unresectable lesions, non-surgical ablative therapies can sometimes be curative with 5-year survival rates approaching 50% (Level IV) (Arii et al. 2000; Sutherland et al. 2006).

15.2.4 Adjuvant and Neoadjuvant Therapies

■ Systemic chemotherapy, hepatic-artery chemotherapy (HAI), TACE, and combinations of these therapies have not clearly demonstrated improved overall or disease-free survival after potentially curative surgery for localized hepatocellular carcinoma (Grade C). In a review of 13 randomized trials with recurrence or survival endpoints reported at 3 years or longer, systemic and hepatic-artery chemotherapy or chemoembolization have not been shown to improve overall or disease-free survival after resection of hepatocellular carcinoma (Level I) (Schwartz et al. 2002). However, there are no definitive trials comparing adjuvant systemic chemotherapy with supportive management.

A meta-analysis of three Japanese studies evaluating adjuvant chemotherapy for resected hepatocellular carcinoma included a total of 108 randomized patients (Level I) (Ono et al. 2001). The authors concluded that adjuvant chemotherapy conferred no significant benefit over supportive care. In a subset analysis, they determined that chemotherapy was associated with significantly lower disease-free and overall survival in the 70 patients with documented cirrhosis. This raises the question of whether patients with cirrhosis can tolerate aggressive adjuvant chemotherapy.

- A phase II randomized trial of PI-88, an agent inhibiting heparinase and VEGF activity, in patients after resection of hepatocellular carcinoma has been recently completed and suggests an improvement in disease-free survival in resected patients (Level III) (Ferro et al. 2007; Gautam et al. 2007).

- Similarly, prevention of recurrence is also important in patients undergoing liver transplantation or ablative therapies. Even after liver transplantation for small hepatocellular carcinoma, metastatic tumor recurrence is not uncommon, and this is in part related to the use of immunosuppressive agents to prevent graft rejection. mTOR inhibitors with dual immunomodulating and anti-cancer effects appear to be particularly useful in this setting; however, additional studies are needed (Pang and Poon 2007).

15.2.5 Treatment of Medically Inoperable or Unresectable Hepatocellular Cancer

- Resectability should be determined using a multidisciplinary approach. Complicated cases should be evaluated at high volume institutions.

Small Unresectable Tumors

- If tumors are small but still unresectable due to tumor location/number or medical comorbidities, ablative therapies include radiofrequency ablation (RFA), ethanol injections, and cryotherapy (Grade C).
  RFA involves the local application of radiofrequency thermal energy to the liver lesion(s). A high frequency alternating current causes ions within the tissue to change direction and results in frictional heating of the tissue. As the temperature rises above 60°C, cells are ablated causing necrosis. RFA provides 5-year survival rates of 33%–40%. In a comprehensive review of 3,670 patients treated with RFA for liver tumors, the mortality was 0.5% and the complication rate was 8.9% (Level I) (Mulier et al. 2002).
  Percutaneous ethanol injections and cryotherapy (alternating freeze-thaw cycles) can also effectively treat small liver lesions; however, they are less common with the widespread application of RFA.

Large Unresectable Tumors

- For large unresectable hepatocellular carcinoma lesions, TACE with chemotherapy, radioembolization (yttrium-90-tagged microspheres), or drug eluting beads can be delivered selectively to the tumor via the hepatic artery (Grade C). These therapies should be used with caution if there is portal vein thrombosis, advanced liver disease (Child-Pugh B/C), biliary obstruction, or if the patient has a poor performance status.

- Hepatocellular carcinoma tumors are supplied primarily by the hepatic artery while the normal liver is supported by the portal vein. With TACE, chemotherapy (adriamycin, cisplatin, or doxorubicin) is suspended in Lipiodol (a lipid contrast taken up by hepatocytes) and injected into the smallest hepatic branch supplying the tumor and sometimes followed with an embolizing agent. Partial responses are reported in 15%–55% of tumors and cause significant delay in tumor progression and vascular invasion. A meta-analysis demonstrated a survival advantage for TACE over no treatment when patients received between three and four TACE treatments per year (Level I) (Llovet and Bruix 2003).

- TheraSpheres (MDS Nordion, Ontario) are insoluble glass microspheres (20–30 μm) and are FDA approved for the treatment of hepatocellular carcinoma. Several activity sizes are available: 3 GBq (81 mCi)-20 GBq (540 mCi). Sir-Spheres SIRT (selective internal radiation therapy) (SIRTex Medical Inc., Australia) are resin-based microspheres impregnated with Y^{90} (20–60 μm) in size and are currently FDA approved for the treatment of colorectal metastasis. Data regarding efficacy in hepatocellular carcinoma patients are limited but emerging (SALEM et al. 2006).

GESCHWIND et al. (2004) reported on 80 patients treated with yttrium-90 microspheres using a segmental, regional, and a whole-liver approach. Pretreatment patients were staged using the Child-Pugh, Okuda, or CLIP scoring systems. The pretreatment CLIP system was superior in stratifying risk. Survival was found to be 628 and 324 days for Okuda I (68%) and II (32%) patients treated with theraspheres, respectively

(Level IV). Currently, a multi-institutional study is being conducted to prospectively evaluate the efficacy of theraspheres in patients with primary and metastatic liver disease.

15.2.6 Radiation Therapy (Conformal and Stereotactic Radiotherapy)

■ There was a historical bias against radiotherapy for liver malignancies because of the low tolerance of whole liver radiation. Radiation-induced liver disease (RILD) can occur in 5% of patients receiving 30–33 Gy of whole liver radiation.

■ Modern techniques including three-dimensional (3D) and intensity-modulated radiation therapy (IMRT) can be recommended for unresectable or inoperable hepatocellular carcinoma and allow for focused partial liver irradiation (Grade B)

Pre-radiation   **6 months Post-radiation**

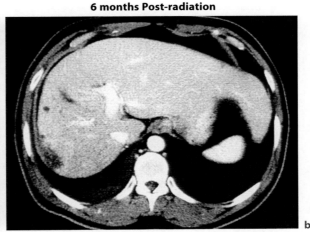

a   b

Fig. 15.2a,b. Radiographic response of hepatocellular carcinoma after conventional radiation. **a** CT scan taken before radiation therapy; **b** 6 months after the completion of radiation therapy (Courtesy of Dr. Theodore Lawrence)

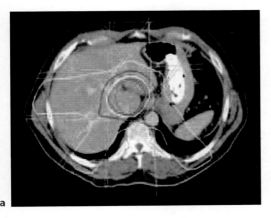

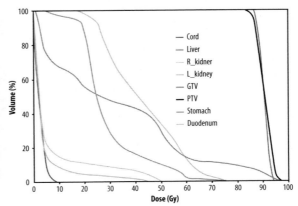

a   b

Fig. 15.3. a,b Intensity-modulated radiation (IMRT) (BEN-JOSEF et al. 2005). Plan to deliver high dose radiation to a HCC lesion

(Figs. 15.2, 15.3). Between 1996 and 2003, 128 patients with primary/metastatic liver cancer and unresectable intrahepatic cholangiocarcinoma were treated at the University of Michigan. Three-dimensional (3-D) conformal individualized radiation therapy was based on the maximum tolerated dose of radiation therapy calculated from the Lyman Normal Tissue Complacation Probability (NTCP) model to be ≤10%–15% risk of developing Radiation Induced Liver Disease (RILD). Radiation therapy (1.5 Gy BID) was given concurrently with intra-arterial 5-FU via a brachial artery catheter. Overall, the median survival for unresectable cholangiocarcinoma and hepatocellular carcinoma was 13.3 and 15.2 months, respectively. Median and progression-free survival of all patients was 21 months vs. 11 months, respectively ($p < 0.05$). Outcome was improved in those lesions treated to > 75 Gy. In field and extrahepatic sites of first disease, progression was similar for hepatocellular carcinoma and cholangiocarcinoma (44%/53% and 36%/40%), respectively. RILD was reported in 4% of patients with one death (Level IV) (BEN-JOSEF et al. 2005).

■ Results of a retrospective series of 50 patients demonstrated that unresectable hepatocellular carcinoma can be safely treated with high doses of twice-daily conformal radiation therapy in combination with TACE and concurrent 5-FU. The overall survival rates at 2 years and 3 years were 38% and 28%, respectively, and the median survival was 17 months (Level IV) (ZHOU et al. 2007).

■ Three-dimensional conformal radiation therapy (3D-CRT) is a practical treatment option in hepatocellular carcinoma patients for whom TACE is ineffective or unsuitable; however, additional studies are necessary to demonstrate efficacy of this regimen (Grade B). One study evaluated 70 patients with unresectable hepatocellular carcinoma who subsequently received 3-D conformal radiation because TACE was ineffective or unsuitable. 3D-CRT was associated with a 54% objective response rate for primary tumors and a 39% objective response rate for patients exhibiting portal venous thrombosis. Both hepatocellular carcinoma and portal venous thrombosis responses were found to be prognostic factors for overall survival (Level IV) (KIM et al. 2008).

■ Stereotactic body radiation therapy (SBRT) is hypofractionated multi-beam conformal radiotherapy delivered to lesions in patients with unresectable hepatocellular carcinoma. With SBRT, tighter margins are used resulting in a smaller volume of normal liver irradiation. Therefore, radioablation with SBRT may result in a lower risk of RILD. SBRT is unique because it is the only potentially non-invasive ablative therapy for the treatment of unresectable hepatocellular carcinoma. In patients with good liver function (Child-Pugh Class A) and small tumors, SBRT appears tolerable (Grade B).

A total of 41 patients with unresectable Child-Pugh A hepatocellular carcinoma ($n = 31$) or intrahepatic carcinoma ($n = 10$) were treated with SBRT delivered in six fractions with a median dose of 36 Gy (range 24–54 Gy) (Level III) (TSE et al. 2008). The median tumor size was 173 ml (9–1, 913 mL). Seven patients (five hepatocellular carcinomas, two intrahepatic carcinomas) had a decline in liver function from Child-Pugh class A to B within 3 months after SBRT. Two patients (5%) with intrahepatic carcinoma developed transient biliary obstruction after the first few fractions, which was alleviated by pre-treatment with dexamethasone. There was no evidence of RILD. Median survival of hepatocellular carcinoma and intrahepatic carcinoma patients was 11.7 months (9.2–21.6 months) and 15 months (6.5–29 months), respectively. With individualized dose allocation, large tumors receive less radiation because of the increased risk of RILD. Therefore, for large tumors the authors recommend the use of radiation sensitizers and protectors to enhance the efficacy of liver SBRT.

The safety and efficacy of hypofractionated SBRT for hepatocellular carcinoma and intrahepatic cholangiocarcinoma were reported in several retrospective and single-institutional prospective phase I/II trials. GUNVEN et al. (2003) evaluated SBRT for recurrent liver lesions and found favorable control rates and that all tumors were locally controlled with complete radiological remission after treatment. Limited side effects were observed after SBRT. Only one patient recurred in the liver (Level IV). Studies by HERFARTH et al. (2001) and WULF et al. (2006) reported no serious toxicity when a selected group of patients were treated with SBRT (Level III). MENDEZ ROMERO et al. (2006) treated 11 hepatocellular carcinoma patients (Child-Pugh A or B, tumor size < 7 cm) with 25 Gy in five fractions, 30 Gy in three fractions, or 37.5 in three fractions (Level III). Some patients were retreated after recurrence and the overall

1-year hepatocellular carcinoma local control rate and survival was 82% and 75%, respectively. One patient developed RILD. Treatment of additional patients with longer follow-up is necessary to determine the efficacy of SBRT for hepatocellular carcinoma and intrahepatic carcinoma.

■ How SBRT affects the tumor and surrounding normal liver is unknown. CUPP et al. (2008) reported on tissue effects after SBRT using CyberKnife (Accuray, Inc., Sunnyvale, CA) on four patients (autopsy) with abdominal malignancies. They found that the pathophysiological mechanisms of radiation-induced normal tissue damage are similar for biologically equivalent single and fractionated doses of radiotherapy (Level IV). How SBRT results in cell death (apoptosis vs. necrosis) and affects normal liver function is currently unknown and requires further study.

15.2.7 Radiation Simulation and 3D Planning

■ CT-based treatment planning is highly recommended for defining the gross tumor volume (GTV) and planning treatment volume (PTV). An individualized immobilization device (e.g., Alpha cradle; Smithers Medical Products, Inc. North Canton, OH) should be used during planning and treatment for reproducible patient set-up. The CT scan should be taken in the supine position with arms placed above the head with 3- to 5-mm-thick CT slices from the level of the carina to L5-S1. Oral and IV contrast should be administered to better identify the stomach and bowel and define the tumor and any adjacent lymph nodes.

■ For unresectable hepatocellular carcinoma, gallbladder cancer, and cholangiocarcinoma, MRI and four-dimensional (4D) CT scans may better determine tumor motion with breathing prior to treatment planning (KIRILOVA et al. 2008).

■ For 3D conformal or IMRT-based radiation planning of primary liver hepatocellular carcinoma or intrahepatic carcinoma, the CTV is GTV plus 1 cm and PTV is CTV plus 0.5-cm margin. In addition, a 0.3- to 3-cm margin should be added for breathing motion (based on dynamic excursion during fluoroscopic/4D simulation). Breathing motion may be decreased and hence smaller margins are needed if it can be controlled by an active breathing control (ABC) device, breathing

exercise programs, and/or body immobilization. For SBRT, breathing motion should be ≤ 5 mm or controlled with external compression or an ABC device. The CTV for SBRT should include the GTV 0.5–1 cm. The PTV should include the CTV + 0.5 cm for set-up uncertainty and an additional margin for breathing motion.

■ For hepatocellular carcinoma fiducials such as gold seeds placed in the tumor by CT or US guidance can sometimes be used to track tumor motion during respiration; however, how fiducials correlate with tumor motion is unknown.

■ SBRT treatment is either isocentric (Linac-based) (TSE et al. 2008) or non-isocentric (CyberKnife) (CASAMASSIMA et al. 2006). Motion secondary to breathing can be controlled by breathing exercises, the ABC device (Linac-based), or a robotic arm (CyberKnife) which moves to track the motion of the tumor (fiducial placed in the tumor) or an external surrogate of breathing motion placed on the patients chest.

■ The tumor volume should be defined by a thin-sliced CT scan, EUS, ERCP, or in some cases an MRI. The utility of a PET/CT scan for the planning of hepatocellular carcinoma, gallbladder cancer, and cholangiocarcinoma is limited (discussed earlier).

■ Normal tissues to be delineated include bilateral kidneys, normal and diseased liver, spinal cord, stomach, and small bowel. Dose volume histograms should be used to outline dose to these structures.

15.2.8 Palliative Options and Chemotherapy

■ Palliative radiation can be offered to patients for pain control (Grade B). A prospective, non-randomized trial of > 100 patients with six different radiation doses and fractionation schedules were evaluated ranging from 21 Gy in seven fractions to 25.6 Gy in 16 fractions. Palliation of pain was achieved in 55% with no difference between treatment regimens (Level III) (BORGELT et al. 1981).

■ Palliative chemotherapy for unresectable and metastatic hepatocellular carcinoma has been largely ineffective. New targeted therapy agents have shown efficacy in palliative treatment of advanced hepatocellular carcinoma and can be recommended (Grade A). Targeted agents such as Sorafenib have shown promising results in a phase II trial (Level III) (Abou-Alfa et al. 2006). In a double-blind, randomized, placebo-controlled phase III trial recently completed, Sorafenib was administered to patients with advanced hepatocellular carcinoma who had no prior systemic therapy. The study enrolled 226 patients from sites in China, Korea, and Taiwan. The primary objectives of the study were to compare overall survival, progression-free survival, and time to progression (TTP) in patients administered Sorafenib 400 mg twice daily versus patients administered placebo. This study was found to prolong survival in HCC patients. Future studies investigating the role of Sorafenib in the adjuvant setting are anticipated. Interpretation of systemic studies is difficult because Asian patients with HCC (younger, cirrhosis due to chronic hepatitis) exhibit a diverse presentation when compared with Western patients (elderly, cirrhosis due to long-term alcohol consumption).

15.3 Management of Gallbladder Cancer

15.3.1 General Principles

■ Gallbladder cancer (GBC) is a rare but fatal malignancy. Fewer than 9,500 new cases are diagnosed in the US yearly. The incidence of incidental GBC is roughly 1 in 100 in patients undergoing cholecystectomy. The poor prognosis stems from the propensity of the disease to spread locoregionally (e.g., lymph nodes), as well as distantly (e.g., lung, liver, peritoneum).

■ Surgical resection alone has resulted in relatively poor survival rates. A complete resection with negative margins seems critical to achieving a favorable outcome.

■ Earlier detection of GBC and integration of novel agents with radiation in the neoadjuvant and adjuvant setting is imperative to improve outcomes.

15.3.2 Curative Resection

■ For patients with preoperatively or intraoperatively diagnosed GBC, a resection that includes a radical cholecystectomy with hepatic resection in conjunction with regional lymph node dissection is recommended (Grade A) (Cubertafond et al. 1999; Ruckert et al. 1996). Contraindications for surgical resection include gross vascular invasion or encasement of major vessels (T4), ascites, diffuse hepatic involvement, distant metastasis, and poor functional status. All patients should be evaluated individually and discussed in a tumor board setting.

The goal for treating GBC is to obtain a margin-negative (R0) resection; however, since most patients present with advanced-stage disease, only a third of patients are potential surgical candidates.

GBC may extend into the hepatic parenchyma, the hepatoduodenal ligament, and adjacent organs (duodenum, transverse colon, stomach, and small bowel). The extent of hepatic resection (e.g., wedge, formal 4b/5 segmentectomy, extended hepatectomy) should be dictated by the patient's anatomy and the extent of the underlying malignant disease.

■ Staging laparoscopy should be considered prior to resection because of the high rate of occult metastatic disease (Grade B). If metastatic disease is found at laparoscopy, tissue biopsy can avoid a non-therapeutic laparotomy and a potential perforation with tumor spread. In a prospective series of 100 patients with extrahepatic biliary carcinoma, the yield of staging laparoscopy was found to approach 50% (Level III) (Weber et al. 2002). FDG-PET scan may also help identify occult metastatic disease in the preoperative setting.

■ Over a 20-year period, one study identified only 38% of patients who were eligible for a curative resection. The cohort that underwent complete resection (all stages considered) rather than palliative surgery had an improved overall survival (31% vs. 13%). As expected, none of the unresectable gallbladder cancer patients were alive at 5-years (Level IV) (Ito et al. 2004).

■ When GBC is discovered incidentally following cholecystectomy and the specimen demonstrates mucosal involvement on microscopic examination (Tis), or there is submucosal or muscular invasion (T1), no further therapy is necessary (Reid et al. 2007). Gallbladder cancers identified at laparoscopic evaluation should be converted to an open procedure and the port sites removed to prevent the potential of port site recurrences (Fong et al. 1993). The expected 5-year survival using this technique for stage 1 cancers approaches

100%; therefore, adjuvant therapy is typically not recommended for these patients (Grade A). Others recommend adjuvant therapy in stage T1b (Level IV) (DE ARETXABALA 1997).

- For patients with T2 or T3 disease, a radical resection including a hepatic resection and lymphadenectomy is indicated.
- Common bile duct resection is not routinely recommended for GBC. Bile duct resection should be performed, however, in the setting of a positive cystic duct margin.
- As noted, the extent of hepatic resection is usually limited to resection of segments IV and V, 2 cm away from the gallbladder bed. This technique is adequate in GBC confined to the subserosal layer but may not be adequate in some T3 and T4 cancers. Therefore, in some cases, extended hepatectomy with or without a caudate lobe resection may be justified.

15.3.3 Neoadjuvant and Adjuvant Treatments

- KOPELSON et al. (1981) reported on 11 gallbladder cancer patients who had curative resection and did not receive adjuvant radiation therapy (RT) or chemotherapy. Of the 11, seven (64%) patients were found to have local-regional failures (Level IV). Poor outcome after surgery alone for gallbladder cancer indicated that adjuvant or neoadjuvant therapy is needed to improve local control rates.
- Prospective phase III studies testing the addition of neoadjuvant or adjuvant chemoradiation to surgery are needed to determine the optimal management of gallbladder cancer. Since gallbladder cancer is rare, it is unlikely these trials will be completed; therefore, only single institution retrospective studies can be referenced.
- There is currently no defined role for neoadjuvant treatment in gallbladder cancer.

Adjuvant Therapy

- Adjuvant RT can be offered to patients with gallbladder cancer with regional lymph node involvement or with positive resection margins (Grade B). In an attempt to improve local-regional control and survival, adjuvant RT alone, or in combination with chemotherapy, has been ex-

plored. The majority of studies evaluating the role of adjuvant radiation therapy +/− chemotherapy are retrospective, and there have been conflicting reports regarding the value of adjuvant RT +/− chemotherapy. This is due to differences in patient selection factors, staging systems, extent of resection, radiation therapy techniques, and chemotherapy regimens used.

- There are several single institution studies evaluating the role of adjuvant therapy for CBC. One recent retrospective report from Duke University described 22 patients with resected and non-metastatic adenocarcinoma of the gallbladder who underwent adjuvant RT between 1980 and 2003 (Level IV) (CZITO et al. 2005). The median dose RT was 45 Gy and 81% received concurrent 5-FU chemotherapy. In this series, margin status did not influence outcome. All seven local failures occurred in the radiation field. The 5-year actuarial overall survival, disease-free survival, metastases-free survival, and local-regional control was 37%, 33%, 36%, and 59%, respectively. Median survival for all patients was 1.9 years. This report advocates a radical resection followed by RT given concurrently with 5-FU. However, the main drawback of this report is the small number of patients included in each group and low RT dose used.
- HOURY et al. (1989) described results of 20 patients who received adjuvant or definitive radiation (mean 42 Gy) +/− chemotherapy (seven patients) for gallbladder cancer between 1977 and 1987 (Level IV). The results are difficult to interpret because of the diverse groups of patients included in the study, however, the authors claim that RT may improve survival in patients with partially resected or unresectable GBC.
- A modern study evaluating the role of radiation in cholangiocarcinoma and gallbladder cancer (n = 28) was recently reported by University of Michigan. The median overall survival and progression-free survival for gallbladder cancer was 14.4 and 11.1 months, respectively. Patients had better outcomes if they underwent a margin-negative resection and received > 45 Gy of radiation. For all patients there was no statistically significant benefit seen with the addition of chemotherapy to radiation although the numbers were small. The treatment was well tolerated overall with nausea and fatigue being the most common symptoms reported (Level IV) (BEN-DAVID et al. 2006).

■ A surveillance epidemiology and end results (SEER) analysis of 3,187 cases of GBC in a Japanese registry from 1992 to 2002 was recently reported (Level III) (Mojica et al. 2007). Of the surgical group, 35% were stage I, 36% were stage II, 6% were stage III, and 21% were stage IV. Adjuvant RT was administered in 17% of the cases. The median survival for those patients who did or did not receive RT was 14 vs. 8 months ($p \leq$ or = 0.001). The survival benefit with RT was seen primarily in those patients with regional spread ($p = 0.0001$) or tumors infiltrating the liver ($p = 0.011$).

■ The use of 5-FU-based chemotherapy concurrent with adjuvant RT can be considered (Grade B). The Mayo Clinic reported on 21 consecutive GBC patients who underwent curative resection followed by adjuvant 5-FU-based chemoradiation between 1985 and 1997. RT fields encompassed the tumor bed and regional lymph nodes (median dose of 54 Gy in 1.8–2.0 Gy fractions). Most patients (n = 20) had stage III–IV disease. The 5-year survival rate for all patients was 33%. For patients with/without residual disease, 5-year survival was 64% vs. 0%, ($p = 0.002$). The 5-year local control rate was 73%. Five-year local control rates were 100% for the six patients who received total radiation therapy doses > 54 Gy. Patients who underwent R0 resections of their gallbladder cancer followed by adjuvant radiation therapy plus 5-FU had a 5-year survival rate of 64% which is superior to 5-year survival rates for historical controls (33%) (Level III) (Kresl et al. 2002). 5-FU is typically given at a dose of 500 mg/m^2/day in bolus fashion for 3 days during weeks 1 and 5 of radiation or by continuous infusion at 225 mg/m^2/day throughout the RT course. Low dose gemcitabine (300–500 mg/m^2) with radiation is also being evaluated.

■ IMRT or conformal radiation should be used in order to decrease the dose to normal adjacent structures and perhaps allow dose escalation of chemotherapy and/or allow for the addition of targeted agents during RT.

■ Intraoperative radiation therapy (IORT) with electrons (IOERT) or high dose/low dose rate brachytherapy (HDR-IORT, LDR-IORT) can sometimes be used to improve local control (Calvo et al. 2006). IORT should be considered in conjunction with neoadjuvant or adjuvant 5-FU-based conformal radiation therapy which has been shown to enhance the likelihood of long-term local control in other sites (Grade C)

(Krempien et al. 2006). This allows for dose escalation to the tumor or tumor bed while limiting the dose to adjacent normal structures.

One non-randomized study evaluated 17 patients undergoing resection for T4N0-1 with gallbladder cancer who received IORT with or without postoperative EBRT. At 3 years, the group receiving IORT had an improved survival compared to resection alone (10% vs. 0%) (Level III) (Todoroki et al. 1991, 1997). Given the limited data, IORT should only be used at experienced centers where patients are at a high risk of undergoing a margin-positive resection.

Adjuvant Chemotherapy

■ Adjuvant chemotherapy may be considered in the treatment of gallbladder cancer, alone or with adjuvant RT depending on the extent of the disease and status of surgical resection margin (Grade B). In a prospective, randomized phase-III trial, Takada et al. (2002) examined the role of adjuvant chemotherapy in 508 patients diagnosed with resectable pancreaticobiliary carcinomas, and 140 had gallbladder cancer. Patients were randomized to receive surgical resection alone or surgery plus adjuvant 5-FU and Mitomycin C. The latter group received Mitomycin C [6 mg/m^2 intravenously (IV)] during the operation and 5-FU (310 mg/m^2 IV) for five consecutive days during the first and third weeks postoperatively, followed by oral 5-FU (100 mg/m^2) starting the fifth postoperative week until tumor recurrence. The 5-year survival rate for patients in the adjuvant treatment group was 26% compared with 14% in the control group ($p = 0.04$) (Level II) (Takada et al. 2002).

As with pancreatic cancer, additional studies are needed to determine which patients may be better treated with adjuvant chemotherapy alone or chemotherapy combined with RT.

15.3.4 Palliative Options (Metastatic and Unresectable Gallbladder Cancer): Radiation and Chemotherapy

■ Patients with advanced unresectable or metastatic gallbladder cancer have a dismal prognosis (5-year survival < 5%). Imaging (MRI, ERCP, and CT scans) can be helpful in determining whether a gallbladder tumor is resectable prior to surgery. However, if the patient's gallbladder cancer is found to be unresectable at the time of surgery, palliative bypass procedures may be considered because of the rate (up to 60%) of gastric and biliary obstruction. Specifically, a Roux-en-Y hepaticojejunostomy +/- a gastrojejunostomy may be performed at the time of exploration.

■ The nonoperative options of percutaneous or endoscopic endobiliary stents plus endoscopic enteric stenting and feeding tubes can be used in patients with locally advanced GBC. This should be considered as primary palliative therapy for patients with poor functional status, limited life expectancy, or significant comorbidities. No controlled trials have compared the use of stents vs. surgical bypass in this patient population; however, patients with metastatic or extensive disease may be better served by stent placement.

■ If the patient has non-metastatic or low burden metastatic disease with an excellent performance status, a definitive course with concurrent 5-FU/gemcitabine-based CRT should be considered (50.4–60 Gy/1.8 fractions). Patients who present with locally advanced metastatic gallbladder cancer who experience pain due to local obstruction should be considered for palliative radiation +/- chemotherapy given over a shorter course (30 Gy/3-Gy fractions).

■ Systemic chemotherapy alone has demonstrated limited benefit in gallbladder cancer; however, most studies are small and typically include other sites such as pancreas and cholangiocarcinoma (Grade C). Objective response rates average between 25%–50%; however, whether these responses influence overall survival is unknown. Recently, several trials have evaluated various chemotherapeutic (gemcitabine, 5-FU) and some targeted therapies (Erlotinib) for metastatic or locally advanced gallbladder cancer (FURUSE et al. 2008; IYER et al. 2007; THOMAS 2007).

15.3.5 Radiation Therapy (Conformal)

Simulation and Field Arrangement, Dose, and Fractionation

■ Adjuvant radiation therapy: 3D conformal or IMRT should be used to treat the tumor bed and local-regional lymph nodes (portohepatic, pericholedochal, celiac, and pancreaticoduodenal) with a 2- to 3-cm margin to a median dose of 45 Gy (range 39.6–45 Gy). Additional radiation therapy is administered using reduced fields to an additional 5.4–9.0 Gy. Patients receive 1.8–2 Gy per fraction daily, 5 days a week. Mixed energy beams (6/15-MV photons) can be used.

■ Historically, external beam doses above 54 Gy should be avoided because of intolerance to adjacent structures including the liver, kidneys, spinal cord, and duodenum. However, with 3D conformal or IMRT doses in excess of 54 Gy can sometimes be delivered if the dose to normal structures, especially bowel, can be limited (Level IV) (BEN-DAVID et al. 2006).

■ MILANO et al. (2004) compared conventional and IMRT plans for six patients with pancreatic or bile duct cancer. Compared with conventional treatment, IMRT reduced the mean dose to the liver, kidneys, stomach, and small bowel. IMRT was well tolerated, with 80% experiencing Grade 2 or less acute upper GI toxicity. In these patients, there did not appear to be any increased risk of local recurrence with IMRT (Level III).

■ The optimal dose of IORT for gallbladder cancer is unknown. In general, the biological effectiveness of single dose IORT is thought to be equivalent to 1.5–2.5 times the same total dose of fractionated EBRT (GUNDERSON et al. 1982). Therefore, adding 15 Gy of IORT to 45 Gy of EBRT is equivalent to an EBRT dose of 75–87.5 Gy, which is the dose range believed to be most effective at controlling microscopic residual disease.

15.4 Management of Cholangiocarcinoma

15.4.1 Curative Resection

■ Cholangiocarcinomas are categorized based on location (intrahepatic, hilar, and distal). For intrahepatic cholangiocarcinoma surgical resection is the only option for cure (Grade A). However, intrahepatic carcinomas are typically large at presentation and, therefore, margin-positive resections are common (Grade A) (WEBER et al. 2001). Standard surgery for intrahepatic carcinoma includes hemi-hepatectomy or extended hepatic resection. Resection may also include bile duct resection, regional lymphadenectomy, and – when indicated – Roux-en-Y hepaticojejunostomy. Whether major vascular resection coupled with these procedures or hepatic transplantation in selected intrahepatic carcinoma patients will improve overall survival is unknown (NAGORNEY and KENDRICK 2006).

- For hilar CC, extended radical resection can be recommended. Extended radical resection offers a chance for cure with a 5-year survival rate of approximately 40% (SEYAMA and MAKUUCHI 2007). In general, routine hepatectomy for hilar CC is advocated to obtain higher rates of margin negative resections and improved survival.

- Pancreaticoduodenectomy with lymphadenectomy is the surgical choice for treatment of distal EHC. Very rarely, for extensive tumors, a major hepatectomy with hepatopancreatoduodenectomy may be necessary. The 5-year survival rate ranges from 24% to 39% after partial resection for middle and distal bile duct cancer (SEYAMA and MAKUUCHI 2007).

15.4.2 Neoadjuvant Treatments

- Patients with large, multi-focal cholangiocarcinoma with vascular involvement typically do poorly following resection and may, therefore, benefit from neoadjuvant therapy (chemotherapy/radiation); however, data is limited (Grade C). BEN-DAVID et al. (2006) found no difference in survival between patients with microscopically positive margins and patients with unresectable disease (Level IV). This stresses the importance of R0 resection and suggests that resection should be attempted only when an R0 resection is likely. Therefore, borderline resectable patients may benefit from neoadjuvant therapy.

- Liver transplantation is considered as an alternative to resection for carefully selected patients with localized, node-negative hilar and distal cholangiocarcinoma (Grade B). The Mayo clinic developed a protocol combining neoadjuvant radiotherapy, chemotherapy, CI 5-FU, IOERT, and orthotopic liver transplantation for patients with stage I and II hilar cholangiocarcinoma between January 1993 and August 2004. A total of 71 patients were considered for the protocol; 54 patients were explored and 26 (48%) eventually underwent liver transplantation, while 28 (52%) had unresectable disease. Patients received 45 Gy with concurrent bolus (5-FU) 500 mg/m^2 daily for the first 3 days of radiation. A boost of radiation was delivered using a transcatheter Iridium-192 brachytherapy wire, with a target dose of 2000–3000 cGy. Following brachytherapy, patients initially continued to receive CI 5-FU or oral capecitabine as tolerated until transplantation. The 1-, 3-, and 5-year patient survival rates were 92%, 82%, and 82% after transplantation. There were few recurrences in the transplant patients (13%) (Level III) (REA et al. 2005).

15.4.3 Adjuvant Treatment

Extrahepatic and Hilar Cholangiocarcinoma

- Adjuvant radiation in patients with resected hilar cholangiocarcinoma should be considered (Grade B). Positive margins were frequently observed after surgical resection, and local recurrence rates were usually unacceptably high after incomplete resections. Positive margins occur in up to 85% of patients with hilar cholangiocarcinoma with a 5-year survival of 9%–40% (NAKEEB et al. 1996). For distal bile duct cancers, the margin-positive rate is lower (25%–40%), most likely due to a more radical resection which includes a pancreaticoduodenectomy and lymph node resection (FRITZ et al. 1994). JARNAGIN et al. (2003) compared recurrence patterns of hilar cholangiocarcinoma and gallbladder cancer (JARNAGIN et al. 2003). In their study, 76 patients had hilar cholangiocarcinoma and 53 (66%) recurred at a follow-up of 24 months. Isolated locoregional recurrences were statistically more common with hilar cholangiocarcinoma vs. gallbladder cancer (59% vs. 15%, $p < 0.001$). Gallbladder cancer patients were statistically more likely to recur distantly compared with hilar cholangiocarcinoma (85% vs. 41%, $p < 0.001$).

■ The European Organization for Research and Treatment of Cancer (EORTC) reported retrospectively on 55 resected patients with cholangiocarcinoma in which 53 had margin-positive resections. A total of 38 received chemoradiation and 17 had surgery only. Adjuvant chemoradiation (no maintenance chemotherapy) was associated with a significant survival benefit (19 vs. 8 months, $p = 0.005$) (Level IV) (GONZALEZ GONZALEZ et al. 1990).

■ GERHARDS et al. (2003) evaluated 41 patients with hilar CC who received RT plus brachytherapy, 30 patients with radiation alone, and 20 who were observed. Only 14% of patients underwent an R0 resection (Level IV). There was a significant benefit with radiation therapy vs. surgery (24 vs. 8 months, $p < 0.01$); however, it is possible that the benefit of adjuvant therapy was secondary to patients undergoing incomplete resections. There was no clear benefit of brachytherapy in this study and these patients experienced more toxicity.

■ Recently, HUGHES et al. (2007) reported a Johns Hopkins retrospective series of adjuvant chemoradiation after partial resection for adenocarcinoma of the distal common bile duct. The median survival was 36.9 months, and the 5-year survival was 35%. Patients with negative lymph nodes lived significantly longer than those with positive lymph nodes ($p < 0.02$). All patients with negative lymph nodes lived at least 5 years, compared with 24% of patients with positive lymph nodes. The outcomes of patients in this study were compared with those of a group of historical controls treated at the same institution at a time before this study when adjuvant therapy was not routinely offered (YEO et al. 1998). The group receiving adjuvant therapy had a significantly longer survival (36.9 months vs. 22 months; $p < 0.05$) (Level IV).

■ In a study by SERAFINI et al. (2001), the mean survival for patients with distal common bile duct tumors who received adjuvant chemoradiation was 41 months compared with 21 months for surgery alone ($p = 0.04$) (Level IV). Disease recurrence occurred in 71% with the site of first recurrence being predominantly metastatic to the liver (83%). The most common site of local recurrence was the portal nodes.

■ The University of Michigan recently reported their series of patients diagnosed with extrahepatic carcinoma (gallbladder 28, distal bile duct 24, hilar 29) between June 1986 and December 2004. A total of 35% underwent potentially curative resection with R0/R1 margins; 64% were unresectable or underwent resection with macroscopic residual disease (R2). All patients received 3D-planned megavoltage radiation therapy. Complete resection (R0) was the only predictive factor significantly associated with increase in both overall survival and progression-free survival ($p = 0.002$), and there was no difference in outcomes between R1 and R2 resections. The first site of failure was predominantly locoregional (69% of all failures). Patients who had complete resection with negative margins followed by adjuvant CRT tended to have a better outcome with 64% surviving 5 years. However, maintenance chemotherapy should be considered because of the high risk of distant failure, which can be as high as 70% in their study (Level IV) (BEN-DAVID et al. 2006).

■ TODOROKI et al. (2000) found that patients who were treated with radiation after resection of hilar carcinoma had significantly higher 5-year survival rates and median survivals than patients who underwent surgery alone: 33.9% and 32 months vs. 13.5% and 10 months, respectively ($p = 0.01$). Patients who were treated with a combination of intraoperative radiation (using electron beam) and postoperative EBRT had the best survival. However, only 3% of patients had negative surgical margins.

■ SAGAWA et al. (2005) reported 69 patients who underwent surgery for hilar cholangiocarcinoma between 1980 and 1998, and 39 patients received adjuvant therapy. Patients treated with adjuvant chemoradiation did not have a significant survival benefit overall ($p = 0.554$); however, there was a significant benefit with pathological stage III or IVA disease after radiation therapy ($p = 0.042$).

■ Local failure is a major problem in extrahepatic carcinoma, suggesting the need for dose escalation and better radiosensitizing strategies. Because R1 resection appears to convey no benefit in survival, it appears that surgery should be contemplated only when an R0 resection is likely. Borderline-resectable patients might be better served by neoadjuvant therapy (WAKAI et al. 2005).

■ Possible treatment fields for hilar cholangiocarcinoma are illustrated in Figure 15.4.

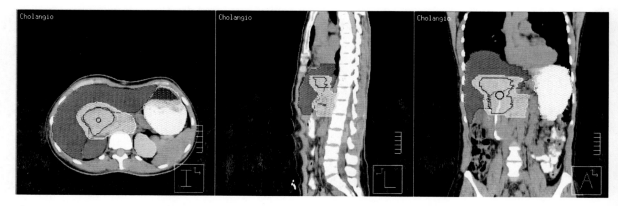

Fig. 15.4. Treatment fields for hilar cholangiocarcinoma (Courtsey of Dr. Joseph M. Herman)

Intrahepatic Cholangiocarcinoma

■ If patients undergo a margin-negative resection (R0), the standard of care is observation (NATIONAL COMPREHENSIVE CANCER NETWORK 2008) or chemotherapy (gemcitabine or 5-FU). If resection margins are positive (R1/R2), then patients should be considered for re-resection, ablative techniques, or receive chemotherapy (gemcitabine or 5-FU) with focused radiation. However, given the small number of patients with intrahepatic carcinoma and limited data, care should be individualized on a case-by-case basis.

15.4.4 Radiation Therapy (Conformal)

Simulation and Field Arrangement, Dose, and Fractionation

■ The techniques of EBRT for cholangiocarcinoma assimilate those used in the treatment of gallbladder cancer.

15.4.5 Palliative Options (Unresectable Cholangiocarcinoma) and Chemotherapy

■ There is limited data on the outcome of primary radiation therapy for unresectable extrahepatic carcinoma. The published retrospective series are typically small and with great heterogeneity in treatment techniques and radiation dose. In general, chemotherapy and radiation should be considered for palliation as described in the gallbladder cancer palliative options (Sect. 15.3.5).

Chemotherapy Alone for Advanced or Metastatic Cholangiocarcinoma

■ The median survival of patients with advanced or metastatic cholangiocarcinoma treated with chemotherapy alone is approximately 5–9 months (BEN-DAVID et al. 2006).

■ In a multicenter phase II study, FURUSE et al. (2008) evaluated the antitumor effect and safety of S-1 (a compound drug consisting of the oral fluoropyrimidine prodrug tegafur and the enzyme inhibitors gimeracil and oteracil) in previously untreated patients with advanced periampullary tumors (Level III). Eligible patients had pathologically proven, unresectable cholangiocarcinoma with no prior chemotherapy or radiotherapy. Patients received S-1 orally at 80 mg/m^2 total daily dose divided twice daily for 28 days followed by 14 days of rest. A total of 40 patients were assessable. The trial included gallbladder ($n = 20$), extrahepatic bile duct ($n = 15$), and the ampulla of Vater ($n = 5$). One patient (2.5%) achieved a complete response, 13 patients (32.5%) had partial responses, 17 patients (42.5%) had no change, seven patients (17.5%) had progressive disease, and two patients (5.0%) were not evaluable. The overall objective response rate was 35.0%. The median overall survival was 9.4 months, and the median time to progression was 3.7 months. S-1 monotherapy should be evaluated in a randomized study.

■ One phase I study evaluated gemcitabine and capecitabine (GemCap) in patients with advanced biliary cancer arising from the intra- and extrahepatic bile ducts or gallbladder with no prior chemotherapy (Level III) (KNOX et al. 2005). Patients were treated on a 3-week cycle consisting of capecitabine at 650 mg/m² orally twice a day for 14 days and gemcitabine at a fixed dose of 1000 mg/m² intravenously over 30 min on days 1 and 8. There were 45 patients enrolled between July 2001 and January 2004. A total of 53% of patients had cholangiocarcinoma, 47% had gallbladder cancer, and 89% had metastatic disease. The overall objective response rate was 31%, 42% stable disease, for a disease control rate of 73%. The median overall survival time was 14 months, and the median progression-free survival time was 7 months. This regimen warrants further evaluation in a randomized study with survival and quality-of-life end points.

15.5 Radiation-Induced Side Effects and Dose Limiting Structures

15.5.1 Radiation-Induced Liver Disease

■ With all hepatobiliary malignancies, normal liver will likely receive some radiation which can lead to radiation-induced liver disease (RILD). The clinical syndrome of RILD includes hepatomegaly, ascites, elevated liver enzymes (AP > transaminases), and jaundice (late effect) which occurs 2 weeks–3 months after radiation therapy. It resembles veno-occlusive disease after transplant resulting in marked venous congestion and hepatocyte atrophy. The pathogenesis is unclear, but is possibly due to selective injury of the vascular endothelial cells rather than hepatocytes. Treatment includes supportive care with diuretics and steroids but can lead to liver failure.

■ Partial liver radiation therapy was first reported by INGOLD et al. (1965) who safely delivered 55 Gy to parts of the liver.

■ EMAMI et al. (1991) suggested that TD5/5 and TD50/5 for 1/3, 2/3, and 3/3 of the liver as 50/50 Gy, 35/45 Gy, and 30/40 Gy, respectively. This data

was based on retrospective reports of "suspected" radiation injury in 27 patients. The volume and dose estimates were "clinical judgments" since detailed dose and volume data were not available (Level IV).

■ The Lyman NTCP model describes the volume dependence of radiation therapy on normal tissue toxicity. It assumes a sigmoidal relationship between dose of uniform radiation given to a volume of an organ and the probability of complications.
DAWSON et al. (2002) analyzed the risk of RILD using the Lyman NTCP model in 203 patients and found the liver radiation therapy exhibits a large volume effect. There was a strong correlation between the normal tissue complication probability and the mean liver dose. No RILD cases were observed when the mean liver dose was < 31 Gy (Level IV).

■ For hepatocellular carcinoma, the RILD risk is predicted to be 5% for an effective liver volume of two-thirds treated to 46 Gy and near 0% if the treated effective liver volume was less than one-third. Thus, it is unlikely that liver tolerance could be exceeded in patients receiving conventional doses of radiotherapy for cholangiocarcinoma or gallbladder cancer. Current estimates of a 15% risk of RILD in hepatocellular carcinoma for the whole liver, 2/3 liver, and 1/3 liver is 32, 47, and 93 Gy, respectively, in 1.5-Gy fractions twice daily. The NTCP for RILD does depend on liver function. Therefore, patients with hepatocellular carcinoma and cirrhosis have a higher risk of RILD when compared to liver metastases (DAWSON et al. 2005).

■ The risk of RILD with hypofractionated SBRT is unknown and is being evaluated in a phase I clinical trial (RTOG 0438). Dose tolerance for various normal structures for SBRT limited by the RTOG 0438 are as follows:

– Normal liver: The normal liver is defined as that portion of liver not radiographically involved by gross tumor (normal liver volume minus GTV). In all patients, it is required that there is at least 1000 cc of normal liver. No more than 30% of the normal liver may receive more than 27 Gy, and no more than 50% of normal liver may receive over 24 Gy.

– Kidney: For patients with only one functioning kidney or creatinine > 2.0 mg/dl, no more than 10% of the functioning kidney(s) may receive 10 Gy or more. For patients with normal creatinine and two functioning kidneys, no more than 33% of the combined renal volume may receive 18 Gy or more.

- Spinal cord: Maximal permitted dose to spinal cord is 34 Gy.
- Small bowel: Maximal permitted dose to small bowel is 37 Gy for any 1 cc volume.
- Stomach: Maximal permitted dose to stomach is 37 Gy for any 1 cc of volume.

The above listed doses were not biologically corrected, and 37 Gy is biologically equivalent to 50 Gy in 2 Gy/fraction using an α/β of 3.

15.5.2 Other Radiation Dose Limiting Structures

- **Kidneys:** Kidney function should be examined prior to treatment. Typically the entire right kidney will receive some radiation even with 3D or IMRT treatment. According to the RTOG 0411 protocol: 2/3 of one kidney should receive less than 18 Gy. The exact radiation tolerance of the kidney is unknown.
- **Stomach and duodenum:** Previously it was reported that 60 Gy to 1/3 of the stomach will give a 5% risk of ulceration and/or perforation (Level IV) (EMAMI et al. 1991). The University of Michigan study of 128 patients treated on the phase I liver protocol (5-FU and radiation) demonstrated a 7% incidence of gastrointestinal bleeding. In this trial the maximum allowed dose to the duodenum or stomach was 68 Gy (BEN-JOSEF et al. 2005). The Mayo clinic analysis involving biliary cancers suggests that doses greater than 55 Gy with radiation (+/– chemotherapy or brachytherapy) resulted in severe gastrointestinal complications in 30%–40% of patients (BUSKIRK et al. 1992). BEN-DAVID et al. (2006) reported that acute toxicity associated with 3D conformal radiotherapy for extrahepatic carcinoma is generally mild. Late gastrointestinal toxicity was also acceptable (five patients, 6%). RILD occurred in two patients with hilar extrahepatic carcinoma who received high-dose radiotherapy (68 Gy and 81 Gy) with concurrent chemotherapy.
- **Arterial:** MANTEL et al. (2007) reported on vascular complications in patients undergoing orthotopic liver transplantation after neoadjuvant chemoradiation for hilar cholangiocarcinoma (MANTEL et al. 2007). Arterial complications arose in 21%, portal venous complications arose in 22%, and overall, 40% developed vascular complications. Late hepatic artery complications occurred more often in living donor recipients transplanted for cholangiocarcinoma compared with the living donor control group ($p = 0.047$). Liver transplantation with neoadjuvant therapy is associated with far higher rates of late arterial and portal venous complications, but these complications do not adversely affect patient and graft survival.

15.6 Post-Treatment Follow-Ups

- Life-long follow-up after definitive treatment of hepatobiliary cancers is usually indicated.

Schedule

- Follow-ups could be scheduled every 3–6 months initially in the first 3 years after treatment, then annually (Grade D) (NATIONAL COMPREHENSIVE CANCER NETWORK 2008).

Table 15.4. Follow-up schedule

Interval	Frequency
First 2 years	Every 3–6 months
Over 3 years	Annually

Work-Ups

- Each follow-up should include a complete history and physical examination. Laboratory tests include complete blood count and multichannel serum chemistry; radiologic imaging or endoscopy may be clinically indicated.
- For HCC, AFP can be performed every 3 months in the first 2 years, if the value was elevated prior to initial treatment (Grade D) (NATIONAL COMPREHENSIVE CANCER NETWORK 2008).
- For gallbladder cancer, imaging studies can be performed every 6 months for 2 years (Grade D) (NATIONAL COMPREHENSIVE CANCER NETWORK 2008).

References

Abou-Alfa GK, Schwartz L, Ricci S, Amadori D, Santoro A, Figer A, De Greve J, Douillard JY, Lathia C, Schwartz B, Taylor I, Moscovici M, Saltz LB (2006) Phase II study of sorafenib in patients with advanced hepatocellular carcinoma. J Clin Oncol 24:4293–4300

de Aretxabala XA, Roa IS, Burgos LA et al. (1997) Curative resection in potentially resectable tumours of the gallbladder. Eur J Surg 163:419–426

Arii S, Yamaoka Y, Futagawa S, Inoue K, Kobayashi K, Kojiro M, Makuuchi M, Nakamura Y, Okita K, Yamada R (2000) Results of surgical and nonsurgical treatment for small-sized hepatocellular carcinomas: a retrospective and nationwide survey in Japan. The Liver Cancer Study Group of Japan. Hepatology 32:1224–1229

Ben-David MA, Griffith KA, Abu-Isa E et al. (2006) External-beam radiotherapy for localized extrahepatic cholangiocarcinoma. Int J Radiat Oncol Biol Phys 66:772–779

Ben-Josef E, Normolle D, Ensminger WD et al. (2005) Phase II trial of high-dose conformal radiation therapy with concurrent hepatic artery floxuridine for unresectable intrahepatic malignancies. J Clin Oncol 23:8739–8747

Borgelt BB, Gelber R, Brady LW et al. (1981) The palliation of hepatic metastases: results of the Radiation Therapy Oncology Group pilot study. Int J Radiat Oncol Biol Phys 7:587–591

Bruix J, Llovet JM (2002) Prognostic prediction and treatment strategy in hepatocellular carcinoma. Hepatology 35(3):519–524

Buskirk SJ, Gunderson LL, Schild SE, Bender CE, Williams HJ Jr, McIlrath DC, Robinow JS, Tremaine WJ, Martin JK Jr (1992) Analysis of failure after curative irradiation of extrahepatic bile duct carcinoma. Ann Surg 215:125–131

Calvo FA, Meirino RM; Orecchia R (2006) Intraoperative radiation therapy first part: rationale and techniques. Crit Rev Oncol Hematol 59:106–115

Cancer of the Liver Italian Program (CLIP) Investigators (2000) Prospective validation of the CLIP score: a new prognostic system for patients with cirrhosis and hepatocellular carcinoma. Hepatology 31:840–845

Casamassima F, Cavedon C, Francescon P, Stancanello J, Avanzo M, Cora S, Scalchi P (2006) Use of motion tracking in stereotactic body radiotherapy: Evaluation of uncertainty in off-target dose distribution and optimization strategies Acta Oncol 45:943–947

Cubertafond P, Mathonnet M, Gainant A, Launois B (1999) Radical surgery for gallbladder cancer. Results of the French Surgical Association Survey. Hepatogastroenterology 46:1567–1571

Cupp JS, Koong AC, Fisher GA, Norton JA, Goodman KA (2008) Tissue effects after stereotactic body radiotherapy using cyberknife for patients with abdominal malignancies. Clin Oncol 20:69–75

Czito BG, Hurwitz HI, Clough RW et al. (2005) Adjuvant external-beam radiotherapy with concurrent chemotherapy after resection of primary gallbladder carcinoma: a 23-year experience. Int J Radiat Oncol Biol Phys 62:1030–1034

Dawson LA, Normolle D, Balter JM et al. (2002) Analysis of radiation-induced liver disease using the Lyman NTCP model. Int J Radiat Oncol Biol Phys 53:810–821

Dawson LA, Ten Haken RK (2005) Partial volume tolerance of the liver to radiation. Semin Radiat Oncol 15:279–283

Emami B, Lyman J, Brown A et al. (1991) Tolerance of normal tissue to therapeutic irradiation. Int J Radiat Oncol Biol Phys 21:109–122

Fattovich G, Giustina G, Schalm SW, Hadziyannis S, Sanchez-Tapias J, Almasio P, Christensen E, Krogsgaard K, Degos F, Carneiro de Moura M (1995) Occurrence of hepatocellular carcinoma and decompensation in western European patients with cirrhosis type B. The EUROHEP Study Group on Hepatitis B Virus and Cirrhosis. Hepatology 21:77–82

Ferro V, Dredge K, Liu L et al. (2007) PI-88 and novel heparan sulfate mimetics inhibit angiogenesis. Semin Thromb Hemost 33:557–568

Fong Y, Brennan MF, Turnbull A, Colt DG, Blumgart LH (1993) Gallbladder cancer discovered during laparoscopic surgery. Potential for iatrogenic tumor dissemination. Arch Surg 128:1054–1056

Fritz P, Brambs HJ, Schraube P, Freund U, Berns C, Wannenmacher M (1994) Combined external beam radiotherapy and intraluminal high dose rate brachytherapy on bile duct carcinomas. Int J Radiat Oncology Biol Phys 29:855–861

Furuse J, Okusaka T, Boku N, Ohkawa S, Sawaki A, Masumoto T, Funakoshi A (2008) S-1 monotherapy as first-line treatment in patients with advanced biliary tract cancer: a multicenter phase II study. Cancer Chemother Pharmacol Jan 23 [Epub ahead of print]

Gautam AM, Wilson EA, Chen PJ et al. (2007) Proc AACR Ann Meet 232:2650

Gerhards MF, van Gulik TM, González González D et al. (2003) Results of postoperative radiotherapy for resectable hilar cholangiocarcinoma. World J Surg 27:173–179

Geschwind JF, Salem R, Carr BI et al. (2004) Yttrium-90 microspheres for the treatment of hepatocellular carcinoma. Gastroenterology 127[5 Suppl 1]:S194–205

Gonzalez Gonzalez D, Gerard JP, Maners AW, De la Lande-Guyaux B, Van Dijk-Milatz A, Meerwaldt JH, Bosset JF, Van Dijk JD (1990) Results of radiation therapy in carcinoma of the proximal bile duct (Klatskin tumor). Semin Liver Dis 10:131–141

Greene F, Page D, Fleming I et al. (2002) AJCC Cancer Staging Manual, 6th edn. Springer, Berlin Heidelberg New York

Gunderson LL, Shipley WU, Suit HD, Epp ER, Nardi G, Wood W, Cohen A, Nelson J, Battit G, Biggs PJ, Russell A, Rockett A, Clark D (1982) Intraoperative irradiation: a pilot study combining external beam photons with „boost" dose intraoperative electrons. Cancer 49:2259–2266

Gunven P, Blomgren H, Lax I (2003) Radiosurgery for recurring liver metastases after hepatectomy. Hepatogastroenterology 50:1201–1204

Herfarth KK, Debus J, Lohr F, Bahner ML, Rhein B, Fritz P, Hoss A, Schlegel W, Wannenmacher MF (2001) Stereotactic single-dose radiation therapy of liver tumors: results of a phase I/II trial. J Clin Oncol 19:164–170

Ho CL, Yu SC, Yeung DW (2003) 11C-acetate PET imaging in hepatocellular carcinoma and other liver masses. J Nucl Med 44:213–221

Houry S, Schlienger M, Huguier M et al. (1989) Gallbladder carcinoma: role of radiation therapy. Br J Surg 76:448–450

Hughes MA, Frassica DA, Yeo CJ, Riall TS, Lillemoe KD, Cameron JL, Donehower RC, Laheru DA, Hruban RH, Abrams RA (2007) Adjuvant concurrent chemoradiation for adenocarcinoma of the distal common bile duct. Int J Radiat Oncol Biol Phys 68:178–182

Ingold JA, Reed GB, Kaplan HS, Bagshaw MA (1965) Radiation hepatitis. Am J Roentgenol Radium Ther Nucl Med 93:200–208

Ito H, Matros E, Brooks DC et al. (2004) Treatment outcomes associated with surgery for gallbladder cancer: a 20-year experience. J Gastrointest Surg 8:183–190

Iyer RV, Gibbs J, Kuvshinoff B, Fakih M, Kepner J, Soehnlein N, Lawrence D, Javle MM (2007) A phase II study of gemcitabine and capecitabine in advanced cholangiocarcinoma and carcinoma of the gallbladder: a single-institution prospective study. Ann Surg Oncol 14:3202–3209

Jarnagin WR, Ruo L, Little SA, Klimstra D, D'Angelica M, DeMatteo RP, Wagman R, Blumgart LH, Fong Y (2003) Patterns of initial disease recurrence after resection of gallbladder carcinoma and hilar cholangiocarcinoma: implications for adjuvant therapeutic strategies. Cancer 98:1689–1700

Jemal A, Siegel R, Ward E, Murray T, Xu J, Thun MJ (2007)) Cancer statistics, 2007. CA Cancer J Clin 57:43–66

Jonas S, Bechstein WO, Steinmuller T, Herrmann M, Radke C, Berg T, Settmacher U, Neuhaus P (2001) Vascular invasion and histopathologic grading determine outcome after liver transplantation for hepatocellular carcinoma in cirrhosis. Hepatology (Baltimore) 33:1080–1086

Kassahun WT, Fangmann J, Harms J et al. (2006) Liver resection and transplantation in the management of hepatocellular carcinoma: a review. Exp Clin Transplant 4:549–558

Kayahara M, Nagakawa T (2007) Recent trends of gallbladder cancer in Japan: an analysis of 4,770 patients. Cancer 110:572–580

Kim JY, Kim MH, Lee TY et al. (2008) Clinical role of 18F-FDG PET-CT in suspected and potentially operable cholangiocarcinoma: a prospective study compared with conventional imaging. Am J Gastroenterol 103:1145–1151

Kirilova A, Lockwood G, Choi P, Bana N, Haider MA, Brock KK, Eccles C, Dawson LA (2008) Three-dimensional motion of liver tumors using cine-magnetic resonance imaging. Int J Radiat Oncol Biol Phys 71:1189–1195

Knox JJ, Hedley D, Oza A, Feld R, Siu LL, Chen E, Nematollahi M, Pond GR, Zhang J, Moore MJ (2005) Combining gemcitabine and capecitabine in patients with advanced biliary cancer: a phase II trial. J Clin Oncol 23:2332–2338

Kopelson G, Galdabini J, Warshaw AL et al. (1981) Patterns of failure after curative surgery for extra-hepatic biliary tract carcinoma: implications for adjuvant therapy. Int J Radiat Oncol Biol Phys 7:413–417

Krempien R, Roeder F, Oertel S, Weitz J, Hensley FW, Timke C, Funk A, Lindel K, Harms W, Buchler MW, Debus J, Treiber M (2006) Intraoperative electron-beam therapy for primary and recurrent retroperitoneal soft-tissue sarcoma. IntJ Radiat Oncol Biol Phys 65:773–779

Kresl JJ, Schild SE, Henning GT et al. (2002) Adjuvant external beam radiation therapy with concurrent chemotherapy in the management of gallbladder carcinoma. Int J Radiat Oncol Biol Phys 52:167–175

Llovet JM, Bruix J (2003) Systematic review of randomized trials for unresectable hepatocellular carcinoma: chemoembolization improves survival. Hepatology 37:429–442

Mantel HT, Rosen CB, Heimbach JK, Nyberg SL, Ishitani MB, Andrews JC, McKusick MA, Haddock MG, Alberts SR Gores GJ (2007) Vascular complications after orthotopic liver transplantation after neoadjuvant therapy for hilar cholangiocarcinoma. Liver Transpl 13:1372–1381

Mendez Romero A, Wunderink W, Hussain SM, De Pooter JA, Heijmen BJ, Nowak PC, Nuyttens JJ, Brandwijk RP, Verhoef C, Ijzermans JN, Levendag PC (2006) Stereotactic body radiation therapy for primary and metastatic liver tumors: a single institution phase I/II study. Acta Oncol 45:831–837

Milano MT, Chmura SJ, Garofalo MC et al. (2004) Intensity-modulated radiotherapy in treatment of pancreatic and bile duct malignancies: toxicity and clinical outcome. Int J Radiat Oncol Biol Phys 59:445–453

Miller G, Schwartz LH, D'Angelica M (2007) The use of imaging in the diagnosis and staging of hepatobiliary malignancies. Surg Oncol Clin N Am 16:343–368

Mojica P, Smith D, Ellenhorn J (2007) Adjuvant radiation therapy is associated with improved survival for gallbladder carcinoma with regional metastatic disease. J Surg Oncol 96:8–13

Mulier S, Mulier P, Ni Y et al. (2002) Complications of radiofrequency coagulation of liver tumours. Br J Surg 89:1206–1222

Nagorney DM, Kendrick ML (2006) Hepatic resection in the treatment of hilar cholangiocarcinoma. Adv Surg 40:159–171

Nakeeb A, Pitt HA, Sohn TA, Coleman J, Abrams RA, Piantadosi S, Hruban RH, Lillemoe KD, Yeo CJ, Cameron JL (1996) Cholangiocarcinoma. A spectrum of intrahepatic, perihilar, and distal tumors. Ann Surg 224:463–473; discussion 473–475

National Comprehensive Cancer Network (2008) Clinical practice guidelines in oncology: hepatobiliary cancer. Version 2.2008. Available at http://www.nccn.org/professionals/physician_gls/PDF/hepatobiliary.pdf. Accessed on March 30, 2008

Oliva MR, Saini S (2004) Liver cancer imaging: role of CT, MRI, US and PET. Cancer Imaging 4 Spec No A:S42–6

Ono T, Yamanoi A, Nazmy El Assal O et al. (2001) Adjuvant chemotherapy after resection of hepatocellular carcinoma causes deterioration of long-term prognosis in cirrhotic patients: metaanalysis of three randomized controlled trials. Cancer 91:2378–2385

Pang RW, Poon RT (2007) From molecular biology to targeted therapies for hepatocellular carcinoma: the future is now. Oncology 72[Suppl 1]:30–44

Pawlik TM, Delman KA, Vauthey JN et al. (2005) Tumor size predicts vascular invasion and histologic grade: implications for selection of surgical treatment for hepatocellular carcinoma. Liver Transpl 11:1086–1092

Pawlik TM, Gleisner AL, Vigano L et al. (2007) Incidence of finding residual disease for incidental gallbladder carcinoma: implications for re-resection. J Gastrointest Surg 11:1478–1487

Piehler JM, Crichlow RW (1978) Primary carcinoma of the gallbladder. Surg Gyn Obstet 147:929–942

Poon RT, Fan ST, Lo CM et al. (2000) Long-term prognosis after resection of hepatocellular carcinoma associated with hepatitis B-related cirrhosis. J Clin Oncol 18:1094–1101

Rea DJ, Heimbach JK, Rosen CB et al. (2005) Liver transplantation with neoadjuvant chemoradiation is more effective than resection for hilar cholangiocarcinoma. Ann Surg 242:451-458; discussion 458-461

Reid KM, Ramos-De la Medina A, Donohue JH (2007) Diagnosis and surgical management of gallbladder cancer: a review. J Gastrointest Surg 11:671–681

Ruckert JC, Ruckert RI, Gellert K, Hecker K, Muller JM (1996) Surgery for carcinoma of the gallbladder. Hepatogastroenterology 43:527–533

Sagawa N, Kondo S, Morikawa T, Okushiba S, Katoh H (2005) Effectiveness of radiation therapy after surgery for hilar cholangiocarcinoma. Surg Today 35:548–552

Salem R, Thurston KG (2006) Radioembolization with yttrium-90 microspheres: a state-of-the-art brachytherapy treatment for primary and secondary liver malignancies: part 3: comprehensive literature review and future direction. J Vasc Interv Radiol 17:1571–1593

Schwartz JD, Schwartz M, Mandeli J et al. (2002) Neoadjuvant and adjuvant therapy for resectable hepatocellular carcinoma: review of the randomised clinical trials. Lancet Oncol 3:593–603

Seo DD, Lee HC, Jang MK et al. (2007) Preoperative portal vein embolization and surgical resection in patients with hepatocellular carcinoma and small future liver remnant volume: comparison with transarterial chemoembolization. Ann Surg Oncol 14:3501–3509

Serafini FM, Sachs D, Bloomston M, Carey LC, Karl RC, Murr MM Rosemurgy AS (2001) Location, not staging, of cholangiocarcinoma determines the role for adjuvant chemoradiation therapy. Am Surg 67:839–843; discussion 843–844

Seyama Y, Makuuchi M (2007) Current surgical treatment for bile duct cancer. World J Gastroenterol 13:1505–1515

Shimada H, Endo I, Fujii Y et al. (2000) Appraisal of surgical resection of gallbladder cancer with special reference to lymph node dissection. Langenbecks Arch Surg 385:509–514

Shimada H, Endo I, Togo S et al. (1997) The role of lymph node dissection in the treatment of gallbladder carcinoma. Cancer 79:892–899

Sutherland LM, Williams JA, Padbury RT, Gotley DC, Stokes B, Maddern GJ (2006) Radiofrequency ablation of liver tumors: a systematic review. Arch Surg 141:181–190

Takada T, Amano H, Yasuda H et al. (2002) Is postoperative adjuvant chemotherapy useful for gallbladder carcinoma? A phase III multicenter prospective randomized controlled trial in patients with resected pancreaticobiliary carcinoma. Cancer 95:1685–1695

Thomas MB (2007) Biological characteristics of cancers in the gallbladder and biliary tract and targeted therapy. Crit Rev Oncol Hematol 61:44–51

Todoroki T, Iwasaki Y, Orii K et al. (1991) Resection combined with intraoperative radiation therapy (IORT) for stage IV (TNM) gallbladder carcinoma. World J Surg 15:357–366

Todoroki T, Kawamoto T, Otsuka M et al. (1997) IORT combined with resection for stage IV gallbladder carcinoma. Front Radiat Ther Oncol 31:165–172

Todoroki T, Ohara K, Kawamoto T, Koike N, Yoshida S, Kashiwagi H, Otsuka M, Fukao K (2000) Benefits of adjuvant radiotherapy after radical resection of locally advanced main hepatic duct carcinoma. Int J Radiat Oncol Biol Phys 46:581–587

Tse RV, Hawkins M, Lockwood G, Kim JJ, Cummings B, Knox J, Sherman M; Dawson LA (2008) Phase I study of individualized stereotactic body radiotherapy for hepatocellular carcinoma and intrahepatic cholangiocarcinoma. J Clin Oncol 26:657–664

Wakai T, Shirai Y, Moroda T, Yokoyama N, Hatakeyama K (2005) Impact of ductal resection margin status on long-term survival in patients undergoing resection for extrahepatic cholangiocarcinoma. Cancer 103:1210–1216

Weber SM, DeMatteo RP, Fong Y et al. (2002) Staging laparoscopy in patients with extrahepatic biliary carcinoma. Analysis of 100 patients. Ann Surg 235:392–399

Weber SM, Jarnagin WR, Klimstra D, DeMatteo RP, Fong Y, Blumgart LH (2001) Intrahepatic cholangiocarcinoma: resectability, recurrence pattern, and outcomes. J Am Coll Surg 193:384–391

Wulf J, Guckenberger M, Haedinger U, Oppitz U, Mueller G, Baier K, Flentje M (2006) Stereotactic radiotherapy of primary liver cancer and hepatic metastases. Acta Oncologica (Stockholm, Sweden) 45:838–847

Yao FY, Ferrell L, Bass NM et al. (2001) Liver transplantation for hepatocellular carcinoma: expansion of the tumor size limits does not adversely impact survival. Hepatology 33:1394–1403

Yeo CJ, Sohn TA, Cameron JL, Hruban RH, Lillemoe KD, Pitt HA (1998) Periampullary adenocarcinoma: analysis of 5-year survivors. Ann Surg 227:821–831

Yoo HY, Patt CH, Geschwind JF (2003) The outcome of liver transplantation in patients with hepatocellular carcinoma in the United States between 1988 and 2001: 5-year survival has improved significantly with time. J Clin Oncol 21:4329–4335

Yoon KT, Kim JK, Kim do Y, Ahn SH, Lee JD, Yun M, Rha SY, Chon CY, Han KH (2007) Role of 18F-fluorodeoxyglucose positron emission tomography in detecting extrahepatic metastasis in pretreatment staging of hepatocellular carcinoma. Oncology 72[Suppl 1]:104–110

Zhou ZH, Liu LM, Chen WW et al. (2007) Combined therapy of transcatheter arterial chemoembolisation and three-dimensional conformal radiotherapy for hepatocellular carcinoma. Br J Radiol 80:194–201

Zimmerman MA, Ghobrial RM, Tong MJ, Hiatt JR, Cameron AM, Hong J, Busuttil RW (2008) Recurrence of hepatocellular carcinoma following liver transplantation: a review of preoperative and postoperative prognostic indicators. Arch Surg 143:182–188; discussion 188

Rectal Cancer

Bradley J. Huth and Luther W. Brady

CONTENTS

B. J. Huth, MD
Department of Radiation Oncology, Drexel University College of Medicine, 216 N. Broad St., 1st Floor Feinstein Building, Mail Stop 200, Philadelphia, PA 19102-1192, USA
L. W. Brady, MD
Department of Radiation Oncology, Drexel University College of Medicine, Broad & Vine Streets, Mail Stop 200, Philadelphia, PA 19102-1192, USA

Introduction and Objectives

Rectal cancers account for approximately 12% of all colorectal cancers diagnosed in the United States. While their histology closely mimics that of colon cancers, their anatomical location below the peritoneal reflection allows them to easily infiltrate the surrounding soft tissues of the pelvis. The close proximity to the anal sphincter and genitourinary structures makes surgical excision more complex with the potential to affect quality of life at early stages of the disease. For these reasons, combined modality therapy plays a vital role in both the neoadjuvant and adjuvant settings.

This chapter examines:

- Recommendations for diagnosis and staging procedures
- The staging systems and prognostic factors
- Treatment recommendations as well as the supporting scientific evidence for surgical excision and neoadjuvant and adjuvant treatment for resectable rectal cancers
- Palliative radiation (external-beam radiation therapy and brachytherapy) for symptomatic control in advanced disease
- Follow-up care and surveillance of survivors

16.1 Diagnosis, Staging, and Prognosis

16.1.1 Diagnosis

Initial Evaluation

- Diagnosis and evaluation of rectal cancer begin with a complete history and physical examination (H&P). Special attention should be given to signs and symptoms specific to rectal cancer, including gross red blood alone, with stool or mucus, changes in stool caliber and bowel habits, including constipation, diarrhea, tenesmus, and incomplete emptying, genitourinary symptoms or pain in the buttocks, perineum or sciatic nerve distribution, personal history of colorectal cancer, colonic polyps, or inflammatory bowel disease.

- Complete physical examination should be performed with attention to the hepatic enlargement or pain and digital rectal exam noting the size, mobility, and distance from the anal verge of any palpable mass. For female patients, a rectovaginal exam should be included.
- Rigid proctoscopy and colonoscopy allow for better characterization, biopsy, and measurement of distance from the anal verge of the primary lesion. A complete colonoscopy should be performed to evaluate for additional lesions within the colon. If a colonoscope cannot be passed by the lesion at the time of diagnosis, then a complete colonoscopy should be performed within a few months following definitive therapy.

Laboratory Tests

- Baseline laboratory tests should include a carcinoembryonic antigen level (CEA), complete blood count, basic blood chemistry, liver function tests, and renal function tests (Table 16.1).

Table 16.1. Imaging and laboratory work-ups for rectal cancer

Imaging studies	Laboratory tests
High-resolution pelvic MRI	CEA
Endoscopic ultrasonography (EUS)	Complete blood count
	Serum chemistry
CT of chest and abdomen	Liver function tests
PET/CT if evaluating oligometastatic disease	Renal function tests

Imaging Studies

- Clinical staging using endoscopic ultrasound or MRI with pelvic or endorectal coils should be performed. Each modality provides excellent guidance in the staging of the primary lesion, but is less effective in staging regional nodal disease. The specific modality selected will vary with an institution's expertise and equipment availability (Table 16.1).
- High-resolution pelvic MRI may be performed to evaluate the depth of invasion and extent of circumferential spread. Evaluation of the regional lymph nodes is slightly less accurate than

EUS. Preoperative pelvic MRI consistently predicts the surgical circumferential margin, leading to appropriate risk stratification of patients (Grade A). Prediction of the radial margin status can be predicted in as much as 94% of cases when high-resolution MR imaging is obtained (Level I) (Lahaye et al. 2005) (Level II) (Brown et al. 2003, Beets-Tan et al. 2001, MERCURY Study Group 2006).

- Endoscopic ultrasonography (EUS) may be performed to determine the lesion's depth of invasion and to evaluate regional lymph nodes for metastatic spread. The sensitivity and specificity of EUS approach 94% and 86% for invasion to the muscularis propria, 90% and 75% for perirectal tissue, and 67% and 78% for lymph nodes (Level I and III) (Bipat et al. 2004; Chun et al. 2006; Massari et al. 1998).
- Interobserver evaluations of T3/4 lesions have been shown to be consistent, while T1/2 lesions display greater variability (Level III) (Burtin et al. 1997).
- CT evaluation of the chest, abdomen, and pelvis with both oral and intravenous contrast is recommended for evaluation of metastasis (Grade A).
- CT evaluation of direct extension to adjacent organs and regional nodal spread, its use in the evaluation of depth of invasion, and circumferential spread are inadequate for preoperative stratification (Level II) (Bipat et al. 2004; Kulinna et al. 2004; Matsuoka et al. 2003; Wolberink et al. 2007).
- PET/CT for the staging of early disease may aid in target delineation, but is experimental and generally not recommended (Grade B) (Level III) (Bassi et al. 2007).

Pathology

- Tissue for pathologic diagnosis can be obtained during initial examination using proctoscopy or endoscopy.
- Pathologic confirmation of rectal cancer is mandatory. More than 90% of rectal cancers are of adenocarcinoma histology. Mucinous variations account for 20%, with 2% being signet ring variants. More rare histologies include squamous cell, carcinoid, lymphomas, and leiomyosarcomas.
- Pathologic margins (proximal, distal, and radial) are key to the treatment and prognosis of rectal cancer. It is unclear if margins ≤2 mm should be considered positive.

16.1.2 Staging

- Rectal cancer may be staged either clinically or pathologically. Clinical staging is based on H&P findings and imaging modalities. Pathologic staging is based on examination of the surgical specimen. The high frequency of neoadjuvant treatment frequently results in pathologic downstaging if more than 7 days elapse between the completion of neoadjuvant therapy and surgery.
- The 2002 American Joint Committee on Cancer Tumor Node Metastasis (TNM) staging system is presented in Table 16.2 (GREENE et al. 2002).
- DUKES (1932) staging was based on the extent of bowel wall penetration and the presence or absence of nodal metastasis. ASTLER and COLLER (1954) staging described specific tumor penetration and nodal metastasis with a later modification specifying adherence to surrounding organs. Both systems are antiquated and do not account for neoadjuvant treat effects.

16.1.3 Prognostic Factors

- TNM stage is the most important prognostic factor in predicting outcome. Patients may be categorized as having low or high risk of recurrence. Low risk includes patient stage T1/T2 through N+ or T3N0. High risk includes patients with stage T3N+ through T4N+. Overall survival and relapse-free survival at 5 years measure 76% and 73% for low risk and 55% and 48% for high risk patients, respectively (INT-0114). Table 16.3 depicts recurrence-free and overall survival at 5 years by AJCC stage.
- T stage predicts response to neoadjuvant treatment with worse prognosis and higher risk of local recurrence in T4 disease, as demonstrated in results of retrospective studies as well as pooled analysis of data from multiple prospective randomized trials (Grade A) (Level III) (STOCCHI et al. 2001; GUNDERSON et al. 2004), and the RTOG 0012 (MOHIUDDIN et al. 2006).
- Nodal stage predicts recurrence risk and survival (Grade A) (Level IV) (STOCCHI et al. 2001; GUNDERSON et al. 2004; KIM et al. 2006) (Table 16.3). The number of nodes analyzed in surgical specimens correlates with time to recurrence and survival in node-negative patients, ranging from 37% for 1–4 nodes to 19% for 8–12 nodes. Evaluating >14 nodes is recommended for determination of nodal stage (Grade B) (Level II and III) (TEPPER et al. 2001; BAXTER and GARCIA-AGUILAR 2005).
- Higher grade and mucinous adenocarcinomas show worse prognosis, specifically with signet ring histology.

Table 16.2. American Joint Committee on Cancer (AJCC) TNM classification of colorectal cancer. [From GREENE et al. (2002) with permission]

Primary tumor (T)	
TX	Primary tumor cannot be assessed
T0	No evidence of primary tumor
Tis	Carcinoma in situ: intraepithelial or invasion of the lamina propria
T1	Tumor invades submucosa
T2	Tumor invades muscularis propria
T3	Tumor invades through the muscularis propria into the subserosa, or into nonperitonealized pericolic or perirectal tissues
T4	Tumor is adherent to or directly invades other organs or structures, and/or perforates the visceral peritoneum
Regional lymph nodes (N)	
NX	Regional lymph node metastasis cannot be assessed
N0	No regional lymph node metastasis
N1	Metastasis to 1–3 regional lymph nodes
N2	Metastasis to 4 or more regional lymph nodes
Distant metastasis (M)	
MX	Distant metastasis cannot be assessed
M0	No distant metastasis
M1	Distant metastasis present
STAGE GROUPING	
0:	Tis N0 M0
I:	T1–2 N0 M0
IIA:	T3 N0 M0
IIB:	T4 N0 M0
IIIA:	T1–2 N1 M0
IIIB:	T3–4 N1 M0
IIIC:	Any T N2 M0
IV:	Any T Any N M1

■ Circumferential margin status at the time of resection predicts local recurrence at the anastomosis and distant metastasis (Grade A). A positive margin following neoadjuvant therapy is more ominous, with a hazard ratio of 6.3 following neoadjuvant treatment versus 2.0 with no prior therapy (Level I) (NAGTEGAAL and QUIRKE 2008).

■ Elevated preoperative CEA predicts relapse with a cut-off of 5 ng/ml (YOON et al. 2007; KIM et al. 2006).

■ Operative method, age, gender, ploidy status, and S-phase fraction in resected specimens have not consistently correlated with recurrence or survival.

■ Locoregional recurrence is the dominant means of failure, with nodal metastasis and deep invasion strongly predicting outcomes.

Table 16.3. The 5-year recurrence-free survival (RFS) and overall survival (OS) by TNM stage. [From O'CONNELL et al. (2004) and PLATELL and SEMMENS (2004)]

	RFS	OS
Stage I	88%	90%
Stage II	62%	72%
Stage III	50%	52%
Stage IV	N/A	7%

16.2 Treatment of Resectable Rectal Cancer

16.2.1 General Principles

■ Surgical resection remains the primary treatment in the management of rectal cancers. Management depends on stage and location of the tumor. Figure 16.1 provides a graphical treatment algorithm.

■ Tis and T1 without high risk features (e.g., LVI, high grade, positive margins) may be locally excised and followed closely.

■ Combined-modality therapy (surgery, radiation, and chemotherapy) is recommended for most patients with Stage II and greater disease (Grade A). While there is general agreement on the use of combined-modality treatment, a specific method and timing are not standardized.

■ Multiple trials evaluating both neoadjuvant and adjuvant radiation with and without chemotherapy have been explored. Local control rates are clearly improved with radiotherapy, while overall survival is effected less.

■ While increasing T-stage generally increases the risk of recurrence, retrospective analyses have shown a subset of patients with T3N0 whose 10 year actuarial recurrence is less than 10% (Level IV) (WILLETT et al. 1999; MERCHANT et al. 1999). Predictors of local recurrence included lymphovascular invasion (LVI) and invasion into perirectal fat ≥ 2 mm in this subset of patients.

16.2.2 Surgical Resection

■ Presentation of most tumors requires extensive resection of mesorectal tissue and all disease, both gross and microscopic.

■ Transanal local excision may be selected for early cancers (T1, <3 cm, well differentiated, within 8 cm of the anal verge, encompassing <30% of rectal wall circumference, and clinically node negative). The specimen should be of full thickness and have ≥ 3-mm negative margin. The 5-year local control rates approach 80% and survival 72% in T1 disease (BAXTER and GARCIA-AGUILAR 2007; NASCIMBENI et al. 2004).

■ Low anterior (LAR) and abdominoperineal resections (APR) with total mesorectal excision (TME) have become the standard of care for radical resection of rectal cancers (Grade A). Overall and cancer-specific survivals for stage II and III patients treated with standardized TME were 70% and 75%, respectively, and 43% and 52% for those treated without standard TME (Level I) (ARBMAN et al. 1996; HAVENGA et al. 1999; BOLOGNESE et al. 2000).

■ The increased difficulty of APR with TME due to thin mesorectal tissue near the anus, close proximity to genitourinary structures, and permanent colostomy detracts from its use.

16.2.3 Preoperative (Neoadjuvant) Treatment

■ While the oncology community agrees on the use of combined modality therapy, great debate rages

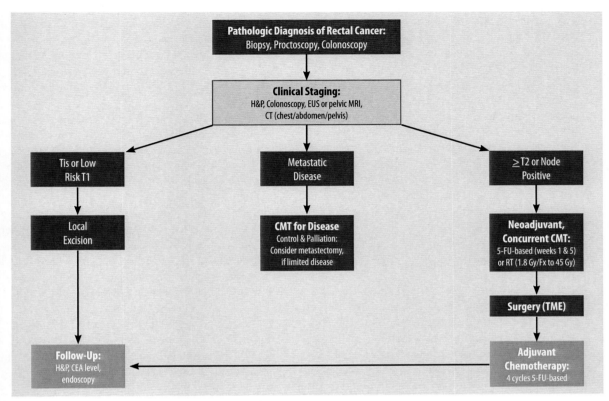

Fig. 16.1. Invasive Rectal Cancer treatment Algorithm

over the use of neoadjuvant versus adjuvant therapy. Proponents of neoadjuvant therapy believe that it improves sphincter preservation and thereby quality of life, allows otherwise unresectable disease to be surgically excised, and delivers improved outcomes of local control. Opponents contend that the surgical procedures are made more difficult following radiation, healing is impaired, and overtreatment of early stage patients occurs.

Preoperative Radiation Therapy

- Neoadjuvant radiation alone effectively improves local control (Grade A). Although neoadjuvant radiation with a biologically effective dose ≥30 Gy provides significant improvement in local failure (odds ratio =0.49) and cancer-specific survival (odds ratio =0.71) at 5 years, it does not improve overall survival or the rate of distant metastasis (Level I) (CAMMÀ et al. 2000; COLORECTAL CANCER COLLABORATIVE GROUP 2001).

The Dutch Colorectal Cancer Group (CKVO 95-04) compared short course, neoadjuvant radiotherapy followed by TME to TME alone in 1861 matched patients with clinically resectable disease. A total dose of 25 Gy in 5-Gy fractions was delivered over 5 days. Initial data at 2 years showed a decrease in local recurrence (8% vs. 2%). This difference remained at 5 years, 5.6% in the RT+TME arm and 10.9% for TME alone. The greatest benefit was seen in patients with midrectal tumor, negative circumferential margins, and positive nodes. There was no benefit in the RT+TME arm as compared to TME alone on overall survival, with 64.2% and 63.5%, respectively (Level II) (KAPITEIJN et al. 2001; PEETERS et al. 2007).

The Swedish Rectal Cancer Trial randomized 1168 patients with resectable, rectal cancers to 25 Gy in five fractions preoperatively versus surgery alone. The 5-year recurrence rates for preoperative RT versus surgery alone were 12% and 27%, respectively. An absolute overall survival benefit of 10% favoring the preoperative RT arm was noted. This trial has been criticized for lacking TME in the surgery only arm, leading to the high failure rate (Level II) (SWEDISH RECTAL CANCER TRIAL 1997; DAHLBERG et al. 1999).

The French Lyon R96-02 trial evaluated T2/T3, Nx, M0 rectal cancers encompassing less than two thirds of the rectum by comparing external-beam radiotherapy (39 Gy in 13 fractions) to the same external beam dose plus a contact X-ray therapy boost to 85 Gy in three fractions. A total of 88 patients were randomized. An increase in the complete response rate was noted between the boost and no boost groups, with 24% versus 2%, respectively. Sphincter preservation was also significantly improved in the boost arm (76% vs. 44%, $p=0.004$). Morbidity, survival, and local control were similar (Level II) (Gerard et al. 2004).

Preoperative (Neoadjuvant) Chemoradiotherapy

- As the specifics of combined-modality treatment evolve, concurrent radiation with a fluoropyrimidine-based chemotherapy regimen is generally recommended (Grade A). The effect of combined preoperative chemoradiation therapy has been demonstrated in a number of randomized trials: The EORTC 22921 trial evaluated neoadjuvant chemotherapy and radiation and the use of adjuvant chemotherapy. In all, 1011 patients with resectable T3 or T4 rectal cancer were randomized to preoperative radiation or chemotherapy, preoperative radiation and chemotherapy, preoperative chemotherapy and radiation with postoperative chemotherapy, or preoperative chemotherapy and postoperative chemotherapy. Radiotherapy consisted of 45 Gy over 5 weeks. Chemotherapy consisted of 5-FU/leucovorin (LV) for 5 days for two cycles of preoperative arms and an additional four cycles in the postoperative arms. The 5-year local recurrence rate in the arms receiving any chemotherapy was approximately 8.5%, while the arm receiving radiation alone was 17% ($p=0.002$). Overall survival was the same (EORTC 22921, Level I) (Bosset et al. 2006).
The German Rectal Cancer Study Group evaluated preoperative versus postoperative chemotherapy and radiation. The trial randomized 823 patients with clinical T3, T4, or node-positive rectal cancer to preoperative radiation (50.4 Gy) with 120-h infusional 5-FU during weeks 1 and 5 of radiation followed by surgery and four cycles of postoperative 5-FU. The postoperative chemoradiation arm included an additional 5.4-Gy boost to the tumor bed. The 5-year overall survival remained the same in the two arms (75%), while local failure was higher in the postoperative than the preoperative arm, at 13% and 6%, respectively. Toxicity was also less in the preoperative arm (German Rectal Cancer Study Group, Level I) (Sauer et al. 2004).
The French rectal cancer trial (FFCD 9203) compared preoperative radiation with preoperative chemoradiation in 733 patients with T3/T4, Nx rectal cancer who were randomized to preoperative radiation (45 Gy over 5 weeks) with or without 5-FU/LV during the 1st and 5th weeks of radiation. All patients were treated with surgery and postoperative 5-FU/LV. At 5 years, the local recurrence rate was lower in the chemoradiation arm than in the radiation arm, with 8% and 16%, respectively. Differences in overall survival and sphincter preservation were not significant (FFCD 9203, Level I) (Gerard et al. 2006).

- The use of oxaliplatin- and capecitabine-based regimens is based on data extrapolated from colon cancer trials. Clinical trials examining their use in rectal cancer are warranted.

16.2.4 Postoperative (Adjuvant) Treatment

Postoperative Radiation Therapy

- Postoperative radiation allows selection only of patients with high-risk features who would benefit from adjuvant care. Drawbacks to adjuvant RT include hypoxia of the post-surgical tumor bed and increased small bowel in the pelvis resulting in increased toxicity.
- Multiple trials have evaluated the timing of radiation in the treatment of rectal cancer. Preoperative radiation shows higher levels of local control and less morbidity, especially when combined with chemotherapy (Grade A).
The Uppsala trial compared short-course preoperative radiation (25.5 Gy over 5 days) to conventional fractionation postoperative treatment (60 Gy over 8 weeks). A total of 471 patients with resectable rectal cancer were randomized. Preoperative treatment was better tolerated. The local recurrence rate was significantly lower after preoperative than after postoperative radiotherapy (12% versus 21%; $p=0.02$) (Level I) (Pahlman and Glimelius 1990).

- The NSABP R-03 and Intergroup 0147 trials were designed to evaluate preoperative versus postoperative therapy, but both closed early due to poor accrual. The NSABP R-03 trial published preliminary 3-year data with 253 of the planned 900 patients that demonstrated improved survival and local control rates in the preoperative treatment arm. This was not statistically significant (NSABP R-03/INT 0147, Level II) (ROH et al. 2004).

- Local excision followed by adjuvant therapy has been explored. CHAKRAVARTI et al. (1999) reported long-term follow-up on 99 patients with transanal excision treated with and without adjuvant radiation. Of the 47 patients treated with adjuvant radiation, 26 also received concurrent 5-FU. Rates for 5-year local control and disease-free survival were 72% and 66%, respectively, for the local excision only group, and 90% and 74%, respectively, for the adjuvant therapy group (Level IV).

Postoperative Chemotherapy

- Based on subset analysis from randomized trials, select T3N0 patients with high rectal tumors and without adverse features may have adequate local control from surgery and may not benefit from further local radiotherapy. This select group may be best treated with surgery and adjuvant chemotherapy (Grade C) (Level IV) (GUNDERSON et al. 2004).

Postoperative Chemoradiotherapy

- The type of chemotherapy administered with radiation remains 5-FU-based; 5-FU with or without LV appears to be equal in efficacy, but bolus 5-FU demonstrated increased hematologic toxicity (Grade A). A sandwich-based regimen is recommended. This consists of two cycles of chemotherapy followed by concurrent chemoradiation (weeks 1 and 5 of RT) and then two final cycles of chemotherapy (Grade B).
Two Intergroup Trials (0114 and 0144) evaluated a postoperative 5-FU-based regimens with adjuvant radiation. Both had similar endpoints and results. Intergroup 0114 examined postoperative adjuvant chemotherapy and radiation therapy in 1695 patients with T3/T4 and node-positive rectal cancer following potentially surgery. Patients were treated by sandwich chemotherapy and radiation, consisting of two cycles of chemotherapy

followed by concurrent chemoradiation (45 Gy with a boost to 50.4–54 Gy) and followed by two final cycles of chemotherapy. The chemotherapy regimens consisted of bolus 5-FU, 5-FU/LV, 5-FU and levamisole, and 5-FU, LV, and levamisole. No difference in overall survival (60%), disease-free survival (52%), and local control (14%) was found (INT 0114/INT 0144, Level I) (TEPPER et al. 2002; SMALLEY et al. 2006).

KROOK et al. (1991) evaluated 204 patients with deeply invasive or node-positive rectal cancers treated with postoperative radiation (45–50.4 Gy) alone or in combination with 5-FU. Patients within the chemoradiation arm received one cycle of 5-FU and semustine before and after radiation. Results at a median follow-up of 7 years were reported. The combined modality arm showed significant improvement in local control and cancer-specific death (Level I) KROOK et al. 1991).

The Gastrointestinal Tumor Study Group (GITSG) protocol GI-7175 evaluated 227 patients with Astler and Colle rectal cancer, randomized to observation, postoperative chemotherapy, postoperative radiotherapy, and combined radiotherapy and chemotherapy. Results of the study showed a significant improvement in combined modality treatment over no adjuvant therapy for time to recurrence ($p=0.005$) and for survival ($p=0.01$) (Level I) (THOMAS et al. 1988).

16.3 Treatment of Locally Advanced Unresectable Rectal Cancer

16.3.1 General Principles

- Current chemotherapy and radiation therapy comprise the standard treatment for locally advanced and surgically unresectable rectal cancer (Grade A).

- The role of surgery after combined modality therapy depends on the likelihood of obtaining clear margins and the patient's willingness to undergo radical treatment.

- Retrospective analysis of 55 patients treated at Memorial Sloan-Kettering with pelvic exenteration showed that 70% of those treated were recurrent, while only 30% had primary colorectal cancer. Most had previous radiotherapy and had a previous APR. In all, 49% received intraoperative radiation at the time of resection, and median survival was 48 months (Level IV) (Jimenez et al. 2003).

■ Using intraoperative radiotherapy (IORT) at Memorial Sloan-Kettering, 68 patients over a 4-year period were treated with neoadjuvant 5-FU/LV followed by surgery and IORT. High-dose-rate IORT consisted of a 10- to 20-Gy fraction delivered using the Harrison-Anderson-Mick applicator. Median follow-up was 17.5 months. Of the minority of primary cases, 81% had local control at 2 years. For patients with recurrent disease, the 2-year local control rate was 63% (Level IV) (Harrison et al. 1998).

16.4 Radiation Therapy

16.4.1 Simulation and Field Arrangement

■ A treatment-planning CT study is recommended for defining gross tumor volume (GTV) and planning target volume (PTV) with the patient in the treatment position.

■ Prone position on a belly board is preferred, although patient mobility may demand supine. Patients should have a full bladder. Radiopaque markers should include anal, vaginal, and perineal skin. Oral and rectal contrasts delineate the small bowel and GTV. If present, the perineal scar should be wired.

■ Photons of 10 MV or higher energy should be used with a three- or four-field box technique. Figure 16.2 details typical prone and supine three-field arrangements.

■ If using 2D technique, posterior-anterior borders include L5–S1 superiorly, 5 cm below the GTV or the inferior aspect of the obturator foramen (whichever is more inferior) inferiorly, and 1.5 cm outside the pelvic inlet laterally. Lateral field borders should be behind the sacrum posteriorly. The anterior border should be 4 cm anterior to the rectum; if T4, the border should be 4 cm anterior to gross disease or anterior to the pubic arch.

■ If using 3D conformal technique, the clinical tumor volume (CTV) should include GTV plus a 2-cm margin and nodal drainage. At risk nodes include the presacral, pelvic mesentery, and in-

ternal iliac nodes. External iliac nodes may be included for T4 disease.

■ A boost field should include the initial GTV plus 2 cm and the sacral hollow.

■ Intensity-modulated radiation therapy is beginning to be explored. Well-designed clinical trials are pending.

16.4.2 Dose and Fraction

■ Continuous course radiation is recommended over split course therapy (Grade A). RTOG 81-15 examined preoperative 5 Gy versus surgery alone. All patients with T3 or node-positive rectal cancer received postoperative RT to 45 Gy. At 5 years overall survival for both groups was 54%. Local recurrence was 26% for patients with preoperative RT and 29% for those with no preoperative RT (Level I) (Sause et al. 1994).

■ Standard fractionation (1.8 Gy/day) up to 45–50.4 Gy is recommended for patients receiving chemoradiation either pre- or postoperatively (Grade A). If postoperative, an additional boost of 5.4–9 Gy is recommended depending on the whole pelvis dose and the amount of small bowel in the field.

■ Hyperfractionated RT (between 1.2 Gy BID and 50.4 Gy) with neoadjuvant chemotherapy was examined by RTOG 00-12, but similar rates of downstaging, tumor response, and toxicity compared to standard fractionation were found (Level I) (Mohiuddin et al. 2006).

■ Short-course, high-dose per fraction RT (25 Gy in five fractions) is viable as neoadjuvant therapy, as mentioned above; however, this regimen has not been evaluated with concurrent chemotherapy (Grade A).

16.4.3 Brachytherapy

■ Intraoperative, interstitial, and endocavitary radiation improves local control in locally advanced and recurrent rectal cancers (Grade B). Doses of 10–20 Gy are generally delivered, with higher doses used for gross residual disease and patients unable to receive external-beam therapy (Level III) (Nuyttens et al. 2004) (Level IV) (Alektiar et al. 2000).

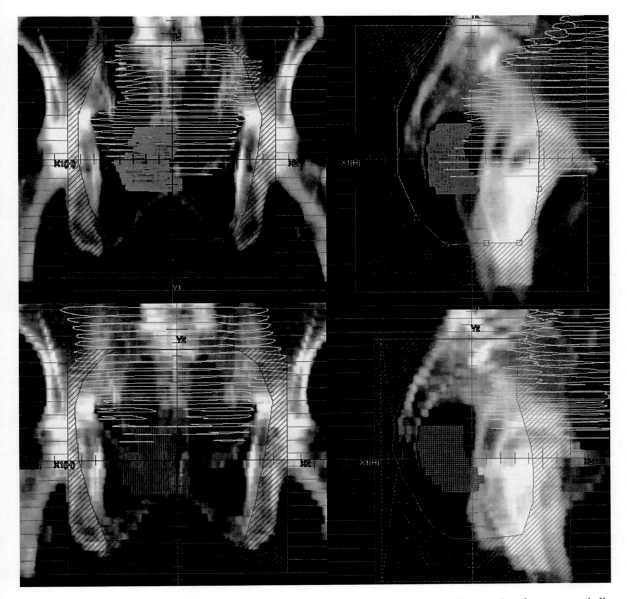

Fig. 16.2. Standard 3-Field PA and Lateral Portals in the same patient simulated supine (*Top Row*) and prone on a belly board (*Bottom Row*). The GTV is contoured in green and small bowel is in yellow

■ Experience with intraoperative electron therapy (IOERT) at Massachusetts General was reported by Nakfoor et al. (1998). They described 73 patients with locally advanced rectal cancer who received IOERT at surgery due to tumor adherence or residual disease. All patients received neoadjuvant RT, most with concurrent 5-FU. At 5 years, local control was associated with the extent of resection. Complete resection and IOERT yielded local control and disease-specific survival of 89% and 63%, respectively, and 65% and 32%, for the 28 patients

undergoing IOERT for residual disease. The 5-year complication rate was 11% (Level IV).

■ Alektiar et al. (2000) described high-dose rate (HDR) intraoperative brachytherapy (IORT) for locally recurrent colorectal cancer at Memorial Sloan-Kettering. They reported on 74 patients treated with surgery and HDR-IORT (10–18 Gy). Less than 50% of the patients received additional external-beam RT or 5-FU-based chemotherapy. All patients received a complete gross resection, 21 of whom had positive microscopic margins.

The dose of HDR-IORT ranged from 10 to 18 Gy. The 5-year local control and overall survival rates were 39% and 23%, respectively (Level IV).

16.4.4 Side Effects and Complications

- Acute radiation-induced side effects and complications are generally mild, but increased severity occurs with combined modality therapy.
- Diarrhea is the most common complaint. Severe diarrhea (Grade 3/4) was reported in 44% of patients treated with 5-FU-based chemotherapy concurrently in INT-0144 (Level I) (SMALLEY et al. 2006).
- Incidence of death related to chemoradiation therapy was $\leq$1% as reported in the GITSG-7175, INT-0114, and NSABP R-02 trials (Level I) (TEPPER et al. 2002; THOMAS and LINDBLAD 1988; WOLMARK et al. 2000).

16.5 Palliative Treatment of Rectal Cancer

16.5.1 General Principles

- Radiotherapy is frequently used to alleviate symptoms of local and distant metastases.
- Rectal stenting of obstructing lesions can provide relief for more than 9 months and have rates of migration $\leq$15% (Level III) (STELZNER 2004).
- Radiopharmaceuticals (samarium-153 and strontium-89) successfully relieve pain in patients with boney metastases active on bone scan (Grade A) (Level I) (BAUMAN et al. 2005).

16.5.2 Resectable Metastatic Disease

- Surgical resection of limited metastatic disease to the liver or lung improves survival. Poor prognostic indicators include the number, size, and laterality of metastases within the organ (Level IV) (IIZAS et al. 2006; ABDALLA et al. 2004).

16.6 Follow-Ups

16.6.1 Post-Treatment Follow-Ups

- Life-long follow-up after definitive treatment of rectal cancer is indicated for detection of local or distant failures.
- Local failure is a major cause of treatment failure, and the rates of locoregional failure range from 25% to 50% after definitive combined modality therapy, most occurring within the first 3 years (PFISTER et al. 2004).

Schedule

- Follow-ups should be scheduled every 3–6 months for 2 years, then every 6 months for 5 years, and annually thereafter (Table 16.4) (NATIONAL COMPREHENSIVE CANCER NETWORK 2008).

Table 16.4. Follow-up schedule after treatment for rectal cancer

Interval	Frequency
First 2 years	Every 3–6 months
Years 3–5	Every 6 months
Over 5 years	Annually

- **Work-Up**
- Each follow-up should include a complete history and physical examination. A CEA should be drawn every 3–7 months for 2 years, then every 6 months for 5 years for lesions $\geq$T2 (Grade B) (NATIONAL COMPREHENSIVE CANCER NETWORK 2008).
- Colonoscopy should be performed 1 year following definitive treatment. If obstruction limited colonoscopy at the time of diagnosis, it should be done within 3–6 months following definitive treatment. Screening exams should be performed every 3–5 years thereafter if normal.
- A proctoscopy is recommended every 6 months for 5 years in patients treated with LAR to evaluate for anastomotic recurrence.
- Diagnostic imaging is warranted if symptomatic or elevations in CEA are noted.

References

Abdalla EK, Vauthey JN, Ellis LM et al (2004) Recurrence and outcomes following hepatic resection, radiofrequency ablation, and combined resection/ablation for colorectal liver metastases. Ann Surg 239:818–825

Alektiar KM, Zelefsky MJ, Paty PB et al (2000) High-dose-rate intraoperative brachytherapy for recurrent colorectal cancer. Int J Radiat Oncol Biol Phys 48:219–226

Arbman G, Nilsson E, Hallböök O et al (1996) Local recurrence following total mesorectal excision for rectal cancer. Br J Surg 83:375–379

Astler VB, Coller FA (1954) The prognostic significance of direct extension of carcinoma of the colon and rectum. Ann Surg 139:846

Bassi MC, Turri L, Sacchetti G et al (2007) FDG-PET/CT imaging for staging and target volume delineation in preoperative conformal radiotherapy of rectal cancer. Int J Radiat Oncol Biol Phys 70:1423–1426

Bauman G, Charette M, Reid R et al (2005) Radiopharmaceuticals for the palliation of painful bone metastasis-a systemic review. Radiother Oncol 75:258–270

Baxter NN, Garcia-Aguilar J (2007) Organ preservation for rectal cancer. J Clin Oncol 25:1014–1020

Baxter NN, Virnig DJ, Rothenberger DA et al (2005) Lymph node evaluation in colorectal cancer patients: a population-based study. J Natl Cancer Inst 97:219–225

Beets-Tan RG, Beets GL, Vliegen RF et al (2001) Accuracy of magnetic resonance imaging in prediction of tumour-free resection margin in rectal cancer surgery. Lancet 357(9255):497–504

Bipat S, Glas AS, Slors FJ et al (2004) Rectal cancer: local staging and assessment of lymph node involvement with endoluminal US, CT, and MR imaging–a meta-analysis. Radiology 232:773–783

Bolognese A, Cardi M, Muttillo IA et al (2000) Total mesorectal excision for surgical treatment of rectal cancer. J Surg Oncol 74:21–23

Bosset JF, Collette L, Calais G. EORTC Radiotherapy Group Trial 22921 (2006) Chemotherapy with preoperative radiotherapy in rectal cancer. N Engl J Med 355:1114–1123

Brown G, Radcliffe AG, Newcombe RG et al (2003) Preoperative assessment of prognostic factors in rectal cancer using high-resolution magnetic resonance imaging. Br J Surg 90:355–364

Burtin P, Rabot AF, Heresbach D et al (1997) Interobserver agreement in the staging of rectal cancer using endoscopic ultrasonography. Endoscopy 29:620–625

Cammà C, Giunta M, Fiorica F et al (2000) Preoperative radiotherapy for resectable rectal cancer: A meta-analysis. JAMA 284:1008–1015

Chakravarti A, Compton CC, Shellito PC et al (1999) Long-term follow-up of patients with rectal cancer managed by local excision with and without adjuvant irradiation. Ann Surg 230:49–54

Chun HK, Choi D, Kim MJ et al (2006) Preoperative staging of rectal cancer: comparison of 3-T high-field MRI and endorectal sonography. AJR Am J Roentgenol 187:1557–1562

Colorectal Cancer Collaborative Group (2001) Adjuvant radiotherapy for rectal cancer: a systematic overview of 8,507 patients from 22 randomised trials. Lancet 358(9290):1291–1304

Czito B, Siddiqi N, Mamon H et al (2007) Gatrointestinal brachytherapy. In: Devlin P (ed) Brachytherapy: Applications and technique. Lippincott Williams & Wilkins, Philadelphia

Dahlberg M, Påhlman L, Bergström R et al (1998) Improved survival in patients with rectal cancer: a population-based register study. Br J Surg 85:515–520

Dukes CE (1932) The classification of cancer of the rectum. J Pathol Bacteriol 35:323

Ellenhorn J, Cullinane C, Coia L et al (2007) Colon, rectal, and anal cancers. In: Cancer management: A multidisciplinary approach. CMP Healthcare Media, LLC, Manhasset, NY

Gerard JP, Chapet O, Nemoz C et al (2004) Improved sphincter preservation in low rectal cancer with high-dose preoperative radiotherapy: the Lyon R96-02 randomized trial. J Clin Oncol 22:2404–2409

Gérard JP, Conroy T, Bonnetain F et al (2006) Preoperative radiotherapy with or without concurrent fluorouracil and leucovorin in T3-4 rectal cancers: results of FFCD 9203. J Clin Oncol 24:4620–4625

Greene F, Page D, Fleming I et al (2002) AJCC cancer staging manual, 6th edn. Springer, Berlin Heidelberg New York

Gunderson LL, Sargent DJ, Tepper JE et al (2004) Impact of T and N substage on survival and disease relapse in adjuvant rectal cancer: a pooled analysis. J Clin Oncol 22:1785–1796

Harrison LB, Minsky BD, Enker WE et al (1998) High dose rate intraoperative radiation therapy (HDR-IORT) as part of the management strategy for locally advanced primary and recurrent rectal cancer. Int J Radiat Oncol Biol Phys 42:325–330

Havenga K, Enker WE, Norstein J et al (1999) Improved survival and local control after total mesorectal excision or D3 lymphadenectomy in the treatment of primary rectal cancer: an international analysis of 1,411 patients. Eur J Surg Oncol 25:368–374

Iizasa T, Suzuki M, Yoshida S et al (2006) Prediction of prognosis and surgical indications for pulmonary metastasectomy from colorectal cancer. Ann Thorac Surg 82:254–260

Jimenez RE, Shoup M, Cohen AM et al (2003) Contemporary outcomes of total pelvic exenteration in the treatment of colorectal cancer. Dis Colon Rectum 46:1619–1625

Kapiteijn E, Marijnen CA, Nagtegaal ID; Dutch Colorectal Cancer Group (2001) Preoperative radiotherapy combined with total mesorectal excision for resectable rectal cancer. N Engl J Med 345:638–646

Kim NK, Baik SH, Seong JS et al (2006) Oncologic outcomes after neoadjuvant chemoradiation followed by curative resection with tumor-specific mesorectal excision for fixed locally advanced rectal cancer: Impact of postirradiated pathologic downstaging on local recurrence and survival. Ann Surg 244:1024–1030

Koh DM, Chau I, Tait D et al (2007) Evaluating mesorectal lymph nodes in rectal cancer before and after neoadjuvant chemoradiation using thin-section T2-weighted magnetic resonance imaging. Int J Radiat Oncol Biol Phys 71:456–461

Krook JE, Moertel CG, Gunderson LL et al (1991) Effective surgical adjuvant therapy for high-risk rectal carcinoma. N Engl J Med 324(11):709–715

Kulinna C, Eibel R, Matzek W et al (2004) Staging of rectal cancer: diagnostic potential of multiplanar reconstructions with MDCT. AJR 183:421–427

Lahaye MJ, Engelen SM, Nelemans PJ et al (2005) Imaging for predicting the risk factors (the circumferential resection margin and nodal disease) of local recurrence in rectal cancer: a meta-analysis. Semin Ultrasound CT MR 26(4):259–268

Massari M, De Simone M, Cioffi U et al (1998) Value and limits of endorectal ultrasonography for preoperative staging of rectal carcinoma. Surg Laparosc Endosc 8(6):438–444

Matsuoka H, Nakamura A, Masaki T et al (2003) A prospective comparison between multidetector-row computed tomography and magnetic resonance imaging in the preoperative evaluation of rectal carcinoma. Am J Surg 185:556–559

Merchant NB, Guillem JG, Paty PB et al (1999) T3N0 rectal cancer: results following sharp mesorectal excision and no adjuvant therapy. J Gastrointest Surg 3(6):642–647

MERCURY Study Group (2006) Diagnostic accuracy of preoperative magnetic resonance imaging in predicting curative resection of rectal cancer: prospective observational study. BMJ 333(7572):779

Mohiuddin M, Winter K, Mitchell E et al (2006) Randomized phase II study of neoadjuvant combined-modality chemoradiation for distal rectal cancer: Radiation Therapy Oncology Group Trial 0012. JCO 24(4):650–655

Nagtegaal ID, Quirke P (2008) What is the role for the circumferential margin in the modern treatment of rectal cancer? JCO 26(2):303–312

Nakfoor BM, Willett CG, Shellito PC et al (1998) The impact of 5-fluorouracil and intraoperative electron beam radiation therapy on the outcome of patients with locally advanced primary rectal and rectosigmoid cancer. Ann Surg 228(2):194–200

Nascimbeni R, Nivatvongs S, Larson DR et al (2004) Long-term survival after local excision for T1 carcinoma of the rectum. Dis Colon Rectum 47(11):1773–1779

National Comprehensive Cancer Network (2008) Clinical practice guidelines in oncology: Rectal cancer, version I.2008. Available at http://nccn.org/professionals/physician_gls/PDF/rectal.pdf.

Nuyttens J, Kolkman-Deurloo IK, Vermaas M et al (2004) High-dose-rate intraoperative radiotherapy for close or positive margins in patients with locally advanced or recurrent rectal cancer. Int J Radiat Oncol Biol Phys 58(1):106–112

O'Connell JB, Maggard MA, Liu JH et al (2004) Are survival rates different for young and older patients with rectal cancer? Dis Colon Rectum 47(12):2064–2069

Påhlman L, Glimelius B (1990) Pre- or postoperative radiotherapy in rectal and rectosigmoid carcinoma. Report from a randomized multicenter trial. Ann Surg 211(2):187–195

Peeters KC, Marijnen CA, Nagtegaal ID et al; Dutch Colorectal Cancer Group (2007) The TME trial after a median follow-up of 6 years: increased local control but no survival benefit in irradiated patients with resectable rectal carcinoma. Ann Surg 246(5):693–701

Pfister DG, Benson AB 3rd, Somerfield MR (2004) Clinical practice. Surveillance strategies after curative treatment of colorectal cancer. N Engl J Med 350(23):2375–2382

Platell CF, Semmens JB (2004) Review of survival curves for colorectal cancer. Dis Colon Rectum 7(12):2070–2075

Roh M, Colangelo L, Wieand S et al (2004) Response to preoperative multimodality therapy predicts survival in patients with carcinoma of the rectum. Proc ASCO 22:14

Sauer R, Becker H, Hohenberger W et al; German Rectal Cancer Study Group (2004) Preoperative versus postoperative chemoradiotherapy for rectal cancer. N Engl J Med 351(17):1731–1740

Sause WT, Pajak TF, Noyes RD et al (1994) Evaluation of preoperative radiation therapy in operable colorectal cancer. Ann Surg 220(5):668–675

Smalley SR, Benedetti JK, Williamson SK et al (2006) Phase III trial of fluorouracil-based chemotherapy regimens plus radiotherapy in postoperative adjuvant rectal cancer: GI INT 0144. J Clin Oncol 24(22):3542–3547

Stelzner M (2004) The 2003 SSAT-AGA-ASGE workshop on "Palliative Therapy of Rectal Cancer." Summary statement. J Gastrointest Surg 8(3):253–258

Stocchi L, Nelson H, Sargent DJ et al; North Central Cancer Treatment Group (2001) Impact of surgical and pathologic variables in rectal cancer: a United States community and cooperative group report. J Clin Oncol 19(18):3895–3902

Swedish Rectal Cancer Trial (1997) Improved survival with preoperative radiotherapy in resectable rectal cancer. N Engl J Med 336(14):980–987

Tepper JE, O'Connell M, Niedzwiecki D et al (2002) Adjuvant therapy in rectal cancer: analysis of stage, sex, and local control–final report of Intergroup 0114. J Clin Oncol 20(7):1744–1750

Thomas PR, Lindblad AS (1988) Adjuvant postoperative radiotherapy and chemotherapy in rectal carcinoma: a review of the Gastrointestinal Tumor Study Group experience. Radiother Oncol 13(4):245–252

Willett CG, Badizadegan K, Ancukiewicz M et al (1999) Prognostic factors in stage T3N0 rectal cancer: do all patients require postoperative pelvic irradiation and chemotherapy? Dis Colon Rectum 42(2):167–173

Wolberink S, Beets-Tan RG, de Haas-Kock D et al (2007) Conventional CT for the prediction of an involved circumferential resection margin in primary rectal cancer. Dig Dis 25:80–85

Wolmark N, Wieand HS, Hyams DM et al (2000) Randomized trial of postoperative adjuvant chemotherapy with or without radiotherapy for carcinoma of the rectum: National Surgical Adjuvant Breast and Bowel Project Protocol R-02. J Natl Cancer Inst 92(5):388–396

Yoon SM, Kim DY, Kim TH et al (2007) Clinical parameters predicting pathologic tumor response after preoperative chemoradiotherapy for rectal cancer. Int J Radiat Oncol Biol Phys 69(4):1167–1172

Cancer of the Anal Canal

Qing Zhang and Andre A. Abitbol

Q. Zhang, MD
Department of Radiation Oncology, The 6th Hospital of Jiao
Tong University, 600 Yi Shan Road, Shanghai 200233, P. R.
China
A. A. Abitbol, MD
Department of Radiation Oncology, Baptist Hospital, 8900
North Kendall Drive, Miami, FL 33176, USA

Introduction and Objectives

Anal cancer is a rare type of gastrointestinal malignancy. Over 80% of anal cancers are of squamous origin and arise from the squamous epithelium of the anal canal and perianal area. Recent evidence has demonstrated that the incidence of squamous cell carcinoma of anal cancer increases in immunocompromised patients. Approximately 10% are adenocarcinoma arising from the glandular mucosa of the upper anal canal or anal glands. Other malignancies of the anal canal, such as melanoma, sarcoma, and lymphoma, are exceedingly rare. Surgery has limited application in the treatment of squamous cell carcinoma of the anal canal. Radiation therapy plays a major role in the treatment of anal cancer, and concurrent chemoradiation therapy is the standard treatment for most cases of locally advanced disease.

This chapter examines:

● Diagnosis and staging procedures of squamous cell carcinoma or adenocarcinoma of the anal canal

● Staging system and prognostic factors

● Recommendations for definitive treatment using radiation therapy or concurrent chemoradiotherapy and supporting peer-reviewed clinical evidence

● Techniques of radiation therapy for definitive treatment of anal cancer

● Definition of persistent and recurrent local disease, as well as their treatment

● Follow-up care and surveillance of survivors

Tumors of the anal margin without involvement of the anal verge are classified and treated as skin cancers, and are discussed in detail in Chapter 36. The management of the rare pathological types of anal malignancies, such as melanoma, soft-tissue sarcoma, and lymphoma, are also not addressed in this chapter.

17.1 Diagnosis, Staging, and Prognoses

17.1.1 Diagnosis

Initial Evaluation

- Diagnosis and evaluation of anal carcinoma start with a complete history and physical examination (H&P). Attention should be paid to anal cancer specific history, signs, and symptoms, including those associated with anal-receptive intercourse and HIV infection.
- Thorough physical examination (including a proctoscopy) should be performed to evaluate the extent of the primary disease and to exclude regional lymph node metastasis. Approximately 10% of patients present with synchronous nodal metastasis in the inguinal area (GERARD et al. 2001). Inguinal and femoral lymph nodes are commonly involved in locally advanced lesions of the anal canal below the dentate line.
- For female patients, a thorough gynecologic examination is indicated to evaluate the extent of the disease and screen for cervical cancer.

Pathology

- Histological confirmation of the diagnosis of anal canal cancer is essential. Treatment strategy of the more commonly diagnosed squamous cell carcinoma is substantially different from those of adenocarcinoma, sarcoma, and melanoma.
- Tissue for pathology diagnosis can be obtained via biopsy of the primary tumor under proctoscopy. Fine-needle biopsy or simple excision of enlarged groin lymph nodes is recommended (WOLFE and BUSSEY 1968). Formal lymph node dissection should not be performed in the initial evaluation of suspicious nodes in the inguinal area.

Imaging Studies

- MRI or CT of the pelvis and abdomen is the most important imaging study for evaluating the extent of local disease.
- Transanal ultrasound may be helpful to identify the depth of tumor penetration and visualize perirectal nodes (TARANTINO and BERNSTEIN 2002).
- PET/CT scan can be recommended for evaluating pelvis lymph nodes and diagnosis of distant metastasis (Grade B). Neither CT nor MRI is reliable for detecting metastasis to internal iliac and superior hemorrhoidal lymph nodes, as approximately 50% of the involved nodes are <0.5 cm (WADE et al. 1989). FDG-PET has been shown to be more sensitive for detecting abnormal inguinal lymph nodes than conventional CT and physical examination (Level III) (COTTER et al. 2006; TRAUTMANN and ZUGER 2005).
- Chest X-ray is usually adequate to rule out lung metastasis, and liver metastasis can be evaluated by CT or MRI of the abdomen. Distant metastases occur in approximately 10% of cases. The most common sites of distant metastasis include liver and lung (MYERSON et al. 1997).
- Bone scan is not routinely recommended except in cases with elevated alkaline phosphatase and symptoms indicating bone metastasis.

Laboratory Tests

- Initial laboratory tests should include a complete blood count, basic blood chemistry, liver, and renal function tests.
- HIV test and CD4 counts are recommended in patients who have a high risk of HIV infection, including homosexual males (Grade B). Patients with HIV infection experience more severe side effects and complications to chemotherapy and radiation therapy (Level IV) (HOFFMAN et al. 1999; KIM et al. 2001; PLACE et al. 2001; STADLER et al. 2004; WEXLER et al. 2007) (Table 17.1).

Table 17.1. Imaging and laboratory work-ups for anal canal cancer

Imaging studies	Laboratory tests
– MRI or CT of pelvis and abdomen – Chest X-ray – FDG-PET or PET/CT scan – Transanal ultrasound (optional) – Bone scan (optional)	– Complete blood count – Serum chemistry – Liver function tests – Renal function tests – Alkaline phosphatase – HIV and CD4 (optional)

17.1.2 Staging

- Anal cancer is usually staged clinically as surgery has a limited role in the definitive treatment of anal cancer. Clinical staging utilizes information from physical examination (including proctoscopy), imaging studies, and laboratory tests.

- The most commonly utilized staging system for anal cancer is the Tumor Node Metastasis (TNM) staging system of the American Joint Committee on Cancer (AJCC) and UICC. The TNM staging system is based on tumor size, invasion of adjacent structures, status of regional lymph nodes, and status of distant metastases (Table 17.2) (GREENE et al. 2002).

17.1.3 Prognostic Factors

- The presenting stage of the disease (including the size and extent of the primary tumor, extent of nodal involvement, and status of distant metastasis) is the most important prognostic factor for anal cancer (CUMMINGS 2001; GREENE et al. 2002).
- When all other factors are equal, male gender, advanced age (65 years or above), and poor performance status before treatment are associated with poor outcome after definitive treatment (Level IV) (BARTELINK et al. 1997; GERARD et al. 1999; PEIFFERT et al. 1997).
- Prognosis of different subtypes of squamous cell carcinoma (keratinizing or non-keratinizing subtypes) is similar. However, patients with well-differentiated disease have more favorable prognosis as compared to those with poorly differentiated disease: the 5-year overall survival rates were 75% versus 25%, respectively (Level IV) (GOLDMAN et al. 1987).
- Side effects and complications of radiation therapy and chemotherapy are more prominent in patients with HIV infection and AIDS, especially when the CD4 count is <200 µl (Level IV) (HOFFMAN et al. 1999; KIM et al. 2001; PLACE et al. 2001; STADLER et al. 2004; WEXLER et al. 2007).

17.2 Treatment of Anal Canal Cancer

17.2.1 General Principles

- Concurrent chemotherapy with radiation therapy is recommended for the definitive treatment of anal canal cancer (Grade A), except for stage

Table 17.2. American Joint Committee on Cancer (AJCC) TNM staging system for anal cancer. [From GREENE et al. (2002) with permission]

Primary tumor (T)	
TX	Primary tumor cannot be assessed
T0	No evidence of primary tumor
Tis	Carcinoma in situ
T1	Tumor 2 cm or less in greatest dimension
T2	Tumor more than 2 cm, but not more than 5 cm in greatest dimension
T3	Tumor more than 5 cm in greatest dimension
T4	Tumor of any size invades adjacent organ(s), e.g., vagina, urethra, bladder [a]

Regional lymph nodes (N)	
NX	Regional lymph nodes cannot be assessed
N0	No regional lymph node metastasis [b]
N1	Metastasis in perirectal lymph node(s)
N2	Metastasis in unilateral internal iliac and/or inguinal lymph node(s)
N3	Metastasis in perirectal and inguinal lymph nodes and/or bilateral internal iliac and/or bilateral internal iliac and/or inguinal lymph nodes

Distant metastasis (M)	
MX	Distant metastasis cannot be assessed
M0	No distant metastasis
M1	Distant metastasis

STAGE GROUPING	
0:	Tis N0 M0
I:	T1 N0 M0
II:	T2 N0 M0, T3 N0 M0
IIIA:	T1 N1 M0, T2 N1 M0, T3 N1 M0, T4 N0 M0
IIIB:	T4 N1 M0, Any T N2 M0, Any T N3 M0
IV:	Any T Any N M1

Histologic grade (G)	
GX	Grade can not be assessed
G1	Well differentiated
G2	Moderately differentiated
G3	Poorly differentiated
G4	Undifferentiated

[a] Direct invasion of the rectal wall, perirectal skin, subcutaneous tissue, or the sphincter muscle(s) is not classified as T4.
[b] Regional lymph nodes for the anal canal include inguinal, perirectal, and internal iliac lymph nodes. Metastasis to other pelvic lymph nodes, including the rectosigmoid, external iliac, and common iliac, or paraaortic lymph nodes, is classified as distant metastasis

T1N0M0 disease, which can be treated with radiation therapy alone.

- Currently there is no evidence to support the use of neoadjuvant and adjuvant chemotherapy in addition to concurrent chemoradiotherapy.
- Surgery as a modality for definitive therapy is usually reserved for selected patients with well-differentiated early-stage (i.e., well-differentiated T1N0M0) squamous cell carcinoma. Abdominal peritoneal resection is reserved for salvage after primary chemoradiotherapy failure (Fig. 17.1).

17.2.2 Combined Radiation Therapy and Chemotherapy

- Radiation therapy with current chemotherapy is the standard treatment for locally advanced (all non-metastatic cases except for T1N0M0) anal canal cancer (Grade A). It has been confirmed that patients who received combined chemotherapy and external-beam radiotherapy had significantly improved local control rates as compared to those who received radiation only. Complete response

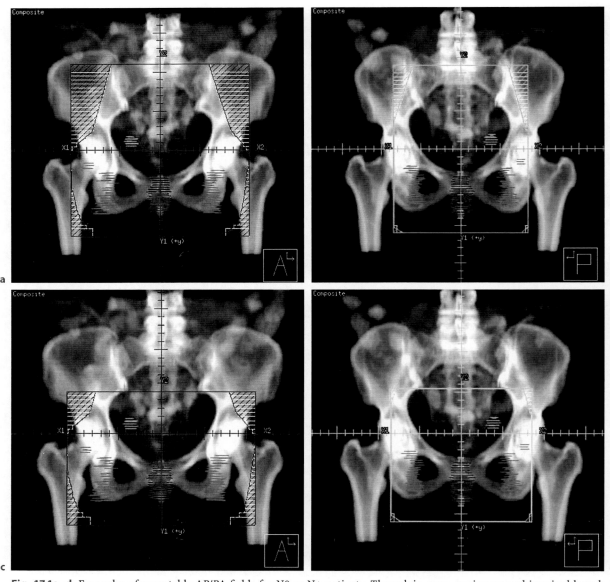

Fig. 17.1a–d. Examples of acceptable AP/PA fields for N0 or N+ patients. The pelvis, anus, perineum and inguinal lymph nodes are treated with AP-PA technique to include lateral inguinal nodes within AP/lateral fields but not PA field. Patient lies supine with a full bladder. Superior border reduced at 30.6 Gy to the level of sacroiliac joint

has been observed in 80%–90% of patients with squamous cell carcinoma of the anal canal after concurrent chemoradiotherapy, and both local control and overall survival rates approached 90%.

In a prospective randomized phase III trial conducted by the UK Coordinating Committee on Cancer Research, a total of 585 patients were randomized to receive either radiation therapy alone (45 Gy in 20 or 25 fractions over 4–5 weeks) or the same regimen of radiotherapy in combination with 5-FU and mitomycin. The results indicated that the addition of chemotherapy gave a reduction of 46% in the risk of local failure in the patients receiving combined treatment ($p<0.0001$). Local control rates were 59% versus 36%, respectively, for patients who received chemoradiotherapy or radiation only. However, the benefit of chemotherapy on overall survival was not observed (UKCCCR, Level I) (UKCCCR 1996).

Similar results were observed in a prospective randomized study from European Organization for Research and Treatment of cancer (EORTC): 101 patients with T3-4N0-3 or T1-2N1-3 anal cancer were randomized to receive either radiation therapy alone (45 Gy at 1.8 Gy per day over 5 weeks) or the same regimen of radiotherapy in combination with 5-FU and mitomycin. Patients who achieved partial or complete response after a rest of 6 weeks were treated with a radiation boost to 20 Gy or 15 Gy, respectively, and non-responders received surgical resection. The addition of chemotherapy to radiotherapy resulted in a significant increase in the complete remission rate from 54% for radiotherapy alone to 80% for combined treatment. The 5-year locoregional control and colostomy-free survival rates were 68% versus 50%, and 72% versus 40%, respectively, both in favor of the combined chemoradiation therapy. Again, no benefit of overall survival was observed (EORTC, Level I) (BARTELINK et al. 1997).

Chemotherapy Regimens

■ Two cycles of concurrent chemotherapy (continuous infusion 5-FU of 1000 mg/m^2 days 1–4 plus mitomycin-C of 10 mg/m^2 bolus on day 1 given in week 1 and 5) and radiation therapy are currently the standard treatment regimen for anal canal cancer (Grade A).

A prospective randomized trial from Radiation Therapy Oncology Group (RTOG) studied the necessity of mitomycin-C in the combined chemo-

radiation regimen. Patients were randomized to receive either radiotherapy (45–50.4 Gy to pelvis) plus concurrent 5-FU, or concurrently with 5-FU and mitomycin-C. At 6 weeks of follow-up, patients with residual tumor on post-treatment biopsy were treated with additional radiation to the pelvis (9 Gy) plus concurrent chemotherapy (5-FU and cisplatin) for salvage. The results showed that although toxicity was significantly higher in patients who received mitomycin-C, colostomy rates (9% vs. 22%; $p=0.002$), colostomy-free survival rates (71% vs. 59%; $p=0.014$), and disease-free survival rates (73% vs. 51%; $p=0.0003$) were significantly improved with the addition mitomycin-C at 4 years. However, a significant difference in overall survival was not observed. (RTOG 87-04, Level I) (FLAM et al. 1996).

■ Currently, there is no evidence to support the use of other chemotherapy combinations as the standard regimen in place of 5-FU and mitomycin-C. An Intergroup phase III randomized trial compared the effects of the standard 5-FU/mitomycin-C regimen to 5-FU/cisplatin (two cycles for induction therapy and two cycles of concurrent treatment) with radiation therapy. No significant differences were observed in the preliminary analyses at 5 years: the estimated disease-free survival and colostomy rates were 56% versus 48% and 10% versus 20%, respectively. The overall survival rate was 69% in both groups. However, grade 3 and 4 hematologic toxicity was significantly higher in the group treated with 5 FU and mitomycin-C (47% versus 67%) (RTOG 98-11, Level I) (AJANI et al. 2006).

Neoadjuvant and Adjuvant Chemotherapy

■ Neoadjuvant chemotherapy is not recommended for anal canal cancer, including locally advanced (T3, T4, or N+) disease (Grade C). Approximately 50% of patients with T3 or T4 disease will require salvage surgery. Neoadjuvant chemotherapy has been shown to be efficacious in approximately 65% of patients in terms of clinical response. However, the advantage of neoadjuvant chemotherapy plus concurrent chemoradiation in comparing with standard concurrent radiation therapy and 5-FU/mitomycin-C has not been confirmed.

In a prospective phase II trial conducted by CALGB, 45 patients with T3, T4, or N2/N3 anal canal cancer were treated with two cycles of infusional 5-FU/cisplatin prior to the standard concurrent chemoradiation regimen. Complete and partial response rates were 18% and 47%, respectively, after induction chemotherapy. At 4 years of follow-up, the overall and disease-free survival rates were 68% and 61%, respectively. The colostomy- and disease-free survival rate were 50% (CALGB 92-81, Level III) (Meropol et al. 1999). In addition, the above-mentioned prospective randomized phase III trial (RTOG 98-11) compared the effects of the concurrent radiation and 5-FU/mitomycin-C to two cycles of neoadjuvant 5-FU/cisplatin chemotherapy followed by concurrent chemoradiation (using 5-FU/cisplatin). There were no significant differences observed in terms of estimated overall, disease-free survival and colostomy rates at 5 years (RTOG 98-11, Level I) (Ajani et al. 2006).

- Currently, there is no evidence to support the use of adjuvant chemotherapy after the completion of definitive concurrent radiation therapy and chemotherapy using a 5-FU and mitomycin-C regimen (Grade D).

17.2.3 Radiation Therapy

External-Beam Radiation Therapy Techniques

- Patients should be treated with equipment with photon energy of 6 MV or greater for pelvic irradiation.
- CT-based planning is recommended (Grade B). Three-dimensional conformal radiation therapy and intensity-modulated radiation therapy (IMRT) have been shown to reduce treatment-induced toxicity in retrospective series (Level IV) (Milano et al. 2005; Salama et al. 2007; Vuong et al. 2007).
- Various treatment techniques of conventional radiation therapy exist for anal cancer treatment, including AP/PA technique, four-field technique, and prone three-field technique (PA and two lateral fields). The more commonly used AP/PA technique is presented here.

Simulation and Field Arrangements

- Patients are simulated in supine position with the bladder filled (to minimize the volume of small bowel in the radiation field) using the AP/PA technique.

- Enlarged inguinal lymph nodes and anal verge (or inferior extent of the tumor, whichever is lower) should be outlined with wire for identification during simulation or on planning CT.
- The borders of the initial pelvic field (for the first 30.6 Gy) are as follows: – Superiorly at L5/S1 to include the common iliac, upper presacral, and rectosigmoid nodes. – Inferiorly at 3 cm below the anal verge or the inferior margin of the tumor (whichever is lower) (Fig. 17.1a). – Laterally to include lateral inguinal nodes as determined by bony landmarks or lymphangiogram for the anterior field (Fig. 17.2) (Level III) (Wang et al. 1996). – Laterally at 1.5 cm lateral to the widest bony margin of the true pelvis for the posterior field (not to include the lateral inguinal region) (Fig. 17.1b)
- After the initial 30.6 Gy, the superior border is lowered to the inlet of the true pelvis at the bottom of the sacroiliac joints for the remaining 14.4 Gy to encompass the internal iliac, perirectal, and lower presacral nodes (Figs. 17.1c,d).
- Supplementary radiation using anterior electron fields to the lateral inguinal region matched with the exit PA field is required to bring the dose of

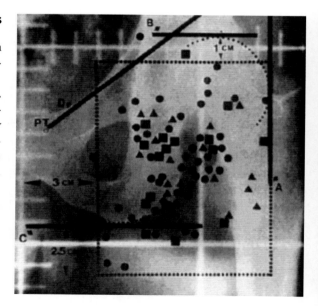

Fig. 17.2. Topographic distribution of inguinal lymph node metastases in patients with carcinoma of the anus and low rectum (circles, $n=50$), vulva vagina-cervix (triangles, $n=17$), and urethra (squares, $n=17$). The field arrangement described provided adequate coverage of 86% of all inguinal lymph nodes (Level III). (Reprinted from Wang et al. (1996) with permission)

the inguinal nodal region to 36 Gy for clinically N0 disease or 45 Gy for N+ disease.

The depth of prescription for electron fields should be determined by CT scan (Grade B). The depth of the femoral vessel ranged from 2.0 to 18.5 cm in one study (Level IV) (KOH et al. 1993).

- Boost field encompassing the primary tumor (and involved inguinal lymph nodes) plus a 2- to 3-cm margin to 9 Gy can be offered to patients with T3, T4, and N+ diseases after 45 Gy to the pelvis (Fig. 17.3) (Grade D).

- The boost treatment for patients with biopsy-proven residual disease at 6 weeks after initial treatment of 45 Gy (concurrent with 5-FU/cisplatin) as described in the RTOG 87-40 protocol is optional (Grade D).

- Conformal technique is recommended to reduce normal tissues toxicities with favorable treatment response (Grade B). In a group of 62 anal cancer patients prospectively treated with 3D conformal radiation therapy, patients were able to complete radiation and chemotherapy without interruption for toxicity, and the local control, freedom from relapse, and overall survival rates were improved (Level IV) (VUONG et al. 2007).

Intensity-Modulated Radiation Therapy (IMRT)

- IMRT is another option to protect normal tissues and deliver an entire course of radiation dose in a single phase of treatment. IMRT has been shown to be effective in the treatment of anal cancer and associated with reduced toxicity, thus less treatment break, when used with concurrent chemotherapy (Level IV) (MILANO et al. 2005; SALAMA et al. 2007).

- Treatment plan should include anorectum and primary disease with a margin, posterior pelvic, internal iliac, and inguinal lymph nodes (Fig. 17.4).

Dose and Fractionation

- External-beam radiation should be delivered as a continuous course at 1.8–2.0 Gy per daily fraction.

- Split course of radiation should not be routinely used in the definitive treatment of anal cancer (Grade B). Treatment break is often necessary for skin intolerance; however, the entire course of radiation should be completed within 5–6.5 weeks, and break of treatment for skin intolerance should not exceed 10 days in total.

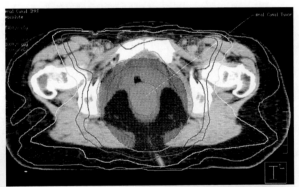

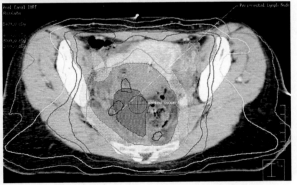

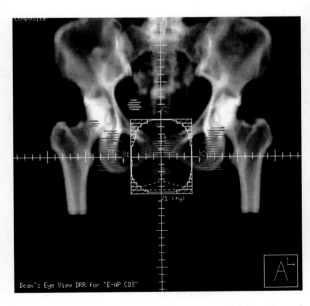

Fig. 17.3. Optional boost field for patients with T3, T4, and N+ disease after 45 Gy

Fig. 17.4. Intensity-modulated Radiation Therapy (IMRT). The planned target volume (PTV) included the gross tumor volume, clinical tumor volume (encompassing both the inguinal and pelvis lymph nodes) in a single phase treatment

Results from a retrospective study of 90 patients treated with chemotherapy and radiation with various lengths of gap revealed that gaps longer than 5 weeks correlated with poorer locoregional control with especially unsatisfactory results observed in younger patients (≤65 years) (Level IV) (WEBER et al. 2001). In addition, increases in radiotherapy dose to 59.4 Gy given in split-course with conventional chemotherapy regimens were not associated with improved local control, according to a phase II trial (RTOG 92-08, Level III) (JOHN et al. 1996).

Side Effects, Complications, and Dose Limiting Structures

- Commonly observed acute effects caused by radiotherapy, especially with concurrent chemotherapy, include skin toxicity, reduced blood count, fatigue, and gastrointestinal and urinary toxicities. Most of the symptoms are self-limited; however, intervention is usually required for skin reactions induced by treatment.
- Dose limitation structures of anal cancer radiation therapy include the bladder, rectum, bone (femoral head and neck), and small bowel. Attention should be paid to limit the amount of small bowel in the treatment field. Radiation dose to the bladder should be limited to 65 Gy, the dose to the femoral head and neck should be limited to 42 Gy, and the dose to the small bowel should be limited to 45 Gy (Level IV) (EMAMI et al. 1991).
- Commonly diagnosed late side effects include anorectal urgency, rectal bleeding, and impotence (Level IV) (ALLAL et al. 1999; VORDERMARK et al. 1999).
- For patients with HIV infection, especially those with CD4 count less than 200/μl, highly active antiretroviral therapy is recommended for the treatment of HIV infection, and reduced radiation field and/or lower dose may be considered (Grade B). Results of numerous retrospective studies confirmed that significant toxicity (especially hematologic toxicities) is usually seen with standard treatment regimens for anal cancer in patients with low CD4 count (Level IV) (HOFFMAN et al. 1999; KIM et al. 2001; PLACE et al. 2001; STADLER et al. 2004; WEXLER et al. 2007). However, outcome after definitive combined treatment for HIV-related anal squamous-cell carcinoma with highly active antiretroviral

therapy seems to be comparable to the outcome in patients without HIV infection (Level IV) (BLAZY et al. 2005; HOFFMAN et al. 1999; WEXLER et al. 2007).

Brachytherapy

- Brachytherapy is not routinely indicated in the definitive treatment of squamous cell carcinoma of the anal canal (Grade C). Results of a collaborative study (retrospective) from France and numerous retrospective studies have shown that the local control rates after brachytherapy following conventionally dosed external beam radiation ranged between 70% and 90% for squamous cell carcinoma of the anal canal (Level IV) (BRUNA et al. 2006; GERARD et al. 1999; KAPP et al. 2001). Substantial improvement in local control disease-free survival rates has not been documented; however, brachytherapy-associated anal necrosis was observed at an average rate of 10%.

17.2.4 Surgery

- The role of surgery is limited in the definitive treatment of anal canal cancer.
- Abdominal perineal resection (APR) is reserved for salvage treatment for irradiated patients who develop locoregional recurrence or persistent disease (Grade B). The long-term overall survival rate for patients who failed primary chemoradiation treated with potentially curative salvage surgery ranged between 30% and 50% in various retrospective series (Level IV) (AKBARI et al. 2004; LONGO et al. 1994; RENEHAN et al. 2005).
- The utilization of local excision is limited to highly selected patients with well-differentiated, small primary disease (T1 N0 M0) and should not be routinely recommended (Grade C). In a retrospective study from the Mayo Clinic, a subset of 12 cases with limited disease was treated with local excision. The overall survival for this group of patients reached 100%, and only one patient developed local recurrence (Level V) (BOMAN et al. 1984). However, results of a smaller series of cases with limited anal canal cancer measuring 2 cm or less in diameter showed that long-term survival was observed in only three of the eight reported cases treated with local excision (Level V) (GREENALL et al. 1985).

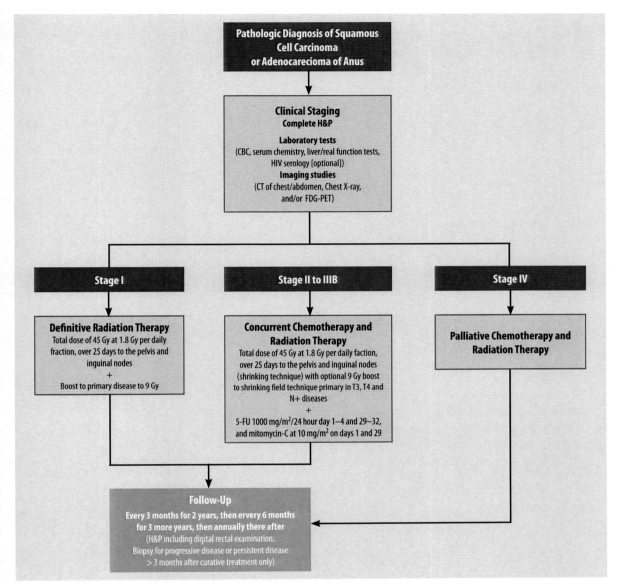

Fig. 17.5. A proposed algorithm for the management of squamous cell carcinoma or adenocarcinoma of the anus

17.3   Follow-Up

17.3.1   Post-Treatment Follow-Up

■ Life-long follow-up is required for all patients with anal canal cancer treated with curative intent.

Schedule

■ Follow-up every 2 months initially in the first 2 years, every 6 months thereafter through year 5, then annually thereafter can be scheduled (Grade D). Most recurrences occur within 3 years after the completion of treatment (Table 17.3).

Work-Up

■ Each follow-up examination should include a complete history and physical examination, including a digital examination (DRE) and proctoscopy. Attention should be paid to the extent of the disease on each examination.

Table 17.3. Follow-up schedule

Interval	Frequency
First follow-up	8 Weeks post-treatment
First 2 year	Every 8 weeks
Year 3–4	Every 6 months
Over 5 years	Annually

■ Biopsy of the residual disease and salvage treatment are not recommended for tumors continuing to decrease in size. Biopsy can be considered for stable residual tumor at 3 months after the completion of treatment and is indicated if a tumor progresses or recurrence after complete response is noticed (Grade B).
Biopsy results from patients who received combined chemoradiation and "salvage" chemoradiation (9 Gy with concurrent 5-FU/cisplatin) from the RTOG 87-04 study revealed that more than 50% of patients can achieve pathologic complete response at 6 weeks after treatment. (FLAM et al. 1996). However, slow regression is common after combined treatment, and complete response may take up to 12 months to achieve (Level III and IV) (CUMMINGS et al. 1991; NIGRO 1984).

■ Imaging studies (CT scan of abdomen and pelvis and FDG-PET) are recommended for progressive disease discovered on DRE or proctoscopy (Grade B) (NATIONAL COMPREHENSIVE CANCER NETWORK 2008).

References

Ajani JA, Winter KA, Gunderson LL et al (2006) Intergroup RTOG 98-11: a phase III randomized study of 5-fluorouracil (5 FU), mitomycin, and radiotherapy versus 5-fluorouracil, cisplatin and radiotherapy in carcinoma of the anal canal. J Clin Oncol 24:4009

Akbari RP, Paty PB, Guillem JG et al (2004) Oncologic outcomes of salvage surgery for epidermoid carcinoma of the anus initially managed with combined modality therapy. Dis Colon Rectum 47:1136–1144

Allal AS, Sprangers MA, Laurencet F et al (1999) Assessment of long-term quality of life in patients with anal carcinomas treated by radiotherapy with or without chemotherapy. Br J Cancer 80:1588–1594

Bartelink H, Roelofsen F, Eschwege F et al (1997) Concomitant radiotherapy and chemotherapy is superior to radiotherapy alone in the treatment of locally advanced anal cancer: results of a phase III randomized trial of the European Organization for Research and Treatment of Cancer Radiotherapy and Gastrointestinal Cooperative Groups. J Clin Oncol 15:2040–2049

Blazy A, Hennequin C, Gornet JM et al (2005) Anal carcinomas in HIV-positive patients: high-dose chemoradiotherapy is feasible in the era of highly active antiretroviral therapy. Dis Colon Rectum 48:1176–1181

Boman BM, Moertel CG, O'Connell MJ et al (1984) Carcinoma of the anal canal. A clinical and pathologic study of 188 cases. Cancer 54:114–125

Bruna A, Gastelblum P, Thomas L et al (2006) Treatment of squamous cell anal canal carcinoma (SCACC) with pulsed dose rate brachytherapy: a retrospective study. Radiother Oncol 79:75–79

Cotter SE, Grigsby PW, Siegel BA et al (2006) FDG-PET/CT in the evaluation of anal carcinoma. Int J Radiat Oncol Biol Phys 65:720–725

Cummings BJ (2001) Anal cancer. In: Gospodarowicz MK, Henson DE, Hutter RV et al (eds) Prognostic factors in cancer, 2nd edn. Wiley-Liss, New York, p 281

Cummings BJ, Keane TJ, O'Sullivan B et al (1991) Epidermoid anal cancer: treatment by radiation alone or by radiation and 5-fluorouracil with and without mitomycin C. Int Radiat Oncol Biol Phys 21:1115–1125

Emami B, Lyman J, Brown A et al (1991) Tolerance of normal tissue to therapeutic irradiation. Int J Radiat Oncol Biol Phys 21:109–122

Flam M, John M, Pajak TF et al (1996) Role of mitomycin in combination with fluorouracil and radiotherapy, and of salvage chemoradiation in the definitive nonsurgical treatment of epidermoid carcinoma of the anal canal: results of a phase III randomized intergroup study. J Clin Oncol 14:2527–2539

Gerard JP, Chapet O, Samiei F et al (2001) Management of inguinal lymph node metastases in patients with carcinoma of the anal canal. Experience in a series of 270 patients treated in Lyon and review of the literature. Cancer 92:77–84

Gerard JP, Mauro F, Thomas L et al (1999) Treatment of squamous cell anal canal carcinoma with pulsed dose rate brachytherapy. Feasibility study of a French cooperative group. Radiother Oncol 51:129–131

Goldman S, Auer G, Erhardt K et al (1987) Prognostic significance of clinical stage, histologic grade, and nuclear DNA content in squamous-cell carcinoma of the anus. Dis Colon Rectum 30:444–448

Greene FL, Page DL, Fleming ID et al (eds) (2002) Anal canal. AJCC Cancer Staging Manual, 6th edn. Springer, New York Heidelberg Berlin

Greenall MJ, Quan SH, Stearns MW et al (1985) Epidermoid cancer of the anal margin. Pathologic features, treatment, and clinical results. Am J Surg 149:95–101

Hoffman R, Welton ML, Klencke B et al (1999) The significance of pretreatment CD4 count on the outcome and treatment tolerance of HIV-positive patients with anal cancer. Int J Radiat Oncol Biol Phys 44:127–131

John M, Pajak T, Flam M et al (1996) Dose escalation in chemoradiation for anal cancer: preliminary results of RTOG 92-08. Cancer J Sci Am 2:205–211

Kapp KS, Geyer E, Gebhart FH et al (2001) Experience with split-course external beam irradiation ± chemotherapy and integrated Ir-192 high-dose-rate brachytherapy in the treatment of primary carcinomas of the anal canal. Int J Radiat Oncol Biol Phys 49:997–1005

Kim JH, Sarani B, Orkin BA et al (2001) HIV-positive patients with anal carcinoma have poorer treatment tolerance and outcome than HIV-negative patients. Dis Colon Rectum 44:1496–1502

Koh WJ, Chiu M, Stelzer KJ et al (1993) Femoral vessel depth and the implications for groin node radiation. Int J Radiat Oncol Biol Phys 27:969–974

Longo WE, Vernava AM 3rd, Wade TP et al (1994) Recurrent squamous cell carcinoma of the anal canal. Predictors of initial treatment failure and results of salvage therapy. Ann Surgery 220:40–49

Meropol NJ, Niedzwicki D, Shank B et al (1999) Combined modality therapy of poor-risk anal canal carcinoma: a phase II study of the Cancer and Leukemia Group B (CALGB). Proc Am Soc Clin Oncol 18:237a

Milano MT, Jani AB, Farrey KJ et al (2005) Intensity-modulated radiation therapy (IMRT) in the treatment of anal cancer: toxicity and clinical outcome. Int J Radiat Oncol Biol Phys 63:354–361

Myerson RJ, Karnell LH, Menck HR (1997) The National Cancer Data Base report on carcinoma of the anus. Cancer 80:805–815

National Comprehensive Cancer Network (2008) Clinical practice guidelines in oncology: Anal carcinoma. Available at http://www.nccn.org/. Accessed on June 23, 2008

Nigro ND (1984) An evaluation of combined therapy for squamous cell cancer of the anal canal. Dis Colon Rectum 27:763–766

Peiffert D, Bey P, Pernot M et al (1997) Conservative treatment by irradiation of epidermoid cancers of the anal canal: prognostic factors of tumoral control and complications. Int J Radiat Oncol Phys 37:313–324

Place RJ, Gregorcyk SG, Huber PJ et al (2001) Outcome analysis of HIV-positive patients with anal squamous cell carcinoma. Dis Colon Rectum 44:506–512

Renehan AG, Saunders MP, Schofield PF et al (2005) Patterns of local disease failure and outcome after salvage surgery in patients with anal cancer. Br J Surg 92:605–614

Salama JK, Mell LK, Schomas DA et al (2007) Concurrent chemotherapy and intensity-modulated radiation therapy for anal canal cancer patients: a multicenter experience. J Clin Oncol 25:4581–4586

Schwarz JK, Siegel BA, Dehdashti F et al (2007) Tumor response and survival predicted by post-therapy FDG-PET/CT in anal cancer. Int J Radiat Oncol Biol Phys [Epub ahead of print]

Stadler RF, Gregorcyk SG, Euhus DM et al (2004) Outcome of HIV-infected patients with invasive squamous-cell carcinoma of the anal canal in the era of highly active antiretroviral therapy. Dis Colon Rectum 47:1305–1309

Tarantino D, Bernstein MA (2002) Endoanal ultrasound in the staging and management of squamous-cell carcinoma of the anal cancer: Potential implications of a new ultrasound staging system. Dis Colon Rectum 45:16–22

Trautmann TG, Zuger JH (2005) Positron emission tomography for pretreatment staging and post-treatment evaluation in cancer of the anal canal. Mol Imaging Biol 7:309–313

UKCCCR (1996) Epidermoid anal cancer: results from the UKCCCR randomised trial of radiotherapy alone versus radiotherapy, 5-fluorouracil, and mitomycin. UKCCCR Anal Cancer Trial Working Party. UK Coordinating Committee on Cancer Research. Lancet 348:1049–1054

Vuong T, Kopek N, Ducruet T et al (2007) Conformal therapy improves the therapeutic index of patients with anal canal cancer treated with combined chemotherapy and external beam radiotherapy. Int J Radiat Oncol Biol Phys 67:1394–1400

Vordermark D, Sailer M, Flentje M et al (1999) Curative-intent radiation therapy in anal carcinoma: quality of life and sphincter function. Radiother Oncol 52:239–243

Wade DS, Herrera L, Castillo NB et al (1989) Metastases to the lymph nodes in epidermoid carcinoma of the anal canal studied by a clearing technique. Surg Gynecol Obstet 169:238–242

Wang CJ, Chin YY, Leung SW et al (1996) Topographic distribution of inguinal lymph nodes metastasis: significance in determination of treatment margin for elective inguinal lymph nodes irradiation of low pelvic tumors. Int J Radiat Oncol Biol Phys 35:133–136

Weber DC, Kurtz JM, Allal AS (2001) The impact of gap duration on local control in anal canal carcinoma treated by split-course radiotherapy and concomitant chemotherapy. Int J Radiat Oncol Biol Phys 50:675–680

Wexler A, Berson AM, Goldstone SE et al (2007) Invasive anal squamous-cell carcinoma in the HIV-positive patient: Outcome in the era of highly active antiretroviral therapy. Dis Colon Rectum [Epub ahead of print]

Wolfe HR, Bussey HJ (1968) Squamous-cell carcinoma of the anus. Br J Surg 55:295–301

Section V:
Tumors of the Genitalurinary System

Kidney and Ureter Cancers

SHEN FU

18

CONTENTS

S. Fu, MD
Department of Radiation Oncology, The 6th Hospital of Jiao
Tong University, 600 Yi Shan Road, Shanghai 200233, P. R.
China

Introduction and Objectives

Renal cell carcinoma (RCC) is the most commonly diagnosed malignancy of the kidney and accounts for approximately 3% of new cancer cases. Surgical resection is the primary treatment for localized renal cell carcinoma, and adjuvant treatment is usually not indicated in the majority of patients after complete resection. Transitional cell carcinoma (TCC) is the most common histological type of cancer of renal pelvis and ureter origin. Synchronous or metachronous involvement of multiple sites of the upper urinary tract is commonly observed, and it frequently metastasizes to regional lymph nodes, especially in high-grade diseases. The management of TCC of the renal pelvis and ureter differs significantly from renal cell carcinoma and usually involves a multi-modality approach.

This chapter examines:

● Recommendations for diagnosis and staging procedures for both renal cell carcinoma and TCC of the renal pelvis and ureter

● The staging systems and prognostic factors

● Unimodal and multimodal regimens based on surgery, radiation therapy, and/or chemotherapy for renal cell carcinoma and TCC of the upper urinary tract

● Techniques of radiation therapy for adjuvant treatment of renal cell carcinoma, as well as definitive and adjuvant treatment of TCC of the renal pelvis and ureter

● Follow-up care and surveillance of survivors

18.1 Diagnosis, Staging, and Prognoses

18.1.1 Diagnosis

Initial Evaluation

■ Diagnosis and evaluation of carcinoma of the upper urinary tract start with a complete patient history and physical examination (H&P). Attention should be paid to signs and symptoms specific to renal cell carcinoma, including gross or microscopic hematuria, palpable mass, and flank pain (the triad of symptoms that occurs in approximately 10% of cases), and to metastatic disease. Symptoms commonly observed with cancer of the renal pelvis and ureter include dysuria, hematuria, flank pain, and a palpable mass caused by hydronephrosis.

■ History of cigarette smoking and exposure to phenacetin-containing analgesics, heavy metals, and asbestos is relevant to renal cell carcinoma and should be recorded.

■ Renal cell carcinoma is associated with paraneoplastic syndromes, including hypertension, anemia, hypercalcemia, liver dysfunction, and fever (SUFRIN et al. 1989).

Laboratory Tests

■ Initial laboratory tests should include a complete blood count, basic blood chemistry, liver and renal function tests, lactate dehydrogenase (LDH), and urinalysis.

Imaging Studies

■ CT scan or MRI of the abdomen and pelvis is required for staging and metastatic workup for renal cell carcinoma, as well as lesions of the renal pelvis and ureter (JOHNSON et al. 1987; SEMELKA et al. 1993). For transitional cell carcinoma of the renal pelvis or ureter, multifocal lesions should be excluded.

■ Intravenous pyelogram (IVP) is recommended for evaluation of tumor mass and organ function.

■ Ultrasound with color-flow Doppler is helpful to identify the tumor thrombus in the renal vein or inferior vena (McCLENNAN 1991).

■ The most common sites of distant metastasis include the lung, bone, and liver. Chest X-ray or CT of the

Table 18.1. Imaging and laboratory work-ups for upper urinary tract cancer

Imaging studies	Laboratory tests
– CT or MRI of abdomen and pelvis – Intravenous pyelogram (IVP) – Chest X-ray or CT of the thorax – Bone scan – Ultrasound with color-flow Doppler (optional) – FDG-PET or PET/CT (optional)	– Complete blood count – Serum chemistry – Liver and renal function tests – Lactate dehydrogenase (LDH) – Urine analysis

thorax is indicated to rule out lung metastasis. Liver metastasis can be evaluated by CT or MRI of the abdomen. Skeletal metastasis occurs in approximately 25%–50% of patients with renal cell cancer, and bone scan should be performed to rule out skeletal metastasis (ALTHAUSEN et al. 1997) (Table 18.1).

■ FDG-PET can be used for detecting and staging of metastatic renal cell carcinoma, but its application in evaluating the primary tumor extension is limited (MARTINEZ et al. 2007; RAMDAVE et al. 2001).

Pathology

■ Histological diagnosis of upper urinary tract cancer is essential. Histological differentiation is significantly associated with prognosis in renal cell carcinoma, transitional cell carcinoma of the renal pelvis, as well as ureteral cancer (COZAD et al. 1995; HALL et al. 1998; HUBEN et al. 1988; ZHANG et al. 2008).

■ Tissue for pathologic diagnosis can be obtained via urine cytology, transurethral biopsy of the suspicious tumor under cystourethroscopy and urethrography, or from metastatic lesions.

■ Pathologic confirmation is often made at the time of curative surgery.

18.1.2 Staging

■ Renal cell carcinoma is staged both clinically and pathologically. Clinical staging relies on results from physical examination, laboratory tests, and imaging studies. Pathologic confirmation of the extent of the disease from resected specimen (kidney including primary tumor, Gerota's fascia, perinephric fat, renal vein, and regional lymph node) is recommended.

■ For renal cell carcinoma, the American Joint Committee on Cancer (AJCC) Staging Classification (Table 18.2) is currently the most commonly used staging system (GREENE et al. 2002). The AJCC staging system is preferred over the historically used Robson's modification of the Flock and Kadesky staging system for renal cell carcinoma, as it more clearly describes the primary and regional tumor extent (SOKOLOFF et al. 1996).

■ For cancers of the renal pelvis and ureter, clinical staging relies on results of physical examination, imaging studies, and laboratory tests. Pathologic

Table 18.2. American Joint Committee on Cancer (AJCC) TNM classification of renal cell carcinoma. [From GREENE et al. (2002) with permission]

Primary tumor (T)	
TX	Primary tumor cannot be assessed
T0	No evidence of primary tumor
T1	Tumor 7 cm or less in greatest dimension, limited to the kidney
T1a	Tumor 4 cm or less in greatest dimension, limited to the kidney
T1b	Tumor more than 4 cm, but not more than 7 cm in greatest dimension, limited to the kidney
T2	Tumor more than 7 cm in greatest dimension, limited to the kidney
T3	Tumor extends into major veins or invades adrenal gland or perinephric tissues, but not beyond Gerota's fascia
T3a	Tumor directly invades adrenal gland or perirenal and/or renal sinus fat but not beyond Gerota's fascia
T3b	Tumor grossly extends into the renal vein or its segmental (muscle-containing) branches, or vena cava below the diaphragm
T3c	Tumor grossly extends into vena cava above diaphragm or invades the wall of the vena cava
T4	Tumor invades beyond Gerota's fascia
Regional lymph nodes (N)[a]	
NX	Regional lymph nodes cannot be assessed
N0	No regional lymph node metastasis
N1	Metastasis in a single regional lymph node
N2	Metastasis in more than one regional lymph node
Distant metastasis (M)	
MX	Distant metastasis cannot be assessed
M0	No distant metastasis
M1	Distant metastasis
STAGE GROUPING	
I:	T1 N0 M0
II:	T2 N0 M0
III:	T1 N1 M0, T2 N1 M0, T3 N0 M0, T3 N1 M0, T3a N0 M0, T3a N1 M0, T3b N0 M0, T3b N1 M0, T3c N0 M0, T3c N1 M0
IV:	T4 N0 M0, T4 N1 M0, Any T N2 M0, Any T Any N M1

[a] Laterality does not affect the N classification.

staging depends on histological examination of the extent of tumor invasion.

■ Both the AJCC Staging Classification (Table 18.3) and the Jewett-Strong classification (originally developed for transitional carcinoma of the bladder) are used for cancer of the renal pelvis and ureter (GREENE et al. 2002).

18.1.3 Prognostic Factors

Renal Cell Carcinoma

■ Presenting stage and histological differentiation (tumor grade) are the most important prognostic factors in renal cell carcinoma and cancers of the renal pelvis or ureter. The estimated 5-year overall survival rates for renal cell carcinoma are 95%, 82%, 65%, and 25%, respectively, for stage I–IV disease (DEVITA et al. 2004). The locoregional treatment failure rates for early stage and low grade cancer of the renal pelvis or ureter are less than 15%, and those of locally advanced or higher grade are more than tripled (COZAD et al. 1995).

■ Presence of tumor thrombus on the level of the renal vein or inferior vena cava is associated with higher tumor grade and stage, and is associated with increased likelihood for distant metastases. In addition, completeness of surgery is prognostically important. The risk of local failure is only 5% after complete resection with radical nephrectomy (RABINOVITCH et al. 1994).

Cancer of the Renal Pelvis and Ureter

■ The stage at presentation and histological differentiation (tumor grade) are the most important prognostic factors for cancers of the renal pelvis and ureter: The average 5-year overall survival rates were >60% for stage I and II, 33% for stage III, and <15% for stage IV diseases, respectively. Those for grade I, II, III, and IV diseases were 85%, 60%, 30%, and <15%, respectively.

■ The number of lesions in multifocal disease, DNA pattern (i.e., heteroploid), and hypermethylation of the promoter region of patients may be adversely related to long-term prognosis (CORRADO et al. 1992).

■ The location of primary tumor may be of prognostic significance in locally advanced disease (Level IV) (WU et al. 2007).

Table 18.3. American Joint Committee on Cancer (AJCC) TNM classification of renal pelvis and ureter. [From Greene et al. (2002) with permission]

Primary tumor (T)	
TX	Primary tumor cannot be assessed
T0	No evidence of primary tumor
Ta	Papillary non-invasive carcinoma
Tis	Carcinoma in situ
T1	Tumor invades subepithelial connective tissue
T2	Tumor invades the muscularis
T3	(For renal pelvis only) Tumor invades beyond muscularis into peripelvic fat or the renal parenchyma
T3	(For ureter only) Tumor invades beyond muscularis into periureteric fat
T4	Tumor invades adjacent organs or through the kidney into the perinephric fat
Regional lymph nodes (N)	
NX	Regional lymph nodes cannot be assessed
N0	No regional lymph node metastasis
N1	Metastasis in a single lymph node, 2 cm or less in greatest dimension
N2	Metastasis in a single lymph node, more than 2 cm, but not more than 5 cm in greatest dimension; or multiple lymph nodes, none more than 5 cm in greatest dimension
N3	Metastasis in a lymph node, more than 5 cm in greatest dimension
Distant metastasis (M)	
MX	Distant metastasis cannot be assessed
M0	No distant metastasis
M1	Distant metastasis
STAGE GROUPING	
0a:	Ta N0 M0
0is:	Tis N0 M0
I:	T1 N0 M0
II:	T2 N0 M0
III:	T3 N0 M0
IV:	T4 N0 M0, Any T N1 M0, Any T N2 M0, Any T N3 M0, Any T Any N M1

18.2 Treatment of Renal Cell Carcinoma

18.2.1 General Principles

■ Surgery is the only curative treatment modality for renal cell carcinoma and is recommended for all resectable and operable cases (Grade A).

■ Neoadjuvant and adjuvant radiation therapy has a limited role for resectable disease or after complete resection and is not routinely recommended (Grade A).

■ Neoadjuvant radiation therapy can be considered in unresectable locally advanced renal cell carcinoma (Grade C). It has been shown to improve the resectability of locally advanced disease, but no significant difference in long-term survival was observed. Adjuvant radiation therapy is indicated in incompletely resected disease. It can also be considered in cases with involved lymph node(s) (Grade C).

■ Neoadjuvant or adjuvant chemotherapy or immunotherapy has no substantial role in the treatment of stage I–III diseases after complete resection (Grade A).

■ Immunotherapy and targeted therapy are the mainstay treatments for metastatic renal cell carcinoma (Grade A). Cytoreductive surgery is recommended prior to systemic immunotherapy and targeted therapy (Grade A). Palliative radiation therapy is a commonly used treatment modality for renal cell carcinoma with brain or bone metastases.

18.2.2 Surgery

■ Radical nephrectomy is the standard treatment for resectable and operable cases of renal cell carcinoma (excluding T1, N0, M0 disease) (Grade A). Radical nephrectomy removes the primary tumor, ipsilateral kidney, ipsilateral adrenal gland (for upper pole disease), Gerota's fascia, perirenal fat, and hilar lymph nodes.

■ Dissection of regional lymph nodes is not routinely recommended for early-stage disease as it is not associated to improved treatment outcome (Grade A). Results from a randomized trial reported by the European Organization for the Research and Treatment of Cancer (EORTC) 30881 revealed that the incidence of unsuspected lymph node metastases was only 3.3%, and complete lymph node dissection did not seem to improve the survival (EORTC 30881, Level I) (BLOM et al. 1999). Therefore, extended lymph node dissection should not be routinely considered, and lymphadenectomy should be limited to perihilar tissue for staging or in selected locally advanced cases.

- Regional dissection during radical nephrectomy can be considered in patients with locally advanced disease (Grade C). The results of a large retrospective review showed that large primary tumor size (>10 cm in largest dimension), T3 disease, high tumor grade, and presence of necrosis were associated with a higher chance of lymph node metastases (Level IV) (BLUTE et al. 2004).

- Partial nephrectomy (nephron-sparing surgery, NSS) can be considered in patients with small primary tumors of less than 7 cm (T1) in largest dimension (Grade A). Results of a number of retrospective studies have indicated that partial nephrectomy was associated with an acceptable local failure rate of less than 5% for T1 disease (Level IV) (LEIBOVICH et al. 2004; PATARD et al. 2004; PERMPONGKOSOL et al. 2006; SAIKA et al. 2003). In addition, preliminary results from an international collaborative Phase III randomized study revealed that NSS partial nephrectomy was of particular importance in patients with bilateral renal cell carcinoma.

- Cytoreductive nephrectomy is recommended for patients with metastatic renal cell cancer prior to immunotherapy or immunotherapy and targeted therapy (Grade A). Results from three intergroup studies completed by the Southwest Oncology Group (SWOG) and the EORTC have confirmed that survival could be improved by cytoreductive surgery performed prior to immunotherapy (SWOG 8949/EORTC, Level I) (FLANIGAN et al. 2001, 2004; MICKISCH et al. 2001; BOORJIAN and BLUTE 2008).

18.2.3 Radiation Therapy

Neoadjuvant Radiation Therapy

- Neoadjuvant radiation therapy is not recommended in patients with resectable renal cell carcinoma (Grade A). Results of two prospective randomized trials published in the 1970s showed that neoadjuvant radiation therapy did not improve the survival after nephrectomy.

The results of a prospective randomized trial reported by JUUSELA et al. (1977) revealed that the overall survival of patients treated with neoadjuvant radiation therapy up to 33 Gy (2.2 Gy per daily fraction) followed by nephrectomy was 47% at 5 years after therapy, whereas for the group treated with nephrectomy it was 63% (Level II).

In an earlier prospective randomized trail, the author found that low-dose neoadjuvant radiation therapy (30 Gy in 15 fractions) was associated with an increased frequency of complete resection in patients with internal and external vein and lymph vessel extension. In addition, the survival at 18 months was significantly higher in the group who received neoadjuvant radiotherapy. However, the overall survival rates were approximately 50% in both groups, with no significant difference (Level II) (VAN DER WERF-MESSING 1973).

- Neoadjuvant radiation can be considered for locally advanced renal cell carcinoma with direct invasion of adjacent organs, especially in cases where complete resection is not feasible (Grade B). In the above mentioned prospective randomized study reported by VAN DER WERF-MESSING (1973), complete resection was more common among patients with tumor involvement of the veins or lymph vessels who received neoadjuvant radiation (Level II).

Adjuvant Radiation Therapy

- Adjuvant radiation therapy is not routinely recommended in renal cell carcinoma after complete resection (Grade A). The local failure rate after complete resection of renal cell carcinoma is approximately 5% in stage I–III diseases. Although retrospective studies have suggested that adjuvant radiotherapy may improve local control in locally advanced diseases, its effect on survival in completely resected cases has not been confirmed by prospective studies:

Results from a number of retrospective or nonrandomized prospective studies have shown that adjuvant radiation therapy may be beneficial for local control of patients with high-risk renal cell carcinoma after nephrectomy. However, survival benefits of adjuvant radiotherapy have not been demonstrated in any of these trials (Level IV)

(GEZ et al. 2002; KAO et al. 1994; STEIN et al. 1992; ULUTIN et al. 2006).

In a prospective randomized trial completed by the Copenhagen Renal Cancer Study Group, 65 patients with stage II and III renal cell carcinoma were randomized and treated with nephrectomy only or nephrectomy followed by adjuvant radiation therapy (50 Gy in 20 fractions). The 5-year survival for the patients who received combined therapy was 38%, as compared to 62% for patients treated with surgery only. Postoperative radiation was associated with an increase of significant complications in nearly half of the patients (Level II) (KJAER et al. 1987).

- Adjuvant radiation should be considered for incompletely resected renal cell cancer including positive margin. It may also improve outcome in patients with positive lymph node(s) (Grade D). In a large single-institutional retrospective review, the outcome of 172 patients with unilateral renal cell carcinoma treated with surgery alone was analyzed. Only six patients developed local failure after complete resection, but 26% of patients developed distant metastasis. Lymph node involvement and renal vein extension were the two independent factors associated to the occurrence of distant metastasis (Level IV) (RABINOVITCH et al. 1994). However, the role of adjuvant radiation therapy in non-metastatic stage IV renal cell carcinoma with nodal involvement has not been specifically addressed in any trials.

Techniques of Radiation Therapy

Simulation and Planning

- CT-based planning is highly recommended for radiation treatment of renal cell cancer, if radiation is indicated, as in preoperative treatment of unresectable disease or cases with residual disease after surgery. Patient should be supine with arms-up position.
- The primary tumor (in preoperative cases), tumor bed (in postoperative cases), vascular extent of tumor, and hilar lymph node should be delineated and included in the treatment portal. Surgical clips should be carefully located and utilized for delineation of the clinical tumor volume (CTV) in postoperative cases.
- Multi-field arrangement can be used to reduce doses to critical tissues and organs, including the liver, contralateral kidney, small intestine, stomach, and spinal cord.

Dose and Schedules

- Total doses of 45–50.4 Gy (1.8 Gy per daily fraction) over 25 or 28 treatments are recommended. In case residual tumor exists, a small field boost to the residual disease with a margin of 2 cm to a total dose of 54–60 Gy is recommended.
- Higher dose of irradiation can be delivered using intensity-modulated radiation therapy (IMRT).

Dose Limiting Structures

- Dose of radiation to the spinal cord should be limited to 45 Gy (1.8–2.0 Gy daily). The dose to the contralateral kidney should be limited to 20 Gy or less, if lateral field(s) is used. The dose to the small intestine should be limited to 40 Gy or less (Level IV) (EMAMI et al. 1991).
- Limited treatment volume and dose to the liver should be considered for tumor of the right kidney and when lateral or oblique fields are applied for the left-sided disease.

18.2.4 Chemotherapy and Immunotherapy

- Neoadjuvant or adjuvant chemotherapy has no substantial role in the treatment of stage I–III diseases after complete resection (Grade A) (YAGODA et al. 1993).
- Immunotherapy [interferon-α or interleukin-2 (IL-2)] is not indicated for the definitive treatment of renal cell carcinoma (Grade A). Results from prospective randomized trials reported by various collaborative research groups aimed to study the efficacy of adjuvant interferon-α or IL-2 on overall survival or relapse-free survival failed to demonstrate their benefits on overall survival (Level I) (ATZPODIEN et al. 2005; CLARK et al. 2003; MESSING et al. 2003; PIZZOCARO et al. 2001).
- Immunotherapy and targeted therapy (with multikinase inhibitor sorafenib or sunitinib, or antiangiogenesis monoclonal antibody bevacizumab) play an important role in the treatment of metastatic renal cell carcinoma and are currently the first-line treatment (Grade A). The effects on progression-free survival (primary end point) of sorafenib, sunitinib, and bevacizumab used with interferon-α have been demonstrated in randomized phase III trials. However, the effects on over-

all survival have not been demonstrated (Level I) (ESCUDIER et al. 2007, 2007; MOTZER et al. 2007).

18.2.5 Radiation Therapy in the Treatment of Metastatic Renal Cell Carcinoma

- Radiation therapy is commonly used for symptomatic control in renal cell cancer with distant metastasis. Lung, bone, and brain are the common sites for distant metastases in renal cell carcinoma (MOTZER et al. 1996).

- Palliative irradiation is recommended for symptomatic bone metastasis in renal cell carcinoma; however, higher dose (BED 50 Gy or higher using $\alpha/\beta=10$) should be considered (Grade C). Although renal cell carcinoma has been considered as "radioresistant," pain palliation is expected in more than two-thirds of patients after radiation therapy:

  In a retrospective study reported by DIBIASE et al. (1997), patients treated with a higher biologically effective dose of radiation had a significantly higher response rate (59%) to radiotherapy, as compared to those who received lower BED (39%) (Level IV). However, the results from a series reported by WILSON et al. (2003) suggested that higher BED did not seem to be a predictor of response or of duration of response in the palliative treatment of renal cell carcinoma. Nevertheless, symptomatic palliation was observed in the majority of patients with metastatic renal cell carcinoma, including patients with painful bone metastasis (Level IV) (WILSON et al. 2003).

- Whole brain irradiation in combination with stereotactic radiosurgery is indicated for patients with single or multiple brain metastases (Grade A). A number of retrospective studies have addressed the effects of combined stereotactic radiotherapy and whole brain radiation on disease control of brain metastasis in renal cell carcinoma: The addition of stereotactic radiosurgery significantly improved the outcome (including overall survival in selected cases) of renal cell cancer patients with brain metastasis, and whole brain irradiation should not be omitted and is associated with an improved local control rate (Level IV) (AMENDOLA et al. 2000; BROWN et al. 2002; FULLER et al. 1992; HERNANDEZ et al. 2002).

18.3 Treatment of Cancer of the Renal Pelvis or Ureter

18.3.1 General Principles

- Surgery is the only curative treatment modality for cancers of the renal pelvis or ureter, and should be considered for all resectable and operable cases (Grade A).

- Adjuvant radiation therapy is recommended for patients with locally advanced disease (stage III or above) or grade 3 and 4 transitional carcinoma of the renal pelvis or ureter (Grade B).

- The effect of adjuvant chemotherapy in the treatment of high-risk patients is largely unknown. Due to the high risk of distant metastasis, adjuvant chemotherapy can be considered for patients after complete resection (Grade D).

- For surgically unresectable or medically inoperable transitional cell carcinoma of the renal pelvis or ureter, definitive chemoradiation therapy can be considered for definitive treatment (Grade D). Regimens utilized in the treatment of transitional cell carcinoma or that of the urinary bladder can be considered because of the similarity of the biological behavior.

18.3.2 Surgery

- For single-site, stage I, and low-grade lesions less than 1.5 cm in largest dimension, partial ureterectomy or nephron-sparing surgery can be considered (Grade B).

- Nephroureterectomy with removal of the bladder cuff is the standard surgical technique for cancer of the renal pelvis or ureter (Grade A). Nephroureterectomy can be performed laparoscopically without compromising the treatment outcome (Level IV) (SHALHAV et al. 2000; GILL et al. 2000; ROUPRÊT et al. 2007).

18.3.3 Radiation Therapy

- The high risk of locoregional treatment failure in locally advanced-stage and higher grade tumors has made adjuvant radiation therapy an important part of definitive treatment of cancer of the renal pelvis or ureter (Grade B). Postoperative radiotherapy has been shown to improve locoregional control and disease-free survival rates in high-risk patients; however, its effect on overall survival has not been consistently demonstrated, partly due to the limited size of reported studies:

In a small retrospective study reported by Cozad et al. (1992), 26 patients with T3, T4, or N+ transitional cell carcinoma of the renal pelvis or ureter were treated with or without adjuvant radiation therapy after surgery. With a median follow-up of 13.5 months, the actuarial 5-year local control rates were 88% and 34%, respectively, for the groups treated with or without adjuvant therapy. The 5-year actuarial survival was 44% with and 24% without adjuvant radiation therapy (p=NS) (Level IV). In a more recently published series with 94 patients with locally advanced disease by Cozad et al. (1995), the effects of adjuvant radiation therapy were again demonstrated. Adjuvant radiation therapy significantly reduced the local recurrence rate. In addition, adjuvant radiotherapy was of borderline significance for significantly improving the survival rate (Level IV).

Techniques of Radiation Therapy

Simulation and Planning

- CT-based planning is highly recommended for external-beam radiotherapy for cancers of the renal pelvis or ureter. The patient should be supine position with arms raised.
- The radiation therapy field after nephroureterectomy should encompass the tumor bed with sufficient margin and regional lymph node (Fig. 18.1) (Grade B). The risk of regional lymph node metastasis can be as high as 60% in high-grade disease (Level IV) (Charbit et al. 1991; Miyao et al. 1998).

  For renal pelvic or upper ureteral disease, coverage of the ipsilateral renal hilar nodes as well as adjacent periaortic or pericaval lymph nodes is recommended. For lower ureteral diseases, coverage of the pelvis lymph node is recommended.
- For unresectable disease, the radiation field should encompass the entire course of the ureter (from the renal fossa to the trigone of the ipsilateral bladder), including the primary tumor bed (Fig. 18.2). However, the parenchyma of the kidney should be spared if possible.

Dose and Schedules

- Total doses of 45–50.4 Gy (1.8 Gy per daily fraction) over 25–28 treatments are recommended. An additional dose to a total of 54–60 Gy to gross or microscopic residual disease is usually recommended if tolerance doses of adjacent normal organs are not exceeded. A higher dose of irradiation can be delivered using IMRT.
- A higher dose of radiation can also be delivered via intraoperative radiation therapy (IORT) for

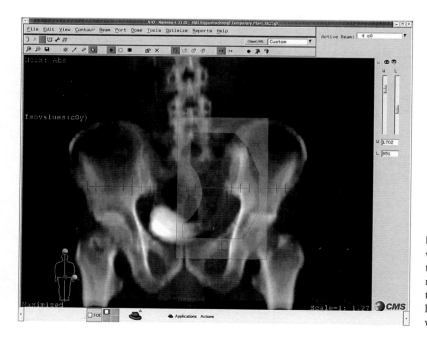

Fig. 18.1. Radiation field for a patient with locally advanced ureter transitional cell cancer of distal ureter after resection. The field encompassed the tumor bed and the ipsilateral pelvis lymph nodes, and was treated to 45 Gy with AP/PA fields

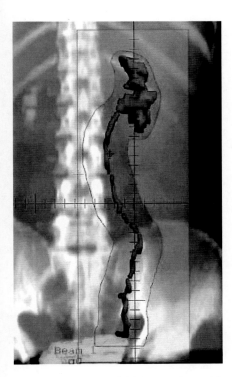

Fig. 18.2. Radiation field for a patient with an unresectable transitional cell cancer of the renal pelvis and upper ureter. The field encompassed the renal pelvis and ureter, and spared most part of the renal parenchyma. Entire ureter was treated up to the insertion in the bladder

ureter cancer (Grade C). The safety and efficacy of IORT have been suggested by a small group of patients treated with nephroureterectomy followed by IORT and external-beam radiation: In a recently published study, ZHANG et al. (2008) prospectively treated 17 patients with locally advanced (T3, T4, or N+) transitional cell carcinoma of the ureter with nephroureterectomy followed by IORT and adjuvant external-beam radiotherapy. The 5-year local control and overall survival rates were 51% and 46%, respectively. In addition, significant side effects and complications associated with high-dose irradiation, including IORT, was not observed (Level III). However, the utilization of IORT on renal pelvic cancer has not been addressed.

Dose Limiting Structures

- The dose of radiation to the spinal cord should be limited to 45 Gy (1.8–2.0 Gy daily). The dose

to the kidneys should be limited to 20 Gy or less; the dose to the small intestine should be limited to 40 Gy or less (Level IV) (EMAMI et al. 1991).

- Limited treatment volume and dose to the bladder should be considered for tumors of the lower ureter, and dose/volume to the liver should be considered if lateral fields are applied.

18.3.4 Adjuvant Chemotherapy

- Platinum-based chemotherapy given concurrently with radiation can be considered in the treatment of locally advanced (T3, T4, N+) transitional cell carcinoma of the upper urinary tract (Grade B). Platinum-based chemotherapy used in an adjuvant setting has been shown to reduce the risk of distant metastases in locally advanced upper urinary tract carcinoma (Level IV) (BAMIAS et al. 2004; KWAK et al. 2006). In addition, results from a retrospective study have indicated that combined chemoradiation therapy in an adjuvant setting was more effective than radiotherapy alone:
  A retrospective study from Massachusetts General Hospital addressed the effects of postoperative concurrent cisplatin-based chemotherapy and radiation therapy. Patients with locally advanced disease (T3, T4, N+) were treated with external beam radiation therapy (median dose: 49.6 Gy), with or without concurrent chemotherapy (methotrexate, cisplatin, and vinblastine). The 5-year actuarial overall and disease specific survival were 27% vs. 67% and 41% vs. 76%, significantly improved with the addition of concurrent chemotherapy (Level IV) (CZITO et al. 2004).

 18.4 Follow-Ups

18.4.1 Post-Treatment Follow-Ups

- Long-term follow-up is required for early detection of recurrence in successfully treated patients with renal cell carcinoma and transitional cell carcinoma of the upper urinary tract. Metachronous recurrence of transitional cell carcinoma in the urinary tract is not uncommon in patients with renal pelvic or ureteral cancer.

Schedule

- For stage I–III renal cell carcinoma, follow-up can be scheduled every 6 months for the first 2 years, then annually for 5 more years (Grade D) (National Comprehensive Cancer Network 2008).

- For transitional cell carcinoma of the renal pelvis or ureter, follow-up can be scheduled every 3–4 months for the first 2 years, then every 6 months for 3 additional years, then annually thereafter (Grade D).

Work-Ups

- Each follow-up examination should include a complete history and physical examination. Laboratory tests, including complete blood count, complete metabolic panel, urine analysis, and LDH, should be performed at each follow-up (Grade D) (National Comprehensive Cancer Network 2008). Cystoscopy should be considered for transitional cell carcinoma of the lower ureter in the first 2 years of follow-up (Grade D).

- For stage I–III renal cell carcinoma, chest X-ray and CT of the abdomen and pelvis should be considered at 4 to 6 months after treatment, then ordered if symptomatically indicated (Grade D) (National Comprehensive Cancer Network 2008).

- For transitional cell carcinoma of the renal pelvis or ureter, in addition to chest X-ray and CT of the abdomen and pelvis, imaging work-ups recommended for bladder cancer for detecting local recurrence can be referenced. Studies should include ureteroscopy, and upper tract imaging (IVP, retrograde pyelogram, CT urography, or MRI urogram) can be performed at 3–12 month intervals (Grade D) (National Comprehensive Cancer Network 2008).

References

Amendola BE, Wolf AL, Coy SR et al (2000) Brain metastases in renal cell carcinoma: management with gamma knife radiosurgery. Cancer J 6:372–376

Althausen P, Althausen A, Jennings LC et al (1997) Prognostic factors and surgical treatment of osseous metastases secondary to renal cell carcinoma. Cancer 80:1103–1109

Atzpodien J, Schmitt E, Gertenbach U et al (2005) Adjuvant treatment with interleukin-2- and interferon-alpha2a-based chemoimmunotherapy in renal cell carcinoma post tumour nephrectomy: results of a prospectively randomised trial of the German Cooperative Renal Carcinoma Chemoimmunotherapy Group (DGCIN). Br J Cancer 92:843–846

Bamias A, Deliveliotis Ch, Fountzilas G et al (2004) Adjuvant chemotherapy with paclitaxel and carboplatin in patients with advanced carcinoma of the upper urinary tract: a study by the Hellenic Cooperative Oncology Group. J Clin Oncol 22:2150–2154

Blom JH, van Poppel H, Marechal JM et al (1999) Radical nephrectomy with and without lymph node dissection: preliminary results of the EORTC randomized Phase III protocol 30881. EORTC Genitourinary Group. Eur Urol 36:570–575

Blute ML, Leibovich BC, Cheville JC et al (2004) A protocol for performing extended lymph node dissection using primary tumor pathological features for patients treated with radical nephrectomy for clear cell renal cell carcinoma. J Urol 172:465–469

Brown PD, Brown CA, Pollock BE et al (2000) Stereotactic radiosurgery for patients with "radioresistant" brain metastases. Neurosurgery 51:656–665; discussion 665–667

Boorjian SA, Blute ML (2008) A prospective randomized EORTC intergroup Phase 3 study comparing the complications of elective nephron-sparing surgery and radical nephrectomy for low stage renal cell carcinoma 26:101–102

Charbit L, Gendreau MC, Mee S et al (1991) Tumors of the upper urinary tract: 10 years of experience. J Urol 146:1243–1246

Clark JI, Atkins MB, Urba WJ et al (2003) Adjuvant high-dose bolus interleukin-2 for patients with high-risk renal cell carcinoma: a cytokine working group randomized trial. J Clin Oncol 21:3133–3140

Corrado F, Mannini D, Ferri C et al (1992) The prognostic significance of DNA ploidy pattern in transitional cell cancer of the renal pelvis and ureter: continuing follow-up. Eur Urol 1[Suppl 21]:48–50

Cozad SC, Smalley SR, Austenfeld M et al (1992) Adjuvant radiotherapy in high stage transitional cell carcinoma of the renal pelvis and ureter. Int J Radiat Oncol Biol Phys 24:743–745

Cozad SC, Smalley SR, Austenfeld M et al (1995) Transitional cell carcinoma of the renal pelvis or ureter: patterns of failure. Urology 46:796–800

Czito B, Zietman A, Kaufman D et al (2004) Adjuvant radiotherapy with and without concurrent chemotherapy for locally advanced transitional cell carcinoma of the renal pelvis and ureter. J Urol 172 (4 pt 1):1271–1275

DeVita VT Jr, Hellman S, Resenberg SA et al (2004) Cancer principles and practice of oncology, 7th edn. Lippincott Williams & Wilkins, Philadelphia

DiBiase SJ, Valicenti RK, Schultz D et al (1997) Palliative irradiation for focally symptomatic metastatic renal cell carcinoma: support for dose escalation based on a biological model. J Urol 158 (3 Pt 1):746–749

Emami B, Lyman J, Brown A et al (1991) Tolerance of normal tissue to therapeutic irradiation. Int J Radiat Oncol Biol Phys 21:109–122

Escudier B, Pluzanska A, Koralewski P et al (2007) Bevacizumab plus interferon alfa-2a for treatment of metastatic renal cell carcinoma: a randomised, double-blind Phase III trial. Lancet 370:2103–2111

Escudier B, Eisen T, Stadler WM et al (2007) Target Study Group. Sorafenib in advanced clear-cell renal-cell carcinoma. N Engl J Med 356:125–134

Flanigan RC, Mickisch G, Sylvester R, et al (2001) Nephrectomy followed by interferon alpha-2b compared with interferon alpha-2b alone for metastatic renal cell carcinoma. N Engl J Med 345:1655–1659

Flanigan RC, Mickisch G, Sylvester R et al (2004) Cytoreductive nephrectomy in patients with metastatic renal cancer: a combined analysis. J Urol 171:1071–1076

Fuller BG, Kaplan ID, Adler J et al (1992) Stereotaxic radiosurgery for brain metastases: the importance of adjuvant whole brain irradiation. Int J Radiat Oncol Biol Phys 23:413–418

Gez E, Libes M, Bar-Deroma R et al (2002) Postoperative irradiation in localized renal cell carcinoma: the Rambam Medical Center experience. Tumori 88:500–502

Gill IS, Sung GT, Hobart MG et al (2000) Laparoscopic radical nephroureterectomy for upper tract transitional cell carcinoma: the Cleveland Clinic experience. J Urol 164:1513–1522

Greene F, Page D, Fleming I et al (2002) AJCC cancer staging manual, 6th edn. Springer, Berlin Heidelberg New York

Hall MC, Womack S, Sagalowsky AI et al (1998) Prognostic factors, recurrence, and survival in transitional cell carcinoma of the upper urinary tract: a 30-year experience in 252 patients. Urology 52:594–601

Hernandez L, Zamorano L, Sloan A et al (2002) Gamma knife radiosurgery for renal cell carcinoma brain metastases. J Neurosurg 97[5 Suppl]:489–493

Huben RP, Mounzer AM, Murphy GP (1988) Tumor grade and stage as prognostic variables in upper tract urothelial tumors. Cancer 62:2016–2020

Johnson CD, Dunnick NR, Cohan RH et al (1987) Renal adenocarcinoma: CT staging of 100 tumors. AJR Am J Roentgenol 148:59–63

Juusela H, Malmio K, Alfthan O et al (1977) Preoperative irradiation in the treatment of renal adenocarcinoma. Scand J Urol Nephrol 11:277–281

Kao GD, Malkowicz SB, Whittington R et al (1994) Locally advanced renal cell carcinoma: low complication rate and efficacy of postnephrectomy radiation therapy planned with CT. Radiology 193:725–730

Kjaer M, Iversen P, Hvidt V et al (1987) A randomized trial of postoperative radiotherapy versus observation in Stage II and III renal adenocarcinoma. A study by the Copenhagen Renal Cancer Study Group. Scand J Urol Nephrol 21:285–289

Kwak C, Lee SE, Jeong IG et al (2006) Adjuvant systemic chemotherapy in the treatment of patients with invasive transitional cell carcinoma of the upper urinary tract. Urology 68:53–57

Leibovich BC, Blute ML, Cheville JC et al (2004) Nephron-sparing surgery for appropriately selected renal cell carcinoma between 4 and 7 cm results in outcome similar to radical nephrectomy. J Urol 171:1066–1070

Martínez de Llano SR, Delgado-Bolton RC, Jiménez-Vicioso A et al (2007) Meta-analysis of the diagnostic performance of 18F-FDG PET in renal cell carcinoma. Rev Esp Med Nucl 26:19–29

McClennan BL (1991) Oncologic imaging. Staging and follow-up of renal and adrenal carcinoma. Cancer 67[4 Suppl]:1199–1208

Messing EM, Manola J, Wilding G et al (2003) Phase III study of interferon alfa-NL as adjuvant treatment for resectable renal cell carcinoma: an Eastern Cooperative Oncology Group/Intergroup trial. J Clin Oncol 21:1214–1222

Mickisch GH, Garin A, van Poppel H et al (2001) Radical nephrectomy plus interferon-alfa-based immunotherapy compared with interferon alfa alone in metastatic renal-cell carcinoma: a randomised trial. Lancet 358:966–970

Miyao N, Masumori N, Takahashi A et al (1998) Lymph node metastasis in patients with carcinomas of the renal pelvis and ureter. Eur Urol 33:180–185

Motzer RJ, Bander NH, Nanus DM (1996) Renal-cell carcinoma. N Engl J Med 335:865–875

Motzer RJ, Hutson TE, Tomczak P et al (2007) Sunitinib versus interferon alfa in metastatic renal-cell carcinoma. N Engl J Med 356:115–124

National Comprehensive Cancer Network (2008) Clinical practice guidelines in oncology: Kidney cancer. Available at http://www.nccn.org/professionals/physician_gls/PDF/kidney.pdf. Accessed on June 24, 2008

Patard JJ, Shvarts O, Lam JS et al (2004) Safety and efficacy of partial nephrectomy for all T1 tumors based on an international multicenter experience. J Urol 171(6 Pt 1):2181–2185

Permpongkosol S, Bagga HS, Romero FR et al (2006) Laparoscopic versus open partial nephrectomy for the treatment of pathological T1N0M0 renal cell carcinoma: a 5-year survival rate. J Urol 176:1984–1988

Pizzocaro G, Piva L, Colavita M et al (2001) Interferon adjuvant to radical nephrectomy in Robson Stages II and III renal cell carcinoma: a multicentric randomized study. J Clin Oncol 19:425–431

Rabinovitch RA, Zelefsky MJ, Gaynor JJ et al (1994) Patterns of failure following surgical resection of renal cell carcinoma: implications for adjuvant local and systemic therapy. J Clin Oncol 12:206–212

Ramdave S, Thomas GW, Berlangieri SU et al (2001) Clinical role of F-18 fluorodeoxyglucose positron emission tomography for detection and management of renal cell carcinoma. J Urol 166:825–830

Rouprêt M, Hupertan V, Sanderson KM et al (2007) Oncologic control after open or laparoscopic nephroureterectomy for upper urinary tract transitional cell carcinoma: a single center experience. Urology 69:656–661

Saika T, Ono Y, Hattori R et al (2003) Long-term outcome of laparoscopic radical nephrectomy for pathologic T1 renal cell carcinoma. Urology 62:1018–1023

Semelka RC, Shoenut JP, Magro CM (1993) Renal cancer staging: comparison of contrast-enhanced CT and gadolinium-enhanced fat-suppressed spin-echo and gradient-echo MR imaging. J Magn Reson Imaging 3:597–602

Shalhav AL, Dunn MD, Portis AJ et al (2000) Laparoscopic nephroureterectomy for upper tract transitional cell cancer: the Washington University experience. J Urol 163:1100–1104

Sokoloff MH, deKernion JB, Figlin RA et al (1996) Current management of renal cell carcinoma. CA Cancer J Clin 46:284–302

Stein M, Kuten A, Halpern J et al (1992) The value of postoperative irradiation in renal cell cancer. Radiother Oncol 24:41–44

Sufrin G, Chasan S, Golio A et al (1989) Paraneoplastic and serologic syndromes of renal adenocarcinoma. Semin Urol 7:158–171

Ulutin HC, Aksu G, Fayda M et al (2006) The value of postoperative radiotherapy in renal cell carcinoma: a single-institution experience. Tumori 92:202–206

van der Werf-Messing B (1973) Proceedings: Carcinoma of the kidney. Cancer 32:1056–1061

Wilson D, Hiller L, Gray L et al (2003) The effect of biological effective dose on time to symptom progression in metastatic renal cell carcinoma. Clin Oncol (R Coll Radiol) 15:400–407

Wu CF, Pang ST, Chen CS et al (2007) The impact factors on prognosis of patients with pT3 upper urinary tract transitional cell carcinoma. J Urol 178:446–450

Yagoda A, Abi-Rached B, Petrylak D (1995) Chemotherapy for advanced renal-cell carcinoma:1983–1993. Semin Oncol 22:42–60

Zhang Q, Fu S, Liu T et al (2008) Adjuvant intra-operative electron radiotherapy and external beam radiotherapy for locally advanced transitional cell carcinoma of the ureter. Urol Oncol (in press) [Epub ahead of print]

Bladder Cancer

JAMES S. BUTLER

CONTENTS

Introduction and Objectives

Bladder cancer is one of the most common malignancies of the urinary tract and is a disease that ranges from localized disease treated with cystoscopy and transurethral tumor resection only to metastatic disease that requires systemic therapy. Although the majority of patients present with superficial disease, approximately one third of patients with bladder cancer will have muscle invasion, and localized invasive disease often requires multidisciplinary management, particularly if bladder preservation is to be attempted.

This chapter examines:

- Recommendations for diagnostic and staging procedures for non-invasive and invasive disease

- The staging system and prognostic factors for recurrence of superficial disease, progression of superficial disease to invasive disease, survival and recurrence of invasive disease, and bladder preservation of invasive disease

- Treatment recommendations with supporting scientific evidence including intravesicular chemotherapy for superficial disease, cystectomy, the potential role of preoperative radiation, neoadjuvant and adjuvant chemotherapy, and bladder preservation therapy

- Radiation therapy techniques and how to combine radiation with chemotherapy and transurethral resection for bladder conservation

- Systemic chemotherapy for metastatic disease

- Treatment recommendations for non-transitional histologies

- Quality of life, follow-up care, and recommendations for surveillance of survivors, including those who have undergone bladder-sparing therapy

J. S. BUTLER, MD
Department of Radiation Oncology, Maimonides Cancer Center, 6300 Eighth Avenue, Brooklyn, NY 11020, USA

19.1 Diagnosis, Staging, and Prognoses

19.1.1 Diagnosis

Initial Evaluation

■ Diagnosis and evaluation of bladder cancer begin with complete history and physical examination. Presenting signs and symptoms depend upon the extent of the tumor. History includes noting symptoms, such as hematuria (the most common symptom, which occurs in approximately 75% of cases), urinary irritative or obstructive symptomatology, decreased appetite, weight loss, bone pain, and pelvic pain.

■ History of carcinogen exposure: tobacco use, occupational history (naphthylamines, benzidines, biphenyl exposure), chemotherapy (cytoxan), catheterization, bladder lithiasis, multiple urinary tract infections, and/or a history of schistosomiasis.

■ Thorough physical examination includes bimanual examination to evaluate for pelvic/bladder mass, abdominal exam for organomegaly, cystoscopy, and boney palpation.

Laboratory Tests

■ Laboratory tests include complete blood count, serum chemistry, liver function tests, renal function tests, and urinalysis, and urine cytology should be performed. Urine cytology has an overall sensitivity of 20–50%, with overall specificity in of 80%–100% (Level I) (Lotan and Roehrborn 2003).

Imaging

■ Diagnostic imaging studies evaluate the extent of disease in the bladder, and for invasive cancer, ruling distant metastases in or out is required.

■ Work-up involves cystoscopy first with imaging of the upper tract collecting system to rule out synchronous primaries. Retrograde pyelography, at the time of the cystoscopy or separately via intravenous pyelography, should be performed.

■ Ultrasonography is useful for detecting bladder masses and can demonstrate the presence of transmural invasion.

■ For patients with invasive cancer, imaging of the upper tract is usually accomplished by CT scan of the abdomen and pelvis with IV contrast. This test also evaluates for adenopathy and metastasis.

■ MRI of the pelvis can be considered if delineation of extravesicular bladder tumor and local extension is desired as MRI can ascertain this better in some circumstances than a CT (Grade B). Staging accuracy in one retrospective study was 85% in differentiating superficial from invasive tumors and 82% in differentiating organ-confined from non-organ-confined tumors (Level III) (Tekes et al. 2005). Results from a prospective study designed to identify prognostic features on MRI before radiotherapy demonstrated that those patients upstaged clinically from T2a to T3b on MRI had a significantly worse outcome (Level III) (Robinson et al. 2000). MRI can be helpful for evaluating less common neoplastic diseases of the bladder, such as urachal carcinoma, and tumors that develop within bladder diverticula (Level III) (Mallampati and Siegelman 2004).

■ Chest X-ray is recommended to rule out pulmonary metastasis in invasive cancer of the bladder. Bone scan is not routinely recommended, but should be ordered for cases with elevated alkaline phosphatase or bone pain.

■ FDG-PET scan is ineffective in evaluating bladder tumors as FDG accumulates in the bladder. However, FDG-PET may be useful for diagnosis of distant or lymphatic metastasis (Grade B). PET imaging identified 17 of 17 patients with metastatic disease as well as two of three patients (67%) with localized lymph node involvement (Level III) (Kosuda et al. 1997). The detection rate for regional nodal disease was 67% in another trial (Level III) (Heicappell et al. 1999).

Table 19.1. Imaging and laboratory work-up for superficial bladder cancer

Imaging studies	Laboratory tests
– Cystoscopy – Intravenous or retrograde pyelography	– Complete blood count – Serum chemistry – Liver function tests – Renal function tests – Alkaline phosphatase – LDH – Urine cytology before and after cystoscopy

Table 19.2. Imaging and laboratory for invasive bladder cancer

Imaging studies	Laboratory tests
– Chest X-ray – Ultrasonagraphy – CT of abdomen and pelvis – MRI (if additional information regarding local tumor extent desired) – Bone scan (if indicated by symptoms or elevated alkaline phosphatase) – FDG-PET (optional for diagnosis of distant metastasis)	– Complete blood count – Serum chemistry – Liver function tests – Renal function tests – Alkaline phosphatase – LDH – Urine cytology before and after cystoscopy

Pathology

■ Because of high specificity of urine cytology, positive cytology is almost always diagnostic of bladder cancer. In 40%–80% of poorly differentiated carcinoma, cytology will be positive, but only 5%–40% of well-differentiated cases will have positive cytology (Level I) (LOTAN and ROEHRBORN 2003). However, it is important to remember that urine cytology cannot differentiate between invasive and superficial disease.

■ Cystoscopy enables direct visualization of the intravesical lesion and provides tissue for histological diagnosis. Transurethral resection of the bladder tumor to a maximum extent should be performed, and random biopsies of the bladder mucosa should be taken to rule out carcinoma in situ.

■ Transitional cell carcinoma (TCC) is the most common type of bladder cancer in North America and Europe. Superficial transitional cell carcinoma comprises 70% of transitional cell carcinomas, and 30% of cases are invasive.

■ Tumors of mixed histology consisting of transitional cell carcinoma with squamous or adenocarcinoma elements are common and were identified in 25% of patients in one large study. These are variants of transitional cell carcinoma and are associated with higher incidence of muscle invasion and extra-vesicle extension, but do not portend a worse survival (Level III) (WASCO et al. 2007). One study demonstrated that these patients have a higher incidence of positive margins after cystectomy (Level IV) (DOTAN et al. 2007).

■ Squamous cell carcinoma is associated with chronic bladder irritation and schistosomiasis infection. Historically, squamous cell carcinoma was the predominant form of bladder cancer in Egypt; however, transitional cell carcinoma has recently become the most frequent type (Level III) (FELIX et al. 2008). Other pathologic types, such as small cell carcinoma, spindle cell carcinoma, and adenocarcinoma, also occur.

19.1.2 Staging

■ Bladder cancer can be staged clinically and pathologically: Clinical staging utilizes information from the history and physical exam, imaging studies, and laboratory tests, as well as findings from cystoscopy and exam under anesthesia. Pathologic staging is based on findings at cystectomy, intraoperative exam, and lymph node dissection.

■ The American Joint Committee on Cancer Tumor Node Metastasis (TNM) staging system for bladder cancer is presented in Table 19.3.

19.1.3 Prognostic Factors

■ The stage at diagnosis is the most important prognostic factor for bladder cancer. Superficial disease is usually not immediately life-threatening as lymph nodes or distant metastases occur only at the invasive stage.

■ Superficial low-grade tumor and papillary configuration predict low risk of recurrence. Higher risk for development of intravesical recurrence of superficial disease includes high-grade disease, carcinoma in situ, multifocal disease, and rapid recurrence post recent transurethral resection. However, these factors do not predict nodal or distant metastasis.

■ If the patient undergoes cystectomy, prognostic groups can be roughly divided according to the stage into organ-confined disease (confined to the wall of bladder with negative nodes, pT2,N0) versus extra-vesicular invasion with negative nodes (pT3-T4,N0) versus patients with metastatic disease to pelvic lymph nodes (pTany, N+).

Table 19.3. American Joint Committee on Cancer (AJCC) TNM Classification of Carcinoma Cancer of the Urinary Bladder. [From GREENE et al. (2002) with permission]

Primary tumor (T)	
TX	Primary tumor cannot be assessed
T0	No evidence of primary tumor
Ta	Non-invasive papillary carcinoma
Tis	Carcinoma in situ: "flat tumor"
T1	Tumor invades subepithelial connective tissue
T2	Tumor invades muscle
pT2a	Tumor invades superficial muscle (inner half)
pT2b	Tumor invades deep muscle (outer half)
T3	Tumor invades perivesical tissue
pT3a	Microscopically
pT3b	Macroscopically (extravesical mass)
T4	Tumor invades any of the following: prostate, uterus, vagina, pelvic wall, abdominal wall
T4a	Tumor invades prostate, uterus, vagina
T4b	Tumor invades pelvic wall, abdominal wall

Regional lymph nodes (N)	
NX	Regional lymph nodes cannot be assessed
N0	No regional lymph node metastasis
N1	Metastasis in a single lymph node, 2 cm or less in greatest dimension
N2	Metastasis in a single lymph node, more than 2 cm, but not more than 5 cm in greatest dimension; or multiple lymph nodes, none more than 5 cm in greatest dimension
N3	Metastasis in a lymph node, more than 5 cm in greatest dimension

Distant metastasis (M)	
MX	Distant metastasis cannot be assessed
M0	No distant metastasis
M1	Distant metastasis

STAGE GROUPING	
0a:	Ta N0 M0
0is:	Tis N0 M0
I:	T1 N0 M0
II:	T2a N0 M0, T2b N0 M0
III:	T3a N0 M0, T3b N0 M0, T4a N0 M0
IV:	T4b N0 M0, Any T N1 M0, Any T N2 M0, Any T N3 M0, Any T Any N M1

Used with permission of the American Joint Committee on Cancer (AJCC), Chicago, IL. The original and primary source for this information is the AJCC Cancer Staging Manual, 6th edn (2002), Springer, New York

- Factors that predict success of bladder preservation are performance of complete transurethral resection, complete regression of disease after radiation and chemotherapy, solitary tumor, lack of ureteral obstruction, or hydronephrosis; T2 is better than T3 (Level IV) (MAMEGHAN et al. 1995; SHIPLEY et al. 1985).
- The hemoglobin level may be prognostic (Level III) (GOSPODAROWICZ et al. 1989).
- Female gender may predict higher chances of positive margins after cystectomy (Level IV) (DOTAN et al. 2007).
- Tumor markers, including p53 status, p21 status, and RB gene status, are being investigated. HER2/neu status has been found to predict reduced complete response, and epidermal growth factor receptor is a predictor of favorable outcome in patients treated with chemoradiation in a review of the RTOG chemoradiation studies (Level III) (CHAKRAVARTI et al. 2005). However, these markers are not ready to be routinely tested for, and their utilization requires further investigation.

19.2 Treatment of Bladder Cancer

19.2.1 Treatment of Superficial Bladder Tumors

- Transurethral resection of the bladder tumor is the standard treatment for superficial bladder tumors (Grade A). However, despite complete resection of the disease, approximately 70% of patients will develop intravesical recurrence, and 15% will progress to invasive recurrence if no further therapy is rendered.
- Patients with superficial bladder tumors can be divided into two risk groups according to the histological characteristics: Low-risk patients include those with low-grade bladder tumor and papillary configuration, and require close cystoscopic surveillance after TURBT. These patients have a 50% probability of developing recurrent bladder tumor with less than a 5% chance of progression to invasive cancer.
- High-risk superficial bladder cancer patients include all others: High-grade disease, carcinoma in situ, multifocal disease, and patients who have

rapid recurrence post recent transurethral resection of bladder tumor. High-risk patients should be considered for installation of intravesicular chemotherapy after transurethral resection (Grade A). Approximately 70% of these patients will develop recurrent bladder tumor, and 30% will progress to invasive disease.

- The types of intravesicular chemotherapy that have been used include Bacillus Calmette-Guerin (BCG), interferon plus BCG, thiotepa, mitomycin-C, doxorubicin, and gemcitabine. Randomized studies and a meta-analysis have demonstrated a decrease in the recurrence of superficial bladder tumors using intravesicular chemotherapy (Level I) (PAWINSKI et al. 1996).

- BCG with or without interferon has been proven to be superior to other types of intravesicular chemotherapy and should be considered an initial treatment (Grade A). A meta-analysis demonstrated that response to BCG was 70% compared to 50% for chemotherapy, and at a median follow-up of 3.6 years, 50% had no evidence of disease compared with 25% who had received chemotherapy (Level I) (SYLVESTER et al. 2005). It is important, however, to note that BCG cannot be used immediately after transurethral resection of the bladder tumor because of risk of systemic absorption.

- Unfortunately, no study has demonstrated that the chances of recurrent disease becoming invasive are reduced. Therefore, particularly for high-risk disease, cystectomy should be considered when a patient has had recurrence, particularly multiple recurrences.

19.2.2 Treatment of Invasive Disease

General Principles

- Cystectomy is considered the standard treatment for invasive transitional cell carcinoma of bladder (Grade B). A selective group of patients is eligible for segmental cystectomy without compromising the treatment outcome and function of the bladder.

- Preoperative radiation therapy is not routinely indicated for patients with invasive bladder cancer (Grade C). However, it may be beneficial for patients with extension to the surrounding organs.

- There is no evidence to support the use of adjuvant radiation therapy after cystectomy, but salvage radiation with chemotherapy should be considered for patients with positive margins based upon the general principle that residual disease will recur without further therapy (Grade D) and based upon the knowledge that these patients have poorer disease-specific survival (Level III) (DOTAN et al. 2007).

- Neoadjuvant chemotherapy can be considered particularly for locally advanced cancers, such as clinical stage T3-4 and/or positive pelvic nodes (Grade C).

- Adjuvant chemotherapy can be considered for patients after cystectomy, particularly for locally advanced disease with extravesical extension and/or positive nodes, and may improve progression-free survival and overall survival (Grade C).

- Maximal TURBT, combined chemoradiation therapy, with or without cystectomy, is currently the standard regimen used in bladder preservation treatment for invasive bladder cancer (Grade A).

Cystectomy

- Cystectomy has been considered standard treatment for invasive bladder cancer in the United States (Grade B). Cystectomy provides the best local control, and the potential of developing second cancers in the bladder is eliminated. A review of 1054 patients at the University of Southern California demonstrates a pelvic recurrence of 7%, a 5-year recurrence-free survival of 68%, and 10-year recurrence-free survival of 66% (Level IV) (STEIN et al. 2001). At the University of Bern, local recurrence was 3% for organ-confined disease, 11% for non-organ-confined node-negative tumors, and 15% for node-positive disease. The 5-year recurrence-free survival was 73%; 5-year overall survival was 62% (Level IV) (MADERSBACHER et al. 2003). At the University of Ulm, local failure was 4% for organ-confined tumors, 16% for non-organ-confined tumors, and 20% for patients with positive lymph nodes (Level IV) (HAUTMANN et al. 2006).

- Radical cystectomy involves cystoprostatectomy and pelvic lymph node dissection in male patients, and consists of pelvic lymph node dissection and an anterior exenteration (removes the bladder, urethra, ventral vaginal wall, and uterus) in female patients.

A minority of patients is eligible for segmental cystectomy. In order to be eligible, the patient needs to have a solitary invasive lesion on an accessible location of the bladder that would afford the patient an opportunity to have complete resection with negative margins. This usually only occurs in the dome of the bladder. In addition, carcinoma in situ must be absent. In such patients, the 5-year overall, disease-specific, and recurrence-free survival rates were 67%, 87%, and 39%, respectively, at M.D. Anderson (Level IV) (Kassouf et al. 2006). At Memorial Sloan Kettering, the overall 5-year survival was 69%, and 67% are disease-free with an intact bladder (Level IV) (Holzbeierlein et al. 2004).

Preoperative Radiation Therapy

Preoperative radiation therapy is not routinely recommended for the treatment of invasive bladder cancer (Grade C). Although it has been considered to be a standard of care previously, available literature fails to consistently support a role for this treatment: A small, prospective, randomized study of 44 patients demonstrated a 61% 5-year survival in patients undergoing surgery only versus 75% in those undergoing radiation followed by surgery (Level II) (Anderstrom et al. 1983). In a larger study of 140 patients, the 5-year survival was 53% in the surgery only group and 43% in the radiation and surgery group (Level II) (Smith et al. 1997). However, the meta-analysis research group reported that the available clinical trial data do not support a role for routine use of preoperative radiation therapy (Level I) (Huncharek 1998).

Preoperative radiation therapy may play a role in bladder cancer patients with extension to adjacent organs and tissues (Grade C). Patients at M.D. Anderson with T3B disease who received preoperative RT had improvement in 5-year local control from 72%–91%, 5-year freedom from distant metastatic of 54%–67%, and overall survival of 40%–52% (Level IV) (Cole et al. 1995). Review of the preoperative radiation therapy literature comprising 1185 patients demonstrates that the addition of preoperative radiation therapy for T3 bladder cancer adds 15%–20% to the 5-year survival (Level IV) (Parsons and Million 1989).

Neoadjuvant Chemotherapy

Neoadjuvant chemotherapy alone is not routinely indicated in the treatment of bladder cancer (Grade C). Multiple studies have demonstrated high response rates to chemotherapy. While local control with cystectomy is high, survival is only 40%–60% secondary to a large percentage developing metastatic disease. Therefore, neoadjuvant chemotherapy should be a promising addition to cystectomy. Unfortunately, neoadjuvant chemotherapy studies have demonstrated limited support for the use of neoadjuvant chemotherapy:

According to the results of a prospective, randomized trial reported by the Medical Research Council and the EORTC, chemotherapy nonsignificantly improved 3-year survival from 50% to 55% (Level I) (MRC/EORTC 1999). An update, presented in abstract form only, demonstrated an improvement in disease-free survival and local-regional progression-free survival (Level II) (Hall 2002). The Nordic cystectomy trial I demonstrated non-significant improvement for chemotherapy (Level I) (Malmstrom et al. 1996). There was, however, a 15% significant improvement in overall survival for patients with stages T3 through T4A disease. Therefore, the Nordic cystectomy trial II included such patients and improved 5-year survival non-significantly from 46% to 53% (Level I) (Sherif et al. 2002).

However, a randomized trial completed by the Southwest Oncology Group demonstrated significant improved median survival from 46 months to 77 months. Improved survival was due to the absence of residual cancer at cystectomy, 15% versus 38% (SWOG, Level I) (Grossman et al. 2003). A meta-analysis demonstrates that survival increased significantly from 45% to 50% at 5 years (Level I) (Advanced Bladder Cancer Meta-Analysis Collaboration 2003).

The results of an RTOG trial randomized 123 patients to receive two cycles of MCV prior to concurrent pelvic radiation with cisplatin versus concurrent radiation and cisplatin alone. There was no difference in any endpoints, and MCV prior to concurrent chemoradiotherapy did not provide any benefit to outcome (RTOG 89-03, Level I) (Shipley et al. 1998).

The probable reason why neoadjuvant chemotherapy has not shown greater benefit is: These studies include patients who have organ-confined lymph-node-negative disease. Such patients achieve 70%–90% recurrence-free survival with cystectomy alone. Patients with non-organ-confined disease, but negative nodes have a 50%–60% chance of recurrence-free survival and those with positive nodes have only about one-third chance of recurrence-free survival (STEIN et al. 2001). The chemotherapy benefit appears to be confined to patients who have no residual at cystectomy, which occurs in about 30% (GROSSMAN et al. 2003; SHERIF et al. 2002).

Adjuvant Chemotherapy

■ There is limited evidence to support the use of adjuvant chemotherapy in bladder cancer (Grade C). There are five small randomized studies addressing the efficacy of adjuvant chemotherapy in the treatment of bladder cancer; however, results of these trials were not consistent: The Swiss Group for Clinical Cancer Research non-significantly improved 5-year survival from 54% to 57% (Level II) (STUDER et al. 1994). The Italian Uro-Oncologic Cooperative Group also found not advantage to adjuvant chemotherapy (Level II) (BONO et al. 1989). At Stanford University, four cycles of CMV significantly improved freedom from progression from 12 months to 37 months. However, median survival was not significantly improved (Level II) (FREIHA et al. 1996). At the University of Southern California, P3, P4, or N+ disease received four cycles of cisplatinum, doxorubicin, cyclophosphamide, or observation. The 3-year time to progression and median survival were both significantly improved from 46% to 70% and 2.4 years to 4.3 years (Level II) (SKINNER et al. 1991). At the University of Mainz, pT3B, pT4A, and/or pN+ received MVAC or MVEC versus observation. An interim analysis closed the study because of significant improvement in progression-free survival (Level II) (STOECKLE et al. 1995). The ABC meta-analysis suggests a 25% relative reduction in risk of death for chemotherapy (Level I) (ADVANCED BLADDER CANCER META-ANALYSIS COLLABORATION 2005).

■ EORTC-30994 will include 1344 patients with pT3 or pT4; N0 or node-positive disease randomized to four cycles of standard MVAC, or high-dose MVAC, or gem-cisplatin versus observation, will hopefully provide higher level evidence for adjuvant chemotherapy.

19.2.3 Bladder Preservation Therapy

Radiation Therapy Alone

■ Historically, radiation therapy alone was used extensively in the 1950s through 1980s before development of modern cystectomy (Grade B). The efficacy of radiotherapy for bladder cancer treatment was repeatedly demonstrated in retrospective trials reported from Europe; however, these older studies demonstrate inferior local control and some inferior survival compared with a cystectomy.

■ The results of a large retrospective series from the University of Edinburgh revealed that 45% of 963 patients treated with radiotherapy achieved local tumor regression (Level IV) (DUNCAN and QUILTY 1986). A 5-year survival of 40% with 41% local control was observed in a retrospective study from the London Hospital in 182 patients with T2 and T3 bladder cancer (Level IV) (JENKINS et al. 1988). At the University of Bergen, Norway, the 5-year and 10-year survival rates were 39% and 23%, respectively, for 90 patients treated with radiotherapy (Level IV) (DAEHLIN et al. 1999). At the Norwegian Radium Hospital, 5-year survival was 22% for 271 patients with T2 through T4 cancer (Level IV) (FOSSA et al. 1996). In 384 patients with T2 through T4 carcinomas, 30%–40% achieved local control (Level IV) (GOFFINET et al. 1975). A total of 470 patients achieved a 5-year survival of 38% and 10-year survival of 22% (Level IV) (GOODMAN et al. 1981). At Princess Margaret Hospital, 247 patients had 10-year survival of 19%, and local control was 32% (Level IV) (CHUNG et al. 2007). At Brescia University, 459 patients had 5-year survival of 36%; failure-free survival was 33% (Level IV) (TONOLI et al. 2006). At City Hospital in Nottingham, UK, 67 patients achieved 5-year survival of 38%, and local control was 42% (Level IV) (BESSEL et al. 1993).

■ There is a subgroup of patients who have high local control with radiation therapy only: clinical stage T2, no ureteral obstruction, complete transurethral resection, complete resolution of disease after radiation therapy, solitary tumors, and patients that do not have T4 disease. These patients can achieve survival and local control in excess of 50%, and radiation only can be considered (Grade B). In 55 patients treated at Massachusetts General with radiation therapy alone,

5-year survival for T2 and T3 versus T4 cancer was 45% versus 9%. Papillary surface histological findings had 63% versus 20% survival for flat tumors. Of these patients, 54% with complete transurethral resection survived versus 17% who had incomplete and 47% without ureteral obstruction versus 14% with survived (Level IV) (SHIPLEY et al. 1985). At the Prince of Wales Hospital in Australia, prognostic factors for higher bladder relapse were tumor multiplicity, presence of ureteric obstruction, and higher T-stage (Level IV) (MAMEGHAN et al. 1995).

Radiation and Chemotherapy

- Maximal TURBT, combined chemoradiation therapy, with or without cystectomy is currently the standard regimen used in bladder preservation treatment for invasive bladder cancer (Grade A). The bladder preservation approach has sought to include patients with as many of the above-mentioned characteristics as possible and also adds chemotherapy to increase the response rate and local control while requiring patients to undergo close cystoscopic surveillance for salvage cystectomy if local invasive failure develops.

- The current scheme for bladder preservation includes maximal TURBT and induction external-beam radiation therapy to 40 Gy at 1.8–2.0 Gy per fraction, with concomitant chemotherapy (preferably cisplatinum 100 mg/m^2 days 1 and 22). Four weeks later, cystoscopy is performed with multiple biopsies and cytology. If this is negative, then a boost of 24 Gy is delivered to the partial bladder or entire bladder with another cycle of chemotherapy. Cystoscopy is performed 4 weeks after completion therapy. If a complete response is achieved, adjuvant chemotherapy could be considered. If at any point there is persistent disease, cystectomy should be performed.

- One of the first studies to utilize this approach was the National Bladder Cancer Group Trial, wherein patients with favorable characteristics were treated with external-beam radiation therapy and cisplatinum. Of the patients, 77% had complete regression of their bladder tumor, and 73% of these patients were alive at 4 years with their bladder intact (Level III) (SHIPLEY et al. 1987). Subsequently, multiple chemoradiation therapy studies have been performed, which have consistently demonstrated survival similar to that reported in cystectomy studies with a high

level of bladder preservation, thereby establishing this treatment as an alternative to cystectomy: RTOG 8512 treated 47 patients with 40 Gy pelvic radiation therapy and cisplatin 100 mg/m^2 days 1 and 22. Of these patients, 66% had complete regression of disease and went on to receive an additional 24 Gy boost with a third dose of cisplatin. Eleven out of 28 evaluable patients remained continuously in remission, eight relapsed in the bladder, and five of these eight cases involved noninvasive tumors. The actual rate of survival was 64% at 3 years (RTOG 85-12, Level III) (TESTER et al. 1993). In RTOG 88-02, 91 patients received two cycles of MCV chemotherapy followed by 39.6 Gy with platinum 100 mg on days 1 and 22. Of these patients, 75% had complete response; 40% of patients required cystectomy either because of incomplete regression of disease or subsequent recurrence. Four-year survival was 62%. Four-year survival with intact bladder was 44% (RTOG 88-02, Level III) (TESTER et al. 1996).

- In RTOG 89-03, 123 patients with stage T2 to T4a NX M0 bladder cancer were randomized to receive two cycles of MCV prior to chemoradiation therapy or to proceed straight to chemoradiation therapy. Chemoradiation therapy was as outlined in RTOG 88-02. The overall 5-year survivals with a functional bladder were 49% and 38% in the two groups, and no significant differences were observed (Level I) (SHIPLEY et al. 1998). A review of 190 patients treated at Massachusetts General who received cisplatin and radiation therapy demonstrated 63% complete response. Five-year survival was 64%, and 10-year survival was 36%. Only 35% underwent radical cystectomy (Level IV) (SHIPLEY et al. 2002). The University of Erlangen treated 415 patients with T2–T3 bladder cancer: 126 with radiation alone, 289 with radiation and cis- or carboplatin. Complete regression of disease was achieved in 72% of patients. Local control after complete response was maintained in 64% of patients. Ten-year disease-free survival was 42% with more than 80% of survivors preserving their bladder (Level IV) (RÖDEL et al. 2002).

- The National Cancer Institute of Canada randomized 99 patients (treated with primary radiation therapy or preoperative radiation therapy) to cisplatin 100 mg/m^2 at 2-week intervals for three cycles or no chemotherapy. Of the cisplatinum-treated patients, 29% had local failure in the pelvis versus 52% of control patients; however, survival, was unchanged (Level II) (COPPIN et al. 1996). The All India Institute randomized 30 patients to radical cystectomy with adjuvant CMV versus 13 patients to two cycles of neoadjuvant CMV chemotherapy followed by concurrent chemoradiation therapy. Equivalent 2-year survival, 56% in the surgery arm and 54% in the chemoradiation arm, was reported (Level III) (HARESH et al. 2007).

Hyperfractionated Radiation and Poly-chemotherapy

■ Altered fractionation radiation with multi-agent chemotherapy may increase the initial response rate and may increase bladder preservation (Grade B). The effect of this dose fractionation in combination with concurrent chemotherapy has been evaluated in a number of phase II clinical trials, mostly from the Radiation Therapy Oncology Group:
The RTOG 95-06 treated 34 patients with cisplatinum and 5-FU with 3 Gy per fraction BID to a dose of 24 Gy, followed by consolidation and the same chemotherapy 2.5 Gy BID to an additional dose of 20 Gy. Of these patients, 67% had complete regression of their disease after the initial chemoradiation therapy. Three-year survival was 83%. Probability of survival with an intact bladder is 66% at 3 years (RTOG 95-06, Level III) (KAUFMAN et al. 2000).
In RTOG 97-06, 43 patients completed 1.8 Gy per fraction in the morning to the pelvis and 1.6 Gy to the tumor in the afternoon for 13 days with cisplatinum 20 mg the first 3 days of each week. Patients were then evaluated cystoscopically several weeks later. The complete regression rate was 74%. These patients received consolidation radiation/chemotherapy. Patients then received adjuvant CMV chemotherapy. Only an additional four patients developed an invasive recurrence. Three-year survival is 61%. However, only 45% of these patients were able to complete the entire therapy (RTOG 97-06, Level III) (HAGAN et al. 2003).
RTOG 99-06, a prospective phase II trial, treated 50 patients with twice-daily irradiation, cisplatin (20 mg/m^2) on the first 2 days of each week and paclitaxel (50 mg/m^2) on the first day of each week. Following induction treatment, 87% of patients had complete resolution of disease, completed consolidation chemoradiation, and then received four cycles of adjuvant cisplatin and gemcitabine chemotherapy. Two-year survival

was 79% for the entire group of patients, and 69% of patients survived with their bladder intact at 2 years (RTOG 99-06, Level III) (KAUFMAN et al. 2005).
The phase II trail completed at the Hôpital Necker at the University of Paris treated 54 patients, wherein patients received 5-FU and cisplatinum and hyperfractionated radiation; 74% of patients had complete regression and went on to receive additional chemo- and radiation therapy. At 3 years, disease-free survival was 62% (Level III) (HOUSSET et al. 1993).

■ Current on-going studies include RTOG 02-33, a randomized phase II trial, in which all patients receive hyperfractionated radiation therapy of 1.6 Gy in the morning to small pelvic fields and a 1.5-Gy boost in the times afternoon for 13 days. Patients are randomized to weekly paclitaxel and cisplatin versus 5-FU and cisplatin every 2 weeks. Patients are evaluated for response with cystoscopy and if their disease has resolved, they receive consolidation radiation with chemotherapy. Patients then go on to receive four cycles of adjuvant chemotherapy.

Brachytherapy

■ Brachytherapy has been promoted by the University of Amsterdam for patients with solitary tumors less than 5 cm in diameter. Their experience has recently been updated: 122 patients received external-beam radiation therapy then underwent cystotomy with the implantation of catheters. Five-year local control is 76% with 73% survival (Level IV) (BLANK et al. 2007).

Radiation Therapy Technique

■ Patients are simulated and treated with an empty bladder. Patients are treated with at least a four-field technique (anteroposterior, posteroanterior, and opposed lateral fields), and the treatment fields are arranged as follows (Fig. 19.1):
- The internal and external iliacs are treated, and common iliacs are treated up to the level of the top of the sacrum.
- The bottom of the field is below the bladder to at least the bottom of the obturator foramen.
- For the anteroposterior and posteroanterior fields, 2 cm of pelvic rim is included.
- For the lateral fields, the bladder needs to be encompassed with at least a 2-cm margin anteri-

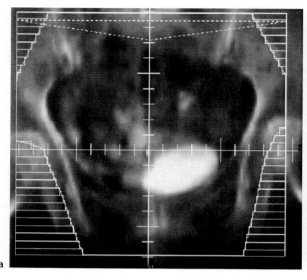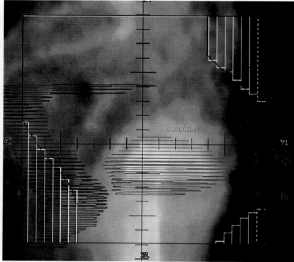

Fig. 19.1a,b. Treatment fields

orly, and the small bowel should be appropriately blocked.

Alternatively, some institutions do not treat pelvic nodes and include only bladder with margin in their initial fields.

■ A total dose of 40 Gy–45 Gy at 1.8 Gy–2 Gy per daily fraction is recommended to the pelvic fields.
■ After cystoscopy reveals no residual tumor, consolidation radiation with an additional 24 Gy at 1.8 Gy–2 Gy per fraction is delivered to the partial bladder, if the tumor can be localized. If not, the whole bladder is treated. Fiducial markers can be implanted, and the dose verification system (DVS) placed on the outside surface of the bladder; then image-guided (via ON Board Imaging) and dose-guided therapies (via DVS) are used to perform partial bladder radiation (Fig. 19.2).

19.2.4 Treatment of Metastatic Transitional Cell Carcinoma

■ Transitional cell carcinoma is a chemosensitive disease, and chemotherapy is recommended for the treatment of patients with metastatic disease (Grade A). Response rates to multi-agent chemotherapy are as high as 60%–70% with as much as 30% complete regression of disease: The results of a retrospective study from the Memorial Sloan Kettering Cancer Center demonstrated a 72% response rate with MVAC-based chemotherapy with 36% complete regression of disease (Level IV) (Sternberg et al. 1989). These findings were confirmed by the results from a Northern California Oncology Group study, which showed a 56% response rate with CMV and a 28% complete response rate (Level III) (Harker et al. 1985). Data from a phase II trial from the Dana-Farber Cancer Institute revealed a 41% response rate to combined chemotherapy with cisplatin and gemcitabine and a 21% rate of complete regression of disease (Level III) (Kaufman et al. 2000). Results of a prospective phase II study from the Herlev University Hospital in Denmark reported a 60% response to docetaxel and cisplatin, and a 26% complete response rate was reported (Level III) (Sengeløv 1998).

■ Newer agents, such as combined cisplatin and gemcitabine, should be considered as an initial treatment regimen (Grade A). The results of a prospective randomized trial have demonstrated that cisplatin and gemcitabine provide similar survival to MVAC, but a better safety profile and tolerability (Level I) (Von der Maase et al. 1998).

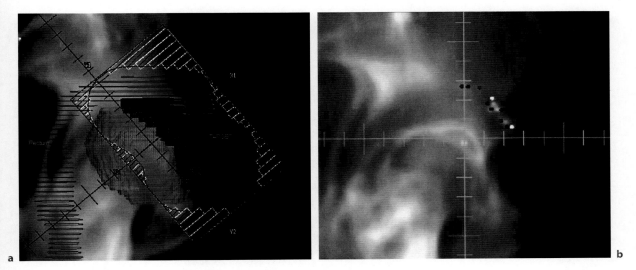

Fig. 19.2a,b. Partial bladder radiation using image- and dose-guided therapy

19.2.5 Treatment of Non-transitional Histologies

Squamous Cell Carcinoma

- Cystectomy is the primary therapy for squamous cell carcinoma of the urinary bladder (Grade B). The overall survival of patients with SCC treated with cystectomy ranged between 30% and 50%. The results from a retrospective study reported by RICHIE et al. (1976) revealed that in 25 patients with SCC of the bladder, the 5-year overall survival was 48% after surgery (Level IV). Another retrospective study reported a 31.5% survival at 4 years in 19 patients with squamous cell carcinoma (Level IV) (SERRETTA et al. 2000). The experience of 35 patients treated at the Cleveland Clinic treated with radical or partial cystectomies revealed a 37% disease-free survival rate (Level IV) (LAGWINSKI et al. 2007).

- Radiation therapy achieves worse local control and survival than cystectomy (Grade B). Results from a retrospective review of 97 patients treated at the University of Glasgow showed an overall 5-year survival rate of 1.9%, and the 5-year survival rates for patients with T2, T3, and T4 disease were 16.7%, 4.8%, and 0%, respectively (Level IV) (RUNDLE et al. 1982). In another study, 49 patients with T3 squamous cancer had 33.7% 3-year local control; survival was only 18.3% at 3 years (Level IV) (QUILTY and DUNCAN 1982). Radiation therapy for patients with clinically staged T3 disease yielded a 5-year survival rate of only 17.7%, which was improved to 34% with radiation followed by cystectomy (Level IV) (JOHNSON et al. 1976).

- Preoperative radiation therapy can be considered in the treatment of locally advanced squamous cell carcinoma and may improve local control and survival (Grade B). A prospective randomized study from Egypt in 92 patients demonstrated an insignificant improvement in survival. However, for patients with high-stage (P3 and P4) and high-grade tumors, there was a significant improvement in survival following preoperative radiation (Level II) (GHONEIM et al. 1985). In addition, a retrospective series from M.D. Anderson of 25 patients treated with preoperative radiation demonstrated a 5-year survival rate of 50%. Ten patients (40%) were down-staged, and no patient whose tumor was down-staged had a recurrence or died of bladder cancer (Level IV) (SWANSON et al. 1990).

- The efficacy of systemic chemotherapy on squamous cell carcinoma of the bladder is unknown, and limited data do not support its routine use (Grade D). A review article has summarized the limited literature that reports poor response of squamous cell carcinoma to chemotherapy (Level IV) (ABOL-ENEIN et al. 2007).

Adenocarcinoma

- Cystectomy or partial cystectomy is the primary treatment of adenocarcinoma of the urinary bladder (Grade C). One study reviewed 15 patients who had a 5-year survival rate of 54% (Level IV) (ANDERSTRÖM et al. 1983). At Tata Memorial Hospital, 48 patients had 5-year survival of 37% (Level IV) (DANDEKAR et al. 1997). At Massachusetts General Hospital, only 1/12 patients with invasive adenocarcinoma of the bladder was alive at more than 5 years. However, two of three patients with invasive urachal adenocarcinoma who had preoperative radiotherapy plus partial cystectomy are free of disease at 38 and 60 months (Level V) (NOCKS et al. 1983).

- Adjuvant radiation can be recommended for the treatment of adenocarcinoma of the bladder (Grade C). Radiation therapy after cystecomy may improve local control and survival: At the National Cancer Institute of Egypt, 69 patients were treated with radical cystectomy and pelvic lymphadenectomy with postoperative radiation versus 123 patients without postoperative radiotherapy. Local control was significantly improved from 53% to 96%. The 5-year disease-free survival rate was improved from 37% to 61% (Level IV) (ZAGHLOUL et al. 2006).

- The efficacy of systemic chemotherapy on adenocarcinoma of the bladder is unknown, and the limited data do not support its routine use (Grade D). A review article has summarized the limited literature that reports poor response of adenocarcinoma to chemotherapy (Level IV) (ABOL-ENEIN et al. 2007).

Small Cell Carcinoma

- Small cell carcinoma of the urinary bladder is considered a systemic disease and should be treated in a similar fashion to other extrapulmonary small cell carcinomas (Grade B). Chemotherapy plays an important role and should be recommended as the initial treatment of small cell carcinoma of the bladder: A retrospective study from M.D. Anderson demonstrated improved survival for patients treated initially with chemotherapy (Level IV) (SIEFKER-RADTKE et al. 2004). Local treatment with involved-field radiation therapy or cystectomy is indicated after systemic chemotherapy (Level IV) (SVED et al. 2004).

19.3 Quality of Life/Side Effects of Therapy

Cystectomy

- Postoperatively, patients can develop infection, bleeding, deep vein thrombosis, pulmonary embolism, or myocardial infarction.

- A major issue for many patients is continence. When a patient has a cystectomy, a segment of ileum, colon, or jejunum is fashioned into either a conduit (for non-continent diversions) or a larger reservoir (for continent diversions). The conduit empties through a stoma on the abdominal wall into a collection device. With a continent diversion, a valve is attached to the abdominal wall, which is catheterized every 4 h. An orthotopic reservoir is attached to the urethra provided that the urethra can be spared. The reservoir is emptied by Valsalva. However, patients also need to intermittently self-catheterize. The postoperative complication rate with the continent diversions is 15%–30% and 10% or less with non-continent diversion.

- Complications after cystectomy include electrolyte abnormalities, acidosis with hyperkalemia, hypercalcemia, or hypomagnesemia. These require treatment with bicarbonate and electrolyte replacement as needed. Patients can develop altered drug metabolism. Drugs that are ordinarily excreted by the kidneys, such as dilantin, can be reabsorbed by the patient's conduit or reservoir. Patients develop renal calculi at rates of 3%–4% with a conduit and 20% with a reservoir. Of the patients, 10%–15% develops bacteremia with urinary tract infection. Neuromechanical complications include retention or hyperperistaltic contractions of the reservoir, which lead to low capacity or incontinence.

- Cystectomy decreases quality of life. At the University of Mainz, patients completed a quality-of-life survey prior to surgery and 1 year post surgery. In areas of physical activity, sexual activity, and emotional well-being, quality of life was decreased (Level III) (HARDT et al. 2000).

- Continent diversion may increase a patient's quality of life (Grade C). At the University Hospital, Lund, Sweden, surveys were completed by 20 patients with a continent cecal reservoir and 40 patients who had a conduit. Continent cecal reservoir was associated with fewer stoma-related problems and allowed greater freedom in social life. Sexual problems, disturbed relations, and emotional problems were common and did not differ between the two groups (Level III) (MÅNSSON et al. 1988). Another study demonstrated that patients with ileal conduits reported a greater impact on their social activities, but fewer problems with the device. All the patients with neobladders had some incontinence, primarily at night, and all patients reported erectile dysfunction (Level III) (RALEIGH et al. 1995). A survey performed by HART et al. (1999) from Stanford University revealed that there was no difference among the urinary diversion subgroups in any quality-of-life area (Level III). At Herlev Hospital, Denmark, daytime leakage was 18% with bladder substitution versus 10% with conduit diversion, and nighttime leakage was 21% versus 3%. However, 58% of the ileal conduit versus 21% of bladder substitution patients reported urinary leakage as their main concern. Also, ileal conduit patients did not retain their body image as well as those with bladder substitution (Level III) (BJERRE et al. 1995).

Radiation Therapy

- Acute side effects include frequency, urgency, dysuria, and occasional incontinence. Patients can develop nausea, vomiting, or diarrhea. These side effects usually resolve.
- Late radiation complications include hematuria, chronic frequency, and contracted bladder in approximately 5% of patients. These symptoms can also occur if the patient develops bladder recurrence. Therefore, these symptoms mandate cystoscopy.
- The majority of patients who undergo bladder preservation therapy and maintain their bladder has normal or near normal function and report quality of life that is superior to that reported by patients who have cystectomy. At the Massachusetts General Hospital, 32 patients returned quality-of-life questionnaires and underwent urodynamic study. In total, 75% percent had normally functioning bladders. The majority of men retained sexual function (Level III) (ZEITMAN et al. 2003). At St. Chiara Hospital, 29 questionnaires from patients treated with radiation and chemotherapy and 30 questionnaires from patients treated with cystectomy were returned.

Quality-of-life scores in the bladder-preservation group were consistently better than in the patients treated with cystectomy. Specifically, bladder preservation patients had higher levels of sexual activity and higher perception of physical well being than cystectomy patients (Level III) (CAFFO et al. 1996). The Karolinska mailed questionnaires to patients treated with radiation therapy, cystectomy, and randomly selected from the population. In all, 58 irradiated patients, 251 who had received cystectomy, and 310 of the population control returned the questionnaires. Of the irradiated patients, 75% reported little or no urinary symptoms, 38% had had intercourse within the previous month, and 57% of these men reported that they had ejaculated. Among cystectomy patients, 13% had had intercourse, and 0% of the men had ejaculated. Of the patients treated with radiation, 32% reported moderate or worse gastrointestinal symptoms versus 24% of the cystectomy patients versus 9% of population controls (Level III) (HENNINGSOHN et al. 2002).

 19.4   Follow-Up

- Superficial bladder cancer should be followed with cystoscopy every 3 months for 2 years along with cytology, then every 6 months for 2 years, and then annually.
- Invasive bladder cancer should be followed with blood work, including complete metabolic panel, liver function tests, electrolytes, and chest X-ray obtained every 6 months. Every 3–6 months, the collecting system needs to be imaged for the first 2 years.
- If a patient has had bladder conservation, he or she needs to have cystoscopy every 3 months for 2 years with cytology, and then every 6 months for 2 years, and then annually. If the patient had cystectomy, he or she needs urine cytology every 6 months. If they had a continent orthotopic diversion, they need a vitamin B12 shot yearly (NATIONAL COMPREHENSIVE CANCER NETWORK 2008).

References

Abol-Enein H, Kava BR, Carmack AJ (2007) Nonurothelial cancer of the bladder. Urology 69 (1 Suppl):93–104

Advanced Bladder Cancer Meta-Analysis Collaboration (2003) Neoadjuvant chemotherapy in invasive bladder cancer: a systematic review and meta-analysis. Lancet 361:1927–1934

Advanced Bladder Cancer (ABC) Meta-Analysis Collaboration (2005) Adjuvant chemotherapy in invasive bladder cancer: a systematic review and meta-analysis of individual patient data. Eur Urol 48:189–199

Anderström C, Johansson S, Nilsson S et al. (1983) A prospective randomized study of preoperative irradiation with cystectomy or cystectomy alone for invasive bladder carcinoma. Eur Urol 9:142–147

Anderström C, Johansson SL, von Schultz L (1983) Primary adenocarcinoma of the urinary bladder. A clinicopathologic and prognostic study. Cancer 52:1273–1280

Bessell EM, Taylor J, Moloney AJ et al. (1993) Regression of transitional cell carcinoma of the bladder with radiotherapy: progression-free control in the bladder at 5 years. Radiother Oncol 29:344–346

Bjerre BD, Johansen C, Steven K (1995) Health-related quality of life after cystectomy: bladder substitution compared with ileal conduit diversion. A questionnaire survey. Br J Urol 75:200–205

Blank LE, Koedooder K, van Os R et al. (2007) Results of bladder-conserving treatment, consisting of brachytherapy combined with limited surgery and external beam radiotherapy, for patients with solitary T1-T3 bladder tumors less than 5 cm in diameter. Int J Radiat Oncol Biol Phys 69:454–458

Bono AV, Benvenuti C, Reali L et al. (1989) Adjuvant chemotherapy in advanced bladder cancer. Italian Uro-Oncologic Cooperative Group. Prog Clin Biol Res 303:533–540

Caffo O, Fellin G, Graffer U et al. (1996) Assessment of quality of life after cystectomy or conservative therapy for patients with infiltrating bladder carcinoma. A survey by a self-administered questionnaire. Cancer 78:1089–1097

Chakravarti A, Winter K, Wu CL et al. (2005) Expression of the epidermal growth factor receptor and Her-2 are predictors of favorable outcome and reduced complete response rates, respectively, in patients with muscle-invading bladder cancers treated by concurrent radiation and cisplatin-based chemotherapy: a report from the Radiation Therapy Oncology Group. Int J Radiat Oncol Biol Phys 62:309–317

Chung PW, Bristow RG, Milosevic MF et al. (2007) Long-term outcome of radiation-based conservation therapy for invasive bladder cancer. Urol Oncol 25:303–309

Cole CJ, Pollack A, Zagars GK et al. (1995) Local control of muscle-invasive bladder cancer: preoperative radiotherapy and cystectomy versus cystectomy alone. Int J Radiat Oncol Biol Phys 32:331–340

Coppin CM, Gospodarowicz MK, James K et al. (1996) Improved local control of invasive bladder cancer by concurrent cisplatin and preoperative or definitive radiation. The National Cancer Institute of Canada Clinical Trials Group. J Clin Oncol 14:2901–2907

Daehlin L, Haukaas S, Maartmann-Moe H et al. (1999) Survival after radical treatment for transitional cell carcinoma of the bladder. Eur J Surg Oncol 25:66–70

Dandekar NP, Dalal AV, Tongaonkar HB et al. (1997) Adenocarcinoma of bladder. Eur J Surg Oncol 23:157–160

Dotan ZA, Kavanagh K, Yossepowitch O et al. (2007) Positive surgical margins in soft tissue following radical cystectomy for bladder cancer and cancer specific survival. J Urol 178:2308–2312

Duncan W, Quilty PM (1986) The results of a series of 963 patients with transitional cell carcinoma of the urinary bladder primarily treated by radical megavoltage X-ray therapy. Radiother Oncol 7:299–310

Felix AS, Soliman AS, Khaled H et al. (2008) The changing patterns of bladder cancer in Egypt over the past 26 years. Cancer Causes Control 19:421–429

Fossa SD, Aass N, Ous S et al. (1996) Survival after curative treatment of muscle-invasive bladder cancer. Acta Oncol 35[Suppl 8]:59–65

Freiha F, Reese J, Torti FM (1996) A randomized trial of radical cystectomy versus radical cystectomy plus cisplatin, vinblastine and methotrexate chemotherapy for muscle invasive bladder cancer. J Urol 155:495–499

Ghoneim MA, Ashamallah AK, Awaad HK et al. (1985) Randomized trial of cystectomy with or without preoperative radiotherapy for carcinoma of the bilharzial bladder. J Urol 134:266–268

Goodman GB, Hislop TG, Elwood JM et al. (1981) Conservation of bladder function in patients with invasive bladder cancer treated by definitive irradiation and selective cystectomy. Int J Radiat Oncol Biol Phys 7:569–573

Goffinet DR, Schneider MJ, Glatstein EJ et al. (1975) Bladder cancer: results of radiation therapy in 384 patients. Radiology 117:149–153

Gospodarowicz MK, Hawkins NV, Rawlings GA et al. (1989) Radical radiotherapy for muscle invasive transitional cell carcinoma of the bladder: failure analysis. J Urol 142:1448–1453

Grossman HB, Natale RB, Tangen CM et al. (2003) Neoadjuvant chemotherapy plus cystectomy compared with cystectomy alone for locally advanced bladder cancer. N Engl J Med 349:859–866

Hagan MP, Winter KA, Kaufman DS et al. (2003) RTOG 97-06: initial report of a phase I–II trial of selective bladder conservation using TURBT, twice-daily accelerated irradiation sensitized with cisplatin, and adjuvant MCV combination chemotherapy. Int J Radiat Oncol Biol Phys 57:665–672

Hall R (2002) On behalf of the International Collaboration of Trialists of the MRC Advanced Bladder Cancer Group: updated results of a randomised controlled trial of neoadjuvant cisplatin (C), methotrexate (M) and vinblastine (V) chemotherapy for muscle-invasive bladder cancer. Proc Am Soc Clin Oncol 21:178(abstract)

Hardt J, Filipas D, Hohenfellner R et al. (2000) Quality of life in patients with bladder carcinoma after cystectomy: first results of a prospective study. Qual Life Res 9:1–12

Haresh KP, Julka PK, Sharma DN et al. (2007) A prospective study evaluating surgery and chemo radiation in muscle invasive bladder cancer. J Cancer Res Ther 3:81–85

Harker WG, Meyers FJ, Freiha FS et al. (1985) Cisplatin, methotrexate, and vinblastine (CMV): an effective chemotherapy regimen for metastatic transitional cell carcinoma of the urinary tract. A Northern California Oncology Group study. J Clin Oncol 3:1463–1470

Hart S, Skinner EC, Meyerowitz BE et al. (1999) Quality of life after radical cystectomy for bladder cancer in patients with an ileal conduit, cutaneous or urethral Kock pouch. J Urol 162:77–81

Hautmann RE, Gschwend JE, de Petriconi RC et al. (2006) Cystectomy for transitional cell carcinoma of the bladder: results of a surgery only series in the neobladder era. J Urol 176:486–492

Heicappell R, Muller-Mattheis V, Reinhardt M et al. (1999) Staging of pelvic lymph nodes in neoplasms of the bladder and prostate by positron emission tomography with 2-[(18)F]-2-deoxy-D-glucose. Eur Urol 36:582–587

Henningsohn L, Wijkström H, Dickman PW et al. (2002) Distressful symptoms after radical radiotherapy for urinary bladder cancer. Radiother Oncol 62:215–225

Holzbeierlein JM, Lopez-Corona E, Bochner BH (2004) Partial cystectomy: a contemporary review of the Memorial Sloan-Kettering Cancer Center experience and recommendations for patient selection. J Urol 172:878–881

Housset M, Maulard C, Chretien Y et al. (1993) Combined radiation and chemotherapy for invasive transitional-cell carcinoma of the bladder: a prospective study. J Clin Oncol 11:2150–2157

Huncharek M, Muscat J, Geschwind JF et al. (1998) Planned pre-operative radiation therapy in muscle invasive bladder cancer; results of a meta-analysis. Anticancer Res 18:1931–1934

Jenkins BJ, Caulfield MJ, Fowler CG et al. (1988) Reappraisal of the role of radical radiotherapy and salvage cystectomy in the treatment of invasive (T2/T3) bladder cancer. Br J Urol 62:343–346

Johnson DE, Schoenwald MB, Ayala AG et al. (1976) Squamous cell carcinoma of the bladder. J Urol 115:542–544

Kassouf W, Swanson D, Kamat AM et al. (2006) Partial cystectomy for muscle invasive urothelial carcinoma of the bladder: a contemporary review of the MD Anderson Cancer Center experience. J Urol 175:2058–2062

Kaufman D, Raghavan D, Carducci M et al. (2000a) Phase II trial of gemcitabine plus cisplatin in patients with metastatic urothelial cancer. J Clin Oncol 18:1921–1927

Kaufman DS, Winter KA, Shipley WU et al. (2000b) The initial results in muscle-invading bladder cancer of RTOG 95-06: phase I/II trial of transurethral surgery plus radiation therapy with concurrent cisplatin and 5-fluorouracil followed by selective bladder preservation or cystectomy depending on the initial response. Oncologist 5:471–476

Kaufman DS, Winter KA, Shipley WU et al. (2005) Muscle-invading bladder cancer, RTOG Protocol 99-06: Initial report of a phase I/II trial of selective bladder-conservation employing TURBT, accelerated irradiation sensitized with cisplatin and paclitaxel followed by adjuvant cisplatin and gemcitabine chemotherapy. J Clin Oncol 2005 ASCO Annual Meeting Proceedings 23[1 Suppl]:4506

Kosuda S, Kison PV, Greenough R et al. (1997) Preliminary assessment of fluorine-18 fluorodeoxyglucose positron emission tomography in patients with bladder cancer. Eur J Nucl Med 24:615–620

Lagwinski N, Thomas A, Stephenson AJ et al. (2007) Squamous cell carcinoma of the bladder: a clinicopathologic analysis of 45 cases. Am J Surg Pathol 31:1777–1787

Lotan Y, Roehrborn CG (2003) Sensitivity and specificity of commonly available bladder tumor markers versus cytology: results of a comprehensive literature review and meta-analyses. Urology 61:109–118

Madersbacher S, Hochreiter W, Burkhard F et a. (2003) Radical cystectomy for bladder cancer today–a homogeneous series without neoadjuvant therapy. J Clin Oncol 21:690–696

Mameghan H, Fisher R, Mameghan J et al. (1995) Analysis of failure following definitive radiotherapy for invasive transitional cell carcinoma of the bladder. Int J Radiat Oncol Biol Phys 31:247–254

Mallampati GK, Siegelman ES (2004) MR imaging of the bladder. Magn Reson Imaging Clin N Am 12:545–555

Malmström PU, Rintala E, Wahlqvist R et al. (1996) Five-year follow-up of a prospective trial of radical cystectomy and neoadjuvant chemotherapy: Nordic Cystectomy Trial I. The Nordic Cooperative Bladder Cancer Study Group. J Urol 155:1903–1906

Månsson A, Johnson G, Månsson W (1988) Quality of life after cystectomy. Comparison between patients with conduit and those with continent caecal reservoir urinary diversion. Br J Urol 62:240–245

MRC/EORTC (1999) Neoadjuvant cisplatin, methotrexate, and vinblastine chemotherapy for muscle-invasive bladder cancer: a randomised controlled trial. International collaboration of trialists. Lancet 354:533–540

National Comprehensive Cancer Network (2008) Clinical practice guidelines in oncology: Bladder cancer. Available at http://www.nccn.org Accessed on 24 February 2008

Nocks BN, Heney NM, Daly JJ (1983) Primary adenocarcinoma of urinary bladder. Urology 21:26–29

Parsons JT, Million RR (1989) Role of planned preoperative irradiation in the management of clinical stage B2-C (T3) bladder carcinoma in the 1980s. Semin Surg Oncol 5:255–265

Pawinski A, Sylvester R, Kurth KH et al. (1996) A combined analysis of European Organization for Research and Treatment of Cancer, and Medical Research Council randomized clinical trials for the prophylactic treatment of stage TaT1 bladder cancer. European Organization for Research and Treatment of Cancer Genitourinary Tract Cancer Cooperative Group and the Medical Research Council Working Party on Superficial Bladder Cancer. J Urol 156:1934–1940

Quilty PM, Duncan W (1986) Radiotherapy for squamous carcinoma of the urinary bladder. Int J Radiat Oncol Biol Phys 12:861–865

Raleigh ED, Berry M, Montie JE (1995) A comparison of adjustments to urinary diversions: a pilot study. J Wound Ostomy Continence Nurs 22:58–63

Richie JP, Waisman J, Skinner DG et al. (1976) Squamous carcinoma of the bladder: treatment by radical cystectomy. J Urol 115:670–672

Robinson P, Collins CD, Ryder WD et al. (2000) Relationship of MRI and clinical staging to outcome in invasive bladder cancer treated by radiotherapy. Clin Radiol 55:301–306

Rödel C, Grabenbauer GG, Kühn R et al. (2002) Combined-modality treatment and selective organ preservation in invasive bladder cancer: long-term results. J Clin Oncol 20:3061–3071

Rundle JS, Hart AJ, McGeorge A et al. (1982) Squamous cell carcinoma of bladder. A review of 114 patients. Br J Urol 54:522–526

Sengeløv L, Kamby C, Lund B et al. (1998) Docetaxel and cisplatin in metastatic urothelial cancer: a phase II study. J Clin Oncol 16:3392–3397

Serretta V, Pomara G, Piazza F et al. (2000) Pure squamous cell carcinoma of the bladder in western countries. Report on 19 consecutive cases. Eur Urol 37:85–89

Sherif A, Rintala E, Mestad O et al. (2002) Neoadjuvant cisplatin-methotrexate chemotherapy for invasive bladder cancer–Nordic cystectomy trial 2. Scand J Urol Nephrol 36:419–425

Shipley WU, Rose MA, Perrone TL et al. (1985) Full-dose irradiation for patients with invasive bladder carcinoma: clinical and histological factors prognostic of improved survival. J Urol 134:679–683

Shipley WU, Prout GR Jr, Einstein AB et al. (1987) Treatment of invasive bladder cancer by cisplatin and radiation in patients unsuited for surgery. JAMA 258:931–935

Shipley WU, Winter KA, Kaufman DS et al. (1998) Phase III trial of neoadjuvant chemotherapy in patients with invasive bladder cancer treated with selective bladder preservation by combined radiation therapy and chemotherapy: initial results of Radiation Therapy Oncology Group 89-03. J Clin Oncol 16:3576–3583

Shipley WU, Kaufman DS, Zehr E et al. (2002) Selective bladder preservation by combined modality protocol treatment: long-term outcomes of 190 patients with invasive bladder cancer. Urology 60:62–67

Siefker-Radtke AO, Dinney CP, Abrahams NA et al. (2004) Evidence supporting preoperative chemotherapy for small cell carcinoma of the bladder: a retrospective review of the MD Anderson cancer experience. J Urol 172:481–484

Skinner DG, Daniels JR, Russell CA et al. (1991) The role of adjuvant chemotherapy following cystectomy for invasive bladder cancer: a prospective comparative trial. J Urol 145:459–464

Smith JA Jr, Crawford ED, Paradelo JC et al. (1997) Treatment of advanced bladder cancer with combined preoperative irradiation and radical cystectomy versus radical cystectomy alone: a phase III intergroup study. J Urol 157:805–807

Stein JP, Lieskovsky G, Cote R et al. (2001) Radical cystectomy in the treatment of invasive bladder cancer: long-term results in 1,054 patients. J Clin Oncol 19:666–675

Sternberg CN, Yagoda A, Scher HI et al. (1989) Methotrexate, vinblastine, doxorubicin, and cisplatin for advanced transitional cell carcinoma of the urothelium. Efficacy and patterns of response and relapse. Cancer 64:2448–2458

Stöckle M, Meyenburg W, Wellek S et al. (1995) Adjuvant polychemotherapy of nonorgan-confined bladder cancer after radical cystectomy revisited: long-term results of a controlled prospective study and further clinical experience. J Urol 153:47–52

Studer UE, Bacchi M, Biedermann C et al. (1994) Adjuvant cisplatin chemotherapy following cystectomy for bladder cancer: results of a prospective randomized trial. J Urol 152:81–84

Sved P, Gomez P, Manoharan M et al. (2004) Small cell carcinoma of the bladder. BJU Int 94:12–17

Swanson DA, Liles A, Zagars GK (1990) Preoperative irradiation and radical cystectomy for stages T2 and T3 squamous cell carcinoma of the bladder. J Urol 143:37–40

Sylvester RJ, van der Meijden AP, Witjes JA et al. (2005) Bacillus calmette-guerin versus chemotherapy for the intravesical treatment of patients with carcinoma in situ of the bladder: a meta-analysis of the published results of randomized clinical trials. J Urol 174:86–91

Tekes A, Kamel I, Imam K et al. (2005) Dynamic MRI of bladder cancer: evaluation of staging accuracy. Am J Roentgenol 184:121–127

Tester W, Porter A, Asbell S et al. (1993) Combined modality program with possible organ preservation for invasive bladder carcinoma: results of RTOG protocol 85-12. Int J Radiat Oncol Biol Phys 25:783–790

Tester W, Caplan R, Heaney J et al. (1996) Neoadjuvant combined modality program with selective organ preservation for invasive bladder cancer: results of Radiation Therapy Oncology Group phase II trial 8802. J Clin Oncol 14:119–126

Tonoli S, Bertoni F, De Stefani A et al. (2006) Radical radiotherapy for bladder cancer: retrospective analysis of a series of 459 patients treated in an Italian institution. Clin Oncol (R Coll Radiol) 18:52–59

Von der Maase H, Hansen SW, Roberts JT et al. (2001) Gemcitabine and cisplatin versus methotrexate, vinblastine, doxorubicin, and cisplatin in advanced or metastatic bladder cancer: results of a large, randomized, multinational, multicenter, phase III study. J Clin Oncol 19:1229–1231

Wasco MJ, Daignault S, Zhang Y et al. (2007) Urothelial carcinoma with divergent histologic differentiation (mixed histologic features) predicts the presence of locally advanced bladder cancer when detected at transurethral resection. Urology 70:69–74

Zaghloul MS, Nouh A, Nazmy M et al. (2006) Long-term results of primary adenocarcinoma of the urinary bladder: a report on 192 patients. Urol Oncol 24:13–20

Zietman AL, Sacco D, Skowronski U et al. (2003) Organ conservation in invasive bladder cancer by transurethral resection, chemotherapy and radiation: results of a urodynamic and quality of life study on long-term survivors. J Urol 170:1772–1776

Prostate Cancer

20

HANS T. CHUNG

Introduction and Objectives

Prostate cancer is the most prevalent cancer and is the second most common cause of cancer death in American men (JEMAL et al. 2007). In the era or PSA screening, the majority of patients are diagnosed prior to the onset of the symptoms. According to the pre-treatment PSA, tumor differentiation (Gleason score) and stage, prostate cancer can be categorized into different risk groups, which can assist in determining treatment strategies.

Management of prostate cancer is largely determined by the characteristics of the patient and the disease. In general, active surveillance, hormones alone, radical prostatectomy, external-beam radiotherapy and brachytherapy are possible options for prostate cancer. For higher risk disease, hormonal therapy and/or brachytherapy may be combined with external-beam radiotherapy to enhance efficacy.

This chapter examines:

● Recommendations for diagnosis and staging procedures

● The staging system, risk groups, and prognostic factors

● Treatment recommendations as well as the supporting scientific evidence for definitive and adjuvant treatment

● The use of surgery, radiation therapy, and hormonal therapy for definitive treatment of limited prostate cancer

● Follow-up care and surveillance of survivors

The most common site for metastatic prostate cancer is the bone. Radiation plays a major role in the treatment of bone metastasis secondary to prostate cancer, and the utilization of both external beam radiotherapy and radioactive isotope for the treatment of bone metastases is detailed in Chapter 43.

H. T. CHUNG, MD, FRCPC
Department of Radiation Oncology, National University Cancer Institute of Singapore, National University Health System, National University of Singapore, 5 Lower Kent Ridge Road, Singapore 119074, Singapore

20.1 Diagnosis, Staging, and Prognosis

20.1.1 Diagnosis

Initial Evaluation

- In the era of PSA screening, most men are asymptomatic at the time of diagnosis.
- History and physical exam focus on local symptoms, such as urinary frequency, urgency, nocturia, weak stream, hesitancy, or hematuria. For more advanced disease, patients may also present with bloody stools or changes in bowel habits. Distant spread is usually to bone and pelvic lymph nodes. Erectile function should also be documented.
- All patients should have a digital rectal exam (DRE), noting the size of the prostate, presence of prostatic nodules, extracapsular extension of nodules, involvement of the seminal vesicles, and the presence of blood on the gloved hand.

Laboratory Tests

- At a minimum, the total prostatic-specific antigen (PSA) level should be measured. If available, this should be compared in the context of all prior PSA measurements to gauge the trend, i.e., PSA velocity. A sudden rise in PSA levels over time is more suggestive of prostate cancer than benign causes.
- While associated with prostate cancer, an elevated PSA is not specific. In general, the higher the PSA level is, the more likely for the cause to be due to prostate cancer. False-positives can arise from inflammation, infection, benign prostatic hypertrophy, recent DRE, and recent ejaculation.
- Strategies to help distinguish between a PSA rise due to malignancy or benign disease include age-adjusted PSA levels, free PSA, PSA density, and PSA velocity, though there is no general consensus on their use.
- A free to total PSA ratio, which is the percentage of PSA that is not bound to proteins in the blood, less than 20% is associated with prostate cancer. The relationship between the probability of prostate cancer and the free to total PSA ratio is inversely proportional (ARCANGELI et al. 1998).

- A complete blood count, basic blood chemistry, liver function tests, renal function tests, total testosterone, and alkaline phosphatase may also be considered.

Imaging Studies

- Imaging studies, such as a bone scan and CT scan of the abdomen and pelvis, are advised for patients with symptoms or signs (e.g., bone pain) suggestive of metastatic disease or for patients with high-risk prostate cancer (Grade D). The American Urology Association guidelines recommend a bone scan if the PSA is >10 ng/ml and a CT scan if the PSA is >20 ng/ml (Level V) (CARROLL et al. 2001).
- A transrectal ultrasound of the prostate can be performed to exclude extracapsular disease and seminal vesicle involvement.
- An MRI with an endorectal coil of the prostate can be suggested for evaluation of local disease (Grade B). The procedure is gaining popularity as it provides superior soft tissue anatomy as compared to CT scans in evaluating for extracapsular extension and/or seminal vesicle involvement (Level IV) (ZHANG et al. 2007).
- Magnetic resonance spectroscopy imaging (MRSI) can be used in staging and post-treatment measurement of efficacy (Grade B). The study combines an MRI with spatial metabolic activity, and its effect has been demonstrated in numerous prospective radiology studies (RAJESH et al. 2007).

Pathology

- A systematic transrectal ultrasound-guided prostate biopsy is used to obtain tissue. At least ten biopsy cores from the entire prostate are recommended.
- The tumor is graded by genitourinary pathologists according to the Gleason scoring system, which is based on 10 points. This consist of two numbers (e.g., $3 + 3 = 6$), with the first number representing the predominant Gleason pattern (scored out of 5) and the second number representing the second most common Gleason pattern. The greater the Gleason score, the higher the grade of the prostate cancer, which is associated with lymph node involvement and distant metastases.

- Among all the biopsy cores, the highest Gleason score is used in determining prognosis and management.
- The limitation of the Gleason scoring system is that it is somewhat subjective, leading to significant inter- and intra-observer variation (ALLSBROOK et al. 2001).
- More than 95% of cancers of the prostate gland are adenocarcinoma. Less common histologies are ductal adenocarcinoma, neuroendocrine tumors, mucinous carcinoma, sarcomatoid carcinoma, endometrioid tumors, adenoid cystic carcinoma, sarcomas, carcinosarcoma, and primary lymphoma.

20.1.2 Staging

- Prostate cancer is clinically staged using the 2003 AJCC TNM system, which is based on DRE findings (Table 20.1).
- Prediction models can be used to help guide treatment (Grade A). A number of risk groups (e.g., D'Amico, MDACC, MSKCC, and Seattle) and nomograms (e.g., MSKCC and Partin table) have been published to predict pathologic stage, biochemical control, prostate cancer-specific mortality, and developing metastases based on retrospective review. Generally, most risk grouping systems classify patients on the basis of PSA, Gleason score, TNM stage, and the percent positive biopsy cores (Level IV) (D'AMICO et al. 1998, 1999, 2002; PARTIN et al. 2001; KATTAN et al. 2000, 2001, 2003; SYLVESTER et al. 2003; ROACH et al. 2000).
- The most commonly used risk grouping system is the one proposed by D'AMICO et al. (1998). These have been adopted by the NCCN guidelines, which divides patients into low-, intermediate-, high-risk, locally advanced and metastatic groups (Table 20.2) (NATIONAL COMPREHENSIVE CANCER NETWORK, VERSION 1.2008).
- The Roach formula can be used to estimate the risk of lymph node involvement (Grade B). The probability of pelvic lymph node involvement = $(2/3) \times PSA + [(Gleason\ score\ -6) \times 10]$ (Level IV) (ROACH 1993).

Table 20.1. American Joint Committee on Cancer (AJCC) TNM Classification of Carcinoma Cancer of the Prostate. [From GREENE et al. (2002) with permission]

Primary tumor (T)	
TX	Primary tumor cannot be assessed
T0	No evidence of primary tumor
T1	Clinically unapparent tumor neither palpable nor visible by imaging
T1a	Tumor incidental histological finding in 5% or less of tissue resected
T1b	Tumor incidental histological finding in more than 5% of tissue resected
T1c	Tumor identified by needle biopsy (e.g., because of elevated PSA)
T2	Tumor confined within prostate
T2a	Tumor involves one-half of one lobe or less
T2b	Tumor involves more than one-half of one lobe, but not both lobes
T2c	Tumor involves both lobes
T3	Tumor extends through the prostate capsule
T3a	Extracapsular extension (unilateral or bilateral)
T3b	Tumor invades seminal vesicle(s)
T4	Tumor is fixed or invades adjacent structures other than seminal vesicles: bladder neck, external sphincter, rectum, levator muscles, and/or pelvic wall
Regional lymph nodes (N)	
NX	Regional lymph nodes were not assessed
N0	No regional lymph node metastasis
N1	Metastasis in regional lymph nodes(s)
Distant metastasis (M)	
MX	Distant metastasis cannot be assessed (not evaluated by any modality)
M0	No distant metastasis
M1	Distant metastasis
M1a	Non-regional lymph node(s)
M1b	Bone(s)
M1c	Other site(s) with or without bone disease
STAGE GROUPING	
I:	T1a N0 M0 G1
II:	T1a N0 M0 G2,3–4, T1b N0 M0 Any G, T1c N0 M0 Any G T1 N0 M0 Any G, T2 N0 M0 Any G
III:	T3 N0 M0 Any G
IV:	T4 N0 M0 Any G, Any T N1 M0 Any G, Any T Any N M1 Any G

Table 20.2. Risk grouping system adopted by the National Comprehensive Cancer Network (NCCN, version 1.2008).

		Disease characteristics		
		Stage	Gleason score	PSA
Risk groups	Low risk	T1–T2a, and	2–6, and	<10 ng/mL
	Intermediate risk	T2b–T2c, or	7, or	10–20 ng/mL
	High risk	T3a, or	8–10, or	>20 ng/mL
	Locally advanced	T3b–T4	Any	Any
	Metastatic	N1 and/or M1	Any	Any

20.1.3 Prognostic Factors

- The risk groupings suggested by D'AMICO et al. (1998) classify patients into low-, intermediate- and high-risk disease. These are useful for prognostication and treatment decisions (Level IV).

- Among intermediate-risk patients, a percent biopsy cores involvement, calculated as the number of cores containing cancer divided by the total number of cores obtained, greater than 50% share similar outcomes as high-risk patients. Another surrogate is the presence of individual biopsy cores containing more than 50% cancer (D'AMICO et al. 2002).

- A PSA velocity, calculated before radical prostatectomy, of >2.0 ng/ml/year has been associated with shorter time to death from prostate cancer and death from any cause. This is in addition to Gleason score 8–10, clinical stage T2, and pretreatment PSA (Level IV) (D'AMICO et al. 2004).

and is an option for asymptomatic, low-volume, low-grade disease in patients with >5-year life expectancy and compliant to regular follow-up (Grade A). No differences in overall survival were observed in multi-institutional randomized trials between watchful waiting and prostatectomy (Level I) (KLOTZ 2004; HOLMBERG et al. 2002; BILL-AXELSON et al. 2005).

- Multi-institutional retrospective study suggests that outcomes after any of the three definitive treatment modalities such as external-beam radiotherapy >72 Gy, brachytherapy, radical prostatectomy yield similar results, with the 5-year PSA progression-free survival of 81%–83% (Level IV) (KUPELIAN et al. 2004).

- For low-risk disease, outcomes of the three treatment options appear to be similar. The differences among the treatment modalities are the logistics, invasiveness of the treatment, side effects, complications, and recovery (Fig. 20.1).

20.2 Treatment Options for Localized Prostate Cancer

20.2.1 General Principles

- To help patients decide on which treatment to select, it is helpful to discuss the natural history of the disease, life expectancy of the patient, treatment outcomes, and its effects on quality of life of all the modalities and early and late toxicities.

- Active surveillance, meaning regular follow-ups with PSA measurements, is indicated for asymptomatic patients with <5-year life expectancy

20.2.2 Low-Dose-Rate Brachytherapy

Treatment Technique

- There are presently two strategies, preplanned and intra-operative planning, in performing LDR brachytherapy. The American Brachytherapy Society has released recommendations on transperineal permanent brachytherapy. Recommended indications for brachytherapy as monotherapy include stage T1–2a, Gleason sum 2–6, and PSA <10 ng/mL. Recommended indications for brachytherapy as a boost to external-beam radiotherapy include stage T2b–c, Gleason 8–10, or PSA >20 ng/ml. Contraindications for brachytherapy include life expectancy <5 years,

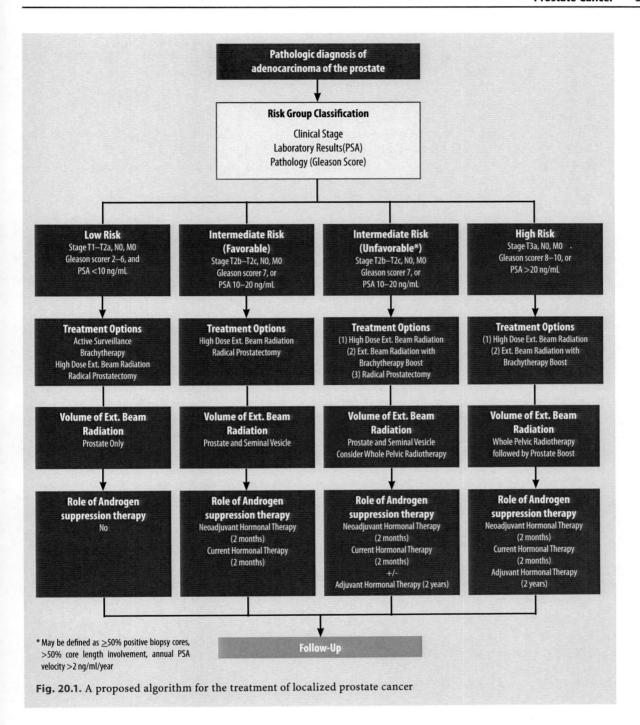

Fig. 20.1. A proposed algorithm for the treatment of localized prostate cancer

large TURP defect, unacceptable operative risks, and distant metastases (Grade D). Relative contraindications for brachytherapy because of higher risk of toxicities include a large median lobe, previous pelvic irradiation, high IPSS score (IPSS >15), history of multiple pelvic surgeries, and severe diabetes with healing problems;

relative contraindications because of inadequate dose coverage include previous TURP, gland size >60 cc at the time of implant (consider in context of pubic arch), prominent median lobe, and positive seminal vesicle invasion (Nag et al. 1999).

■ The preplanned technique, advocated by the Seattle Prostate Institute, involves two separate visits for the patient. In the first visit, a volume study is performed. In the dorsal lithotomy position, a transrectal ultrasound, mounted onto a brachytherapy stepper, is used to capture sequential axial images of the prostate in 5-mm increments. Aerated jelly is inserted into the urethra during the procedure to visualize the urethra on the ultrasound images. These images are transferred to a laptop computer loaded with a brachytherapy planning software. Afterwards, planning is done offline to determine an optimal seed implantation pattern. Once finalized, the seeds are ordered. Usually, the actual implant is performed approximately 1–2 weeks after the volume study.

- The intraoperative planning approach consolidates the two visits into a single sitting, i.e., planning and implantation of seeds can be done at the same time as the volume study. Advantages include patient convenience, less use of hospital resources, and minimal change in patient positioning. However, doing it in one sitting adds an extra layer of complexity (Zelefsky et al. 2007).
- Neoadjuvant hormones may be considered for large prostate glands (>60 cc) in the hopes of downsizing the prostate.
- Patients should be counseled on radiation protection issues, such as how to retrieve and dispose of seeds that have passed in the urine, minimizing radiation exposure to small children and pregnant women, wearing condoms for the initial period, cremation issues, and the issuance of a card that describes the amount of radiation and the procedure for security checkpoint purposes.

Isotope and Dose

- The ABS recommends monotherapy prescription doses for I-125 and Pd-103 to be 145 Gy and 125 Gy, respectively (Grade B). For external-beam radiotherapy with I-125 or Pd-103 prostate boost, the ABS recommended boost doses of 100–110 Gy and 90–100 Gy, respectively (Grade B) (Rivard et al. 2007).
- The dose response using post-implant dosimetry with a CT scan taken 30 days after I-125 prostate brachytherapy was analyzed using retrospective data. Freedom from biochemical failure was associated with the D90 (dose delivered to 90% of the prostate gland): at 5 years, 68% for D90 <140 Gy, 97% for 140–<160 Gy, 98% for 160–<180 Gy, and 95% for ≥180 Gy (p=0.0025). Post-treatment

prostate biopsies taken at 2 years were positive in 22% for D90 <160 Gy and 9% for D90 ≥160 Gy (Level IV) (Stock et al. 2002).

Post-Implant Dosimetry

- The American Brachytherapy Society convened a panel discussion in 2004 regarding critical organ dosimetry. Among the recommendations, they reiterated that postimplant dosimetry is critical for quality assurance, provides prognostic information, and may identify systematic technical errors. The urethra should be delineated as a volume, either with fusion with ultrasound images or with a catheter in place during the CT scan. The dosimetric endpoints that should be recorded include the V150%, D5%, and D30%. The inner and outer wall of the rectum should be contoured on all CT slices where seeds are identified; the dosimetric parameters are V100% and V150% (Grade B) (Crook et al. 2005).
- A CT scan performed after implant is used to assess the quality of the implant. The interval between the implant and the CT scan may be variable, but this should be considered when comparing the quality of the implant as prostate edema may still be significant if scanned early. In general, the CT scan can be performed on the same day up to 30 days post-implant.
- Some centers have studied CT-MRI fusion, which addresses the CT image artifact from the seeds and the difficulty in identifying the prostate base and apex (Crook et al. 2002).

Outcomes

- A multi-institutional study of long-term results after LDR brachytherapy for 2,693 men with T1-2 prostate cancer was recently published. Median follow-up was 63 months. Patients with a prostate D90 ≥130 Gy had an 8-year PSA relapse-free survival of 93% versus 76% for patients with a D90 <130 Gy (p< 0.001). PSA nadir was associated with PSA control; 8-year PSA relapse-free survival was 92%, 86%, 79%, and 67% for PSA nadirs of < 0.5, 0.5–0.99, 1.0–1.99, and >2.0 ng/ml, respectively (Level IV) (Zelefsky et al. 2007).
- The long-term outcomes of a single-institution's experience in 1,266 cases of permanent seeds brachytherapy for stage T1-2 disease showed that 5-year PSA disease-free survival and cause-specific survival was 76% and 98%, respectively, in

the entire cohort. Median follow-up was 4.1 years. Multivariate analyses found that the presence of Gleason score $\geq$7, PSA $\geq$10, or clinical T stage $\geq$T2b significantly increased the risk of PSA failures from 1.4 to 2.9 times. The hazard ratio for cause-specific survival was also significantly increased for Gleason score $\geq$7 and PSA $\geq$10, ranging from 4.7 to 6.4 (Level IV) (Beyer et al. 2003).

- In a retrospective study from the Seattle Prostate Institute, 10-year PSA progression-free survival of I-125 brachtherapy as monotherapy for early stage disease was 87% (Level IV) (Grimm et al. 2001).

20.2.3 External-Beam Radiotherapy

Treatment Technique

Simulation

- CT simulation is performed in the supine position with arms on the chest. Scan slice thickness should be 3 mm or less. The bladder should be comfortably full to displace the bowel away from the prostate. The rectum should be empty, which may be achieved with a bowel preparation or modification of diet.
- Immobilization using alpha cradles, knee sponge, and ankle rests may be considered.
- To assist in identifying the prostatic apex, an urethrogram is suggested; other techniques include MRI fusion and intraprostatic fiducial markers. Fiducial markers should be implanted by transrectal ultrasound guidance at least 1–2 weeks before the CT simulation.

Beam Energy and Dose Calculation

- A minimum of 10-MV photon beams should be used.

Field Arrangement

- For both 3DCRT and IMRT, a five- to seven-beam iso-centric technique is used to minimize radiation to nearby critical organs, such as the rectum, bladder, penile bulb, and femoral heads (Fig. 20.2).
- The CTV includes the entire prostate gland. The PTV margin should account for inter- and intra-

fraction organ motion and setup variation, which will vary between centers depending on the use of any image-guidance technique. Examples of image-guided radiotherapy (IGRT) include the implantation of three to four intraprostatic fiducial markers (Pouliot et al. 2003), B-mode acquisition and targeting (BAT) ultrasound (Lattanzi et al. 1999), and cone-beam CT (Moseley et al. 2007).

Whole Pelvic Treatment

- Traditionally, conventional field placement using bony landmarks has been used in placing a four-field box. The superior border is placed at the L5–S1 interspace. The inferior border is at the inferior aspect of the ischium. The posterior border is at the S2–3 interspace. The anterior border is at the anterior aspect of the pubic symphysis. The lateral borders are 2 cm lateral to the widest point of the pelvic brim.
- IMRT can be considered for the treatment of pelvic lymph nodes (Grade B). Many centers have migrated to IMRT for the pelvic nodes, though this requires significant knowledge of pelvic anatomy. The CTV includes the distal common iliac, internal iliac, and external iliac nodal regions. The corresponding vessels should be used as a guide in delineating these nodal regions. In a comparison between 3DCRT and IMRT for the first treatment phase (45 Gy in 25 fractions) of whole-pelvic radiotherapy in high-risk patients, IMRT significantly improved the coverage of the nodes at risk (D95 46.0 vs. 27.4 Gy, $p<0.01$), while significantly sparing the rectum (V45 Gy), small bowel (V45 Gy), and bladder (V45 Gy) (Level III) (Wang-Chesebro et al. 2006).
- In a study of lymphotropic nanoparticles, draining nodal patterns of the prostate were mapped and formed the recommendations for delineation of the pelvic nodes. The proposed guidelines suggested that the pelvic nodal clinical target volume should include a 2-cm radial margin around the distal common iliac, proximal internal iliac, and proximal external iliac vessels. This volume would cover 94.5% of the pelvic nodes at risk in the study's cohort of 18 patients with node-positive disease (Level III) (Shih et al. 2005).
- At ASCO 2008 GU Symposium, Lawton et al. presented the RTOG consensus guidelines on CTV nodal delineation for high-risk patients. The guideline will be published on the RTOG website.

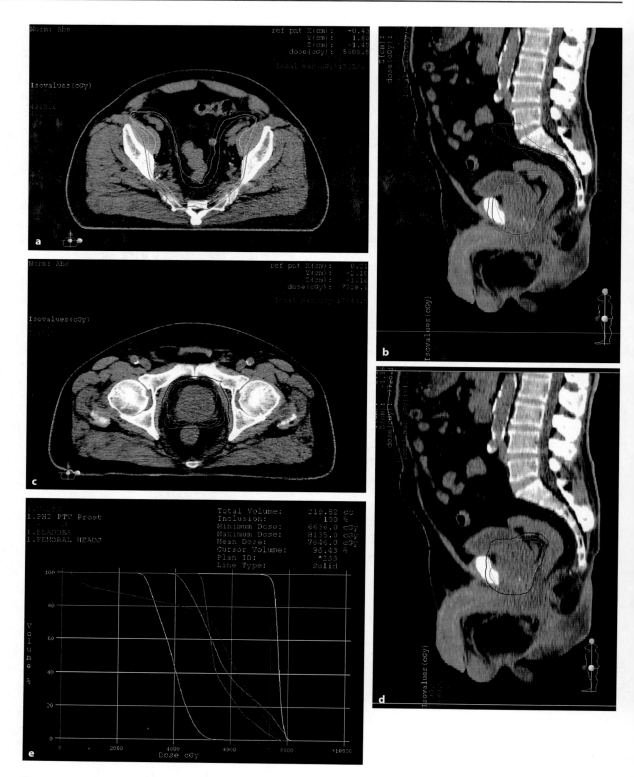

Fig. 20.2a–e. Isodose curves of an inverse IMRT plan using seven gantry angles delivered with conventional MLC for a patient with high-risk adenocarcinoma of the prostate. **a** Axial view of IMRT phase 1 isodose lines covering the PTV nodes (*yellow line*); **b** sagittal view of IMRT phase 1 isodose lines covering the PTV nodes (*purple line*) and PTV prostate and seminal vesicles (*magenta line*); **c** axial view of IMRT composite plan of isodose lines covering the PTV prostate (*green line*); **d** sagittal view of IMRT composite plan of isodose lines covering the PTV prostate (*magenta line*); **e** DVH of composite plan

Dose and Fractionation

Dose Escalation

- The recommended minimum dose to the prostate is at least 72 Gy to the PTV, which can be delivered in 1.8 to 2.0 Gy per fraction. The choice of total dose will vary from center to center and is based on the availability and type of targeting systems, IMRT, and physician comfort level. With image-guided radiotherapy, the minimum dose should be escalated further to at least 78 Gy (Grade A). Generally, there are two prescription methods used in the dose-escalation trials. Some studies prescribe to the isocenter (i.e., 100%), which means that the minimum dose to the PTV is lower (usually 95%). Other studies prescribe a minimum dose to the PTV, which means that the maximum dose within the PTV will be higher. It is imperative to highlight this difference when comparing trials.

- Dose-escalation (>72 Gy) is considered standard based on several phase III trials. When analyzed by risk groups, the benefit of dose escalation is not consistently positive, which may be due to inadequate power, short follow-up, or the use of different definitions of PSA relapse. Unless specified, the studies below excluded the use of hormones.

- In a phase III study comparing 70 and 78 Gy in T1–3 disease, 8-year PSA control was 59% and 78%, respectively (p=0.004). The benefit was seen in low-risk disease, but in intermediate- and high-risk disease only patients with a PSA >10 ng/ml benefited (Level I) (POLLACK et al. 2002; KUBAN et al. 2008).

- In a phase III trial comparing 70.2 versus 79.2 Gy in T1b–T2b disease and PSA <15 ng/ml, protons were used for the prostate boost phase in both arms. The 5-year PSA control rate was 61.4% and 80.4%, respectively (p< 0.001). The benefit was seen in both low- (60.1% and 80.5%, p<0.001) and intermediate-risk patients (62.7% vs. 81.0%, p=0.02) (Level I) (ZIETMAN et al. 2005).

- The phase III trial of 68 versus 78 Gy using 3DCRT found that 5-year freedom from failure was 54% and 64%, respectively (p=0.02). Depending on the estimated risk of seminal vesicle involvement, the seminal vesicles were included in the treatment fields. Twenty-one percent of patients received (neo)adjuvant hormones, of which 55% received long-term (3 years) hormones. No difference was seen in the low-risk patients. Intermediate-risk patients significantly benefited from 78 Gy, whereas in high-risk patients there was a trend towards 78 Gy (Level I) (PEETERS et al. 2006).

- Initial results of the MRC RT01 randomized trial comparing 64 and 74 Gy to the prostate were recently published. Eight hundred forty-three men with cT1b–3N0 prostate cancer received 3–6 months of neoadjuvant androgen suppression until completion of radiation. Whole-pelvic radiotherapy was not given. The dose was prescribed to isocenter. Accrued patients had the following characteristics: median pre-treatment PSA 12.8 ng/ml, 13% had Gleason score 8–10, and 18% had cT3 disease. Median follow-up was 63 months. The 5-year PSA control (71% vs. 60%, p=0.0007) was significantly higher with high-dose radiotherapy. No differences in overall survival, cause-specific survival, and distant metastases were noted. Escalated dose was associated with more late RTOG grade $\geq$2 (p=0.005) and $\geq$3 (p=0.055) bowel toxicities, but not urinary toxicities (Level I) (DEARNALEY et al. 2007).

- The earliest phase 1–2 study of dose escalation from 64.8 to 86.4 Gy using 3DCRT and IMRT showed that higher doses were associated with improved PSA control. When comparing dose groups of 64.8–70.2 Gy and 75.6–86.4 Gy, the 5-year PSA control rates were improved in favorable (77% vs. 90%, p=0.05), intermediate (50% vs. 70%, p=0.001), and unfavorable risk (21% vs. 47%, p=0.002). Lower doses were associated with a greater likelihood of positive postradiation prostate biopsies. In separate analyses of the subgroup who received 81 Gy with IMRT, 8-year PSA control rates were 85%, 76%, and 72% for favorable, intermediate, and unfavorable risk groups (Level II) (ZELEFSKY et al. 2001, 2006).

- Retrospective study of 839 patients treated with 3DCRT showed a significant positive correlation between radiation dose and biochemical failure between the <72 Gy, 72–75.9 Gy, and $\geq$76 Gy dose groups for intermediate-, but not low- and high-risk patients. In multivariate analyses, dose was a significant predictor of biochemical failure (Level IV) (POLLACK et al. 2004).

- The results of a prospective dose-escalation study with 3DCRT from 68 to 79 Gy showed that when stratified by PSA and radiation dose, patients with a PSA >10 ng/ml or PSA >20 ng/ml did not benefit from dose escalation. However, among patients with a PSA of 10–20 ng/ml, there was a clear dose-escalation advantage seen with 8-year PSA control increasing from 19% to 84% (Level II) (HANKS et al. 2002).

- In a large multi-institutional retrospective study of 1,325 patients with T1–2 disease, the 5-year PSA control rate was higher in the cohort given at least 72 Gy than the cohort given less than 72 Gy (63% vs. 69%, $p=0.046$). Dose was also significant in multivariate analyses (Level IV) (KUPELIAN et al. 2005).

Hypofractionation

- Unlike most tumors, recent studies suggest that the alpha-beta ratio of prostate cancers may be low, like late-responding normal tissues (Level IV) (BRENNER et al. 1999, 2002; FOWLER et al. 2001; KING et al. 2001). Higher dose per fraction, or hypofractionation, may be more effective for prostate cancer (Grade B). This has the added advantage of patient convenience because of a shorter overall treatment time. However, the worry is that this may lead to more late rectal and bladder toxicities. Longer follow-up and a large-scale multi-institutional phase III trial will be needed before hypofractionation becomes standard.

- Results are described from a retrospective, single-institution study of 70 Gy in 28 fractions over 5.5 weeks (2.5 Gy/fraction) to the prostate ± seminal vesicles with IMRT. Neoadjuvant or adjuvant hormones were given to 60% of patients, of whom 18% received more than 6 months of treatment; 34%, 28%, and 38% had low-, intermediate-, and high-risk disease. The 5-year PSA control was 94%, 83%, and 72% for low-, intermediate-, and high-risk groups, respectively. Daily target localization was performed using daily transabdominal ultrasound. Severe acute and late toxicities occurred in 1% and 1.5% of patients, respectively (Level IV) (KUPELIAN et al. 2007).

- Preliminary results of a single-institution phase II trial of 60 Gy in 20 fractions over 4 weeks (3.0 Gy/fraction) with IMRT for T1c–2c disease found that the 14-month PSA control rate was 97%. Of the 92 patients, 85 had low- or intermediate-risk disease. Eight of 92 patients received adjuvant hormones. Daily target localization was performed using intraprostatic markers. There was one case of severe acute toxicities and no cases of severe late toxicities (Level III) (MARTIN et al. 2007).

- Phase I/II study of 33.5 Gy in five fractions (6.7 Gy/fraction) delivered with non-coplanar, confor-mal beams and daily target localization using intraprostatic fiducial markers reported a 4-year rate of biochemical freedom from relapse of 70% (ASTRO definition) and 90% (RTOG-Phoenix definition). Acute grade 1–2 toxicities were 48.5% and 39% for GU and GI, respectively. Only one case of acute grade 3 toxicity (GU) was seen. No late grade 3–5 toxicities were seen, but late grade 2 GU and GI toxicities were 20% and 7.5%, respectively (Level III) (MADSEN et al. 2007).

- In a randomized trial of 76 Gy in 38 fractions over 7.5 weeks versus 70.2 Gy in 26 fractions over using IMRT in intermediate- and high-risk patients, preliminary results show that one and four patients, respectively, experienced severe acute genitourinary toxicities during radiation. No patients experienced severe acute urinary toxicities at 3 months post-treatment (Level II) (POLLACK et al. 2006).

External-Beam Radiotherapy and

Brachytherapy Boost

- Based on the results of multiple retrospective studies, the American Brachytherapy Society recommendations for brachytherapy as a boost to external-beam radiotherapy include stage T2b–c, Gleason 8–10, or PSA >20 ng/ml (Grade B) (NAG et al. 1999). The combination of external-beam radiotherapy and brachytherapy prostate boost is usually reserved for higher risk patients, where the risks of extracapsular extension and/or seminal vesicle invasion are deemed unacceptably high, and brachytherapy alone may not be able to encompass the disease. A second indication for adding external-beam radiotherapy is for suboptimal brachytherapy dose distribution.

- There is no consensus on the external-beam radiotherapy volume. It can range from treating only the peri-prostatic tissues to the entire true pelvis. The decision on how much to treat will depend on the estimated risk of disease extension beyond the capsule and to the lymph nodes. By virtue of a larger volume of irradiated tissue, GI and GU toxicities will be higher, though still acceptable. The recommended dose is 45 Gy in 25 fractions.

- The brachytherapy boost can be given with either LDR or HDR. HDR has been traditionally given for locally advanced disease, where LDR may have difficulty in encompassing the at-risk volume. Advantages of HDR are conformal dose distribution, accurate dosimetry, and no radiation exposure to the patient's family members and hospital staff as the Ir-192 seeds are placed in an afterloading technique. Also, if the prostate cancer does indeed behave like late tissue, such that the alpha-beta ratio is closer to 3, the large dose fraction sizes of HDR may be beneficial. For external-beam radiotherapy with I-125 or Pd-103 prostate boost, the recommended LDR boost doses are 100–110 Gy and 90–100 Gy, respectively. As there is no consensus in the HDR dose fractionation, it is suggested to review the current literature (RIVARD et al. 2007).

■ Long-term results (median follow-up 7.25 years) from a single institution (*n*=209) of external-beam radiotherapy (36 Gy in 20 fractions to the peri-prostatic tissue) and HDR brachytherapy (total 22–24 Gy) are described. Two implants were performed 1 week apart, with two HDR fractions given ≥6 h apart during each implant (four HDR fractions, 5.5–6.0 Gy each). No hormones were given before radiotherapy. The 10-year PSA progression-free survival for low-, intermediate-, and high-risk patients was 90%, 87%, and 69%, respectively. Among the high-risk patients, none had local failure. The median PSA nadir was 0.1 ng/ml, and the median time to reach the nadir was 3.5 years. The PSA nadir was a significant predictor of PSA progression-free survival. Of the patients, 6.7% developed a urinary stricture requiring surgical intervention, and 3.8% developed urinary incontinence (Level IV) (DEMANES et al. 2005).

■ In a phase I/II study from William Beaumont Hospital, the outcomes of 197 patients with intermediate- and high-risk disease who also received external-beam radiotherapy to the pelvis and 2–3 HDR boost were analyzed. HDR dose fractionation was progressively increased over the study period and is grouped into a "low-dose" group that received a mean prostate BED of 88.2 Gy and a "high-dose" group that received a mean prostate BED of 116.8 Gy (alpha-beta ratio of 1.2). The HDR dose ranged from 5.5 Gy × 3 fractions to 11.5 Gy × 2 fractions. At 5 years, the biochemical failure, cause-specific survival, and overall survival were 21.6%, 98.3%, and 92.9%, respectively, for the entire cohort. When stratified by dose group, the "high-dose" group had superior 5-year biochemical failure (32.7% vs. 14.0%, *p*=0.006), locoregional failure (8.6% vs. 3.5%, *p*=0.3), distant failure (9.1% vs. 2.7%, *p*=0.05), cause-specific survival (95.4% vs. 100%, *p*=0.02) and overall survival (86.2% vs. 97.8%, *p*=0.002). No difference was seen in the GU and GI toxicity profile between the two dose groups. Overall, the incidence of grade 3–4 GI and GU toxicities was 2% for both, which included rectal ulceration requiring surgery and urinary diversion. Grade 3 rectal bleeding occurred in <1% (Level III) (VARGAS et al. 2006).

■ The long-term outcomes in a cohort of 223 men with T1–3 disease treated at the Seattle Prostate Institute with external-beam radiotherapy (45 Gy "mini-pelvis" field) and permanent LDR brachytherapy boost were reported. No hormones were given unless for failure. The brachytherapy doses were ~100 Gy with Pd-103 (NIST 99) and 108 Gy with I-125 (TG-43), and implanted a median of 4 weeks after completing external-beam radiotherapy. Median follow-up was 9.4 years. The 15-year PSA relapse-free survival was 86%, 80%, and 68% for low-, intermediate-, and high-risk diseases, respectively (Level IV) (SYLVESTER et al. 2007).

■ A retrospective analysis of 64 intermediate- and high-risk patients treated at University of California San Francisco with an HDR boost was recently published. Patients received 2 months of neoadjuvant hormones, concurrent hormones, and with or without 2 years of adjuvant for high-grade disease (Gleason score >7). Whole-pelvic radiotherapy (45 Gy in 25 fractions) was indicated for 40 patients with >15% risk estimated nodal involvement; otherwise, peri-prostate volume was irradiated. The HDR implant was performed 1 week after completing external-beam radiotherapy, delivering a total of 18 Gy in three fractions separated by at least 6 h. The 4-year disease-free survival was 92%. Two patients had peri-operative hematuria, with one requiring a blood transfusion. There were no late grade ≥3 GU toxicities. One patient had a late grade 4 GI toxicity with subsequent bowel obstruction (Level IV) (HSU et al. 2005).

Prophylactic Pelvic Nodal Radiotherapy

■ Prophylactic pelvic nodal radiation can be considered in the treatment of high-risk patients (Grade C). However, after the initial then updated results of RTOG 9413, the concept of whole-pelvic radiotherapy for patients considered at high-risk of harboring microscopic disease in the pelvic nodes is controversial. Critics cite the suboptimal dose (70.2 Gy) used in RTOG 9413, which is inadequate for prostate tumor eradication. Of note, all prior RTOG studies of high-risk patients gave WPRT. Surgical data from Johns Hopkins suggest that an extended as compared to a limited node dissection for high-risk patients may improve PSA outcomes (Level IV) (ALLAF et al. 2004).

■ RTOG 9413 was a phase III, four-armed study with a 2×2 randomization schema. A total of 1,292 men with an estimated pelvic node involvement of >15% or cT2c-4 and Gleason score ≥6 were randomized to either 4 months of neoadjuvant and concurrent (NCHT) or 4 months of adjuvant (AHT) androgen suppression therapy, and whole-pelvic radiotherapy (WPRT) or prostate-only radiotherapy (PORT). At the time of study design, no interaction was assumed between hormone timing and radiotherapy volume; therefore, the study was not powered to compare the four arms individually. The total prostate dose in all four arms was 70.2 Gy in 1.8 Gy fractions. In the WPRT arms, 50.4 Gy was given to the entire pelvis, followed by 19.8 Gy to the prostate. Concerning patient characteristics, the 4-year progression-free survival was 54% and 47% for the WPRT and PORT arms, respectively ($p=0.02$). No difference in 4-year progression-free survival was seen between the NCHT and AHT arms ($p=0.56$). When analyzed separately, the NCHT+WPRT arm had superior 4-year progression-free survival than the other three arms (60% vs. 44–50%, $p=0.008$). Severe (RTOG grade ≥3), acute (2% vs. 1%, $p=0.06$), and late (1.7% vs. 0.6%, $p=0.09$) GI toxicities were borderline higher in the WPRT than PORT arms, but no difference was seen in acute or late GU toxicities (Level I) (ROACH et al. 2003).

■ In a secondary analysis of RTOG 9413, two of the four arms were re-analyzed by stratifying based on field size. The NCHT+WPRT and NCHT+PORT arms were chosen to eliminate the treatment completion time bias with the two arms that received AHT. The NCHT+PORT arm was divided into the subgroup that received "mini-pelvis," defined as a field size of >10×11 cm, or "prostate-only," defined as a field size of <10×11 cm. The field size of 10×11 cm was chosen because it was the median in the NCHT+PORT arm. A significant association between larger field sizes and 4-year progression-free survival was detected ($p=0.024$). As expected, acute grade 2 or greater GI toxicities were more frequent with larger fields (WPRT, "mini-pelvis," prostate-only: 46.6%, 36.7%, 20.2%, $p<0.001$). Late grade 3 or greater GI toxicities were also more frequent with larger fields (5-year WPRT, "mini-pelvis," prostate-only: 4.3%, 1.2%, 0%, $p=0.006$) (Level I) (ROACH et al. 2006).

■ In an update of RTOG 9413, the median follow-up increased from 59.5 to 79 months. The significant improvement in progression-free survival seen in the WPRT versus the PORT arms in the initial analysis was no longer significant with increased follow-up ($p=0.99$). No difference was seen between the NCHT and AHT arms ($p=0.59$). When analyzed separately and adjusted for multiple pairwise comparisons (significant p-value <0.008), there was no significant difference between the four arms for progression-free survival. Late severe GU toxicities were similar in the four arms, though severe GI toxicities were more frequent in the NCHT+WPRT arm versus the other three arms (5% vs. 1%–2%, $p=0.002$) (Level I) (LAWTON et al. 2007).

■ In the French GETUG-01 phase 3 trial, 444 patients with T1b-3N0 with any PSA and any Gleason score were randomized to WPRT or PORT. "High-risk" patients (defined as the presence of any of the following: T3, Gleason score ≥7, or PSA >12) received 4–8 months of neoadjuvant and concurrent androgen suppression. The total prostate dose was 66–70 Gy. In the trial, 54% had an estimated lymph node involvement of less than 15%, median PSA was 11.5, and 50% had Gleason score <7. Preliminary results after a median follow-up of 42 months were presented. There was no significant difference in 5-year progression-free survival between the WPRT and PORT arm for the high-risk (59.8% vs. 63.4%, $p=0.2$) and low-risk (83.9% vs. 75.1%, $p=0.21$) patients, respectively. Multi-variate analyses suggested that the addition of hormones and estimated nodal risk were significant predictors, but field size and radiation dose were not. No difference was seen in acute and late rectal toxicities. In comparing this study with RTOG 9413, this study did not treat the entire pelvis as the upper border was taken at S1–2, which may miss as much as 20% of draining lymph nodes based on the nanoparticles study. Second, 60% of patients received less than 70 Gy, which is considered sub-optimal and may have led to inadequate tumor eradication in the prostate. Third, these results represent preliminary data (Level II) (POMMIER et al. 2007).

20.2.4 Androgen Suppression Therapy

- Androgen suppression therapy consists of an LHRH agonist (e.g., goserelin and leuprolide) and an anti-androgen (e.g., flutamide and bicalutamide).
- The trials supporting the combination of hormones and external-beam radiotherapy all used prostate doses of 70 Gy or less. In contrast, most dose-escalation trials did not use hormones. Thus, it is unclear whether hormones are beneficial in the setting of dose escalation.
- Whole-pelvic radiotherapy was not given in the two contemporary trials of intermediate-risk disease. In the studies of high-risk patients, all but one study treated the pelvis in both arms.
- Hormonal therapy is not recommended as an addition to definitive treatment for low-risk disease.

Intermediate-Risk Disease

- For intermediate-risk disease, the recommended hormone timing and duration are 2 months of neoadjuvant then concurrent hormones with external-beam radiotherapy (Grade A). A phase III trial randomized 206 patients with prostate cancer to radiotherapy alone or radiotherapy with 6 months of androgen suppression therapy. Patient characteristics were: median PSA of 11 ng/ml; clinical T1 (48%) and T2 (52%); Gleason score <7 (27%), 7 (58%), and 8–10 (15%). The radiotherapy was directed to the prostate only with a dose of 70 Gy in 35 fractions using 3D conformal radiotherapy. At a median follow-up of 4.52 years, 5-year overall survival (88% vs. 78%, $p=0.04$), cause-specific survival (100% vs. 94%, $p=0.02$), and PSA control (79% vs. 55%, $p<0.001$) were significantly better in the radiotherapy with a hormone arm. Updated results after a median follow-up of 7.6 years showed that all-cause mortality was significantly greater in the radiotherapy alone arm (HR 1.8, $p=0.01$). Subgroup analyses suggest that the significant difference was primarily in patients with no or minimal comorbidity (HR 4.2, $p<0.001$) (Level I) (D'AMICO et al. 2004, 2008).
- A phase III trial from Australia randomized 818 patients with prostate cancer to one of three arms: radiotherapy alone, radiotherapy with 3 months of androgen suppression therapy (started 2 months before radiotherapy), or radiotherapy with 6 months of androgen suppression therapy (started 5 months before radiotherapy). Radiotherapy was to the prostate and seminal vesicles to a total dose of 66 Gy in 33 fractions. Patient characteristics included: clinical T2 (60%), T3–4 (40%); median PSA 15; Gleason score <7 (44%), 7 (38%), and 8–10 (17%). Median follow-up was 5.9 years. Compared to the control arm of radiotherapy only, 3 months of hormones significantly improved biochemical control (HR 0.70, $p=0.002$), and disease-free survival (HR 0.65, $p=0.0001$). Compared to the control arm, 6 months of hormones significantly improved biochemical control (HR 0.58, $p<0.0001$), disease-free survival (HR 0.56, $p<0.0001$), distant failure (HR 0.67, $p=0.046$), and prostate cancer-specific survival (HR 0.56, $p=0.04$) (TROG 9601, Level I) (DENHAM et al. 2005).

High-Risk Disease

- For high-risk disease, the recommended hormone timing and duration is 2 months of neoadjuvant, concurrent, and 2–3 years of adjuvant hormones with external-beam radiotherapy (Grade A).
- Long-term results of a phase III trial from Sweden of 91 patients with locally advanced disease randomized to external-beam radiotherapy with or without orchiectomy were recently updated. The pelvis received a dose of 50 Gy and the prostate a mean dose of 65 Gy. At 14–19 years after enrollment, deaths from any cause (87% vs. 76%, $p=0.03$) and prostate cancer mortality (57% vs. 36%, $p=0.02$) were significantly higher for the radiotherapy only arm. The survival advantage appeared to be limited to the 39 patients with node-positive disease as detected by lymphadenectomy (Level I) (GRANFORS et al. 2006).
- Long-term results (median follow-up 66 months) of the landmark EORTC 22961 phase 3 trial of external-beam radiotherapy with or without immediate androgen suppression therapy were recently reported. Hormones were started on the first day of radiotherapy. Up to 50 Gy was given to the whole pelvis, followed by 20 Gy to the prostate and seminal vesicles. Accrued patients had T3 (82%), T4 (9%); Gleason score 7–10 (35%); PSA >20 (57%). The 5-year locoregional failure (16.4% vs. 1.7%, $p<0.0001$) and distant metastases (29.2% vs. 9.8%, $p<0.0001$) were significantly reduced with immediate hormones. The 5-year biochemical disease-free survival (76% vs. 45%, $p<0.0001$), overall survival (76% vs. 62%, $p=0.0002$), and cause-specific

survival (94% vs. 79%, $p=0.0001$) continued to be significantly better in the immediate hormones arm (Level I) (BOLLA et al. 2002).

■ RTOG 8531 randomized 977 men with clinical stage T3 and/or nodal involvement either by histological or radiographic evidence, or pT3a–b disease after radical prostatectomy, to either radiotherapy alone (with hormones at relapse) or radiotherapy with androgen suppression therapy started in the last week of radiation and continued indefinitely. Except in post-prostatectomy patients, whole pelvic radiation (44–46 Gy) was followed by prostate boost of 20–25 Gy for all other patients. Gleason score 8–10 (central review) was present in 32%, positive nodes in 28%, and post-prostatectomy in 15% of patients. Median follow-up was 5.6 years. The 8-year local failure (23% vs. 37%, $p<0.0001$), distant metastases (27% vs. 37%, $p<0.0001$), and PSA control less than 1.5 ng/ml (32% vs. 8%, $p<0.0001$) were significantly in favor of the radiotherapy with immediate hormones. Overall, there was no difference in overall survival or cause-specific survival. In subgroup analyses, a significant improvement in overall survival ($p=0.036$) and cause-specific mortality ($p=0.019$) was observed in the cohort of patients who received immediate hormones and had Gleason score 8–10 and did not undergo prostatectomy (Level I) (LAWTON et al. 2001).

■ RTOG 8610 randomized 456 men to either 2 months of neoadjuvant and concurrent androgen suppression therapy with radiotherapy or radiotherapy alone. The study included bulky primary tumors, clinical stage T2–4, and involved pelvic nodes. Pelvic nodes received 44–46 Gy, followed by a prostate boost to a total of 65–70 Gy. Positive nodes were present in 8%, clinical stage T3–4 70%, and Gleason score 8–10 in 28% of patients. Median follow-up was 6.7 years. The 8-year local failure (30% vs. 42%, $p=0.016$), distant metastases (34% vs. 45%, $p=0.04$), PSA control less than 1.5 ng/ml (16% vs. 3%, $p<0.0001$), and cause-specific mortality (23% vs. 31%, $p=0.05$) were significantly improved in the arm that received hormones and radiotherapy. Subset analyses found that the benefit of hormones was primarily in patients with centrally reviewed Gleason score 2–6 for all endpoints including overall survival (70% vs. 52%, $p=0.015$), but not in patients with centrally reviewed Gleason score 8–10 (Level I) (PILEPICH et al. 2001).

■ RTOG 9202 randomized 1,554 men with clinical stage T2c–4 disease and treated with 2 months of neoadjuvant and concurrent hormones with radiotherapy to either no adjuvant hormones or 24 months of adjuvant hormones. The whole-pelvis received 44–50 Gy, and the prostate received 65–70 Gy. The median follow-up was 5.8 years. Patient characteristics were: clinical stage T2c (45%), T3 (51%), T4 (4%); median PSA 19.9–20.8 ng/ml; Gleason score 7 (34%), 8–10 (26%). The 5-year disease-free survival (28.1% vs. 46.4%, $p<0.0001$), distant metastases (17.0% vs. 11.5%, $p=0.0035$), local progression (12.3% vs. 6.4%, $p=0.0001$), and cause-specific survival (91.2% vs. 94.6%, $p=0.006$) were significantly in favor of the arm that received adjuvant hormones. No difference in overall survival was found ($p=0.7$). In subset analyses, all endpoints, including overall survival, were significantly improved in the adjuvant hormones arm for patients who had a Gleason score of 8–10 (Level I) (HANKS et al. 2003).

■ The Canadian phase III trial randomized 378 men with T1c–4, any PSA, and any Gleason score to either 3 or 8 months of neoadjuvant androgen suppression therapy prior to radiotherapy (66–67 Gy to the prostate). Patients with an estimated nodal involvement of >10–15% received whole-pelvic radiotherapy (45–46 Gy). Median follow-up was 44 months. Patient characteristics included: clinical stage T1c–2a (53%), T2b–2c (34%), and T3–4 (13%); Gleason score 7 (38%) and 8–10 (11%); low- (25%), intermediate- (43%), and high-risk (31%); median PSA 8.9–10.1 ng/ml. There was no significant difference between the two arms in terms of freedom from biochemical failure ($p=0.36$), local failure, or distant failure. Of patients who had a prostate biopsy done 2 years after treatment, there was no difference in the distribution of results ($p=0.34$) (Level I) (CROOK et al. 2004).

■ In a randomized study from Quebec, 481 patients with clinical stage T2–3 disease were enrolled in one of two successive studies. The first study (L-101) randomized patients to external-beam radiotherapy alone, 3 months of neoadjuvant hormones and radiotherapy, or neoadjuvant, concomitant, and adjuvant hormones for a total of 10 months with radiotherapy. The second study (L-200) randomized patients to neoadjuvant and concurrent hormones for a total of 5 months with radiotherapy, and neoadjuvant, concomitant and adjuvant hormones for a total of 10 months with radiotherapy. The total prostate dose was 64 Gy, and the pelvic nodes were not treated. In L-101, ~30% had T3 disease, median PSA was 9.2–12, and 20–29% had Gleason score 7–10. The 7-year PSA relapse-free survival was 42%, 66% (p=0.009) and 69% (p=0.003), respectively. In L-200, 12–15% had T3 disease, 26–30% had Gleason score 7–10, and the median PSA was 11.9–12.7. The 4-year PSA control was 70% in both arms (Level I) (LAVERDIERE et al. 2004).

■ RTOG 9413 was a phase 3, four-armed study with a 2×2 randomization schema. A total of 1,292 men with an estimated pelvic node involvement of >15% or cT2c–4 and Gleason score ≥6 were randomized to either four months of neoadjuvant and concurrent (NCHT) or 4 months of adjuvant (AHT) androgen suppression therapy, and whole-pelvic radiotherapy (WPRT) or prostate-only radiotherapy (PORT). Please see the "Prophylactic Pelvic Nodal Radiotherapy" section (Level I) (ROACH et al. 2003).

20.2.5 Radical Prostatectomy

■ When technically feasible, nerve-sparing radical prostatectomy should be done to improve potency preservation (Grade A). The nerves are located in the posterolateral aspect of the prostate gland and innervate the corpora cavernosa. Potency preservation can be as high as 70%. Two other techniques gaining acceptance is the laparoscopic approach and robotics microsurgery. Both reduce blood loss, postoperative pain, and a quicker return to regular activities. The extent of lymph node dissection is controversial. These can be broadly divided into three categories based on extent: minimal (obturator fossa), limited (external iliac and obturator fossa), and extended (internal and external iliac and obturator). The decision for which one to perform is based on estimation of lymph node involvement.

■ Updated long-term results of 3,478 consecutive cases (1983–2003) of retropubic radical prostatectomy from a single surgeon at Washington University showed that 10-year PSA progression-free survival, cancer-specific survival, and overall survival to be 68%, 97%, and 83%, respectively (Level IV) (ROEHL et al. 2004).

■ In a large series of 2,404 retropubic radical prostatectomy cases (1982–1999) from Johns Hopkins,

10-year recurrence-free survival, cancer-specific survival was 74% and 96%, respectively (Level IV) (HAN et al. 2001).

■ From MSKCC, 10-year progression-free survival and cancer-specific survival after retropubic radical prostatectomy (1,000 cases from 1983–1998) were 75% and 98%, respectively (Level IV) (HULL et al. 2002).

Adjuvant and Salvage Therapy

20.3.1 Adjuvant Radiation Therapy

■ Supported by three phase III trials detailed below, postoperative radiotherapy to the prostate bed is indicated for extracapsular extension, positive surgical margins, or seminal vesicle invasion (Grade A). The benefit of postoperative radiotherapy is the relative reduction of PSA relapse by roughly 50%. Longer follow-up is needed to see whether a survival advantage is present. The risk of late toxicities is more with adjuvant radiotherapy, but nonetheless is small.

■ The SWOG study randomized 425 men with any of positive surgical margins, extracapsular extension, or seminal vesicle invasion to immediate radiotherapy (60–64 Gy) or observation. Radiotherapy was directed to the prostatic bed, and no adjuvant hormonal therapy was given. Immediate radiotherapy led to fewer metastases (35.1% vs. 43.1%, HR =0.75, p=0.06) and PSA relapse-free survival (HR 0.43, p<0.001). This came at a cost of increased urethral strictures (17.8% vs. 9.5%), total urinary incontinence (6.5% vs. 2.8%), and rectal complications (3.3% vs. 0%). Adjuvant radiotherapy reduced local failures from 22% to 8% and 16% to 7% (SWOG, Level I) (THOMPSON et al. 2006; SWANSON et al. 2007).

■ In the largest phase III trial of adjuvant radiotherapy, 1,005 men with pT3a-b and/or positive surgical margins were randomized to adjuvant radiotherapy or expectant management. Adjuvant radiotherapy (60 Gy in 30 fractions) was given within 90 days after surgery. In the expectant management arm, locoregional failure was four times greater than distant failure (73 vs. 18), whereas in the adjuvant radiotherapy arm, locoregional and distant failures were similar (23 vs. 19, respectively). The 5-year PSA progression-free survival improved from 52.6% to 74.0% (p<0.0001) with adjuvant radiotherapy. The 5-year locoregional failure rates also decreased significantly with adjuvant radiotherapy (15.4% vs. 5.4%, p<0.0001). At 5 years, severe late toxicities were more common with adjuvant radiotherapy (2.6% vs. 4.2%, p=0.07) (EORTC, Level I) (BOLLA et al. 2005).

■ Secondary analysis of the EORTC study showed that margin status was the strongest predictor of biochemical disease-free survival with immediate radiotherapy. With positive margins, the hazard ratio for immediate radiotherapy was 0.38 (95% CI 0.26–0.54), whereas with negative margins, it was 0.88 (95% CI 0.53–1.46) (EORTC, Level I) (VAN DER KWAST et al. 2007).

■ A third randomized study that has been presented in abstract form only included 385 patients with pT3 or positive surgical margins to adjuvant radiotherapy (60 Gy in 30 fractions) or observation. When analyzed by treatment received, 4-year progression-free survival was 81% and 61% in favor of adjuvant radiotherapy (p<0.0001). In patients who achieved an undetectable post-surgery PSA, adjuvant radiotherapy significantly improved progression-free survival (p<0.0001). Adjuvant radiotherapy was well tolerated; the acute grade 3 bladder toxicity rate was 3%, and no acute grade rectal toxicities were observed. Late grade 3 bladder and rectal toxicities were 2% and 0%, respectively (Level I) (WIEGEL et al. 2005).

■ Outcomes from a multi-institutional cohort of 1,540 patients who received salvage radiotherapy were compiled to create a nomogram in predicting disease progression after salvage radiotherapy. Neoadjuvant and/or concurrent androgen suppression therapy was given to 14% of patients for a median of 4.1 months. Median follow-up after completing salvage radiotherapy was 53 months. The overall 6-year progression-free survival was 32%. Pre-radiotherapy PSA was a significant predictor of progression-free survival, with 48% at 6 years for PSA ≤0.5 ng/ml and 18–40% for PSA >0.5 ng/ml. In the nomogram, statistically significant variables included pre-radiotherapy PSA, prostatectomy Gleason grade, PSA doubling time, surgical margins, neoadjuvant/concurrent hormones, and lymph node metastases (Level III) (STEPHENSON et al. 2007).

20.3.2 Salvage Radiation Therapy

■ While there are no phase III trials in guiding eligibility, salvage radiotherapy is indicated if the estimated risk of persistent local disease is sufficiently high, and the risk of distant metastases low (Grade B). The absence of adequate diagnostic tools to detect disease at such low PSA levels precludes any certainty in the site of failure. Predictors favoring local disease include: positive surgical margin, disease-free interval as measured by an undetectable PSA of >1 year, Gleason score <8, postoperative PSA doubling time >10 months, and pre-radiotherapy PSA <1 ng/ml (HAYES et al. 2005).

■ Work-up investigations may include a bone scan, CT scan of the abdomen and pelvis, prostate bed biopsy, and/or a ProstaScint scan. These will largely depend on what the current PSA level is.

20.3.3 Treatment Technique

Simulation

■ CT simulation is performed in the supine position with arms on the chest. Scan slice thickness should be 3 mm or less. The bladder should be comfortably full to displace the bowel away from the prostate. The rectum should be empty, which can be achieved with a bowel preparation or a modification of diet. To identify the pelvic floor and thus the prostatic fossa above, an urethrogram is suggested.

■ Immobilization using alpha cradles, knee sponge, and ankle rests may be considered.

■ Implantation of fiducial markers into the prostatic fossa may be considered to reduce setup error. The positional errors were measured in ten consecutive patients treated at the University of California, San Francisco, and the study found that the mean (± standard deviation) prostate bed motion was 0.3±0.9 mm, 0.4±2.4 mm, and -1.1±2.1 mm in the left-right (LR), superior-inferior (SI), and anterior-posterior (AP) axes, respectively. Mean total positioning error was 0.2±4.5 mm, 1.2±5.1 mm, and -0.3±4.5 mm in the LR, SI, and AP axes, respectively. Total positioning errors >5 mm occurred in 14.1%, 38.7%, and 28.2% of all fractions in the LR, SI, and AP axes, respectively (Level III) (SCHIFFNER et al. 2007).

Beam Energy and Dose Calculation

- A minimum of 10-MV photon beams should be used.

Field Arrangement

- For both 3DCRT and IMRT, a five to seven beam iso-centric technique is used to minimize radiation to nearby critical organs, such as the rectum, bladder, penile bulb, and femoral heads.
- At the ASCO 2008 GU Symposium, MICHALSKI et al. presented the RTOG consensus guidelines on prostatic fossa CTV for post-prostatectomy patients. Inferiorly, the CTV should extend 8–12 mm below the vesicourethral anastomosis. Superiorly, the CTV should extend to the level of the caudal vas deferens remnant. Above the pubic symphysis, the anterior border should include the posterior 1–2 cm of the bladder wall, the posterior border at the mesorectal fascia, and the lateral border at the sacrorectogenitopubic fascia. Below the superior aspect of the pubic symphysis, the anterior border is placed at the posterior aspect of the pubis, the posterior border to the anterior aspect of the rectum, and lateral border at the levator ani. The seminal vesicle remnant may be included if involved. These will be published on the RTOG website.
- The PTV margin should account for inter- and intra-fraction organ motion and setup variation, which will vary between centers depending on the use of any image-guidance technique.

Whole-pelvic Treatment

- The same treatment volume as used in definitive external-beam radiotherapy is recommended (see Sect. 20.2.3). 3DCRT or IMRT may be used.
- In a retrospective study of a cohort of 114 patients considered to have high risk of nodal involvement (Gleason score 8–10, PSA >20 ng/ml, pT3a–b disease, and pathologic nodal involvement) and receiving either adjuvant or salvage whole-pelvic or prostate-only radiotherapy, 5-year PSA relapse-free survival was significantly better in the subgroup that received whole-pelvic radiotherapy (47% vs. 21%; p=0.008). The addition of total androgen suppression therapy was only beneficial in the subgroup that received WPRT (Level IV) (SPIOTTO et al. 2007).
- At the ASCO 2008 GU Symposium, LAWTON et al. presented the RTOG consensus guidelines on CTV nodal delineation for high-risk patients (Grade D). Although these guidelines were developed for patients receiving definitive external-beam radiotherapy, it is probably reasonable to apply them to the post-operation setting. These will be published on the RTOG website.

Dose and Fractionation

- For adjuvant radiotherapy, the recommended dose is 64–66 Gy to the prostate bed. Whole-pelvic radiotherapy (45–50 Gy) and androgen suppression therapy may be considered for patients with high-risk features, such as Gleason score 8–10, PSA >20 ng/ml, pT3a-b disease, and pathologic nodal involvement. For salvage radiotherapy, the recommended dose is 68–70 Gy to the prostate bed. Whole-pelvic radiotherapy (45–50 Gy) and androgen suppression therapy may be considered for patients with high-risk features, such as Gleason score 8–10, PSA >20 ng/ml, pT3a-b disease, and pathologic nodal involvement (Grade B).
- A retrospective study of 122 pathologic node-negative patients who received salvage radiotherapy was performed to see whether a dose-response exists. The median prostate bed dose was 67.8 Gy in the overall cohort; 31% and 69% of patients received a median of 60 Gy (range 60–64 Gy) and 70 Gy (range 67.8–70 Gy). Whole-pelvic radiotherapy (50 Gy) was to 59% of patients, and 4 months of neoadjuvant and concurrent androgen suppression therapy was given to 56% of patients. Pre-radiotherapy PSA was ≤1.0 ng/ml in 63% and >1.0 ng/ml in 37%. Median follow-up was >5 years. The median time to PSA failure after salvage radiotherapy was 1.2 years. The 5-year PSA relapse-free survival was 25% and 58% for the 60 Gy and 70 Gy groups (p<0.0001). Among patients who did not receive hormones, the 5-year PSA relapse-free survival was significantly improved in the 70 Gy group (17% vs. 55%, p=0.016). Multivariate analyses found that a prostate bed dose of 70 Gy, pre-radiotherapy PSA ≤1.0 ng/ml, and lack of seminal vesicle invasion were independent predictors of PSA relapse-free survival (KING et al. 2008).

Androgen Suppression Therapy

- In the retrospective study of patients with high risk of nodal involvement (Gleason score 8–10, PSA >20 ng/ml, pT3a–b disease, and pathologic nodal involvement) and receiving either adjuvant or salvage whole-pelvic or prostate-only radiotherapy, the addition of total androgen suppression therapy was only beneficial in the subgroup that received WPRT ($p=0.04$) (Level IV) (SPIOTTO et al. 2007).

■ Limited to postoperative patients receiving adjuvant radiotherapy, a secondary subset analysis of RTOG 8531 showed that adding hormones improved 5-year PSA progression-free survival (65% vs. 42%, $p=0.002$) (Level I) (CORN et al. 1999).

■ RTOG 9601 is a phase III, randomized controlled trial comparing radiotherapy to the prostate bed (64.8 Gy in 36 fractions) with 2 years of bicalutamide 150 mg daily or with placebo for patients with pT3N0 or positive margins after radical prostatectomy. The results of this trial are pending.

20.4 Side Effects and Complications

■ For external-beam radiotherapy, the acute toxicities include hematuria, dysuria, irritative urinary symptoms, diarrhea, and proctitis. Potential late toxicities include increased frequency of bowel movements, change in stool caliber, urinary incontinence, rectal ulceration and bleeding, erectile dysfunction, and proctitis. Rectal toxicities may be reduced with IMRT.

■ In the acute phase, the toxicities of LDR brachytherapy include perineal and rectal bleeding, perineal pain, perineal edema, hematuria, dysuria, irritative and obstructive urinary symptoms, and passing of the implanted radioactive seeds. Potential late toxicities include seed migration (usually to the lungs), urinary retention, hematuria, urinary incontinence, rectal ulceration and bleeding, erectile dysfunction, and dysuria.

20.5 Follow-Up

■ After definitive treatment, the NCCN guidelines recommend a PSA every 6–12 months for 5 years,

then yearly thereafter. A DRE is recommended annually (Grade D) (NCCN v1.2008).

■ The recommendations of the RTOG-ASTRO Phoenix Consensus Conference (the "Phoenix definition") stated that *after* radiotherapy, a PSA rise of 2 ng/ml or more above the PSA nadir is considered a biochemical recurrence (Grade D) (ROACH et al. 2006).

■ After a radical prostatectomy, the PSA should be less than 0.2 ng/ml. Persistent elevations suggest residual disease, either local or distant. A recurrence is suggested if the PSA rises on two subsequent measurements.

References

Allaf ME, Palapattu GS, Trock BJ et al. (2004) Anatomical extent of lymph node dissection: impact on men with clinically localized prostate cancer. J Urol 172:1840–1844

Allsbrook WC Jr, Mangold KA, Johnson MH et al. (2001) Interobserver reproducibility of Gleason grading of prostatic carcinoma: urologic pathologists. Hum Pathol 32:74–80

Arcangeli CG, Humphrey PA, Smith DS et al. (1998) Percentage of free serum prostate-specific antigen as a predictor of pathologic features of prostate cancer in a screening population. Urology 51:558–564

Bill-Axelson A, Holmberg L, Ruutu M et al. (2005) Radical prostatectomy versus watchful waiting in early prostate cancer. N Engl J Med 352:1977–1984

Bolla M, Collette L, Blank L et al. (2002) Long-term results with immediate androgen suppression and external irradiation in patients with locally advanced prostate cancer (an EORTC study): a phase III randomised trial. Lancet 360:103–106

Bolla M, van Poppel H, Collette L et al. (2005) Postoperative radiotherapy after radical prostatectomy: a randomised controlled trial (EORTC trial 22911). Lancet 366(9485):572–578

Beyer DC, Thomas T, Hilbe J et al. (2003) Relative influence of Gleason score and pretreatment PSA in predicting survival following brachytherapy for prostate cancer. Brachytherapy 2:77–84

Brenner DJ, Hall EJ (1999) Fractionation and protraction for radiotherapy of prostate carcinoma. Int J Radiat Oncol Biol Phys 43:1095–1101

Brenner DJ, Martinez AA, Edmundson GK et al. (2002) Direct evidence that prostate tumors show high sensitivity to fractionation (low alpha/beta ratio), similar to late-responding normal tissue. Int J Radiat Oncol Biol Phys 52:6–13

Carroll P, Coley C, McLeod D et al. (2001) Prostate-specific antigen best practice policy–part II: prostate cancer staging and post-treatment follow-up. Urology 57:225–229

Corn BW, Winter K, Pilepich MV (1999) Does androgen suppression enhance the efficacy of postoperative irradiation? A secondary analysis of RTOG 85-31. Radiation Therapy Oncology Group. Urology 54:495–502

Crook J, Milosevic M, Catton P et al. (2002) Interobserver variation in postimplant computed tomography contouring affects quality assessment of prostate brachytherapy. Brachytherapy 1:66–73

Crook J, Ludgate C, Malone S et al. (2004) Report of a multicenter Canadian phase III randomized trial of 3 months vs 8 months neoadjuvant androgen deprivation before standard-dose radiotherapy for clinically localized prostate cancer. Int J Radiat Oncol Biol Phys 60:15–23

Crook JM, Potters L, Stock RG et al. (2005) Critical organ dosimetry in permanent seed prostate brachytherapy: defining the organs at risk. Brachytherapy 4:186–194

D'Amico AV, Whittington R, Malkowicz SB et al. (1998) Biochemical outcome after radical prostatectomy, external beam radiation therapy, or interstitial radiation therapy for clinically localized prostate cancer. JAMA 280:969–974

D'Amico AV, Whittington R, Malkowicz SB et al. (1999) Pretreatment nomogram for prostate-specific antigen recurrence after radical prostatectomy or external-beam radiation therapy for clinically localized prostate cancer. J Clin Oncol 17:168–172

D'Amico AV, Cote K, Loffredo M et al. (2002) Determinants of prostate cancer-specific survival after radiation therapy for patients with clinically localized prostate cancer. J Clin Oncol 20:4567–4573

D'Amico AV, Keshaviah A, Manola J et al. (2002) Clinical utility of the percentage of positive prostate biopsies in predicting prostate cancer-specific and overall survival after radiotherapy for patients with localized prostate cancer. Int J Radiat Oncol Biol Phys 53:581–587

D'Amico AV, Chen MH, Roehl KA et al. (2004) Preoperative PSA velocity and the risk of death from prostate cancer after radical prostatectomy. N Engl J Med 351(2):125–135

D'Amico AV, Manola J, Loffredo M et al. (2004) Six-month androgen suppression plus radiation therapy vs radiation therapy alone for patients with clinically localized prostate cancer: a randomized controlled trial. JAMA 292:821–827

D'Amico AV, Chen MH, Renshaw AA et al. (2008) Androgen suppression and radiation vs radiation alone for prostate cancer: a randomized trial. JAMA 299:289–295

Dearnaley DP, Sydes MR, Graham JD et al. (2007) Escalated-dose versus standard-dose conformal radiotherapy in prostate cancer: first results from the MRC RT01 randomised controlled trial. Lancet Oncol 8:475–487

Demanes DJ, Rodriguez RR, Schour L et al. (2005) High-dose-rate intensity-modulated brachytherapy with external beam radiotherapy for prostate cancer: California endocurietherapy's 10-year results. Int J Radiat Oncol Biol Phys 61:1306–1316

Denham JW, Steigler A, Lamb DS et al. (2005) Short-term androgen deprivation and radiotherapy for locally advanced prostate cancer: results from the Trans-Tasman Radiation Oncology Group 96.01 randomised controlled trial. Lancet Oncol 6:841–850

Fowler J, Chappell R, Ritter M. (2001) Is alpha/beta for prostate tumors really low? Int J Radiat Oncol Biol Phys 50:1021–1031

Granfors t, Modig H, Damber JE et al. (2006) Long-term follow-up of a randomized study of locally advanced prostate cancer treated with combined orchiectomy and external radiotherapy versus radiotherapy alone. J Urol 176:544–547

Grimm PD, Blasko JC, Sylvester JE et al. (2001) 10-year biochemical (prostate-specific antigen) control of prostate cancer with (125)I brachytherapy. Int J Radiat Oncol Biol Phys 51:31–40

Han M, Partin AW, Pound CR et al. (2001) Long-term biochemical disease-free and cancer-specific survival following anatomic radical retropubic prostatectomy. The 15-year Johns Hopkins experience. Urol Clin North Am 28:555–565

Hanks GE, Hanlon AL, Epstein B et al. (2002) Dose response in prostate cancer with 8–12 years' follow-up. Int J Radiat Oncol Biol Phys 54:427–435

Hanks GE, Pajak TF, Porter A et al. (2003) Phase III trial of long-term adjuvant androgen deprivation after neoadjuvant hormonal cytoreduction and radiotherapy in locally advanced carcinoma of the prostate: the Radiation Therapy Oncology Group Protocol 92-02. J Clin Oncol 21:3972–3978

Hull GW, Rabbani F, Abbas F et al. (2002) Cancer control with radical prostatectomy alone in 1,000 consecutive patients. J Urol 167:528–534

Hayes SB, Pollack A (2005) Parameters for treatment decisions for salvage radiation therapy. J Clin Oncol 23:8204–8211

Holmberg L, Bill-Axelson A, Helgesen F et al. (2002) A randomized trial comparing radical prostatectomy with watchful waiting in early prostate cancer. N Engl J Med 347:781–789

Hsu IC, Cabrera AR, Weinberg V et al. (2005) Combined modality treatment with high-dose-rate brachytherapy boost for locally advanced prostate cancer. Brachytherapy. 4:202–206

Jemal A, Siegel R, Ward E, Murray T, Xu J, Thun MJ (2007) Cancer statistics, 2007. CA Cancer J Clin 57:43–66

Kattan MW, Zelefsky MJ, Kupelian PA et al. (2000) Pretreatment nomogram for predicting the outcome of three-dimensional conformal radiotherapy in prostate cancer. J Clin Oncol 18:3352–3359

Kattan MW, Potters L, Blasko JC et al. (2001) Pretreatment nomogram for predicting freedom from recurrence after permanent prostate brachytherapy in prostate cancer. Urology 58:393–399

Kattan MW, Zelefsky MJ, Kupelian PA et al. (2003) Pretreatment nomogram that predicts 5-year probability of metastasis following three-dimensional conformal radiation therapy for localized prostate cancer. J Clin Oncol 21:4568–4571

King CR, Fowler JF (2001) A simple analytic derivation suggests that prostate cancer alpha/beta ratio is low. Int J Radiat Oncol Biol Phys 51:213–214

King CR, Spiotto MT (2008) Improved outcomes with higher doses for salvage radiotherapy after prostatectomy. Int J Radiat Oncol Biol Phys 71:23–27

Klotz L (2004) Active surveillance with selective delayed intervention: using natural history to guide treatment in good risk prostate cancer. J Urol 172:S48–50

Kuban DA, Tucker SL, Dong L et al. (2008) Long-term results of the M. D. Anderson randomized dose-escalation trial for prostate cancer. Int J Radiat Oncol Biol Phys 70:67–74

Kupelian P, Kuban D, Thames H et al. (2005) Improved biochemical relapse-free survival with increased external radiation doses in patients with localized prostate cancer: the combined experience of nine institutions in patients treated in 1994 and 1995. Int J Radiat Oncol Biol Phys 61:415–419

Kupelian PA, Potters L, Khuntia D et al. (2004) Radical prostatectomy, external beam radiotherapy <72 Gy, external beam radiotherapy ≥72 Gy, permanent seed implantation, or combined seeds/external beam radiotherapy for stage T1–T2 prostate cancer. Int J Radiat Oncol Biol Phys 58:25–33

Kupelian PA, Willoughby TR, Reddy CA et al. (2007) Hypofractionated intensity-modulated radiotherapy (70 Gy at 2.5 Gy per fraction) for localized prostate cancer: Cleveland Clinic experience. Int J Radiat Oncol Biol Phys 68:1424–1430

Lattanzi J, McNeeley S, Pinover W et al. (1999) A comparison of daily CT localization to a daily ultrasound-based system in prostate cancer. Int J Radiat Oncol Biol Phys 43:719–725

Laverdiere J, Nabid A, De Bedoya LD et al. (2004) The efficacy and sequencing of a short course of androgen suppression on freedom from biochemical failure when administered with radiation therapy for T2–T3 prostate cancer. J Urol 171:1137–1140

Lawton CA, DeSilvio M, Roach M 3rd et al. (2007) An update of the phase III trial comparing whole pelvic to prostate only radiotherapy and neoadjuvant to adjuvant total androgen suppression: updated analysis of RTOG 94-13, with emphasis on unexpected hormone/radiation interactions. Int J Radiat Oncol Biol Phys 69:646–655

Lawton CA, Winter K, Murray K et al. (2001) Updated results of the phase III Radiation Therapy Oncology Group (RTOG) trial 85-31 evaluating the potential benefit of androgen suppression following standard radiation therapy for unfavorable prognosis carcinoma of the prostate. Int J Radiat Oncol Biol Phys 49:937–946

Madsen BL, Hsi RA, Pham HT et al. (2007) Stereotactic hypofractionated accurate radiotherapy of the prostate (SHARP), 33.5 Gy in five fractions for localized disease: first clinical trial results. Int J Radiat Oncol Biol Phys 67:1099–1105

Martin JM, Rosewall T, Bayley A et al. (2007) Phase II trial of hypofractionated image-guided intensity-modulated radiotherapy for localized prostate adenocarcinoma. Int J Radiat Oncol Biol Phys 69:1084–1089

Moseley DJ, White EA, Wiltshire KL et al. (2007) Comparison of localization performance with implanted fiducial markers and cone-beam computed tomography for online image-guided radiotherapy of the prostate. Int J Radiat Oncol Biol Phys 67:942–953

Nag S, Beyer D, Friedland J et al. (1999) American Brachytherapy Society (ABS) recommendations for transperineal permanent brachytherapy of prostate cancer. Int J Radiat Oncol Biol Phys 44:789–799

Partin AW, Mangold LA, Lamm DM et al. (2001) Contemporary update of prostate cancer staging nomograms (Partin Tables) for the new millennium. Urology 58:843–848

Peeters ST, Heemsbergen WD, Koper PC et al. (2006) Dose response in radiotherapy for localized prostate cancer: results of the Dutch multicenter randomized phase III trial comparing 68 Gy of radiotherapy with 78 Gy. J Clin Oncol 24:1990–1996

Pilepich MV, Winter K, John MJ et al. (2001) Phase III radiation therapy oncology group (RTOG) trial 86-10 of androgen deprivation adjuvant to definitive radiotherapy in locally advanced carcinoma of the prostate. Int J Radiat Oncol Biol Phys 50:1243–1252

Pollack A, Hanlon AL, Horwitz EM et al. (2004) Prostate cancer radiotherapy dose response: an update of the fox chase experience. J Urol 171:1132–1136

Pollack A, Zagars GK, Starkschall G et al. (2002) Prostate cancer radiation dose response: results of the MD Anderson phase III randomized trial. Int J Radiat Oncol Biol Phys 53:1097–1105

Pollack A, Hanlon AL, Horwitz EM et al. (2006) Dosimetry and preliminary acute toxicity in the first 100 men treated for prostate cancer on a randomized hypofractionation dose escalation trial. Int J Radiat Oncol Biol Phys 64:518–526

Pommier P, Chabaud S, Lagrange JL et al. (2007) Is there a role for pelvic irradiation in localized prostate adenocarcinoma? Preliminary results of GETUG-01. J Clin Oncol 25:5366–5373

Pouliot J, Aubin M, Langen KM et al. (2003) (Non)-migration of radiopaque markers used for on-line localization of the prostate with an electronic portal imaging device. Int J Radiat Oncol Biol Phys 56:862–866

Rajesh A, Coakley FV, Kurhanewicz J (2007) 3D MR spectroscopic imaging in the evaluation of prostate cancer. Clin Radiol 62:921–929

Rivard MJ, Butler WM, Devlin PM et al. (2007) American Brachytherapy Society recommends no change for prostate permanent implant dose prescriptions using iodine-125 or palladium-103. Brachytherapy 6:34–37

Roach M (1993) Re: The use of prostate specific antigen, clinical stage and Gleason score to predict pathological stage in men with localized prostate cancer. J Urol 150:1923–1924

Roach M, Lu J, Pilepich MV et al. (2000) Four prognostic groups predict long-term survival from prostate cancer following radiotherapy alone on Radiation Therapy Oncology Group clinical trials. Int J Radiat Oncol Biol Phys 47:609–615

Roach M, DeSilvio M, Lawton C et al. (2003) Phase III trial comparing whole-pelvic versus prostate-only radiotherapy and neoadjuvant versus adjuvant combined androgen suppression: Radiation Therapy Oncology Group 9413. J Clin Oncol 21:1904–1911

Roach M, DeSilvio M, Valicenti R et al. (2006) Whole-pelvis, "mini-pelvis," or prostate-only external beam radiotherapy after neoadjuvant and concurrent hormonal therapy in patients treated in the Radiation Therapy Oncology Group 9413 trial. Int J Radiat Oncol Biol Phys 66:647–653

Roach M 3rd, Hanks G, Thames H Jr et al. (2006) Defining biochemical failure following radiotherapy with or without hormonal therapy in men with clinically localized prostate cancer: recommendations of the RTOG-ASTRO Phoenix Consensus Conference. Int J Radiat Oncol Biol Phys 65:965–974

Roehl KA, Han M, Ramos CG et al. (2004) Cancer progression and survival rates following anatomical radical retropubic prostatectomy in 3,478 consecutive patients: long-term results. J Urol 172:910–914

Schiffner DC, Gottschalk AR, Lometti M et al. (2007) Daily electronic portal imaging of implanted gold seed fiducials in patients undergoing radiotherapy after radical prostatectomy. Int J Radiat Oncol Biol Phys 67:610–619

Shih HA, Harisinghani M, Zietman AL et al. (2005) Mapping of nodal disease in locally advanced prostate cancer: rethinking the clinical target volume for pelvic nodal irradiation based on vascular rather than bony anatomy. Int J Radiat Oncol Biol Phys 63:1262–1269

Spiotto MT, Hancock SL, King CR (2007) Radiotherapy after prostatectomy: improved biochemical relapse-free survival with whole pelvic compared with prostate bed only for high-risk patients. Int J Radiat Oncol Biol Phys 69:54–61

Stephenson AJ, Scardino PT, Kattan MW et al. (2007) Predicting the outcome of salvage radiation therapy for recurrent prostate cancer after radical prostatectomy. J Clin Oncol 25:2035–2041

Stock RG, Stone NN, Dahlal M et al. (2002) What is the optimal dose for 125I prostate implants? A dose-response analysis of biochemical control, posttreatment prostate biopsies, and long-term urinary symptoms. Brachytherapy 1:83–89

Swanson GP, Hussey MA, Tangen CM et al. (2007) Predominant treatment failure in postprostatectomy patients is local: analysis of patterns of treatment failure in SWOG 8794. J Clin Oncol 25:2225–2229

Sylvester JE, Blasko JC, Grimm PD et al. (2003) Ten-year biochemical relapse-free survival after external beam radiation and brachytherapy for localized prostate cancer: the Seattle experience. Int J Radiat Oncol Biol Phys 57:944–952

Sylvester JE, Grimm PD, Blasko JC et al. (2007) Fifteen-year biochemical relapse free survival in clinical stage T1–T3 prostate cancer following combined external beam radiotherapy and brachytherapy; Seattle experience. Int J Radiat Oncol Biol Phys 67:57–64

Thompson IM, Tangen CM, Paradelo J et al. (2006) Adjuvant radiotherapy for pathologically advanced prostate cancer: a randomized clinical trial. JAMA 296:2329–2335

Van der Kwast, Bolla M, Van Poppel H et al. (2007) Identification of patients with prostate cancer who benefit from immediate postoperative radiotherapy: EORTC 22911. J Clin Oncol 25:4178–4186

Vargas CE, Martinez AA, Boike TP et al. (2006) High-dose irradiation for prostate cancer via a high-dose-rate brachytherapy boost: results of a phase I to II study. Int J Radiat Oncol Biol Phys 66:416–423

Wiegel T, Willich N, Piechota H et al. (2005) Phase III results of adjuvant radiotherapy (RT) versus "wait and see" (WS) in patients with pT3 prostate cancer following radical prostatectomy (RP). J Clin Oncol 23 (Suppl):4513

Wang-Chesebro A, Xia P, Coleman J et al. (2006) Intensity-modulated radiotherapy improves lymph node coverage and dose to critical structures compared with three-dimensional conformal radiation therapy in clinically localized prostate cancer. Int J Radiat Oncol Biol Phys 66:654–662

Zelefsky MJ, Fuks Z, Hunt M et al. (2001) High dose radiation delivered by intensity modulated conformal radiotherapy improves the outcome of localized prostate cancer. J Urol 166:876–881

Zelefsky MJ, Chan H, Hunt M et al. (2006) Long-term outcome of high dose intensity modulated radiation therapy for patients with clinically localized prostate cancer. J Urology 176:1415–1419

Zelefsky MJ, Kuban DA, Levy LB et al. (2007) Multi-institutional analysis of long-term outcome for stages T1–T2 prostate cancer treated with permanent seed implantation. Int J Radiat Oncol Biol Phys 67:327–333

Zelefsky MJ, Yamada Y, Cohen GN et al. (2007) Five-year outcome of intraoperative conformal permanent I-125 interstitial implantation for patients with clinically localized prostate cancer. Int J Radiat Oncol Biol Phys 67:65–70

Zhang JQ, Loughlin KR, Zou KH et al. (2007) Role of endorectal coil magnetic resonance imaging in treatment of patients with prostate cancer and in determining radical prostatectomy surgical margin status: report of a single surgeon's practice. Urology 69:1134–1137

Zietman AL, DeSilvio ML, Slater JD et al. (2005) Comparison of conventional-dose vs high-dose conformal radiation therapy in clinically localized adenocarcinoma of the prostate: a randomized controlled trial. JAMA 294:1233–1239

Testicular Cancer

21

Bin S. Teh, Arnold C. Paulino, and E. Brian Butler

CONTENTS

Introduction and Objectives

Radiotherapy plays an important role in the management of early-stage seminoma. Other options for adjuvant treatment after radical orchiectomy for stage I seminoma are surveillance and chemotherapy. The radiotherapy field is also evolving from an infra-diaphragmatic (dogleg) approach encompassing paraaortic and ipsilateral pelvic lymphatics to a paraaortic lymphatics-alone approach.

This chapter examines:

● Recommendations for diagnosis and staging procedures

● Staging system and prognostic factors

● Treatment recommendations for stage I, II and III seminoma as well as the supporting scientific evidence

● Radiotherapy guidelines for stage I and II seminoma

● Follow-up recommendations

As radiation therapy has a limited role in their treatment of non-seminoma except for palliation, the management is not detailed in this chapter.

21.1 Diagnosis, Staging, and Prognosis

21.1.1 Diagnosis

Initial Evaluation

■ Diagnosis and evaluation of testicular cancer start with a complete patient history and physical examination. Attention should be paid to history of cryptorchidism, prior history of testicular malignancy, gonadal dysgenesis, and family history of testicular malignancy.

■ The most common clinical presentation is a painless testicular mass. However, associated pain,

B. S. Teh, MD
A. C. Paulino, MD
E. B. Butler, MD
Department of Radia tion Oncology, The Methodist Hospital, Cornell University/Weill Medical College, 6565 Fannin Street, DB1-077, Houston, TX 77030, USA

discomfort, and swelling suggesting orchitis or epididymitis can be seen in up to 45% of patients.

- Other presentations include infertility, gynecomastia, signs and symptoms of metastatic lymph node disease, including a mass from supraclavicular lymphadenopathy, respiratory problems from mediastinal lymphadenopathy, gastrointestinal/back pain from retroperitoneal lymphadenopathy, and others.

Laboratory Tests

- Initial laboratory tests should include a complete blood count, basic blood chemistry, liver function tests, renal function tests, serum tumor markers, including α-fetoprotein (AFP), β-human chorionic gonadotropin (hCG), and lactate dehydrogenase (LDH).
- These serum markers are important to diagnose, prognosticate, and evaluate treatment response and outcome. They should be assessed before, during, and after treatment.
- AFP (half-life of 5–7 days), produced by nonseminomatous cells, is not elevated in pure seminoma.
- β-hCG (half-life of 1–3 days) and LDH may be elevated in both seminoma and nonseminoma.

Imaging Studies

- Testicular ultrasound, although optional, is performed in most cases for evaluation of both testicles.
- Chest X-ray and CT scans of the abdomen and pelvis are performed. CT scan of the chest is recommended if CXR is abnormal or abdomino-pelvic CT shows retroperitoneal lymphadenopathy.

Table 21.1. Imaging and laboratory workups for diagnosis and evaluation of seminoma

Imaging studies	Laboratory tests
– CT of abdomen and pelvis – Testicular ultrasound – Chest X-ray or CT of the thorax	– Complete blood count – Serum chemistry – Liver and renal function tests – Lactate dehydrogenase (LDH) – Tumor markers including AFP and β-hCG

Pathology

- In total, 95% of testicular malignancies are comprised of germ cell tumors (GCT). GCT is the most common solid tumor in men aged 15–35.
- GCT is further classified as seminoma (40%) and nonseminoma (60%).
- The subtypes of seminoma are classic or typical, anaplastic and spermatocytic.
- Nonseminomas include embryonal cell carcinoma, teratoma, choriocarcinoma, yolk sac tumor, and mixed GCT.
- Non GCT includes stromal tumors (Sertoli's cell, Leydig's cell, etc.), lymphoma, sarcoma, and melanoma.

21.1.2 Staging

- Pure seminomas tend to remain localized or involve only lymph nodes, while nonseminomas are more likely to have hematogenous spread.
- A total of 85% of patients with pure seminoma present with localized disease. The disease usually spreads in an orderly pattern to retroperitoneal lymph nodes (Stage II), then proximally to mediastinal and supra-clavicular lymph nodes (Stage IIIA). Lung (Stage IIIA) and non-pulmonary (bone, liver and brain) (Stage IIIC) involvement is rare and usually late in the disease progression.
- The AJCC (2002) TNM staging system (Table 21.2), incorporating anatomic and non-anatomic (serum markers) prognostic factors, is the recommended staging system (Greene 2002). Nodal staging (N1-N3) is based on the size of regional lymph nodes, i.e., <2 cm, 2–5 cm, and >5 cm, classified as N1, N2, and N3 or stage grouping IIA, IIB, and IIC, respectively. S0 signifies normal serum markers, and S1-S3 is classified based on the levels of LDH, beta-hCG, and AFP. Metastatic disease is divided into M1a (involvement of non-regional nodes or lung) and M1b (non-pulmonary metastases).
- The modified Royal Marsden Hospital staging system (Table 21.3) was another staging system adopted at a consensus conference on testicular cancer held in England in 1989.
- The International Germ Cell Cancer Collaborative Group Consensus Classification has been incorporated into the AJCC system. Patients with seminomas and nonseminomas were divided into either two (good or intermediate) or three (good, intermediate or poor) prognostic groups, respectively (International Germ Cell Consensus 1997).

Table 21.2. American Joint Committee on Cancer (AJCC) TNM classification of carcinoma cancer of testis. [From GREENE et al. (2002) with permission]

Primary tumor (T)	
pTX	Primary tumor cannot be assessed
pT0	No evidence of primary tumor (e.g., histologic scar in testis)
pTis	Intratubular germ cell neoplasia (carcinoma in situ)
pT1	Tumor limited to the testis and epididymis without vascular/lymphatic invasion; tumor may invade into the tunica albuginea, but not the tunica vaginalis
pT2	Tumor limited to the testis and epididymis with vascular/lymphatic invasion, or tumor extending through the tunica albuginea with involvement of the tunica vaginalis
pT3	Tumor invades the spermatic cord with or without vascular/lymphatic invasion
pT4	Tumor invades the scrotum with or without vascular/lymphatic invasion

Regional lymph nodes (N)	
Clinical	
NX	Regional lymph nodes cannot be assessed
N0	No regional lymph node metastasis
N1	Metastasis with a lymph node mass 2 cm or less in greatest dimension; or multiple lymph nodes, none more than 2 cm in greatest dimension
N2	Metastasis with a lymph node mass more than 2 cm, but not more than 5 cm in greatest dimension; or multiple lymph nodes, any one mass greater than 2 cm but not more than 5 cm in greatest dimension
N3	Metastasis with a lymph node mass more than 5 cm in greatest dimension
Pathological	
pNX	Regional lymph nodes cannot be assessed
pN0	No regional lymph node metastasis
pN1	Metastasis with a lymph node mass 2 cm or less in greatest dimension and less than or equal to 5 nodes positive, none more than 2 cm in greatest dimension
pN2	Metastasis with a lymph node mass more than 2 cm, but not more than 5 cm in greatest dimension; or more than 5 nodes positive, none more than 5 cm; or evidence of extranodal extension of tumor
pN3	Metastasis with a lymph node mass more than 5 cm in greatest dimension

Distant metastasis (M)	
MX	Distant metastasis cannot be assessed
M0	No distant metastasis
M1	Distant metastasis
M1a	Non-regional nodal or pulmonary metastasis
M1b	Distant metastasis other than to non-regional lymph nodes and lungs

Serum tumor markers (S)	
SX	Marker studies not available or not performed
S0	Marker study levels within normal limits
S1	LDH $< 1.5 \times N^a$ and hCG (mIu/ml) <5,000 and AFP (ng/ml) <1,000
S2	LDH 1.5-10 $\times$ N or hCG (mIu/ml) <5,000–50,000 or AFP (ng/ml) 1,000–10,000
S3	LDH >10 $\times$ N or hCG (mIu/ml) >50,000 or AFP (ng/ml) >10,000

STAGE GROUPING	
0:	pTis N0 M0 S0
I:	pT1-4 N0 M0 SX
IA:	pT1 N0 M0 S0
IB:	pT2 N0 M0 S0, pT3 N0 M0 S0, pT4 N0 M0 S0
IS:	Any pT/Tx N0 M0 S1-3
IIA:	Any pT/Tx N1 M0 S0, Any pT/Tx N1 M0 S1
IIB:	Any pT/Tx N2 M0 S0, Any pT/Tx N2 M0 S1
IIC:	Any pT/Tx N3 M0 S0, Any pT/Tx N3 M0 S1
III:	Any pT/Tx Any N M1 SX
IIIA:	Any pT/Tx Any N M1a S0, Any pT/Tx Any N M1a S1
IIIB:	Any pT/Tx N1-3 M0 S2, Any pT/Tx Any N M1a S2
IIIC:	Any pT/Tx N1-3 M0 S3, Any pT/Tx Any N M1a S3, Any pT/Tx Any N M1b Any S

^{a}N indicates the upper limit of normal for LDH assay.

Table 21.3. Modified Royal Marsden Hospital staging system

Stage I	No clinical evidence of metastases beyond the testicle
Stage II	Infra-diaphragmatic lymph node metastases IIA Maximum diameter <2 cm IIB Maximum diameter >2 but <5 cm IIC Maximum diameter >5 but <10 cm IID Maximum diameter >10 cm
Stage III	Supra-diaphragmatic nodal involvement
Stage IV	Parenchymal metastatic disease

21.1.3 Prognosis

- In general, patients with pure seminoma have a better prognosis than those with nonseminoma. Specifically, the prognosis is associated with TNMS (tumor, nodal, metastasis, and serum tumor markers) stage.
- Tumor size and rete testes invasion have been shown to be important for predicting relapse risk. Results from a retrospective series of 638 patients showed that tumor size of ≤4 cm or >4 cm is an important predictor for recurrence (hazard ratio [HR] 2.0, 95% [CI] 1.3–3.2], as was the invasion of the rete testis (hazard ratio [HR] 1.7, 95% [CI] 1.1–2.6) (Level IV) (WARDE et al. 2002). Vascular invasion may be an important prognostic factor for nonseminoma, but its significance was not demonstrated on multivariate analysis.
- Retroperitoneal nodal size has been shown to be associated with the risk of recurrence.

21.2 Treatment of Seminoma

21.2.1 General Principles and Treatment Options

- Radical orchiectomy with high ligation (or inguinal orchiectomy) is the primary treatment of seminoma. Orchiectomy is both diagnostic and therapeutic.
- Sperm banking needs to be discussed prior to treatment.
- Open inguinal biopsy of the contralateral testes is considered if there is a suspicious finding of intratesticular malignancies on ultrasound, marked testicular atrophy, and undescended testes
- For stage I seminoma, the risk of nodal relapse in the paraaortics and pelvics is 15%–20% and less than 5%, respectively.
- Adjuvant treatment for stage 1 seminoma after orchiectomy includes radiotherapy, active surveillance, and chemotherapy.
- A proposed treatment algorithm for seminoma is shown in Figure 21.3.

21.2.2 Radical Orchiectomy

- Surgical approach is through an inguinal incision to avoid interruption of testicular lymphatics.
- The testicular vessels and vas deferens are mobilized and a non-crushing clamp is placed across the cord structure to decrease the risk of tumor spreading by manipulation.
- Pathologic determination of seminoma or nonseminoma follows.

21.2.3 Active Surveillance

- Active surveillance can be offered for patients who cannot undergo radiotherapy in cases of prior radiotherapy, active inflammatory bowel disease, and horseshoe kidney.
- However, patients who choose an active surveillance approach need to understand that frequent and long-term follow-up with imaging and laboratory tests is required (Grade B). In a pooled analysis including 638 patients with stage I seminoma followed up by surveillance, the 5- and 10-year recurrence-free survivals were 82.3% and 78.7%, respectively. Although close to 70% of recurrences occurred within the first 2 years after surgery, 7% of recurring cases occurred after 6 years of follow-up. Tumor markers, chest X-ray, and abdominal/pelvic CT every 3–4 months for years 1–3, every 6 months for years 4–7, and then annually are required (Level IV) (WARDE et al. 2002).

21.2.4 Radiation Therapy

- Radiotherapy has a long track record as an effective adjuvant therapy. An infradiaphragmatic field encompassing paraaortic and ipsilateral pelvic lymph nodes (dogleg) has been used for many years
- Adjuvant radiation therapy can be recommended after radical orchiectomy with high ligation (Grade A). The cancer-specific survivals for stage I and II A–B seminoma after radical orchiectomy and radiotherapy of 99%–100% and 93%–100%, respectively, have been repeatedly demonstrated in prospective randomized trials and retrospective series. The relapse-free survivals are more than 95% and 85%, respectively.

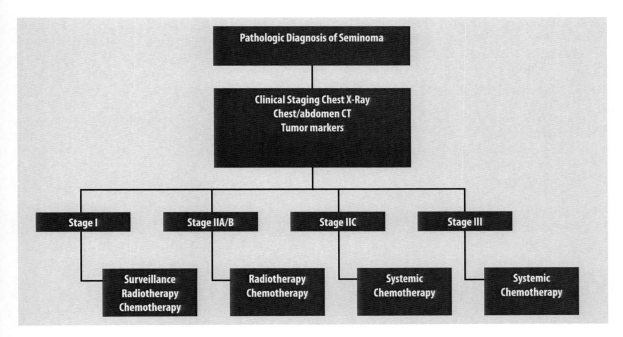

Fig. 21.3. A proposed treatment algorithm for testicular seminoma

Simulation and Field Arrangement

■ The patient is simulated and treated in a supine position. The kidneys are delineated and shielded. A clamshell is placed on the remaining testicle.

■ Figure 21.1 shows the "dogleg" field arrangement from the top of T11 (superior border) to the top of the obturator foramen (inferior border). Figure 21.2 demonstrates the paraaortic-only field arrangement from the top of T11 (superior border) to the bottom of L5 (inferior border). Laterally, the field edge is placed at the tips of the transverse processes, which may be expanded to include the left renal hilum for left-sided tumors. For stage I seminoma, the paraaortic field is recommended for adjuvant irradiation (Grade A). A MRC randomized trial showed that there is no difference in 3-year relapse-free survival/overall survival for patients treated with dogleg (97%/96%) when compared to paraaortic-only radiotherapy (99%/100%). However, there is a slight decrease in 3-year pelvic relapse-free survival in the paraaortic (98%) when compared to the dogleg group (100%) (MRC, Level 1) (FOSSA et al. 1999).

■ Approximately 15%–20% of patients are diagnosed with stage II seminoma, and standard dogleg fields are recommended for stage IIA and IIB diseases to treat the paraaortic and ipsilateral pelvic lymph nodes. The field width is expanded accordingly with a 2-cm margin to encompass the lymph node mass.

Dose and Fractionation

■ There is a range of acceptable doses and fractionation with 25–25.5 Gy in 15–20 fractions (Grade A). Stage IIA and IIB lymph nodes can be boosted to 30 Gy and 36 Gy, respectively. An MRC randomized trial showed no difference between patients receiving 30-Gy vs. 20-Gy radiotherapy doses in terms of 5-year RFS (MRC/EORTC, Level I) (JONES et al. 2005).

Side Effects and Complications

■ Radiation-induced side effects and complications are generally very mild and infrequent with low-dose irradiation.

■ Acute side effects may include nausea, vomiting, diarrhea, and transient decline in blood counts. Anti-emetics are recommended 1 hour prior to radiotherapy.

■ Late complications may include:

– Gastro-intestinal: peptic ulcer disease, small bowel obstruction, and chronic diarrhea.

- Gonadal: with the dogleg treatment and the use of testicular shield, the contralateral remaining testicle will receive about 1%–2% of the prescribed dose, which can lead to temporary reduction in spermatogenesis and fertility. About half of the patients have sub-fertile sperm counts on presentation or after surgery. Fertility usually restored within 2–3 years in those who were fertile before radiotherapy. The patients are also advised to avoid fatherhood for 6–12 months after radiotherapy.
- Second malignancy: a small risk in the 10–15 years after radiotherapy, largely gastrointestinal cancers and sarcoma (Level IV) (TRAVIS et al. 2005).

21.2.5 Chemotherapy

- A single cycle of carboplatin can be used as an alternative to adjuvant radiotherapy (Grade B). However, there is only one randomized trial with limited follow-up time, and longer term follow-up is required: The MRC randomized trial compared adjuvant radiotherapy (87% paraaortic-only field,

the remainder paraaortic and ipsilateral pelvic field) and one cycle of single-agent carboplatin. The 3-year relapse-free survival rates were similar at 95.9% and 94.8%, respectively (MRC, Level I) (OLIVER et al. 2005).
- Chemotherapy is usually recommended for stage IIC and higher disease, usually comprised of etoposide/cisplatin (EP) or bleomycin/ etoposide/cisplatin (BEP) (Grade A).

21.3　Treatment of Nonseminoma

- Treatment of nonseminoma is beyond the scope of this chapter as radiotherapy plays a limited role in this disease. After radical orchiectomy and staging work-up, the treatment options include observation, retroperitoneal lymph node dissection, or systemic chemotherapy, usually comprised of bleomycin/etoposide/cisplatin (BEP) or etoposide/cisplatin (EP) (Fig. 21.3).

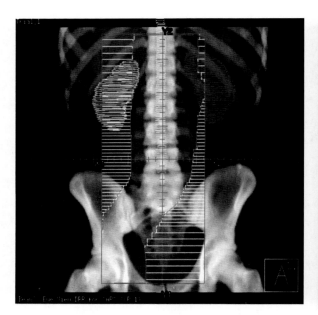

Fig. 21.1. Classic dogleg field encompasses both paraaortic and ipsilateral pelvic nodes. The superior border is at the T10/11 interspace and the inferior border just above the obturator foramen. The lateral borders of the paraaortic field are at the tips of the lumbar transverse processes

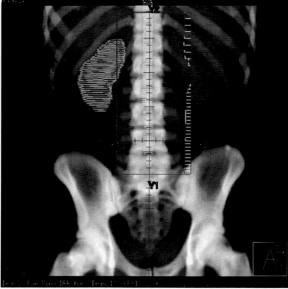

Fig. 21.2. Paraaortic fields extend from the T10/11 interspace to the inferior border of L5. Laterally, the field edge is placed at the tips of the transverse processes, but may be expanded at the left renal hilum for left-sided tumors

<table>
<tr><td>

21.4 Follow-Up

21.4.1 Surveillance

- For patients undergoing active surveillance, frequent follow-up with complete history and physical examinations, laboratory tests of tumor markers, imaging studies with chest X-ray, CT of the abdomen and pelvis every 3–4 months for year 1–3, every 6 months for year 4–7, and then annually are recommended (Grade B) (Level IV) (WARDE et al. 2002).

21.4.2 Post-Treatment Follow-Up

- After infradiaphragmatic (dogleg) radiotherapy, the patient should undergo history and physical examination, chest X-ray, and tumor markers every 3–4 months for year 1, every 6 months for year 2, and then annually thereafter (Grade D).
- After paraaortic-only radiotherapy, the patient will need pelvic CT annually for 3 years in addition to the above (Grade B). The results from a number of retrospective series indicated that the paraaortic-only radiation therapy changed the pattern of recurrence. Pelvic recurrence was observed only in patients receiving paraaortic irradiation (Level IV) (POWER et al. 2005).

</td><td>

References

Fossa SD, Horwich A, Russell JM et al. (1999) Optimal planning target volume for stage I testicular seminoma: A Medical Research Council randomized trial. Medical Research Council Testicular Tumor Working Group. J Clin Oncol 17:1146

Greene F, Page D, Fleming I et al. (2002) AJCC cancer staging manual, 6th edn. Springer, Heidelberg Berlin New York

International Germ Cell Consensus Classification (1997) A prognostic factor-based staging system for metastatic germ cell cancers. International Germ Cell Cancer Collaborative Group. J Clin Oncol 15:594–603

Jones WG, Fossa SD, Mead GM et al. (2005) Randomized trial of 30 versus 20 Gy in the adjuvant treatment of stage I testicular seminoma: a report on Medical Research Council Trial TE18, European Organisation for the Research and Treatment of Cancer Trial 30942 (ISRCTN18525328). J Clin Oncol 23:1200–1208

Oliver RT, Mason MD, Mead GM et al. (2005) Radiotherapy versus single-dose carboplatin in adjuvant treatment of stage I seminoma: a randomised trial. Lancet 366:293–300

Power RE, Kennedy J, Crown J et al. (2005) Pelvic recurrence in stage I seminoma: a new phenomenon that questions modern protocols for radiotherapy and follow-up. Int J Urol 12:378–382

Travis LB, Fossa SD, Schonfeld SJ et al. (2005) Second cancers among 40, 576 testicular cancer patients: focus on long-term survivors. J Natl Cancer Inst 97:1354–1365

Warde P, Specht L, Horwich A et al. (2002) Prognostic factors for relapse in stage I seminoma managed by surveillance: a pooled analysis. J Clin Oncol 20:4448–4452

</td></tr>
</table>

Section VI:

Gynaecological Cancers

Ovarian and Fallopian Tube Cancers

22

Subhakar Mutyala and Aaron H. Wolfson

CONTENTS

S. Mutyala, MD
Department of Radiation Oncology, Montefiore Medical Center, 1565 Poplar St., Bronx, NY 10461, USA
A. H. Wolfson, MD
Department of Radiation Oncology, University of Miami Miller School of Medicine, 1475 NW, 12th Avenue, Miami, FL 33136, USA

Introduction and Objectives

Ovarian cancer and fallopian tube cancer typically fail in the abdomen, along with the pelvis, making them more systemic diseases. With this consideration, effective chemotherapy has slowly replaced the use of whole abdominal radiation.

Fallopian tumor cancer is the most rarely diagnosed gynecological malignancy. As such, no prospective trial is available, and recommendations on diagnosis and treatment are based on retrospective trials (i.e., level IV evidence).

This chapter examines:
- Recommendations for diagnosis and staging procedures
- The staging systems and prognostic factors
- Treatment recommendations, as well as the supporting scientific evidence for adjuvant treatment for the different stages of ovarian cancer and fallopian tube cancer
- Follow-up care and surveillance of survivors

22.1 Diagnosis, Staging, and Prognoses

22.1.1 Diagnosis

Initial Evaluation

- Diagnosis and evaluation of ovarian cancer starts with a complete history and physical examination (H&P), with focus on bimanual pelvic exam. Early-stage disease usually presents as a palpable adnexal mass on pelvic exam. Advanced disease presents with abdominal pain and increasing abdominal girth, and/or urinary frequency or rectal pressure from the abdominal mass.
- There is no effective screening program for ovarian cancer. One prospective study attempted to use transvaginal ultrasound and CA-125 to screen for ovarian cancer. The study found the two

screening tests to be very non-sensitive (<50%) and to have a high false-negative rate (Level III) (Stirling et al. 2005).

Laboratory Tests

- Initial laboratory tests should include a complete blood count, basic blood chemistry, renal function tests, liver function tests, and alkaline phosphatase.
- CA-125 should be tested as the preoperative CA-125 level has been found to be an independent prognostic factor (Grade B). CA-125 is elevated in 50% of cases. The normal level of CA-125 is <35 U/ml. For patients >50, level >35 u/ml is 98.5% specific and for patients <50, 94.5% specific (Level IV) (Einhorn et al. 1992), and level >65 U/ml is 97% specific and 78% sensitive (Level IV) (Zurawski et al. 1987).

  In a retrospective study, the preoperative value of CA-125 for epithelial ovarian cancer was compared to outcome. An association of increasing CA-125 level was found between decreased disease-free survival, high grade, and higher stage, but not the ability to have cytoreductive surgery (Level IV) (Cooper et al. 2002).
- Other tumor markers, including CEA, CA 19-9, β-HCG, and AFP, can be considered; however, their sensitivity and specificity are usually limited:
  - CEA is elevated in 60% of cases of ovarian cancer.
  - CA 19-9 is useful for mucinous cystadenoma of the ovary.
  - β-HCG and AFP are useful for patients <30 for germinoma.

Imaging Studies

- Transvaginal or transabdominal ultrasound is carried out by an operator with gynecologic imaging experience (Grade B). Results of a prospective study demonstrated that transvaginal ultrasound (TVUS) is sensitive for tumor size (sensitivity of 87%), ascites (97%), invasion of adjacent organs (>98%), and peritoneal carcinomatosis (96%), but not for detection of malignant lymph nodes (sensitivity of 8%) (Level III) (Henrich et al. 2007).
- A randomized control trial compared routine ultrasound and an ultrasound by an expert in gynecologic imaging. The number of diagnostic surgeries and procedures was reduced with better imaging. The correct histological diagnosis was made after ultrasound in 99% of patients with expert ultrasonography and 52% with routine ultrasonography (Level II) (Yazbek et al. 2008).
- CT of the abdomen and pelvis to evaluate the primary mass, as well as to detect metastatic disease, is commonly recommended. MRI of the pelvis should be considered to evaluate the primary mass (Grade C). The Radiology Diagnostic Oncology Group compared MRI, ultrasound, and CT scan in the evaluation of ovarian cancer. MRI has been shown to be superior to ultrasound and CT for diagnosis of adnexal masses. Ultrasound was found to be the most sensitive in diagnosing abdominal spread (Level IV) (Kurtz et al. 1999).

  A prospective study evaluated the ability of MRI to differentiate benign and malignant adnexal masses. The results were 87% accuracy, 86% sensitivity, and 88% specificity (Level III) (Chen et al. 2006).
- FDG-PET or PET/CT can be used to evaluate a suspicious ovarian mass for malignancy and to detect distant metastasis (Grade B). A prospective trial showed that PET/CT is very sensitive (100%) and specific (92.5%) in diagnosing ovarian malignancies (Level III) (Risum et al. 2007). PET/CT has been shown to be more specific (100%–61%) than TVUS and more sensitive than CT for diagnosis and staging of ovarian cancer (Level III) (Castellucci et al. 2007).
- Chest X-ray to evaluate for metastatic disease and pleural effusion is recommended (Table 22.1).

Pathology

- Tissue diagnosis is imperative prior to the initiation of any treatment for ovarian cancer. Treatments for various pathologic types of ovarian malignancy differ substantially.
- Epithelial tumors (90%) from the ovarian surface include:

Table 22.1. Imaging and laboratory work-ups for ovarian cancer

Imaging studies	Laboratory tests
– Transvaginal or trans-abdominal ultrasound	– Complete blood count
– CT of abdomen/pelvis	– Serum chemistry
– Chest X-ray	– Liver function tests
– MRI of pelvis (optional)	– Renal function tests
– PET or PET/CT (optional)	– Alkaline phosphatase
	– Tumor markers: CA-125, CEA, CA 19-9, β-BCG, AFP

- Serous tumors, resembling fallopian tube.
- Mucinous tumors, resembling endocervix.
- Endometrioid tumors, resembling endometrium.
- Clear cell tumor, resembling endometrial glands during pregnancy.
- Undifferentiated carcinoma.

■ Approximately 15% of ovarian tumors are of borderline malignant potential.

■ Germ cell tumors account for 5% of all ovarian tumors and include dysgerminoma and nondysgerminoma.

■ Other malignancies of the ovaries include sex cord-stromal tumors (3%), extragonadal germ cell tumors, and metastatic cancer from endometrial cancer, GI tumors, or breast cancer.

22.1.2 Staging

■ Ovarian cancer is staged by TNM and FIGO surgical staging. Staging depends on the extent and success of surgery.

■ The 2007 American Joint Committee on Cancer Tumor Node Metastasis (TNM) staging system is presented in Table 22.2.

22.1.3 Prognostic Factors

■ Stage at diagnosis is the most important prognostic factor of ovarian cancer. Advanced stage is associated with decreased survival. The statistics published by the National Cancer Institute report a 5-year overall survival for stage I of 90%, stage II 80%, stage III 20%, and stage IV < 5% (Level IV) (NATIONAL CANCER INSTITUTE 1986).

■ The preoperative CA-125 level has been found to be an independent prognostic factor. The results of a retrospective study reported by COOPER et al. (2002) detailed the above demonstrated association of increasing CA-125 level with decreased disease-free survival, high grade, higher stage, but not the ability to have cytoreductive surgery (Level IV).

■ Tumor differentiation is a significant prognostic factor. Results from a retrospective review that combined two GOG studies revealed that tumor grade was an independent prognostic factor, with higher grade leading to higher recurrence and decreased survival for early-stage ovarian cancer

Table 22.2. Staging for ovarian cancer (TNM and FIGO-surgical staging)

TNM	FIGO	
T0		No evidence of primary tumor
T1a	IA	Tumor limited to one ovary: capsule intact, no tumor on ovarian surface, negative ascites/peritoneal washings
T1b	IB	Tumor limited to both ovaries: capsules intact, no tumor on ovarian surface, negative ascites/peritoneal washings
T1c	IC	Tumor limited to one or both ovaries: capsule ruptured, tumor on ovarian surface, and/or positive ascites/peritoneal washings
T2a	IIA	Extension and/or implants on uterus and/or tubes, negative ascites/peritoneal washings
T2b	IIB	Extension to other pelvic tissues, negative ascites/peritoneal washings
T2c	IIC	Pelvic extension (2a or 2b), positive ascites/peritoneal washings
T3a	IIIA	Microscopic peritoneal metastasis beyond the pelvis
T3b	IIIB	Macroscopic peritoneal metastasis beyond the pelvis <2 cm in greatest dimension
T3c/ N1	IIIC	Peritoneal metastasis beyond the pelvis >2 cm in greatest dimension and/or regional lymph node metastasis
M1	IV	Distant metastasis excluding peritoneal metastasis
N0		No regional lymph node metastasis
N1		Regional lymph node metastasis (external iliac, internal iliac, paraaortic, hypogastric/obturator, inguinal, lateral sacral)
M0		No distant metastasis
M1		Distant metastasis (excludes peritoneal metastasis)

STAGE GROUPING	
0:	Tis N0 M0
IA:	T1a N0 M0
IB:	T1b N0 M0
IC:	T1c N0 M0
IIA:	T2a N0 M0
IIB:	T2b N0 M0
IIC:	T2c N0 M0
IIIA:	N0 M0
IIIB:	T3b N0 M0
IIIC:	T3c N0 M0, Any T N1 M0
IV:	Any T Any N M1

(Level IV) (CHAN et al. 2008). Another retrospective series did a multivariate analysis on stage I–III with optimal debulking. Grade, independent of histology and residuum, carries weight as an independent prognostic factor (Level IV) (CAREY et al. 1993).

■ Residual disease after surgical resection is also associated with treatment outcome. A prospective randomized GOG trial compared the addition of chemotherapy to suboptimally debulked patients. On subset analysis, patients with residual disease <2 cm had a much higher overall survival than patients with residual disease >2 cm (40% versus 20%). There was no statistical difference in the amount of residual disease (2–4 vs. 4–6, etc.) (Level II) (HOSKINS et al. 1994). A recent meta-analysis of GOG data confirmed these results showing that less residual disease after surgery has better survival (Level I) (WINTER et al. 2008).

■ Histology does not have prognostic significance independent of stage and grade (Level IV) (CAREY et al. 1993).

22.2 Treatment of Low-Risk Early-stage Ovarian Cancer

22.2.1 General Principles

■ Low-risk early-stage ovarian cancer includes borderline or low-malignant-potential ovarian tumor at stage IA–IB, grade 1–2.

■ For low-risk early-stage ovarian cancer, usually TAH/BSO and full surgical staging are the mainstay of treatment.

22.2.2 Surgical Staging

■ Optimal surgical staging is required (Grade A). Results from an EORTC randomized trial demonstrated that for patients with early stage ovarian cancer treated with surgery only, optimal staging was associated with a statistically significant improvement in overall survival (HR = 2.31) and recurrence-free survival (HR = 1.82) (EORTC, Level I) (TRIMBOS et al. 2003).

■ Surgical staging and resection of the low-risk early-stage ovarian tumor should include the following procedures: midline incision; peritoneal washings from the abdomen, pelvis and gutters; extrafascial TAH/BSO; maximal tumor debulking; infracolic omentectomy; palpitation of all intraperitoneal surfaces; biopsy of peritoneal surfaces; biopsy of undersurface of diaphragm; pelvic and paraaortic lymph node sampling.

■ The need for second-look laparotomy for washings, lymph node sampling, multiple biopsies of the peritoneum, and resection of residual disease is questionable (Grade C). A recent GOG trial compared second-look laparotomy (SLL) and early salvage treatment versus no SLL and salvage treatment when disease had clinically failed. The results showed no improvement in survival for SLL (Level III) (GREER et al. 2005).

22.2.3 Adjuvant Chemotherapy

■ Adjuvant chemotherapy is not indicated for low-risk patients after full surgical staging (Grade A). The results of a phase III GOG trial for stage IA–IB grade 1–2 ovarian cancer after TAH/BSO and full staging were randomized to adjuvant melphalan versus observation. The chemotherapy arm did not show any benefit in either 5-year DFS or OS (Level I) (YOUNG et al. 1990).

■ For patients who have not been optimally staged, chemotherapy is indicated (Grade A). Platinum-based chemotherapy has been shown to have a benefit for local control, disease-free and overall survival compared to observation (EORTC, Level I) (TRIMBOS et al. 2003)

22.3 Treatment of High-Risk Early-stage Ovarian Cancer

22.3.1 General Principles

■ High-risk early-stage ovarian cancers include stage IA–IB grade 3, stage IC, stage Ia–IC clear cell, and stage II any grade.

- For high-risk early-stage ovarian cancer, full surgical staging and adjuvant treatment are generally recommended (Grade A).

22.3.2 Adjuvant Chemotherapy

- Carboplatin- and paclitaxel-based chemotherapy for three to six cycles is recommended for adjuvant treatment after surgery (Grade B). The results of a prospective randomized trial for stage IA–IB grade 2–3 ovarian cancer after full surgical staging were randomized to observation versus cisplatin chemotherapy. The cisplatin arm had statistically improved DFS (83% versus 63%), but OS was similar (83% versus 82%) (Level II) (Bolis et al. 1995). GOG-157 was a prospective randomized trial comparing surgery and either carboplatin/paclitaxel and six cycles versus three for stage IA–IB, grade 2–3, stage IC, and stage II. A trend toward improved local control benefit was found for six cycles of carboplatin/paclitaxel compared to three cycles, but the difference was not statistically significant (Level II) (Bell et al. 2006).
- Chemotherapy is preferred over whole abdominal radiation (WAR) as the adjuvant treatment of choice after surgery (Grade A). The efficacies of WAR and chemotherapy have been compared in a number of prospective randomized trials, and most studies did not demonstrate any significance between the two treatments in terms of overall survival. The use of whole abdominal radiation has been largely replaced by chemotherapy for epithelial ovarian cancers. In a prospective randomized trial completed by the National Cancer Institute of Canada, 257 patients with stage I, IIA "high-risk" ovarian carcinoma, IIB, and III (disease confined to the pelvis) were randomized to: (1) total abdominal radiotherapy (22.5 Gy in 20 daily fractions), (2) chemotherapy with melphalan (8 mg/m^2/day every 4 weeks for 18 courses), or (3) intraperitoneal chromic phosphate (10–20 mCi). All patients were initially treated with pelvic radiotherapy to bring the pelvic dose to 45 Gy. The results showed a marginally significant difference in disease-free survival with melphalan chemotherapy as compared to whole abdominal radiation. The 5-year survival rates are 62%, 61%, and 66% for the WAR-, chemotherapy-, and IP chro-

mic phosphate-treated groups, respectively. No significant difference in survival was observed (NCIC, Level II) (Klaassen et al. 1988). A prospective randomized trial compared surgery plus cisplatin and cyclophosphamide chemotherapy versus surgery followed by whole abdominal radiation. The chemotherapy arm tended toward higher overall survival and relapse-free survival; however, there was poor compliance to WAR (Level II) (Chiara et al. 1994). Except for the results published by Dembo et al. (1979), which showed a significantly improved 10-year relapse-free survival with WAR as compared to pelvic radiotherapy with or without chlorambucil, results from three more randomized trials all revealed no significant differences in overall survival (Level II) (Smith et al. 1975; Sell et al. 1990).

- A prospective randomized trial compared platinum-based chemotherapy to intraperitoneal P^{32}. Although not statistically significant, the trend toward lower recurrence rate with chemotherapy and lower toxicity recommends the use of platinum-based chemotherapy regimens (Level II) (Young et al. 2003).

22.3.3 Radiation Therapy

Whole Abdominal Radiation

- Indications for radiation therapy as an alternative to chemotherapy include stage I–II with high-risk features or completely debulked stage III ovarian cancer (as detailed below in Sect. 22.4.2).
- When radiation therapy is utilized, whole abdominal radiation is the technique of choice. Pelvic irradiation is usually not recommended in the treatment of epithelial ovarian cancer. A prospective randomized trial compared pelvic radiation to WAR. WAR was found to be superior in overall survival (51%–78%, 5-year) and local control (Level II) (Dembo et al. 1979).
- The total dose of WAR is 30 Gy delivered in 20 daily fractions (1.5 per daily fraction).

Field Arrangement

- Anteroposterior and posteroanterior fields are commonly used. The field borders are set up as follows:

- Superior: 1 cm above diaphragm at maximal expiration (can watch breathing under fluoroscopy)
- Inferior: ischial tuberosities
- Lateral: 1.5 cm to peritoneal reflection
■ Kidneys (from CT) should be blocked in the PA field during the entire treatment or in both the AP and PA after 15 Gy of irradiation.
  Liver block can be considered at 25.5 Gy during irradiation (not required by GOG trials).
  Femoral heads should be blocked to limit the radiation dose.

Side Effects and Complications

■ Acute toxicity induced by whole abdominal radiation includes GI toxicity (nausea, vomiting, and diarrhea), which occurs in 61% of cases. Myelosuppression (especially thrombocytopenia) occurs in 11%. Overall, approximately 10% of patients are unable to complete treatment due to acute treatment-induced toxicities.
■ Commonly observed treatment-induced chronic toxicities include small bowel obstruction (4.2%) and radiation hepatitis (44%). However, treatment-caused death is rare and occurs in less than 1% of cases.

22.4   Treatment of Advanced-stage Ovarian Cancer

22.4.1 General Principles

■ Initial treatment of advanced-stage ovarian cancer is full surgical staging, attempting to remove all gross disease. Advanced-stage ovarian cancer can be differentiated into stage III with optimally debulked ($\leq$2 cm residual) or stage III suboptimally debulked (>2 cm residual).
■ Chemotherapy is indicated as an adjuvant treatment (Grade A). The most frequently used chemotherapy option for ovarian cancer is carboplatin AUC 6 and paclitaxel 175 mg/m^2.
  A meta-analysis of 37 trials showed that platinum containing first-line regimens have a 5% 2- and 5-year overall survival advantage compared to non-platinum-containing first-line regimens. The analysis also compared the use of cisplatin

to carboplatin. The two chemotherapy drugs are considered equivalent in terms of tumor control (Level I) (AABO et al. 1998).
■ The treatment for suboptimally debulked stage III patients is identical to patients with stage IV diseases.

22.4.2 Stage III, Optimally Debulked (<2 cm Residual)

■ Adjuvant chemotherapy is indicated for patients with optimally debulked stage III ovarian cancer (Grade A). Adjuvant intraperitoneal (IP) chemotherapy has been shown to be superior to intravenous chemotherapy.
  The results of a prospective randomized trial revealed that for optimally debulked (<2 cm residual) stage III and IV diseases, patients randomized to receive cyclophosphamide and IP cisplatin had superior outcome than those treated with IV cyclophosphamide and cisplatin in terms of increased median survival (49–41 months) and decreased toxicity (tinnitus, hearing loss, and neuromuscular toxicity) (Level II) (ALBERTS et al. 1996).
  Results from another prospective randomized trial compared IV carboplatin and IP paclitaxel + cisplatin versus IV cisplatin and paclitaxel. The IP arm had statistically improved progression-free survival and a trend towards overall survival (Level I) (MARKMAN et al. 2001).
  Results from a more recently published prospective randomized multi-institution trial also demonstrated an improved survival for IP cisplatin and paclitaxel compared to IV cisplatin and paclitaxel (Level I) (ARMSTRONG et al. 2006).
  The effect of IP chemotherapy over IV chemotherapy was further confirmed by a meta-analysis. The analysis combined the seven randomized studies comparing IP chemotherapy versus IV chemotherapy. The results show an increase in overall survival [relative risk 0.88, 95% (CI) 0.81–0.95]. However, severe adverse events and catheter-related complications with intraperitoneal chemotherapy were significantly more common (Level I) (ELIT et al. 2007).
■ Chemotherapy plus WAR has been shown to be superior to chemotherapy alone (Grade B) in a small prospective randomized trial. In that trial, stage III patients with no residual disease were treated with cisplatin and epirubicin, followed

by WAR or observation. The chemotherapy plus WAR arm had statistically significantly improved disease-free survival (77% vs. 54% at 2 years and 45% vs. 19% at 5 years) and overall survival (88% vs. 58% at 2 years and 59% vs. 26% at 5 years) (Level II) (PICKEL et al. 1999).

- In a prospective phase II trial, carboplatin has been shown to be safe and efficacious to administer intraperitoneally. However, the outcomes have not been directly compared to IP cisplatin (Level III) (NAGAO et al. 2008)

22.4.3 Stage III, Suboptimally Debulked (>2 cm Residual), or Stage IV

- Adjuvant carboplatin and paclitaxel chemotherapy is indicated for patients with suboptimally debulked stage III or stage IV ovarian cancer (Grade A). Paclitaxel has been found to be more responsive than cyclophosphamide. A prospective randomized trial compared cisplatin and cyclophosphamide versus cisplatin and paclitaxel. The cisplatin and paclitaxel combination had an improved clinically complete rate (31% versus 51%) as well as median survival (24 months versus 38 months) (GOG 111, Level II) (McGUIRE et al. 1996).

- Carboplatin has been shown to be superior to cisplatin in a prospective randomized trial. Patients with stage III suboptimally debulked and stage IV were randomized to cisplatin and cyclophosphamide versus carboplatin and cyclophosphamide. Although no significant tumor response was detected, carboplatin was found to be less toxic for neurotoxicity, nausea/vomiting, alopecia, and renal toxicity (Level II) (HANNIGAN et al. 1993).

22.5 Fallopian Tube Cancer

22.5.1 Presentation and Diagnosis

- Diagnosis and evaluation of fallopian tube cancer start with a complete history and physical examination (H&P).

- Presenting symptoms can include all three of the following (Latzko's triad, present in 15% of patients):
- Pelvic pain
- Pelvic mass
- Serosanguineous vaginal discharge
- Hydrops turbans profluens presents in 5% of patients. Colicky lower abdominal pain is alleviated with the release of a sporadic, yellowish vaginal discharge.
- Criteria for diagnosis of primary fallopian tube carcinoma has been defined by SEDLIS et al. (1978)
- Main tumor is in the tube and has papillary serous histology.
- Tubal mucosa is involved with the primary.
- There should be a transition from benign, dysplastic to malignant epithelium.
- If endometrium and/or ovaries are involved, it should be only minimal compared to the fallopian tube.
- Up to 25% of fallopian tube cancers present as bilateral disease.

22.5.2 Laboratory Tests, Imaging Studies, and Pathology

- In addition to the routine laboratory tests including complete blood count and serum chemistry, CA-125 and CA 19-9 are usually indicated (Grade B). These tumor markers can be specific if elevated at the time of diagnosis: CA-125 is elevated in 80%, and 87% of tumors have been found to stain pathologically with CA-125 (Level IV) (PULS et al. 1993).
- Transvaginal ultrasound with Doppler can be considered for diagnosis and evaluation, and is considered as the most sensitive and specific test (Grade D) (Level V) (YAMAMOTO et al. 1988).
- CT has been described as able to show the mass, however unable to differentiate it from an endometrial or ovarian primary (Level V) (KAWAKAMI et al. 1993). The use of MRI has been described in identifying primary fallopian tube carcinoma and helps to differentiate the adnexal mass from the ovarian primary (Level V) (WANG et al. 1998; KURACHI et al. 1999).
- Pap smear and endometrial biopsy are usually required, but are insensitive for diagnosis of fallopian tube cancers. Hysteroscopy or hystero-

salpingography can be utilized to visualize the tumor (Level V) (HINTON et al. 1988).

- A relationship has been found with BRCA1 or BRCA2. A total of 16% of cases reported in Ontario were found to be BRCA1- or BRCA2-positive (Level IV) (AZIZ et al. 2002).

22.5.3 Staging

- Staging of fallopian tube tumors is presented in Table 22.3.

22.5.4 Prognostic Factors

- Stage at diagnosis is the most important prognostic factor. In a multivariate analysis, higher stage was the only prognostic indicator, compared to age and depth of invasion (Level IV) (ALVARADO-CABRERO et al. 1999).
- The 5-year survival by stage is: stage I, 95%, stage II, 75%, stage III, 69%, and stage IV, 45% (Level IV) (KOSARY and TRIMBLE 2002).
- Depth of wall invasion is of prognostic significance, as suggested in case studies (Level V) (ROSE et al. 1990).
- Tumor differentiation is associated with prognosis. Results of a retrospective review revealed that higher grade is associated with inferior outcome (Level IV) (CORMIO et al. 1996).
- Residual tumor >2 cm is associated adversely with the prognosis. Surgical series have shown that extent of disease and optimal surgery have improved survival (Level V) (BENEDET et al. 1977; PETERS et al. 1988; ROSEN et al. 1993).
- Lymph node involvement is associated with inferior survival. There are incidences of lymph node involvement at early-stage (Level V) (DI RE et al. 1996), with paraaortic nodes as frequent as pelvic nodes (Level V) (TAKESHIMA and HASUMI 2000).
- CA-125 level has been found to be an independent risk factor for disease-free survival and overall survival (Level IV) (HEFLER et al. 2000).
- Angiolymphatic invasion was suggested to be related to poor outcome after treatment, according to the results from two retrospective series (Level IV) (TAMINI and FIGGE 1981; ASMUSSEN et al. 1988).

- The patterns of failure for this disease are predominantly within the region encompassed by whole abdominal radiation therapy, and distant failure occurs in no more than 15% of cases (Level IV) (WOLFSON et al. 1998).

Table 22.3. Staging for fallopian tube cancer

TNM	FIGO	
Tis	0	Carcinoma *in situ* (limited to the tubal mucosa)
T1a	IA	Tumor limited to one tube without penetrating the serosal surface and no ascites
T1b	IB	Tumor limited to both tubes without penetrating the serosal surface and no ascites
T1c	IC	Tumor limited to one or both tubes with extension onto or through the tubal serosa, or with malignant cells in ascites or peritoneal washings
T2a	IIA	Tumor extension and/or metastasis to the uterus and/or ovaries
T2b	IIB	Tumor extension to other pelvic structures
T2c	IIC	Tumor with pelvic extension and malignant cells in ascites or peritoneal washings
T3a	IIIA	Microscopic peritoneal metastasis outside the pelvis
T3b	IIIB	Macroscopic peritoneal metastasis outside the pelvis <2 cm in greatest dimension
T3c/ N1	IIIC	Peritoneal metastasis >2 cm in diameter and/or positive regional lymph nodes
M1	IV	Distant metastases (excludes peritoneal metastasis)
N1		Regional lymph node metastasis (paraaortic, common iliac, internal iliac, external iliac, inguinal nodes)
M1		Distant metastasis (liver, lungs)
STAGE GROUPING		
0:		Tis N0 M0
IA:		T1a N0 M0
IB:		T1b N0 M0
IC:		T1c N0 M0
IIA:		T2a N0 M0
IIB:		T2b N0 M0
IIC:		T2c N0 M0
IIIA:		T3a N0 M0
IIIB:		T3b N0 M0
IIIC:		T3c N0 M0, Any T N1 M0
IV:		Any T Any N M1

22.5.5 Treatment of Fallopian Tube Cancer

■ Surgery is the mainstay treatment of fallopian tube cancer, and surgical staging and treatment similar to that used for ovarian cancer are used. Procedures include TAH/BSO, omentectomy, and peritoneal washings; biopsies of the peritoneum, diaphragm, and bowel are required. Lymph node dissection should also be considered (Grade D). Results from a small series showed that improved median survival was observed in patients with lymph node dissection (43 months versus 21 months) (Level V) (KLEIN et al. 1999).

■ For disease confined to the fallopian tube, adjuvant chemotherapy or radiation therapy is not routinely indicated after surgery (Grade B). One retrospective review found that for disease confined to the tube, a single-agent chemotherapy or pelvis radiation did not improve survival (Level IV) (PETERS et al. 1988).

■ Cisplatin-based chemotherapy can be considered for advanced disease (Grade B). Results from phase II trials showed safe use of cisplatin-based chemotherapy regimens (Level III) (BARAKAT et al. 1991; PECTASIDES et al. 1994; WAGENAAR et al. 2001; MORRIS et al. 1990).

■ As locoregional failure is common after surgery for fallopian tube cancer, whole abdominal radiation can be considered (Grade B). Intra-abdominal failure is a common mode of recurrence in patients with stage II, III, and IV disease. In a retrospective series of 21 patients reported from Yale University, adjuvant treatment is recommended as most patients who died of disease did so within the first 2 years after diagnosis. In addition, negative second-look surgery did not provide assurance of permanent remission (Level IV) (BROWN et al. 1985). These findings were supported by the results of a multi-institutional retrospective series of 72 patients demonstrating that 18%, 36%, and 19% of treatment failures occurred in the pelvis, abdomen, or distant sites. Upper abdominal failures were more frequently found in stages II/III/IV (29%) than in stage I (7%) (p=0.03). Relapses solely outside of what would be included in standard whole abdominal radiotherapy portals occurred in only 15% of patients with failures (Level IV) (WOLFSON et al. 1998). Both authors suggested the use of whole abdominal radiation for adjuvant therapy.

■ If used, the treatment techniques of whole abdominal radiation are similar to those used in advanced ovarian cancers. However, the effect of radiotherapy has not been compared to chemotherapy in any studies.

22.6 Follow-Ups

▦ Follow-up is recommended in patients with ovarian cancer or fallopian tube cancer after treatment for early detection of disease recurrence and treatment-induced side effects and complications.

▦ No recommendation specific to fallopian tube cancer can be concluded, but a follow-up scheme similar to those used for ovarian cancer is reasonable (Table 22.4).

▦ Post-treatment follow-ups could be scheduled every 2–4 months initially in the first 2 years after treatment, then every 6 months thereafter through year 5. Annual follow-up is recommended for long-term survivors after 5 years (Grade D) (NATIONAL COMPREHENSIVE CANCER NETWORK 2008).

Work-Ups

▦ Each follow-up examination should include a complete history and physical examination, a pelvic exam, and Pap smear at each visit.

▦ CA-125 should be tested at each visit if the level is initially elevated (Grade B). Close to 90% of recurrences were noted with an elevated CA-125 prior to clinical or radiological confirmation of disease (Level IV) (HEFLER et al. 2000).

▦ Imaging studies (including annual chest X-ray, CT of the abdomen and pelvis, and PET/CT scan) can be considered if clinically necessary. Laboratory tests, including complete blood count and serum chemistry, can be done if indicated (Grade D) (NATIONAL COMPREHENSIVE CANCER NETWORK 2008).

Table 22.4. Follow-up schedule

Interval	Frequency
First 2 years	Every 2–4 months
Years 3–5	Every 6 months
Over 5 years	Annually

References

Aabo K, Adams M, Adnitt P et al. (1998) Chemotherapy in advanced ovarian cancer: four systematic meta-analyses of individual patient data from 37 randomized trials. Advanced Ovarian Cancer Trialists' Group. Br J Cancer 78:1479–1487

Alberts DS, Liu PY, Hannigan EV, O'Toole R, Williams SD, Young JA, Franklin EW, Clarke-Pearson DL, Malviya VK, DuBeshter B (1996) Intraperitoneal cisplatin plus intravenous cyclophosphamide versus intravenous cisplatin plus intravenous cyclophosphamide for stage III ovarian cancer. N Engl J Med 335:1950–1955

Alvarado-Cabrero I, Young RH, Vamvakas EC, Scully RE (1999) Carcinoma of the fallopian tube: a clinicopathological study of 105 cases with observations on staging and prognostic factors. Gynecol Oncol 72:367–379

Armstrong DK, Bundy B, Wenzel L, Huang HQ, Baergen R, Lele S, Copeland LJ, Walker JL, Burger RA (2006) Gynecologic Oncology Group. Intraperitoneal cisplatin and paclitaxel in ovarian cancer. N Engl J Med 354:34–43

Asmussen M, Kaern J, Kjoerstad K, Wright PB, Abeler V (1988) Primary adenocarcinoma localized to the fallopian tubes: report on 33 cases. Gynecol Oncol 30:183–186

Aziz S, Kuperstein G, Rosen B, Cole D, Nedelcu R, McLaughlin J, Narod SA (2001) A genetic epidemiological study of carcinoma of the fallopian tube. Gynecol Oncol 80:341–345

Barakat RR, Rubin SC, Saigo PE et al. (1991) Cisplatin-based combination chemotherapy in carcinoma of the fallopian tube. Gynecol Oncol 42:156–160

Bell J, Brady MF, Young RC, Lage J, Walker JL, Look KY, Rose GS, Spirtos NM; Gynecologic Oncology Group (2006) Randomized phase III trial of three versus six cycles of adjuvant carboplatin and paclitaxel in early stage epithelial ovarian carcinoma: a Gynecologic Oncology Group study. Gynecol Oncol 102:432–439. Epub 2006 Jul 24

Benedet JL, White GW, Fairey RN, Boyes DA (1977) Adenocarcinoma of the fallopian tube–Experience with 41 patients. Obstet Gynecol 50:654–657

Bolis G, Colombo N, Pecorelli S et al. (1995) Adjuvant treatment for early epithelial ovarian cancer: results of two randomised clinical trials comparing cisplatin to no further treatment or chromic phosphate (32P). GICOG: Gruppo Interregionale Collaborativo in Ginecologia Oncologica. Ann Oncol 6:887–893

Brown MD, Kohorn EI, Kapp DS, Schwartz PE, Merino M (1985) Fallopian tube carcinoma. Int J Radiat Oncol Biol Phys 11:583–590

Carey MS, Dembo AJ, Simm JE, Fyles AW, Treger T, Bush RS (1993) Testing the validity of a prognostic classification in patients with surgically optimal ovarian carcinoma: a 15-year review. Int J Gynecol Cancer 3:24–35

Castellucci P, Perrone AM, Picchio M, Ghi T, Farsad M, Nanni C, Messa C, Meriggiola MC, Pelusi G, Al-Nahhas A, Rubello D, Fazio F, Fanti S (2007) Diagnostic accuracy of 18F-FDG PET/CT in characterizing ovarian lesions and staging ovarian cancer: correlation with transvaginal ultrasonography, computed tomography, and histology. Nucl Med Commun 28:589–595

Chan JK, Tian C, Monk BJ, Herzog T, Kapp DS, Bell J, Young RC (2008) Prognostic factors for high-risk early stage epithelial ovarian cancer: a gynecologic oncology group study. Cancer. Epub 2008 Mar 17

Chen M, Wang WC, Zhou C, Zhou NN, Cai K, Yang ZH, Zhao WF, Li SY, Li GZ (2006) Differentiation between malignant and benign ovarian tumors by magnetic resonance imaging. Chin Med Sci J 21:270–275

Chiara S, Conte P, Franzone P et al. (1994) High-risk early stage ovarian cancer. Randomized clinical trial comparing cisplatin plus cyclophosphamide versus whole abdominal radiotherapy. Am J Clin Oncol 17:72–76

Cooper BC, Sood AK, Davis CS, Ritchie JM, Sorosky JI, Anderson B, Buller RE (2002) Preoperative CA 125 levels: an independent prognostic factor for epithelial ovarian cancer. Obstet Gynecol 100:59–64

Cormio G, Maneo A, Gabriele A, Rota SM, Lissoni A, Zanetta G (1996) Primary carcinoma of the fallopian tube. A retrospective analysis of 47 patients. Ann Oncol 7:271–275

Cormio G, Maneo A, Gabriele A et al. (1997) Treatment of fallopian tube carcinoma with cyclophosphamide, adriamycin, and cisplatin. Am J Clin Oncol 20:143–145

Dembo AJ, Bush RS, Beale FA, Bean HA, Pringle JF, Sturgeon J, Reid JG (1979) Ovarian carcinoma: improved survival following abdominopelvic irradiation in patients with a completed pelvic operation. Am J Obstet Gynecol 134:793–800

Di Re E, Grosso G, Raspagliesi F, Baiocchi G (1996) Fallopian tube cancer: incidence and role of lymphatic spread. Gynecol Oncol 62:199–202

Einhorn N, Sjövall K, Knapp RC, Hall P, Scully RE, Bast RC Jr, Zurawski VR Jr (1992) Prospective evaluation of serum CA 125 levels for early detection of ovarian cancer. Obstet Gynecol 80:14–18

Elit L, Oliver TK, Covens A, Kwon J, Fung MF, Hirte HW, Oza AM (2007) Intraperitoneal chemotherapy in the first-line treatment of women with stage III epithelial ovarian cancer: a systematic review with metaanalyses. Cancer 109:692–702. Review

Greer BE, Bundy BN, Ozols RF, Fowler JM, Clarke-Pearson D, Burger RA, Mannel R, DeGeest K, Hartenbach EM, Baergen RN, Copeland LJ (2005) Implications of second-look laparotomy in the context of optimally resected stage III ovarian cancer: a non-randomized comparison using an explanatory analysis: a Gynecologic Oncology Group study. Gynecol Oncol 99:71–79

Hannigan EV, Green S, Alberts DS, O'Toole R, Surwit E (1993) Results of a Southwest Oncology Group phase III trial of carboplatin plus cyclophosphamide versus cisplatin plus cyclophosphamide in advanced ovarian cancer. Oncology 50 (Suppl 2):2–9

Hefler LA, Rosen AC, Graf AH, Lahousen M, Klein M, Leodolter S, Reinthaller A, Kainz C, Tempfer CB (2000) The clinical value of serum concentrations of cancer antigen 125 in patients with primary fallopian tube carcinoma: a multicenter study. Cancer 89:1555–1560

Henrich W, Fotopoulou C, Fuchs I, Wolf C, Schmider A, Denkert C, Lichtenegger W, Sehouli J (2007) Value of preoperative transvaginal sonography (TVS) in the description of tumor pattern in ovarian cancer patients: results of a prospective study. Anticancer Res 27:4289–4294

Hinton A, Bea C, Winfield AC et al. (1988) Carcinoma of the fallopian tube. Urol Radiol 10:113–115

Hoskins WJ, McGuire WP, Brady MF, Homesley HD, Creasman WT, Berman M, Ball H, Berek JS (1994) The effect of diameter of largest residual disease on survival after primary cytoreductive surgery in patients with suboptimal residual epithelial ovarian carcinoma. Am J Obstet Gynecol 170:974–979; discussion 979–980

Kawakami S, Togashi K, Kimura I et al. (1993) Primary malignant tumor of the fallopian tube: appearance at CT and MR imaging. Radiology 186:503–508

Klaassen D, Shelley W, Starreveld A et al. (1988) Early stage ovarian cancer: a randomized clinical trial comparing whole abdominal radiotherapy, melphalan, and intraperitoneal chromic phosphate: a National Cancer Institute of Canada Clinical Trials Group report. J Clin Oncol 6:1254–1263

Klein M, Rosen AC, Lahousen M, Graf AH, Rainer A (1999) Lymphadenectomy in primary carcinoma of the fallopian tube. Cancer Lett 147:63–66

Kosary C, Trimble EL (2002) Treatment and survival for women with fallopian tube carcinoma: a population-based study. Gynecol Oncol 86:190–191

Kurachi H, Maeda T, Murakami T, Tsuda K, Narumi Y, Nakamura H, Miyake A, Murata Y (1999) A case of fallopian tube carcinoma: successful preoperative diagnosis with MR imaging. Radiat Med 17:63–66

Kurtz AB, Tsimikas JV, Tempany CM, Hamper UM, Arger PH, Bree RL, Wechsler RJ, Francis IR, Kuhlman JE, Siegelman ES, Mitchell DG, Silverman SG, Brown DL, Sheth S, Coleman BG, Ellis JH, Kurman RJ, Caudry DJ, McNeil BJ (1999) Diagnosis and staging of ovarian cancer: comparative values of Doppler and conventional US, CT, and MR imaging correlated with surgery and histopathologic analysis–report of the Radiology Diagnostic Oncology Group. Radiology 212:19–27

Markman M, Bundy BN, Alberts DS, Fowler JM, Clark-Pearson DL, Carson LF, Wadler S, Sickel J (2001) Phase III trial of standard-dose intravenous cisplatin plus paclitaxel versus moderately high-dose carboplatin followed by intravenous paclitaxel and intraperitoneal cisplatin in small-volume stage III ovarian carcinoma: an intergroup study of the Gynecologic Oncology Group, Southwestern Oncology Group, and Eastern Cooperative Oncology Group. J Clin Oncol 19:1001–1007

McGuire WP, Hoskins WJ, Brady MF, Kucera PR, Partridge EE, Look KY, Clarke-Pearson DL, Davidson M (1996) Cyclophosphamide and cisplatin compared with paclitaxel and cisplatin in patients with stage III and stage IV ovarian cancer. N Engl J Med 334:1–6

Morris M, Gershenson DM, Burke TW, Kavanagh JJ, Silva EG, Wharton JT (1990) Treatment of fallopian tube carcinoma with cisplatin, doxorubicin, and cyclophosphamide. Obstet Gynecol 76:1020–1024

Nagao S, FUjiwara K, Ohishi R, Nakanishi Y, Iwasa N, Shimizu M, Goto T, Shimoya K (2008) Combination chemotherapy of intraperitoneal carboplatin and intravenous paclitaxel in suboptimally debulked epithelial ovarian cancer. Int J Gynecol Cancer. Epub 2008 Feb 15

National Cancer Institute, Division of Cancer Prevention and Control (1986) Cancer statistics review, NIH publication no. 87-2789.National Cancer Institute, Bethesda, MD

National Comprehensive Cancer Network (2008) Clinical practice guidelines in oncology: Ovarian cancer. Version I.2008. Available at http://www.nccn.org/professionals/physician_gls/PDF/ovarian.pdf . Accessed on March 30, 2008

Pectasides D, Barbounis V, Sintila A et al. (1994) Treatment of primary fallopian tube carcinoma with cisplatin-containing chemotherapy. Am J Clin Oncol 17:68–71

Peters WA, Anderson WA, Hopkins MP, Kumar NB, Morley GW (1988) Prognostic features of carcinoma of the fallopian tube. Cancer 71:757–762

Pickel H, Lahousen M, Petru E, Stettner H, Hackl A, Kapp K, Winter R (1999) Consolidation radiotherapy after carboplatin-based chemotherapy in radically operated advanced ovarian cancer. Gynecol Oncol 72:215–219

Puls LE, Davey DD, DePriest PD, Gallion HH, van Nagell JR Jr, Hunter JE, Pavlik EJ (1993) Immunohistochemical staining for CA-125 in fallopian tube carcinomas. Gynecol Oncol 48:360–363

Risum S, Høgdall C, Loft A, Berthelsen AK, Høgdall E, Nedergaard L, Lundvall L, Engelholm SA (2007) The diagnostic value of PET/CT for primary ovarian cancer – a prospective study. Gynecol Oncol 105:145–149. Epub 2007 Jan 16

Rose PG, Piver MS, Tsukada Y (1990) Fallopian tube cancer. The Roswell Park experience. Cancer 66:2661–2667

Rosen AC, Klein M, Lahousen M, Graf AH, Rainer A, Vavra N (1993) Primary carcinoma of the fallopian tube–A retrospective analysis of 115 patients. Br J Cancer 68:605–609

Sedlis A (1978) Carcinoma of the fallopian tube. Surg Clin North Am 58:121–129

Sell A, Bertelsen K, Andersen JE et al. (1990) Randomized study of whole-abdomen irradiation versus pelvic irradiation plus cyclophosphamide in treatment of early ovarian cancer. Gynecol Oncol 37:367–373

Smith JP, Rutledge FN, Delclos L (1975) Postoperative treatment of early cancer of the ovary: a random trial between postoperative irradiation and chemotherapy. Natl Cancer Inst Monogr 42:149–153

Stirling D, Evans DG, Pichert G, et al. (2005) Screening for familial ovarian cancer: failure of current protocols to detect ovarian cancer at an early stage according to the International Federation of Gynecology and Obstetrics system. J Clin Oncol 23:5588–5596

Tamini HK, Figge DC (1981) Adenocarcinoma of the uterine tube. Potential for lymph node metastases. Am J Obstet Gynecol 141:132–137

Takeshima N, Hasumi K (2000) Treatment of fallopian tube cancer. Review of the literature. Arch Gynecol Obstet 264:13–19. Review

Trimbos JB, Vergote I, Bolis G, Vermorken JB, Mangioni C, Madronal C, Franchi M, Tateo S, Zanetta G, Scarfone G, Giurgea L, Timmers P, Coens C, Pecorelli S; EORTC-ACTION collaborators. European Organisation for Research and Treatment of Cancer-Adjuvant Chemo-Therapy in Ovarian Neoplasm (2003) Impact of adjuvant chemotherapy and surgical staging in early-stage ovarian carcinoma: European Organisation for Research and Treatment of Cancer-Adjuvant Chemotherapy in Ovarian Neoplasm trial. J Natl Cancer Inst 95(2):113–125

Wagenaar HC, Pecorelli S, Vergote I, Curran D, Wagener DJ, Kobierska A, Bolis G, Bokkel-Huinink WT, Lacave AJ, Madronal C, Forn M, de Oliveira CF, Mangioni C, Nooij MA, Goupil A, Kerbrat P, Marth CH, Tumolo S, Herben MG, Zanaboni F, Vermorken JB. Phase II study of a combination of cyclophosphamide, adriamycin and cisplatin in advanced fallopian tube carcinoma. An EORTC gynecological cancer group study. European Organization for Research and Treatment of Cancer. Eur J Gynaecol Oncol 22:187–193

Wang PH, Lee RC, Chao KC, Chao HT, Yuan CC, Ng HAT (1998) Preoperative diagnosis of primary fallopian tube carcinoma by magnetic resonance imaging: a case report. Zhonghua Yi Xue Za Zhi (Taipei) 61):755–759

Winter WE 3rd, Maxwell GL, Tian C, Sundborg MJ, Rose GS, Rose PG, Rubin SC, Muggia F, McGuire WP; Gynecologic Oncology Group (2008) Tumor residual after surgical cytoreduction in prediction of clinical outcome in stage IV epithelial ovarian cancer: a Gynecologic Oncology Group Study. J Clin Oncol 26:83–89. Epub 2007 Nov 19

Wolfson AH, Tralins KS, Greven KM, Kim RY, Corn BW, Kuettel MR, Phillippart C, Raub WA, Randall ME (1998) Adenocarcinoma of the fallopian tube: Results of a multi-institutional retrospective analysis of 72 patients. Int J Radiat Oncol Biol Phys 40:71–76

Yamamoto K, Katoh S, Nakayama S, Kijima S, Takahashi K, Murao F, Kitao M (1988) Ultrasonic evaluation of fallopian tube carcinoma. Gynecol Obstet Invest 25:202–208

Yazbek J, Raju SK, Ben-Nagi J, Holland TK, Hillaby K, Jurkovic D (2008) Effect of quality of gynaecological ultrasonography on management of patients with suspected ovarian cancer: a randomised controlled trial. Lancet Oncol 9:124–131

Young RC, Walton LA, Ellenberg SS, Homesley HD, Wilbanks GD, Decker DG, Miller A, Park R, Major F Jr (1990) Adjuvant therapy in stage I and stage II epithelial ovarian cancer. Results of two prospective randomized trials. N Engl J Med 322:1021–1027

Young RC, Brady MF, Nieberg RK, Long HJ, Mayer AR, Lentz SS, Hurteau J, Alberts DS (2003) Adjuvant treatment for early ovarian cancer: a randomized phase III trial of intraperitoneal 32P or intravenous cyclophosphamide and cisplatin – a gynecologic oncology group study. J Clin Oncol 21:4350–4355

Zurawski VR Jr, Broderick SF, Pickens P, Knapp RC, Bast RC Jr (1987) Serum CA 125 levels in a group of nonhospitalized women: relevance for the early detection of ovarian cancer. Obstet Gynecol 69:606–611

Endometrial Cancer

23

Khai Mun Lee

CONTENTS

K. Mun Lee, MD
Department of Radiation Oncology, National University Cancer Institute of Singapore, National University Health System, National University of Singapore, 5 Lower Kent Ridge Road, Singapore 119074, Singapore

Introduction and Objectives

Endometrial cancer is the most common gynecological cancer in the United States, and its incidence is expected to rise worldwide. Approximately 70%–80% of patients with endometrial cancer present with FIGO stage I disease confined to the uterus. Surgery is the mainstay of evaluation for risk of extra-uterine spread as well as definitive treatment. Multidisciplinary management, including radiation therapy, plays an important role as adjuvant treatment for patients with high risk of recurrence determined by surgical-pathological staging. In addition, patients who are medically or surgically inoperable can also be treated with radiotherapy with either radical or palliative intent.

This chapter examines:

● Recommendations for diagnosis and staging procedures
● The staging systems and prognostic factors
● Treatment recommendations as well as the supporting scientific evidence, including the complementary role of surgical staging and pelvic lymph node dissection
● The role of adjuvant external pelvic radiotherapy and vaginal-cuff brachytherapy, as well as radiation techniques
● The role of chemotherapy and hormonal therapy in advanced disease
● Palliative radiation for symptomatic control in advanced diseases
● Radiation-induced side effects and complications
● Follow-up care and surveillance of survivors

23.1 Diagnosis, Staging, and Prognoses

23.1.1 Diagnosis

Initial Evaluation

■ Diagnosis and evaluation of endometrial cancer start with a complete history and physical examination (H&P). Attention should be paid to duration and severity of disease-related signs and symptoms, especially vaginal bleeding, the most commonly observed presenting sign of endometrial cancer.

■ Known risk factors, including obesity, hypertension, diabetes mellitus, history of unopposed estrogen use or endometrial atypical hyperplasia, and past history of breast cancer and treatment with tamoxifen, are pertinent to endometrial adenocarcinoma and should be recorded.

■ Thorough physical examination should be performed with attention to the abdomen, pelvic examination of the cervix and vagina, and palpation of lymph nodes in the inguinal and supraclavicular regions.

Laboratory Tests

■ Initial laboratory tests should include a complete blood count, basic blood chemistry, renal function tests, liver function tests, and alkaline phosphatase (Table 23.1).

Imaging Studies

■ Transvaginal ultrasound for assessment of endometrial thickness is usually recommended for initial diagnosis and evaluation (Grade B). The results of a Nordic multicenter study showed that the risk of finding pathologic endometrium at curettage when the endometrium was ≤4 mm as measured by transvaginal ultrasonography was 5.5%. Using a threshold of 5 mm for women presenting with postmenopausal bleeding, this procedure has a sensitivity of 94% and specificity of 78% for endometrial cancer (Level III) (KARLSSON et al. 1995).

■ CT of the abdomen and pelvis is recommended to assess extra-uterine disease and regional lymph node involvement if locally advanced disease is suspected (Grade B). CT is not routinely recommended for patients with clinical stage I disease

Table 23.1. Imaging and laboratory work-ups for esophageal cancer

Imaging studies	Laboratory tests
– Transvaginal ultrasound	– Complete blood count
– CT of pelvis and abdomen	– Serum chemistry
– MRI of pelvis (if indicated)	– Renal function tests
– Chest X-ray and/or	– Liver function tests
– CT of thorax	– Alkaline phosphatase
– Bone scan (optional)	

when surgery is planned. However, CT scan has limited value in evaluating the extent of myometrial invasion of the tumor and detection of minor parametrial, lymph nodal, or local extrauterine invasion (Level IV) (DORE et al. 1987).

■ Like CT of the pelvis, MRI is not routinely recommended for patients with clinical stage I disease when surgery is planned. MRI of the pelvis is recommended for assessment of the extent of primary tumor if local invasion into adjacent pelvic organs is suspected (Grade B). MRI with IV contrast is more accurate for detecting myometrial invasion and cervical involvement (i.e., FIGO stage II diseases). The sensitivity, specificity, and diagnostic accuracy for evaluation of myometrial invasion were 87%, 91%, and 89%, respectively; those for cervical infiltration were 80%, 96%, and 92%, respectively. However, the sensitivity was 50% for lymph node assessment (Level III) (MANFREDI et al. 2004).

■ Chest X-ray is recommended to exclude lung metastasis. CT scan of the thorax can be ordered if the result of the chest X-ray is equivocal.

■ Bone scan is not routinely indicated except in patients with elevated alkaline phosphatase or if bone pain is reported.

Pathology

■ Tissue diagnosis is imperative prior to the initiation of any treatment for confirmation of endometrial cancer that comprises mainly endometrioid carcinoma (75%–80%), histological grading of tumor, and exclusion of the more aggressive sub-types, such as papillary serous carcinoma (<10%), clear cell carcinoma (<5%), and uterine sarcoma (<5%).

■ Tissue for pathology diagnosis can be obtained by standard dilatation and curettage (D&C), Pipelle biopsy, or hysteroscopic biopsy of the endometrium.

■ Treatment decision and prognosis are often determined by pathological diagnosis, including differentiation in addition to tumor stage.

23.1.2 Staging

■ Complete surgical staging, including selective pelvic and para-aortic lymph node dissection or sampling, is recommended by the 1988 International Federation of Gynecology and Obstetrics (FIGO) staging system for endometrial cancer. The FIGO staging is based on the surgical and pathological findings. The value of lymphadenectomy and the extent of lymphadenectomy are debatable; however, lymphadenectomy is of treatment value for endometrial cancer.

- The 1988 International Federation of Gynecology and Obstetrics staging system is the most commonly used based on surgical-pathologic tumor assessment (Table 23.2).

23.1.3 Prognostic Factors

- The prognosis of patients with endometrial cancer is directly related to age, tumor stage, including the extent of myometrial invasion, histological grade, capillary space invasion, and cell type (GOG, Level III) (MORROW et al. 1991), (Level IV) (GREVEN et al. 1997).

Table 23.2. Federation of Gynecology and Obstetrics (FIGO) surgical staging system for endometrial carcinoma (1988)

Stage and Grade	Description
IA (G1,2,3)	Tumor limited to endometrium
IB (G1,2,3)	Invasion limited to <50% of the myometrium
IC (G1,2,3)	Invasion of >50% of the myometrium
IIA (G1,2,3)	Endocervical glandular involvement only
IIB (G1,2,3)	Cervical stromal invasion
IIIA (G1,2,3)	Tumor invades serosa and/or adnexa and/or positive peritoneal cytology
IIIB (G1,2,3)	Vaginal metastases
IIIC (G1,2,3)	Metastases to pelvic and/or para-aortic lymph nodes
IVA (G1,2,3)	Tumor invasion to bladder and/or bowel mucosa
IVB (G1,2,3)	Distant metastases including intra-abdominal and/or inguinal lymph nodes
FIGO histologic grading	
G1	<5% non-squamous or non-morular solid growth pattern
G2	5%–50% non-squamous or non-morular solid growth pattern
G3	>50% non-squamous or non-morular solid growth pattern

- Myometrial invasion and histological grade are strongly correlated, but both have been shown to be independent prognostic factors for tumor recurrence and patient survival (GOG, Level III) (MORROW et al. 1991). Deep myometrial invasion, especially into the outer one third of the myometrium, is particularly associated with higher recurrence rate. Furthermore, the pattern of myometrial invasion is of prognostic significance: diffuse infiltration into the deep myometrium carries worse prognosis than tumor expansion into the myometrium (Level IV) (SUZUKI et al. 2003). Results from most studies demonstrated that the histological grade is of greater significance than the depth of myometrial invasion in predicting the treatment outcome.

- The risk of regional lymph node metastases is a direct function of tumor stage, as well as depth of myometrial invasion and tumor grade in stage I disease: The probability for pelvic lymph node metastases is 0%, 3%, and 18% for patients with grade 1 disease without myometrial invasion, myometrial invasion of < 50% or grade 2/3 disease, and deep invasion, respectively (GOG, Level III) (CREASEMAN et al. 1987).

- Lymphovascular space invasion (LVSI) is of prognostic significance and is associated with lymph node metastasis and distant recurrence. The 5-year recurrence rates for stage I-III endometrial cancer patients with and without LVSI were approximately 40% and 20%, respectively, and those for stage I patients were approximately 30% and 15%, respectively (Level IV) (BRIËT et al. 2005).

23.2 Treatment of Early-Stage Endometrial Cancer

23.2.1 General Principles

- Total abdominal hysterectomy and bilateral salpingoooophorectomy (TAH-BSO) are the mainstay of clinical management for the complete extirpation of tumor, as well as pathological assessment of tumor extent and risk factors for recurrence (Grade A). Patients with FIGO stage I–II endometrial cancer have highly curable tumors with overall and disease-free survival rates at 5 years in the order of 75%–85% and 65%–80%, respectively.

- Adjuvant radiation therapy can be considered in patients deemed at risk of recurrence based on surgical-pathological factors (Grade B). The role of adjuvant radiotherapy with either external-beam pelvic irradiation, brachytherapy, or a combination is to improve locoregional tumor control at the pelvis and vagina. It would be just as important to identify patients with low risk of recurrence so as to avoid irradiation and the attending side effects with little gain.
- Patients who are medically unfit for surgery should be considered for radical radiotherapy involving external-beam pelvic irradiation and brachytherapy (Grade B).
- The role of chemotherapy in the management of early-stage endometrial cancer is investigational and is not routinely recommended (Grade B). However, for histologically aggressive tumors (e.g., papillary serous and clear cell carcinomas), which carry a high risk of extra-uterine spread, chemotherapy should be considered.

23.2.2 Surgical Resection

- Total abdominal hysterectomy and bilateral salpingooophorectomy (TAH-BSO) are the main treatment modality for stage I and II endometrial cancer.
- For suspected or clinical FIGO stage II disease, radical hysterectomy and bilateral salpingo-oophorectomy (TAH-BSO) should be performed in view of tumor extension to the cervix and possible para-cervical spread. A review of 203 patients with stage II endometrial cancer showed that survival rates by surgical procedure were 79% if simple hysterectomy was used and 94% if radical hysterectomy was used at 5 years and 74% and 94%, respectively, at 10 years (Level IV) (SARTORI et al. 2001). In a more recently published retrospective series from Turkey, patients treated with simple hysterectomy followed by radiation therapy achieved outcomes similar to those who received radical hysterectomy: The 5-year disease-free and overall survival rates for patients treated with simple hysterectomy plus radiation were 81% and 83%, respectively, as compared to 85% and 90%, respectively, for those treated with radical hysterectomy without adjuvant therapy. Survival rates were not significantly different from both groups (Level IV) (AYHAN et al. 2004).

- Pelvic and para-aortic lymph node dissection and inspection of pelvic and intra-abdominal structures, as well as peritoneal lavage, or cytology are needed for complete surgical staging. In addition to staging and prognostication, there are reports of therapeutic benefits of pelvic and para-aortic lymphadenectomy (Level IV) (KILGORE et al.1995; PODRATZ et al. 1998; MARIANI et al. 2000a). However, its value in stage I disease with grade 1 and 2 pathology has been questioned (Level IV) (MARIANI et al. 2000b).
- Currently, there is no strong evidence to recommend the extent of lymphadenectomy. The extent of lymphadenectomy often varies with institutional practice and also takes into consideration the patient's performance status to undergo more extensive surgery.

23.2.3 Adjuvant Radiotherapy

- Adjuvant radiotherapy should be considered for all patients with outer myometrial invasion and/or grade 3 histology to improve locoregional control (Grade C). The efficacy of adjuvant radiation therapy for local control has been demonstrated in three major prospective randomized trials; however, a survival benefit has not been confirmed. The Norwegian trial published by AALDERS et al. (1980) randomized 540 patients with stage I endometrial cancer after hysterectomy and postoperative vaginal brachytherapy to observation or adjuvant pelvis radiotherapy. The local recurrence rate was reduced with the addition of pelvic radiation (2% versus 5%); however, no difference in overall survival was observed (Level I). Subgroup analysis with a limited number of patients with deep myometrial invasion with grade 3 pathology revealed that these patients may benefit from adjuvant pelvic irradiation for both local control and overall survival. In the Postoperative Radiation Therapy in Endometrial Carcinoma (PORTEC) trial, patients with stage 1 endometrial cancer (G1 with >50% myometrial invasion, G2 with any myometrial invasion and G3 with <50% myometrial invasion) were randomized to adjuvant pelvic radiotherapy or observation after TAH-BSO without lymphadenectomy. The results revealed that patients who received adjuvant radiation achieved a significantly reduced locoregional recurrence rate of 4% at 5 years after treatment, as compared to 14% in the observation arm. However, the overall survival rates were not significantly different (Level I) (CREUTZBERG et al. 2000). In a subsequent report of the PORTEC trial, the 8-year actuarial overall survival rates were reportedly 71% and 77%, respectively, for the radiation and control groups ($p=0.18$). The majority of the locoregional relapses were located in the vagina, mainly in the vaginal vault, and survival after treatment for recurrence was significantly better in the patient group without previous radiation. Treatment for vaginal relapse was effective, with 89% complete response and 65% 5-year survival in the control group, while there was no difference in survival between patients with pelvic relapse and those with distant metastases. The author concluded that as pelvic radiation was shown to improve locoregional control significantly, but without a survival benefit, its use should be limited to those patients who had 15% or more risk (i.e., high-risk category with two of the three major risk factors including grade 3, outer 50% myometrial invasion, and age 60 or above) for recurrence in order to maximize local control and relapse-free survival (Level I) (CREUTZBERG et al. 2003). The results from a randomized trial from GOG demonstrated very similar findings to those of the PORTEC study. Patients with stage IB, IC, or IIA were differentiated according to the characteristics of the disease and patient (Table 23.3) and were treated with TAH-BAO with lymphadenectomy followed by observation or adjuvant radiation. The overall cumulative incidence recurrence rates at 2 years was 12% in the observation group and 3% in the radiotherapy group. The reduction on recurrence rate with adjuvant radiotherapy was more evident for the high-intermediate risk patients from 26% to 6%. However, the estimated overall survival at 4 years was not significantly different (GOG 99, Level I) (KEYS et al. 2004).

Table 23.3. Risk groups defined by the GOG-99 trial

Risk factors	High-intermediate risk group
– Age: <50 vs. <70 vs. >70 – Grade: grade 1 vs. 2–3 – Depth of invasion: inner 2/3 or outer 1/3 – Lymphovascular space invasion: absent vs. present	– Age ≥70 and one other factor – Age ≥50 and two other factors – Any age and all other factors

- Adjuvant radiotherapy should be offered to patients with FIGO stage II disease, especially those with features of cervical stromal invasion, capillary-lymphatic space invasion, and older age group of >65 years in view of the higher risk of relapse (Grade B). The disease-free and overall survival after surgery and adjuvant radiation therapy is approximately 70% and 80%, respectively, according to the results from a number of retrospective trials using combined treatment (Level IV) (LANCIANO et al. 1990; FELTMATE et al. 1999; PITSON et al. 2002).

- A more recently published large retrospective population-based study on more than 21,000 patients suggested a survival benefit of 10%–20% at 10 years with the use of adjuvant radiotherapy for stage IC, grade 1, and grade 3 or 4 endometrial cancer (SEER, Level IV) (LEE et al. 2006).

External-Beam Radiation Therapy

- Postoperative irradiation is usually given using a fractionated course of external-beam radiotherapy (45 Gy to 50.4 Gy at 1.8 Gy per daily fraction over 25–28 fractions to the pelvis). External-beam pelvic radiotherapy with 8–10 MV photons is usually given using the standard four-field technique encompassing the entire pelvis from the L5-S1 junction superiorly to the lower borders of the obturator forminae inferiorly targeting the previous site of the uterus and adnexae, parametria, upper two-thirds of the vagina, and regional lymphatics (Fig. 23.1a,b).

Intensity-Modulated Radiation Therapy

- Intensity-modulated radiation therapy (IMRT) can be considered for adjuvant treatment of endometrial cancer if available (Grade B). Results from treatment planning studies have demonstrated the advantage of IMRT over conventional radiotherapy: the dose to critical organs, including the small bowel, rectum, and bone marrow, can be significantly reduced (Level III) (HERON et al. 2003; LUJAN et al. 2003; MUNDT et al. 2002). Preliminary results from clinical trials have demonstrated that modest reduction of radiation-induced acute and late toxicities can be expected with the use of IMRT for pelvic irradiation for gynecologic malignancies (Level III) (BRIXEY et al. 2002; MUNDT et al. 2002, 2003).

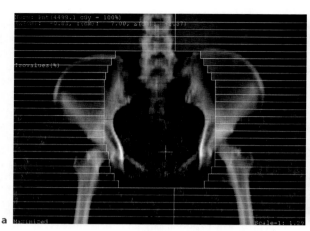 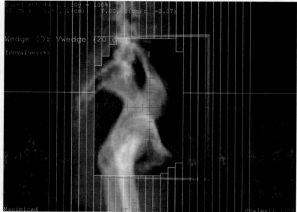

Fig. 23.1a,b. Digitally reconstructed radiographs of anteroposterior (**a**) and lateral pelvic (**b**) fields

■ Figures 23.2 and 23.3 depict the comparison of whole pelvic radiation therapy plans using IMRT and conventional radiation for a representative patient. Doses to the small bowel and bone marrow were significantly reduced with the use of IMRT in the pelvis irradiation.

Vaginal-Cuff Brachytherapy

■ If the pelvic lymph node involvement has been surgically excluded or the risk is low, radiation therapy can be delivered by vaginal-cuff brachytherapy using a cylindrical applicator with low dose rate (LDR) or high dose rate (HDR) irradiation (Grade B). The long-term results from a prospective trial revealed that for patients with stage I, grade 1–2, with < 50% myometrial invasion treated with hysterectomy (without formal staging pelvic and periaortic lymph node sampling or lymphadenectomy) and postoperative vaginal brachytherapy without external-beam radiation, an overall survival of close to 95% can be expected (Level III) (ELTABBAKH et al. 1997). The findings from a similarly arranged prospective study of patients with surgically staged IB, IC and II endometrial cancer using HDR brachytherapy also revealed that relatively optimal outcome can be expected: the 5-year overall and disease-free survivals both approached 90% (Level III) (HOROWITZ et al. 2002). Similar findings were reported by a large retrospective series of 382 patients with stage IB and IIB diseases that had undergone surgical staging and lymph node sampling (Level IV) (ALEKTIAR et al. 2005).

■ With HDR brachytherapy alone, a wide range of dose and fractions has been used (e.g., 21 Gy in three fractions or 25 Gy in five fractions prescribed at 0.5 cm depth encompassing the upper two-thirds of the vagina). A lower dose of 10–12 Gy in two to three fractions prescribed at 0.5 cm depth is recommended by the American Brachytherapy Society consensus on brachytherapy for endometrial cancer when HDR brachytherapy is combined with external-beam radiotherapy (Level IV).

■ A combination of both external-beam pelvic radiotherapy and of vaginal-cuff brachytherapy is often used depending on the extent of surgical staging performed and the practice favored by individual radiotherapy centers (Grade C). A retrospective study had showed that vaginal-cuff recurrence was significantly higher when adjuvant external-beam radiotherapy was not combined with brachytherapy (Level IV). However, other series have raised questions on the benefit of the brachytherapy boost (Level IV) (GREVEN et al. 1999).

23.2.4 Adjuvant Chemotherapy

■ Adjuvant chemotherapy is not recommended in the treatment of early-stage endometrial cancer, with the exception of those with aggressive histology subtypes (Grade B). The results of a randomized trial from GOG aimed at evaluating the effect of doxorubicin did not demonstrate any survival benefits of doxorubicin-based single-agent adjuvant chemotherapy to high-risk stage I and II endometrial cancer (GOG, Level I) (MORROW et al. 1990).

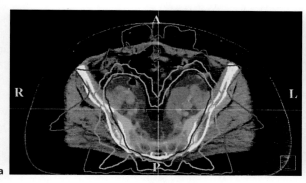
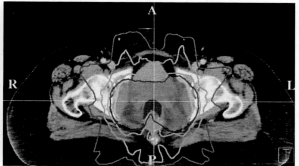

Fig. 23.2a,b. Isodose curves from an IM-WPRT plan superimposed on an axial CT slice through the upper pelvis (**a**) and lower pelvis (**b**). The small bowel and PTV are shaded in orange and green, respectively in (**a**). The bladder, rectum, and PTV are shaded in yellow, light blue, and green, respectively in (**b**). Highlighted are the 100% (*red*), 90% (*green*), 70% (*light blue*), and 50% (*dark blue*) isodose curves. [From Mundt AJ, Lujan AE, Rotmensch J et al. (2002) Intensity-modulated radiotherapy in women with bynecologic malignancies. By permission from publisher]

Fig. 23.3a–c. Axial CT slice for representative patient showing 100%, 70%, 50%, and 40% isodose lines for (**a**) BMS IM-WPRT in which all isodose lines bend medially away from BM, (**b**) IM-WPRT without BM as a constraint, and (**c**) four-field WPRT showing BM almost entirely enclosed by 40% isodose line. PTV shown in green and BM indicated in red. [From Lujan AE, Mundt AJ, Yamada SD et al. (2003) Intensity-modulated radiotherapy as a means of reducing dose to bone marrow in gynecologic patients receiving whole pelvic radiotherapy. By permission from publisher]

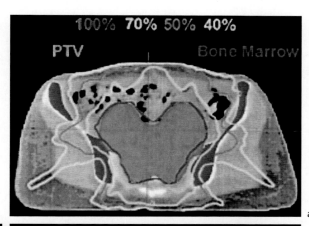
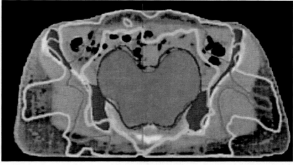
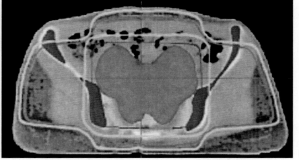

23.2.5 Treatment of Medically Inoperable Disease

■ Definitive radical radiation therapy comprising external-beam irradiation and intracavitary brachytherapy should be offered to patients who have clinically early-stage tumors, but are inoperable for medical reasons (Grade B). Results from a retrospective case-controlled study showed that cancer-specific survival rates of 80%–85% at 5 years can be expected with radiation as exclusive treatment (Level IV) (FISHMAN et al. 1996).

■ External-beam pelvic radiation techniques are similar to those described for adjuvant treatment.

■ Brachytherapy for definitive treatment requires an intra-uterine source channel together with upper vaginal sources for a dose distribution that covers the entire uterus.

Radiotherapy-Induced Side Effects

- Radiotherapy to the pelvic region can result in clinically significant side effects. This is often aggravated when radiotherapy is combined with other modalities of treatment, namely surgery and chemotherapy. For example, routine pelvic lymph-node dissections as part of surgical staging followed by pelvic radiotherapy for patients with high-risk endometrial cancer may result in an increase in risk of lower limb lymphoedema.

- The increasing use of chemotherapy in combination with radiotherapy has also resulted in higher rates of hematological and gastrointestinal toxicities while achieving better tumor control and survival.

- Radiotherapy side effects can be classified as "acute/early," which are common, symptomatically treatable, and usually reversible, or "late," which may be chronic and non-reversible (Table 23.4). Risk of severe late side effects from radiotherapy should not exceed 5% with careful planning and delivery of irradiation.

23.3 Treatment of Locoregionally Advanced Endometrial Cancer

23.3.1 General Principles

- Patients with locally advanced surgical-pathological FIGO stages (III–IVA) require postoperative pelvic irradiation for locoregional control of

disease in view of the higher risk of recurrence (Grade B).

- Patients who have FIGO stage IIIA disease with positive peritoneal cytology may not benefit from adjuvant therapy in the absence of other adverse factors (such as myometrial invasion) (Grade B). Radiation therapy is usually recommended for patients with high-grade stage IIIA disease with serosal or adnexal involvement (Grade C).

- Patients who have unresectable disease (e.g., stage IVA) should be considered for radical radiotherapy with a combination of external-beam radiotherapy and intracavitary brachytherapy as described for those medically unfit for surgery.

- Para-aortic lymphadenopathy should be treated with extended–field radiotherapy to include the para-aortic lymphatics.

- Adjuvant chemotherapy with cisplatin and adriamycin should be considered for those with good performance status (Grade A).

23.3.2 Adjuvant Radiotherapy

- Patients with locally advanced surgical-pathological FIGO stages (III–IVA) require postoperative pelvic irradiation for locoregional control of disease in view of the higher risk of recurrence (Grade C). In a retrospective series of 57 patients with pathological stage III disease treated with surgery plus pre- or postoperative radiotherapy, the 5-year overall and disease-free survivals observed for all patients were 43.5 and 46.2%, respectively (Level IV) (GRIGSBY et al. 1987). In

Table 23.4. Potential radiation-induced side effects or complications by site

Sites	Side effects or complications	
Skin	Early:	Erythema, dry and moist desquamation
	Late:	Subcutaneous edema and fibrosis
Bowel	Early:	Acute ileitis, colitis, proctitis (colic and diarrhea)
	Late:	Ulceration, stricture, and fistula
Bladder	Early:	Acute cystitis, urinary tract infection (frequency, urgency, dysuria)
	Late:	Ureteric stricture, chronic cystitis, and bladder fibrosis
Vulva/vagina	Early:	Acute vaginitis, thrush
	Late:	Adhesions, fibrosis, stenosis
Ovary	Early/late:	Radiation-induced menopause

a multicenter retrospective series, 105 patients with stage III endometrial cancer were reviewed. All patients received adjuvant radiotherapy to the pelvis or pelvis and paraaortic regions for pathologically positive paraaortic nodes. The 5-year disease-free survival rate for all patients was 64%, and the overall 5-year pelvic recurrence rate was 21% (Level IV) (GREVEN et al. 1993). Results of a retrospective review from Harvard University demonstrated that pelvic external-beam radiotherapy did not provide any survival benefit for patients with stage IIIA or IIIB diseases; however, stage IIIC patients had increased disease-free survival and a trend for increased survival with pelvic radiation (Level IV) (SCHORGE et al. 1996).

■ Patients who have FIGO stage IIIA disease because of positive peritoneal cytology may not benefit from adjuvant therapy in the absence of other adverse factors (such as adnexal involvement) (Grade B). Results from a number of retrospective studies demonstrated that the outcome of patients with positive peritoneal cytology only (cytologic stage IIIA) assimilated patients with stage I disease (Level IV) (KADAR et al. 1992; KASAMATSU et al. 2003; MARIANI et al. 2002; TEBEU et al. 2004).

■ Postoperative irradiation is usually given using a fractionated course of external-beam radiotherapy (45–50.4 Gy in 25–28 fractions to the pelvis).

■ External-beam pelvic radiotherapy with 8–10 MV photons is usually given using the standard four-field technique encompassing the entire pelvis from the L5-S1 junction superiorly to the lower borders of the obturator forminae inferiorly, targeting the previous site of the uterus and adnexae, parametria, upper two-thirds of the vagina, and regional lymphatics. The treatment technique is similar to that used for early-stage endometrial cancer.

■ A combination of both external-beam pelvic radiotherapy and two to three applications of vaginal-cuff brachytherapy is often used depending on the practice favored by individual radiotherapy centers.

23.3.3 Adjuvant Chemotherapy and Hormonal Therapy

■ Adjuvant doxorubicin-cisplatin-based chemotherapy is recommended for patients with locally advanced endometrial cancer (Grade A). A GOG randomized trial studied the effect of whole abdominopelvic irradiation versus doxorubicin-cisplatin-based chemotherapy for locally advanced (stage III and IV non-metastatic) endometrial cancer. The results found that chemotherapy significantly improved progression-free and overall survival rates, but at the costs of increased toxicities and a higher rate of initial pelvic failure. At 60 months after treatment, 55% of chemotherapy patients were predicted to be alive compared with 42% of irradiated patients (GOG 122, Level I) (RANDALL et al. 2006). A more recent EORTC randomized study for patients with high-risk stage I–III disease reported in abstract form has demonstrated an improved 5-year progression-free survival of 82% with adjuvant chemoradiation over 75% with adjuvant radiotherapy alone. Although doxorubicin-cisplatin-based chemotherapy is effective in improving overall survival of locally advanced endometrial cancer, the sequence of adjuvant radiotherapy, which is significant for improving local control, and adjuvant double-agent chemotherapy has not been addressed.

■ The effect of adjuvant chemotherapy versus adjuvant combined chemoradiation therapy has not been addressed in any prospective randomized clinical trials. An RTOG study has been initiated to compare the outcome of adjuvant chemoradiotherapy and radiation alone.

■ Adjuvant hormonal treatment is not routinely recommended for endometrial cancer (Grade A). Although grades 1 and 2 endometrial cancer are usually positive for progesterone receptors, and more than 20% of metastatic cases of endometrial adenocarcinoma show response to progesterone treatment, the value of adjuvant hormonal treatment on survival has not been demonstrated: The results of a meta-analysis of six randomized trials with more than 3500 patients with endometrial cancer failed to demonstrate a benefit in overall survival for those received progesterone treatment (Level I) (MARTIN-HIRSCH et al. 1996). In addition, a more recently published Cochrane Database Systemic Review also confirmed that post-surgical progesterone treatment has no significant effect on overall survival (Level I) (MARTIN-HIRSCH et al. 2000).

23.4 Treatment of Uterine Sarcoma

23.4.1 General Principles

■ Uterine sarcoma is a group of rare uterine tumors comprising malignant mixed mullerian tumor or carcinosarcoma, leiomyosarcoma, and endometrial stromal sarcoma.

■ Uterine sarcoma is generally considered to be aggressive with a high risk of relapse and metastatic potential favoring the need for adjuvant treatment with pelvic radiation and adriamycin- or ifosfamide-based chemotherapy.

■ Radiotherapy is recommended in the treatment of uterine sarcoma as adjuvant treatment for locoregional control (Grade B). Results from a number of retrospective trials have demonstrated that radiotherapy can reduce pelvic recurrence, especially in locoregionally advanced disease with reported improvement of locoregional control: A prospective randomized trial aimed at determining the efficacy of doxorubicin on uterine sarcoma was conducted between 1973 and 1982. It studied 225 women with stage I or II uterine sarcoma, and patients were randomized to either 60 mg/m^2 of doxorubicin every 3 weeks for eight courses or no further therapy. Adjuvant radiation therapy was optional in the study. The results showed that chemotherapy provided no advantage to the progression-free survival and overall survival. However, those who received radiation therapy had significantly lower locoregional recurrence (Level III) (HORNBACK et al. 1986). Results from a non-randomized series of 60 patients with carcinosarcoma revealed that the addition of radiotherapy significantly reduced the local recurrence rate from 55% to 3%. Adjuvant radiotherapy reduced the risk of distant failure and death in patients with disease confined to the uterus, but did not impact distant recurrence or survival in stage III patients (Level IV) (GERSZTEN et al. 1998). A small retrospective series from Sweden reported an improved outcome in overall survival with the use of adjuvant radiotherapy following surgery for endometrial stromal sarcoma. Adjuvant radiotherapy seems to be of benefit in high-grade tumors, and the 5-year survival rate after surgery and radiation therapy was 73%, which exceeds most reported results (Level IV) (LARSON et al.

1990a). Similar findings were reported in 147 patients with stage I uterine mixed mullerian tumors treated with adjuvant radiation. A lower local failure rate and improved overall survival were demonstrated with surgery followed by combined radiotherapy (intracavitary + external irradiation) as compared to surgery in combination with either intracavitary or external irradiation (Level IV) (LARSON 1990b). However, the effect of adjuvant radiotherapy was not demonstrated in another retrospective review of 208 patients with leiomyosarcoma of the uterus (Level IV) (GIUNTOLI et al. 2003). Although limited evidence has supported the use of adjuvant radiation therapy for locally advanced uterine sarcomas, stage III uterine sarcomas are usually referred for postoperative radiotherapy as well as chemotherapy in view of the high risk of locoregional and systemic relapse.

23.4.2 Adjuvant Radiotherapy

■ Radiotherapy and brachytherapy techniques for uterine sarcoma are similar to those described for endometrial cancer

23.5 Treatment of Recurrent/Metastatic Endometrial Cancer

23.5.1 General Principles

■ Patients with isolated pelvic or vaginal recurrence after previous surgery can be treated with salvaging radical radiation therapy (Grade B). Long-term overall survival rates of isolated lower 1/3 vaginal, vaginal vault, and pelvic recurrences of 50%, 45%, and 24%, respectively, have been reported (Level IV) (POULSON and ROBERTS 1988).

■ Patients with stage IV disease who are symptomatic from distant metastases should be treated systemically with palliative chemotherapy (for aggressive tumors) or hormones (for well-differentiated tumors), e.g., progestins or tamoxifen (Grade A) (KAUPPILA 1989). Chemotherapy regimens usually comprise cisplatin and adriamycin. The addition of paclitaxel to the cisplatin and adriamycin combination has not been shown to be more superior (GOG, Level I) (FLEMING et al. 2004).

■ Symptoms due to locoregional disease, e.g., vaginal bleeding and discharge, can be palliated with local radiotherapy

23.5.2 Radiotherapy Technique

■ Salvage radical radiotherapy for isolated pelvic or vaginal recurrence should be initially targeted at the whole pelvis with a dose of 45–50.4 Gy in 25–28 fractions, as described above, followed by a boost to a total dose of 60–66 Gy to the recurrent tumor using CT-planning 3D conformal technique to limit the dose to adjacent normal organs, such as the bladder, rectum, and small bowels.

■ Patients with advanced disease requiring palliative radiotherapy for control of local symptoms, e.g., bleeding and pain, require a short course of tumor-directed external-beam pelvic radiotherapy to a dose of 30 Gy in ten fractions or equivalent.

■ Vaginal brachytherapy as described above can also be used for palliation with superficial vaginal recurrences.

23.6 Follow-Ups

23.6.1 Post-Treatment Follow-Ups

■ Life-long follow-up after definitive treatment of endometrial cancer is usually indicated for detection of local or distant failures. Follow-up is also necessary for the assessment of long-term treatment-related side effects, such as ileitis, proctitis, bladder fibrosis, lymphoedema, vaginal adhesions, and stenosis.

■ Ideally, patients should have access to a feminine care clinic with trained staff to advise and manage problems related to vaginal care, sexual function, menopausal and fertility issues.

Follow-Up Schedule

■ Follow-ups can be scheduled every 3–6 months for 2 years, then every 6–12 months thereafter (Grade D) (NCCN 2008).

Work-Ups

■ Each follow-up should include a complete history and physical examination, including a pelvic examination. CA-125 can be considered at each follow-up.

■ Vaginal cytology should be checked every 6 months for 2 years, and annually thereafter (Grade D) (NCCN 2008).

■ CT scan of the abdomen and pelvis and chest X-ray can be considered annually during follow-up or ordered based on relevant symptoms and clinical findings.

Table 23.5. Follow-up schedule after treatment for esophageal cancer

Interval	Frequency
First 2 years	Every 3–6 months
Over 2 years	Every 6 months or annually

References

Aalders J, Abeler V, Kolstad P et al (1980) Postoperative external irradiation and prognostic parameters in stage I endometrial carcinoma: clinical and histopathologic study of 540 patients. Obstet Gynecol 56:419–427

Alektiar KM, Venkatraman E, Chi DS et al. (2005) Intravaginal brachytherapy alone for intermediate-risk endometrial cancer. Int J Radiat Oncol Biol Phys 62:111–117

Ayhan A, Taskiran C, Celik C et al (2004) The long-term survival of women with surgical stage II endometrioid type endometrial cancer. Gynecol Oncol 93:9–13

Brixey CJ, Roeske JC, Lujan AE et al (2002) Impact of intensity-modulated radiotherapy on acute hematologic toxicity in women with gynecologic malignancies. Int J Radiat Oncol Biol Phys 54:1388–1396

Briët JM, Hollema H, Reesink N et al (2005) Lymphvascular space involvement: an independent prognostic factor in endometrial cancer. Gynecol Oncol 96:799–804

Creasman WT, Morrow CP, Bundy BN et al (1987) Surgical pathologic spread patterns of endometrial cancer. A Gynecologic Oncology Group Study. Cancer 60[8 Suppl]:2035–2041

Creutzberg CL, van Putten WL, Koper PC et al (2000) Surgery and postoperative radiotherapy versus surgery alone for patients with stage-1 endometrial carcinoma: multicentre randomised trial. PORTEC Study Group. Post Operative

Radiation Therapy in Endometrial Carcinoma. Lancet 355:1404–1411

Creutzberg CL, van Putten WL, Koper PC et al (2003) Survival after relapse in patients with endometrial cancer: results from a randomized trial. Gynecol Oncol 89:201–209

Dore R, Moro G, D'Andrea F et al (1987) CT evaluation of myometrium invasion in endometrial carcinoma. J Comput Assist Tomogr 11:282–289

Eltabbakh GH, Piver MS, Hempling RE et al (1997) Excellent long-term survival and absence of vaginal recurrences in 332 patients with low-risk stage I endometrial adenocarcinoma treated with hysterectomy and vaginal brachytherapy without formal staging lymph node sampling: report of a prospective trial. Int J Radiat Oncol Biol Phys 38:373–380

Feltmate CM, Duska LR, Chang Y et al (1999) Predictors of recurrence in surgical stage II endometrial adenocarcinoma. Gynecol Oncol 73:407–411

Fishman DA, Roberts KB, Chambers JT et al (1996) Radiation therapy as exclusive treatment for medically inoperable patients with stage I and II endometrioid carcinoma with endometrium. Gynecol Oncol 61:189–196

Fleming GF, Filiaci VL, Bentley RC et al (2004) Phase III randomized trial of doxorubicin + cisplatin versus doxorubicin + 24-h paclitaxel + filgrastim in endometrial carcinoma: a Gynecologic Oncology Group study. Ann Oncol 15:1173–1178

Gerszten K, Faul C, Kounelis S et al (1998) The impact of adjuvant radiotherapy on carcinosarcoma of the uterus. Gynecol Oncol 68:8–13

Giuntoli RL 2nd, Metzinger DS, DiMarco CS et al (2003) Retrospective review of 208 patients with leiomyosarcoma of the uterus: prognostic indicators, surgical management, and adjuvant therapy. Gynecol Oncol 89:460–469

Greven KM, Lanciano RM, Corn B et al (1993) Pathologic stage III endometrial carcinoma. Prognostic factors and patterns of recurrence. Cancer 71:3697–3702

Greven KM, Corn BW, Case D et al (1997) Which prognostic factors influence the outcome of patients with surgically staged endometrial cancer treated with adjuvant radiation? Int J Radiat Oncol Biol Phys 39:413–418

Grigsby PW, Perez CA, Kuske RR et al (1987) Results of therapy, analysis of failures, and prognostic factors for clinical and pathologic stage III adenocarcinoma of the endometrium. Gynecol Oncol 27:44–57

Heron DE, Gerszten K, Selvaraj RN et al (2003) Conventional 3D conformal versus intensity-modulated radiotherapy for the adjuvant treatment of gynecologic malignancies: a comparative dosimetric study of dose-volume histograms. Gynecol Oncol 91:39–45

Hornback NB, Omura G, Major FJ (1986) Observations on the use of adjuvant radiation therapy in patients with stage I and II uterine sarcoma. Int J Radiat Oncol Biol Phys 12:2127–2130

Horowitz NS, Peters WA 3rd, Smith MR et al (2002) Adjuvant high dose rate vaginal brachytherapy as treatment of stage I and II endometrial carcinoma. Obstet Gynecol 99:235–240

Kadar N, Homesley HD, Malfetano JH (1992) Positive peritoneal cytology is an adverse factor in endometrial carcinoma only if there is other evidence of extrauterine disease. Gynecol Oncol 46:145–149

Kauppila A (1989) Oestrogen and progestin receptors as prognostic indicators in endometrial cancer. A review of the literature. Acta Oncol 28:561–566

Kasamatsu T, Onda T, Katsumata N et al (2003) Prognostic significance of positive peritoneal cytology in endometrial carcinoma confined to the uterus. Br J Cancer 88:245–250

Karlsson B, Granberg S, Wikland M et al (1995) Transvaginal ultrasonography of the endometrium in women with postmenopausal bleeding–a Nordic multicenter study. Am J Obstet Gynecol 172:1488–1494

Keys HM, Roberts JA, Brunetto VL et al. (2004) A phase III trial of surgery with or without adjunctive external pelvic radiation therapy in intermediate risk endometrial adenocarcinoma: a Gynecologic Oncology Group study. Gynecol Oncol 92:744–751

Kilgore LC, Partridge EE, Alvarez RD et al (1995) Adenocarcinoma of the endometrium: survival comparisons of patients with and without pelvic node sampling. Gynecol Oncol 56:29–33

Lanciano RM, Curran WJ Jr, Greven KM et al (1990) Influence of grade, histologic subtype, and timing of radiotherapy on outcome among patients with stage II carcinoma of the endometrium. Gynecol Oncol 39:368–373

Larson B, Silfverswärd C, Nilsson B et al (1990a) Endometrial stromal sarcoma of the uterus. A clinical and histopathological study. The Radiumhemmet series 1936–1981. Eur J Obstet Gynecol Reprod Biol 35:239–249

Larson B, Silfverswärd C, Nilsson B et al (1990b) Mixed mullerian tumours of the uterus–prognostic factors: a clinical and histopathologic study of 147 cases. Radiother Oncol 17:123–132

Lee CM, Szabo A, Shrieve DC et al. (2006) Frequency and effect of adjuvant radiation therapy among women with stage I endometrial adenocarcinoma. JAMA 295:389–397

Lujan AE, Mundt AJ, Yamada SD et al (2003) Intensity-modulated radiotherapy as a means of reducing dose to bone marrow in gynecologic patients receiving whole pelvic radiotherapy. Int J Radiat Oncol Biol Phys 57:516–521

Manfredi R, Mirk P, Maresca G et al (2004) Local-regional staging of endometrial carcinoma: role of MR imaging in surgical planning. Radiology 231:372–378

Mariani A, Webb MJ, Galli L et al (2000a) Potential therapeutic role of para-aortic lymphadenectomy in node-positive endometrial cancer. Gynecol Oncol 76:348–356

Mariani A, Webb MJ, Keeney GL et al (2000b) Low-risk corpus cancer: is lymphadenectomy or radiotherapy necessary? Am J Obstet Gynecol 182:1506–1519

Mariani A, Webb MJ, Keeney GL et al (2002) Assessment of prognostic factors in stage IIIA endometrial cancer. Gynecol Oncol 86:38–44

Martin-Hirsch PL, Lilford RJ, Jarvis GJ (1996) Adjuvant progestagen therapy for the treatment of endometrial cancer: review and meta-analyses of published randomised controlled trials. Eur J Obstet Gynecol Reprod Biol 65:201–207

Martin-Hirsch PL, Jarvis G, Kitchener H et al (2000) Progestagens for endometrial cancer. Cochrane Database Syst Rev 2000(2):CD001040

Morrow CP, Bundy BN, Homesley HD et al (1990) Doxorubicin as an adjuvant following surgery and radiation therapy in patients with high-risk endometrial carcinoma, stage I and occult stage II: a Gynecologic Oncology Group Study. Gynecol Oncol 36:166–171

Morrow CP, Bundy BN, Kurman RJ et al (1991) Relationship between surgical-pathological risk factors and outcome in clinical stage I and II carcinoma of the endometrium: a Gynecologic Oncology Group study. Gynecol Oncol 40:55–65

Mundt AJ, Lujan AE, Rotmensch J et al (2002) Intensity-modulated whole pelvic radiotherapy in women with gynecologic malignancies. Int J Radiat Oncol Biol Phys 52:1330–1337

Mundt AJ, Mell LK, Roeske JC (2003) Preliminary analysis of chronic gastrointestinal toxicity in gynecology patients treated with intensity-modulated whole pelvic radiation therapy. Int J Radiat Oncol Biol Phys 56:1354–1360

Pitson G, Colgan T, Levin W et al (2002) Stage II endometrial carcinoma: prognostic factors and risk classification in 170 patients. Int J Radiat Oncol Biol Phys 53:862–867

Podratz KC, Mariani A, Webb MJ (1998) Staging and therapeutic value of lymphadenectomy in endometrial cancer. Gynecol Oncol 70:163–164

Poulsen MG, Roberts SJ (1988) The salvage of recurrent endometrial carcinoma in the vagina and pelvis. Int J Radiat Oncol Biol Phys 15:809–813

Randall ME, Filiaci VL, Muss H et al (2006) Randomized phase III trial of whole-abdominal irradiation versus doxorubicin and cisplatin chemotherapy in advanced endometrial carcinoma: a Gynecologic Oncology Group Study. J Clin Oncol 24:36–44

Sartori E, Gadducci A, Landoni F et al (2001) Clinical behavior of 203 stage II endometrial cancer cases: the impact of primary surgical approach and of adjuvant radiation therapy. Int J Gynecol Cancer 11:430–437

Schorge JO, Molpus KL, Goodman A et al (1996) The effect of postsurgical therapy on stage III endometrial carcinoma. Gynecol Oncol 63:34–39

Suzuki C, Matsumoto T, Sonoue H et al (2003) Prognostic significance of the infiltrative pattern invasion in endometrioid adenocarcinoma of the endometrium. Pathol Int 53:495–500

Tebeu PM, Popowski Y, Verkooijen HM et al (2004) Positive peritoneal cytology in early-stage endometrial cancer does not influence prognosis. Br J Cancer 91:720–724

Cervical Cancer

24

SUBHAKAR MUTYALA and AARON H. WOLFSON

CONTENTS

Introduction and Objectives

Cervical cancer is a malignancy occurring worldwide. In developing countries, cervical cancer can be epidemic and is higher in incidence and prevalence than in this country due to Pap smear screening. If the disease process is found early, many patients can be diagnosed with CIN and be treated without ever developing invasive cancer. As the disease progresses to invasive cancer, even advanced stages can be treated and cured.

Cervical cancer is a disease process that requires multidisciplinary management, especially in the locally advanced stages. Chemotherapy, radiation therapy, and surgery are important treatment modalities in the curative treatment for cervical cancer.

This chapter examines:

● Recommendations for diagnosis and staging procedures

● The staging systems and prognostic factors

● Treatment recommendations as well as the supporting scientific evidence for definitive and adjuvant treatment for early stage cervical cancer

● The use of combined chemotherapy and radiotherapy for definitive treatment of locally advanced disease

● Side effects and complications of treatment

● Follow-up care and surveillance of survivors

● Radiation therapy techniques for the treatment of pituitary tumors

● Follow-up care and surveillance after treatment

S. MUTYALA, MD
Department of Radiation Oncology, Montefiore Medical Center, Albert Einstein College of Medicine, 1625 Poplar St., Bronx, NY 10461, USA
A. H. WOLFSON, MD
Department of Radiation Oncology, University of Miami Miller School of Medicine, 1475 NW 12 Avenue, D-31, Miami, FL 33136, USA

24.1.1 Diagnosis

Initial Evaluation

- Cervical cancer can be detected in its early stage by annual Pap smear screening. Annual Pap tests are recommended for sexually active women and/or those 21–70 years of age by the American College of Obstetrics and Gynecology.
- Diagnosis and evaluation of cervical cancer start with a complete history and physical examination (H&P). The most common presenting symptom is vaginal bleeding, such as postcoital spotting, inter-menstrual bleeding, menorrhagia, or anemia. Advanced disease can present with pain from sidewall disease or bladder or rectal symptoms.
- Abnormal Pap results should be followed with colposcopy with directed and/or random biopsies. Conization should be performed if the transition zone is not visualized, disagreement exists between the Pap smear and biopsies, or for CIN 3 or CIS.
- Full pelvic exam using a speculum and bimanual exam to assess for pelvic sidewall disease and vaginal extension is required, as is examination under anesthesia with biopsies and cystoscopy and proctoscopy.

Laboratory Tests

- Initial laboratory tests should include a complete blood count, basic blood chemistry, alkaline phosphatase, and liver and renal function tests (Table 24.1).

Table 24.1. Imaging and laboratory work-ups for cervical cancer

Imaging studies	Laboratory tests
– CT and MRI of abdomen/pelvis	– Complete blood count
– Chest X-ray	– Serum chemistry
– Lymphangiogram (optional)	– Liver function tests
– FDG-PET scan or PET/CT (optional)	– Renal function tests
– Bone scan (optional)	– Alkaline phosphatase

Imaging Studies

- CT of the abdomen and pelvis or IVP is necessary to evaluate for hydronephrosis. Lymphangiogram can be utilized to evaluate for nodal disease.
- MRI of the pelvis is recommended for evaluation of the extent of local disease (Grade B). MRI has been shown to provide better definition of the extent of local disease and to be a better tool for prognostic indicators than clinical staging using the staging system of the Federation of Gynecology and Oncology (FIGO) (Level III) (Sethi et al. 2005). Although MRI scanning is not yet accepted by FIGO for staging purposes, one retrospective study demonstrated that MRI-derived size assessments correlated with pelvic nodal involvement and progression-free survival (Level IV) (Wagenaar et al. 2001).
- Chest X-ray is recommended to rule out metastatic pulmonary disease. Bone scan is not routinely performed for staging unless indicated by elevated alkaline phosphatase or bone pain.
- Positron emission tomography (PET) scan is not required or included for staging (Grade B). Current use of PET combined with CT has increased detection of nodal disease for locally advanced disease $\geq$IB. Sensitivity is 75% and specificity 96% for PET detection of pelvic adenopathy, and sensitivity is 100% and specificity 99% for PET detection of para-aortic adenopathy (Level III) (Loft et al. 2007). For early stage disease, the sensitivity and specificity of PET CT were about 73% and 97%, respectively (Level III) (Sironi et al. 2006).

Pathology

- Histological diagnosis is mandatory for the diagnosis of cervical cancer prior to any treatment. Tissue for pathology diagnosis can be obtained via biopsy of the primary tumor.
- The most common type of malignancy of the uterine cervix is squamous cell carcinoma, which accounts for more than 80% of all cases of cervical cancer. Adenocarcinoma of the cervix accounts for 15% of all cervical cancer cases.
- Clear cell carcinoma, a rare variant of cervical adenocarcinoma, is linked with prenatal exposure to diethylstilbestrol (DES), a medication used in the 1940s to prevent miscarriages (Herbst et al. 1979).
- Staging laparotomy for histological conformation of metastatic lymph nodes is not necessary.

24.1.2 Staging

■ Cervical cancer is usually staged clinically by the by FIGO staging system. Table 24.2 illustrates the FIGO and Tumor-Node-Metastases (TNM) surgical staging systems for cervical cancer.

■ The FIGO staging system allows physical exam, exam under anesthesia, IVP, cytoscopy, proctoscopy, and barium enema for the staging of cervical cancer. Information from CT of the abdomen and pelvis (except for hydronephrosis), MRI, lymphangiogram, or FDG-PET (or PET/CT) is not to be utilized in the FIGO clinical staging.

Table 24.2. International Federation of Gynecology and Obstetrics (FIGO) and Tumor Node Metastases (TNM) surgical staging systems for carcinoma of the uterine cervix. [Reprinted from Benedet et al. (2000) with permission]

FIGO stages	Clinical and/or surgical-pathologic findings	TNM categories
	Primary tumor cannot be assessed	TX
	No evidence of primary tumor	T0
0	Carcinoma in situ (preinvasive carcinoma)	Tis
I	Cervical carcinoma confined to uterus (extension to the corpus should be disregarded)	T1
IA	Invasive carcinoma diagnosed only by microscopy All macroscopically visible lesions, even with superficial invasion, are stage IB/T1b	T1a
IA1	Stromal invasion 3.0 mm or less in depth and 7.0 mm or less in horizontal spread	T1a1
IA2	Stromal invasion more than 3.0 mm and not more than 5.0 mm with a horizontal spread of 7.0 mm or less[a]	T1a2
IB	Clinically visible lesion confined to the cervix or microscopic lesion greater than IA2/T1a2	T1b
IB1	Clinically visible lesion 4.0 cm or less in greatest dimension	T1b1
IB2	Clinically visible lesion more than 4.0 cm in greatest dimension	T1b2
II	Tumor invades beyond the uterus, but not to pelvic wall or lower third of the vagina	T2
IIA	Without parametrial invasion	T2a
IIB	With parametrial invasion	T2b
III	Tumor extends to pelvic wall and/or involves lower third of vagina and/or causes hydronephrosis or nonfunctioning kidney	T3
IIIA	Tumor involves lower third of vagina, no extension to pelvic wall	T3a
IIIB	Tumor extends to pelvic wall and/or causes hydronephrosis or nonfunctioning kidney	T3b
IVA	Tumor invades mucosa of bladder or rectum, and/or extends beyond true pelvis. The presence of bullous edema is not sufficient to classify a tumor as T4	T4
IVB	Distant metastasis	
Regional lymph nodes (N)		
NX	Regional lymph nodes cannot be assessed	
N0	No regional lymph node metastasis	
N1	Regional lymph node metastasis	
Distant metastasis (M)		
MX	Distant metastasis cannot be assessed	
M0	No distant metastasis	
M1	Distant metastasis	

[a] The depth of invasion should not be more than 5 mm taken from the base of the epithelium, either surface or glandular, from which it originates. The depth of invasion is defined as the measurement of the tumor from the epithelial–stromal junction of the adjacent most superficial epithelial papilla to the deepest point of invasion. Vascular space involvement, venous or lymphatic, does not affect classification.

24.1.3 Prognostic Factors

■ Extent of disease at diagnosis (stage) is the most important prognostic factor of cervical cancer. Decrease of survival with advanced stage has been repeatedly demonstrated: The overall 5-year survivals are as follows (Level IV) (Perez et al. 1986):
  – Carcinoma in situ (CIS) – 100%
  – Stage IA1 – 100%
  – Stage IA2 – 95%
  – Stage IB1 – 85%
  – Stage IB2 – 75%
  – Stage IIA – 70%
  – Stage IIB – 65%
  – Stage III – 45%
  – Stage IVA – 20%
  – Stage IVB – 5%

■ Large tumor diameter (>4 cm according to the Gynecologic Oncology Group definition), depth of invasion, presence of capillary-lymphatic space involvement or parametrial extension, and advanced age are associated with pelvic lymph node involvement (GOG, Level III) (Delgado et al. 1989).

■ Para-aortic lymph node metastasis is the most important prognostic factor for both tumor recurrence and overall survival of patients treated with radiation therapy. The significance of tumor size and pelvis lymph node involvement is significant only in patients without para-aortic adenopathy, according to a retrospective review of three prospective trials from GOG (Level IV) (Stehman et al. 1991).

■ The impact of the histological type of cervical cancer on prognosis is debatable. The prognosis of patients with adenocarcinoma was reportedly worse in some series, especially in early stage diseases after hysterectomy (Level IV) (Eifel et al. 1995; Look et al. 1996). However, other series found that prognoses of patients with squamous cell carcinoma or adenocarcinoma have no significant differences (Level IV) (Takeda et al. 2002; Shingleton et al. 1995).

■ Total treatment time of radiation therapy has a significant prognostic impact: Prolonging the course of radiation therapy for definitive treatment beyond 8 weeks is adversely associated with regional control. Accelerated repopulation of cervical cancer has been demonstrated (Level IV) (Withers et al. 1988). The estimated

increment of pelvic recurrence was approximately 0.5%–1% for every additional day after 7 weeks (Level III, IV) (Fyles et al. 1992; Lanciano et al. 1993; Petereit et al. 1995; Perez et al. 1995).

■ Average level of hemoglobin (Hgb) during radiation therapy is associated with the treatment outcome. Results from early retrospective studies suggested that the presence of anemia in patients was associated with adverse outcome after radiation (Level IV) (Bush 1986; Girinski et al. 1989). Two studies further demonstrated the importance of Hgb levels during radiation therapy of cervical cancer and revealed that an Hgb level of 11–12 g/dl should be maintained during irradiation (Level IV) (Grogan et al. 1999; Kapp et al. 2002).

24.2 Treatment of Early-Stage Cervical Cancer

24.2.1 General Principles

■ Treatment of cervical malignancy depends on the extent of the presenting disease and patient preference.

■ Pre-invasive diseases are usually managed by local excision (loop excision or cervical conization) or ablation (laser ablation or cryotherapy). Hysterectomy can be considered in the treatment of pre-invasive cervical lesions for patients who have high-grade dysplasia and no plan for childbearing.

■ Surgery is the treatment of choice for patients with microinvasive disease (i.e., FIGO Stage IA) and limited localized disease (i.e., FIGO Stages IB and IIA). The extent of surgery (simple or radical hysterectomy) depends on the stage at presentation (Grade A).

■ Radiation therapy is the mainstay treatment for patients with more advanced diseases (Grade A). Radiation is also recommended in the treatment of stage IA–IIA cervical cancer patients who are medically inoperable.

■ Combined chemoradiation therapy is the standard treatment for locally advanced cervical cancer (Grade A).

24.2.2 Surgery

- Surgery alone is a curative treatment modality for early stage (FIGO Stages IA1–II) cervical cancer.
- For stage IA1, a simple extrafascial hysterectomy can be performed (Grade B). A conization with close follow-up can be considered for maintenance of fertility. An overall survival rate of close to 100% can be expected after definitive treatment of stage IA cervical cancer (Level IV) (KOLSTAD 1989).
- For stage IA2–IB1 diseases, a radical hysterectomy (or modified radical) with pelvic lymph node dissection is the surgery of choice (Grade B). Limited surgery for stage IA2 cervical cancer is not recommended, as the probability of regional lymph nodal involvement is approximately 5%–10% (Level IV) (BURGHARDT and PICKEL1978).
- Adjuvant radiation therapy is often indicated after surgery (as described below). Outcome after surgery (followed by adjuvant radiation therapy if indicated) is comparable to that from definitive radiation therapy, in the range of 90% at 5 years after treatment, according to a prospective randomized trial from Italy. However, more toxicity is expected in patients treated with surgery and adjuvant radiation as compared to those treated with radiation alone (Level I) (LANDONI et al. 1997).

24.2.3 Radiation Therapy

Adjuvant Radiation

- Postoperative adjuvant radiation therapy is indicated when the negative prognostic factors listed below are found on pathology (Grade A). Adjuvant radiation therapy has been shown to improve local control, disease-free survival (DFS), and overall survival (OS) for pathologically proven deep stromal invasion, bulky disease, or positive lymphovascular invasion.
  The results of a prospective randomized trial show that for "intermediate risk" patients with at least two risk factors, i.e., tumor diameter >4 cm, deep stromal involvement (> 1/3), or capillary lymphatic space involvement, adjuvant radiation therapy provided a statistically significant reduction in local recurrence (from 28%–15%). The recurrence-free rates at 2 years were 88% versus

79% for patients with or without adjuvant radiation, respectively. The addition of adjuvant radiation increases the chance of grade 3 and 4 complication by 6%, as compared to those who received surgery only (Level I) (SEDLIS et al. 1999).
- Radiation therapy alone is not recommended, and combined chemoradiation therapy should be considered for stage IA2, IB, and IIA cervical cancer patients with the risk factors described below.

Adjuvant Combined Chemoradiation Therapy

- Postoperative radiation therapy with concurrent cisplatin-containing chemotherapy is recommended for early stages (IA2, IB, and IIA) with more than one positive pelvis lymph node, positive margins, and parametrium involvement on pathology (Grade A). The results of an intergroup, prospectively randomized phase III trial has demonstrated that for IA(2), IB, and IIA cervical cancer patients with the above-mentioned factors on pathology, adjuvant chemoradiotherapy significantly improved the treatment outcome. The 4-year progression-free survivals and overall survival rates were 63% versus 80% and 71% versus 81%, respectively, for patients who received radiation therapy only or combined chemoradiation as adjuvant treatment (Intergroup, Level I) (PETERS et al. 2000).
  A retrospective analysis of the 268 patients involved in the above-mentioned Intergroup study further revealed that the effect of additional chemotherapy to radiation is not significant in patients when only one lymph node is positive or when the tumor size is < 2 cm (Level IV) (MONK et al. 2005).

Definitive Radiation

- Radiation therapy is the treatment of choice for patients with early stage, but medically inoperable cervical cancer and for patients who decline surgery.
  For stage IA1 diseases, intercavitary brachytherapy alone can be used. For stage IA2 or IB1 disease, whole pelvic RT followed by intercavitary brachytherapy should be considered.
- Radiation therapy compared to surgery (with radiation for higher risk patients) has been shown to be equally effective (Grade A). The above-mentioned randomized trial from Italy compared

radical hysterectomy and pelvic lymph node dissection to radical radiation for stage IB–IIA. The 5-year DFS was 76% and 78% and OS 84% and 88% for surgery and radiation, respectively. Neither was found to be statistically significant (Level I) (LANDONI et al. 1997).

- Monitoring of hemoglobin level during radiation therapy is recommended (Grade B). An Hgb level of 10 g/dl (by transfusion if needed) should be maintained during treatment.

Radiation Technique

- Whole pelvic radiation therapy (using 10 MV photons) is the field arrangement of choice for adjuvant treatment after radical hysterectomy. Simulation, beam energy, and dose calculation are similar to the whole pelvis, with those utilized in definitive radiation for locally advanced cervical cancer described below.
- When intercavitary brachytherapy alone is used for stage IA1 disease, a tandem and ovoid should be used as described below to an LDR equivalent dose of 65–75 Gy to point A.
- For stage IA2 and IB diseases, combined external-beam radiation (whole pelvic irradiation) with a tandem and ovoid should be used as described below to a cumulative total dose of 75–80 Gy to point A.

24.2.4 Adjuvant Chemotherapy

- There is no evidence to support the use of chemotherapy alone after surgery or definitive chemoradiation therapy.

24.3 Treatment of Locally Advanced Cervical Cancer

24.3.1 General Principles

- A combination of cisplatin-containing chemotherapy and radiation therapy is the treatment of choice for patients with locally advanced cervical cancer (Grade A). Radiation therapy and chemotherapy should be delivered concurrently.

- The role of induction chemotherapy before and consolidation chemotherapy after concurrent chemoradiation are not yet proven and should not be routinely utilized.
- Surgery after definitive chemoradiation therapy is not routinely recommended (Grade C).
- There is no evidence to support the use of chemotherapy alone after surgery or definitive chemoradiation therapy.

24.3.2 Concurrent Chemotherapy and Radiation Therapy

- Concurrent chemotherapy and radiation therapy are considered as the standard treatment combination for locally advanced cervical cancer (Grade A). The efficacy of concurrent chemoradiation over radiotherapy only in the definitive treatment of locally advanced cervical cancer has been repeatedly demonstrated by prospective randomized trials:

In a GOG/SWOG trial, 368 patients with stage IIB, III, and IV squamous cell carcinoma, adenocarcinoma, or adenosquamous cell carcinoma were randomized and received either radiation therapy with concurrent hydroxyurea or concurrent radiation and chemotherapy (5-FU and cisplatin). The results showed that progression-free survival (PFS) and overall survival were both statistically significantly improved in the group that received chemoradiation therapy ($p = 0.033$) (GOG/SWOG, Level I) (WHITNEY et al. 1999).

A similar GOG trial randomized 526 patients with stage IIB, III, or IVA cervical cancer without involvement of the para-aortic lymph nodes to: (1) cisplatin 40 mg/m^2 weekly for 6 weeks; (2) cisplatin 50 mg/m^2 on days 1 and 29, followed by 5-FU 4 g/m^2 given as a 96-h infusion on days 1 and 29, and hydroxyurea 2 g/m^2 twice weekly for 6 weeks; or (3) oral hydroxyurea 3 g/m^2 twice weekly for 6 weeks. After a median follow-up of 3 years, the overall survival rate and relative risks of disease progression or death were significantly improved in the two groups receiving cisplatin-based chemotherapy. However, there was no difference in the 2-year progression-free survival, overall survival, local control, and lung metastasis rates between the two chemotherapy arms (Level I) (ROSE et al. 1999).

A larger randomized multi-institution trial, RTOG 90-01, compared the effect of radiation therapy to the para-aortic lymph nodes and pelvis (45 Gy to both areas in 25 daily fractions) and concurrent chemotherapy and pelvic irradiation (45 Gy in 25 daily fractions). The results revealed that the addition of chemotherapy to pelvic radiation produced a significant improvement in 5-year disease-free survival (67% versus 40%), overall survival (73% versus 58%), and distant relapse (14% versus 33%) rates, as compared to patients treated with extended field radiation therapy only (Level I) (MORRIS et al. 1999). Mature analysis with a median follow-up of more than 6 years confirmed that the addition of fluorouracil and cisplatin to radiotherapy significantly improved the survival rate of women with locally advanced cervical cancer without increasing the rate of late treatment-related side effects (Level I) (EIFEL 2004).

■ The effect of preoperative chemoradiation therapy has also been shown to be superior to radiation alone. In a GOG study, women with bulky stage IB cervical cancers (tumor ≥4 cm in diameter) were randomly assigned to receive radiotherapy alone or in combination with cisplatin (40 mg/m^2 weekly for up to six doses; maximal weekly dose 70 mg), followed in all patients by adjuvant hysterectomy. The results showed that the rates of both progression-free survival ($p < 0.001$) and overall survival ($p = 0.008$) were significantly higher in the combined-therapy group at 4 years (Level I) (KEYS et al. 1999). However, although the long-term follow-up further confirmed the benefit of combined chemoradiation therapy to hysterectomy, this practice (tri-modality that includes surgery) has been discontinued due to the results of other studies (STEHMAN et al. 2007).

24.3.3 Chemotherapy Regimens

■ Current chemotherapy recommendations are for weekly cisplatin 40 mg/m^2 (Grade A). In the above-mentioned randomized trial from GOG, the outcome in terms of 2-year progression-free survival, overall survival, local control, and lung metastasis rates between the two chemotherapy arms was not significantly different for the two cisplatin-based chemotherapy regimens with or without 5-FU and hydroxyurea (Level I) (ROSE et al. 1999).

24.4 Radiation Therapy Techniques

24.4.1 External-Beam Radiation Therapy

Simulation

■ CT-based planning is recommended, and the CT scan should be taken in the treatment position with 3-mm-thick slices in the treatment position (Grade B). A prospective study showed that fields based solely on bony landmarks had at least one inadequate margin in 95.4% or an excess margin in 55.8% of patients (Level III) (FINLAY et al. 2006).

■ Intravenous contrast can be used for planning CT, or a fusion of CT with contrast may be needed if IV contrast is necessary for vessel delineation.

■ Intensity-modulated radiation therapy (IMRT) should be considered experimental at this point and should not be routinely recommended without further data (Grade D). IMRT for definitive cervical cancer has been studied only in small series from single institutions (Level IV) (MUNDT et al. 2002). Currently, IMRT for post hysterectomy is being studied under the RTOG 04-18 phase II protocol.

Beam Energy and Dose Calculation

■ A megavoltage accelerator with a minimum source to an isocenter distance of 100 cm is recommended.

■ Higher energy photons beams, 10–18 MV, should be used if possible to reduce the dose to normal tissue.

■ Doses are to be calculated without heterogeneity correction, i.e., no correction is to be made for density differences between air in the bowel and fluid in the bladder.

■ Four fields should be used for maximal sparing of normal tissue (especially small bowel and sciatic nerve).

Field Arrangement

Whole Pelvis Fields

■ Whole pelvic radiation therapy (using 10 MV photons) using a four-field arrangement can be considered for definitive treatment or adjuvant treatment after surgery. This field arrangement aims to encompass the internal iliac, external iliac, and common iliac nodal stations along with the tumor bed to a dose of 45–50 Gy at 1.8 Gy per fraction. A midline block should be added if delivering a dose above 45 Gy. In case bulky tumor is present and utilization of the lateral fields may block the posterior tumor region, anterior and posterior opposed fields with high energy (≥15 MV) can be considered to treat the whole pelvis. Total dose to the whole pelvis using the AP/PA technique should not exceed 40–45 Gy.

■ Field arrangement is described as follows (Fig. 24.1):

– The superior border is set at the L4–5 interspace to encompass common iliac lymph nodes.

– The inferior border is set below the obturator foramen or 3 cm inferior to distal disease, whichever is lower.

– The lateral border of the anteroposterior or posteroanterior field is set at 1.5–2 cm lateral to the pelvic brim with sparing of the medial aspect of the femoral heads.

– The anterior border of the lateral field is set anterior to the pubic symphysis with small bowel block.

– The posterior border of the lateral field is set posterior to the sacrum (see Fig. 24.1, anteroposterior and lateral simulation fields of the pelvic field).

Parametrial Boost Fields

■ Parametrial boost is indicated in patients with bulky primary disease. An additional dose of 5.4–9.0 Gy can be considered for parametrial boost after 45–50.4 Gy to the whole pelvis.

■ Parametrial boost is usually delivered using AP/PA arrangements. The fields for the parametrial boost are set as follows:

– The superior border is set at 1 cm superior to the bottom of the SI joint.

– The lateral and inferior borders are identical to the AP/PA field of the whole pelvic setting.

– A midline block of 4–5 cm in diameter blocks bladder and rectum hotspots from brachytherapy. A customized midline shielding can be contoured using a point A isodose line and is associated with fewer complications (Level III) (Wolfson et al. 1997).

■ The small bowel should be visualized by CT to ensure that the dose does not exceed 45 Gy.

Para-aortic Fields

■ Irradiation to the para-aortic nodal region is indicated in patients with stage III B cervical cancer with pelvic and para-aortic nodal involvement (Fig. 24.2). Para-aortic irradiation is not recommended routinely if para-aortic adenopathy is absent.

■ Para-aortic irradiation can be delivered using AP/PA and opposed lateral (four-field) arrangements. The fields for the parametrial boost are set as follows:

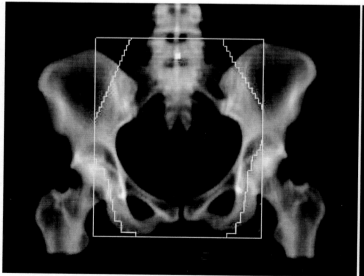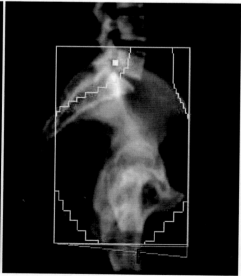

Fig. 24.1. Anteroposterior and lateral simulation fields of the pelvic field

Fig. 24.2. Simulation film of extended field for external irradiation of pelvic and para-aortic lymph nodes

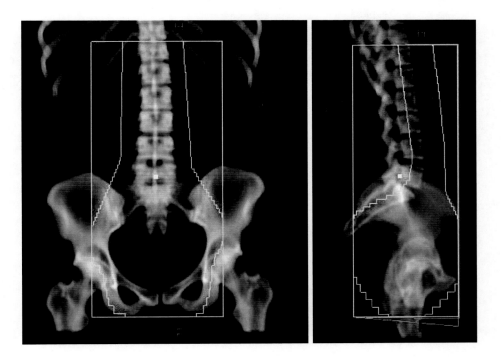

– For the AP/PA fields, the superior border of the AP/PA fields is set at the T11 and T12 interspace; the inferior border of the AP/PA fields is set at the L4–5 interspace (if separating from pelvic fields) or continues with the AP/PA fields of the pelvic portal; the lateral border is set at lateral aspects of transverse processes.

– For the lateral fields, the anterior border is set at 2 cm anterior to vertebral bodies; the posterior border should split the vertebral bodies.

■ Kidneys should be visualized by CT to ensure 2/3 of each kidney is blocked.

Dose and Fractionation

■ The whole pelvic field should be treated to 45–50.4 Gy with conventional fractionation (1.8 Gy or 2.0 Gy per fraction).

■ If the para-aortic field is added, the para-aortic field should be treated with up to 45 Gy at 1.5–1.8 Gy per fraction.

■ Parametrial boost should be treated with 5.4–9.0 Gy at 1.8 Gy per fraction.

■ The approximate average total dose to point A with the LDR brachytherapy implant should deliver 35–45 Gy as described below.

24.5   Brachytherapy

■ Brachytherapy is an important component of the treatment of cervical cancer, with or without EBRT, for definitive or adjuvant radiotherapy.

■ For stage IA1 or selected cases of IA2 cervical cancer, intracavitary tandem and ovoid/ring brachytherapy alone can be sufficient treatment.

■ For more advanced stages, external-beam radiotherapy up to 45–50 Gy plus intracavitary brachytherapy is indicated. Treatment is usually delivered using with tandem and ovoid/ring; for patients with persistent vaginal disease, tandem and cylinder can be considered.

■ Brachytherapy can be initiated prior to the completion of external-beam radiation to the pelvis.

■ For more advanced disease, an interstitial implant might be indicated: Patients should complete external-beam radiation therapy and be re-assessed with examination under anesthesia. Interstitial implant is indicated if persistent disease is observed, including: sidewall disease, cervical os that is not palpable, or vaginal disease thicker than 5 mm.

Dosing of Brachytherapy

- High dose rate (HDR) and low dose rate (LDR) have been found to be effective in the treatment of cervical cancer, and both can be considered (Grade A). The effects from HDR and LDR are reportedly equivalent in prospective randomized trials: A randomized prospective trial comparing HDR and LDR brachytherapy revealed no difference in 5-year local control or OS for stage I–III cervical cancer: 73% versus 78% for stage I, 62% versus 64% for stage II, and 50% versus 43% for stage III (Level I) (Patel et al. 1994). These findings were supported in a single institutional randomized trial, which indicated that the 10-year cause-specific survival and failure pattern was not different between HDR and LDR for stage I–III cervical cancer (Level II) (Teshima et al. 1993).

- The International Commission on Radiation Units and Measurements (ICRU 1985) Report No. 38 defined the dose and volume specifications for reporting of brachytherapy for gynecologic cancers.

- The dose of brachytherapy is prescribed to point A at 2 cm superior to the cervical os and 2 cm lateral to tandem according to the GOG definition (Fig. 24.3). Dose recommendations (to point A) for both LDR and HDR brachytherapy for different stages are as follows. The dose used in HDR was one of the recommended dose arrangements recommended by the American Brachytherapy Society Consensus on HDR brachytherapy for cervical cancer (Level V) (Nag et al. 2000):

  - IA1–2, small IB1 (brachytherapy only): 60–70 Gy for LDR; 7 Gy for seven fractions for HDR.
  - IB1–IIIB: 35–45 Gy LDR (total 80–90 Gy); 6 Gy for five fractions HDR.
  - Parametrial boost if persistent parametrial disease is present for additional 5.4–9.0 Gy.

- Dose to point B, at 2 cm superior to the cervical os and 5 cm lateral to the patient midline, should be recorded for locally advanced disease (i.e., stage IB2 or higher).

- The bladder point is set using a Foley balloon with 7 cc of contrast and water, and the center of the balloon on AP film and posterior of the surface of the Foley balloon along the AP line drawn through the center. The bladder point dose should be kept to <90% of point A or a total of <75 Gy (±5%) (ICRU 1985).

- The rectum point is set at the lower end of tandem or midpoint of ovoids on AP film and 0.5 cm behind the posterior vaginal wall, defined by packing. Rectum dose should be kept up to <80% of point A or total <70 Gy (±5%) (ICRU 1985).

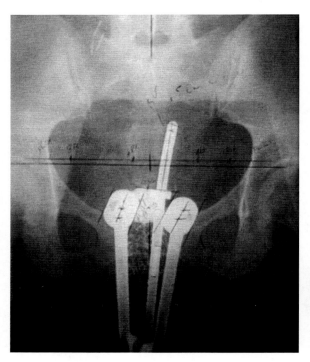
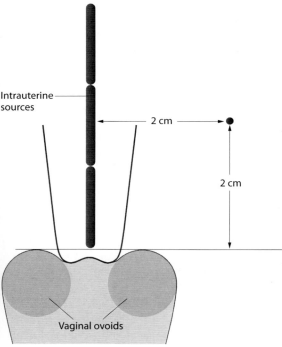

Fig. 24.3. Location of point A using the method recommended in ICRU 38

24.6 Side Effects and Complications

24.6.1 Surgical Complications

- Acute surgical complications secondary to hysterectomy are not common, postoperative mortality is less than 1%, and wound infection is expected in less than 5% of cases.
- Late surgical complications include urinary dysfunction, which is the most common complication (including partial denervation of the detrusor muscle that causes urinary retention and loss of bladder sensation) and is seen in approximately 20% of cases.
- Other late surgical complications include ureteral stricture, lymphocele (20% by imaging, 2% clinically), and menopausal symptoms.

24.6.2 Radiation-Induced Side Effects and Complications

Acute Complications

- Commonly observed acute radiation-induced complications include enteritis (diarrhea and/or abdominal cramping), proctitis (anorectal discomfort, tenesmus, or rectal bleeding), and cystourethritis (frequency, dysuria, and/or nocturia). Most of these symptoms can be medically treated.
- Late complications from radiation therapy and treatment are described as follows.

- Vaginal stenosis can be prevented and treated with a vaginal dilator.
- Vaginal ulceration or necrosis occurs in approximately 7% of patients typically at 6–12 months after treatment. Supportive measures are recommended, and the symptoms usually subside in 1–6 months.
- Late gastrointestinal complications can occur for up to 19 months, and late genitourinary complications can occur for up to 2 years.
- Ureteral stricture can be observed especially in patients treated with a standard 4-cm midline block for parametrial boost. Customized midline shielding should be considered to prevent the occurrence of ureteral stricture (Level III) (WOLFSON et al. 1997) (Table 24.3).

24.7 Follow-Ups

24.7.1 Post-Treatment Follow-Ups

- Life-long follow-up is required for all patients with cervical cancer treated with curative intent. However, there is no definitive study or uniform agreement to support the optimal follow-up practice for cervical cancer.

Schedule

- Follow-up could be scheduled every 3 months initially in the 1st year after treatment, then every

Table 24.3. Dose limiting structures

Organ	Class	Injury	TD$_{5/5}$	TD$_{50/5}$	Whole or part
Intestine	I	Ulcer, perforation	45 Gy	55 Gy	400 cm^2
		Hemorrhage	50 Gy	65 Gy	100 cm^2
Rectum	II	Ulcer, stricture	60 Gy	75 Gy	75 cm^2
Bladder	II	Contracture	60 Gy	80 Gy	Whole
Ureters	II	Stricture	75 Gy	100 Gy	5–10 cm
Ovary	II	Sterilization	2–3 Gy	6–12 Gy	Whole
Uterus	III	Necrosis, perforation	>100 Gy	>200 Gy	Whole
Vagina	III	Ulcer, fistula	90 Gy	>100 Gy	Whole

4 months in the 2nd year, and every 6 months for 3 additional years. Annual follow-up is recommended for long-term survivors after 5 years (Grade D) (Table 24.4).

Table 24.4. Follow-up schedule

Interval	Frequency
First year	Every 3 months
Second year	Every 4 months
Year 3–5	Every 6 months
Over 5 years	Annually

Work-Ups

- Each follow-up examination should include a complete history and physical examination, pelvic exam, and Pap smear at each visit (Grade D) (NCCN 2008).
- Chest X-ray can be performed annually (Grade D) (NCCN 2008). Other imaging studies and laboratory workups are optional, and routine use is not recommended. However, recent evidence supports the use of FDG-PET scanning beginning at 3–4 months for follow-up after treatment (Grade B) (Level IV) (GRIGSBY 2003, 2004).

References

Benedet JL, Bender H, Jones H 3rd et al. (2000) FIGO staging classifications and clinical practice guidelines in the management of gynecologic cancers. FIGO Committee on Gynecologic Oncology. Int J Gynaecol Obstet 70:209–262

Burghardt E, Pickel H (1978) Local spread and lymph node involvement in cervical cancer. Obstet Gynecol 52:138–145

Bush R (1986) The significance of anemia in clinical radiation therapy. Int J Radiat Oncol Biol Phys 12:2047–2050

Delgado G, Bundy BN, Fowler WC Jr et al (1989) A prospective surgical pathological study of stage I squamous carcinoma of the cervix: a Gynecologic Oncology Group Study. Gynecol Oncol 35:314–320

Eifel PJ, Winter K, Morris M et al (2004) Pelvic irradiation with concurrent chemotherapy versus pelvic and paraaortic irradiation for high-risk cervical cancer: an update of radiation therapy oncology group trial (RTOG) 90-01. J Clin Oncol 22:872–880

Finlay MH, Ackerman I, Tirona RG et al (2006) Use of CT simulation for treatment of cervical cancer to assess the adequacy of lymph node coverage of conventional pelvic fields based on bony landmarks. Int J Radiat Oncol Biol Phys 64:205–209

Fyles A, Keane TJ, Barton M et al (1992) The effect of treatment duration in the local control of cervix cancer. Radiother Oncol 25:273–279

Girinski T, Pejovic-Lenfant MH, Bourhis J et al (1989) Prognostic value of hemoglobin concentrations and blood transfusions in advanced carcinoma of the cervix treated by radiation therapy: results of a retrospective study of 386 patients. Int J Radiat Oncol Biol Phys 16:37–42

Grigsby PW, Siegel BA, Dehdashti F et al (2003) Posttherapy surveillance monitoring of cervical cancer by FDG-PET. Int J Radiat Oncol Biol Phys 55:907–913

Grigsby PW, Siegel BA, Dehdashti F et al (2004) Posttherapy [18F] fluorodeoxyglucose positron emission tomography in carcinoma of the cervix: response and outcome. J Clin Oncol 22:2167–2171

Grogan M, Thomas GM, Melamed I et al (1999) The importance of hemoglobin levels during radiotherapy for carcinoma of the cervix. Cancer 86:1528–1536

Herbst AL, Cole P, Norusis MJ et al (1979) Epidemiologic aspects and factors related to survival in 384 registry cases of clear cell adenocarcinoma of the vagina and cervix. Am J Obstet Gynecol 135:876–886

International Commission of Radiation Units and Measurements (1985) Dose and volume specifications for reporting intracavitary therapy in gynecology. ICRU Report 38.International Commission on Radiation Units, Bethesda, MD

Kapp KS, Poschauko J, Geyer E et al (2002) Evaluation of the effect of routine packed red blood cell transfusion in anemic cervix cancer patients treated with radical radiotherapy. Int J Radiat Oncol Biol Phys 54:58–66

Keys HM, Bundy BN, Stehman FB et al (1999) Cisplatin, radiation, and adjuvant hysterectomy compared with radiation and adjuvant hysterectomy for bulky stage IB cervical carcinoma. N Engl J Med 340:1154–1161

Kolstad P (1989) Follow-up study of 232 patients with stage Ia1 and 411 patients with stage Ia2 squamous cell carcinoma of the cervix (microinvasive carcinoma). Gynecol Oncol 33:265–272

Lanciano RM, Martz K, Coia LR et al (1993) Tumor and treatment factors improving outcome in stage III–B cervix cancer. Int J Radiat Oncol Biol Phys 20:95–100

Landoni F, Maneo A, Colombo A et al (1997) Randomised study of radical surgery versus radiotherapy for stage Ib–IIa cervical cancer. Lancet 350:535–540

Loft A, Berthelsen AK, Roed H et al (2007) The diagnostic value of PET/CT scanning in patients with cervical cancer: a prospective study. Gynecol Oncol 106:29–34

Look KY, Brunetto VL, Clarke-Pearson DL et al (1996) An analysis of cell type in patients with surgically staged stage IB carcinoma of the cervix: a Gynecologic Oncology Group study. Gynecol Oncol 63:304–311

Monk BJ, Wang J, Im S et al (2005) Rethinking the use of radiation and chemotherapy after radical hysterectomy: a clinical-pathologic analysis of a Gynecologic Oncology Group/Southwest Oncology Group/Radiation Therapy Oncology Group trial. Gynecol Oncol 96:721–728

Morris M, Eifel PJ, Lu J et al (1999) Pelvic radiation with concurrent chemotherapy compared with pelvic and paraaortic radiation for high-risk cervical cancer. N Engl J Med 340:1137–1143

Mundt AJ, Lujan AE, Rotmensch J et al (2002) Intensity-modulated whole pelvic radiotherapy in women with gynecologic malignancies. Int J Radiat Oncol Biol Phys 52:1330–1337

Nag S, Erickson B, Thomadsen B et al (2000) The American Brachytherapy Society recommendations for high-dose-rate brachytherapy for carcinoma of the cervix. Int J Radiat Oncol Biol Phys 48:201–211

National Comprehensive Cancer Network (2007) Clinical practice guidelines in oncology: Cervical vancer, version 1.2008. Available at http://www.nccn.org/professionals/physician_gls/PDF/cervical.pdf. Last accessed on 8 March 2008

Patel FD, Sharma SC, Negi PS et al (1994) Low dose rate vs. high dose rate brachytherapy in the treatment of carcinoma of the uterine cervix: a clinical trial. Int J Radiat Oncol Biol Phys 28:335–341

Perez CA, Camel HM, Kuske RR et al (1986) Radiation therapy alone in the treatment of carcinoma of the uterine cervix: a 20-year experience. Gynecol Oncol 23:127–140

Perez CA, Grigsby PW, Castro-Vita H et al (1995) Carcinoma of the uterine cervix. I. Impact of prolongation of overall treatment time and timing of brachytherapy on outcome of radiation therapy. Int J Radiat Oncol Biol Phys 32:1275–1288

Peters WA, Liu PY, Barrett RJ et al (2000) Concurrent chemotherapy and pelvic radiation therapy after radical surgery in high-risk early-stage cancer of the cervix. J Clin Oncol 18:1606–1613

Petereit DG, Sarkaria JN, Chappell R et al (1995) The adverse effect of treatment prolongation in cervical carcinoma. Int J Radiat Oncol Biol Phys 32:1301–1307

Rose PG, Bundy BN, Watkins EB et al (1999) Concurrent cisplatin-based radiotherapy and chemotherapy for locally advanced cervical cancer. N Engl J Med 340:1144–1153

Sedlis A, Bundy BN, Rotman MZ et al (1999) A randomized trial of pelvic radiation therapy versus no further therapy in selected patients with stage IB carcinoma of the cervix after radical hysterectomy and pelvic lymphadenectomy: A Gynecologic Oncology Group Study. Gynecol Oncol 73:177–183

Sethi TK, Bhalla NK, Jena AN et al (2005) Magnetic resonance imaging in carcinoma cervix–does it have a prognostic relevance. J Cancer Res Ther 1:103–107

Shingleton HM, Bell MC, Fremgen A et al (1995) Is there really a difference in survival of women with squamous cell carcinoma, adenocarcinoma, and adenosquamous cell carcinoma of the cervix? Cancer 76(10 Suppl):1948–1955

Sironi S, Buda A, Picchio M et al (2006) Lymph node metastasis in patients with clinical early-stage cervical cancer: detection with integrated FDG PET/CT. Radiology 238:272–279

Stehman FB, Bundy BN, DiSaia PJ et al (1991) Carcinoma of the cervix treated with radiation therapy. I. A multi-variate analysis of prognostic variables in the Gynecologic Oncology Group. Cancer 67:2776–2785

Stehman FB, Ali S, Keys HM et al (2007) Radiation therapy with or without weekly cisplatin for bulky stage 1B cervical carcinoma: follow-up of a Gynecologic Oncology Group trial. Am J Obstet Gynecol 197:503. e1–6

Takeda N, Sakuragi N, Takeda M et al (2002) Multivariate analysis of histopathologic prognostic factors for invasive cervical cancer treated with radical hysterectomy and systematic retroperitoneal lymphadenectomy. Acta Obstet Gynecol Scand 81:1144–1151

Teshima T, Inoue T, Ikeda H et al (1993) High-dose rate and low-dose rate intracavitary therapy for carcinoma of the uterine cervix. Final results of Osaka University Hospital. Cancer 72:2409–2414

Wagenaar HC, Trimbos JB, Postema S et al (2001) Tumor diameter and volume assessed by magnetic resonance imaging in the prediction of outcome for invasive cervical cancer. Gynecol Oncol 82:474–482

Whitney CW, Sause W, Bundy BN et al (1999) Randomized comparison of fluorouracil plus cisplatin versus hydroxyurea as an adjunct to radiation therapy in stage IIB-IVA carcinoma of the cervix with negative para-aortic lymph nodes: a Gynecologic Oncology Group and Southwest Oncology Group study. J Clin Oncol 17:1339–1348

Withers HR, Taylor JM, Maciejewski B (1988) The hazard of accelerated tumor clonogen repopulation during radiotherapy. Acta Oncol 27:131–146

Wolfson AH, Abdel-Wahab M, Markoe AM et al (1997) A quantitative assessment of standard versus customized midline shield construction for invasive cervical carcinoma. Int J Radiat Oncol Biol Phys 37:237–242

Carcinoma of the Vulva

25

Stephanie C. Han

CONTENTS

Introduction and Objectives

Carcinoma of the vulva is a relatively uncommon malignancy and accounts for 3%–5% of all gynecologic malignancies in the United States. Preservation of function, as well as anatomy, can be paramount in the decision-making process for the treatment of vulvar cancer. Except for diseases with very limited volume and extent that can be treated with surgical excision only, the majority of cases require multidisciplinary management. Radiation therapy plays a major role in the treatment of vulva cancer. Adjuvant radiotherapy is indicated in patients with certain risk factors of locoregional recurrence after surgery. For locally advanced disease or lesions with extension to the midline structures, concurrent chemotherapy +/− surgery is usually the preferred treatment choice.

This chapter examines:

● Recommendations for diagnosis and staging procedures for carcinoma of the vulva
● The FIGO/AJCC staging systems and prognostic factors
● The management of vulvar cancer using unimodal and multimodal regimens based on surgery, radiation therapy, and chemotherapy
● Treatment recommendations as well as the supporting scientific evidence
● Techniques of radiation therapy
● Follow-up care and surveillance of survivors

25.1 Diagnosis, Staging, and Prognoses

25.1.1 Diagnosis

Initial Evaluation

■ Diagnosis and evaluation of vulva carcinoma start with a complete history and physical ex-

S. C. Han
Department of Radiation Oncology, Maimonides Cancer Center, 6300 Eighth Avenue, Brooklyn, NY 11220, USA

amination (H&P). Attention should be paid to vulvar cancer-specific history, signs, and symptoms, such as pruritus, pain, spotting or bleeding, and discharge.

- Thorough physical examination should be performed to evaluate the extent of the primary disease and regional lymph node metastasis. Most lesions involve the labia majora; less commonly, lesions originate on the labia minora and the clitoris. Direct extension can involve the vagina, perineum, clitoris, and anus. The frequency of inguinofemoral nodal involvement is dependent on the size of the primary tumor and depth of stromal invasion (HACKER et al. 1984; HOFFMAN et al. 1983). For lesions <1 cm, the incidence is 5%. For lesions >4 cm, the incidence is 30%–50% (WHARTON et al. 1974; BOYCE et al. 1985). Lateralized lesions drain to the ipsilateral groin. Midline lesions can drain to either groin. Pelvic lymph node involvement is rare unless more than three inguinofemoral nodes are involved (ANDREWS et al. 1994). Inguinal and femoral lymph nodes are commonly involved in locally advanced lesions of the vulva.
- A thorough gynecologic examination with Pap smear of the cervix is indicated to evaluate the extent of the disease and screen for cervical cancer.
- EUA, cystoscopy, and sigmoidoscopy should be used as needed depending on the extent of the primary tumor.

Pathology

- Histological confirmation of vulvar cancer is essential. Approximately 85% of vulvar cancers are squamous cell type. The remaining, less common histologies are melanoma, basaloid, adenocarcinoma (usually arising in the Bartholin's glands), neuroendocrine carcinoma (Merkel cell), and sarcoma.
- Diagnosis of vulva cancer requires biopsy of the primary tumor. This is performed under local anesthesia.
- Fine-needle aspirate of enlarged groin lymph nodes should be done to determine nodal involvement (Grade A). Approximately 22% of patients with clinically positive groin nodes have negative nodes pathologically (Level IV) (CROSBY et al. 1989; WAY 1960; MORLEY 1976; IVERSEN et al. 1980; RUTLEDGE et al. 1970; MORRIS 1977). Likewise, approximately 20% of clinically negative groin nodes harbor subclinical metastasis (KOH et al. 1993).

Imaging Studies

- MRI or CT of the pelvis and abdomen are important imaging studies for evaluating the extent of local disease and detecting nodal involvement.
- FDG-PET can be considered for evaluating the extent of regional disease and staging of vulvar cancer (Grade B). It has been shown to be more sensitive for detecting abnormal inguinal lymph nodes than conventional CT. FDG-PET has been shown to have sensitivity of 67%–80% and specificity of 90%–95% in detecting lymph node metastasis (Level III) (COHN et al. 2002).
- Chest X-ray is usually adequate to rule out lung metastasis, and liver metastasis can be evaluated by CT or MRI of the abdomen.
- Bone scan is not routinely recommended except in cases with elevated alkaline phosphatase or symptoms indicating bone metastasis.
- Cystoscopy and proctoscopy may be helpful depending on the location and extent of the primary lesion.

Laboratory Tests

- Initial laboratory tests should include a complete blood count, basic blood chemistry, alkaline phosphatase, liver and renal function tests. Table 25.1 lists the recommended imaging studies and laboratory test for the diagnosis and evaluation of vulvar cancer.

25.1.2 Staging

- Clinical staging utilizes information from physical examination and imaging studies. As described above, palpation of inguinal lymph nodes is associated with 20% false-positive and false-negative rates.

Table 25.1. Imaging and laboratory work-ups for vulva cancer

Imaging studies	Laboratory tests
– MRI or CT of pelvis and abdomen – Chest X-ray – FDG-PET scan (optional)	– Complete blood count – Serum chemistry – Liver function tests – Renal function tests – Alkaline phosphatase

- The International Federation of Gynecology and Obstetrics (FIGO) and the American Joint Committee on Cancer (AJCC) have adopted a standard surgical staging for vulvar cancer. The TNM staging system is based on tumor size, invasion of adjacent structures, status of regional lymph nodes, and status of distant metastases (Table 25.2). According to the AJCC, inguinofemoral nodes are considered regional spread, whereas pelvic nodes are considered distant metastasis.

25.1.3 Prognosis

- The presenting stage of the disease (including the size and extent of the primary tumor, extent of nodal involvement, and status of distant metastasis), depth of invasion, and lymphovascular space invasion are the most important prognostic factor for vulva cancer (ANDREASSON and NYBOE 1985; BINDER et al. 1990; BOYCE et al. 1984; DONALDSON et al. 1980; HOMESLEY et al. 1993; IVERSEN et al. 1980; PODRATZ et al. 1983).
- Local relapse is associated with positive or close surgical margins (<8 mm), lymphovascular space invasion, deep stromal invasion (>5 mm), and large primary tumor size (Level III) (HOMESLEY et al. 1991); (Level IV) (RUTLEDGE et al. 1991; ROUZIER et al. 2002; HEAPS et al. 1991).
- Patients with one groin node involvement have lower risk of recurrence than patients with two or more nodes involved (HOMESLEY et al. 1991). Patients with unilateral groin nodal involvement have better survival than those with bilateral nodal involvement (CURRY et al. 1980).

25.2 Treatment of Vulvar Cancer

25.2.1 Surgery

- Historically, en bloc radical vulvectomy and regional lymphadenectomy were uniformly applied to all patients regardless of the stage of their disease (WAY 1948).
- Wide local excision (also referred to as radical local excision, radical wide excision, and modified radical vulvectomy) is now used to treat T1 and early T2 vulvar cancer not located near critical midline structures. Obtaining a minimum histopathological margin of 8 mm (equivalent to 1-cm clinical margin) around the tumor is essential to minimize the risk of local recurrence (Level IV) (BURKE et al. 1990). The incision should be carried down to the inferior fascia of the urogenital diaphragm.
- Radical vulvectomy and bilateral groin dissection are recommended to treat large T2 and T3 lesions (Grade B) (BURKE et al. 1995; BURRELL et al. 1988). Triple separate incisions for the vulva and groin instead of en bloc resection are used to reduce the risks of wound breakdown (HACKER et al. 1981). Recurrence within the skin bridge is rare.
- Inguinal lymph node dissection is an important treatment to reduce the mortality of early vulvar cancer and is usually recommended for all cases with invasive disease of more than 1 mm depth (Grade B). The risk of groin node metastasis is related to the size of the primary tumor, depth of invasion, and the presence of lymphovascular space invasion (Level IV) (WILKINSON et al. 1982; KNEALE et al. 1982; KRUPP et al. 1975). Disease spread to contralateral groin nodes without ipsilateral nodal involvement occurs in <15% of patients with metastases to groin nodes, according to a retrospective series of 195 patients who had extended vulvectomy and bilateral inguinal and pelvic lymphadenectomy (Level IV) (KRUPP and BOHM 1978).

In GOG 88, patients with IB–III disease treated with radical vulvectomy were randomized to bilateral inguinal femoral lymph node dissection or external radiation to the groin. If pelvic lymph nodes were involved, then patients received radiation to bilateral inguinal and pelvic nodes. This study was closed after interim analysis of only 58 patients revealed that five patients in the surgery group had positive nodes without any groin failures, and five of 27 patients (18.5%) in the radiation group suffered groin failure. The 2-year overall survival rate favored the surgery group (90% vs. 70%) (GOG 88, Level II) (STEHMAN et al. 1992). Criticisms include poor radiation techniques of radiation dose prescription to a depth of 3 cm, resulting in all inguinal nodes that recurred receiving less than the prescribed dose. KOH et al. (1993) studied a series of patients' CT scans and concluded that the average depth of the femoral vessels was 6 cm below the skin (Level III).

Table 25.2. American Joint Committee on Cancer (AJCC) TNM classification of carcinoma cancer of the Vulva. [From Greene et al. (2002) with permission]

Primary tumor (T)		
TX		Primary tumor cannot be assessed
T0		No evidence of primary tumor
Tis	0	Carcinoma in situ
T1	I	Tumor confined to the vulva or vulva and perineum, 2 cm or less in greatest dimension
T1a	IA	Tumor confined to the vulva, or vulva and perineum, 2 cm or less in greatest dimension, and with stromal invasion no greater than 1 mm
T1b	IB	Tumor confined to the vulva, or vulva and perineum, 2 cm or less in greatest dimension, and with stromal invasion greater than 1 mm
T2	II	Tumor confined to the vulva, or vulva and perineum, more than 2 cm in greatest dimension
T3	III	Tumor of any size with contiguous spread to the lower urethra and/or vagina or anus
T4	IVA	Tumor invades any of the following: upper urethra, bladder mucosa, rectal mucosa, or is fixed to the pubic bone
Regional lymph nodes (N)		
NX		Regional lymph nodes cannot be assessed
N0		No regional lymph node metastasis
N1	III	Unilateral regional lymph node metastasis
N2	IVA	Bilateral regional lymph node metastasis
Distant metastasis (M)		
MX		Distant metastasis cannot be assessed
M0		No distant metastasis
M1	IVB	Distant metastasis (including pelvic lymph node metastasis)
FIGO/AJCC STAGE GROUPING	
0:	Tis N0 M0
I:	T1 N0 M0
IA:	T1a N0 M0
IB:	T1b N0 M0
II:	T2 N0 M0
III:	T1 N1 M0, T2 N1 M0, T3 N0 M0, T3 N1 M0
IVA:	T1 N2 M0, T2 N2 M0, T3 N2 M0, T4 Any N M0
IVB:	Any T Any N M1

- Preoperative radiation or combined chemoradiation therapy should be considered for tumors close to the clitoris, vagina, urethra, or rectum (<5 mm) when preservation of these structures may not be possible with upfront surgery (Grade B). Response to preoperative chemoradiation therapy can be observed in approximately 90% of cases (Level III) (Lupi et al. 1996). The effect of preoperative chemoradiation therapy has been supported by results of a phase-II GOG study, as detailed below (Level III) (Moore et al. 1998).

- Extended radical vulvectomy and bilateral groin dissection or pelvic exenteration may be required for tumors involving the rectum, vagina, or urethra (Cavanagh and Shepherd 1982; Phillips et al. 1981). Preoperative radiation or combined chemoradiation therapy, or definitive chemoradiation, should be considered for organ preservation.

- Sentinel lymph node evaluation is a promising staging technique in the absence of suspicious inguinal lymph nodes, but the false-negative rate is not well defined (Level III) (Sliutz et al. 2002; DeCicco et al. 2000; de Hullu et al. 2000; Moore et al. 2003; Puig-Tintore et al. 2003). Further clinical studies are needed before it can be routinely applied.

25.2.2 Radiation Therapy

Preoperative Radiation Therapy

- Preoperative radiation or preoperative chemoradiation followed by inguinal lymph node dissection and resection of residual primary tumor should be considered for locally advanced lesions and/or clinically matted/fixed/ulcerated lymph nodes (Grade B). 5-FU, cisplatin and mitomycin-C are the most common chemotherapy agents used with radiation.

- A phase-II GOG study of patients with stage III–IV squamous cell vulvar carcinoma examined the feasibility and outcomes of preoperative chemoradiation (47.6 Gy with concurrent cisplatin and 5-FU) in reducing the need for more radical surgery; 46.5% of patients completing treatment had no visible vulvar cancer at the time of planned surgery, and only 2.8% had residual unresectable disease. In only three patients was it not possible to preserve urinary and/or gastrointestinal continence (GOG, Level III) (Moore et al. 1998).

Postoperative Radiation Therapy

■ Postoperative radiation is used when limited surgery has been performed for organ preservation or when adverse pathologic features, such as large tumor (>4 cm), positive, or close (<8 mm) surgical margin, lymphovascular space invasion, and depth of stromal invasion >5 mm, are present (Grade B). Surgical margin is the most powerful predictor of local vulvar recurrence, and a margin less than 8 mm is associated with a 50% chance of recurrence (Level IV) (Heaps et al. 1990).

■ Results of a retrospective study of 50 patients with primary or recurrent vulvar cancer treated with combined surgery and radiation showed that wide local tumor excision and radiation therapy or irradiation alone in T1-2 tumors is an alternative treatment to radical vulvectomy in controlling vulvar carcinoma, with significantly less morbidity (Level IV) (Perez et al. 1993).

■ Postoperative radiation is also indicated in patients with two or more involved inguinal nodes (Grade A), extracapsular extension, or gross residual nodal disease (Grade B).
In GOG 37, patients with involved inguinal nodes after radical vulvectomy and bilateral inguinal node dissection were randomized to pelvic node dissection versus postoperative radiotherapy. Radiation was delivered bilaterally to the pelvic and inguinal nodes while shielding the central vulva area; 45–50 Gy was prescribed to the midplane using anterior and posterior opposing fields. The trial was closed after 114 patients were accrued after interim analysis revealing a significant survival advantage for patients receiving radiotherapy (2-year survival 68% vs. 54%, p=0.03) due to lower rate of relapse in the radiotherapy arm (5% vs. 24%, p=0.02). Subset analysis suggested this survival advantage was particularly noted in patients presenting with clinically suspicious or fixed ulcerated groin nodes or two or more positive groin nodes. There was no difference in pelvic recurrence (Level I) (Homesley et al. 1986). As a result of this study, pelvic lymph node dissection is not indicated, and adjuvant radiation has become the standard of care for patients with the above two major poor prognostic factors present (Grade A).

■ The radiation volume should encompass the primary tumor bed and surgical bed (Grade C). Radical vulvectomy has been considered sufficient for treatment for vulvar carcinoma, and postoperative radiation can be directed only to the lymph nodes. However, results from a retrospective study suggested that the application of a midline block to protect the radiosensitive vulva resulted in a 48% central recurrence rate (versus less than 10% reported historically). Postoperative radiation volumes should be tailored to the individual patient (Level IV) (Dusenbery et al. 1994).

■ The additional benefit of concurrent chemotherapy with postoperative radiation in patients with high-risk features for relapse is unclear.

Definitive Chemoradiation Therapy

■ Definitive chemoradiation is indicated for unresectable or medically inoperable vulvar cancers. It is also indicated in locally advanced vulvar cancer for organ preservation (Grade B). High response rates have been reported, and the majority of patients achieving complete response have durable local control. In a small series of 14 patient treated with definitive chemotherapy (cisplatin and 5-FU) and radiation therapy, a total response rate of 92% was reported, and 64% of patients achieved complete response (Level III) (Cunningham et al. 1997). Similar results have been demonstrated in other non-randomized prospective trials (Level III, IV) (Akl et al. 2000; Han et al. 2000; Montana et al. 2000; Gerszten et al. 2005).

■ Although the efficacy of combined chemoradiotherapy as compared to radiotherapy has not been studied in prospective randomized trials, retrospective data suggest the superiority of chemoradiation compared to radiation alone (Level III).

External-Beam Radiation Therapy Techniques

■ Patients must be treated with equipment with photon energy of 6 MV or greater for pelvic irradiation.

■ CT-based planning is essential to obtain the depth of inguinal nodes (Grade B). The average depth of femoral lymph nodes is 6 cm, but can range from 2.0 cm to 18.5 cm (Level III) (Koh et al. 1993). Delineation of the femoral lymph nodes is critical for adequate coverage of the inguinal nodes. The location of the inguinofemoral nodes is depicted in Figure 25.1 (Level III) (Wang et al. 1996).

- Various treatment techniques of conventional radiation therapy are available for vulvar cancer treatment:
- A wide AP field that includes the pelvic and inguinal regions, with a narrow PA field covering only the pelvis and sparing the femoral heads; the dose to inguinal regions is supplemented by separate anterior electron fields matched to the pelvic field (Fig. 25.2). This technique is described in detail below.
  - A wide AP field and narrow PA field with a partial transmission block placed in the central portion of the AP field. The desired dose at a specific depth is delivered to the inguinal nodes through the AP field (Kalend et al. 1990).
  - Matched AP/PA fields to include the primary and the pelvic nodes and treating the groins through separate anterior electron fields (Fig. 25.3).

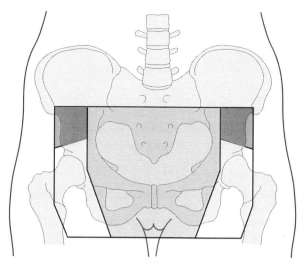

Fig. 25.2. Treatment borders demonstrating the wide anterior field (*outer border*) and the narrow posterior field (*shaded region*). The pelvis, vulva, perineum and inguinal lymph nodes will be treated with AP-PA technique to include lateral inguinal nodes within AP fields but not PA fields. Patient lies supine with a full bladder

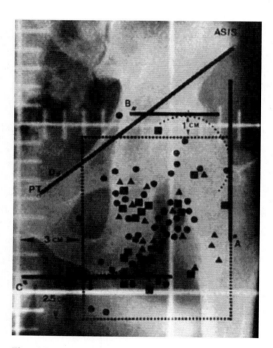

Fig. 25.1. Topographic distribution of inguinal lymph node metastases in patients with carcinoma of the anus and low rectum (circles, n=50), vulva vagina-cervix (triangles, n=17), and urethra (squares, n=17). The field arrangement described provided adequate coverage of 86% of all inguinal lymph nodes (Level III) (Reprinted from Wang et al. (1996) with permission

- The use of a midline block to shield the radiosensitive vulva is controversial and should be avoided to reduce the probability of local recurrence (Grade C). In the study by Dusenbery et al. (1994), 27 patients with stage III/IV vulvar cancer with involved inguinal lymph nodes were treated with postoperative radiation with a midline block after surgical resection. The use of a midline block was associated with 48% central recurrence rate (Level IV).
- Intensity-modulated radiation therapy (IMRT) can be considered in the treatment of vulvar cancer (Grade B). Early results from a comparative dosimetric study revealed an optimal clinical response and a reduction of doses to normal structures, including the rectum, bladder, small bowel, and femoral heads in retrospective studies (Level III) (Ahmad et al. 2004; Beriwal et al. 2006). However, long-term results after IMRT for preoperative, definitive, or postoperative treatment of vulva cancer are lacking.

Simulation and Field Arrangements

- Patients are simulated in supine, frog-leg position (to minimize the bolus effect from skin folds) with the bladder full (to minimize the volume of small bowel in the radiation field) with custom immobilization.

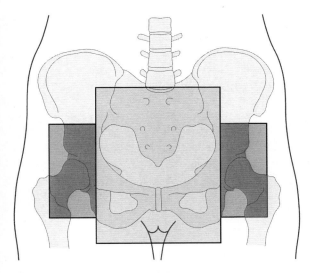

Fig. 25.3. Treatment borders demonstrating the matched AP/PA fields to include the primary and the pelvic nodes only. The inguinal lymph nodes will be treated throught separate anterior electron firles (*shaded areas*)

- Enlarged inguinal lymph nodes, vulva tumor, scars, and anal verge should be outlined with wire for identification on planning CT.
- The borders of the pelvic field are as follows (Fig. 25.2):
- Superiorly: mid SI joint to include external and internal iliac lymph nodes; if there is suspected or proven internal or external iliac node involvement, the superior border at L4/5 should include the common iliac nodes.
- Inferiorly: flash the entire vulva or inferior margin of the tumor (whichever is lower).
- Laterally: 2 cm beyond the widest point of the pelvic inlet on the PA field and greater trochanter to include inguinal lymph nodes in the AP field.

- Supplemental radiation using anterior electron fields to the lateral inguinal region matched with the exit PA field is required to bring the dose to the inguinal nodal region to 45 Gy.
- It is a common practice to include the inguinal node dissection scars in the radiation field.
- Bolus material should be used to ensure adequate dose to the superficial portions of the groin.
- Cone down fields encompassing the primary tumor (and involved inguinal lymph nodes) plus a 2- to 3-cm margin after 45 Gy to the pelvis.

Dose and Fractionation

- Preoperative radiation dose for the area of the primary and the lymph nodes should be 45–50 Gy (Grade B). Response to radiation alone in this dose range can be expected in close to 90% of patients (ACOSTA et al. 1978; HACKER et al. 1984). External-beam radiation should be delivered as a continuous course at 1.7–2.0 Gy per daily fraction.
- Postoperative radiation dose for possible residual microscopic disease is 50 Gy. If there is extracapsular extension of tumor in the lymph nodes, the dose to the groins should be 50–60 Gy. If there is gross residual disease, the dose should be 65–70 Gy.
- For definitive chemoradiation with appropriate field reduction, the dose should be brought up to 60–65 Gy as tolerated by the patient.

Side Effects, Complications, and Dose Limiting Structures

- The most significant acute toxicity of radiation alone or in combination with chemotherapy is the skin reaction in the vulva-perineal region and inguinal folds. Moist desquamation by the 3rd to 5th weeks of treatment is common. A treatment break is almost always necessary. Diarrhea and cystitis are other common acute side effects.
- Acute hematologic toxicity is common and depends on the type and intensity of the chemotherapy used.
- Common late toxicities include telangiectasia, atrophy of skin, fibrosis, dryness, and shortening and narrowing of the vagina. Avascular necrosis of the femoral head has been reported (ANDERSON et al. 1988). Femoral neck fracture is associated with osteoporosis and smoking.
- Dose limiting structures in vulvar radiation include the bladder, rectum, femoral heads, small bowel, and lower vagina. Attention should be paid to limit the amount of small bowel in the treatment field. The radiation dose to the bladder should be limited to 60 Gy, to the femoral head and neck to 45 Gy, to the small bowel to 45-50 Gy, and to the lower vagina to 75-80 Gy.
- Treatment of vulvar cancer is also associated with significant psychosexual consequences, relating to sexual function and body image (Level IV) (ANDERSEN and HACKER 1983).

Intensity-Modulated Radiation Therapy (IMRT)

- Intensity-modulated radiation therapy (IMRT) has been shown to offer an advantage over 3D CRT for vulvar cancer by reducing the dose to normal structures, such as the bladder, rectum, small bowel, and femoral heads, and eliminating dose modulation across the overlapping region (Level III) (AHMAD et al. 2004; BERIWAL et al. 2006).
- If used, the clinical tumor volume (CTV) should include a 1- to 2-cm margin around the entire vulvar region and a 1- to 2-cm margin around the bilateral external iliac, internal iliac, and inguinofemoral nodes. The planning tumor volume (PTV) is defined as a 1-cm margin beyond CTV. Normal tissue constraints include the small bowel, bladder, rectum, and femoral heads (BERIWAL et al. 2006).

25.2.3 Chemotherapy

Preoperative

- Single-agent chemotherapy is mostly ineffective as a preoperative treatment for advanced vulvar cancer. Combination chemotherapy is recommended for preoperative treatment (Grade B). Multidrug chemotherapy has been shown to provide better a response rate, but is associated with significant toxicity. The response rate to neoadjuvant bleomycin (B), methotrexate (M), and CCNU (C) was 56% according to a phase II study from EORTC (Level III) (DURRANT et al. 1990; WAGENAAR et al. 2001). The results of a recently reported retrospective study combining chemotherapy with 5-FU and cisplatin provided a response rate of 100% in a small group of patient treated in neoadjuvant fashion (Level IV) (GEISLER et al. 2006). Most trials studying combined chemoradiation have been performed using 5-FU alone or in combination with cisplatin or mitomycin-C (AKL et al. 2000; CUNNINGHAM et al. 1997; EIFEL et al. 1995; HAN et al. 2000; LUPI et al. 1996; MOORE et al. 1998).
- Chemotherapy combined with radiation to potentiate the effectiveness of radiation is rapidly becoming the standard of care for tumors close to the clitoris, vagina, urethra, or rectum (<5 mm) when preservation of these structures may not be possible with upfront surgery (Grade B). A total response of 90% can be expected after neoadjuvant chemoradiation therapy, and its efficacy has been demonstrated in a prospective phase II trial detailed above (Level III) (LUPI et al. 1996; MOORE et al. 1998).
- Bleomycin alone is not recommended in the preoperative setting with combined radiation therapy (Grade B). Results of two prospective trials using radiation with concurrent bleomycin have been disappointing (Level III) (IVERSEN 1982; SCHEISTRÖEN and TROPÉ 1993).

Postoperative

- Concurrent chemoradiation can be recommended for patients with high-risk pathological features, such as close/involved surgical margins, lymphovascular space invasion, and involved lymph nodes (Grade C). However, the effect of combined chemoradiation therapy versus radiation therapy alone given after surgery has not yet been demonstrated in any prospective trials. Results from small retrospective series have not demonstrated the additive effect of chemotherapy to radiation in the adjuvant setting (Level IV) (HAN et al. 2000).

Chemotherapy for Recurrent or Metastatic Disease

- Chemotherapy for recurrent or metastatic vulvar cancer is recommended; however, its use has not been extensively studied or proven to be of great benefit. Responses have been low in phase II trials (Level III) (DEPPE et al. 1979).

25.3 Follow-Ups

25.3.1 Post-Treatment Follow-Ups

- Life-long follow-up is required for all patients with vulvar cancer treated with curative intent for early detection of tumor recurrence and second primary gynecological malignancies (Grade B). The risk of second primary cancer other than vulvar, such as cervical, is also noted to be a reason for routine long-term follow-up (Level IV) (CHOO 1982).

Schedule

■ Follow-up should be every 3 months initially in the first 2 years, every 6 months thereafter through year 5, then annually thereafter (Table 25.3) (Grade D). Most recurrences occur within 3 years after the completion of treatment. Distant spread occurs late in the course of the disease. Sites of hematogenous spread include bone and lung.

Work-Ups

■ Each follow-up examination should include a complete history and physical examination, including a pelvic examination. Chest X-ray should be obtained annually for 5 years.

■ Imaging studies (CT scan of abdomen and pelvis or FDG-PET) are indicated for suspected recurrent disease discovered on physical examination or laboratory studies.

Table 25.3. Follow-up schedule

Interval	Frequency
First 2 years	Every 3 months
Years 3–5	Every 6 months
Over 5 years	Annually

References

Acosta AA, Given FT, Frazier AB et al. (1978) Preoperative radiation therapy in the management of squamous cell carcinoma of the vulva: preliminary report. Am J Obstet Gynecol 132:198–206

Ahmad M, Song H, Moran M et al. (2004) IMRT of whole pelvis and inguinal nodes: evaluation of dose distributions produced by an inverse treatment planning system. Int J Radiat Oncol Biol Phys 60:484–485

Akl A, Akl M, Boike G et al. (2000) Preliminary results of chemoradiation as a primary treatment for vulvar carcinoma. Int J Radiat Oncol Biol Phys 48:415–420

Andersen BL, Hacker NF (1983) Psychosexual adjustment after vulvar surgery. Obstet Gynecol 62:457–462

Anderson BL, Turnquist D, LaPolla J et al. (1988) Sexual functioning after treatment of in situ vulvar cancer: preliminary report. Obstet Gynecol 71:15–19

Andreasson B, Nyboe J (1985) Value of prognostic parameters in squamous cell carcinoma of the vulva. Gynecol Oncol 22:341–351

Andrews SJ, Williams BT, DePriest PD et al. (1994) Therapeutic implications of lymph nodal spread in lateral T1 and T2 squamous cell carcinoma of the vulva. Gynecol Oncol 55:41–46

Beriwal S, Heron DE, Kim H et al. (2006) Intensity-modulated radiotherapy for the treatment of vulvar carcinoma: a comparative dosimetric study with early clinical outcome. Int J Radiat Oncol Biol Phys 64:1395–1400

Binder SW, Huang I, Fu YS et al. (1990) Risk factors for the development of lymph node metastasis in vulvar squamous cell carcinoma. Gynecol Oncol 37:9–16

Boyce J, Fruchter RG, Kasambilides E et al. (1985) Prognostic factors in carcinoma of the vulva. Gynecol Oncol 20:364–377

Burke TW, Stringer CA, Gershenson DM et al. (1990) Radical wide excision and selective inguinal node dissection for squamous cell carcinoma of the vulva. Gynecol Oncol 38:328–332

Burke TW, Levenback C, Coleman RL et al. (1995) Surgical therapy of T1 and T2 vulvar carcinoma: further experience with radical wide excision and selective inguinal lymphadenectomy. Obstet Gynecol 57:215–220

Burrell MO, Franklin EW 3rd, Campion MJ et al. (1988) The modified radical vulvectomy with groin dissection: an eight-year experience. Am J Obstet Gynecol 159:715–722

Cavanagh D, Shepherd JH (1982) The place of pelvic exenteration in the primary management of advanced carcinoma of the vulva. Obstet Gynecol 13:318–322

Choo YC (1982) Invasive squamous carcinoma of the vulva in young patients. Gynecol Oncol 13:158–164

Cohn DE, Dehdashti F, Gibb RK et al. (2002) Prospective evaluation of positron emission tomography for the detection of groin node metastases from vulvar cancer. Gynecol Oncol 85:179–184

Crosby JH, Bryan AB, Gallup DG et al. (1989) Fine-needle aspiration of inguinal lymph nodes in gynecologic practice. Obstet Gynecol 73:281–284

Cunningham MJ, Goyer RP, Gibbons SK et al. (1997) Primary radiation, cisplatin, and 5-fluorouracil for advanced squamous carcinoma of the vulva. Gynecol Oncol 66:258–261

Curry SL, Wharton JT, Rutledge F (1980) Positive lymph nodes in the vulvar squamous carcinoma. Gynecol Oncol 9:63–67

DeCicco C, Sideri M, Bartolomei M et al. (2000) Sentinel node biopsy in early vulvar cancer. Br J Cancer 82:295–299

de Hullu JA, Hollerna H, Piers DA et al. (2000) Sentinel lymph node procedure is highly accurate in squamous cell carcinoma of the vulva. J Clin Oncol 18:2811–2816

Deppe G, Cohen CJ, Bruckner HW (1979) Chemotherapy of squamous cell carcinoma of the vulva: a review. Gynecol Oncol 7:345–348

Donaldson ES, Powell DE, Hanson MB et al. (1981) Prognostic parameters in invasive vulvar cancer. Gynecol Oncol 11:184–190

Durrant KR, Mangioni C, Lacave AJ et al. (1990) Bleomycin, methotrexate, and CCNU in advanced inoperable squamous cell carcinoma of the vulva: a phase II study of the EORTC Gynecological Cancer Cooperative Group (GCCG). Gynecol Oncol 37:359–362

Dusenbery KE, Carlson JW, LaPorte RM et al. (1994) Radical vulvectomy with postoperative irradiation for vulvar cancer: therapeutic implications of a central block. Int J Radiat Oncol Biol Phys 29:989–998

Eifel PJ, Morris M, Burke TW et al. (1995) Prolonged continuous infusion cisplatin and 5-fluorouracil with radiation for locally advanced cancer of the vulva. Gynecol Oncol 59:51–56

Geisler JP, Manahan KJ, Buller RE (2006) Neoadjuvant chemotherapy in vulvar cancer: avoiding primary exenteration. Gynecol Oncol 100:53–57

Gerszten K, Selvaraj RN, Kelley J et al. (2005) Preoperative chemoradiation for locally advanced carcinoma of the vulva. Obstet Gynecol 99:640–644

Greene F, Page D, Fleming I et al. (2002) AJCC Cancer Staging Manual, 6th edn. Springer, Berlin Heidelberg New York

Hacker NF, Leuchter RS, Berek JS et al. (1981) Radical vulvectomy and bilateral inguinal lymphadenectomy through separate groin incisions. Obstet Gynecol 58:574–579

Hacker NF, Berek JS, Juillard GJ et al. (1984) Preoperative radiation therapy for locally advanced vulvar cancer. Cancer 54:2056–2061

Hacker NF, Berek JS, Lagasse LD et al. (1984) Individualization of treatment for stage I squamous cell vulvar carcinoma. Obstet Gynecol 63:155–162

Han SC, Kim DH, Higgins SA et al. (2000) Chemoradiation as primary or adjuvant treatment for locally advanced carcinoma of the vulva. Int J Radiat Oncol Biol Phys 47:1235–1244

Heaps JM, Fu YS, Montz FJ et al. (1990) Surgical-pathologic variables predictive of local recurrence in squamous cell carcinoma of the vulva. Gynecol Oncol 38:309–314

Hoffman JS, Kumar NB, Morley GW (1983) Microinvasive squamous carcinoma of the vulva: search for a definition. Obstet Gynecol 61:615–618

Homesley HD, Bundy BN, Sedlis A et al. (1986) Radiation therapy versus pelvic node resection for carcinoma of the vulva with positive groin nodes. Obstet Gynecol 68:733–740

Homesley HD, Bundy BN, Sedlis A et al. (1991) Assessment of current International Federation of Gynecology and Obstetrics staging of vulvar carcinoma relative to prognostic factors for survival (a Gynecologic Oncology Group study). Am J Obstet Gynecol 164:997–1003

Homesley HD, Bundy BN, Sedlis A et al. (1993) Prognostic factors for groin node metastasis in squamous cell carcinoma of the vulva (a Gynecologic Oncology Group study). Gynecol Oncol 49:279–283

Iversen T (1982) Irradiation and bleomycin in the treatment of inoperable vulval carcinoma. Acta Obstet Gynecol Scand 61:195–197

Iversen T, Aalders JG, Christensen A et al. (1980) Squamous cell carcinoma of the vulva: a review of 424 patients 1956–1974. Gynecol Oncol 9:271–279

Kalend AM, Park TL, Wu A et al. (1990) Clinical use of a wing field with transmission block for the treatment of the pelvis including the inguinal node. Int J Radiat Oncol Biol Phys 19:153–158

Kneale BLG, Elliott PM, McDonald IA (1981) Microinvasive carcinoma of the vulva: Clinical features and management. In: Coppleson M (ed) Gynecologic Oncology. Edinburgh, Churchill Livingstone, p 320

Koh WJ, Chiu M, Stelzer KJ et al. (1993) Femoral vessel depth and the implications for groin node radiation. Int J Radiat Oncol Biol Phys 27:969–974

Krupp PJ, Bohm JW (1978) Lymph gland metastases in invasive squamous cell carcinoma of the vulva. Am J Obstet Gynecol 130:943–952

Krupp PJ, Lee FY, Bohm JW et al. (1975) Prognostic parameters and clinical staging criteria in epidermoid carcinoma of the vulva. Obstet Gynecol 46:84–88

Lupi G, Raspagliesi F, Zucali R et al. (1996) Combined preoperative chemoradiotherapy followed by radical surgery in locally advanced vulvar carcinoma. A pilot study. Cancer 77:1472–1478

Montana GS, Thomas GM, Moore DH et al. (2000) Preoperative chemoradiation for carcinoma of the vulva with N2/N3 nodes: a gynecologic oncology group study. Int J Radiat Oncol Biol Phys 48:1007–1013

Moore DH, Thomas GM, Montana GS et al. (1998) Preoperative chemoradiation for advanced vulvar cancer: A phase II study of the Gynecologic Oncology Group. Int J Radiat Oncol Biol Phys 42:79–85

Moore RG, Depasquale SE, Steinhoff MM et al. (2003) Sentinel node identification and the ability to detect metastatic tumor to inguinal lymph nodes in vulvar malignancies. Gynecol Oncol 89:475–479

Morley GW (1976) Infiltrative carcinoma of the vulva: results of surgical treatment. Am J Obstet Gynecol 124:874–888

Morris JM (1977) A formula for selective lymphadenectomy: its application to cancer of the vulva. Obstet Gynecol 50:152–158

Perez CA Grigsby PW, Galakatos A et al. (1993) Radiation therapy in management of carcinoma of the vulva with emphasis on conservation therapy. Cancer 71:3707–3716

Phillips B, Buchsbaum HJ, Lifshitz S (1981) Pelvic exenteration for vulvovaginal carcinoma. Am J Obstet Gynecol 141:1038–1044

Podratz KC, Symmonds RE, Taylor WF et al. (1983) Carcinoma of the vulva: analysis of treatment and survival Obstet Gynecol 61:63–74

Puig-Tintore LM, Ordi J, Vidal-Sicart S et al. (2003) Further data on the usefulness of sentinel lymph node identification and ultrastaging in vulvar squamous cell carcinoma. Gynecol Oncol 88:29–34

Rutledge FN, Mitchell MF, Munsell MF et al. (1991) Prognostic indicators for invasive carcinoma of the vulva. Gynecol Oncol 42:239–244

Rouzier R, Haddad B, Plantier F et al. (2002) Local relapse in patients treated for squamous cell vulvar carcinoma: incidence and prognostic value. Obstet Gynecol 100:1159–1167

Rutledge F, Smith JP, Franklin EW (1970) Carcinoma of the vulva. Am J Obstet Gynecol 106:1117–1130

Scheiströen M, Tropé C (1993) Combined Bleomycin and irradiation in preoperative treatment of advanced squamous cell carcinoma of the vulva. Acta Oncol 32:657–661

Sliutz G, Reinthaller A, Lantzsch T et al. (2002) Lymphatic mapping of sentinel nodes in early vulvar cancer. Gynecol Oncol 84:449–452

Stehman FB, Bundy BN, Thomas G et al. (1992) Groin dissection versus groin radiation in carcinoma of the vulva: a Gynecologic Oncology Group study. Int J Radiat Oncol Biol Phys 24:389–396

Wagenaar HC, Colombo N, Vergote I et al. (2001) Bleomycin, methotrexate, and CCNU in locally advanced or recurrent, inoperable, squamous cell carcinoma of the vulva: an EORTC Gynecological Cancer Cooperative Group Study, European Organization for Research and Treatment of Cancer. Gynecol Oncol 81:348–354

Wang, CJ, Chin, YY, Leung SW et al. (1996) Topographic distribution of inguinal lymph nodes metastasis: significance in determination of treatment margin for elective inguinal lymph nodes irradiation of low pelvic tumors. Int J Radiat Oncol Biol Phys 35:133–136

Way S (1948) The anatomy of the lymphatic drainage of the vulva and its influence on the radical operation. Ann R Coll Surg Engl 3:1159–1164

Way S (1960) Carcinoma of the vulva. Am J Obstet Gynecol 79:692–697

Wharton JT, Gallager S, Rutledge FN (1974) Microinvasive carcinoma of the vulva. Am J Obstet Gynecol 118:159–162

Wilkinson EJ, Rico MJ, Pierson KK (1982) Microinvasive carcinoma of vulva. Int J Gynecol Pathol 1:29–39

Vaginal Cancer

26

Hiram A. Gay and Ron R. Allison

CONTENTS

Introduction and Objectives

Carcinomas of the vagina are uncommon tumors comprising 2% of gynecologic malignancies. Malignancy of epithelial origin is the most commonly diagnosed entity, and the clinical characteristics of vaginal intraepithelial neoplasia (VaIN) or invasive squamous cell carcinoma of vagina differ significantly from those of adenocarcinoma and malignant melanoma. Radiotherapy plays a central role in the management of invasive vaginal carcinoma.

This chapter focuses on the management of vaginal carcinoma, particularly VaIN, invasive squamous cell carcinoma, invasive adenocarcinoma, and melanoma, and examines:

● Recommendations for diagnostic and staging procedures

● The staging systems and prognostic factors

● Treatment recommendations for VaIN, invasive squamous cell carcinoma, invasive adenocarcinoma, and melanoma, as well as the supporting peer-reviewed scientific evidence

● Follow-up care and surveillance of survivors

The management of vaginal sarcomas, lymphomas, and other rare vaginal tumors are not the focus of this chapter.

H. A. GAY, MD
Department of Radiation Oncology, The Brody School of Medicine at ECU, 600 Moye Blvd., Greenville, NC 27834, USA
R. R. ALLISON, MD
Department of Radiation Oncology, The Brody School of Medicine at ECU, 600 Moye Blvd., Greenville, NC 27834, USA

26.1 Diagnosis, Staging, and Prognoses

26.1.1 Diagnosis

Initial Evaluation

- Diagnosis and evaluation of vaginal cancer starts with a complete history and physical examination. Careful bimanual and rectovaginal clinical examination should be performed in all cases, preferably by an experienced examiner and under anesthesia.
- Most lesions of vaginal cancer occur in the upper vagina. Anterior and posterior lesions, especially in the lower two-thirds of the vagina, can be easily missed since the blades of the speculum obscure this area. Therefore, the speculum should be slowly withdrawn so that the entire vaginal mucosa is visualized. A light source adaptable transparent plastic speculum may facilitate visualization of the entire vaginal mucosa.
- Definitive diagnosis is accomplished by biopsy of the suspected lesion. Cervical and vulvar cancer primaries should be excluded, and may require multiple biopsies of these areas. Examination of the perianal area to rule out a synchronous anal cancer should be performed.
- If a lesion is not visualized in the presence of abnormal cytologic results, colposcopy of the cervix and vagina must be performed with acetic acid followed by Lugol's iodine stain (Schiller's test).

Table 26.1. Imaging and laboratory work-ups for vaginal cancer

Imaging studies	Laboratory tests
– Chest X-ray	– Complete blood count
– CT or MRI scan of abdomen and pelvis[a]	– Liver function tests
	– Renal function tests
– FDG-PET scan (for detection of metastatic disease, particularly in locoregionally advanced disease)	– HIV (if clinically suspected or if patient is at high risk)

[a] MRI yields the most useful information for guiding locoregional treatment.

Laboratory Tests

- Initial laboratory tests should include a complete blood count, and liver and renal function tests. (see Table 26.1).

- HIV testing should be performed if clinically suspected or if patient is at high risk due to intravenous drug use since 1985 or sexual risk behaviors (e.g., having ever had more than 5 sexual partners, traded sex for drugs or money, or engaged in sex with a male injecting drug user or a man known or suspected to be HIV-infected).

Imaging Studies

- An abdominal and pelvic MRI using a pelvic phased array is recommended for staging of locoregional disease (Grade C) (see Table 26.1). T2-weighted images acquired using a pelvic phased array coil provided the best detail for staging. Most tumors are of iso-intense signal to muscle on T1-weighted images and hyper-intense to muscle on T2-weighted images. In a retrospective study of 25 patients with primary vaginal carcinoma stage I–IV, MRI identified over 95% of the tumors. Bladder, ureter, urethra, rectal, muscle, cervix, and pelvic sidewall involvement were visualized in various patients. The authors proposed an MRI staging system based on the FIGO staging; however, there was no pathologic confirmation of the findings (Level IV) (TAYLOR et al. 2007).
- FDG-PET is recommended for evaluation of lymph node metastases (Grade C). In a prospective registry study of 23 consecutive patients stage II–IVA with carcinoma of the vagina, FDG-PET identified abnormal uptake in 21 intact primary tumors (100%), compared to nine (43%) visualized on CT. Abnormal uptake was found in the groin lymph nodes in four patients, pelvic lymph nodes in two, and both groin and pelvic lymph nodes in two patients (eight of 23, 35%). The sensitivity and specificity of FDG-PET for the detection of lymph node metastases could not be determined since there was no pathologic confirmation of groin or pelvic lymph nodes with abnormal uptake on FDG-PET (Level III) (LAMOREAUX et al. 2005).

Pathology

- Secondary malignancy of the vagina is far more frequent than primary vaginal malignancy.
- Most vaginal cancers occur in post-menopausal or elderly women.
- In the United States, primary vaginal cancer falls predominantly in the invasive carcinoma (66%) and in situ carcinoma (25%) categories. The majority of invasive cancers are squamous

(79%), followed by adenocarcinoma (14%), melanoma, sarcoma, and others in order of frequency (Level IV) (CREASMAN et al. 1998).

- The percentage of invasive squamous cell carcinomas increases with age, from 14% in ages 0–19, to 86% in patients older than 80. On the other hand, the percentage of in situ carcinomas and adenocarcinomas decreases with age (Level IV) (CREASMAN et al. 1998).

- The histologic distinction between squamous cell carcinoma and adenocarcinoma is important because the two types represent distinct diseases with different clinical behaviors.

Table 26.2. FIGO staging system for carcinoma of the vagina. [Adapted with permission from the International Federation of Gynecology and Obstetrics (FIGO); the original source of the FIGO information is from: Beller U, Benedet JL, Creasman WT, Ngan HYS, Quinn MA, Maisonneuve PA et al. (2006) Carcinoma of the vagina. Int J Gynecol Obstet 95(Suppl 1):S29-S42]

FIGO	AJCC	FIGO description
	TX	Primary tumor cannot be assessed
	T0	No evidence of primary tumor
Stage 0	Tis	Carcinoma in situ; intraepithelial neoplasia grade 3[a]
Stage I	T1	The carcinoma is limited to the vaginal wall
Stage II	T2	The carcinoma has involved the subvaginal[b] tissue but has not extended to the pelvic wall
Stage III	T3	The carcinoma has extended to the pelvic wall[c]
Stage IV	T4	The carcinoma has extended beyond the true pelvis or has involved the mucosa of the bladder or rectum; bullous edema as such does not permit a case to be allotted to stage IV
IVA		Tumor invades bladder and/or rectal mucosa and/or direct extension beyond the true pelvis
IVB		Spread to distant organ

[a] Only FIGO makes the distinction "intraepithelial neoplasia Grade 3."
[b] The AJCC Cancer Staging Manual, 6th Edition, uses the word "paravaginal" instead of subvaginal.
[c] The AJCC Cancer Staging Manual, 6th Edition, defines pelvic wall as muscle, fascia, neurovascular structures, or skeletal portions of the bony pelvis

26.1.2 Staging

- Vaginal cancer is usually staged clinically and both FIGO (Table 26.2) and AJCC (Table 26.3) staging for vaginal cancer are clinical. The following examinations are allowed for clinical staging: palpation, inspection, colposcopy, endocervical curettage, hysteroscopy, cystoscopy, proctoscopy, intravenous urography, and X-ray examination of the lungs and skeleton. Findings from laparoscopy and other imaging modalities are of value for planning therapy, but should not be the basis of clinical staging (GREENE et al. 2002).

- Since secondary malignancy of the vagina is more frequent than primary vaginal malignancy, a careful metastatic work-up is necessary. A growth that involves the cervix, including the external os, should always be assigned to carcinoma of the cervix. Tumors present in the vagina as secondary growths, from either genital or extra-genital sites should not be included (GREENE et al. 2002). The vagina can be a common site of metastatic disease through direct extension of cervical and vulvar tumors, or lymphatic or vascular spread from other cancers.

Table 26.3. American Joint Committee on Cancer (AJCC) stage grouping for carcinoma of the vagina. [Used with the permission of the American Joint Committee on Cancer (AJCC), Chicago, Illinois. The original source for this material is the AJCC Cancer Staging Manual, Sixth Edition (2002) published by Springer Science and Business Media LLC, HYPERLINK "http://www.springerlink.com" www.springerlink.com]

Regional lymph nodes (N)	
NX	Regional nodes cannot be assessed
N0	No regional lymph node metastasis
N1	Pelvic or inguinal lymph node metastasis
Distant metastasis (M)	
MX	Distant metastasis cannot be assessed
M0	No distant metastasis
M1	Distant metastasis
STAGE GROUPING	
0:	Tis[a] N0 M0
I:	T1 N0 M0
II:	T2 N0 M0
III:	T3 N0 M0, T1–T3 N1
IVA:	T4 Any N M0
IVB:	Any T Any N M1

[a] See Table 26.2 for the (T) definitions

26.1.3 Prognostic Factors

- Stage at presentation is the most important prognostic factor of vaginal cancer. Advanced stages are associated with worse disease-specific survival (DSS) (Frank et al. 2005) and cause-specific survival (CSS) (Level IV) (KIRKBRIDE et al. 1995).
- The size of the primary tumor is of prognostic significance: Tumors > 4 cm in largest dimension have worse DSS (Frank et al. 2005) and CSS as compared to those ≤ 4 cm (Level IV) (KIRKBRIDE et al. 1995).
- Non-diethylstilbestrol (DES)-associated adenocarcinoma of the vagina (NDAV) has worse overall survival, pelvic disease control rate, and higher likelihood of developing distant metastases when compared to patients with squamous cell carcinoma (Level IV) (FRANK et al. 2007).
- Histology, tumor grade, age, lymph node status, overall treatment time, length of vaginal involvement, tumor site, parametrial dose, prior hysterectomy, and hemoglobin level have been statistically significant prognostic factors in some series. However, findings from various reports were inconsistent (Level IV) (TRAN et al. 2007).

26.2 Treatment of Vaginal Intraepithelial Neoplasia

26.2.1 General Principles

- Since the natural history of VaIN has not been fully characterized, treatment of vaginal intraepithelial neoplasia (VaIN) is recommended given the potential of some lesions to progress to invasive carcinoma (Grade B). A large proportion of VaIN lesions are multifocal, and approximately one half of the lesions are associated with concomitant cervical or vulvar intraepithelial neoplasia (VIN). These lesions can progress to invasive carcinoma, persist, or regress (Level IV) (AHO et al. 1991). The upper third of the vagina is the most frequently involved site.
- The choice of therapy for VaIN depends on the presence or absence of: multifocal disease, medical comorbidities, desire to preserve sexual function, previous treatment failures, and the certainty with which invasive disease has been excluded.

- Patients with HIV have more vulvar, vaginal, and perianal intraepithelial lesions compared with HIV-uninfected women (Level III) (JAMIESON et al. 2006). HIV testing should be performed if clinically indicated.
- Prophylactic vaccine for HPV 16 and 18 might be effective in reducing the incidence of VaIN2/3. HAMPL et al. (2006) reported that seven of eleven VaIN2/3 samples were positive for HPV 16 (Level IV).

26.2.2 Treatment Options

Non-radiotherapy Treatment Options

- A variety of non-radiotherapy treatment options are available for therapy of VaIN including: excision (Grade B), CO_2 ablation (Grade B), and topical 5-fluorouracil (5-FU) chemotherapy (Grade B) with recurrence rates after the first treatment ranging from approximately 0% to 60% depending on the series. An evidence-based comparison of these modalities is beyond the scope of this book.
- No treatment modality, including radiotherapy, provides complete protection against recurrence, persistence, or progression to invasion.

Brachytherapy

- High dose rate (HDR, > 1200 cGy/h) and medium dose rate (MDR, 200–1200 cGy/h) brachytherapy has been primarily used in the treatment of VaIN 3. Low dose rate (LDR, 40–200 cGy/h) brachytherapy has been used to treat stage 0 (VaIN but the grade was not specified) vaginal cancer. There is insufficient evidence to recommend an optimal HDR or MDR fractionation scheme or technique for VaIN 3.
- Some factors to be considered when choosing a prescription depth, length, and technique are: the degree of certainty that there is no invasive cancer, tumor location, prior therapy, and multifocality.

LDR Brachytherapy in the Treatment of Stage 0 Vaginal Cancer

- A retrospective series of 301 patients with vaginal carcinoma included 37 stage 0 patients. Most patients (n = 33) were treated with intracavitary radiotherapy with a vaginal surface dose between 70 and 80 Gy (mean 78.8 Gy). Intracavitary radiotherapy consisted of either a vaginal cylinder, ovoids, or a uterine tandem as appropriate. Six patients experienced local failure (Level IV) (CHYLE et al. 1996).

MDR Brachytherapy in the Treatment of VaIN 3

■ In one MDR brachytherapy retrospective series of 22 patients with VaIN 3, 21 patients were treated with one or two ovoids. Since the typical dose rate was 150–160 cGy/h, LDR might be more appropriate for describing the study although some patients fit the MDR definition. Doses were prescribed to a point lateral to the center of one ovoid at a distance of 0.5 cm from the surface of the ovoid. Seven patients received one fraction ranging from 22.2 to 26.4 Gy. With a follow-up ranging from 32 to 220 months, one of the seven patients progressed to vaginal cancer. Two patients developed RTOG grade 3 vaginal stenosis. In all, 15 patients received two fractions with a total dose ranging from 41.3 to 49.9 Gy. With a follow-up ranging from 14 to 203 months, one patient developed residual/recurrent VaIN 3, one recurrent VaIN 3 with a subsequent focus of invasive carcinoma, and one invasive vaginal carcinoma. Two patients developed RTOG grade 3 vaginal stenosis, one grade 3 urethral stricture requiring intermittent self-catheterization, and one grade 4 vaginal ulceration (Level IV) (GRAHAM et al. 2007).

HDR Brachytherapy in the Treatment of VaIN 3

■ It is suggested that the dose should be prescribed to the vaginal surface for lesions of the wall and at a depth of 0.5–1 cm for lesions of the vault to take into account the vaginal epithelium sequestered above the hysterectomy suture line (Grade D). The largest retrospective series of HDR brachytherapy for VaIN 3 treated 14 patients with doses ranging from 34 to 45 Gy in 4.5 to 8.5 Gy fractions to the vaginal mucosa with 2.5–4 cm diameter cylinders. The whole residual length of the vagina was treated. At a median follow-up of 46 months, one patient progressed to invasive carcinoma of the vagina; in another patient, VaIN 3 persisted; both patients had received 45 Gy in 4.5 Gy fractions. None of the nine patients receiving 42.5 Gy in 8.5 Gy fractions failed. Two patients had RTOG grade 3 toxicity with prominent vaginal atrophy and stenosis (Level III) (MACLEOD et al. 1997). Another retrospective series included six patients who received 15–30 Gy in 5 Gy fractions. One pa-

tient received 20 Gy of brachytherapy plus 20 Gy of external-beam radiotherapy (EBRT). Lesions of the vaginal stump were treated with ovoids, and the dose was calculated at a point 1 cm superior to the vaginal apex. For lesions distal to the vaginal apex, doses were calculated 1 cm beyond the plane of the vaginal cylinder. With a follow-up ranging from 51 to 125 months, there were no recurrences. Rectal bleeding occurred in the only patient receiving 30 Gy (Level III) (OGINO et al. 1998).

26.3 Treatment of Invasive Squamous Cell Carcinoma, Stage I–IVA

26.3.1 General Principles

■ Radiation therapy is the treatment of choice for most patients with invasive squamous cell carcinoma (Grade B) (Fig. 26.1).

■ Surgery has a limited role in part because of the close proximity of the bladder and rectum.

26.3.2 Surgery

■ In young patients who require radiotherapy, pretreatment laparotomy may allow ovarian transposition, surgical staging, and resection of any bulky positive lymph nodes (Grade C) (FIGO 2006).

■ Surgery is mainly limited to disease for stage I patients involving the upper posterior vagina. In patients with an intact uterus, upper vaginectomy to achieve at least 1-cm margins, and pelvic lymphadenectomy may be performed (Grade C) (FIGO 2006).

■ In patients with a prior hysterectomy, radical upper vaginectomy and pelvic lymphadenectomy may be an option (Grade C) (FIGO 2006).

■ In patients with Stage IVA disease, especially if a recto-vaginal or vesico-vaginal fistula is present, primary pelvic exenteration with pelvic lymphadenectomy or pre-operative radiation is an option. If the lower third of the vagina is involved, bilateral groin dissection should be considered (Grade C) (FIGO 2006).

■ In patients with a central recurrence after radiation therapy, pelvic exenteration may be necessary (Grade C) (FIGO 2006).

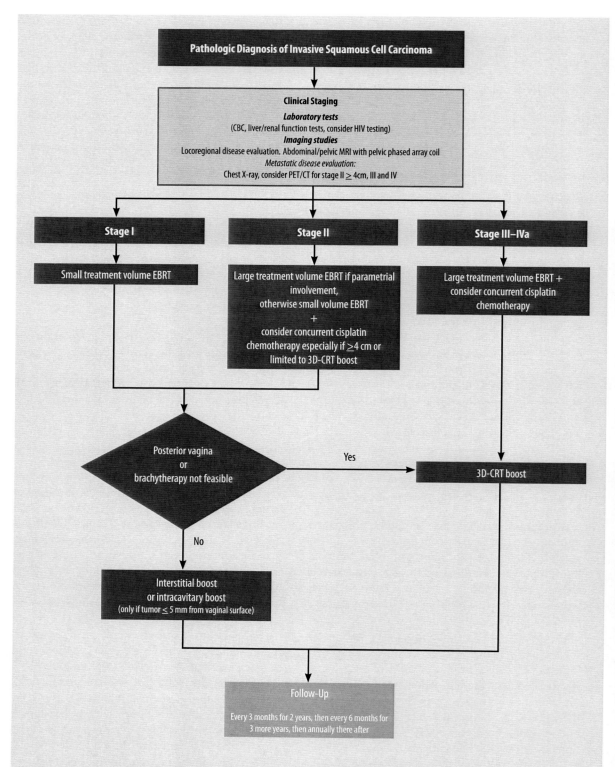

Fig. 26.1. Proposed treatment algorithm for invasive vaginal squamous cell carcinoma

26.3.3 Chemotherapy

■ Concurrent cis-platinum chemotherapy should be considered for stage II–IVA vaginal cancer (Grade C). A retrospective review of six stage II, four stage III, and two stage IVA vaginal cancer patients treated with concurrent weekly cis-platinum (5 weeks at a dose of 40 mg/m^2) and radiotherapy had 5-year overall survival, progression-free survival, and locoregional progression-free survival rates of 66%, 75%, and 92%, respectively. Patients received pelvic EBRT (median dose 45 Gy; range 40–55 Gy) and a LDR interstitial or HDR intracavitary brachytherapy boost (median dose 30 Gy; range 15–42 Gy). Two out of 10 patients undergoing interstitial brachytherapy developed fistulae requiring surgery, one of which subsequently had ongoing gastrointestinal complications and died of a bowel obstruction. The authors concluded that it is feasible to deliver concurrent weekly cis-platinum chemotherapy with high-dose radiation (Level IV) (SAMANT et al. 2007). The extremely high local control despite six patients having stage III or IVA disease and two patients with adenocarcinoma, which is associated with a worse prognosis, was very encouraging.

26.3.4 Radiation Therapy

■ EBRT is recommended for the treatment of posterior vaginal wall lesions (Grade C). The largest single institution retrospective study in squamous cell carcinoma of the vagina is from M. D. Anderson Cancer Center. Between 1970 and 2000, a total of 193 patients were treated with definitive radiation. At 5 years, disease-specific survival (DSS) rates were 85% for the 50 patients with stage I, 78% for the 97 patients with stage II, and 58% for the 46 patients with stage III–IVA disease. Of the 193 patients, 181 received EBRT: 58 EBRT and intracavitary, 61 EBRT and interstitial, and 62 EBRT only. The 5-year and 10-year cumulative rates of major (i.e., grade 3 or 4) complications were 10% and 17%, respectively. In all, 20 patients had a total of 25 major complications. Eight of 11 patients (73%) with major rectal complications had had tumors that involved the posterior vaginal wall (Level IV) (FRANK et al. 2005).

Figure 26.2 demonstrates The University of Texas M. D. Anderson Cancer Center treatment guidelines.

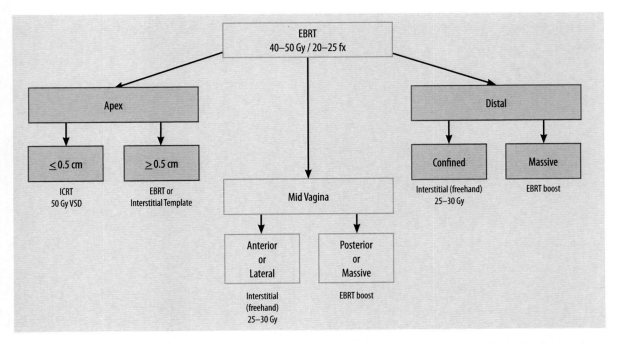

Fig. 26.2. M. D. Anderson Cancer Center guidelines for tailoring definitive radiation therapy on the basis of tumor location, tumor size, and the tumor response to treatment. EBRT = external-beam radiation therapy; fx = fractions; ICRT = intracavitary radiation therapy; VSD = vaginal surface dose. [Reprinted from Frank SJ, Jhingran A, Levenback C, Eifel PJ (2005) Definitive radiation therapy for squamous cell carcinoma of the vagina. Int J Radiat Oncol Biol Phys 62(1):138–147, with permission from Elsevier.]

Treatment Technique

Field Coverage and Arrangement

■ For stages I–IIA (IIA = FIGO II), a "small treatment volume" four-field technique with the superior edge at the bottom of the SI joints is recommended (Figs. 26.3 and 26.4). For stages IIB–IVA (IIB = FIGO II with parametrial involvement) a "large treatment volume" four-field technique is recommended (Figs. 26.5 and 26.6) (Grade C). A retrospective review of 65 patients with squamous cell carcinoma of the vagina who received definitive radiotherapy observed that the primary failure sites were the vagina ($n = 6$), the paracolpal tissues ($n = 4$), and the inguinal nodes ($n = 2$). A "small treatment volume" or "large treatment volume" technique was used based on physician preference. Based on the patterns of failure, the authors made suggestions regarding the optimal treatment volume for each stage. Since the inguinal failures were within 10 cm of midline, the authors advised only elective treatment of the medial inguinal nodes (Level IV) (Yeh et al. 2001).

■ In the case of locoregionally advanced disease or lack of CT planning, a two-field anteroposterior-

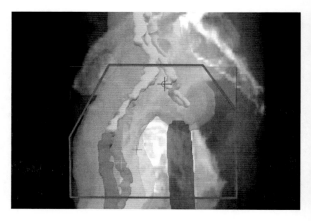

Fig. 26.4. Small treatment volume left lateral pelvic field. The arterial 2-cm volume expansion (*light purple*) helps ensure adequate coverage of the external iliac nodes when designing the blocks

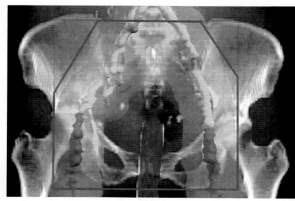

Fig. 26.5. Large treatment volume anterior pelvic field. The upper border is at L5/S1

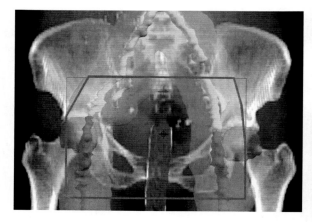

Fig. 26.3. Small treatment volume anterior pelvic field outlined in *red*. Blocked areas in the treatment field are *green*. The upper border of the field is at the bottom of the sacroiliac joints. The common iliac, external iliac, and internal iliac arteries are outlined in *light blue*, while the femoral arteries are *purple*. A 2-cm volume expansion on the arteries (*light purple*) helps define the lateral margin of the treatment field at the level of the external and internal iliac arteries. At the level of the femoral arteries, the lateral margins are tighter because the goal is elective coverage of the medial inguinal nodes which are medial to the femoral artery. A vaginal cylinder (dark blue) helps identify the vagina and location of the vaginal cuff

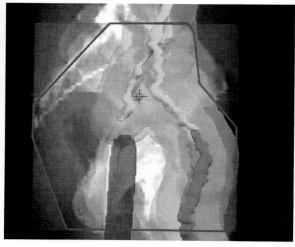

Fig. 26.6. Large treatment volume right lateral pelvic field. Avoid shielding presacral, perirectal, or anterior external iliac nodes

posteroanterior technique is advisable to avoid missing the external iliac lymph nodes. However, a four-field box technique should be used to minimize treating the small bowel.

■ Shrinking field techniques, and three-dimensional conformal radiotherapy (3D-CRT) can be used to dose escalate if brachytherapy is not feasible. With careful attention to treatment volumes and motion, intensity-modulated radiation therapy and image-guided radiation therapy (IMRT/IGRT) could emerge as a feasible treatment alternative.

■ For posterior vaginal tumors, an EBRT boost is recommended to minimize the risk of rectal complications from an interstitial or intracavitary brachytherapy boost (Grade C).

■ Careful evaluation at the top border of the field is needed if the lesion arises in the vaginal apex in order to avoid a marginal miss.

Simulation

■ Margins of 15–20 mm from vessel to field edge are reasonable when designing pelvic fields. CT simulation with vessel contouring as a surrogate for lymph node localization provides more precise and individualized field delineation (Grade D) (Level IV) (FINLAY et al. 2006).

■ The open or "frog leg" position is useful when treating the inguinal area to minimize skin reactions from skin folds.

■ A small radio-opaque marker seed inserted in the distal portion of the tumor may help when designing the treatment fields.

■ Several maneuvers could be used to minimize marginal misses including:

– Instilling a fixed volume of saline in the bladder for simulation and daily treatment using a Foley catheter (FRANK et al. 2005).

– Creating a vaginal/tumor internal target volume (ITV) by fusing the vaginal contour when the bladder is empty and full.

■ Elective irradiation of the inguinal nodes is recommended for tumors involving the lower third of the vagina (Grade B), and the rates of inguinal failure are less than 1% with this practice (Level IV) (FRANK et al. 2005).

■ Unexpected nodal drainage is possible and should at least be considered when designing treatment fields and evaluating diagnostic scans. A study of 14 women with newly diagnosed vaginal cancer who underwent pretreatment lymphatic mapping and sentinel lymph node identification showed

that, of the four women with lesions located in the upper third of the vagina, two had a sentinel node in the inguinal triangle (Level IV) (FRUMOVITZ et al. 2008).

■ If the inguinal lymph nodes are involved, the modified segmental boost technique (Figs. 26.7–26.10) can minimize dose inhomogeneity compared to traditional techniques (Grade D) (MORAN et al. 2004).

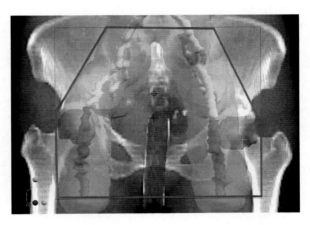

Fig. 26.7. Segmental boost technique anterior field out of four fields (MORAN et al. 2004). The inguinal field takes into consideration the potential location of ingunal nodes based on a topographic study of inguinal metastases (WANG et al. 1996). In an actual patient, the legs should be in the open-leg position to minimize skin reactions. The open-leg position could necessitate altering the treatment fields to ensure adequate inguinal node coverage

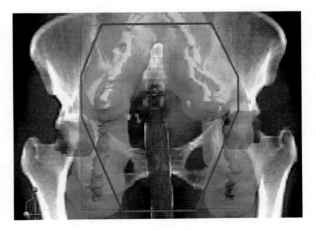

Fig. 26.8. Segmental boost technique posterior field

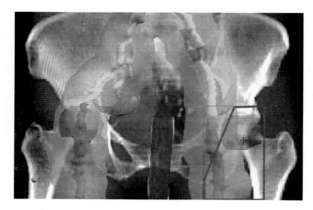

Fig. 26.9. Segmental boost technique left anterior oblique field. The right anterior oblique field is not illustrated

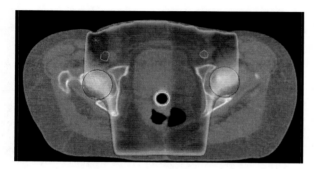

Fig. 26.10. Segmental boost technique coronal dose distribution. Note how the femoral heads and normal tissues receive less dose than in a conventional anteroposterior-posteroanterior two-field technique

Dose and Fractionation

■ A dose–response effect in squamous cell carcinoma of the vagina has been reported (Level IV) (PEREZ et al. 1999). In a series reported by CHYLE et al. (1996), patients treated to doses below 55 Gy had a 5-year local recurrence rate of 53% (Level IV).

■ Pelvic EBRT is usually delivered first to doses of 40–50 Gy in 1.8- to 2-Gy fractions (Grade C). Table 26.4 provides an overview of potential doses for different clinical situations (FRANK et al. 2005; YEH et al. 2001; PEREZ et al. 1999).

■ Following EBRT, a boost is administered with interstitial brachytherapy, intracavitary brachytherapy, or 3D-CRT. Although higher doses can usually be achieved with brachytherapy, there is no evidence that boost with EBRT is a substandard modality when compared to a brachytherapy boost (Level IV) (CHYLE et al. 1996; OTTON et al. 2004).

■ Careful attention should be paid to doses delivered to the introitus in order to avoid skin necrosis, in particular with brachytherapy.

Radiation-Induced Late Side Effects and Complications

■ Observed late gastrointestinal treatment complications include: rectal ulceration, stricture, proctitis, or proctitis requiring transfusion; small bowel obstruction or necrosis; large bowel obstruction; chronic diarrhea and chronic diarrhea resulting in death; recto-vaginal fistula. Observed late genitourinary complications include: vaginal ulceration, necrosis, narrowing, or complete vaginal stenosis; incontinence or hemorrhagic cystitis; urethral stricture; vesico-peritoneal fistula; vesico-vaginal fistula; vesico-cutaneus fistula; uretero-vaginal fistula; osteonecrosis of the pubis; ureteric stenosis with hydronephrosis (Level IV) (FRANK et al. 2005; CHYLE et al. 1996; DE CREVOISIER et al. 2007; STOCK et al. 1995).

■ At the M. D. Anderson Cancer Center, the 5- and 10-year cumulative rates of major (i.e., grade 3 or 4) complications was 10% and 17%, respectively (FRANK et al. 2005), which is similar to rates experienced in other institutions in the treatment of vaginal cancer.

■ Ideally, vaginal cancers should be treated in experienced centers given the potentially serious late complications from treatment.

Table 26.4. Doses for stage I–IVA invasive squamous cell carcinoma

Target	Modality	Dose
Pelvis	Pelvic EBRT	40–50 Gy
Primary	Boost to primary:	
	Intracavitary LDR VSD (≤ 5 mm deep) (40–60 cGy/h)	50 Gy for apical lesion
	Interstitial LDR (40–60 cGy/h)	25–30 Gy
	3D CRT	60–70 Gy (total dose)
Additional dose considerations	Parametrial involvement	65 Gy
	Pelvic side wall involvement	60 Gy
	Medial inguinal nodes (elective)	45–50 Gy
	Involved inguinal nodes	60 Gy

EBRT, external-beam radiotherapy; LDR, low dose rate; VSD, vaginal surface dose; CRT, conformal radiotherapy.

26.4 Treatment of Adenocarcinoma of Vagina

26.4.1 General Principles

- Diethylstilbestrol (DES) clear cell adenocarcinoma (CCA) and non-diethylstilbestrol associated adenocarcinoma of the vagina (NDAV) are two different entities with different prognosis and clinical behavior:
- The 5-year survival for NDAV is 34% (Level IV) (FRANK et al. 2007), versus 84% for CCA (Level IV) (WAGGONER et al. 1994).
- NDAV is more likely than CCA to present with, or later develop, lung metastases or metastases to supraclavicular nodes (WAGGONER et al. 1994). NDAV can also metastasize to the liver and bone (FRANK et al. 2007).
- The mean age at diagnosis is approximately 20 years for both NDAV and CCA (WAGGONER et al. 1994). However, the median age in one NDAV series was 54 (FRANK et al. 2007).
- There is insufficient evidence to make recommendations regarding the optimal management of CCA or NDAV. However, the role of radiotherapy will be briefly discussed.

26.4.2 Radiotherapy Considerations

Non-diethylstilbestrol-Associated Adenocarcinoma of the Vagina

- One retrospective series of 26 patients with NDAV confirmed by central pathologic review treated with EBRT followed by brachytherapy or EBRT alone reported a 5-year overall survival of 34%, with a pelvic disease control of 31%. The authors concluded that more aggressive treatments, possibly including chemotherapy or novel systemic biologic agents, may be needed to improve cure rates. The authors also recommended pelvic EBRT even for superficial stage I adenocarcinomas (Level IV) (FRANK et al. 2007).

Clear Cell Adenocarcinoma

- One retrospective series supports the role of adjuvant radiotherapy after local therapy for stage I CCA (Level IV) (SENEKJIAN et al. 1987) and another primary radiotherapy for stage II CCA (Level IV) (SENEKJIAN et al. 1988).

26.5 Treatment of Melanoma of Vagina

26.5.1 General Principles

- Vaginal melanomas account for 3%–4% of all vaginal malignancies. About 78% of melanomas are diagnosed in patients older than 60. The overall 5-year relative survival rate is 14% and decreases with increasing Clark's level of invasion (Level IV) (CREASMAN et al. 1998).
- The management of melanoma is beyond the scope of this chapter, but the role of radiotherapy will be briefly discussed.

26.5.2 Radiotherapy Considerations

- In a retrospective study of 14 patients with vaginal melanoma, three of seven patients (43%) with tumors < 3 cm survived longer than 5 years compared to none of seven patients with tumor size > 3 cm. The three long-term survivors with tumors < 3 cm also received primary radiotherapy, or surgery and adjuvant radiotherapy. The authors concluded that radiotherapy may be of value as an alternative to surgery or as an adjunct modality in patients with lesions < 3 cm in diameter (Level IV) (PETRU et al. 1998).
- Some authors recommend fractions > 400 cGy for vaginal melanoma to improve local control based on limited experience (Level V) (IRVIN et al. 1998). The long-term toxicity and efficacy, as well as the optimal hypofractionated scheme remain to be evaluated in a larger number of patients.

Follow-Ups

26.6.1 Post-Treatment Follow-Ups

■ Life-long follow-up after definitive treatment of vaginal carcinoma is recommended for detecting recurrence, secondary tumors, or other long-term complications of treatment.

■ Long-term surveillance is necessary since vaginal cancer patients may develop metachronous gynecologic cancers during their lifetime.

■ A retrospective, non-randomized study of 70 women who were treated with intracavitary irradiation with or without EBRT for cervical or endometrial cancer showed that, of the 35 patients using a vaginal stent (dilator) daily for 1 year, 11% had evidence of vaginal stenosis. In contrast, 57% of the 35 patients who did not use a dilator and were advised to have sexual intercourse developed stenosis. The four patients who developed stenosis in the stent group were non-compliant from confusion, perceived lack of information on the use of the dilator, and fear of vaginal injury (Level IV) (DECRUZE et al. 1999).

■ A survey among nurse specialists and radiotherapy centers in the UK on vaginal dilation with pelvic radiotherapy showed some areas of consensus (Level IV) (WHITE and FAITHFULL 2006):
- Acceptability of use established prior to instruction
- Continue intercourse during radiation therapy
- Resume intercourse post radiation therapy
- Dilator insertion depth as comfort permits
- Inform patient on the management of discomfort associated with insertion and the significance of minimal vaginal bleeding
- 5–10 min duration for individual insertions
- Use lubricant with dilators

Schedule

■ Follow-ups could be scheduled every 3 months for 2 years, then every 6 months for 3 additional years, then annually thereafter (Grade D).

Work-Ups

■ Each follow-up should include a complete history and physical examination.

■ Chest X-ray annually for 5 years can be performed to rule out metastatic recurrence in lungs.

Acknowledgments

Thanks to Darin Noble, medical dosimetrist, for his exceptional assistance planning the segmental boost technique and creating the treatment figures.

References

Aho M, Vesterinen E, Meyer B et al. (1991) Natural history of vaginal intraepithelial neoplasia. Cancer 68:195–197

Beller U, Benedet JL, Creasman WT, Ngan HYS, Quinn MA, Maisonneuve PA et al (2006) Carcinoma of the vagina. Int J Gynecol Obstet 95[Suppl 1];S29–S42

Chyle V, Zagars GK, Wheeler JA et al. (1996) Definitive radiotherapy for carcinoma of the vagina: outcome and prognostic factors. Int J Radiat Oncol Biol Phys 35:891–905

Creasman WT, Phillips JL, Menck HR (1998) The National Cancer Data Base report on cancer of the vagina. Cancer 83:1033–1040

de Crevoisier R, Sanfilippo N, Gerbaulet A et al. (2007) Exclusive radiotherapy for primary squamous cell carcinoma of the vagina. Radiother Oncol 85:362–370

Decruze SB, Guthrie D, Magnani R (1999) Prevention of vaginal stenosis in patients following vaginal brachytherapy. Clin Oncol (R Coll Radiol) 11:46–48

FIGO (2006) Staging classifications and clinical practice guidelines for gynaecologic cancers. FIGO Committee on Gynecologic Oncology, 2006. (Accessed February 3, 2008, at http://www.figo.org/publications_annual.asp.)

Finlay MH, Ackerman I, Tirona RG et al. (2006) Use of CT simulation for treatment of cervical cancer to assess the adequacy of lymph node coverage of conventional pelvic fields based on bony landmarks. Int J Radiat Oncol Biol Phys 64:205–209

Frank SJ, Jhingran A, Levenback C et al. (2005) Definitive radiation therapy for squamous cell carcinoma of the vagina. Int J Radiat Oncol Biol Phys 62:138–147

Frank SJ, Deavers MT, Jhingran A et al. (2007) Primary adenocarcinoma of the vagina not associated with diethylstilbestrol (DES) exposure. Gynecol Oncol 105:470–474

Frumovitz M, Gayed IW, Jhingran A et al. (2008) Lymphatic mapping and sentinel lymph node detection in women with vaginal cancer. Gynecol Oncol 108:478–481

Graham K, Wright K, Cadwallader B et al. (2007) 20-Year retrospective review of medium dose rate intracavitary brachytherapy in VaIN3. Gynecol Oncol 106:105–111

Greene FL, Page DL, Fleming ID et al. (2002) American Joint Committee on Cancer, American Cancer Society. AJCC Cancer Staging Manual. 6th ed. Springer, Berlin Heidelberg New York

Hampl M, Sarajuuri H, Wentzensen N et al. (2006) Effect of human papillomavirus vaccines on vulvar, vaginal, and anal intraepithelial lesions and vulvar cancer. Obstet Gynecol 108:1361–1368

Irvin WP Jr, Bliss SA, Rice LW et al. (1998) Malignant melanoma of the vagina and locoregional control: radical surgery revisited. Gynecol Oncol 71:476–480

Jamieson DJ, Paramsothy P, Cu-Uvin S et al. (2006) Vulvar, vaginal, and perianal intraepithelial neoplasia in women with or at risk for human immunodeficiency virus. Obstet Gynecol 107:1023–1028

Kirkbride P, Fyles A, Rawlings GA et al. (1995) Carcinoma of the vagina – experience at the Princess Margaret Hospital (1974–1989). Gynecol Oncol 56:435–443

Lamoreaux WT, Grigsby PW, Dehdashti F et al. (2005) FDG-PET evaluation of vaginal carcinoma. Int J Radiat Oncol Biol Phys 62:733–737

MacLeod C, Fowler A, Dalrymple C et al. (1997). High-dose-rate brachytherapy in the management of high-grade intraepithelial neoplasia of the vagina. Gynecol Oncol 65:74–77

Moran M, Lund MW, Ahmad M et al. (2004) Improved treatment of pelvis and inguinal nodes using modified segmental boost technique: dosimetric evaluation. Int J Radiat Oncol Biol Phys 59:1523–1530

Ogino I, Kitamura T, Okajima H et al. (1998) High-dose-rate intracavitary brachytherapy in the management of cervical and vaginal intraepithelial neoplasia. Int J Radiat Oncol Biol Phys 40:881–887

Otton GR, Nicklin JL, Dickie GJ et al. (2004) Early-stage vaginal carcinoma – an analysis of 70 patients. Int J Gynecol Cancer 14:304–310

Perez CA, Grigsby PW, Garipagaoglu M et al. (1999) Factors affecting long-term outcome of irradiation in carcinoma of the vagina. Int J Radiat Oncol Biol Phys 44:37–45

Petru E, Nagele F, Czerwenka K et al. (1998) Primary malignant melanoma of the vagina: long-term remission following radiation therapy. Gynecol Oncol 70:23–26

Samant R, Lau B, E C et al. (2007) Primary vaginal cancer treated with concurrent chemoradiation using Cis-platinum. Int J Radiat Oncol Biol Phys 69:746–750

Senekjian EK, Frey KW, Anderson D et al. (1987) Local therapy in Stage I clear cell adenocarcinoma of the vagina. Cancer 60:1319–1324

Senekjian EK, Frey KW, Stone C et al. (1988) An evaluation of Stage II vaginal clear cell adenocarcinoma according to substages. Gynecol Oncol 31:56–64

Stock RG, Chen AS, Seski J (1995) A 30-year experience in the management of primary carcinoma of the vagina: analysis of prognostic factors and treatment modalities. Gynecol Oncol 56:45–52

Taylor MB, Dugar N, Davidson SE et al. (2007) Magnetic resonance imaging of primary vaginal carcinoma. Clin Radiol 62:549–555

Tran PT, Su Z, Lee P et al. (2007) Prognostic factors for outcomes and complications for primary squamous cell carcinoma of the vagina treated with radiation. Gynecol Oncol 105:641–649

Waggoner SE, Mittendorf R, Biney N et al. (1994) Influence of in utero diethylstilbestrol exposure on the prognosis and biologic behavior of vaginal clear-cell adenocarcinoma. Gynecol Oncol 55:238–244

Wang CJ, Chin YY, Leung SW et al. (1996) Topographic distribution of inguinal lymph nodes metastasis: significance in determination of treatment margin for elective inguinal lymph nodes irradiation of low pelvic tumors. Int J Radiat Oncol Biol Phys 35:133–1336

White ID, Faithfull S (2006) Vaginal dilation associated with pelvic radiotherapy: a UK survey of current practice. Int J Gynecol Cancer 16:1140–1146

Yeh AM, Marcus RB Jr, Amdur RJ et al. (2001) Patterns of failure in squamous cell carcinoma of the vagina treated with definitive radiotherapy alone: what is the appropriate treatment volume? Int J Cancer 96[Suppl]:109–116

Section VII:
Lymphomas

Non-Hodgkin's Lymphoma

Theodore E. Yaeger, Jiade J. Lu, and Luther W. Brady

Introduction and Objectives

Non-Hodgkin's lymphoma (NHL) is generally considered a systemic disease process in 80%–85% of patients. The majority are of B-cell origin, with a wide variety of clinical phenotypes. A multi-disciplinary approach for management is appropriate for most cases. Chemotherapy is the mainstay of treatment in the majority of symptomatic presentations. External-beam radiation therapy is an important treatment modality for limited, localized indolent NHL, as well as in stage I and II aggressive diseases. Immunotherapy (rituximab) is often added to chemotherapy either concurrently or sequentially for CD20-positive disease. This chapter focuses on the management of indolent and aggressive non-Hodgkin's lymphoma, particularly follicular lymphoma, marginal zone lymphoma, gastric MALT, and diffuse large-cell lymphoma, and examines:

● Recommendations for diagnoses and staging procedures
● The staging systems and prognostic factors
● Treatment recommendations for indolent NHL and the supporting peer-reviewed scientific evidence
● Treatment recommendations for gastric MALT and the supporting peer-reviewed scientific evidence
● The use of systemic chemotherapy and immunotherapy in combination with localized radiation therapy for definitive treatment of stage I and II aggressive NHL
● Follow-up care and surveillance of survivors

The management of ocular and orbital lymphoma, CNS lymphoma, cutaneous lymphoma, and NK/T cell lymphoma is not the focus of this documentation and is detailed in other chapters.

T. E. Yaeger, MD
Caldwell Memorial Hospital, 321 Mulberry Street SW, P.O. Box 1890, Lenior, NC 28645, USA
J. J. Lu, MD, MBA
Department of Radiation Oncology, National University Cancer Institute of Singapore, National University Health System, National University of Singapore, 5 Lower Kent Ridge Road, Singapore 119074, Singapore
L. W. Brady, MD
Department of Radiation Oncology, Drexel University College of Medicine, Broad & Vine Streets, Mail Stop 200, Philadelphia, PA 19102–1192, USA

27.1 Diagnosis, Staging, and Prognoses

27.1.1 Diagnosis

Initial Evaluation

■ Diagnosis and evaluation of non-Hodgkin's lymphoma (NHL) usually start with a complete history and physical examination. Attention should be paid to NHL-associated signs and symptoms: unexplained weight loss of more than 10% over 6 months prior to diagnosis, unexplained fever >38°C, and/or drenching night sweats that require change of bedclothes ("B" symptoms), shortness of breath, hemoptysis, pruritus, recent onset of alcohol beverage intolerance, and unusual fatigue.

■ History that reveals exposure to toxic chemicals – solvents, benzene compounds, and tobacco use/exposure is relevant and should be recorded.

■ A thorough physical examination special attention should be focused on externally palpable nodal sites, the liver, spleen, skin, oral cavity, and oral pharynx. NHL commonly presents as an enlarged, non-tender, rubbery, moveable lymph node within a typical node-bearing area, an enlarged nodular liver, enlarged non-tender spleen, or enlarged non-ulcerated tonsil.

■ The examination should include epitrochlear, axillary, supraclavicular node areas, and Waldeyer's ring as they are the commonly involved areas.

Laboratory Tests

■ Initial laboratory tests should include a complete blood count, basic blood chemistry, liver and renal function tests, alkaline phosphatase, lactate dehydrogenase (LDH), and erythrocyte sedimentation rate (ESR) (GREENE et al. 2002).

Imaging Studies

■ CT scans of the chest, abdomen, and pelvis are required to appropriately evaluate and stage NHL.

■ FDG-PET scan is recommended for diagnosis and staging of NHL (Grade A). Results from a number of retrospective trials have shown that FDG-PET has significantly higher site and patient sensitivity for NHL of all histological types (except

for small lymphocytic lymphoma and marginal zone lymphoma) than gallium-27 scintigraphy (Level III) (TSUKAMOTO et al. 2007; WIRTH et al. 2002; ELSTROM et al. 2003).

■ Fluorine-18 fluorodeoxyglucose positron emission tomography (FDG-PET) in combination with a concurrent CT scan has become an approved study for baseline systemic staging as well as for restaging when failure is suspected (WIRTH et al. 2002).

■ Gallium-67 scanning is important for initial staging for NHL. Tumor response on subsequent gallium-67 scanning is also prognostically important: 70% of patients who achieved complete response on gallium-67 scan at midcourse of chemotherapy were alive and disease-free at 3-year follow-up, as compared to 41% for those who had partial response (KAPLAN et al. 1990). Gallium-67 scan is recommended if FDG-PET is not available, but it has been gradually replaced by FDG-PET scan for diagnosis and staging.

■ In the absence of neurological symptoms, a CT or MRI of the brain is not routinely recommended. Bone scan is indicated (if FDG-PET is not available) for patients with bone pain or elevated alkaline phosphatase.

Pathology

■ Histological confirmation is critical to determine the type, histopathology, and immunophenotyping for diagnosis and treatment determination of non-Hodgkin's lymphoma (Table 27.1).

■ Typically, fine-needle aspiration of a suspected lymph node, soft tissue nodule/organ mass, cytological spin of an effusion, or a bone marrow biopsy (bilateral) will yield sufficient cells to analyze (JEFFERS et al. 1998; SADDIK et al. 1997).

Table 27.1. Imaging and laboratory work-ups for non-Hodgkin's lymphoma

Imaging studies	Laboratory tests
– CT scan of chest, abdomen, and pelvis	– Complete blood count
– FDG-PET scan or PET/CT	– Serum chemistry
– Gallium-67 scan (if PET unavailable)	– Lactate dehydrogenase (LDH)
– MRI or CT of the brain (if symptomatically indicated)	– Liver function tests
– Bone scan (if symptomatically indicated)	– Renal function tests
	– Erythrocyte sedimentation rate (ESR)

- Immunophenotyping is an important diagnostic modality and is crucial for the classification of non-Hodgkin's lymphoma. Certain markers, such as the CD-20 receptor, have become crucial for treatment as newer biologic agents have utilized this receptor therapeutically (FISHER et al. 2005).
- Bone marrow biopsy (bilateral) is recommended for all cases of NHL because of the high probability of bone marrow involvement for the commonly diagnosed NHL in North America: 70% in small lymphocytic lymphoma, 50% in follicular lymphoma, and >10% in diffuse large-cell lymphoma or marginal zone lymphoma.
- Cytological examination of cranial spinal fluid (CSF) is indicated for stage IV disease with bone marrow, testis, and parameningeal involvement (GREENE et al. 2002).
- The Working Formulation for Clinical Usage has been the most widely utilized classification of lymphoma in North America. It differentiates various histological subtypes of lymphoma into clinically relevant grades (low, intermediate, and high), which directs treatment strategy selection (Table 27.2) (THE NHL PATHOLOGIC CLASSIFICATION PROJECT 1982).
- The WHO classification, which is derived from the Revised European-American Classification of Lymphoid Neoplasms (REAL), now recognizes three major sub-types of lymphomas: B-cell, T-cell, and Hodgkin's disease. The WHO classification describes cytological, morphologic, immunophenotypic, and genetic features of different types of lymphoma (JAFFE et al. 2001).

27.1.2 Staging

- Non-Hodgkin's lymphoma is usually staged clinically based on results of physical examination, laboratory tests, imaging studies, and bone marrow biopsy.
- Departing from past experience, laparotomy and pathologic staging is no longer considered a standard of care and is rarely beneficial. If needed, a laparoscopy can be performed for biopsy to assess the presence of abdominal disease or to define histological microscopic disease extent in the abdomen, or when no peripheral site is available.
- The Ann Arbor Staging System is used for both Hodgkin's disease and non-Hodgkin's lymphomas (Table 27.3) (GREENE et al. 2002).

Table 27.2. Working formulation of commonly diagnosed non-Hodgkin's lymphoma

Low-grade (indolent)
Follicular small cleaved
Follicular mixed, small cleaved, and large cell (grade I and II follicular lymphoma)
Small lymphocytic

Intermediate-grade (aggressive)
Diffuse large cell
Diffuse mixed small and large cell
Follicular large cell (grade III follicular lymphoma)
Diffuse small cleaved cell differentiated lymphocytic

High-grade (highly aggressive)
Small noncleaved: Burkitt's, non Burkitt's
Lymphoblastic
Large cell immunoblastic

Table 27.3. The Ann Arbor Staging Classification for Hodgkin's Disease and Non-Hodgkin's Lymphoma. [From GREENE et al. (2002) with permission]

Stage I:	Involvement of a single lymph node regions (I) or single extralymphatic organ or site in the absence of any lymph node involvement (IE)
Stage II:	Involvement of two or more lymph node regions on the same side of the diaphragm (II) or localized involvement of an extralymphatic organ or site in association with regional lymph node involvement with or without involvement of other lymph node regions on the same side of the diaphragm (IIE)
Stage IV:	Involvement of lymph node regions on both sides of the diaphragm (III), which also may be accompanied by extralymphatic extension in association with adjacent lymph node involvement (IIIE) or by involvement of the spleen (IIIS) or both (IIIS,E)
Stage IV:	Diffuse or disseminated involvement of one or more extra lymphatic organs with or without associated lymph node involvement, or isolated lymph node involvement, but in conjunction with disease in distant site(s). Any involvement of the liver or bone marrow, or nodular involvement of the lung(s)

Waldeyer's ring, thymus, spleen, appendix, and Peyer's patches of the small intestine are considered lymphatic tissue and not stage 'E' involvement

Prognostic Factors

- Histology subtype of lymphoma is the most important determinant of prognosis of non-Hodgkin's lymphoma.
- NHL of certain origins, such as primary CNS lymphoma and testicular NHL, have particularly poor outcome after treatment.
- The presenting stage is an important prognostic factor. For example, the 10-year cause-specific survival for patients with stage I, II, III, and IV follicular cell type are 68%, 56%, 42%, and 18%, respectively (GOSPODAROWICZ et al. 1984).
- "B" symptoms, including unexplained weight loss >10% over 6 months prior to diagnosis, unexplained fever >38°C, and/or drenching night sweats are associated with poor outcome (GREENE et al. 2002).
- Other significant prognostic factors include patient age (younger or older than 60 years), gender (female gender has a better prognosis in low grade lymphoma), tumor size (less or more than 10 cm in diameter), performance status, level of serum lactate dehydrogenase (LDH), extent of extranodal involvement, beta-2 microglobulin, and S-phase fraction.
- The International Prognostic Index (IPI) for aggressive NHL includes five of the above-mentioned significant risk factors to predict overall survival (Table 27.4): stage (I or II vs. III or IV), serum LDH (normal vs. abnormal), extranodal site involvement (0 or 1 vs. >1), age of the patient (younger than 60 vs. older than 60), and performance status (ECOG 0 or 1 vs. 2–4). The IPI risk groups are determined by the numerical summation of the number of adverse risk factors (0 to 5), and a higher number of adverse risk factors are associated with poor prognosis (Table 27.4) (INTERNATIONAL NON-HODGKIN'S LYMPHOMA PROGNOSTIC FACTORS PROJECT 1993).
- Diffuse large-cell lymphomas that transformed from follicular lymphomas do not respond to conventional chemotherapy as in diffuse large-cell disease.

Table 27.4. International prognostic index for aggressive non-Hodgkin's lymphoma

Risk group	IPI score	5-Year survival (%)
Low-risk	0–1	73%
Low-intermediate	2	51%
High-intermediate	3	43%
High-risk	4–5	26%

27.2 Treatment of Low-Grade (Indolent) Non-Hodgkin's Lymphoma

27.2.1 General Principles

- Radiation therapy is the standard treatment of stage I and II follicular lymphoma (Grade I and II disease), marginal zone lymphoma, and small lymphocytic lymphoma (Grade A). Chemotherapy is not indicated in the treatment of localized (stage I and II) follicular follicle center cell lymphoma or small lymphocytic lymphoma (Grade A).
- For stage III indolent NHL, comprehensive lymphatic irradiation is indicated in patients with good performance status, no "B" symptoms, and a limited number (less than five) of involved regions or sites (Grade C).
- More advanced stage III and stage IV low-grade diseases are generally incurable, and treatment (chemotherapy or chemotherapy plus immunotherapy) can be deferred until symptomatic. Chemotherapy usually does not affect the natural history of advanced-stage (stage III and IV) indolent lymphomas and is usually not recommended for asymptomatic patients (Grade B).
- The effect of rituximab (anti-CD20 monoclonal antibody) in combination with chemotherapy on stage III and IV indolent NHL has been reported and is recommended as the first-line treatment for patients with indication (Grade A).
- Radiation therapy is an effective treatment modality for symptomatic palliation in advanced or recurrent disease.
- The radiolabeled anti-CD20 antibodies, Y^{90} ibritumamab-Zevalin and I^{131} tositumomab-Bexxar, have become an important treatment option for consolidation treatment after initial chemo-immunotherapy or for recurrent/persistent disease after chemotherapy and/or non-radiolabeled immunotherapy (Grade A) (CHESON 2003; WITZIG et al. 2002).
- Surgery has no role in the definitive treatment of indolent non-Hodgkin's lymphoma. The utilization of surgery is limited to obtaining tissue for diagnosis or orthopedic stabilization.

27.2.2 Treatment of Stage I and II Indolent NHL

Radiation Therapy

■ Radiation therapy is the mainstay treatment of stage I and II grade I and II follicular lymphoma, marginal zone lymphoma (non-gastric), and small lymphocytic lymphoma (Grade A). Follicle lymphoma is the most common type of indolent NHL, and approximately 20%–30% of patients present with stage I or II disease; however, less than 10% of patients with small lymphocytic lymphomas have truly localized disease without bone marrow involvement. Patients treated with definitive radiation therapy can usually achieve long-term disease control: The overall survival rate at 5 years is 80%–100% after IFRT (ARMITAGE and WEISSENBURGER 1998).

■ Long-term results of a large retrospective study reported by the British National Lymphoma Investigation (BNLI) revealed that the complete response after radiation therapy was achieved in 98% of the 208 patients with early-stage low-grade NHL, and 10-year disease-free and cause-specific survival rates were 47% and 71%, respectively, for this group of patients (Level III) (VAUGHAN et al. 1994). These results were in accordance with those observed in a retrospective review from Stanford University: For patients with follicular cell histology who were treated with definitive radiation therapy [IFRT or extended-field radiation therapy (EFRT)], the actuarial survival rates at 5, 10, 15, and 20 years were 82%, 64%, 44%, and 35%, respectively, and the recurrence-free survival rates at 5, 10, 15, and 20 years were 55%, 44%, 40%, and 37%, respectively (Level III) (MACMANUS and HOPPE 1996).

■ Significant difference in recurrence-free survival rates between stage I and II indolent lymphoma has not been observed in the above-mentioned studies (Level III) (MACMANUS and HOPPE 1996; VAUGHAN et al. 1994).

Field Arrangement

■ IFRT is the standard technique for the treatment of indolent NHL (Grade A). There is no clear evidence that extended field treatment offers any survival advantage:

■ The results of an early retrospective study reported by CHEN et al. (1979) revealed that successful radiotherapy for all stages of non-Hodgkin's lymphoma of all histologies was not correlated with extended versus involved fields. Distant metastasis was the cause of treatment failure in close to 90% of cases (Level III). In addition, in the above-mentioned retrospective study from Stanford University, although relapse-free survival was improved with the utilization of large field (to both sides of the diaphragm) irradiation, no significant survival benefit was observed (Level III) (MACMANUS and HOPPE 1996).

■ IFRT delivers treatment to the clinically involved region, with or without irradiation of the first echelon uninvolved lymph node region. Attention should be paid to minimize dose to critical structures in the treatment field (Fig. 27.1).

■ Complete response or partial response can be achieved after chemotherapy; initially, involved lymph nodes are often resolved or normally sized. In these cases, a CTV (clinical target volume) that encompasses the initial volume of the lymph node(s) before chemotherapy should be contoured (Grade D). However, normal structures that have been displaced (not infiltrated) by the enlarged lymph node(s) or disease(s) are not included in the irradiated volume (e.g., muscle displaced by cervical lymph nodes or lung displaced by mediastinal lymph nodes).

Dose

■ A radiation dose between 36 Gy and 40 Gy delivered in conventional fractionation is recommended for the treatment of low-grade NHL with curative intent, and a dose higher than 40 Gy may be required for bulky disease (Grade B). Low-grade lymphomas are generally radio-responsive diseases. It has been demonstrated that doses ranged from 30–35 Gy delivered in conventional fractions have produced control rates of close to 80% in follicular lymphoma (Level III) (FUKS and KAPLAN 1973).

Chemotherapy

■ Chemotherapy is usually not indicated in the treatment of early-stage indolent non-Hodgkin's lymphoma (Grade A). Prospective randomized trials have failed to demonstrate the efficacy of adjuvant chemotherapy on overall survival when used in combination with radiation therapy:

■ A number of prospective randomized trials, including an EORTC trial, compared the efficacy of combined CVP (cyclophosphamide, vincristine,

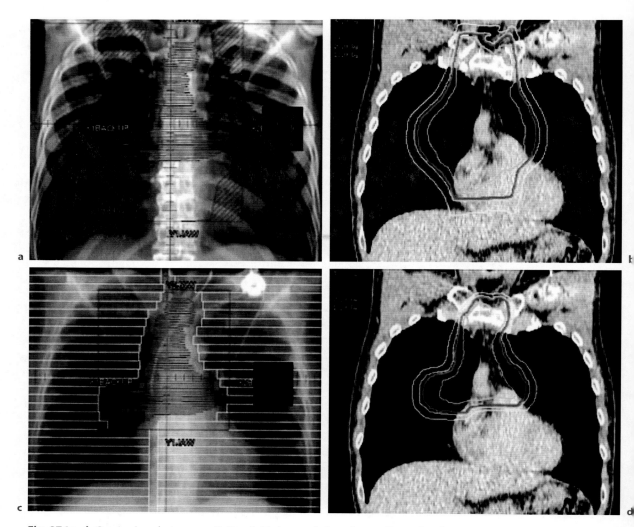

Fig. 27.1a–d. Comparison between radiation field sizes and the volume of heart irradiation using either IFRT with (**a** and **b**) or without (**c** and **d**) irradiating the first echelon lymph nodes for Hodgkin's disease or NHL in the mediastinum (From: Girinsky T, van der Maazen R, Specht L et al. (2006) Involved-node radiotherapy in patients with early Hodgkin lymphoma: Concepts and guidelines. By permission of the publisher)

and prednisone)-based chemotherapy and radiotherapy versus radiotherapy alone for stage I and II non-Hodgkin's lymphoma. The results repeatedly demonstrated that recurrence-free survival may be prolonged by the addition of chemotherapy to radiation; however, no improvement in overall survival was observed in the subgroup of patients with indolent lymphoma in any of these trials (Level I or II) (CARDE et al. 1984; NISSEN et al. 1983; MONFARDINI et al. 1980).

■ Additionally, the therapeutic effect of the more commonly used chemotherapy regimen in intermediate-grade NHL CHOP [cyclophosphamide, doxorubicin (hydroxydaunomycin), vincristine (Oncovin), and prednisone] used after radiation therapy was not

demonstrated in a single institutional randomized study (Level II) (YAHALOM et al. 1993).

27.2.3 Treatment of Stage III Indolent Lymphoma

Radiation Therapy

■ Total lymphatic irradiation (TLI) can be recommended for a selected group of patients with stage III indolent NHL (Grade B). Patients with fewer than five sites of disease involvement (non-bulky) and no signs of "B" symptoms may benefit from total lymphatic irradiation. However, the difference of outcome between patients treated with radiation therapy (with or without chemotherapy) or watchful waiting has not been systematically addressed:

- Results from the long-term follow-up of a group of patients with stage III follicular lymphoma from Stanford University revealed that definitive radiation therapy produced 88% freedom from relapse (FFR) and 100% cause-specific survival rates in patients with limited stage III (lack of "B" symptoms, < 5 sites of involvement, and < 10 cm in longest dimension of disease) follicular lymphoma. Adjuvant chemotherapy did not significantly alter the treatment outcome (Level III) (MURTHA et al. 2001).
- In a retrospective study including 34 patients with stage III low-grade NHL, the actuarial overall, disease-free, and cause-specific survival rates at 15 years are 28%, 40%, and 46%, respectively, after central lymphatic irradiation (CLI). Disease-free survival was significantly improved in patients with five or fewer sites of involvement (Level III) (JACOBS et al. 1993). The efficacy of CLI was also demonstrated in a single-arm prospective trial that reported the results of 47 patients with follicular lymphoma (including five patients with follicular large cell lymphoma and 28 patients with stage III disease) prospectively treated with CLI (mantle, whole abdomen, and pelvic radiation fields with a 1-month break after each field). The total doses ranged between 30 Gy to 30.6 Gy at 1.5–1.8 Gy/fraction followed by a boost of 9 Gy to the areas with gross disease. All patients with grade I and II diseases achieved complete response after radiation, and CLI was well tolerated. The 5-year overall survival and FFP were 94% and 53%, respectively (Level III) (HA et al. 2003).
- Additionally, the results of a prospective randomized trial compared CVP-based chemotherapy plus radiation (IFRT or total lymphoid irradiation) versus CVP chemotherapy alone revealed that the overall survival (OS) and event-free survival (EFS) of patients with stage III and IV follicular lymphoma who received adjuvant radiation therapy were significantly improved with minimal toxicity. The overall survival rates at 20-years were 71% versus 89% for patients received chemotherapy or combined chemoradiotherapy, respectively (Level II) (AVILÉS et al. 2002).
- In another series from M.D. Anderson Cancer Center, the actuarial 5- and 10-year overall sur-

vival rates were 65% and 42%, and the 5- and 10-year freedom-from progression (FFP) rates were 42% and 26%, respectively, for patients with stage III follicular lymphoma after chemotherapy or chemoradiation therapy. Although no differences were observed for the group of patients who received chemotherapy or combined chemoradiation in terms of overall survival, a trend of improved 5-year overall FFP with the addition of adjuvant radiation therapy (43% vs. 56%, $p = 0.06$) was found. Less than 75% of the patients received subtotal or central lymphatic irradiation in this study (Level III) (HA et al. 2003).

- The role of chemotherapy used in combination with radiation therapy has not been determined, and routine use of chemotherapy in the treatment of stage III low-grade NHL is controversial. In the above-mentioned study from Stanford University, adjuvant chemotherapy did not significantly alter the treatment outcome (Level III) (MURTHA et al. 2001).

Field Coverage

- The radiation portal of total lymphatic irradiation encompassing cervical, supraclavicular, axillary, mediastinal, paraaortic, mesenteric, pelvic, and femoral lymphatics can be considered for patients with stage III indolent NHL (Fig. 27.2) (Grade D).

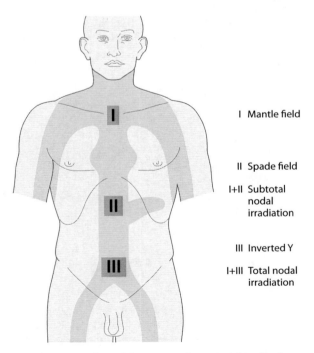

I   Mantle field

II   Spade field

I+II Subtotal
      nodal
      irradiation

III Inverted Y

I+III Total nodal
      irradiation

Fig. 27.2. Lymph nodal coverage in comprehensive lymphatic irradiation (Adopted from the SEER's Training Website http://training.seer.cancer.gov)

Dose

- Radiation dose of approximately 30 Gy with or without a boost to the gross tumor delivered in 1.5–1.8 Gy per fraction as used in various studies can be considered if total lymphatic irradiation is offered (Grade D). A treatment break after irradiation to each field (i.e., mental field, abdominal field, or pelvic/femoral field) can reduce potential side effects and complications induced by radiation.

27.2.4 Treatment of Stage IV Indolent Lymphoma

- Asymptomatic patients with more advanced stage III or stage IV low-grade NHL can be closely monitored (watchful waiting) (Grade A). Intense, multiagent chemotherapy is associated with a high response rate, but also with a continuous risk of relapse and long-term bone marrow suppression. Treatment can be deferred until symptoms develop (WINTER et al. 2004).
- HORNING and ROSENBERG (1984) studied the outcome of 83 low-grade lymphoma patients who were initially managed without active treatment and reported that the actuarial risk of transformation among the initially untreated patients was similar to those who were treated immediately after diagnosis. The incidence and time to histological transformation were not affected by the time of treatment initiation (Level III).
- Rituximab is a "humanized" anti-CD20 monoclonal antibody that can be recommended for the treatment of indolent non-Hodgkin's lymphoma (CD20 positive), and its efficacy in the treatment of relapsed or refractory indolent NHL has been repeatedly demonstrated (PLOSKER and FIGGITT 2003).
- Combined rituximab and chemotherapy should be recommended for indolent NHL patients who have indication for treatment (Grade A). Indications for treatment include active symptoms, cytopenias, progression of disease, or potential organ compromises. Results from phase III trials comparing R-CHOP to CHOP and R-CVP to CVP revealed that overall chemoimmunotherapy appears to be superior to chemotherapy alone, for both chemotherapy-naive patients and those who have been previously treated for indolent follicular lymphoma (Level I) (HIDDEMANN et al. 2003; MARCUS et al. 2003) (Fig. 27.3).

- Single-agent fludarabine, alkylators, or upfront radioimmunotherapy can be considered as an alternate to external-beam radiation when symptoms are not imminently threatening or for patients with contraindications for a more intensive treatment (Grade B) (KAMINSKI et al. 2005).
- Radiation therapy can be used for palliation for symptomatic patients with stage IV indolent lymphoma.

27.3 Treatment of Gastric Mucosa-Associated Lymphoid Tumors (MALT)

27.3.1 General Principles

- For *H. Pylori*-positive stage IE gastric MALT, antibiotic treatment of *H. Pylori* should be used as the initial treatment (Grade A). Radiation therapy is an effective modality for definitive treatment of localized (stage IE or II) gastric MALT and is recommended for *H. Pylori*-negative cases, as well as for patients with deep invasion, active symptoms, or disease progression after antibiotic treatment (Grade A).
- For stage III or IV gastric MALT, chemotherapy and/or rituximab should be considered (Grade A). Radiation therapy is indicated for local symptomatic control.
- Treatment strategy of the more commonly diagnosed large B-cell lymphoma of the stomach (comprises approximately 60% of all gastric lymphoma cases) is identical to that of the intermediate-grade NHL.

27.3.2 Treatment of Stage IE/II Gastric MALT

- Eradication of *H. Pylori* with antibiotics should be recommended as the sole initial treatment of MALT confined to the stomach (Grade A). Any of the effective anti-Helicobacter antibiotic regimens can be selected. Treatment of *H. Pylori*-positive stage IE gastric MALT with antibiotics is successful in approximately 70% of cases. In addition, the 3-year local recurrence rate is

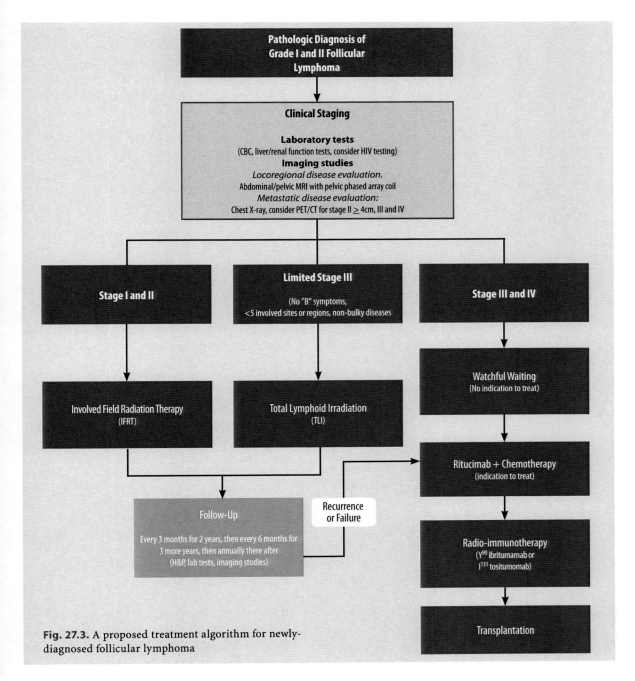

Fig. 27.3. A proposed treatment algorithm for newly-diagnosed follicular lymphoma

approximately 15% in patients achieving complete response (MALT Lymphoma Study Group, Level II) (SACKMANN et al. 1997).

■ Surgery has a limited role in the treatment of gastric MALT, and surgery alone does not alter overall relapse-free survival rates (Grade A). The overall survival after conservative treatment, chemotherapy, or radiation therapy with or without surgery is approximately 85% (Level II, III) (D'AMORE et al. 1994; KOCH et al. 2001; KOCH

et al. 2005). In addition, no difference in overall survival was observed after surgery, radiation therapy, or chemotherapy according to the results of a prospective randomized trial (Level II) (AVILÉS et al. 2005).

Radiation Therapy

■ IFRT is the mainstay treatment of stage IE/II gastric MALT in *H. Pylori*-negative cases or for patients who fail antibiotic treatment (Grade A). The complete response rate after IFRT was 95%, and the cause-specific survival and overall rates approached 100% and 90%, respectively (Level II, III) (Avilés et al. 2005; Koch et al. 2001; Koch et al. 2005).

- Radiation portal of IFRT should encompass the entire stomach and perigastric nodes, as gastric MALT is usually a multifocal disease (Wotherspoon et al. 1992).
- Doses ranging from 30 Gy to 40 Gy in conventional fractionation, as reported in the above-mentioned studies, can be considered.

27.3.2 Treatment of Stage III and IV Gastric MALT

- Chemotherapy and immunotherapy (with rituximab) are indicated for patients with advanced disease (Grade B). The efficacy of alkylating agents (such as cyclophosphamide 100 mg/day or chlorambucil 6 mg/day) has been reported, and a long-term survival rate of approximately 75% at 5 years can be expected (Level III) (Hammel et al. 1995).
- The effect of rituximab has been demonstrated in a phase II trial for untreated and recurrent MALT (including 15 gastric cases): the overall response rate of patients treated with rituximab was approximately 73%. However, the effect of rituximab on long-term survival and disease control remains unknown (IESLG, Level II) (Conconi et al. 2003).
- Radiation therapy can be offered for consolidation or symptomatic control in cases of poor response to chemotherapy and/or immunotherapy.

27.4　Treatment of Intermediate-Grade (Aggressive) Non-Hodgkin's Lymphoma

27.4.1 General Principles

- Treatment strategies of the more commonly diagnosed aggressive NHL, including diffuse large B-cell lymphoma, grade III follicular lymphoma,

peripheral T-cell lymphoma, and mantle-cell lymphoma, follow similar recommendations.

- For stage I and II aggressive NHL, CHOP-based chemotherapy followed by adjuvant IFRT is the standard treatment. Rituximab is indicated for CD20-positive large-cell non-Hodgkin's lymphoma (Grade A).
- For stage III and IV aggressive NHL, CHOP-based chemotherapy is the mainstay treatment. Rituximab is indicated for CD20 positive large-cell non-Hodgkin's lymphoma. The role of adjuvant radiation therapy is not clear. However, radiation therapy may improve treatment outcome in bulky diseases (> 10 cm in diameter) (Grade A).
- The radiolabeled anti-CD20 antibodies, Y^{90} ibritumamab and I^{131} tositumomab, have become an important treatment option for consolidative treatment after initial chemo-immunotherapy or for recurrent/persistent disease after chemotherapy and/or non-radiolabeled immunotherapy (Grade A) (Cheson 2003).

27.4.2 Treatment of Stage I and II Aggressive NHL

Combined Chemoradiation Therapy

- Multiagent chemotherapy is the mainstay treatment of early-stage intermediate-grade non-Hodgkin's lymphoma (Grade A). Six to eight cycles of CHOP-based chemotherapy are recommended for early-stage NHL.
- Radiation therapy alone is curative in approximately 40%–50% of patients (Level III) (Jones et al. 1973; Chen et al. 1979). The efficacy of chemotherapy followed by radiation therapy (IFRT or extended-field radiation therapy) over definitive radiotherapy alone on recurrence-free and/or overall survival rates has been repeatedly demonstrated in prospective randomized studies, although the sample sizes of most of these trials were limited (Level II) (Monfardini et al. 1980; Nissen et al. 1983; Yahalom et al. 1993).
- Rituximab, an immunotherapy agent (anti-CD20) used in combination with CHOP chemotherapy (the R-CHOP regimen), is recommended to patients with stage I or II diffuse large B-cell lymphoma (Grade B): In a European cooperative trial reported by the MabThera International Trial Group, patients with stage I (bulky disease)

to IV diffuse large B-cell lymphoma were treated with six cycles of CHOP-like or R-CHOP-like regimens. Patients with bulky and extranodal sites also received additional radiotherapy. The 3-year event-free survival and overall survival rates were 79% versus 59% and 93% versus 84%, respectively, significantly improved with the use of rituximab (MInT study, Level I) (PFREUNDSCHUH et al. 2006).

Radiation Therapy

- Adjuvant IFRT is part of the standard regimen for the treatment of stage I and II aggressive NHL (Grade A). The effects of radiation therapy on overall survival and long-term failure-free survival have been suggested by numerous retrospective and single-arm prospective trials, and have been confirmed by two prospective randomized trials completed by the Southwest Oncology Group (SWOG) and the Eastern Cooperative Oncology Group (ECOG):
- In the SWOG trial, 401 patients were randomized and treated with either eight cycles of CHOP chemotherapy or three cycles of CHOP chemotherapy followed by IFRT using the prechemotherapy tumor volume (most patients received 45–50 Gy in conventional fractionation, but doses ranging from 40–55 Gy were allowed). The results showed that combined treatment significantly improved the progression-free survival rate (64%–77%) and the overall survival rate (72% vs. 82%) (SWOG, Level I) (MILLER et al. 1998).
- In the ECOG trial, 352 patients were randomized and treated with eight cycles of CHOP chemotherapy with or without IFRT. Patients in the combined treatment arm who achieved complete response after chemotherapy received 30 Gy of IFRT, and those who had partial response were irradiated to 40 Gy. The 6-year disease-free survival rates were 73% and 56%, respectively, in favor of the combined chemoradiotherapy arm ($p = 0.05$). However, there is no significant difference in the overall survival rates (ECOG E1484, Level I) (HORNING et al. 2004).
- The effect of adjuvant radiation therapy on treatment outcome when used in combination with R-CHOP-based chemotherapy or more aggressive chemotherapy regimen is not clear. In a randomized trial from France, 647 patients with localized aggressive lymphoma were randomized and treated with CHOP followed by IFRT- or ACVBP-

based chemotherapy (without radiation). The results revealed that treatment outcome was significantly superior in patients treated with ACVBP chemotherapy (Level I) (REYES et al. 2005).
- However, no randomized investigation has been reported on the effects of radiation when used in combination with the aggressive chemotherapy or chemoimmunotherapy regimens. Further investigation is required before any change of the standard chemoradiation combination can be revised.

Field Arrangement

- IFRT is the standard technique for the treatment of stage I and II intermediate-grade NHL (Grade A). Although no randomized trial comparing IFRT versus extended-field radiation therapy (EFRT) has been performed, the efficacy of IFRT delivered after chemotherapy has been repeatedly demonstrated in retrospective or prospective trials. The long-term overall survival of patients treated with chemotherapy followed by IFRT ranges between 70% and 100% (Level I) (HORNING et al. 2004; MILLER et al. 1998).
- The field arrangement is detailed above in the Section 27.2.2.

Dose

- The optimal dose of consolidation radiation therapy has not been determined, and dose ranges used in the above-mentioned SWOG and ECOG trials can be referenced: For patients with complete response (CR) after three to eight cycles of chemotherapy (as confirmed by FDG-PET, PET CT, or gallium-67 scanning), consolidation radiation therapy with a dose of 30–40 Gy can be recommended; however, higher doses ranging from 40–55 Gy are recommended for patients who achieved less than a CR after chemotherapy.

27.4.3 Treatment of Stage III and IV Aggressive NHL

Chemotherapy

- CHOP-based chemotherapy is the mainstay treatment of stage III and IV aggressive NHL (Grade A). The complete response and long-term cure rates after definitive chemotherapy using the CHOP regimen are approximately 65% and 33%, respectively (KIMBY et al. 2001).

■ Although more intensive chemotherapy regimens were tried for the treatment of advanced stage aggressive NHL, their efficacy over the conventional CHOP regimen has not been demonstrated. In a prospective randomized trial completed by SWOG, more than 900 patients were randomized and received CHOP chemotherapy, or other chemotherapy combinations (m-BACOD, ProMACE/cytaBOM, or MACOP-B). The 3-year disease-free survival and overall survival rates were 44% and 52%, respectively, for the entire group, and no significant differences were detected (SWOG, Level I) (FISHER et al. 1993).

■ Rituximab, used in combination with CHOP chemotherapy (R-CHOP regimen), should be recommended to patients with advanced stage aggressive NHL (CD20 positive) (Grade A). In the above-mentioned MInT cooperative trial, patients with stage II to IV diffuse large B-cell lymphoma were treated with CHOP-like or R-CHOP-like regimens. The 3-year FFS and overall survival rates were 79% versus 59% and 93% versus 84%, respectively, in favor of R-CHOP treatment (MInT study, Level I) (PFREUNDSCHUH et al. 2006).

■ The value of rituximab used with CHOP chemotherapy in the treatment of elderly patients with advanced large B-cell lymphoma was further demonstrated in a French cooperative (Groupe d'Etudes des Lymphomes de l'Adulte) trial. A total of 399 elderly patients (>60 years) with advanced disease was randomized and received CHOP chemotherapy alone or a R-CHOP regimen. The 5-year overall survival and FFS rates were 58% versus 45% and 54% versus 30%, respectively, both in favor of R-CHOP treatment (GELA, Level I) (FEUGIER et al. 2005).

Radiation Therapy

■ Consolidation radiation therapy is commonly used in North America and can be recommended in advanced-stage aggressive NHL with bulky disease or an incomplete response after chemotherapy (Grade A). Radiation is frequently used for incomplete responders. Also, radiation is still considered an effective induction regimen for patients presenting with severe symptoms such as superior vena cava syndrome, spinal cord/epidural masses, brain lesions, bulky nodal masses with obstruction, painful or risky bone lesions, etc (Grade A). The effect of adjuvant radiation

therapy in stage III or IV intermediate-grade NHL has been demonstrated in both retrospective and randomized trials from Europe and South America:

■ In a phase III trial from Mexico, 218 patients with stage IV diffuse large cell lymphoma were treated with chemotherapy [CEOP-bleo regimen (cyclophosphamide, epirubicin, vincristine, prednisone, bleomycin) alternating with DAC (dexamethasone, Ara C, and cisplatin) regimens]. Among all patients who achieved complete response, 88 patients who presented with bulky tumor (>10 cm in largest dimension) were randomized to IFRT (40–50 Gy in conventional fractionation) or observation. The 5-year disease-free and overall survival rates were 72% versus 35% and 81% versus 55%, respectively, for patients treated with chemotherapy or combined chemoradiation, in favor of the irradiated group ($p<0.01$) (Level II) (AVILÉS 1994). The same research group reported a follow-up study with larger sample size: 341 patients with stage IV aggressive diffuse large cell lymphoma with bulky nodal disease but who achieved pathologic complete response after chemotherapy were randomized and treated with IFRT (40 Gy) or observation. The results confirmed the efficacy of IFRT on both event-free survival (EFS) and overall survival (OS). The 5-year EFS and OS rates were 82% versus 55% and 87% versus 66%, and significantly improved with the addition of consolidation radiation (Level I) (AVILÉS et al. 2004).

■ In a retrospective review from Italy, 94 patients with stage III or IV diffuse large-cell lymphoma and bulky (≥10 cm) or semibulky (6–9 cm) disease who achieved complete response after chemotherapy were treated with radiation therapy (30–46 Gy) or observed. Consolidation radiation therapy significantly prolonged the time to recurrence (TTR) time (41+ months vs. 18 months) and improved the 5-year overall survival (73% vs. 57%) (Level III) (FERRERI et al. 2000) (Fig. 27.4).

■ The effect of radiation therapy after high-dose chemotherapy with stem-cell transplantation was suggested in a retrospective trial from France. Patients who received consolidation radiotherapy following chemotherapy had superior outcome in terms of event-free survival, as compared to those received radiation therapy at the time of recurrence (Level III) (FOUILLARD et al. 1998).

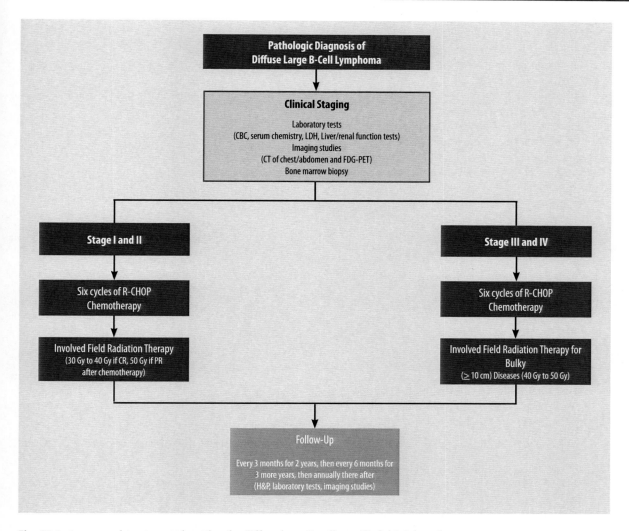

Fig. 27.4. A proposed treatment algorithm for diffuse large B-cell non-Hodgkin's lymphoma

27.5 Follow-Ups

27.5.1 Post-Treatment Follow-Ups

■ Life-long follow-up after definitive treatment of NHL is recommended for detecting recurrence, secondary tumors, or other long-term complications of radiation therapy or chemotherapy (Table 27.5).

Schedule

■ Follow-up could be scheduled every 3 months for 2 years, then every 6 months for 3 additional years, then annually thereafter (Grade D) (ESMO 2007).

Work-Ups

■ Each follow-up should include a complete history and physical examination.
■ Complete blood count and LDH at 3, 6, 12 and 24 months then ordered when clinically indicated are recommended; CT of the chest and/or abdomen at 6, 12, and 24 months after the completion of treatment are usually recommended (Grade D) (ESMO 2007).
■ Evaluation of thyroid function with thyroid-stimulating hormone (TSH) in patients receiving radiation therapy to the neck and/or upper chest should be performed at years 1, 2, and 5.
■ For gastric MALT after treatment, a strict endoscopic follow-up with multiple biopsies taken 2–3 months after treatment to document H. *Py-*

lori eradications and subsequently at least twice annually for 2 years to monitor the histologic regression of the disease is indicated (Grade D) (ESMO 2007).

■ For female patients who received radiation therapy prior to menopause, especially at an age younger than 25 years, screening for secondary breast cancers should be considered.

Table 27.5. Follow-up schedule after treatment of non-Hodgkin's lymphoma

Interval	Frequency
First 2 years	Every 3 months
Years 3–5	Every 6 months
Over 5 years	Annually

Reference

Armitage JO, Weisenburger DD (1998) New approach to classifying non-Hodgkin's lymphomas: clinical features of the major histologic subtypes. Non-Hodgkin's Lymphoma Classification Project. J Clin Oncol 16:2780–2795

d'Amore F, Brincker H, Grønbaek K et al (1994) Non-Hodgkin's lymphoma of the gastrointestinal tract: a population-based analysis of incidence, geographic distribution, clinicopathologic presentation features, and prognosis. Danish Lymphoma Study Group. J Clin Oncol 12:1673–1684

Avilés A, Delgado S, Nambo MJ et al (1994) Adjuvant radiotherapy to sites of previous bulky disease in patients with stage IV diffuse large cell lymphoma. Int J Radiat Oncol Biol Phys 30:799–803

Avilés A, Delgado S, Fernández R et al (2002) Combined therapy in advanced stages (III and IV) of follicular lymphoma increases the possibility of cure: results of a large controlled clinical trial. Eur J Haematol 68:144–149

Avilés A, Fernándezb R, Pérez F et al (2004) Adjuvant radiotherapy in stage IV diffuse large cell lymphoma improves outcome. Leuk Lymphoma 45:1385–1389

Avilés A, Nambo MJ, Neri N et al (2005) Mucosa-associated lymphoid tissue (MALT) lymphoma of the stomach: results of a controlled clinical trial. Med Oncol 22:57–62

Carde P, Burgers JM, van Glabbeke M et al (1984) Combined radiotherapy-chemotherapy for early stages non-Hodgkin's lymphoma: the 1975–1980 EORTC controlled lymphoma trial. Radiother Oncol 2:301–312

Chen MG, Prosnitz LR, Gonzalez-Serva A et al (1979) Results of radiotherapy in control of stage I and II non-Hodgkin's lymphoma. Cancer 43:1245–1254

Cheson BD (2003) Radioimmunotherapy of non-Hodgkin lymphomas. Blood 101:391–398

Conconi A, Martinelli G, Thiéblemont C et al (2003) Clinical activity of rituximab in extranodal marginal zone B-cell lymphoma of MALT type. Blood 102:2741–2745

Elstrom R, Guan L, Baker G et al (2003) Utility of FDG-PET scanning in lymphoma by WHO classification. Blood 101:3875–3876

European Society for Medical Oncology. Clinical recommendations. Newly diagnosed non-Hodgkin's lymphoma: ESMO clinical recommendations for diagnosis, treatment and follow-up. Ann Oncol 18(S2):ii55–ii64

Ferreri AJ, Dell'Oro S, Reni M et al (2000) Consolidation radiotherapy to bulky or semibulky lesions in the management of stage III–IV diffuse large B cell lymphomas. Oncology 58:219–226

Feugier P, van Hoof A, Sebban C et al (2005) Long-term results of the R-CHOP study in the treatment of elderly patients with diffuse large B-cell lymphoma: a study by the Groupe d'Etude des Lymphomes de l'Adulte. J Clin Oncol 23:4117–4126

Fisher RI, LeBlanc M, Press OW et al (2005) New Treatment Options have changed the survival of patients with follicular lymphoma. J Clin Oncol 23:8447–8452

Fouillard L, Laporte JP, Labopin M et al (1998) Autologous stem-cell transplantation for non-Hodgkin's lymphomas: the role of graft purging and radiotherapy posttransplantation–results of a retrospective analysis on 120 patients autografted in a single institution. J Clin Oncol 16:2803–2816

Fuks Z, Kaplan HS (1973) Recurrence rates following radiation therapy of nodular and diffuse malignant lymphomas. Radiology 108:675–684

Gospodarowicz MK, Bush RS, Brown TC et al (1984) Prognostic factors in nodular lymphomas: a multivariate analysis based on the Princess Margaret Hospital experience. Int J Radiat Oncol Biol Phys 10:489–497

Greene FL, Page DL, Fleming ID et al (2002) American Joint Committee on Cancer, American Cancer Society. AJCC cancer staging manual, 6th edn. Springer, Berlin Heidelberg, New York

Girinsky T, van der Maazen R, Specht L et al (2006) Involved-node radiotherapy in patients with early Hodgkin lymphoma: concepts and guidelines. Radiother Oncol 79:270–277

Ha CS, Kong JS, McLaughlin P et al (2003) Stage III follicular lymphoma: long-term follow-up and patterns of failure. Int J Radiat Oncol Biol Phys 57:748–754

Ha CS, Kong JS, Tucker SL et al (2003) Central lymphatic irradiation for stage I–III follicular lymphoma: report from a single-institutional prospective study. Int J Radiat Oncol Biol Phys 57:316–320

Hammel P, Haioun C, Chaumette MT et al (1995) Efficacy of single-agent chemotherapy in low-grade B-cell mucosa-associated lymphoid tissue lymphoma with prominent gastric expression. J Clin Oncol 13:2524–2529

Hiddemann W, Dreyling MH, Forstpointer R et al (2003) Combined immuno-chemotherapy (R-CHOP) significantly improves time to treatment failure in first line therapy of follicular lymphoma–results of a prospective randomized trial of the German Low Grade Lymphoma Study Group (GLSG). Blood 102:104a

Horning SJ, Rosenberg SA (1984) The natural history of initially untreated low-grade non-Hodgkin's lymphomas. N Engl J Med 311:1471–1475

Horning SJ, Weller E, Kim K et al (2004) Chemotherapy with or without radiotherapy in limited-stage diffuse aggressive non-Hodgkin's lymphoma: Eastern Cooperative Oncology Group study 1484. J Clin Oncol 22:3032–3038

The International Non-Hodgkin's Lymphoma Prognostic Factors Project (1993) A predictive model for aggressive non-Hodgkin's lymphoma. The International Non-Hodgkin's Lymphoma Prognostic Factors Project. N Engl J Med 329:987–994

Jacobs JP, Murray KJ, Schultz CJ et al (1993) Central lymphatic irradiation for stage III nodular malignant lymphoma: long-term results. J Clin Oncol 11:233–238

Jaffe ES, Harris NH, Stein H et al (2001) Pathology and genetics of tumors of hematopoietic and lymphoid tissues. World Health Organization Classification of Tumors. Lyon, France: IARC Press

Jeffers MD, Milton J, Herriot R et al (1998) Fine-needle aspiration cytology in the investigation on non-Hodgkin's lymphoma. J Clin Pathol 51:189–196

Jones S, Fuks Z, Bull M et al (1973) Non-Hodgkin's lymphomas. IV. Clinicopathologic correlation in 405 cases. Cancer 31:806–823

Kaminski MS, Tuck M, Estes J et al (2005) 131I-tositumomab therapy as initial treatment for follicular lymphoma. N Engl J Med 352:441–449

Kaplan WD, Jochelson MS, Herman TS et al (1990) Gallium-67 imaging: a predictor of residual tumor viability and clinical outcome in patients with diffuse large-cell lymphoma. J Clin Oncol 8:1966–1970

Kimby E, Brandt L, Nygren P et al (2001) A systematic overview of chemotherapy effects in aggressive non-Hodgkin's lymphoma. Acta Oncol 40:198–212

Koch P, del Valle F, Berdel WE et al (2001) Primary gastrointestinal non-Hodgkin's lymphoma: II. Combined surgical and conservative or conservative management only in localized gastric lymphoma–results of the prospective German Multicenter Study GIT NHL 01/92. J Clin Oncol 19:3874–3883

Koch P, Probst A, Berdel WE et al (2005) Treatment results in localized primary gastric lymphoma: data of patients registered within the German multicenter study (GIT NHL 02/96). J Clin Oncol 23:7050–7059

MacManus MP, Hoppe RT (1996) Is radiotherapy curative for stage I and II low-grade follicular lymphoma? Results of a long-term follow-up study of patients treated at Stanford University. J Clin Oncol 14:1282–1290

Marcus R, Imrie K, Belch A et al (2003) An international, multicentre, randomized, open-label, phase III trial comparing rituximab added to CVP chemotherapy to CVP chemotherapy alone in untreated stage III/IV follicular non-Hodgkin's lymphoma. Blood 102:28a

Miller TP, Dahlberg S, Cassady JR et al (1998) Chemotherapy alone compared with chemotherapy plus radiotherapy for localized intermediate- and high-grade non-Hodgkin's lymphoma. N Engl J Med 339:21–26

Monfardini S, Banfi A, Bonadonna G et al (1980) Improved 5-year survival after combined radiotherapy-chemotherapy for stage I–II non-Hodgkin's lymphoma. Int J Radiat Oncol Biol Phys 6:125–134

Murtha AD, Rupnow BA, Hansosn J et al (2001) Long-term follow-up of patients with Stage III follicular lymphoma treated with primary radiotherapy at Stanford University. Int J Radiat Oncol Biol Phys 49:3–15

Nissen NI, Ersbøll J, Hansen HS et al (1983) A randomized study of radiotherapy versus radiotherapy plus chemotherapy in stage I–II non-Hodgkin's lymphomas. Cancer 52:1–7

Plosker GL, Figgitt DP (2003) Rituximab: a review of its use in non-Hodgkin's lymphoma and chronic lymphocytic leukemia. Drugs 63:803–843

Pfreundschuh M, Trumper L, Osterborg A et al (2006) CHOP-like chemotherapy plus rituximab versus CHOP-like chemotherapy alone in young patients with good-prognosis diffuse large-B-cell lymphoma: a randomised controlled trial by the MabThera International Trial (MInT) Group. Lancet Oncol 7:379–391

Reyes F, Lepage E, Ganem G et al (2005) ACVBP versus CHOP plus radiotherapy for localized aggressive lymphoma. N Engl J Med 352:1197–1205

Sackmann M, Morgner A, Rudolph B et al (1997) Regression of gastric MALT lymphoma after eradication of Helicobacter pylori is predicted by endosonographic staging. MALT Lymphoma Study Group. Gastroenterology 113:1087–1090

Saddik M, el Dabbagh L, Mourad WA (1997) Ex vivo fine-needle aspiration cytology and flow cytometric phenotyping in the diagnosis of lymphoproliferative disorders: a proposed algorithm for maximum resource utilization. Diagn Cytopathol 16:126–131

Tsukamoto N, Kojima M, Hasegawa M et al (2007) The usefulness of (18)F-fluorodeoxyglucose positron emission tomography (18)F-FDG-PET) and a comparison of (18) F-FDG-pet with (67)gallium scintigraphy in the evaluation of lymphoma: relation to histologic subtypes based on the World Health Organization classification. Cancer 110:652–659

Vaughan HB, Vaughan HG, MacLennan KA et al (1994) Clinical stage I non-Hodgkin's lymphoma: long-term follow-up of patients treated by the British National Lymphoma Investigation with radiotherapy alone as initial therapy. Br J Cancer 69:1088–1093

Winter JN, Gascoyne RD, Van Besien K (2004) Low-grade lymphoma. Hematology Am Soc Hematol Educ Program:203–220

Wirth A, Seymour JF, Hicks RJ et al (2002) Fluorine-18 fluorodeoxyglucose positron emission tomography, gallium-67 scintigraphy, and conventional staging for Hodgkin's disease and non-Hodgkin's lymphoma. Am J Med 112:262–268

Witzig TE, Gordon LI, Cabanillas F et al (2002) Randomized controlled trial of yttrium-90-labeled ibritumomab tiuxetan radioimmunotherapy versus rituximab immunotherapy for patients with relapsed or refractory low-grade, follicular, or transformed B-cell non-Hodgkin's lymphoma. J Clin Oncol 20:2453–2463

Wotherspoon AC, Doglioni C, Isaacson PG (1992) Low-grade gastric B-cell lymphoma of mucosa-associated lymphoid tissue (MALT): a multifocal disease. Histopathology 20:29–34

Yahalom J, Varsos G, Fuks Z et al (1993) Adjuvant cyclophosphamide, doxorubicin, vincristine, and prednisone chemotherapy after radiation therapy in stage I low-grade and intermediate-grade non-Hodgkin lymphoma. Results of a prospective randomized study. Cancer 71:2342–2350

Hodgkin's Lymphoma

B-Chen Wen and Kelly LaFave

CONTENTS

Introduction and Objectives

Approximately 8,000 cases of Hodgkin's lymphoma occur annually in the United States. It is a chemo- and radio-sensitive disease. Early-stage Hodgkin's lymphoma can be cured with radiotherapy or chemotherapy. Advances in radiation technique, radiological imaging, understanding of prognostic factors, and development of less toxic chemotherapy regimens have allowed for better tailoring of treatment and aim to improve the complication-free survival for Hodgkin's lymphoma.

This chapter examines:

● Recommendations for initial evaluation, laboratory studies, and imaging studies

● Staging system, pathology, and prognostic factors

● Treatment recommendations for early stage favorable and unfavorable and advanced Hodgkin's lymphoma in adult patients accompanied by supporting literature

● Radiation therapy technique including field arrangement and dose for the treatment of adult Hodgkin's lymphoma

● Discussion of treatment-related toxicities and follow-up care

The etiology and management of Hodgkin's lymphoma in children differ significantly from those in adults. The management of pediatric Hodgkin's lymphoma is detailed in Chapter 39.

B-C. Wen, MD
Department of Radiation Oncology, Sylvester Comprehensive Cancer Center, University of Miami, 1475 N.W. 12th Avenue, D-31, Miami, FL 33136, USA
K. LaFave, MD
Department of Radiation Oncology, Sylvester Comprehensive Cancer Center, University of Miami, 1475 N.W. 12th Avenue, D-31, Miami, FL 33136, USA

28.1 Diagnosis, Staging, and Prognosis

28.1.1 Diagnosis

Initial Evaluation

- Evaluation of Hodgkin's lymphoma/disease (HL) begins with a complete history and physical examination with special attention to disease-related signs and symptoms. Fever of 38°C or higher for 3 consecutive days, drenching night sweats, and unexplained weight loss >10% over 6 months prior to diagnosis (the "B" symptoms) should be documented. Patients presenting with fever and weight loss have a worse prognosis (CRNKOVICH et al. 1987). Pel-Ebstein fever is the classical descriptor for the waxing and waning fever of HL (GOOD and DINUBILE 1995). Other commonly observed symptoms of HL include pruritus, painless lymphadenopathy, respiratory difficulty, alcohol-induced pain, and fatigue.
- Thorough examination of all lymphoid regions including the spleen and the liver is required. In total 80% of patients present with cervical lymphadenopathy, while 50% present with mediastinal lymphadenopathy. Involvement of Waldeyer's ring or mesenteric lymph nodes is rare (<5%). HL spreads in an orderly, contiguous pattern through lymph nodes (Level IV) (ROSENBERG and KAPLAN 1966). As the disease advances, hematogenous metastasis may occur to liver and bone.

Laboratory Tests

- Laboratory studies should include CBC with differential, lactate dehydrogenase (LDH), albumin, renal and liver function tests, erythrocyte sedimentation rate (ESR), and alkaline phosphatase. β_2-microglobulin may also be helpful.
- For reproductive females, a pregnancy test is essential as well as consideration for reproductive counseling and oophoropexy, especially if pelvic RT is planned. MRI may be helpful in the staging of pregnant patients. Male patients may be offered semen cryopreservation if chemotherapy or pelvic RT is a possibility.
- An HIV test is recommended for patients with risk factors. Patients with HIV/AIDS usually have advanced presentation, atypical clinical presentation, and an aggressive clinical course (RUBIO 1994).

Imaging Studies

- Diagnostic imaging studies, including chest X-ray [posteroanterior (PA) and lateral views] and CT scan of the thorax, abdomen, and pelvis are required for staging and evaluation of the bulk of disease, as well as determining the extent of the radiation treatment field. CT scan of the neck area is indicated for cervical and upper mediastinal diseases.
- Bulky mediastinal disease denotes poor prognosis and has been defined in three different ways on imaging studies:
- Maximum mass width (MMW) divided by maximum intrathoracic diameter (MTD) equal to or greater than 1/3 on PA chest X-ray by the German Hodgkin Lymphoma Study Group (GHSG)
- Mediastinal mass (MM) greater than 10 cm on imaging by the Stanford University regimen (HUGHES-DAVIES et al. 1997)
- Mediastinal mass (MM) divided by the thoracic diameter (TD) at T5-6 equal to or greater than 1/3 on PA chest X-ray by the European Organization of Research and Treatment of Cancer (EORTC)
- Compared to staging laparotomy, CT of the abdomen and pelvis is less likely to detect small lesions in the liver, spleen, or mesenteric LN (Level III) (CASTELLINO et al. 1984).
- PET/CT should be considered if CT is equivocal for stage I or II patients (Grade B). PET/CT has increased accuracy as compared to CT and also changes the stage and treatment in approximately 20% of patients (Level III) (NAUMANN et al. 2004; PARTRIDGE et al. 2000; LANG et al. 2001).
- Bone scan is not routinely recommended, but should be performed in patients with an elevated alkaline phosphatase or presenting with bone pain.
- Staging laparotomy is no longer considered the standard diagnostic procedure because most patients receive systemic chemotherapy, and diagnostic testing and understanding of prognostic factors have improved. For patients prepared for radiation therapy alone, staging laparotomy may be informative, as shown in the EORTC 6F trial (Level III) (CARDE et al. 1993; DIEHL et al. 2004).

Pathology

- Tissue diagnosis is required prior to the determination of any treatment. Tissue can be obtained by surgical nodal or extranodal biopsy. Any effusion can be considered for cytological examination.

- Bone marrow biopsy should be considered in patients with advanced stage or "B" symptoms.

- HL is classified into two main categories and five total subtypes by the World Health Organization (HARRIS et al. 1999) (Table 28.1):

- Classical HL (CHL)

- Nodular sclerosis (NSHL) is the most common HL and commonly presents with mediastinal LN. One-third present with "B" symptoms. Prognosis is less favorable than NLPHL.

- Mixed cellularity (MCHL) may present in older patients. Retroperitoneal LN involvement and more advanced stage are common. Prognosis is less favorable than NSHL.

- Lymphocyte depleted (LDHL) is the rarest HL presenting with "B" symptoms, advanced stage, and in older patients. LDHLs have the least favorable prognosis of all the HL subtypes.

- Lymphocyte-rich classical HL (LRCHL) can present in older patients with localized peripheral lymph nodes and is the most favorable group in CHL.

- Nodular lymphocyte predominant HL (NLPHL) is seen in younger patients, presenting in early stage with a solitary lymph node. "B" symptoms are uncommon. NLPHL is the most favorable HL with an indolent course.

Table 28.1. Classical Hodgkin's lymphoma and NLPHL group characteristics (HERBST et al. 1991; HALUSKA et al. 1994)

	Classical HL	**NLPHL**
Characteristic cell	Reed-Sternberg cell	Lymphocytic and histiocytic cell "popcorn cells"
Surface antigens	CD15+,CD30+, CD20+/–, CD45–, EMA–	CD15–, CD30–, CD20+, CD45+, EMA+
EBV	+EBV in 50%	EBV–

28.1.2 Staging

- Patients with HL are clinically staged. Treatment recommendations are based on staging as well as prognostic factors (Table 28.2).

Table 28.2. Ann Arbor staging system for Hodgkin's lymphoma. [Modified from CARBONE et al. (1971) with permission]

Ann Arbor staging system	
Stage I	Involvement of single lymph node (I) or extralymphatic site (IE)
Stage II	Involvement of two or more involved lymph node sites on the same side of the diaphragm (II) or localized involvement of one extralymphatic organ or site plus one or more lymph node regions on the same side of diaphragm (IIE)
Stage III	Involvement of lymph node regions on both sides of diaphragm (III), which can also include involvement of the spleen (IIIS) or localized extralymphatic site or organ extension (IIIE) or both (IIISE)
Stage IV	Diffuse (multifocal) involvement of one or more extralymphatic organs or sites
Descriptors	A=No "B" symptoms B=Unexplained fever >38°C, weight loss >10% in previous 6 months, drenching night sweats X=Bulky disease

28.1.3 Prognosis

Prognostic Factors for Early-Stage Hodgkin's Lymphoma Treated with Radiation Therapy Alone

- In patients treated with radiation alone, risk factors for increased relapse include the following: men, advanced age, mixed cellularity, lymphocyte-depleted, "B" symptoms, bulky mediastinal disease, large number of involved LN, and elevated ESR (WIRTH et al. 1999; TUBIANA et al. 1989). Patients with risk factors could be considered for combined treatment with chemotherapy and radiation therapy.

- Early-stage HL can be divided into favorable and unfavorable groups based on various prognostic factors. Patients with fewer of these poor prognostic factors can be considered for less intensive therapy. Different criteria have been used to define the criteria for the unfavorable group (see Table 28.3).

Unfavorable Prognostic Factors for Advanced Hodgkin's Lymphoma

- The International Prognostic Factors Project evaluated 5141 patients with advanced disease treated with chemotherapy ± radiotherapy at 25 centers.

Table 28.3. Comparison of prognostic factors in four major research groups

Factor	EORTC	GHSG	NCIC[a]	Stanford
Mediastinum	MM >35% of TD at T5/6 on PA CXR	MMW/MTD ≥ 1/3 on PA CXR	MMW/MTD >1/3 on PA CXR	MM >10 cm OR MMW/MTD >1/3 on PA CXR
ESR/ "B" symptoms	ESR ≥30 w/"B" symptoms ESR ≥50 w/o "B" symptoms	ESR ≥30 w/"B" symptoms ESR ≥50 w/o "B" symptoms	ESR ≥50 or "B" symptoms	"B" symptoms
Nodal sites	≥4 Sites	≥3 Sites	≥4 Sites	
Others	Age ≥50	Extranodal site	Age ≥40 or MCHL/LDHL	

[a]National Cancer Institute of Canada.

Several prognostic factors were identified on multivariate analyses (Table 28.4) (HASENCLEVER and DIEHL 1998).

- Each factor reduces the 5-year freedom from progression of disease by approximately 8% (HASENCLEVER and DIEHL 1998) (Table 28.5).

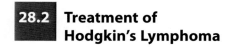

28.2 Treatment of Hodgkin's Lymphoma

28.2.1 General Principles

- ABVD containing multidrug regimen(s) is the treatment of choice for HL (Grade A). Multidrug chemotherapy is superior to single drug regimens, and ABVD-containing regimens produce improved disease-free survival as compared to MOPP alone (Level I) (CANELLOS et al. 1992; SOMERS et al. 1990) (Table 28.6). Furthermore, ABVD has less sterility and hematological toxicity, but more pulmonary and cardiac toxicity.
  Brief and dose-intense chemotherapy regimens (Stanford V regimen) plus radiation therapy to bulky disease sites for locally extensive and advanced-stage Hodgkin's disease have produced acceptable outcomes, according to the long-term follow-up of a non-randomized prospective trial (Level III) (HORNING et al. 2002). BEACOPP is an option for unfavorable or advanced presentations (EORTC/IPFP, Level I) (HASENCLEVER and DIEHL 1998; NOORDIJK et al. 2005).
- Radiation is the single most effective therapeutic agent in controlling locoregional HL. Radiation fields should be based on anatomical structures and the extent of the tumor.

Table 28.4. Unfavorable prognostic factors for advanced Hodgkin's lymphoma

Age ≥45
Male
Albumin <4 g/dl
Hemoglobin <10.5 g/dl
Stage IV disease
WBC ≥15×10³/mm³
Lymphocyte <600/mm³ or lymphocyte <8% of WBC

Table 28.5. Prognostic score for advanced Hodgkin's disease (HASENCLEVER and DIEHL 1998)

Factors	5-year freedom from progression	5-year overall survival
0	84%	89%
1	77%	90%
2	67%	81%
3	60%	78%
4	51%	61%
≥5	42%	56%

Table 28.6. Chemotherapy regimens for the treatment of Hodgkin's lymphoma

Regimens	Chemotherapy agents
MOPP	Nitrogen mustard, Oncovin (vincristine), procarbazine, prednisone. Every 3 weeks
ABVD	Adriamycin, bleomycin, vinblastine, dacarbazine. Every 4 weeks
MOPP/ABVD	MOPP/ABVD. Every 8 weeks
Stanford V	Mechlorethamine, doxorubicin, etoposide, vincristine, vinblastine, bleomycin, prednisone. Every 4 weeks
BEACOPP	Bleomycin, etoposide, adriamycin, cyclophosphamide, vincristine, procarbazine, prednisone. Every 3 weeks. Increased dose BEACOPP is given every 22 days

- The current direction is to use the smallest effective radiation dose with the smallest effective field size to minimize toxicities.
- Chemoradiation therapy should be given in a sequential fashion. Systemic chemotherapy is usually given first to reduce the bulk of disease, thus the irradiation field size. In addition, chemotherapy is important to treat any disseminated disease earlier and in decreasing the significance of radiation-induced bone marrow suppression.

28.2.2 Treatment of Stage I–IIA Favorable Hodgkin's Lymphoma

- Four cycles of ABVD-based chemotherapy followed by involved-field radiation (20–30 Gy) or two cycles of Stanford V (8 weeks) followed by involved-field radiation (30 Gy) to start within 3 weeks after chemotherapy can be recommended (Grade A). The efficacy of various chemotherapy combinations has been demonstrated in randomized phase III trials.
  Alternatively, six cycles of ABVD-based chemotherapy can be suggested, only if complete response (CR) or unconfirmed complete response (CRu) at restaging after four cycles of ABVD (Grade B).
- Chemotherapy followed by involved-field radiation therapy is currently the standard treatment recommendation (Grade A). Results from multiple randomized trials have confirmed the superiority of sequential chemotherapy followed by radiation therapy over radiation therapy alone or chemotherapy alone. Freedom from treatment failure and overall survival rates are 90%–95%.
  The GHSG HD7 evaluated favorable stage I–II patients with extended-field radiation therapy (EFRT) of 30 Gy plus 10 Gy boost versus ABVD for two cycles and the same EFRT 30 Gy plus 10 Gy boost. Results showed improvement in freedom from treatment failure (FFTF) at 7 years of 67% vs. 88% for the combined modality with similar overall survival (OS) 92 vs. 94% (GHSG HD7, Level I) (ENGERT et al. 2007).
  SWOG 9133/Intergroup study confirmed the superiority of sequential chemotherapy (adriamycin + vinblastine × 3) followed by STLI (36–40 Gy) to STLI alone (FFTF 94% vs. 81%). There was no difference in OS at 3 years (98% vs. 96%) (Level I) (PRESS et al. 2000).

EORTC H7F randomized patients to STLI alone versus EBVP (epirubicin, bleomycin, vinblastine, and prednisone) + IFRT. Results at 5 years showed improvement in recurrence-free survival (92% vs. 81%) with similar OS (98% vs. 95%) (Level I) (CARDE et al. 1997). Combined regimens were superior to radiation alone in the EORTC H8F trial comparing STLI (36–40 Gy) vs. MOPP/ABV × 3 followed by IFRT (36–40 Gy). The combined group was superior over RT alone in event-free survival (EFS) (93% vs. 68%) and OS (97% vs. 92%) at 10 years (Level I) (FERME et al. 2007).

- Combined chemoradiation therapy should be considered, and chemotherapy alone should not be routinely recommended (Grade A). The EORTC H9F randomized stage I–II CR patients after EBVP × 6 to no RT, IFRT 20 Gy, or IFRT 36 Gy. At 4 years the EFS was statistically significant with no RT vs. RT (70%, 84%, and 87%). When using EBVP chemotherapy, IFRT should be strongly considered following complete response (Level I) (NOORDIJK et al. 2005).
  In a NCIC trial, early-stage patients were randomized to subtotal nodal irradiation (STNI) of 35 Gy plus two cycles of ABVD for the unfavorable group vs. ABVD × 4–6. The 5-year FFP and overall survival rates were improved in the radiation-containing groups. In the favorable group, subset analyses comparing STNI of 35 Gy vs. ABVD × 4–6 showed similar results for FFP and OS at 5 years (MEYER et al. 2005).
- Reduced dose chemotherapy and reduced dose irradiation should be considered (Grade A). The efficacy of reduced intensity chemotherapy and radiation were found to be equally effective in randomized trials and a meta-analysis. GHSG HD 10 is a four-arm study comparing four versus two cycles of ABVD with 30 Gy and 20 Gy of IFRT. Results at 2 years show no difference in FFTF (96.6%) or OS (98.5%). However, longer follow-up is needed for the data to mature (Level II) (DIEHL et al. 2005).
  GHSG HD 7, 10, and 13 were designed to evaluate the effect of less intensive chemotherapy with involved-field radiation therapy. A total of 42 patients were identified with treatment failure among the 1129 patients enrolled. Analysis of patients involved in these trials revealed that failure after ABVD × 2, ABV × 2, VD × 2, or AV × 2 followed by IFRT 30 Gy is rare (Level IV) (SIENIAWSKI et al. 2007).

■ IFRT should be considered the treatment field of choice for stage I and II patients (Grade A). The Milan trial enrolled stage I–II favorable and unfavorable patients to four cycles of ABVD followed by either STLI (36–40 Gy) or IFRT (36–40 Gy). The results revealed no differences at 12 years in freedom from progression rate (93% versus 94%) and overall survival rate (96% versus 94%) (Level I) (BONADONNA et al. 2004).

Results of patients with stage I–IIA favorable group treated with two cycles of Stanford V regimen followed by IFRT to a total dose of 30 Gy produced 95% freedom from progression rate at 3 years (Level IV) (DIEHL et al. 2004).

■ If a patient is unable to tolerate chemotherapy, radiation therapy alone can be used for definitive treatment:

For supradiaphragmatic disease STNI is preferred, including a mantle field followed by a 2- to 3-week break and then a paraortic-splenic field. For subdiaphragmatic disease, staging laparotomy is preferred prior to RT, and the treatment volume depends on the findings. The dose for gross disease is 39.6 Gy/22 fractions (or 40 Gy/20), and for microscopic disease, 30.6 Gy/17 fractions (or 30 Gy/15 fractions).

28.2.3 Treatment of Stage IA–IIB Unfavorable Hodgkin's Lymphoma

■ Chemotherapy followed by IFRT should be recommended for patients with non-bulky stage IA–IIB HL with unfavorable features (Grade B). Several regimens can be considered: (1) a total of four cycles of ABVD followed by IFRT of 30 Gy, (2) two cycles of Stanford V (8 weeks) followed by IFRT 30 Gy, or (3) four cycles of BEACOPP followed by IFRT 30 Gy (Grade B). FFP and OS for these patients is 80%–90% at 10 years.

Alternatively, six cycles of ABVD-based chemotherapy can be suggested only if there is complete response (CR) or unconfirmed complete response (CRu) at restaging after four cycles of ABVD (Grade C).

■ Chemotherapy followed by IFRT should be recommended for patients with bulky stage IA–IIB HL with unfavorable features (Grade B). Several regimens can be considered: (1) a total of six cycles of ABVD followed by IFRT of 30–36 Gy, (2) three cycles of Stanford V (12 weeks) followed

by IFRT 36 Gy to initial bulky disease (>5 cm), or (3) four cycles of BEACOPP followed-by IFRT 30 Gy (Grade B). FFP and OS for these patients is 80%–90% at 10 years.

■ IFRT should be considered as the standard field arrangement for patients with unfavorable stage IA–IIB HL (Grade A). IFRT is equally effective with less toxicity as compared to subtotal lymphoid irradiation: EORTC H8U randomized early stage unfavorable patients to MOPP/ABV × 6 + IFRT (36–40 Gy) or MOPP/ABV × 4 + IFRT or MOPP/ABV × 4 + STLI (36–40 Gy). There was no difference in 10-year EFS (82% vs. 80% vs. 80%) and 10-year OS (88% vs. 85% vs. 84%) (Level I) (FERME et al. 2007).

A Milan trial compared stage I–II favorable and unfavorable patients with four cycles of ABVD followed by either STLI (36 Gy–40 Gy) or IFRT (36–40 Gy), revealing no differences at 12 years in freedom from progression rate (93% vs. 94%) and OS (96% vs. 94%) (Level I) (BONADONNA et al. 2004).

GHSG HD8 randomly compared COPP/ABVD × 2 + EFRT vs. COPP/ABVD × 2 + IFRT (same dose). The 5-year FFTF (86% vs. 84%) and OS (91% vs. 92%) showed no difference between the groups. Toxicity was less in the IFRT group (ENGERT et al. 2003).

■ Lower dose irradiation to a total dose of 20 Gy could be considered for adjuvant therapy; however, longer follow-up is needed before it can be considered standard (Grade B). The GHSG HD11 randomized early-stage unfavorable patients in a four-arm fashion to four cycles of ABVD followed by IFRT 30 Gy, four cycles of ABVD followed by IFRT 20 Gy, or four cycles of BEACOPP followed by IFRT 30 Gy or 4 cycles of BEACOPP followed by IFRT 20 Gy. The early 2-year results show no differences in the FFTF (90%) and OS rates (97%) (Level II) (KLIMM et al. 2005).

■ ABVD-based chemotherapy is considered the standard regimen for the treatment of stage I and II HL with unfavorable features; however, certain newer chemotherapy regimens, such as Stanford V, can also be considered (Grade B). Early-stage I and II patients with extensive mediastinal involvement were treated with Stanford V for 12 weeks followed by 36 Gy IFRT to the initial sites >5 cm. The 5-year FFP (89%) and OS (96%) show the effectiveness of this regimen (HORNING et al. 2002).

■ The EORTC H9U evaluated early-stage unfavorable patients comparing six cycles of ABVD, four cycles of ABVD, or four cycles of BEACOPP followed by IFRT to 30 Gy. Results showed similar 4-year EFS rates (94% vs. 89% vs. 91%) and 4-year OS rates (96% vs. 95% vs. 93%). However, there was greater toxicity with BEACOPP without any further benefits in EFS or OS (Level I) (NOORDIJK et al. 2005).

■ Two ongoing trials comparing different chemotherapy regimens need to be noted: The ECOG 2496 is currently ongoing to further evaluate the Stanford V regimen. This trial compares ABVD × 6 + IFRT 36 Gy (initial bulky sites >5 cm) versus Stanford V × 3 + IFRT 36 Gy to bulky sites (DIEHL et al. 2004).
GHSG HD 14 is currently ongoing and aims to compare four cycles of ABVD chemotherapy followed by IFRT (30 Gy) to two cycles of BEACOPP escalated plus two cycles of ABVD chemotherapy followed by IFRT to the same dose (DIEHL et al. 2004).

28.2.4 Treatment of Stage III–IV Hodgkin's Lymphoma

■ Systemic chemotherapy is currently the standard treatment of choice for stage III and IV HL (Grade B). Six to eight cycles of ABVD or eight cycles of BEACOOP can be considered for definitive treatment. Restaging is performed after four cycles. Typically, two more cycles are given after CR/CRu is achieved. For the ABVD group, 30–36 Gy of IFRT is given for bulky sites or partial response (PR) and for the BEACOPP group, consolidative IFRT 30–40 Gy is given to initial sites >5 cm or after partial response (Grade A). The 5-year FFTF ranges from 65%–85%, while 5-year OS is between 70% and 90%.

■ ABVD-containing regimens show superiority over MOPP chemotherapy and are considered the mainstay treatment regimen (Grade A). A trial reported by CALGB compared advanced-stage patients to six to eight cycles of MOPP, 12 cycles of MOPP/ABVD, or six to eight cycles of ABVD. The ABVD and MOPP/ABVD had improved 10-year FFS (55%, 50%) versus MOPP (38%). ABVD alone was found equally effective as compared to the MOPP/ABV hybrid. The overall survival rates were similar among the three groups (Level I) (CANELLOS et al. 1992).

■ IFRT for consolidative treatment should be considered for bulky disease or partial response after initial chemotherapy (Grade B). In a prospective randomized trial, patients with stage III–IV HL were treated with six to eight cycles of MOPP/ABVD chemotherapy. Patients in complete remission after chemotherapy were randomized between no further treatment and IFRT. Those in partial response after six cycles received IFRT (30 Gy to originally involved nodal areas and 18 Gy to 24 Gy to extranodal sites with or without a boost). Non-random comparison showed that the addition of IFRT 30 Gy to MOPP/ABV × 6–8 in patients with PR improved the EFS to the level of the CR with or without RT (Level III) (ALEMAN et al. 2007).

■ Consolidative radiation is not routinely recommended in patients who achieved complete response after initial chemotherapy (Grade C). In the above-mentioned study, patients who achieved CR to MOPP/ABVD chemotherapy demonstrated similar EFS and OS rates without radiation, as randomly compared to those who received IFRT (Level II) (ALEMAN et al. 2007). A prospective randomized trial reported by EORTC evaluated MOPP/ABV × 6–8 followed by IFRT 24 Gy versus no further treatment for complete responders and showed that the addition of RT did not improve the 5-year EFS or OS. However, patients who achieved partial response may benefit from the addition of adjuvant radiation therapy (EORTC 20884, Level I) (ALEMAN et al. 2003).

■ Increased dose intensity for chemotherapy is recommended for advanced HL and is associated with improved survival (Grade A). GHSG HD9 compared COPP-ABVD × 8 versus BEACOPP standard × 8 versus BEACOPP increased dose × 8. Radiation therapy was recommended for bulky or residual disease (30 Gy and 40 Gy, respectively). Results showed improvement in 10-year FFTF (64% versus 70% versus 82%) and overall survival (75% versus 80% versus 85%) rates for the BEACOPP increased dose group (Level I) (DIEHL et al. 2007).
BEACOPP given in 14-day intervals (BEACOPP-14) was analyzed in a phase II clinical trial. BEACOPP-14 for eight cycles with or without adjuvant radiation therapy provided a FFTF and overall survival rates of 90% and 97%, respectively, at 34 months after treatment (Level III) (SIEBER et al. 2003). The GHSG HD 12 trial randomly compared four groups of patients with advanced HL: (1) BEACOPP escalated for eight cycles with adjuvant radiotherapy of 30 Gy for bulky/residual disease, (2) BEACOPP escalated for eight cycles without radia-

tion, (3) BEACOPP escalated for four cycles plus + BEACOPP for four cycles with RT 30 Gy for bulky/residual disease, and (4) BEACOPP escalated for four cycles plus BEACOPP for four cycles without RT. The radiation arm versus the no radiation arm showed no difference in FFTF (95% vs. 88%). However, 10% of patients in the no-RT group had RT due to minor response or residual disease after chemotherapy (Level I) (EICHT et al. 2007).

■ Newer chemotherapy regimens include ChIVPP/EVA, VAPEC-B, and Stanford V. The Stanford V regimen has been evaluated in a phase II trial. Stanford V × 3 + IFRT to initial sites of bulky disease >5 cm showed a 5-year FFP of 89% and OS of 96% (Level III) (HORNING et al. 2002). ChIVPP/EVA was found to be superior to VAPEC-B in the 5-year freedom-from progression rate (82% versus 62%) and overall survival rate (89% versus 79%) (Level I) (RADFORD et al. 2002).

■ Two ongoing trials for advanced HL need to be noted: The ECOG 2496 mentioned above is currently ongoing to further evaluate the Stanford V regimen. This trial compares six to eight cycles of ABVD followed by IFRT of 36 Gy for initial bulky sites >5 cm versus three cycles of Stanford V chemotherapy followed by IFRT of 36 Gy to bulky sites (DIEHL et al. 2004).
GHSG HD 15 is another ongoing trial aimed at comparing BEACOPP escalated for eight cycles, BEACOPP escalated for six cycles, and BEACOPP-14 for eight cycles. Radiation therapy is used only in patients with positive FDG-PET after chemotherapy (DIEHL and FUCHS 2007).

28.3 Treatment of Nodular Lymphocyte-Predominant Hodgkin's Lymphoma (NLPHL)

■ NLPHL is a relatively rare entity, and there are limited data to guide management.

■ Stage IA NLPHL can be treated with IFRT to a total dose of 30–36 Gy (Grade B). EFRT or combined chemotherapy and radiation therapy provide no further benefit (Level IV) (NOGOVA et al. 2005). A German Hodgkin's Lymphoma Study Group (GHSG) phase II study is ongoing using rituximab (anti-CD20 monoclonal antibody) in stage IA NLPHL patients (NOGOVA et al. 2008).

■ Stage IIA NLPHL can be treated with definitive radiation therapy alone or chemotherapy followed by IFRT (Grade D).

■ Stage IB or IIB diseases should be treated with combined chemotherapy followed by IFRT (Grade D).

■ Patients with stage IIIA or IVA diseases can be observed or treated with chemotherapy with or without radiation (Grade D). Rituximab is recommended for patients who cannot tolerate chemotherapy.

■ Patients with stage IIIB or IVB diseases are usually treated with chemotherapy with or without radiation therapy (Grade D). Rituximab is recommended for patients who cannot tolerate chemotherapy.

■ For relapsed and refractory disease, rituximab can be considered (Grade B). Results of a phase II trial have demonstrated excellent response rates of 94% (Level III) (SCHULZ et al. 2008).

28.4 Radiation Therapy Fields and Dose

■ Radiation is commonly utilized in combination with definitive chemotherapy. In such a regimen, IFRT is usually performed. Definitions of various radiation treatment fields are as follows (YAHALOM et al. 2007) (Fig. 28.1):
  - IFRT: includes clinically involved lymph node site.
  - Regional field (RF): IFRT + additional adjacent uninvolved lymph node.
  - Extended field (EF): Includes IFRT + several additional lymph node groups. Examples include mantle field and "inverted Y."
  - Total nodal irradiation (TNI): Mantle + inverted Y field.
  - Subtotal lymphoid irradiation (STLI): TNI – pelvic field.

■ Involved lymph node field can be elected for the treatment of localized HL. Involved nodal field encompasses involved node and a margin of 1–2 cm (YAHALOM 2007).

■ When treating a subdiaphragmatic field, careful consideration is necessary for oophoropexy in women and use of a testes shield for men.

■ Mantle field irradiation is indicated in patients with early-stage HL who cannot tolerate or who decline chemotherapy.

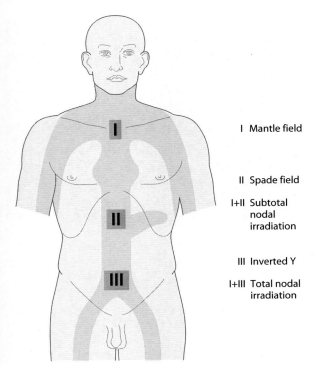

I   Mantle field

II   Spade field

I+II   Subtotal nodal irradiation

III   Inverted Y

I+III   Total nodal irradiation

Fig. 28.1. Various irradiation fields for lymph nodal coverage in the treatment of Hodgkin's lymphoma or non-Hodgkin's lymphoma (Adopted from the SEER's Training Website http://training.seer.cancer.gov)

28.4.1 Arrangement and Simulation for Involved Field Radiation

■ CT simulation for three-dimensional conformal radiation therapy is highly recommended to determine doses to normal structure and further delineate tumor volume, especially in the abdomen, axilla, and mediastinum (YAHALOM et al. 2007; HOPPE 2008). Intensity-modulated radiation therapy (IMRT) may be considered for high cervical fields to reduce the parotid dose.

■ *Unilateral Cervical Field.* The unilateral cervical field encompasses cervical and supraclavicular (SCV) lymph nodes:

- Superior border: 1–2 cm above the tip of the mastoid and mid-point through the mandible.
- Inferior border: 1–2 cm below the clavicle.
- Medial border: (1) At the ipsilateral transverse process if there is no SCV or medial cervical LN. (2) At the contralateral vertebral body if there is no SCV LN, but a positive medial cervical LN. (3) At the contralateral transverse process if there is positive SCV LN.

- Lateral border: Includes the medial two thirds of the clavicle.
- Modifiers: Block oral cavity. Consider a laryngeal block at 20 Gy, if it will not block disease. Consider a spinal cord block especially if cord dose is >40 Gy. Consider blocking the larynx and vertebral bodies above the larynx if stage I and no medial nodes.

■ *Pelvic Field.* In oophoropexy the ovaries are moved by laparoscopy to either behind the uterus or to the iliac wings.

- Superior border: L4/5 or 2-cm margin on LN, whichever is larger.
- Inferior border: Lesser trochanter or 2 cm below LN, whichever is more inferior.
- Lateral border: 1.5–2.0 cm lateral of the pelvis.
- Midline blocks: Use a gonadal shield. A 10 half-value layer is added to block the ovaries identified by a radiopaque clip. The block needs to cover the ovaries by 2 cm to reduce the dose to 8% (LE FLOCH et al. 1976). A testes shield reduces the dose to 0.75%–3%.

■ *Axilla Field.*

- Position: Supine position, arms akimbo, or arms up.
- Superior border: C5/6
- Inferior border: Tip of the scapula or 2 cm below the tumor volume, whichever is lower.
- Medial border: Ipsilateral cervical transverse process. If the SCV is involved, then include the entire vertebral body.
- Lateral border: At the lateral border of the humeral head.
- Blocks: Block humeral head and lung.

■ *Paraaortic Field.*

- Superior border: Top of T11 or 2 cm above the pre-chemotherapy volume, whichever is superior.
- Inferior border: L4/L5 or 2 cm below the pre-chemotherapy volume, whichever is lower.
- Lateral borders: Include the transverse processes or 2 cm on the post-chemotherapy volume, whichever is larger.

■ If the spleen is to be treated, use a margin of 1.5–2 cm of the post-chemotherapy volume taking into account the respiratory movement of the spleen by either fluoroscopy or CT inspiration/expiration images. Kidneys should be shielded bilaterally.

■ *Inguinal Field.*

- Superior border: Mid-sacroiliac joint. If common iliac is involved the superior border should be increased to L4/5 or 2 cm above the pre-chemotherapy tumor volume.

- Inferior border: 5 cm below the lesser trochanter.
- Medial border: Medial edge of obturator foramen or 2 cm margin on LN, whichever is larger.
- Lateral border: Greater trochanter or 2 cm margin on LN, whichever is larger.
- ■ *Inverted Y Field.* Includes paraaortic, bilateral pelvic, and inguinofemoral with or without treating the spleen. Inverted Y field is rarely used.
- ■ *Mediastinal Field.*
- Position: Arms may be down if not treating the axilla. Includes bilateral hilar and mediastinal LN. The axilla is only included if involved. The medial SCV is included if no SCV involved. The entire SCV is included if involved and part of the cervical region.
- Superior border: At C5/6 including the medial part of the SCV.
- Inferior border: 5 cm below the carina or 2 cm below the pre-chemotherapy volume, whichever is inferior.
- Hilar border: If hilum initially involved, add a margin of 1.5 cm and 1 cm if not involved.
- Mediastinal border: Post-chemotherapy volume + 1.5-cm margin.
- If supraclavicular lymph nodes are involved, then the superior border is at the top of the larynx with the lateral border at the medial two-thirds of the clavicle.

28.4.2 Arrangement and Simulation for Mantle Field Radiation

- ■ *Mantle Field.* The Mantle field encompasses submandibular, cervical, supraclavicular, infraclavicular, axillary, mediastinal, subcarinal, and hilar lymph nodes (Fig. 28.2) (YAHALOM et al. 2007; HOPPE et al. 2008):
- ■ Position: Simulate supine, neck fully extended. Simulating with arms up allows the axillary lymph nodes to be pulled from the chest and therefore more lung blocking. If arms are down or akimbo, this allows the humeral head to be blocked and fewer skin folds.
- ■ Superior border: Bisect the mandible and mastoid.
- ■ Inferior border: Inferior border of the axilla is the tip of the scapula or follows the posterior 6th rib. Inferior border of the mediastinal field is usually T10–11, but should be 5 cm below the extent of disease.

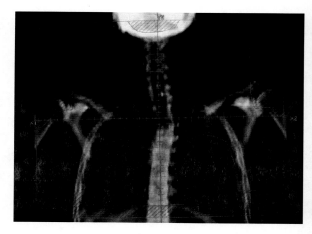

Fig. 28.2. Typical mantle radiation field with shielding of the lungs, humeral heads, larynx, and oral cavity (see text for detailed description]

- ■ Lateral border: At the lateral border of the humeral head.
- ■ Blocks: Block the larynx anteriorly, spinal cord posteriorly, and humeral heads. The radiation dose and the extent of disease determine whether a block would be beneficial as it may not be necessary if the dose is low and should not be used if it blocks disease. Lung block should allow a 1-cm margin around mediastinal disease and inclusion of the hilum bilaterally. Superior lung block should allow a 1-cm margin of the clavicle and follows along the posterior rib tapered laterally. The heart should be blocked 5 cm below the carina after 30 Gy in order to reduce the heart dose if there is no residual disease. Block the apex of the heart at 15 Gy if you are treating the entire heart for pericardial or mediastinal disease.
- ■ *The mini-mantle field* encompasses the mantle field without encompassing mediastinum, subcarinal, and hilar regions.
- ■ *Modified mantle field* encompasses the mantle field without axilla.

28.4.3 Radiation Dose

- ■ For definitive radiation therapy for HL, a total dose of 35–44 Gy is recommended to the involved region of disease. The uninvolved region should be treated to 30–36 Gy.
- ■ For adjuvant radiation therapy following definitive multi-drug chemotherapy, 30–36 Gy is rec-

ommended for bulky disease (stage I–IV), and 20–30 Gy is recommended for non-bulky diseases (stage I–IV). A total of 30 Gy can be recommended for excised NLPHL.

■ Fraction size of 1.5–2.0 Gy per daily fraction is usually used.

28.5 Chemotherapy- or Radiotherapy-Induced Side Effects and Toxicities

■ Information regarding long-term toxicity of radiation is from older data when doses of radiation were approximately 40 Gy and field sizes were larger. These data are not necessarily applicable to modern day IFRT with smaller doses.

■ With smaller radiation fields, lower radiation doses and less toxic chemotherapy regimens, long-term complications may be reduced (Level V) (MAUCH et al. 2005).

28.5.1 Acute and Subacute Complications

■ Acute side effects from irradiation depend on the area treated, but usually include mild dermatitis, myelosuppression, hair loss, nausea, diarrhea, dry mouth, changes in taste, sore throat, fatigue, cough, and shortness of breath.

■ Subacute adverse effects induced by radiotherapy may include radiation pneumonitis, which may occur 6–12 weeks after the completion of radiotherapy in 5% of mantle-treated patients. The risk of radiation pneumonitis is increased with bleomycin. L'Hermitte's syndrome presents with paraesthesia caused by neck flexion 12 months after mantle radiation therapy. L'Hermitte's syndrome resolves spontaneously.

28.5.2 Late Complications

■ Subclinical hypothyroidism, evident by normal T4 and elevated TSH, is found in 30% of long-term survivors treated with standard mantle RT.

■ Xerostomia can occur if Waldeyer's ring is irradiated, and scheduled dental care is required.

■ Infertility is a concern for patients treated with subdiaphragmatic radiation. Sperm, oocyte, and embryo cryopreservation should be discussed with patients concerned with infertility. If a testes shield is used, azoospermia is usually transient. MOPP and BEACOPP have alkylating agents and procarbazine, which can cause sterility in men. Even with oophoropexy in women, the small scatter dose can still cause infertility. Early menopause can occur with pelvic radiation, as well as with alkylating agents.

■ Secondary malignancies after HL are divided into three groups: leukemia, lymphomas, and solid tumors. Alkylating agents or procarbazine increase the risk of leukemia. Non-Hodgkin's lymphoma may develop in 1.2%–2.1% of patients at 15 years due to immunosuppression. The two most common secondary solid tumors are lung and breast cancer. Smoking, chest radiation dose, and alkylating chemotherapy dose increase the risk of lung cancer. A case controlled study showed chemotherapy alone resulted in twice the risk of developing lung cancer in comparison to radiation therapy alone. Age of chest irradiation younger than 30 and increased radiation dose increase the breast cancer risk.

■ Cardiovascular risk is increased with chest radiation, especially when combined with doxorubicin. Decreasing the cardiac radiation dose decreases the mortality from cardiac disease.

28.6 Treatment of Residual Disease

■ Patients with an unconfirmed complete response (CRu) with a positive FDG-PET scan or less than a CRu after definitive chemotherapy should be individualized for their treatment. Treatment options include chemotherapy, radiation therapy, and high-dose chemotherapy.

■ In progressive or stable disease with no obvious response to chemotherapy, a biopsy may be performed to confirm the lack of response. High-dose chemotherapy with or without IFRT followed by autologous hematopoietic stem cell transplant (AHSCT) can be considered for refractory disease, as detailed below.

28.7 Treatment of Refractory and Recurrent Hodgkin's Lymphoma

- Restaging including bone marrow biopsy should be performed in all patients after a biopsy-proven recurrence.
- Treatment recommendation for recurrent HL is based on prior therapy. Patients with recurrence after radiation therapy alone may be salvaged with standard chemotherapy. Additional IFRT of 15–25 Gy can be considered depending on the tolerance of surrounding structures (Grade D).
- In patients with stage IA–IIA HL treated with chemotherapy alone, failure at the initial site of presentation needs individualized salvage treatment strategy.
- In patients with prior combination chemoradiation therapy, AHSCT is recommended, especially if there has been a long disease-free interval (Grade A). Results of a number of prospective randomized trials have confirmed that high-dose chemotherapy followed by transplantation of autologous hematopoietic stem cells (BEAM-HSCT) improves FFTF in patients with recurrent Hodgkin's disease irrespective of the length of initial remission (Level I) (Schmitz et al. 2002; Sureda et al. 2008). Approximately 50% of these can be salvaged (Armitage et al. 2007).

  A recently published prospective non-randomized series demonstrated that the 5-year EFS and OS rates were both 83% after total lymphoid irradiation and high-dose chemotherapy with autologous stem-cell transplantation (Level II) (Evens et al. 2007).
- Radiation to previously unirradiated areas may be considered since relapse rates are high with salvage high-dose chemotherapy alone.

28.8 Follow-Up

28.8.1 Post-Treatment Follow-Ups

- Life-long follow-up after definitive treatment of HL is recommended for detecting recurrence, secondary tumors, or other long-term complications of radiation therapy or chemotherapy.

Schedule

- Follow-ups could be scheduled every 3–4 months for 2 years, then every 6 months for 3 additional years, then annually thereafter (Grade D) (Table 28.7).

Work-Up

- Each follow-up should include a complete history and physical examination. Counseling should take place regarding cardiovascular and skin cancer risk as well as psychosocial issues.
- Complete blood count, ESR, and alkaline phosphatase can be ordered every 3–4 months for 2 years, every 6 months for an addition 3 years, then annually thereafter (Grade D). Evaluation of thyroid function with thyroid-stimulating hormone (TSH) in patients receiving radiation therapy to the neck and/or upper chest should be performed annually (Grade D) (Level IV) (Mauch et al. 2005).
- Chest X-ray or CT of the thorax every 3–6 months for the first 2–3 years, then annually up to 5 years can be recommended. Afterwards chest imaging annually should be performed only for patients with high risk factors such as chest radiation and bleomycin. Abdominal/pelvic CT every 6 months for the first 2–3 years, then annually up to 5 years can be considered (Grade D).
- Counseling regarding self-breast examination should be offered to all female patients. Mammography should be done annually for RT above the diaphragm 5–8 years after treatment or at age 40, whichever comes first (Grade D) (Level IV) (Mauch et al. 2005). In addition to mammography, breast MRI is recommended by the American Cancer Society.
- Annual influenza vaccine is necessary, particularly if the patient is high risk or received chest RT or bleomycin. If the patient had splenic RT or splenectomy, pneumococcal, H. influenza, and meningococcal vaccines are recommended every 5–7 years.
- Due to increased risk of cardiac toxicity, resting and stress echocardiography is recommended annually 10 years after treatment.

Table 28.7. Follow-up schedule after treatment for non-Hodgkin's lymphoma

Interval	Frequency
First 2 years	Every 3–4 months
Year 3–5	Every 6 months
Over 5 years	Annually

References

Aleman BM, Raemaekers JM, Tirelli U et al (2003) Involved-field radiotherapy for advanced Hodgkin's lymphoma. N Engl J Med 348:2396–2406

Aleman BM, Raemaekers JM, Tomisic R et al (2007) Involved-field radiotherapy for patients in partial remission after chemotherapy for advanced Hodgkin's lymphoma. Int J Radiat Oncol Biol Phys 67:19–30

Armitage JO et al (2007) Role of hematopoietic stem-cell transplantation in Hodgkin lymphoma. In: Hoppe RT, Armitage JA, Diehl V et al (eds) Hodgkin lymphoma. Lippincott Williams & Wilkins, Philadelphia, pp 281–292

Bonadonna G, Bonfante V, Viviani S et al (2004) ABVD plus subtotal nodal versus involved-field radiotherapy in early-stage Hodgkin's disease: long-term results. J Clin Oncol 22:2835–2841

Canellos GP, Anderson JR, Propert KJ et al (1992) Chemotherapy of advanced Hodgkin lymphoma with MOPP, ABVD, or MOPP alternating with ABVD. N Engl J Med 327:1478–1484

Carbone PP, Kaplan HS, Musshoff K et al (1971) Report of the Committee on Hodgkin's Disease Staging Classification. Cancer Res 31:1860–1861

Carde P, Hagenbeek A, Hayat M et al (1993) Clinical staging versus laparotomy and combined modality with MOPP versus ABVD in early-stage Hodgkin's disease: the H6 twin randomized trials from the European Organization for Research and Treatment of Cancer Lymphoma Cooperative Group. J Clin Oncol 11:2258–2272

Carde P, Hagenbeek A, Hayat M et al (1997) Superiority of EBVP chemotherapy in combination with involved field irradiation over subtotal nodal irradiation in favorable clinical stage I–II Hodgkin's disease: the EORTC-GPMC H7F randomized trial. Proc ASCO 16:13

Castellino RA, Hoppe RT, Blank N et al (1984) Computed tomography, lymphography, and staging laparotomy: correlations in initial staging of Hodgkin disease. AJR Am J Roentgenol 143:37–41

Castellino RA, Blank N, Hoppe RT et al (1986) Hodgkin disease: contributions of chest CT in the initial staging evaluation. Radiology 160:603–605

Crnkovich MJ, Leopold K, Hoppe RT et al (1987) Stage I to IIB Hodgkin disease: the combine experience at Stanford University and the Joint Center for Radiation Therapy. J Clin Oncol 5:1041–1049

Diehl V, Harris NL, Mauch PM (2004) Hodgkin lymphoma. In: Devita VT, Hellman S, Rosenberg SA (eds) Cancer: Principles and practice of oncology. Lippincott Williams & Wilkins, Philadelphia, pp 2020–2075

Diehl V, Brillant C, Engert A et al (2005) HD10: Investigating reduction of combined modality treatment intensity in early stage Hodgkin's lymphoma. Interim analysis of a randomized trial of the German Hodgkin Study Group (GHSG). ASCO:6506

Diehl V, Franklin J, Pfistner B et al (2007) Ten-year results of a German Hodgkin Study Group randomized trial of standard and increased dose BEACOPP chemotherapy for advanced Hodgkin lymphoma (HD9). J Clin Oncol 2007 ASCO Annual Meeting Proceedings Part I. 25:LBA8015

Diehl V, Franklin J, Pfreundschuh M et al (2003) Standard and increased-dose BEACOPP chemotherapy compared with COPP-ABVD for advanced Hodgkin's disease. N Engl J Med 348:2386–2395

Diehl V, Fuchs M (2007) Early, intermediate and advanced Hodgkin's lymphoma: modern treatment strategies. Ann Oncol 18:ix71–79

Eich HT, Gossmann A, Engert A et al (2007) A contribution to solve the problem of the need for consolidative radiotherapy after intensive chemotherapy in advanced stages of Hodgkin's lymphoma – analysis of a quality control program initiated by the radiotherapy reference center of the German Hodgkin Study Group (GHSG). Int J Radiat Oncol Biol Phys 69:1187–1192

Engert A, Franklin J, Eich HT et al (2007) Two cycles of doxorubicin, bleomycin, vinblastine, and dacarbazine plus extended-field radiotherapy is superior to radiotherapy alone in early favorable Hodgkin's lymphoma: final results of the GHSG HD7 trial. J Clin Oncol 25:3495–3502

Engert A, Schiller P, Josting A et al (2003) Involved-field radiotherapy is equally effective and less toxic compared with extended-field radiotherapy after four cycles of chemotherapy in patients with early-stage unfavorable Hodgkin's lymphoma: results of the HD8 trial of the German Hodgkin's Lymphoma Study Group. J Clin Onco 21:3601–3608

Evens AM, Altman JK, Mittal BB et al (2007) Phase I/II trial of total lymphoid irradiation and high-dose chemotherapy with autologous stem-cell transplantation for relapsed and refractory Hodgkin's lymphoma. Ann Oncol 18:679–688

Fermé C, Eghbali H, Meerwaldt JH et al (2007) Chemotherapy plus involved-field radiation in early-stage Hodgkin's disease. N Engl J Med 357:1916–1927

Good GR, DiNubile MJ (1995) Images in clinical medicine. Cyclic fever in Hodgkin's disease (Pel-Ebstein fever). N Engl J Med 332:436

Haluska FG, Brufsky AM, Canellos GP (1994) The cellular biology of the Reed-Sternberg cell. Blood 84:1005–1019

Harris NL, Jaffe ES, Diebold J et al (1999) World Health Organization classification of neoplastic diseases of the hematopoietic and lymphoid tissues: report of the Clinical Advisory Committee meeting-Airlie House, Virginia 1997. J Clin Oncol 17:3835–3849

Hasenclever D, Diehl V (1998) A prognostic score for advanced Hodgkin's disease. International Prognostic Factors Project on Advanced Hodgkin's Disease. N Engl J Med 339:1506–1514

Herbst H, Dallenbach F, Hummel M et al (1991) Epstein-Barr virus latent membrane protein expression in Hodgkin and Reed-Sternberg cells. Proc Natl Acad Sci USA 88:4766–4770

Hoppe RT (2008) Hodgkin lymphoma. In: Perez CA, Brady LW (eds) Brady's principle and practice of radiation oncology. Lippincott Williams & Wilkins, Philadelphia, pp 1721–1738

Hoppe RT, Advani RH, Bierman PJ et al (2006) Hodgkin disease/lymphoma. Clinical practice guidelines in oncology. J Natl Compr Canc Netw 4:210–230

Horning SJ, Hoppe RT, Breslin S et al (2002) Stanford V and radiotherapy for locally extensive and advanced Hodgkin's disease: mature results of a prospective clinical trial. J Clin Oncol 20:630–637

Hughes-Davies L, Tarbell NJ, Coleman CN et al (1997) Stage IA–IIB Hodgkin's disease: management and outcome of extensive thoracic involvement. Int J Radiat Oncol Biol Phys 39:361–369

Klimm BC, Engert A, Brillant C et al (2005) Comparison of BEACOPP and ABVD chemotherapy in intermediate stage Hodgkin's lymphoma: results of the fourth interim analysis of the HD 11 trial of the GHS. J Clin Oncol 2005 ASCO Annual Meeting Proceedings 23:6507

Lang O, Bihl H, Hültenschmidt B, Sautter-Bihl ML (2001) Clinical relevance of positron emission tomography (PET) in treatment control and relapse of Hodgkin's disease. Strahlenther Onkol 177:138–144

Le Floch O, Donaldson SS, Kaplan HS (1976) Pregnancy following oophoropexy and total nodal irradiation in women with Hodgkin's Disease. Cancer 38:2263–2268

Mauch P, Ng A, Aleman B et al (2005) Report from the Rockefellar Foundation Sponsored International Workshop on reducing mortality and improving quality of life in long-term survivors of Hodgkin's disease: July 9–16, 2003, Bellagio, Italy. Eur J Haematol Suppl 75:68–76

Meyer RM, Gospodarowicz MK, Connors JM et al (2005) Randomized comparison of ABVD chemotherapy with a strategy that includes radiation therapy in patients with limited-stage Hodgkin's lymphoma: National Cancer Institute of Canada Clinical Trials Group and the Eastern Cooperative Oncology Group. J Clin Oncol 23:4634–4642

Naumann R, Beuthien-Baumann B, Reiss A et al (2004) Substantial impact of FDG PET imaging on the therapy decision in patients with early-stage Hodgkin's lymphoma. Br J Cancer 90:620–625

Nogová L, Reineke T, Eich HT et al (2005) Extended field radiotherapy, combined modality treatment or involved field radiotherapy for patients with stage IA lymphocyte-predominant Hodgkin's lymphoma: a retrospective analysis from the German Hodgkin Study Group (GHSG). Ann Oncol 16:1683–1687

Nogová L, Reineke T, Brillant C et al (2008) Lymphocyte-predominant and classical Hodgkin's lymphoma: a comprehensive analysis from the German Hodgkin Study Group. J Clin Oncol 26:434–439

Noordijk EM, Carde P, Dupouy N et al (2006) Combined-modality therapy for clinical stage I or II Hodgkin's lymphoma: long-term results of the European Organization for Research and Treatment of Cancer H7 randomized controlled trials. J Clin Oncol 24:3128–3135

Noordijk EM, Thomas J, Fermé C et al (2005) First results of the EORTC-GELA H9 randomized trials: the H9-F trial (comparing three radiation dose levels) and H9-U trial (comparing three chemotherapy schemes) in patients with favorable or unfavorable early stage Hodgkin's lymphoma (HL). J Clin Oncol 2005 ASCO Annual Meeting Proceedings 23:6505

Partridge S, Timothy A, O'Doherty MJ et al (2000) 2-Fluorine-18-fluoro-2-deoxy-D glucose positron emission tomography in the pretreatment staging of Hodgkin's disease: influence on patient management in a single institution. Ann Oncol 11:1273–1279

Press OW, LeBlanc M, Lichter AS et al. (2001) Phase III randomized intergroup trial of subtotal lymphoid irradiation versus doxorubicin, vinblastine, and subtotal lymphoid irradiation. J Clin Oncol 19:4238–4244

Radford JA, Rohatiner AZ, Ryder WD et al (2002) ChlVPP/EVA hybrid versus the weekly VAPEC-B regimen for previously untreated Hodgkin's disease. J Clin Oncol 20:2988–2994

Rosenberg S, Kaplan HS (1966) Evidence of an orderly progression in the spread of Hodgkin disease. Cancer Res 26:1225–1231

Rubio R (1994) Hodgkin's disease associated with human immunodeficiency virus infection. A clinical study of 46 cases. Cooperative Study Group of Malignancies Associated with HIV Infection of Madrid. Cancer 73:2400–2407

Schmitz N, Pfistner B, Sextro M et al (2002) Aggressive conventional chemotherapy compared with high-dose chemotherapy with autologous haemopoietic stem-cell transplantation for relapsed chemosensitive Hodgkin's disease: a randomised trial. Lancet 359:2065–2071

Sureda A, Robinson S, Canals C et al (2008) Reduced-intensity conditioning compared with conventional allogeneic stem-cell transplantation in relapsed or refractory Hodgkin's lymphoma: an analysis from the Lymphoma Working Party of the European Group for Blood and Marrow Transplantation. J Clin Oncol 26:455–462

Schulz H, Rehwald U, Morschhauser F et al (2008) Rituximab in relapsed lymphocyte-predominant Hodgkin lymphoma: long-term results of a phase 2 trial by the German Hodgkin Lymphoma Study Group (GHSG). Blood 111:109–111

Sieber M, Bredenfeld H, Josting A et al (2003) Fourteen-day variant of the bleomycin, etoposide, doxorubicin, cyclophosphamide, vincristine, procarbazine, and prednisone regimen in advanced-stage Hodgkin's lymphoma: results of a pilot study of the German Hodgkin's Lymphoma Study Group. J Clin Oncol 21:1734–1739

Sieniawski M, Franklin J, Nogova L et al (2007) Outcome of patients experiencing progression or relapse after primary treatment with two cycles of chemotherapy and radiotherapy for early-stage favorable Hodgkin's lymphoma. J Clin Oncol 25:2000–2005

Somers R, Carde P, Henry-Amar M et al (1994) A randomized study in stage IIIB and IV Hodgkin's disease comparing eight courses of MOPP versus an alteration of MOPP with ABVD: a European Organization for Research and Treatment of Cancer Lymphoma Cooperative Group and Groupe Pierre-et-Marie-Curie controlled clinical trial. J Clin Oncol 12:279–287

Tubiana M, Henry-Amar M, Carde P et al (1989) Toward comprehensive management tailored to prognostic factors of patients with clinical stages I and II in Hodgkin's disease. The EORTC Lymphoma Group controlled clinical trials: 1964–1987. Blood 73:47–56

Wirth A, Chao M, Corry J et al (1999) Mantle irradiation alone for clinical stage I–II Hodgkin's disease: long-term follow-up and analysis of prognostic factors in 261 patients. J Clin Oncol 17:230–240

Yahalom J (2007) The lymphomas. In: FM Khan (ed) Treatment planning in radiation oncology. Lippincott Williams & Wilkins, Minneapolis, pp 343–356

Multiple Myeloma and Plasmacytoma

Wee Joo Chng and Jiade J. Lu

CONTENTS

Introduction and Objectives

Multiple myeloma is a malignancy of post-germinal center B-cells characterized by accumulation of abnormal clonal plasma cell secreting monoclonal proteins in the bone marrow. In many instances, it is preceded by monoclonal gammopathy of undetermined significance (MGUS), a pre-malignant stage that is present in approximately 3% of individuals above 50, or a more advanced stage of clonal expansion where the patient is still asymptomatic, called smoldering myeloma.

Solitary plasmacytoma is the localized disease that can arise from the bone (solitary plasmacytoma of the bone) or in the soft tissue (extramedullary plasmacytoma). All plasma cell tumors are highly radiosensitive. However, while radiation is the primary and potentially curative treatment in solitary plasmacytoma, it has only a palliative role in the management of multiple myeloma.

This chapter examines:

● Recommendations for diagnosis and staging procedures

● The staging systems and prognostic factors

● Treatment recommendations for multiple myeloma, osseous plasmacytoma, and extramedullary plasmacytoma, as well as the supporting scientific evidence,

● Maintenance therapy and supportive therapy for multiple myeloma

● Follow-up care and surveillance of survivors

W. J. Chng, MD
Department of Hematology Oncology, National University Cancer Institute of Singapore, National University Health System, National University of Singapore, 5 Lower Kent Ridge Road, Singapore 119074, Singapore
J. J. Lu, MD, MBA
Department of Radiation Oncology, National University Cancer Institute of Singapore, National University Health System, National University of Singapore, 5 Lower Kent Ridge Road, Singapore 119074, Singapore

29.1 Diagnosis, Staging, and Prognoses

29.1.1 Diagnosis

Initial Evaluation

- The aim of initial evaluation is to establish the diagnosis and stage the patients for prognosis. Diagnosis should be made according to the diagnostic criteria established by the INTERNATIONAL MYELOMA WORKING GROUP (2003) (Table 29.1). It is important to exclude other potential causes of M-proteins, such as AL amyloidosis, B-cell non-Hodgkin lymphoma (including Waldenstrom macroglobulinemia), and chronic lymphocytic leukemia.

Laboratory Tests

- Initial laboratory tests should include a complete blood count, basic serum electrolytes and urea, creatinine, and calcium, albumin, and β-2 microglobulin, liver and renal function tests, alkaline phosphatase, and lactate dehydrogenase (LDH) (Tables 29.2, 29.3).
- Quantification of serum M-protein by densitometry on the monoclonal peak on serum or urine protein electrophoresis should be performed. Immunochemical measurement of the total immunoglobulin isotype level can also be used and is particularly useful for IgA and IgD M-proteins. The type of M-protein should be confirmed by immunofixation.

Table 29.1. Diagnostic criteria for MGUS, SMM, MM, and solitary plasmacytoma

Monoclonal gammopathy of unknown significance
– Serum M-protein <30 g/l
– Bone marrow clonal plasma cells <10%
– Absence of myeloma-related organ or tissue impairment (Table 29.2)
– No clinical or laboratory features of amyloidosis or light-chain deposition disease
Smoldering multiple myeloma
– Serum M-protein >30 g/l and/or bone marrow clonal plasma cells >10%
– Absence of myeloma-related organ or tissue impairment
Multiple myeloma
– M-protein in serum and/or urine (no specific level required form diagnosis)
– Bone marrow clonal plasma cells or biopsy proven plasmacytoma
– Any myeloma-related organ or tissue impairment
Solitary plasmacytoma
– Biopsy-proven monoclonal plasmacytoma of bone in a single site only. X-rays and MRI must be negative outside the primary site
– Primary lesion may be associated with small serum and/or urine M-component (serum IgG <3.5 g/dl; serum IgA <2.0 g/dl; urine monoclonal kappa or lambda <1.0 g/24 h)
– Bone marrow clonal plasma cells <10%
– No myeloma-related organ or tissue impairment
Extramedullary plasmacytoma
– Biopsy-proven extramedullary tumor of clonal plasma cells.
– Normal skeletal survey
– May be associated with small serum and/or urine M-component (serum IgG <3.5 g/dl; serum IgA <2.0 g/dl; urine monoclonal kappa or lambda <1.0 g/24 h)
– Bone marrow clonal plasma cells <10%
– No myeloma-related organ or tissue impairment

Table 29.2. Myeloma-related organ or tissue impairment

Increase calcium levels	Corrected serum calcium >0.25 mmol/l above the upper limit of normal or >2.75 mmol/l
Renal insufficiency	Attributable to myeloma
Anemia	Hemoglobin 2 g/dl below the lower limit of normal or hemoglobin <10 g/dl
Bone lesions	Lytic lesions or osteoporosis with compression fractures
Other	Symptomatic hyperviscosity, amyloidosis, recurrent bacterial infections (more than two episodes in 12 months)

Table 29.3. Imaging and laboratory work-ups for multiple myeloma

Imaging studies	Laboratory tests
– Skeletal survey	– Complete blood count
– CT scan (to clarify ambiguous lesions)	– Serum electrolytes, urea, creatinine, calcium, albumin, and β-2 microglobulin
– MRI (for spine lesions and if cord compression suspected)	– Serum and urine protein electrophoresis and immunofixation
	– Quantification of immunoglobulins
	– Bone marrow aspirate and trephine with cytogenetic and FISH (if available)

- Quantification of serum-free immunoglobulin light chain levels and the κ/λ ratio is useful in the monitoring and diagnosis of light chain only myeloma and non-secretory myeloma in which the serum and urine are negative on immunofixation (Grade B) (Level III) (BRADWELL et al. 2003; DRAYSON et al. 2001).
- Bone marrow aspirate and biopsy are required.
- Serum β-2 microglobulin and albumin, which constitute the international staging system (Table 29.4), should be measured.
- Cytogenetics and FISH for t(4;14) and 17p13 deletion should be performed on the aspirate where facilities are available.

Imaging Studies

- Skeletal survey should be performed in newly diagnosed myeloma patients and should include a postero-anterior (PA) view of the chest, antero-posterior (AP) and lateral views of the cervical spine, thoracic spine, lumbar spine, humeri, and femora, AP and lateral view of the skull, and AP view of the pelvis. Any symptomatic areas should be specifically visualized.
- CT scan should be used to clarify the significance of ambiguous plain radiographic findings, especially in parts of the skeleton that are difficult to visualize on plain radiographs, such as ribs, sternum, and scapulae, or symptomatic areas of the skeleton where no pathological lesion is found on skeletal survey. However, CT scan should not be used for routine screening for lytic lesions.
- MRI of the spine is recommended for suspected solitary plasmacytoma of the vertebral body (Grade A). More than one third of cases of solitary plasmacytoma of the vertebral body diagnosed using standard diagnostic procedures have multiple osteolytic lesions on MRI of the spine (Level III) (GHANEM et al. 2006; MOULOPOULOS et al. 1993; WILDER et al. 2002).
- Urgent MRI is the diagnostic procedure of choice to assess suspected cord compression in myeloma patients even in the absence of vertebral collapse.

29.1.2 Staging

- The International Staging System (Table 29.4) is currently the preferred system (Grade B). The Durie-Salmon staging system, which is a surrogate for tumor load, was commonly used in the past. However, the distribution of patients into the different stages is not even, and it is based on a large number of criteria, making its use more cumbersome.

In a large international study including American, European and Asian centers, in patients treated with standard chemotherapy and stem cell transplantation, a staging system comprising two routinely measured laboratory parameters, albumin and β-2 microglobulin, was found to segregate patients into three groups with distinctly different survival rates. Importantly, the index was derived using statistically rigorous methods in a test cohort and validated in an independent cohort, and is equally applicable to patients from different geographical regions and patients treated with both chemotherapy and stem cell transplantation. (Level III) (GREIPP et al. 2005).

29.1.3 Prognostic Factors

- The presenting stage defined by the International Staging System is the most important prognostic factor for multiple myeloma.
- Karyotypically defined hypodiploidy and chromosome 13 deletion are associated with poor prognosis. These findings are consistently reported across a large number of studies including patients entered into clinical trials (FONSECA et al. 2004; WU et al. 2007). These are also among the genetic abnormalities proposed by the Mayo Clinic to define high-risk myeloma (STEWART et al. 2007).
- t(4;14) and 17p13 deletions detected by fluorescent in-situ hybridization (FISH) are associated with poor survival independent of the ISS staging (AVET-LOISSEAU et al. 2007). Progression-free survival of patients with t(4;14) and 17p13 deletion is less than 1 year after stem cell transplantation (GERTZ et al. 2005).

Table 29.4. The international staging system for multiple myeloma

Stage	Criteria	Median survival
I	Serum β-2 microglobulin <3.5 mg/l and serum albumin >35 g/l	62 months
II	Neither I nor III	45 months
III	Serum β-2 microglobulin >5.5 mg/l	29 months

- Many other prognostic factors have been proposed in myeloma, including serum LDH (Jacobson et al. 2003), the number of bone lesions on MRI (Walker et al. 2007), plasmablastic morphology (Greipp et al. 1998), centrosome amplification (Chng et al. 2007), plasma cell labeling index (Greipp et al. 1993), and p53 mutation (Chng et al. 2007), but these were either shown in limited studies or cumbersome assays, and hence are not recommended in routine clinical practice.

29.2 Treatment of Multiple Myeloma

29.2.1 General Principles

- Therapeutic intervention is only warranted in patients with symptomatic myeloma (Grade A). Early intervention in asymptomatic myeloma has shown no benefit in two randomized controlled trials (Level I) (Hjorth et al. 1993; Riccardi et al. 2000).
- The main aim of treatment is to achieve a complete response at the end of the treatment as this has been consistently shown to be associated with longer survival. For patients who require treatment, their eligibility for high-dose therapy (HDT) followed by autologous stem cell transplantation (ASCT) should be determined.
- Acute and subacute complications, such as spinal cord compression, acute renal failure, hypercalcemia, anemia, bone pain, and impending fracture, should be vigorously treated. Radiation therapy plays an important role in symptomatic palliation.

29.2.2 Upfront Chemotherapy and Targeted Therapy

- For patients who are not candidates for high-dose therapy and transplant, the treatment of choice at diagnosis is the melphalan-prednisolone-thalidomide (MPT) regimen (Grade A), which has been shown in two randomized trials to produce superior response, progression-free survival, and overall survival rates compared to the former standard melphalan and prednisolone (MP) regimen (Level I) (Palumbo et al. 2006; Facon et al. 2007).

- Prednisolone is preferred over dexamethasone as the steroid of choice in these patients (Grade A). Three randomized studies showed that the use of dexamethasone instead of prednisolone resulted in greater toxicity without improving efficacy (Level I) (Shustik et al. 2007; Facon et al. 2006; Hernandez et al. 2004).
- For candidates of HDT and ASCT, thalidomide with dexamethasone is the initial treatment of choice (Grade A). This combination has been shown to produce a significantly higher response rate compared to high-dose dexamethasone (Level I) (Rajkumar et al. 2006). Case-control comparison from Italy has shown that thalidomide and dexamethasone had significantly better response compared to vincristine-doxorubicin-dexamethasone (VAD) and comprise a well-tolerated oral regimen (Level II) (Cavo et al. 2005). As the aim of the initial therapy is to achieve rapid cytoreduction without affecting stem cell mobilization, alkylating agents such as melphalan should be avoided as this will affect stem cell collection.
- If thalidomide is not available or contraindicated, VAD or pulsed dexamethasone alone is an acceptable and well-studied frontline option prior to ASCT (Grade B). VAD produces a response rate of 60%–70%, although complete remission is relatively rare. Pulse high-dose dexamethasone, which produces response rates of about 40%–50%, is a reasonable alternative to VAD. A historical comparison from the Mayo Clinic compared outcomes in 35 patients who received pulsed high-dose dexamethasone with 72 patients who received VAD as initial therapy. The response rate was 63% with pulsed high-dose dexamethasone and 74% with VAD ($p=0.25$), but no significant differences were observed in the progression-free and OS at 1-year post-transplant (Level II) (Kumar et al. 2004)
- Duration of treatment prior to HDT and ASCT is generally 4–6 months, which achieves maximal response in the majority of patients. There is no evidence that achievement of complete response prior to transplant is important for overall survival.

29.2.3 Stem Cell Transplantation

- Autologous stem cell transplantation (ASCT) after high-dose therapy (HDT) is the treatment of choice in eligible patients (Grade A). Although not unanimous, the majority of the five prospective randomized trials comparing standard therapy with HDT for newly diagnosed MM patients up to age 65 years favors HDT:

- The IFM90 study reported by the InterGroupe Francophone du Myélome (IFM) randomized 200 patients to standard therapy or HDT with ASCT. Response, progression-free survival (PFS), and overall survival (OS) were all significantly better in the HDT arm (IFM 90, Level I) (ATTAL et al. 1996). The MRC trial compared the ABCM regimen (adriamycin, bleomycin, cyclophosphomide, and mitomycin-C) with C-VAMP followed by HDT and showed significantly longer event-free survival (EFS) and OS in the HDT arm (Level I) (CHILD et al. 2003). The French MAG91 study showed a significant prolongation of EFS, but not OS, possibly due to the use of HDT as salvage for patients in the chemotherapy arm. These results held when updated at a median follow-up of 10 years (Level I) (FERMAND et al. 2005). Results from two randomized trials did not demonstrate the superiority of HDT with ASCT. The US intergroup trials comparing melphalan 140 mg/m^2 plus total body irradiation with combination chemotherapy did not detect any difference in response, PFS, and OS (BARLOGIE et al. 2006). Similarly, the Spanish PATHEMA trial did not show any benefit in EFS or OS in favor of HDT. However, in this trial, only patients responding to the first four cycles of chemotherapy were randomized (BLADE et al. 2005).

- High-dose therapy is usually performed upfront rather than at relapse (Grade C). The results of a French randomized trial did not observe any difference in overall survival in patients treated with upfront HDT or at relapse (Level I) (FERMAND et al. 1998). If transplant is not performed as a planned primary strategy, additional therapy, including maintenance therapy, is usually required with associated toxicity. Furthermore, the major impact of the transplant is deferred.

- Melphalan 200 mg/m^2 should be used as the conditioning regimen (Grade A). A randomized study from IFM comparing melphalan 200 mg/m^2 with total body irradiation (TBI) 8 Gy plus melphalan 140 mg/m^2 showed that TBI was associated with increased toxicity, and although EFS was comparable in the two arms, OS was shorter in the TBI arm (Level I) (MOREAU et al. 2002).

- Purging is not recommended (Grade A). While it is effective in reducing tumor contamination of the stem cell graft, purging does not prolong time to progression or relapse and should not be used (Level I) (STEWART et al. 2001; BOURHIS et al. 2007).

- A second melphalan 200 mg/m^2 with ASCT should be given within 3 months of the first HDT, especially in patients who did not attain at least 90% reduction in M-protein after the first HDT (Grade A) (Level I) (ATTAL et al. 2006a; CAVO et al. 2007)

HDT in Elderly

- HDT can be safely performed up to the age of 70, although the upper age limit of all the randomized studies was 60 or 65 years (Grade B). A number of single-center series suggest that the results of HDT in selected patients >65 years old are similar to those in younger patients (Level II) (SIEGEL et al. 1999; SIROHI et al. 2000; TERPOS et al. 2003; REECE et al. 2003; JANTUNEN et al. 2006).

HDT in Renal Failure

- HDT and ASCT may be considered for patients with severe renal impairment (creatinine clearance/GFR < 30 ml/min), including those on dialysis, but the dose of melphalan should be reduced to 140 mg/m^2 (Grade B), and the procedure should be carried out in a center with special expertise. Several studies have shown that non-hematologic toxicity and treatment-related mortality are higher in this group of patients than in patients with normal renal function (Level II) (SAN MIGUEL et al. 2000; KNUDSEN et al. 2005; SIROHI et al. 2001).

- The largest series was published by the University of Arkansas. Significant non-hematologic toxicities were observed in patients with renal failure on dialysis (GFR <30 ml/min) when treated with melphalan 200 mg/m^2, leading researchers to reduce the dose in subsequent patients to 140 mg/m^2. These data were extended in a subsequent report, showing a treatment-related mortality (TRM) of 19%. However, reversibility of renal failure was observed in 24% of patients who became dialysis-independent (Level II) (BADROS et al. 2001; LEE et al. 2004).

Allogeneic Stem Cell Transplant (Allo-SCT)

- Allo-SCT using conventional conditioning and human leukocyte antigen (HLA)-matched sibling donors can be considered in patients up to the age of 50 years who have achieved at least a partial response after initial therapy. The procedure should preferably be performed as part of a clinical trial (Grade B). Allo-SCT is a potentially curative therapy with about a third of patients attaining molecular remission with a low risk of relapse (CORRADINI et al. 2003).

- Allo-SCT following reduced-intensity condition (RIC) should be considered in patients up to 65 years who have HLA-matched siblings. The procedure would usually follow an initial ASCT, should be done early in the disease phase, and should be done as part of a clinical trial (Grade C). The aim of RIC Allo-SCT is to induce a GvM effect while reducing the toxicity of conditioning. However, two randomized trials have produced conflicting results:
In a randomized study from Italy, patients with a HLA donor (who were randomized to HDT with ASCT followed by RIC allo-SCT) have significantly longer survival than those without (who were randomized to tandem ASCT) regardless of risk categories, and the TRM is similar in both arms. However, the study is hampered by the relatively small study size, the unusually high percentage of patients having HLA-matched siblings, and the low percentage of patients completing the assigned treatment (BRUNO et al. 2007). In contrast, the study from IFM showed that RIC allo-SCT after an initial HDT with ASCT is not better than a tandem HDT procedure in high-risk patients (GARBAN et al. 2006).

29.2.4 Maintenance Therapy

- Maintenance therapy with thalidomide should be given in patients who do not achieve very good partial response (VGPR) or complete response after HDT (Grade A). An IFM randomized study comparing thalidomide to placebo and pamidronate showed that thalidomide leads to prolonged relapse-free survival (Level I) (ATTAL et al. 2006b).
- Interferon is not recommended for maintenance therapy in the treatment of multiple myeloma (Grade A). A meta-analysis has evaluated individual patient data on 1,543 patients in 12 trials where patients were randomized to receive interferon after induction therapy and a further 2,469 patients in 12 trials where patients were randomized to receive interferon in the induction phase, and showed improvement in PFS and

OS by less than 6 months, but at the cost of significant toxicity (Level I) (MYELOMA TRIALISTS' COLLABORATIVE GROUP 2001).

29.2.5 Therapy of Refractory or Relapse Disease

- For refractory disease, an alternative regimen known to be active in multiple myeloma and comprising largely different drugs should be utilized.
- For relapsed disease, if good response (very good partial response or complete response) was achieved to initial therapy, the same regimen, including salvage HDT with ASCT, can be utilized at recurrence. Alternatively, an alternate regimen or novel therapeutic agents, including bortezomib, lenalidomide, liposomal doxorubicin, and thalidomide either as single-agent or part of a multi-agent regimen, can be used (Grade A). A number of novel agents with significant activity have been demonstrated in multiple myeloma:
In a large randomized study comprising 669 patients with relapse myeloma, single-agent bortezomib, a proteasome inhibitor, was shown to produce significantly better response rate (38% versus 18%, $p<0.001$) compared to high-dose dexamethasone. Median time to progression (6.2 versus 3.5 months, $p<0.001$) and 1-year survival rate (80% versus 66%, $p=0.03$) were also superior in patients treated with bortezomib (Level I) (RICHARDSON et al. 2005). Updated results show that the median survival is 29.8 months versus 23.7 months in favor of bortezomib (Level I) (RICHARDSON et al. 2007).
In two large randomized studies of similar design from North America and Europe, lenalidomide plus dexamethasone was shown to be significantly better than placebo plus dexamethasone in terms of response rate, time to progression, and OS in relapse patients (Level I) (WEBER et al. 2007; DIMOPOULOS et al. 2007).
A trial comparing bortezomib plus pegylated liposomal doxorubicin with bortezomib monotherapy in 646 relapse or refractory multiple myeloma patients showed that the addition of pegylated liposomal doxorubicin results in significant prolongation of time to progression and overall survival (Level I) (ORLOWSKI et al. 2007).
- Thalidomide has never been studied in a phase III setting in recurrent myeloma. A systematic review of 42 phase II trials comprised of 1,629 relapse

or refractory multiple myeloma patients showed that 29% of patients achieve either complete or partial response with single-agent thalidomide. The dose used ranges from 50 mg to 800 mg, but the median tolerated dose is 400 mg. There is no convincing evidence of a dose-response relationship (Level II) (GLASMACHER et al. 2006).

29.2.6 Management of Acute Complications and Supportive Measures

Spinal Cord Compression

■ A total of 8–16 mg/day of dexamethasone should be given immediately in suspected cases of spinal cord compression, and radiation therapy is the treatment of choice and should be commenced within 24 h of diagnosis, as detailed below.
■ Surgery is indicated when there is spinal instability.

Renal Impairment or Failure

■ Adequate hydration should be ensured, and nephrotoxic agents, including intravenous radiological contrast, must be avoided.
■ Hypercalcemia should be corrected with rehydration, if present. If hypercalcemia does not respond to rehydration, intravenous bisphosphonates should be administered.
■ A nephrologist should be consulted if there is no improvement in renal function by 48 h.
■ There is no conclusive evidence regarding the use of plasma exchange in MM patients presenting with acute renal failure; thus, it should be performed in a trial setting. Current available evidence has been obtained from small randomized studies that have produced conflicting results (ZUCCHELLI et al. 1998; JOHNSON et al. 1990; CLARK et al. 2005).

Bone Disease and Use of Bisphosphonates

■ Intravenous bisphosphonates (pamidronate or zoledronic acid) should be given to myeloma patients with lytic bone lesions, compression fracture, or osteopenia (Grade A). A Cochrane Review of bisphosphonates use in myeloma included data from ten placebo-controlled trials and concluded that the addition of bisphosphonates to the treatment of myeloma reduces vertebral fractures and

pain, but not mortality (Level I) (DJULBEGOVIC et al. 2002). Pamidronate may be preferred to zoledronic acid as the latter is associated with a 9.5-fold greater risk of developing osteonecrosis of the jaw (ZERVAS et al. 2006).
■ It is recommended that therapy continues for 2 years, after which time it can be stopped and recommended if a new skeletal event develops (Grade C) (KYLE et al. 2007). An IFM study showed that there was no difference in the proportion of skeletal events in the pamidronate maintenance arm (21% vs. 18%) compared with no maintenance (24%) after 29 months of follow-up (Level II) (ATTAL et al. 2006).
■ The dose of zoledronic acid should be reduced in patients with mild to moderate renal impairment (creatinine clearance 30–60 ml/min, checked before each dose), and zoledronic acid should not be used in patients with severe renal impairment. Pamidronate 90 mg administered over 4 to 6 h is recommended for patients with severe renal impairment.
■ Albuminuria should be screened at 3- to 6-monthly intervals. In patients experiencing unexplained albuminuria (defined as >500 mg/24 h of urinary albumin), discontinuation of the drug is advised until the renal problems are resolved. When the renal function returns to baseline, pamidronate therapy should be reinstituted at a slower infusion rate.
■ Osteonecrosis of the jaw is a rare but serious complication of bisphosphonate therapy. All patients should have a comprehensive dental examination before commencing treatment. Active oral infections should be treated, and the patient should maintain excellent oral hygiene and avoid invasive dental procedures if possible.
■ Bisphosphonate therapy is not indicated for solitary plasmacytoma, smoldering multiple myeloma, or MGUS.

Management of Anemia with Erythropoietin (EPO)

■ A therapeutic trial of EPO should be considered in multiple myeloma patients with symptomatic anemia receiving chemotherapy; however, it is usually not recommended before response to therapy has been assessed in newly diagnosed patients.
■ EPO should be used with caution in patients treated with thalidomide or lenalidomide and doxorubicin or corticosteroids, as EPO further increases the risk of thromboembolic complications (Level II) (BENNETT et al. 2006).

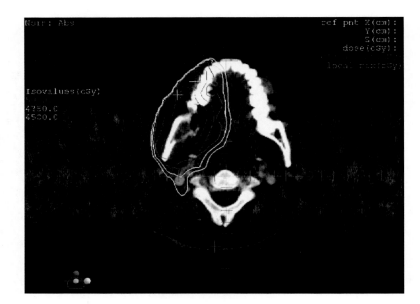

Fig. 29.1. Dose distribution of irradiation for a solitary osseous plasmacytoma of the mandible. The lesion extended to the surrounding tissue. The 95% isodose line (47.5 Gy, *yellow line*) covers the gross tumor volume (*thin red line*) with a margin of 2 cm, without elective irradiation to draining lymph nodes

29.2.7 Palliative Radiation Therapy

- Palliative radiotherapy is indicated for bone pain or neurological compression in multiple myeloma (Grade A). Approximately 40% of patients with multiple myeloma require palliative radiotherapy during their course of disease (FEATHERSTONE et al. 2005).
- Treatment for recurrence of bone pain after initial radiation therapy is required in about 5% of patients.
- Radiation therapy can be utilized for pathologic fracture or impending pathologic fracture after orthopedic stabilization and symptomatic soft-tissue mass.
- Palliative radiotherapy and chemotherapy can be given sequentially, and concurrent chemoradiotherapy is not routinely recommended (Grade C). In a retrospective series reported by LEIGH et al. (1993) detailed below, no significant difference in pain relief was found when radiation was given with or without concurrent chemotherapy (Level III). However, results from an earlier retrospective report showed that radiation given during melphalan and prednisone treatment is more effective in pain palliation (80% versus 31.8% response rate) (Level III) (ADAMIETZ et al. 1991).

Simulation and Treatment Volume

- Conventional planning is usually adequate for simulation for palliative treatment to long bone or spine. CT-based planning may help to define accurately the treatment volume if a soft-tissue mass is present.
- For lesion(s) of the long bone, involved-field external beam radiation to the radiographic lesion(s) with 2-cm margins is the standard field arrangement (Grade B). Irradiation of the entire bone is usually not needed for the lesions in the long bone. A retrospective series of 163 patients with multiple myeloma compared the effects of irradiation to either the entire long bone or involved field of symptomatic portion of the bone. The results revealed that limited-field irradiation did not compromise outcome. Symptomatic recurrence out of the irradiated field is uncommon and can be effectively treated (Level III) (CATELL et al. 1998).
- For lesion(s) of the vertebra, margins should include the entire vertebra (including transverse processes) and one or two vertebral bodies above and below.
- Hemibody radiation used for consolidation treatment after chemotherapy is not recommended (Grade A). The durations of relapse-free survival and overall survival were both significantly reduced with the addition of consolidation hemibody radiation, as compared to chemotherapy for consolidation, according to a phase III prospective randomized trial completed by Southwest Oncology Group (SWOG). Consolidation radiation reduced the durations of overall survival from 43 months to 29 months and relapse-free survival from 26 months to 20 months (SWOG, Level I) (SALMON et al. 1990).

Dose of Radiation

▪ Lower dose radiation therapy (e.g., 25 Gy in 10 fractions at 2.5 Gy/fraction or 30 Gy in 15 fractions at 2 Gy/fraction) is recommended for most cases of multiple myeloma for bone pain palliation (Grade B). Multiple myeloma is highly radioresponsive. Low-dose irradiation is effective in bone pain palliation, has limited toxicities to bone marrow, and allows for potential re-irradiation for local recurrence of symptoms. Retreatment of symptomatic recurrence is required in approximately 6% of patients after low-dose radiation. Multiple retrospective studies have confirmed the efficacy of low-dose radiation therapy in bone pain palliation. In a retrospective trial reported by MILL and GRIFFITH (1980), more than 80% of patients achieved complete or partial pain relief after radiotherapy. Subjective pain alleviation could be noticed after as low as 5 Gy of radiation, and the median dose for subjective pain relief was between 10 to 15 Gy. Re-irradiation is required for 6% of patients after radiation therapy, and no association between the radiation doses and symptomatic recurrence was found (Level III). The retrospective series reported by LEIGH et al. (1993) involved 101 patients and 306 symptomatic sites. Approximately 97% of the patients presenting with bone pain achieved complete (26%) or partial response (71%) after palliative radiation to a mean dose of 25 Gy. No difference in symptomatic relief was noticed among patients treated to lower than 10 Gy or above 10 Gy. In addition, concurrent chemotherapy did not increase the rate of complete response, and only 6% of patients developed local symptomatic recurrence (Level III).

▪ Total dose of 20 Gy or more may be required for both pain palliation and healing of lytic lesion(s) caused by multiple myeloma (Grade C). Results from several retrospective studies revealed that low dose radiation may palliate bone pain caused by multiple myeloma, but no objective radiographic improvement of lytic lesions is associated to lower dose (in the range of 10 Gy) treatment (Level III) (BOSCH et al. 1988; MILL and GRIFFITH 1980). However, such a finding was not supported in the above-mentioned study from Leigh, which found that radiation doses of less than or more than 10 Gy were equally effective (Level III).

▪ A higher dose of irradiation in the range of 30 Gy or above delivered in an extensive-course is required for spinal cord compression caused by multiple myeloma (Grade B). The results of a multicenter retrospective study from Germany concluded that the improvement of motor function within 1 year after treatment was significantly better in patients receiving long-course radiation (37.5 Gy in 15 fractions, 30 Gy in 10 fractions, or 20 Gy in 10 fractions), as compared to those receiving shorter courses (20 Gy in 5 fractions or 8 Gy in 1 fraction). In addition, subgroup analysis revealed no difference in functional outcome for patients receiving different doses and fractionations of long-course radiation (Level III) (RADES et al. 2006).

Side Effects and Complications

▪ Severe acute or late toxicity secondary to radiation therapy (unless in re-irradiation for symptomatic recurrences) is not common due to the limited irradiation dose and size of the treatment field.

▪ Anemia and leukopenia (secondary to radiation-induced bone marrow toxicity) and fatigue are probable side effects for large-field radiation.

▪ Attention should be paid to the amount of bone marrow included in radiation field(s) if a large field or multiple sites are irradiated, especially when bone marrow transplant is planned.

 29.3 Treatment of Solitary Plasmacytoma of Bone (Osseous Plasmacytoma)

29.3.1 General Principles

▪ Radiation therapy is the standard treatment for solitary plasmacytoma of the bone (Grade A).

▪ Surgery should be reserved only for treatment of pathological fracture or stabilization of bone with impending fracture.

▪ For patients who received gross tumor excision for diagnosis, definitive dose irradiation is indicated after surgery (Grade B). In a large multicenter retrospective series of 206 cases, five patients underwent gross tumor excision alone without radiation, and four patients developed local recurrence (Rare Cancer Network Study, Level IV) (KNOBEL et al. 2006).

■ Adjuvant chemotherapy should not be routinely recommended for the treatment of solitary plasmacytoma of the bone after definitive radiation (Grade C). However, some evidence has shown that adjuvant chemotherapy may postpone the transformation of solitary plasmacytoma of bone to multiple myeloma.

29.3.2 Radiation Therapy

Dose and Fractionation

■ External-beam radiation up to 40–50 Gy in conventional fractionation over 4–5 weeks is recommended for the treatment of solitary plasmacytoma of bone (Grade C). Local control (defined as absence of disease progression on imaging studies in the treated field) can be achieved in 90% to 100% of patients after radiation therapy. However, the optimal dose for treatment has not yet been defined.
The results of a multicenter retrospective study of 206 patients with solitary plasmacytoma of bone showed that the 5-year overall survival and local control rates were 70% and 88%, respectively. The 10-year local control rate was 79%. A radiation dose of 30 Gy or higher is associated with improved local control; however, no further dose-response relationship was observed for doses at 30 Gy or higher (Rare Cancer Network Study, Level III) (Knobel et al. 2006). Experience from the Princess Margaret Hospital from 46 patients with solitary plasmacytoma revealed that a dose of less than 35 Gy was not associated with higher risk of local recurrence. However, tumor size larger than 5 cm had a worse local control (Level III).
Conversely, in a retrospective study of 81 patients with solitary plasmacytoma reported by Mendenhall et al. (1980), local control was achieved in 94% of patients irradiated to 40 Gy or higher dose, as compared to 64% of patients treated to doses less than 40 Gy (Level III). Similar results were concluded in a retrospective analysis of 43 patients reported by Mill and Griffith (1980) in which all patients treated to 40 Gy or higher dose achieved local control (Level III).

Simulation and Treatment Volume

■ Involved-field external beam radiation to the radiographic lesion(s) defined by MRI and/or FDG-PET scan with a generous margin (2–3 cm from gross tumor) can be recommended for definitive treatment (Grade D) (Fig. 29.2).
■ For lesion(s) located in the vertebral body, margins should include the entire vertebra and one or two vertebral bodies above and below.
■ Elective nodal irradiation is not recommended for solitary plasmacytoma of bone (Grade A). Results from numerous clinical trials indicated that the probability of regional nodal failure is less than 5% after involved-field radiation therapy (Level III) (Knobel et al. 2006).

29.3.3 Adjuvant Chemotherapy

■ Adjuvant chemotherapy should not be routinely recommended for the treatment of solitary plas-

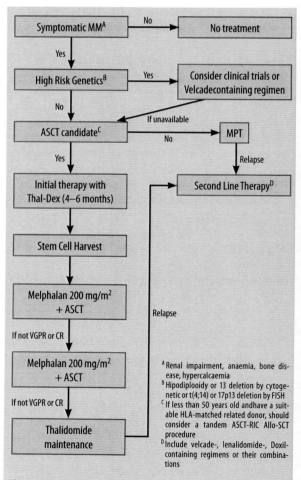

Fig. 29.2. A proposed treatment algorithm for multiple myeloma

macytoma of bone after definitive radiation (Grade C). However, the results of a randomized study reported by AVILES et al. (1996) showed that in 53 patients with solitary plasmacytoma of the bone, 54% of those in the radiotherapy arm had progressed compared to only 12% of those given adjuvant melphalan and predniso-lone for 3 years after radiotherapy. Consistent with this, the overall survival of patients given adjuvant chemotherapy was significantly longer (Level III). However, results from this small trial need to be confirmed before chemotherapy can be routinely recommended.

29.4 Treatment of Extramedullary Plasmacytoma

29.4.1 General Principles

- Radiation therapy is the standard treatment for extramedullary plasmacytoma (Grade A). Radiation therapy alone is equivalent to surgery alone in terms of local control.
- Surgery is curative for small lesions; however, post-surgical radiation therapy is indicated for most patients with larger tumors.

29.4.2 Radiation Therapy

Dose and Fractionation

- External-beam radiation up to 40–50 Gy in conventional fractionation over 4–5 weeks is recommended for the treatment of extramedullary plasmacytoma (Grade B). Higher dose in the range of 50 Gy or above may be needed for bulky disease. In the above-mentioned retrospective study of 81 patients with solitary plasmacytoma reported by MENDENHALL et al. (1980), local control was achieved in 94% of patients irradiated to 40 Gy or higher dose. However, all cases of local failure in this dose range were extramedullary plasmacytoma (Level III). In addition, the results of the study reported by MILL and GRIFFITH (1980) suggested the optimal radiation dose for extramedullary plasmacytoma is above 50 Gy (Level III).

Simulation and Treatment Volume

- Involved-field external beam radiation to the radiographic lesion(s) defined by MRI and/or FDG-PET scan with a generous margin (2–3 cm from gross tumor) can be recommended for definitive radiotherapy (Grade D) (Fig. 29.1).
- Elective nodal irradiation is not recommended for extramedullary plasmacytoma, including those located in the aerodigestive system (Grade B). Results from a review of published literature that included 800 cases of extramedullary plasmacytoma revealed that collectively the incidence of lymph node metastases was less than 10% for diseases located in the aerodigestive tract and less for diseases originating in non-aerodigestive locations (Level IV) (ALEXIOU et al. 2000) However, clinical trials aimed to determine the efficacy of prophylactic irradiation to the regional nodal areas is lacking.

29.4.3 Adjuvant Chemotherapy

- Adjuvant chemotherapy should not be routinely recommended for the treatment of extramedullary plasmacytoma after definitive radiation (Grade B). The incidence of progression to multiple myeloma from extramedullary plasmacytoma was approximately 15%, and the local recurrence rate was 22% after definitive radiation therapy, surgery, or their combination, according to the extensive review of 800 cases reported by ALEXIOU et al. (2000) (Level IV). Significant improvement in local and distant control is not likely with the addition of adjuvant chemotherapy.

29.5 Follow-Ups

29.5.1 Post-Treatment Follow-Ups

- Long-term follow-up is required for all patients treated for multiple myeloma as none of the current treatments (except allo-SCT) is curative, and most patients will invariably relapse.
- Long-term follow-up is required for all patients treated for solitary plasmacytoma of bone and extramedullary plasmacytoma (Grade B). More

than 50% of cases with solitary plasmacytoma of bone progress to multiple myeloma at 5 years (KNOBEL et al. 2006), and approximately 15% of patients with extramedullary plasmacytoma progress to multiple myeloma at 10 years after treatment (ALEXIOU et al. 2000)

■ Recently, uniform criteria for treatment response and relapse have been published, and should be used during follow-up of patients to determine disease status (Table 29.5) (DURIE et al. 2006).

Schedule

■ A suggested follow-up schedule for patients with multiple myeloma and plasmacytoma is presented in Table 29.6.

Work-Ups

■ Each follow-up examination should include a complete history and physical examination, testing quantitative immunoglobulin and quantification of M-protein, complete blood count, and serum urea, creatinine and calcium. Skeletal survey should be performed annually or when patients have developed new areas of bone pain.

■ For extramedullary plasmacytoma, MRI should be performed 8 weeks after the completion of radiation or surgery (Grade D). Repeated MRI can be done every 4–6 months to assess the response to treatment. Surveillance imaging is not recommended after the complete resolution of the tumor or for stable residual tumor on consecutive studies.

Table 29.5. Uniform response criteria for multiple myeloma after treatment

Response subcategory	Response criteria
Strict complete response (sCR)	CR as defined below plus normal FLC ratio and absence of clonal cells in bone marrow by immunohistochemistry or immunofluorescence.
Complete response (CR)	Negative immunofixation on the serum and urine and disappearance of any soft tissue plasmacytomas and ≤5% plasma cell in bone marrow.
Very good partial response (VGPR)	Serum and urine M-protein detectable by immunofixation, but not on electrophoresis, or 90% or greater reduction in serum M-protein plus urine M-protein level <100 mg/24 h.
Partial response (PR)	≥50% Reduction of serum M-protein and reduction in 24-h urinary M-protein by ≥90% or to <200 mg/24 h. If the serum and urine M-protein are unmeasurable, a ≥50% decrease in the difference between involved and uninvolved FLC levels is required in place of the M-protein criteria. If the serum and urine M-protein are unmeasurable, and serum FLC assay is also unmeasurable, ≥50% reduction in plasma cells is required in place of M-protein, provided baseline bone marrow plasma cell percentage was ≥30%. In addition to the above-listed criteria, if present at baseline, a ≥50% reduction in the size of soft tissue plasmacytomas is also required .
Stable disease (SD)	Not meeting criteria for CR, VGPR, PR, or progressive disease.
Progressive disease (PD)	PD requires any one of the following: Increase of ≥25% from baseline in serum M-protein and/or the absolute increase must be ≥0.5 g/dl. Urine M-protein and/or the absolute increase must be ≥200 mg/24 h. Only in patients without measurable serum and urine M-protein levels: the difference between involved and uninvolved FLC levels. The absolute increase must be >10 mg/dl. Bone marrow plasma cell percentage: the absolute % must be ≥10%. Definite development of new bone lesions or soft tissue plasmacytomas or definite increase in the size of existing bone lesions or soft tissue plasmacytomas. Development of hypercalcemia (corrected serum calcium >11.5 mg/dl or 2.65 mmol/l) that can be attributed solely to the plasma cell neoplasm.
Relapse from CR	Any one or more of the following: Reappearance of serum or urine M-protein by immunofixation or electrophoresis. Development of ≥5% plasma cells in the bone marrow. Appearance of any other sign of progression (i.e., new plasmacytoma, lytic lesion, or hypercalcaemia).

■ For multiple myeloma and solitary plasmacytoma of bone, imaging studies after the completion of radiation are not suggested to assess the extent of response, as persistent abnormality in affected bone is expected in follow-up imaging studies (Grade D).

Table 29.6. Follow-up schedule for patients with multiple myeloma and plasmacytoma

Interval	Frequency
First year	1–2 monthly
Second year	3 monthly
Years 3–4	6 monthly
Over 5 years	Yearly

References

Adamietz IA, Schöber C, Schulte RW, et al (1991) Palliative radiotherapy in plasma cell myeloma. Radiother Oncol 20:111–116

Alexiou C, Kau RJ, Dietzfelbinger H, et al (1999) Extramedullary plasmacytoma: Tumor occurrence and therapeutic concepts. Cancer 85:2305–2314

Avilés A, Huerta-Guzmán J, Delgado S, et al (1996) Improved outcome in solitary bone plasmacytomata with combined therapy. Hematol Oncol 14:111–117

Attal M, Harousseau JL, Stoppa JM, et al (1996) A prospective, randomized trial of autologous bone marrow transplantation and chemotherapy in multiple myeloma. Intergroupe Français du Myélome. New Engl J Med 335:91–97

Attal M, Harousseau JL, Facon T, et al (2006a) Single versus double autologous stem-cell transplantation for multiple myeloma. New Engl J Med 349:2495–2502

Attal M, Harousseau JL, Leyvraz S, et al. (2006b) Maintenance therapy with thalidomide improves survival in patients with multiple myeloma. Blood 108(10): 3289–3294

Avet-Loisseau H, Attal M, Moreau P, et al (2007) Genetic abnormalities and survival in multiple myeloma: the experience of the Intergroupe Francophone du Myelome. Blood 109:3489–3495

Badros A, Barlogie B, Morris C, et al (2001) Results of autologous stem cell transplant in multiple myeloma patients with renal failure. Br J Haematol 114:822–829

Barlogie B, Kyle RA, Anderson KC, et al (2006) Standard chemotherapy compared with high-dose chemoradiotherapy for multiple myeloma: final results of phase III US Intergroup Trial S9321. J Clin Oncol 24:929–936

Bennett CL, Angelotta C, Yarnold PR, et al (2006) Thalidomide- and lenalidomide-associated thromboembolism among patients with cancer. JAMA 296:2558–2560

Blade J, Rosinol L, Sureda A, et al (2005) High-dose therapy intensification compared with continued standard chemotherapy in multiple myeloma patients responding to the initial chemotherapy: long-term results from a prospective randomized trial from the Spanish cooperative group PETHEMA. Blood 106:3755–3759

Bosch A, Frias Z (1988) Radiotherapy in the treatment of multiple myeloma. Int J Radiat Oncol Biol Phys 15:1363–1369

Bourhis JH, Bouko Y, Koscielny S, et al (2007) Relapse risk after autologous transplantation in patients with newly diagnosed myeloma is not related with infused tumor cell load and the outcome is not improved by CD34+ cell selection: long-term follow-up of an EBMT phase III randomized study. Hematologica 92:1083–1090

Bradwell AR, Carr-Smith HD, Mead GP, Harvey TC, Drayson MT. (2003) Serum testing for assessing patients with Bence Jones myeloma. Lancet 361(9356):489–491

Bruno B, Rotta M, Patriarca F, et al (2007) A comparison of allografting with autografting for newly diagnosed myeloma. New Engl J Med 356:1110–1120

Catell D, Kogen Z, Donahue B, et al (1998) Multiple myeloma of an extremity: must the entire bone be treated? Int J Radiat Oncol Biol Phys 40:117–119

Cavo M, Zamagni E, Tosi P, et al (2005) Superiority of thalidomide and dexamethasone over vincristine-doxorubicindexamethasone (VAD) as primary therapy in preparation for autologous transplantation for multiple myeloma. Blood 106:35–39

Cavo M, Tosi P, Zamagni E, et al (2007) Prospective, randomized study of single compared with double autologous stem-cell transplantation for multiple myeloma: Bologna 96 clinical study. J Clin Oncol 25:2434–2341

Child JA, Morgan GJ, Davies FE, et al (2003) High-dose chemotherapy with hematopoietic stem-cell rescue for multiple myeloma. New Engl J Med 348:1875–1883

Chng WJ, Ahmann GJ, Henderson K, et al (2006) Clinical implication of centrosome amplification in plasma cell neoplasm. Blood 107:3669–3675

Chng WJ, Price-Troska T, Gonzalez-Paz N, et al (2007) Clinical significance of TP53 mutation in myeloma. Leukaemia 21:582–584

Clark WF, Stewart AK, Rock GA, et al (2005) Plasma exchange when myeloma presents as acute renal failure: a randomized, controlled trial. Ann Intern Med 143:777–784

Corradini P, Cavo M, Lokhorst M, et al (2003) Molecular remission after myeloablative allogeneic stem cell transplantation predicts a better relapse-free survival in patients with multiple myeloma. Blood 102:1927–1929

Dimopoulos M, Spencer A, Attal M, et al (2007) Lenalidomide plus dexamethasone for relapsed or refractory multiple myeloma. New Engl J Med 357:2123–2132

Djulbegovic B, Wheatley K, Ross J, et al (2002) Bisphosphonates in multiple myeloma. Cochrane Database Syst Rev CD003188

Drayson M, Tang LX, Drew R, Mead GP, Carr-Smith H, Bradwell AR (2001) Serum free light chain measurements for identifying and monitoring patients with nonsecretory multiple myeloma. Blood 97:2900–2902

Durie BGM, Harousseau JL, Miguel JS, et al (2006). International uniform response criteria for multiple myeloma. Leukemia 20:1467–1473

Facon T, Mary JY, Pergourie B, et al (2006) Dexamethasone-based regimens versus melphalan-prednisone for elderly multiple myeloma patients ineligible for high-dose therapy. Blood 107:1292–1298

Facon T, Mary JY, Hulin C, et al (2007). Melphalan and prednisone plus thalidomide versus melphalan and prednisone alone or reduced-intensity autologous stem cell transplantation in elderly patients with multiple myeloma (IFM 99-06): a randomised trial. Lancet 370(9594):1209–1218

Featherstone C, Delaney G, Jacob S, et al (2005) Estimating the optimal utilization rates of radiotherapy for hematologic malignancies from a review of the evidence: part II-leukemia and myeloma. Cancer 103:393–401

Fermand JP, Ravaud P, Chevret S, et al (1998) High-dose therapy and autologous peripheral blood stem cell transplantation in multiple myeloma: up-front or rescue treatment? Results of a multicenter sequential randomized clinical trial. Blood 92:3131–3136

Fermand JP, Katsahian S, Divine M, et al (2005) High-dose therapy and autologous blood stem-cell transplantation compared with conventional treatment in myeloma patients aged 55 to 65 years: long-term results of a randomized control trial from the Group Myelome-Autogreffe. J Clin Oncol 23:9227–9233

Fonseca R, Barlogie B, Bataille R, et al (2004). Genetics and cytogenetics of multiple myeloma: a workshop report. Cancer Res 64:1546–1558

Garban F, Attal M, Michallet M, et al (2006) Prospective comparison of autologous stem cell transplantation followed by dose-reduced allograft (IFM99-03 trial) with tandem autologous stem cell transplantation (IFM99-04 trial) in high-risk de novo multiple myeloma. Blood 107:3474–3480

Gertz MA, Lacy M. Dispenzieri A, et al (2005) Clinical implications of t(11;14)(q13;q32), t(4;14)(p16.3;q32), and -17p13 in myeloma patients treated with high-dose therapy. Blood 106:2837–2840

Ghanem N, Lohrmann C, Engelhardt M, et al (2006) Whole-body MRI in the detection of bone marrow infiltration in patients with plasma cell neoplasms in comparison to the radiological skeletal survey. Eur Radiol 16:1005–1014

Glasmacher A, Hahn C, Hoffmann F, et al (2006) A systematic review of phase-II trials of thalidomide monotherapy in patients with relapsed or refractory multiple myeloma. Br J Haematol 132:584–593

Greipp PR, Lust JA, O'Fallon WM, Katzmann JA, Witzig TE, Kyle RA (1993) Plasma cell labeling index and beta 2-microglobulin predict survival independent of thymidine kinase and C-reactive protein in multiple myeloma. Blood 81:3382–3387

Greipp PR, Leong T, Bennett JM, et al (1998) Plasmablastic morphology–an independent prognostic factor with clinical and laboratory correlate: Eastern Cooperative Oncology Group (ECOG) myeloma trial E9486 report by the ECOG myeloma laboratory group. Blood 91:2501–2507

Greipp PR, San Miguel J, Durie BG, et al (2005). International staging system for multiple myeloma. J Clin Oncol 23:3412–3420

Hernandez JM, Garcia-Sanz R, Golvano E, et al (2004) Randomized comparison of dexamethasone combined with melphalan versus melphalan with prednisone in the treatment of elderly patients with multiple myeloma. Br J Haematol 127:159–164

Hjorth M, Hellquist L, Holmberg E et al (1993) Initial versus deferred melphalan-prednisone therapy for asymptomatic multiple myeloma stage I – a randomized study.

Myeloma Group of Western Sweden. Eur J Haematol 50:95–102

Jacobson JL, Hussain MA, Barlogie B, et al (2003) A new staging system for multiple myeloma patients based on the Southwest Oncology Group (SWOG) experience. Br J Haematol 122:441–450

Jantunen E, Kuittinen T, Penttila K, Lehtonen P, Mahlamaki E, Nousiainen T (2006) High-dose melphalan (200 mg/m2) supported by autologous stem cell transplantation is safe and effective in elderly (≥65 years) myeloma patients: comparison with younger patients treated on the same protocol. Bone Marrow Transplant 37:917–922

Johnson WJ, Kyle RA, Pineda AA, O'Brien PC, Holley KE (1990) Treatment of renal failure associated with multiple myeloma. Plasmapheresis, hemodialysis, and chemotherapy. Arch Intern Med 150:863–869

Knobel D, Zouhair A, Tsang RW, et al (2006) Prognostic factors in solitary plasmacytoma of the bone: a multicenter Rare Cancer Network study. BMC Cancer 6:118

Knudsen LM, Nielsen B, Gimsing P, Geisler C (2005) Autologous stem cell transplantation in multiple myeloma: outcome in patients with renal failure. Eur J Haematol 75:27–33

Kumar S, Lacy MQ, Dispenzieri A, et al (2004) Single agent dexamethasone for pre-stem cell transplant induction therapy for multiple myeloma. Bone Marrow Transplant 34:485–490

Kyle RA, Yee GC, Somerfield MR, et al (2007) American Society of Clinical Oncology 2007 clinical practice guideline update on the role of bisphosphonates in multiple myeloma. J Clin Oncol 25:2464–2472

Lee CK, Zangari M, Barlogie B, et al (2004) Dialysis-dependent renal failure in patients with myeloma can be reversed by high-dose myeloablative therapy and autotransplant. Bone Marrow Transplant 33:823–828

Leigh BR, Kurtts TA, Mack CF, et al (1993) Radiation therapy for the palliation of multiple myeloma. Int J Radiat Oncol Biol Phys 25:801–804

Mendenhall CM, Thar TL, Million RR (1980) Solitary plasmacytoma of bone and soft tissue. Int J Radiat Oncol Biol Phys 6:1497–1501

Mill WB, Griffith R (1980) The role of radiation therapy in the management of plasma cell tumors. Cancer 45:647–652

Moreau P, Facon T, Attal M, et al (2002) Comparison of 200 mg/m2 melphalan and 8 Gy total body irradiation plus 140 mg/m2 melphalan as conditioning regimens for peripheral blood stem cell transplantation in patients with newly diagnosed multiple myeloma: final analysis of the Intergroupe Francophone du Myélome 9502 randomized trial. Blood 99:731–735

Moulopoulos LA, Dimopoulos MA, Weber D, et al (1993) Magnetic resonance imaging in the staging of solitary plasmacytoma of bone. J Clin Oncol 11:1311–1315

Myeloma Trialists' Collaborative Group (2001) Interferon as therapy for multiple myeloma: an individual patient data overview of 24 randomized trials and 4012 patients. Br J Haematol 113:1020–1034

Orlowski RZ, Nagler A, Sonneveld P, et al (2007) Randomized phase III study of pegylated liposomal doxorubicin plus bortezomib compared with bortezomib alone in relapsed or refractory multiple myeloma: combination therapy improves time to progression. J Clin Oncol 25:3892–3901

Ozsahin M, Tsang RW, Poortmans P, et al (2006) Outcomes and patterns of failure in solitary plasmacytoma: a multicenter Rare Cancer Network study of 258 patients. Int J Radiat Oncol Biol Phys 64:210–217

Palumbo A, Bringhen S, Caravita T, et al (2006) Oral melphalan and prednisone chemotherapy plus thalidomide compared with melphalan and prednisone alone in elderly patients with multiple myeloma: randomised controlled trial. Lancet 367(9513):825–831

Rades D, Hoskin PJ, Stalpers LJ, et al (2006) Short-course radiotherapy is not optimal for spinal cord compression due to myeloma. Int J Radiat Oncol Biol Phys 64:1452–1457

Rajkumar SV, Blood E, Vesole D, et al (2006) Phase III clinical trial of thalidomide plus dexamethasone compared with dexamethasone alone in newly diagnosed multiple myeloma: a clinical trial coordinated by the Eastern Cooperative Oncology Group. J Clin Oncol 24:431–436

Reece DE, Bredeson C, Perez WS, et al (2003) Autologous stem cell transplantation in multiple myeloma patients <60 vs ≥60 years of age. Bone Marrow Transplant 32:1135–1143

Riccardi A, Mora O, Tinelli C, et al (2000) Long-term survival of stage I multiple myeloma given chemotherapy just after diagnosis or at progression of the disease: a multicentre randomized study. Cooperative Group of Study and Treatment of Multiple Myeloma. Br J Cancer 82:1254–1260

Richardson PG, Sonneveld P, Schuster M, et al (2005) Bortezomib or high-dose dexamethasone for relapsed multiple myeloma. New Engl J Med 52:2487–2498

Richardson PG, Sonneveld P, Schuster M, et al (2007) Extended follow-up of a phase 3 trial in relapsed multiple myeloma: Final time-to-event results of the APEX trial. Blood 110:3557–3560

Salmon SE, Tesh D, Crowley J, et al (1990) Chemotherapy is superior to sequential hemibody irradiation for remission consolidation in multiple myeloma: a Southwest Oncology Group study. J Clin Oncol 8:1575–1584

San Miguel J, Lahuerta JJ, Garcia-Sanz R, et al (2000) Are myeloma patients with renal failure candidates for autologous stem cell transplantation? Haematol J 1:28–36

Shustik C, Belch A, Robinson S, et al (2007) A randomised comparison of melphalan with prednisone or dexamethasone as induction therapy and dexamethasone or observation as maintenance therapy in multiple myeloma: NCIC CTG MY.7. Br J Haematol 136:203–211

Siegel DS, Desikan KR, Mehta J, et al (1999) Age is not a prognostic variable with autotransplants for multiple myeloma. Blood 93:51–54

Sirohi B, Powles R, Traleaven J, et al (2000) The role of autologous transplantation in patients with multiple myeloma aged 65 years and over. Bone Marrow Transplant 25:533–539

Sirohi B, Powles R, Mehta J, et al (2001) The implication of compromised renal function at presentation in myeloma: similar outcome in patients who receive high-dose therapy: a single-center study of 251 previously untreated patients. Med Oncol 18:39–50

Stewart AK, Vescio R, Schiller G, et al (2001) Purging of autologous peripheral-blood stem cells using CD34 selection does not improve overall or progression-free survival after high-dose chemotherapy for multiple myeloma: results of a multicenter randomized controlled trial. J Clin Oncol 19:3771–3779

Stewart AK, Bergsagel PL, Greipp P, et al (2007). A practical guide to defining high-risk myeloma for clinical trials, patients counseling and choice of therapy. Leukaemia 21:529–534

Susnerwala SS, Shanks JH, Banerjee SS, et al (1997) Extramedullary plasmacytoma of the head and neck region: clinicopathological correlation in 25 cases. Br J Cancer 75:921–927

Terpos E, Apperley JF, Samson D, et al (2003) Autologous stem cell transplantation in multiple myeloma: improved survival in nonsecretory multiple myeloma but lack of influence of age, status at transplant, previous treatment and conditioning regimen. A single-centre experience in 127 patients. Bone Marrow Transplant 31:163–170

The International Myeloma Working Group (2003) Criteria for the classification of monoclonal gammopathies, multiple myeloma and related disorders: a report of the International Myeloma Working Group. Br J Haematol 121:749–757

Tsang RW, Gospodarowicz MK, Pintilie M, et al (2001) Solitary plasmacytoma treated with radiotherapy: impact of tumor size on outcome. Int J Radiat Oncol Biol Phys 50:113-120

Walker R, Barlogie B, Haessler J, et al (2007) Magnetic resonance imaging in multiple myeloa: diagnostic and clinical implications. J Clin Oncol 25:1121–1128

Weber DM, Chen C, Niesvizky R, et al (2007) Lenalidomide plus dexamethasone for relapsed multiple myeloma in North America. New Engl J Med 357:2133–2142

Wilder RB, Ha CS, Cox JD, et al (2002) Persistence of myeloma protein for more than 1 year after radiotherapy is an adverse prognostic factor in solitary plasmacytoma of bone. Cancer 94:1532–1537

Wu KL, Beverloo B, Lokhorst HM, et al (2007) Abnormalities of chromosome 1p/q are highly associated with chromosome 13/13q deletions and are an adverse prognostic factor for the outcome of high-dose chemotherapy in patients with multiple myeloma. Br J Haematol 136:615–623

Zervas K, Verrou E, Teleioudis Z, et al (2006) Incidence, risk factors and management of osteonecrosis of the jaw in patients with multiple myeloma: a single-centre experience in 303 patients. Br J Haematol 134:620–623

Zucchelli P, Pasquali S, Cagnoli L, Ferrari G (1988) Controlled plasma exchange trial in acute renal failure due to multiple myeloma. Kidney Int 33:1175–1180

Cutaneous T-Cell and Extranodal NK/T-Cell Lymphoma

Yexiong Li and Jiade J. Lu

CONTENTS

Introduction and Objectives

Skin is the most common site of extranodal non-Hodgkin's lymphoma (NHL). Mycosis fungoides, or its variants, account for approximately 50% of cutaneous lymphoma, and are highly sensitive to radiation therapy. Radiation plays an important role in the definitive treatment of localized disease, as well as in palliating disseminated cutaneous, nodal, or visceral lesions.

Extranodal NK/T-cell lymphoma of nasal type is a rare disease entity in North America, but is relatively common in Asian countries. The nasal cavity is the most common site for this malignancy, and nasal NK/T-cell lymphoma is the prototype of the disease. Radiation therapy plays a major role in the treatment of localized nasal NK/T-cell lymphoma.

This chapter focuses on the management of cutaneous lymphoma, particularly mycosis fungoides, and nasal and nasal-type NK/T-cell lymphoma and examines:

- Recommendations for diagnoses and staging procedures of mycosis fungoides and nasal NK/T-cell lymphoma
- The staging systems and prognostic factors
- Treatment recommendations for mycosis fungoides and the supporting peer-reviewed scientific evidence
- Treatment technique of total skin electron-beam therapy (TSEBT) for nonlocalized or disseminated cutaneous disease of mycosis fungoides
- Treatment recommendations for nasal and nasal-type NK/T-cell lymphoma and the supporting peer-reviewed scientific evidence
- Follow-up care and surveillance of survivors

Y. X. Li, MD
Department of Radiation Oncology, Cancer Hospital, Chinese Academy of Medical Sciences and Peking Union Medical College, P. O. Box 2258, Beijing 100021, P. R. China
J. J. Lu, MD, MBA
Department of Radiation Oncology, National University Cancer Institute of Singapore, National University Health System, National University of Singapore, 5 Lower Kent Ridge Road, Singapore 119074, Singapore

30.1 Diagnosis, Staging, and Prognoses of Mycosis Fungoides

30.1.1 Diagnosis

Initial Evaluation

- Diagnosis and evaluation of mycosis fungoides start with a complete history and physical examination. A thorough physical examination with special attention to skin and lymph nodes, as well as an evaluation of liver and spleen for hepatosplenomegaly are required.
- The characteristics of the cutaneous lesion(s), including size, number of lesions, distribution, and extension, as well as the presence of adenopathy should be recorded. The percentage of skin involvement is important for staging of mycosis fungoides, and is of prognostic value.

Laboratory Tests

- Initial blood tests should include a complete blood count with differential, basic blood chemistry, liver function tests, renal function tests, and lactate dehydrogenase (LDH).
- Flow cytometry of peripheral blood for CD2, CD3, CD4, CD5, CD7, CD8, CD20, and CD45RO is required. An expanded population of CD4+, CD7–, or CD45RO+ lymphocytes, or an elevated CD4:CD8 ratio indicates probable blood involvement.

Imaging Studies

- For patients with stage I mycosis fungoides, chest X-ray can be used to rule out lung involvement. As the probability of pulmonary metastasis is exceedingly low in patients with early stage mycosis fungoides, CT scan of the chest is usually not recommended in most cases (Grade B) (Level IV) (BASS et al. 1993).
- CT scan of the chest, abdomen, and pelvis is indicated to evaluate the status of node and visceral involvement for patients with more advanced disease (Grade B). CT findings in cutaneous T-cell lymphoma were found to be important to predict pathophysiological features of the disease, and is important for the staging of mycosis fungoides (Level IV) (BASS et al. 1993; MIKETIC et al. 1993).

- The value of FDG-PET in the initial diagnosis and staging of cutaneous T-cell lymphoma including mycosis has not been confirmed and should not be routinely recommended (Grade B). In a retrospective study aimed at comparing the sensitivity of FDG-PET and CT scan for initial staging of mycosis fungoides, the sensitivity of FDG-PET was 80% for distant disease, as compared to 100% with CT scan (Level IV) (KUMAR et al. 2006).
- The required imaging and laboratory work-ups for mycosis fungoides are listed in Table 30.1.

Table 30.1. Imaging and laboratory work-ups for mycosis fungoides

Imaging studies	Laboratory tests
– Chest X-ray for localized (stage I) disease – CT scan of the chest, abdomen, and pelvis for more advanced disease	– Complete blood count and differential count – Serum chemistry – Liver/renal function tests – Lactate dehydrogenase (LDH) – Flow cytometry of peripheral blood – PCR for T-cell receptor gene rearrangement

Pathology

- Pathological evaluation of tissue biopsy including skin and large lymph nodes is required. Immunophenotyping and T-cell receptor gene rearrangement should be performed. Mycosis fungoides is typically positive for the pan T-cell markers (CD2+, CD3+, CD5+), helper T-cell marker (CD4+), memory T-cell marker (CD45RO+), and cutaneous lymphoid antigen (CLA+), and negative for the cytotoxic T-cell marker (CD8–) and activated T-cell marker (CD30–).
- Bone marrow aspirate and biopsy is usually not indicated, unless patients present with unexplained cytopenias.
- Sézary syndrome is a distinct disease entity within the realm of cutaneous T-cell lymphoma according to the EORTC-WHO classification for cutaneous lymphomas (WILLEMZE et al. 2005). Sézary syndrome is defined as generalized erythroderma with evidence of malignant circulating T cells. Its pathological association with mycosis fungoides has not been confirmed, although the two disease entities were often discussed together historically.

30.1.2 Staging

- Mycosis fungoides is staged clinically based on the extent and characteristics of skin lesions, status of lymph node involvement, presence of visceral disease, as well as presence of circulating atypical cells (Sézary cells) (Greene et al. 2002).
- The Tumor Node Metastasis (TNM) staging system of the American Joint Committee on Cancer (AJCC) for mycosis fungoides is outlined in Table 30.2.

Table 30.2. American Joint Committee on Cancer (AJCC) TNM classification of cutaneous lymphoma. [From Greene et al. (2002) with permission]

Primary tumor (T)	
T1	Patches and/or plaques involving < 10% body surface area
T2	Patches and/or plaques involving ≥ 10% body surface area
T3	One or more cutaneous tumors
T4	Generalized erythroderma
Regional lymph nodes (N)	
N0	Lymph nodes clinically uninvolved
N1	Lymph nodes clinically enlarged but histologically uninvolved
N2	Lymph nodes clinically nonpalpable but histologically involved
N3	Lymph nodes clinically enlarged and histologically involved
Distant metastasis (M)	
M0	No visceral disease present
M1	Visceral disease present
B0	No circulating atypical cells (< 1,000 Sézary cells [CD4 CD7-]/ μL)
B1	Circulating atypical cells present (> 1,000 Sézary cells [CD4 CD7-]/μL) (The B descriptor is not considered in stage classification.)
STAGE GROUPING	
IA:	T1 N0 M0
IB:	T2 N0 M0
IIA:	T1-2 N1 M0
IIB:	T3 N0-1 M0
IIIA:	T4 N0 M0
IIIB:	T4 N1 M0
IVA:	T1-4 N2-3 M0
IVB:	T1-4 N0-3 M1

30.1.3 Prognostic Factors

- Stage at diagnosis is the most important prognostic factor in mycosis fungoides: The long-term (30-year) survival of patients with stage IA disease is similar to the expected survival of a race-, age-, and gender-matched control population, according to a series reported from Stanford University (Level IV) (Kim et al. 1996). The median survival time of patients with T2 disease is more than 10 years, versus less than 5 years for patients with T3 or T4 diseases. Presence of extracutaneous disease (i.e., N+ and/or M+) is associated with poor prognosis and a median survival of approximately 1 year (Level IV) (de Coninck et al. 2001; Ysebaert et al. 2004).
- The survival rate is adversely associated with B1 classification (> 1000 Sézary cells in circulation) (Level IV) (Kim 1995; Scarisbrick et al. 2001).
- Like other types of NHL, advanced age (65 years or older) and elevated serum LDH are associated with poor outcome after treatment (Level IV) (Kim et al. 1995; Diamandidou et al. 1999). Elevated soluble interleukin-2 receptor levels, identical T-cell clone in the skin and peripheral blood, T-cell clonality in dermatopathic lymph nodes and within the cutaneous infiltrate detected by PCR have also been reported to adversely affect the prognosis of mycosis fungoides.

30.2 Treatment of Mycosis Fungoides

30.2.1 General Principles

- For stage IA (T1 N0 M0) mycosis fungoides, localized and superficial electron-beam radiation therapy is a reasonable first-line treatment (Grade B).
- For more extensive disease (T2–T4 diseases), total skin electron-beam therapy (TSEBT) can be recommended as a primary treatment (Grade B). The efficacy of TSEBT as compared to that of other treatment modalities has not been studied prospectively.
- Topical therapies including steroids, mechlorethamine, carmustine, psoralen plus ultraviolet A (PUVA), and ultraviolet B are effective for cutaneous mycosis fungoides as initial treatment. Their efficacy as compared to superficial skin ir-

radiation has not been studied in any prospective trials.

- Systemic chemotherapy or immunotherapy is not indicated in the treatment of early-stage mycosis fungoides, and is usually reserved for refractory cutaneous disease or disease with visceral metastasis (Grade A).

30.2.2 Radiation Therapy

Stage IA Mycosis Fungoides

- Local and superficial radiation therapy is a reasonable first-line treatment of limited and isolated patches and/or plaques (stage IA) (Grade B). The prognosis of patients with stage IA mycosis fungoides after definitive radiation therapy is favorable, and long-term disease-free survival approaching 90% can be expected.
- The efficacy of radiation therapy has not been prospectively compared with other forms of treatment, such as topical steroids, mechlorethamine, or PUVA. Results from a retrospective series from Stanford University showed that patients treated with radiation (TSEBT) achieved a more favorable freedom-from-relapse outcome than those treated with topical mechlorethamine hydrochloride (nitrogen mustard). However, no significant difference in survival was observed between the two treatment groups (Level IV) (KIM et al. 1996).
- Involved-field radiation therapy using electron-beam or superficial X-ray to the disease area with a margin of 2–3 cm, with sufficient coverage to a depth of 4 mm is usually sufficient. A single radiation field should be used whenever possible for small lesions. For lesions of the convex or concave skin surface (such as scalp, axilla, hand, or foot), a single radiation field may not be feasible and matched abutting fields can be applied. Feathering of the junction of the fields should be considered on a weekly basis for dose homogeneity.
- Radiation dose of 30 Gy or more delivered at 1.2–2 Gy per daily fraction is recommended for definitive treatment of stage IA mycosis fungoides (Grade B). Mycosis fungoides is highly sensitive to radiotherapy with little ability for radiation-induced sublethal damage repair. Results of retrospective studies have indicated that a dose-response relationship exists for localized super-

ficial treatment of mycosis fungoides, and doses higher than 30 Gy were associated with improved disease control:

In a group of 20 patients with 191 lesions of mycosis fungoides treated with various doses of radiation for palliation, a significant dose response to radiotherapy (superficial X-ray, Cobalt-60, or electron-beam) was observed. In-field recurrence occurred in approximately 40% of the lesions treated to 10 Gy or less, ~ 30% for those treated to 10–20 Gy, ~ 20% for those irradiated to 20–30 Gy, and none in lesions treated to 30 Gy or higher (Level IV) (COTTER et al. 1983). Additionally, experience from Yale University revealed that the disease-free survival and local control rates reached 91% after superficial radiotherapy for patients with stage IA mycosis fungoides irradiated to > 20 Gy; however, 20% of patients treated with 20 Gy or less experienced local treatment failure (Level IV) (WILSON et al. 1998).

In a retrospective review of 18 patients with unilesional mycosis fungoides reported by MICAILY et al. (1998), all patients except one were treated to 30.6 Gy or more with superficial radiation therapy. Complete response was observed in all patients within 4–8 weeks, and no in-field recurrence was observed. The actuarial relapse-free and overall survival rates at 10 years were 86.2% and 100%, respectively (Level IV).

Stage IB, II, and III Mycosis Fungoides

- TSEBT can be recommended for definitive treatment of stage IB–III mycosis fungoides (Grade B). The efficacy of TSEBT (with or without boost treatment for cutaneous tumors) in the treatment of mycosis fungoides has been repeatedly demonstrated. A complete response rate of > 70% can be expected for stage IB, II, or III disease after TSEBT (Level IV) (CHINN et al. 1999; JONES et al. 2002; QUIRÓS et al. 1996, 1997).
  Despite its efficacy, the palliative effect of TSEBT has not been prospectively compared to other treatment modalities.
- Before delivering TSEBT, a "boost" treatment to symptomatic areas using electron-beam radiation therapy can be considered at 1–2 weeks prior to the administration of TSEBT (Grade D). A single dose of 4–6 Gy using electron-beam therapy of appropriate energy can produce substantial improvement in symptoms (EORTC, Level IV) (JONES et al. 2002).

■ The target volume of stage IB and II diseases should include the epidermis and dermis, whereas the target volume of stage III (cutaneous tumors) disease may also include the full depth of the tumors. A total dose of at least 26 Gy should be prescribed to a depth of 4 mm in truncal skin as recommended by the EORTC guidelines for TSEBT (Table 30.3) (JONES et al. 2002). The surface dose is 31–36 Gy using 4- to 6-MeV electron beams (Grade B).

Results from two retrospective studies demonstrated a dose–response relationship of mycosis fungoides to TSEBT: a retrospective review of 176 patients treated at Stanford University showed that the complete response rate approached 95% with a total dose of 30–36 Gy, as compared to 75% or less with doses lower than 30 Gy (Level IV) (HOPPE et al. 1977). Similar findings were observed in a more recently published study. The complete response rate reached 85% for patients irradiated to 36 Gy, as compared to 64% for those who received 30 Gy or less for TSEBT (Level IV) (JONES et al. 1994).

■ For T3 lesions (cutaneous tumors) that extend deeper than 4 mm from the skin surface, boost irradiation using higher voltage electron-beam therapy to an additional 10–20 Gy over five to ten fractions can be given with minimal margins (Grade D) (EORTC, Level IV) (JONES et al. 2002).

■ TSEBT can be delivered for a second time for symptomatic palliation in recurrent mycosis fungoides (Grade B). Complete and partial response rates ranging from 50% to 85% have been reported after ~ 23 Gy prescribed to the skin surface (Level IV) (BECKER et al. 1995; WILSON et al. 1996).

Treatment Schedule and Technique

■ TSEBT should be delivered on 36 treatment days (1 Gy per day, 4 days per week) over 9 weeks. Six treatment positions are used: anteroposterior (AP), right anterior oblique (RAO), left anterior oblique (LAO), posteroanterior (PA), right posterior oblique (RPO), and left posterior oblique (LPO) (Fig. 30.1).
Treatment fields include AP/RPO/LPO on day 1 and PA/RAO/LAO on day 2. This 2-day treatment cycle is repeated twice weekly over 4 days (Fig. 30.2). The geometric arrangement of the symmetrical dual-field treatment technique is illustrated in

Table 30.3. EORTC guidelines for total skin electron-beam therapy

– Dose inhomogeneity in air at treatment distance should be < 10% within vertical and lateral dimensions
– 80% Isodose line should be > 4 mm deep to the skin surface to ensure that the epidermis and dermis fall within the high dose region
– 80% Isodose line should receive a minimum total dose of 26 Gy
– 20% Isodose line should be < 20 mm from the skin surface to minimize dose to underlying structures
– 30–36 Fractions should be used to minimize acute side effects
– Total dose to bone marrow from photon contamination should be less than 0.7 Gy
– Patch treatments should be utilized to underdosed areas such as the perineum, scalp, and soles of feet
– Internal and external eye shields should be used to ensure that the dose to the globe is not more than 15% of the prescribed skin surface dose

Figure 30.3. Each of the six treatment positions is treated with both an upper and a lower field to maximize dose homogeneity.

■ Patch treatment is recommended to the underdosed area (Grade B). TSEBT using the six-position technique can maximize the skin unfolding and ensure the homogeneity of dose distribution. However, the soles of feet are usually not treated, as well as other parts that may be underdosed with TSEBT, including scalp, inframammary, pannicular, perianal, buttocks/thighs, inner thighs, and perineal skin regions. Analysis of the in vivo dosimetric data of patients treated with TSEBT demonstrated that the dose inhomogeneity throughout the skin surface is approximately 15% (Level IV) (ANACAK et al. 2003).

TSEBT-Induced Side Effects and Complications

■ Commonly observed toxicities are usually limited to skin reaction secondary to TSEBT and include erythema, dry desquamation, hypohidrosis, pruritus, xerosis, bullae of the feet, alopecia, and loss of fingernails and toenails.
Radiation-induced toxicities to bone marrow is minimal from TSEBT, and cytopenias are usually not expected.
Patients at reproductive age should be informed about toxicities to the testis or ovaries. Severe

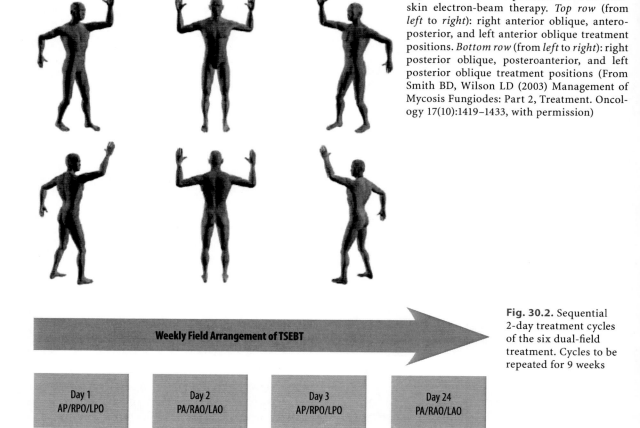

Fig. 30.1. Treatment positions used in total-skin electron-beam therapy. *Top row* (from *left* to *right*): right anterior oblique, antero-posterior, and left anterior oblique treatment positions. *Bottom row* (from *left* to *right*): right posterior oblique, posteroanterior, and left posterior oblique treatment positions (From Smith BD, Wilson LD (2003) Management of Mycosis Fungiodes: Part 2, Treatment. Oncology 17(10):1419–1433, with permission)

Fig. 30.2. Sequential 2-day treatment cycles of the six dual-field treatment. Cycles to be repeated for 9 weeks

long-term toxicity or complication rarely occur, but may include radiation-induced second primary cancer.

30.2.3 Other Treatments for Mycosis Fungoides

- Other treatment modalities effective for the initial treatment of mycosis fungoides include interferon-α-2a, psoralen plus ultraviolet A (PUVA) and ultraviolet B, photopheresis, topical steroids, mechlorethamine, rexinoids, and carmustine.
- Adjuvant treatment can be considered after TSEBT and may improve disease-free survival for advanced mycosis fungoides (Grade B). In a retrospective study reported by Quirós et al. (1997), PUVA was used as an adjuvant therapy for a group of patients with T1 or T2 cutaneous T-cell lymphoma after TSEBT. The results

of the study revealed that adjuvant PUVA significantly extended the median disease-free survival; however, overall survival was not affected (Level IV). The efficacy of topical nitrogen mustard as adjuvant treatment after TSEBT for disease control was also demonstrated in a retrospective study in patients with T2 or T3 mycosis fungoides (Level IV) (Chinn et al. 1999). Other adjuvant therapy modalities after TSEBT such as photopheresis, interferon-α, or bexarotene were also reported to be effective.
- Systemic chemotherapy is not recommended for initial treatment of mycosis fungoides, and is reserved for the treatment of refractory disease or visceral disease (Grade A). Although the addition of systemic chemotherapy to radiation could improve the complete response rate, the overall treatment outcome was not altered. The long-term follow-up results of a randomized trial aimed at comparing the outcome after sequential topical therapy and combined TSEBT plus chemotherapy did not demonstrate any significant

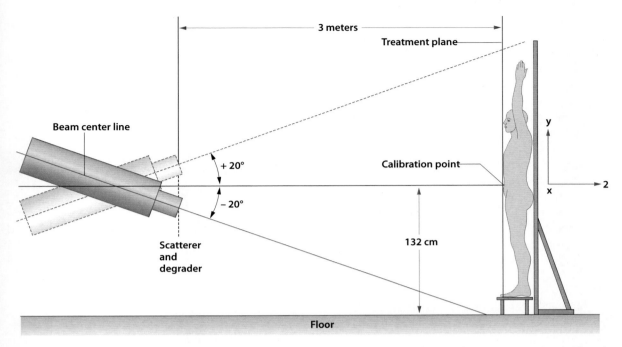

Fig. 30.3. Geometrical arrangement of the symmetrical dual-field treatment technique. Equal exposures are given with each beam. The calibration point dose is at (x=0, y=0) in the treatment plane

difference between disease-free or overall survival (Level I) (Kaye et al. 1989).

■ Systemic chemotherapy and immunotherapy play an important role in the treatment of refractory mycosis fungoides.

30.3 Follow-Ups

30.3.1 Post-Treatment Follow-Ups

■ Long-term follow-up after treatment of mycosis fungoides is recommended for early detection of recurrence and treatment complications (Grade D).

Schedule and Work-Ups

■ Patients should be followed-up every 3 months by their radiation oncologists or dermatologists (Grade D).

– Each follow-up should include a complete history and physical examination with attention to the lesion(s) treated and new cutaneous lesion(s).

Biopsy of any suspicious lesion(s) should be performed.

– Complete blood count and other laboratory tests can be ordered if clinically indicated. Serum LDH, IL-2 receptor levels and CD4:CD8 ratio should be monitored in patients with abnormal values at diagnosis.

– Imaging studies are usually not needed in follow-up unless indicated by clinical symptoms (Grade D).

30.4 Diagnosis, Staging, and Prognoses of Nasal NK/T-Cell Lymphoma

30.4.1 Diagnosis

Initial Evaluation

■ Diagnosis and evaluation of nasal NK/T-cell lymphoma start with a complete history and physical examination. A thorough physical examination with special attention to the disease area and neck lymph nodes is important.

- A careful examination of the facial skin is warranted as this disease shows a propensity to skin involvement at presentation and during progression and recurrence.
- All patients should be examined with special focus on the upper aerodigestive tract including nasopharynx, oropharynx, palate, base of the tongue, tonsil, hypopharynx, and larynx for exclusion of multifocal disease.
- Patients' performance status and "B" symptoms are of prognostic significance and should be evaluated and recorded.

Laboratory Tests

- Initial blood tests should include a complete blood count with differential, basic blood chemistry, liver and renal function tests, and lactate dehydrogenase (LDH).
- EBV serology may be useful for predicting the prognosis for patients with EBV+ nasal-type NK/T-cell lymphoma.

Imaging Studies

- MRI and CT scan of the head and neck area are recommended in all cases of nasal NK/T-cell lymphoma, as paranasal extension into the adjacent organs or tissues and metastasis to the neck nodes is common (Grade B). The disease usually presents as a soft tissue mass of the nasal cavity with bone erosion or destruction on imaging studies; however, the findings on MRI and/or CT scan are usually nonspecific, as confirmed in three small retrospective studies (Level IV) (Ooi et al. 2000; KING et al. 2000; Ou et al. 2007).
- CT scan of the chest, abdomen, and pelvis is recommended to evaluate the status of organ involvement.
- FDG-PET/CT has not been extensively studied and its value for local disease evaluation has not been confirmed. In a small study of 41 patients with extranodal T-cell and NK-cell lymphomas, eight patients with nasal-type NK/T-cell lymphoma showed 100% positive rate (Level IV) (KAKO et al. 2007). In another study of seven patients with 30 involved sites, ^{18}F-FDG-PET identified all disease sites (100%) (Level IV) (TSUKAMOTO et al. 2007). The value of FDG-PET for evaluating distant me-

tastasis from nasal NK/T-cell lymphoma has not been documented either.

- The required imaging and laboratory work-ups for diagnosis and staging of nasal NK/T-cell lymphoma are listed in Table 30.4.

Table 30.4. Imaging and laboratory work-ups for nasal NK/T-cell lymphoma

Imaging studies	Laboratory tests
– Chest X-ray – MRI or CT scan of the head and neck, preferably MRI – CT scan of the chest, abdomen, and pelvis	– Complete blood count and differential count – Serum chemistry – Liver and renal function tests – Lactate dehydrogenase (LDH) – Peripheral EBV serology

Pathology

- Pathologic diagnosis of extranodal NK/T-cell lymphoma of nasal and nasal type is required before determining the treatment strategy. The primary treatment of nasal NK/T-cell lymphoma differs significantly from other types of NHL occurring in the same region.
- Repeated biopsy is usually required to obtain sufficient tissue for pathologic diagnosis, due to extensive necrosis of the affected area and small sample sizes.
- According to the WHO classification, extranodal NK/T-cell lymphoma consists of at least two major subtypes: nasal NK/T-cell lymphoma and nasal-type NK/T-cell lymphoma. The nasal cavity is the most common and prototypic site of involvement. The term "nasal NK/T-cell lymphoma" is used only for those cases presenting in the nasal cavity. Tumors with an identical morphology and phenotype occur in the extra-nasal sites, mostly in the Waldeyer's ring, skin, gastrointestinals, and soft tissue, and should be referred to as nasal-type.
- The typical phenotype of nasal and nasal-type NK/T-cell lymphoma is CD2+CD56+, surface CD3– and cytoplasmic CD3+, CD20–/CD79α, cytotoxic molecule (TIA, Granzyme B, Perforin)+, and EBV+. Other NK and T-cell markers are usually negative: CD4, CD8, CD16, and TCR. CD43, CD45RO, Fas (CD95) and Fas ligand are commonly expressed (HARRIS et al. 2000; JAFFE et al. 1996; CHAN et al. 2001).
- EBV infection is observed in more than 90% of nasal NK/T-cell lymphoma cases. In contrast,

EBV expression is relatively low (40%–76%) for nasal-type NK/T-cell lymphoma outside the nasal cavity (Level IV) (Ko et al. 2004; Kanavaros et al. 1993; van Gorp et al. 1994; Arber et al. 1993; Chan et al. 1994; Hahn et al. 2002).

30.4.2 Staging

- Extranodal NK/T-cell lymphoma of nasal type is usually clinically staged using information from physical examination, laboratory tests, and bone marrow biopsy.
- The Ann Arbor Staging System for both NHL and Hodgkin's disease is commonly used for the staging of extranodal NK/T-cell lymphoma of nasal type (Table 27.3).
- To assess the prognostic value of paranasal extension, Ann Arbor Stage IE can be subclassified into limited- and extensive-stage IE (Grade B). Limited-stage IE tumors were confined to the nasal cavity, whereas extensive-stage IE tumors extended beyond the nasal cavity and into the neighboring structures without any dissemination (Level IV) (Li et al. 1998, 2006).

30.4.3 Prognostic Factors

- Prognosis of nasal NK/T-cell lymphoma varied from series to series. Variations in patient population and selection of initial treatment modality (i.e., chemotherapy vs. radiation therapy) significantly affected the reported outcome.
- Stage at diagnosis is one of the most important prognostic factors for nasal NK/T-cell lymphoma. The 5-year overall survival rate was 40%–86% for stage IE and IIE diseases, whereas long-term survival in stage III or IV diseases is rarely observed. Patients with stage IE had a much better prognosis as compared to those with stage IIE, with 5-year overall survival rates of about 70% for stage IE and less than 50% for stage II, respectively (Level IV) (Aviles et al. 2000; Cheung et al. 2002; Chim et al. 2004; Huang et al. 2008; Kim et al. 2001; Ko et al. 2004; Koom et al. 2004; Li et al. 2004; Li et al. 2006; You et al. 2004).
- The survival rate is adversely associated with paranasal extension, "B" symptoms, poor performance, elevated LDH, and regional lymph nodes

(Level IV) (Kim et al. 2005; Lee et al. 2006; Li et al. 2006).

- The prognostic value of the international prognostic index (IPI) for aggressive lymphoma or modified IPI (stage II as adverse factor) was largely confirmed in many recent studies (Li et al. 2006; Chim et al. 2004; Li et al. 2004; Na et al. 2007; Kim TM et al. 2005; Pagano et al. 2006), but not in other studies (Kim et al. 2007; Aviles et al. 2000; Cheung et al. 2002). A prognostic model for nasal and nasal-type NK/T-cell lymphoma was suggested. The adverse prognostic factors include B symptoms, LDH, and regional lymph nodes (Level IV) (Lee et al. 2006).
- Nasal-type NK/T-cell lymphoma of the extra-upper aerodigestive tract has a highly aggressive clinical course with a worse prognosis as compared to those occur in the nasal cavity. The median survival for these patients was only 3.5–19 months (Level IV) (Bekkenk et al. 2004; Mraz-Gernhard et al. 2001; Lee et al. 2005a,b; Lee et al. 2006).
- The expression of EBV, Ki-67 and COX-2, and p53 mutation were associated with poor outcome (Level IV) (Hahn et al. 2002; Ko et al. 2004; Kim et al. 2007; Shim et al. 2007).

30.5 Treatment of Nasal NK/T-Cell Lymphoma

30.5.1 General Principles

- For localized extranodal NK/T-cell lymphoma originating from the nasal area (nasal NK/T-cell lymphoma) (stage IE and IIE), radiation therapy is the primary treatment of choice (Grade A).
- Chemotherapy has a limited role in the definitive treatment of stage IE and IIE NK/T-cell lymphoma and does not prolong overall survival in early-stage disease. Chemotherapy should not be utilized as an initial treatment prior to the completion of definitive radiation therapy (Grade A).
- The optimal treatment for stage III and IV nasal NK/T-cell lymphoma is largely unknown. Patients with advanced nasal NK/T-cell lymphoma should be encouraged to participate in prospective clinical trials. These patients usually carry a very poor prognosis, even after aggressive chemotherapy.
- The treatment strategy of extranodal nasal-type NK/T-cell lymphoma located in other sites has

30.5.2 Radiation Therapy of Early-Stage Disease

Radiation Therapy

■ Radiation therapy is the mainstay treatment of stage I and II disease (Grade A). Five large retrospective studies have demonstrated that the outcome with primary radiotherapy was superior to initial chemotherapy or chemotherapy alone. A definite advantage of primary radiotherapy has been ascertained and confirmed in two large studies: In a series of 105 patients with stage I and II nasal NK/T-cell lymphoma receiving primary radiotherapy, the 5-year OS and PFS were 71% and 59% for stage I and II disease combined (78% and 63% for stage IE disease, and 46% and 40% for stage IIE disease, respectively) (Level IV) (Li et al. 2006).These finding confirmed the previously reported data from Mexico, which showed that in 108 patients with early-stage nasal NK/T-cell lymphoma treated with radiotherapy followed by four cycles of CHOP-bleo, the 8-year OS and DFS was 86% (Level IV) (Aviles et al. 2000).

In addition, in a study of 82 patients with localized NK/T-cell lymphoma of the upper aerodigestive tract (77% of nasal NK/T-cell lymphoma), stage IE disease, 18 patients receiving up-front radiotherapy (radiotherapy alone or radiotherapy followed by chemotherapy) had significantly better overall survival and disease-free survival compared to that of 28 patients receiving initial chemotherapy (5-year OS 90% vs. 48.9%, p = 0.012; 5-year DFS 78.7% vs. 39.9%, p = 0.021) (Level IV) (Huang et al. 2008).

Results from a number of other retrospective trials also confirmed that the overall survival of patients with stage I and II nasal NK/T-cell lymphoma treated with radiotherapy were in the range of 80%, whereas those treated with chemotherapy as primary treatment were less than 30% (Level IV) (Chim et al. 2004; Li et al. 2004; You et al. 2004).

Radiation Technique

■ An "extended" involved field is recommended to irradiate the early-stage nasal NK/T-cell lymphoma. The clinical target and radiation fields have been investigated previously in several studies (Level IV) (Li et al. 1998, 2006; Isobe et al. 2006; Koom et al. 2004). In general, the clinical target is suggested to cover all gross tumor and adjacent organs and structures. For patients with primary tumor confined to the nasal cavity (limited-stage IE), clinical target encompassed the bilateral nasal cavity, hard plate, ipsilateral maxillary sinus, and bilateral anterior ethmoid sinuses. It also included the nasopharynx when the primary tumor was close to the posterior nasal aperture. For those patients with extensive-stage IE and stage IIE, the clinical target volume was extended to the involved paranasal organs/tissues or cervical lymph nodes. A higher local failure with small radiation target volume was observed in a retrospective study. In a study of 35 patients with stage I and II nasal and nasal-type NK/T-cell lymphoma who were treated with radiotherapy, 27 patients received radiotherapy that included all macroscopic lesions and sites of potential contiguous spread, such as all paranasal sinuses, palate, and the nasopharynx with adequate margins, whereas the remaining eight patients encompassed all lesions with generous margins (small field). The 5-year local control probability was 71.9% versus 41.7%, respectively (p = 0.007) (Level IV) (Isobe et al. 2006). Similarly, Li et al. (2004) reported that in 56 patients with stage I and II nasal NK/T-cell lymphoma, the radiation fields included the involved primary with adequate margins and radiation dose was 40–50 Gy. Of these patients, 24 (43%) developed local failure (Level IV).

■ For stage IE disease confined to the nasal cavity (limited-stage IE), a single anterior port including the nasal cavity and the ipsilateral maxillary/ethmoid sinuses was used, whereas for patients with extensive disease or limited-stage IE disease close to the choanae, two lateral opposing fields and an anteroposterior port were used, which extended to encompass involved paranasal tissues, nasopharynx, and other adjacent structures or organs. For those with stage IIE disease, the fields were extended to encompass also the involved cervical lymph nodes (Fig. 30.4). Three-dimensional conformal radiotherapy (3D-CRT) can be used for better dose distribution; the effects of intensity-modulated radiotherapy (IMRT) are being studied.

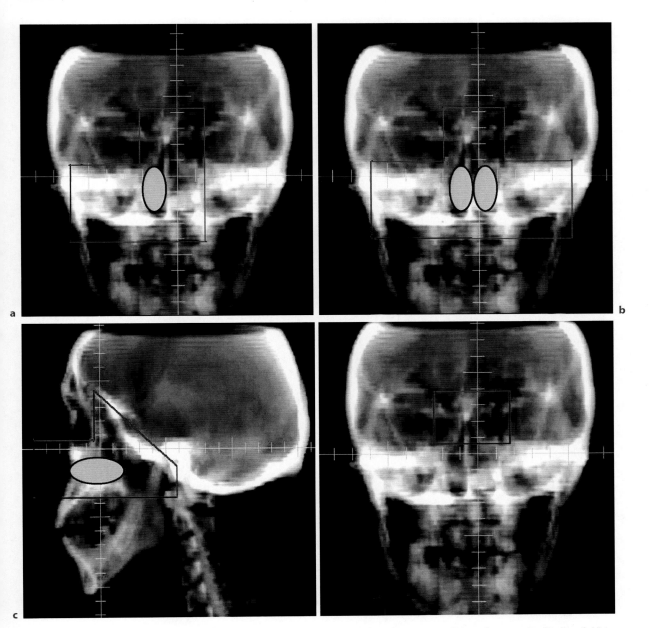

Fig. 30.4a–c. Proposed radiation field arrangement for the treatment of nasal NK/T-cell lymphoma. **a** Radiation field in patients with tumor involving the right nasal cavity; **b** radiation field in patients with tumor involving bilateral nasal cavity; **c** radiation field in patients with tumor close to the posterior nasal aperture or extended into the nasopharynx

■ Prophylactic cervical node irradiation was not necessary for patients with stage IE nasal NK/T-cell lymphoma (Grade A). The most common sites of failure are extranodal metastases, especially in the skin, whereas relapse in the cervical lymph nodes (< 5%) is uncommon: Lı et al. (1998) reported that in 175 patients with nasal lymphoma (majority of which were NK/T-cell-type), prophylactic neck irradiation was not used in 106 of 133 stage IE patients, two of whom (2%) developed progression in the cervical lymph nodes, whereas none of the remaining 27 stage IE patients treated with prophylactic neck irradiation developed cervical progression or recurrence (Level IV) (Lı et al. 1998). Similarly, only one of 46 (2%) stage IE patients with nasal and nasal-type NK/T-cell lymphoma who did not receive elective neck radiotherapy developed regional lymph node recurrence as reported in another retrospective trial (Level IV) (Koom et al. 2004).

■ Radical radiation dose in a range between 50 Gy and 55 Gy at 1.8–2 Gy per fraction, with a boost of 5–10 Gy to the residual tumor is recommended for definitive treatment (Grade A). Nasal NK/T-cell lymphoma is a radiosensitive disease and complete response can be achieved at lower doses; however, lower total dose of irradiation (< 50 Gy) and small field size (i.e., tumor bed plus a margin without surrounding tissues as described) has resulted in higher local failure in several studies. With the large radiation fields and high doses (median dose of 50 Gy) to the nasal cavity and neighboring organs or structures, a local failure of 7.8% was observed in 102 patients with nasal NK/T-cell lymphoma receiving radiotherapy. Due to the small numbers of patients receiving low doses of 40–45 Gy or high doses of > 55 Gy, a dose–response relationship between local failure and optimal radiation dose was not defined in this series (Level IV) (Li et al. 2006). In another large study of 102 patients with stage I–II nasal and nasal-type NK/T-cell lymphoma of the head and neck areas, a median dose of 45 Gy was given. The complete response (CR) rate was 72% after radiotherapy, whereas the local failure was 47% for all patients. The local failure was 64% for < 45 Gy as compared to 38% for ≥ 45 Gy ($p = 0.02$) (Level IV) (Koom et al. 2004). Although this study demonstrated a dose–response relation within the range of 20–54 Gy with a plateau at doses in excess of approximately 54 Gy, it should be pointed out that radiation dose of 45 Gy is not optimal for radical radiotherapy and may contribute to extremely high local failure in this series. You et al. (2004) administered higher radiotherapy doses of 54–60 Gy and achieved a 5-year failure-free survival rate of 83.3% (Level IV). In another study of 74 stage I and II patients receiving radiotherapy, the 5-year OS and DFS were 75.5% and 46.1% for ≥ 54 Gy, as compared to 60.3% and 33.4% for < 54 Gy ($p < 0.05$) (Level IV) (Huang et al. 2008). Shikama et al. (2001) reported that the 5-year local control was significantly higher with a total dose of ≥ 50 Gy as compared to < 50 Gy (100% vs. 67%, $p = 0.013$) for patients with nasal lymphomas (Level IV). In agreement with this data, Isobe et al. (2006) reported a local failure rate of 67% for < 50 Gy and 27% for ≥ 50 Gy in 35 patients with nasal and nasal-type NK/T-cell lymphoma ($p = 0.038$) (Level IV).

Chemotherapy

■ Chemotherapy is not recommended for primary treatment in stage IE and IIE nasal NK/T-cell lymphoma (Grade B). Results of a number of retrospective trials have demonstrated that chemotherapy has no effect on both disease-free and overall survival rates. In addition, nasal NK/T-cell lymphoma is refractory to conventional chemotherapy. The reported complete response rate ranged from 8% to 59% after chemotherapy, the majority being below 40% (Ribrag et al. 2001; Kim et al. 2001; Kim et al. 2001; Kim et al. 2005; Yong et al. 2006; Guo et al. 2008; Huang et al. 2008). The low response rate and poor prognosis after chemotherapy alone reflect the resistance to conventional combination chemotherapy and is associated with P53 mutation and MDR expression (Level IV) (Yamaguchi et al. 1995; Quintanilla-Martinez et al. 2001; Takahara et al. 2004; Li et al. 2000).

■ Adjuvant chemotherapy is not recommended for early-stage nasal NK/T-cell lymphoma (Grade A). The addition of chemotherapy to radiotherapy does not improve the survival: In the above-mentioned study of 105 patients with stage I and II nasal NK/T-cell lymphoma, 31 patients were treated with radiotherapy alone, 34 with radiotherapy followed by chemotherapy, and 37 patients with a short course of combination chemotherapy (one to four cycles) followed by radiotherapy, and only three patients with chemotherapy alone. The 5-year OS and PFS were 76% and 61% for combined modality therapy as compared to 66% and 61% for radiotherapy alone ($p = 0.6433$ for OS, $p = 0.8391$ for PFS) (Level IV) (Li et al. 2006). There was no statistically significant difference in OS and PFS between the two groups. For stage IE patients, the 5-year OS and PFS with combined modality therapy were 80% and 64%, while those with radiotherapy alone were 73% and 63%, respectively ($p = 0.9274$ for OS and $p = 0.8533$ for PFS).

Several recent large series have also reported no convincing clinical benefit by adding conventional chemotherapy to radiotherapy: Kim et al. (2001) reported that in a series of 143 Korean patients with stage I and II angiocentric lymphoma of the head and neck area, 104 patients were treated with radiotherapy alone and 39 with chemotherapy followed by radiotherapy. The CR rate was much higher with radiotherapy than those with chemotherapy (69% versus 8%); for patients receiving initial chemotherapy, an overall CR rate of 67% could be achieved after salvage radiotherapy. However, no statistically significant difference in survival was observed between RT alone and CMT (5-year OS, 35% versus 38%). CHEUNG et al. (2002) reported that in a series of 79 Chinese patients with stage I and II nasal NK/T-cell lymphoma, the majority of patients were treated with chemotherapy followed by radiotherapy (actually radiotherapy as salvage therapy in the latter group). The 5-year OS and DFS for all patients were 37.9% and 35.5%, respectively. The 5-year OS and DFS were 40.3% and 35.8% for CMT as compared to 29.8% and 30.5% for radiotherapy alone ($p = 0.693$ for OS and $p = 0.795$ for DFS). Of 61 patients receiving initial chemotherapy, 31 (51%) had disease progression and 17 of them progressed locoregionally. Nine of the latter patients were successfully salvaged with further radiotherapy. However, of 18 patients receiving radiotherapy, 14 patients (78%) achieved a CR, whereas none of the remaining four patients, who had disease progression, were salvaged with chemotherapy. Another Korean study reported on 53 patients with stage I and II nasal and nasal-type NK/T-cell lymphoma, 33 patients were treated with radiotherapy and 20 patients with chemotherapy and radiotherapy. The 5-year OS was 76% for radiotherapy alone and 59% for CMT, respectively ($p = 0.27$) (KIM et al. 2005).

■ The high local progression or relapse after chemotherapy alone or initial chemotherapy was observed in several studies of patients with early-stage disease, and some of those patients can be successfully salvaged with radiotherapy (KIM et al. 2003; LEE KW et al. 2006; KIM et al. 2006; CHEUNG et al. 2002). Again, the low rate of complete response and high local failure with chemotherapy and successful salvage with radiotherapy indicate the important role of radiotherapy as primary therapy for early stage patients.

■ Conventional CHOP-based chemotherapy combined with L-asparaginase or oral nitrosourea was evaluated in a few studies. Its value was not confirmed as all these patients received salvage radiotherapy following initial chemotherapy (YONG 2006; GUO et al. 2008).

A new chemotherapeutic regimen, IMEP (ifosfamide, methotrexate, etoposide and prednisolone), was evaluated in a study of 26 patients with nasal or upper aerodigestive tract localization (LEE et al. 2006). The CR rate after IMEP was observed in 12 of 22 (55%) evaluable patients. Of the 14 patients with stage I and II diseases, 11 (79%) achieved CR with chemotherapy alone, and seven developed local recurrence.

30.5.3 Treatment of Stage III and IV Disease

■ Conventional chemotherapy is the primary treatment for patients with stage III and IV disease. However, patients with extensive diseases have an extremely poor prognosis and survival of more than 5 years is rare. The poor prognosis and extranodal progression observed in patients with stage III–IV disease clearly illustrates the need for innovative systemic treatments.

■ Palliative radiotherapy can be used for these patients.

■ The data on autologous stem cell transplantation for nasal NK/T-cell lymphoma is limited and further investigation is needed. Successful treatment with autologous stem cell transplantation has been reported in several studies with small numbers of patients (Level IV) (AU et al. 2003; TAKENAKA et al. 2001; LIANG et al. 1997; SASAKI et al. 2000).

30.6 Follow-Ups

30.6.1 Post-Treatment Follow-Ups

■ Long-term follow-up after definitive treatment of nasal NK/T-cell lymphoma is recommended for early detection of recurrence (Grade D).

Schedule and Work-Ups

■ Follow-ups could be scheduled every 3 months for 2 years, then every 6 months for 3 additional years, then annually thereafter (Grade D). The incidence of late relapse is uncommon, but has been reported in the literature.

■ Each follow-up should include a complete history and physical examination, complete blood count, and LDH. CT scanning of the head and neck, abdomen and pelvis can be performed at each follow-up session for symptomatic patients; however, the effect of routine use of imaging studies during follow-on survival is not confirmed.

References

Anacak Y, Arican Z, Bar-Deroma R et al. (2003) Total skin electron irradiation: evaluation of dose uniformity throughout the skin surface. Med Dosim 28:31–34

Arber DA, Weiss LM, Albujar PF et al. (1993) Nasal lymphomas in Peru. High incidence of T-cell immunophenotype and Epstein-Barr virus infection. Am J Surg Pathol 17:392–399

Au WY, Lie AKW, Liang R et al. (2003) Autologous stem cell transplantation for nasal NK/T-cell lymphoma: a progress report on its value. Ann Oncol 14:1673–1676

Aviles A, Diaz NR, Neri N et al. (2000) Angiocentric nasal T/natural killer cell lymphoma: a single center study of prognostic factors in 108 patients. Clin Lab Haematol 22:215–220

Bass JC, Korobkin MT, Cooper KD et al. (1993) Cutaneous T-cell lymphoma: CT in evaluation and staging. Radiology 186(1):273–278

Becker M, Hoppe RT, Knox SJ. (1995) Multiple courses of high-dose total skin electron beam therapy in the management of mycosis fungoides. Int J Radiat Oncol Biol Phys 32:1445–1449

Bekkenk MW, Jansen PM, Meijer CJLM et al. (2004) CD56+ hematological neoplasms presenting in the skin: a retrospective analysis of 23 new cases and 130 cases from the literature. Ann Oncol 15:1097–1108

Chan JK, Yip TT, Tsang WY et al. (1994) Detection of Epstein-Barr viral RNA in malignant lymphomas of the upper aerodigestive tract. Am J Surg Pathol 18:938–946

Chan JKC, Jaffe ES, Ralfkiaer E (2001) Extranodal NK/T-cell lymphoma, nasal type. In: Jaffe ES, Harris NL, Stein H, Vardiman JW (eds) World Health Organization classification of tumours: pathology and genetics of tumours of haematopoietic and lymphoid tissues. IARC Press, Lyon, pp 204–207

Chim CS, Ma SY, Au WY et al. (2004) Primary nasal natural killer cell lymphoma: long-term treatment outcome and relationship with the international prognostic index. Blood 103:216–221

Chinn DM, Chow S, Kim YH et al. (1999) Total skin electron beam therapy with or without adjuvant topical nitrogen mustard or nitrogen mustard alone as initial treatment of T2 and T3 mycosis fungoides. Int J Radiat Oncol Biol Phys 43:951–958

Cheung MM, Chan JK, Lau WH et al. (2002) Early stage nasal NK/T-cell lymphoma: clinical outcome, prognostic factors, and the effect of treatment modality. Int J Radiat Oncol Biol Phys 54:182–190

Cotter GW, Baglan RJ, Wasserman TH et al. (1983) Palliative radiation treatment of cutaneous mycosis fun-

goides – a dose response. Int J Radiat Oncol Biol Phys 9:1477–1480

de Coninck EC, Kim YH, Varghese A et al. (2001) Clinical characteristics and outcome of patients with extracutaneous mycosis fungoides. J Clin Oncol 19:779–784

Diamandidou E, Colome M, Fayad L et al. (1999) Prognostic factor analysis in mycosis fungoides/Sézary syndrome. J Am Acad Dermato 40(6 Pt 1):914–924

Greene F, Page D, Fleming I et al. (2002) AJCC Cancer Staging Manual, 6th edn. Springer, Berlin Heidelberg New York

Guo Y, Lu JJ, Ma X et al. (2008) Combined chemoradiation for the management of nasal natural killer (NK)/T-cell lymphoma: elucidating the significance of systemic chemotherapy. Oral Oncol 44:23–30

Hahn JS, Lee ST, Min YH et al. (2002) Therapeutic outcome of Epstein-Barr Virus positive T/NK cell lymphoma in the upper aerodigestive tract. Yonsei Med J 43:175–182

Harris NL, Jaffe ES, Diebold J et al. (2000) The World Health Organization classification of neoplastic diseases of the haematopoietic and lymphoid tissues: report of the clinical advisory committee meeting, Airlie House, Virginia, November 1997. Histopathology 36:69–86

Hoppe RT, Fuks Z, Bagshaw MA. (1977) The rationale for curative radiotherapy in mycosis fungoides. Int J Radiat Oncol Biol Phys 2:843–851

Huang MJ, Jiang Y, Liu WP et al. (2008) Early or up-front radiotherapy improved survival of localized extranodal NK/T-cell lymphoma, nasal-type in the upper aerodigestive tract. Int J Radiat Oncol Biol Phys 70:166–174

Isobe K, Uno T, Tamaru JI et al. (2006) Extranodal natural killer/T-cell lymphoma, nasal type. Cancer 106:609–615

Jaffe ES, Chan JK, Su IJ et al. (1996) Report of the workshop on nasal and related extranodal angiocentric T/natural killer cell lymphomas: definitions, differential diagnosis and epidemiology. Am J Surg Pathol 20:103–111

Jones GW, Tadros A, Hodson DI et al. (1994) Prognosis with newly diagnosed mycosis fungoides after total skin electron radiation of 30 or 35 GY. Int J Radiat Oncol Biol Phys 28:839–845

Jones GW, Kacinski BM, Wilson LD et al. (2002) Total skin electron radiation in the management of mycosis fungoides: Consensus of the European Organization for Research and Treatment of Cancer (EORTC) Cutaneous Lymphoma Project Group. J Am Acad Dermatol 47:364–370

Kako S, Izutsu K, Ota Y et al. (2007) FDG-PET in T-cell and NK-cell neoplasms. Ann Oncol 18:1685–1690

Kanavaros P, Lescs MC, Briere J et al. (1993) Nasal T-cell lymphoma: a clinicopathologic entity associated with peculiar phenotype and with Epstein-Barr virus. Blood 81:2688–2695

Kaye FJ, Bunn PA Jr, Steinberg SM et al. (1989) A randomized trial comparing combination electron-beam radiation and chemotherapy with topical therapy in the initial treatment of mycosis fungoides. N Engl J Med 321:1784–1790

Kim BS, Kim TY, Kim CW et al. (2003) Therapeutic outcome of extranodal NK/T-cell lymphoma initially treated with chemotherapy – result of chemotherapy in NK/T-cell lymphoma. Acta Oncol. 42:779–783

Kim GE, Lee SW, Chang SK et al. (2001) Combined chemotherapy and radiation versus radiation alone in the management of localized angiocentric lymphoma of the head and neck. Radiother Oncol 61:261-269

Kim K, Chie EK, Kim CW et al. (2005) Treatment outcome of angiocentric T-cell and NK/T-cell lymphoma, nasal type: radiotherapy versus chemoradiotherapy. Jpn J Clin Oncol 35:1-5

Kim SJ, Kim BS, Choi CW et al. (2006) Treatment outcome of front-line systemic chemotherapy for localized extranodal NK/T cell lymphoma in nasal and upper aerodigestive tract. Leuk Lymphoma 47:1265-73

Kim SJ, Kim BS, Choi CW et al. (2007) Ki-67 expression is predictive of prognosis in patients with stage I/II extranodal NK/T-cell lymphoma, nasal type. Ann Oncol 18:1382-1387

Kim TM, Park YH, Lee SY et al. (2005) Local tumor invasiveness is more predictive of survival than International Prognostic Index in stage IE/IIE extranodal NK/T cell lymphoma, nasal type. Blood 106:3785-3790

Kim YH, Bishop K, Varghese A et al. (1995) Prognostic factors in erythrodermic mycosis fungoides and the Sézary syndrome. Arch Dermatol 131:1003-1008

Kim YH, Jensen RA, Watanabe GL et al. (1996) Clinical stage IA (limited patch and plaque) mycosis fungoides. A long-term outcome analysis. Arch Dermatol 132:1309-1313

King AD, Lei KIK, Ahuja AT et al. (2000) MR imaging of nasal T-cell/natural killer cell lymphoma. AJR Am J Roentgenol 174:209-211

Ko YH, Cho EY, Kim JE et al. (2004) NK and NK-like T-cell lymphoma in extranasal sites: a comparative clinicopathological study according to site and EBV status. Histopathol 44:480-489

Koom WS, Chung EJ, Yang WI et al. (2004) Angiocentric T-cell and NK/T-cell lymphomas: radiotherapeutic viewpoints. Int J Radiat Oncol Biol Phys 59:1127-1137

Kumar R, Xiu Y, Zhuang HM et al. (2006) 18F-fluorodeoxyglucose-positron emission tomography in evaluation of primary cutaneous lymphoma. Br J Dermatol 155:357-363

Lee J, Kim WS, Park YH et al. (2005a) Nasal-type NK/T cell lymphoma: clinical features and treatment outcome. Brit J Caner 92:1226-1230

Lee J, Park YH, Kim WS et al. (2005b) Extranodal nasal type NK/T-cell Lymphoma: Elucidating clinical prognostic factors for risk-based stratification of therapy. Eur J Cancer 41:1402-1408

Lee J, Suh C, Park YH et al. (2006) Extranodal natural killer T-cell lymphoma, nasal-type: a prognostic model from a retrospective multicenter study. J Clin Oncol 24:612-618

Lee KW, Yun T, Kim DW et al. (2006) First-line ifosfamide, methotrexate, etoposide and prednisolone chemotherapy ± radiotherapy is active in stage I/II extranodal NK/T-cell lymphoma. Leuk Lymphoma 47:1274-1282

Li CC, Tien HF, Tang JL et al. (2004) Treatment outcome and pattern of failure in 77 patients with sinonasal natural killer/T-cell or T-cell lymphoma. Cancer 100:366-375, 2004

Li T, Hongyo T, Syaifudin M et al. (2000) Mutations of the p53 gene in nasal T/NK-cell lymphoma. Lab Invest 80:493-499

Li YX, Coucke PA, Li JY et al. (1998) Primary non-Hodgkin's lymphoma of the nasal cavity: prognostic significance of paranasal extension and the role of radiotherapy and chemotherapy. Cancer 83:449-456

Li YX, Yao B, Jin J et al. (2006) Radiotherapy as primary treatment for stage IE and IIE nasal natural killer/T cell lymphoma. J Clin Oncol 24:181-189. In reply, 24:2684-2686

Liang R, Chen F, Lee CY et al. (1997) Autologous bone marrow transplantation for primary nasal T/NK cell lymphoma. Bone Marrow Transplant 19:91-93

Micaily B, Miyamoto C, Kantor G et al. (1998) Radiotherapy for unilesional mycosis fungoides. Int J Radiat Oncol Biol Phys 42:361-364

Miketic LM, Chambers TP, Lembersky BC (1993) Cutaneous T-cell lymphoma: value of CT in staging and determining prognosis. AJR Am J Roentgenol 160:1129-1132

Mraz-Gernhard S, Natkunam Y, Hoppe RT et al. (2001) Natural killer/natural killer-like T-cell lymphoma, CD56+, presenting in the skin: an increasingly recognized entity with an aggressive course. J Clin Oncol 19:2179-2188

Na II, Kang HJ, Park YH et al. (2007) Prognostic factors for classifying extranodal NK/T cell lymphoma, nasal type, as lymphoid neoplasia. Eur J Haematol 79:1-7

Ooi GC, Chim CS, Liang R et al. (2000) Nasal T-cell/natural killer cell lymphoma: CT and MR imaging features of a new clinicopathologic entity. AJR Am J Roentgenol 174:1141-1145

Ou CH, Chen CC, Ling JC et al. (2007) Nasal NK/T-cell lymphoma: computed tomography and magnetic resonance imaging findings. J Chin Med Assoc 70:207-712

Pagano L, Gallamini A, Trape G et al. (2006) NK/T-cell lymphomas 'nasal type': an Italian multicentric retrospective survey. Ann Oncol 17:794-800

Quintanilla-Martinez L, Kremer M, Keller G et al. (2001) p53 mutations in nasal natural killer/T-cell lymphoma from Mexico: association with large cell morphology and advanced disease. Am J Pathol 159:2095-2105

Quirós PA, Kacinski BM, Wilson LD (1996) Extent of skin involvement as a prognostic indicator of disease free and overall survival of patients with T3 cutaneous T-cell lymphoma treated with total skin electron beam radiation therapy. Cancer 77:1912-1917

Quirós PA, Jones GW, Kacinski BM et al. (1997) Total skin electron beam therapy followed by adjuvant psoralen/ultraviolet-A light in the management of patients with T1 and T2 cutaneous T-cell lymphoma (mycosis fungoides). Int J Radiat Oncol Biol Phys 38:1027-1035

Ribrag V, Ell Hajj M, Janot F et al. (2001) Early locoregional high-dose radiotherapy is associated with long-term disease control in localized primary angiocentric lymphoma of the nose and nasopharynx. Leukemia 15:1123-1126

Sasaki M, Matsue K, Takeuchi M et al. (2000) Successful treatment of disseminated nasal NK/T cell lymphoma using double autologous peripheral blood stem cell transplantation. Int J Hematol 71:75-78

Scarisbrick JJ, Whittaker S, Evans AV et al. (2001) Prognostic significance of tumor burden in the blood of patients with erythrodermic primary cutaneous T-cell lymphoma. Blood 97:624-630

Shikama N, Ikeda H, Nakamura S et al. (2001) Localized aggressive non-Hodgkin's lymphoma of the nasal cavity: a survey by the Japan Lymphoma Radiation Therapy Group. Int J Radiat Oncol Biol Phys 51:1228-1233

Shim SJ, Yang WI, Shin E et al. (2007) Clinical significance of cyclooxygenase-2 expression in extranodal natural killer

(NK)/T-cell lymphoma, nasal type. Int J Radiat Oncol Biol Phys 67:31–38

Takahara M, Kishibe K, Bandoh N et al. (2004) P53, N- and K-Ras, and β-Catenin gene mutations and prognostic factors in nasal NK/T-cell lymphoma from Hokkaido, Japan. Hum Pathol 35:86–95

Takenaka K, Shinagawa K, Maeda Y et al. (2001) High-dose chemotherapy with hematopoietic stem cell transplantation is effective for nasal and nasal-type CD56+ natural killer cell lymphomas. Leuk Lymphoma 42:1297–1303

Tsukamoto N, Kojima M, Hasegawa M et al. (2007) The usefulness of ^{18}F-fluorodeoxyglucose positron emission tomography (^{18}F-FDG-PET) and a comparison of ^{18}F-FDG-pet with 67gallium scintigraphy in the evaluation of lymphoma. Cancer 110:652–659

van Gorp J, Doornewaard H, Verdonck LF et al. (1994) Epstein-Barr virus in nasal T-cell lymphomas (polymorphic reticulosis/midline malignant reticulosis) in western China. J Pathol 173:81–87

Willemze R, Jaffe ES, Burg G et al. (2005) WHO-EORTC classification for cutaneous lymphomas. Blood 105:3768–3785

Wilson LD, Quiros PA, Kolenik SA et al. (1996) Additional courses of total skin electron beam therapy in the treatment of patients with recurrent cutaneous T-cell lymphoma. J Am Acad Dermatol 35:69–73

Wilson LD, Kacinski BM, Jones GW (1998) Local superficial radiotherapy in the management of minimal stage IA cutaneous T-cell lymphoma (Mycosis Fungoides). Int J Radiat Oncol Biol Phys 40:109–115

Yamaguchi M, Kita K, Miwa H et al. (1995) Frequent expression of P-glycoprotein/MDR1 by nasal T-cell lymphoma cells. Cancer 76:2351–2356

Yong W, Zheng W, Zhu J et al. (2006) Midline NK/T-cell lymphoma nasal-type: treatment outcome, the effect of L-asparaginase based regimen, and prognostic factors. Hematol Oncol 24:28–32

You JY, Chi KH, Yang MH et al. (2004) Radiation therapy versus chemotherapy as initial treatment for localized nasal natural killer (NK)/T-cell lymphoma: a single institute survey in Taiwan. Ann Oncol 15:618–625

Ysebaert L, Truc G, Dalac S et al. (2004) Ultimate results of radiation therapy for T1-T2 mycosis fungoides (including reirradiation). Int J Radiat Oncol Biol Phys 58:1128–1134

Primary Central Nervous System Lymphoma

Evan M. Landau and Marnee M. Spierer

CONTENTS

E. M. Landau, MD
M. M. Spierer, MD
Department of Radiation Oncology, Montefiore Medical
Center, 111 East 210th Street, Bronx, NY 10467, USA

Introduction and Objectives

Primary central nervous system lymphoma (PCNSL) is a rare type of non-Hodgkin's lymphoma. Chemotherapy is the mainstay curative treatment for PCNSL. Radiation therapy plays an important role as both an adjuvant treatment and as palliation for patients who are not candidates for curative chemotherapy. The neurotoxicities of combined modality treatment can be severe. The data for treatment of this disease consist of phase II trials and retrospective analyses. The patient populations among these trials are heterogeneous, and comparison between studies is limited. As such, definitive clinical evidence is limited.

This chapter examines:

● Recommendation for diagnosis and evaluation
● Staging and prognostic scoring system
● Treatment recommendations and the available supporting scientific evidence
● Techniques of radiation therapy
● Follow-up and surveillance for survivors

31.1 Diagnosis, Staging, and Prognoses

31.1.1 Diagnosis

Initial Evaluation

■ Diagnosis of primary central nervous system lymphoma (PCNSL) begins with a detailed history and physical. Of particular importance are the neurological, ophthalmologic, including a slit-lamp eye exam, and lymph node examination. A testicular examination should be performed on males of advanced age.

■ The most common presenting symptoms of PCNSL include focal neurological deficits, neuropsychiatric symptoms, or symptoms related to increased intracranial pressure. This is in contrast to systemic lymphoma, which can present with B symptoms of fever, weight loss, and night sweats (Level IV) (BATAILLE et al. 2000). Uveitis is present in 10%–20% of patients at diagnosis (Level IV) (BESSEL et al. 2007).

- Age and performance status should be recorded in each patient as they are widely quoted prognostic factors and may affect therapeutic decisions. This recommendation is based on the consensus of the standardized guidelines for the baseline evaluation and response assessment of PCNSL (Grade D) (ABREY et al. 2005).

- The consensus also recommends a mini-mental status exam (MMSE) to be assessed prior to treatment (Grade D). The MMSE is used to establish a baseline for response to therapy and a framework to understand future neurocognitive toxicities (ABREY et al. 2005).

- Steroids should be withheld, if possible, prior to the diagnostic procedure, as responses to steroid are usually fast in onset and can mask the signs on imaging studies (Grade D) (BATCHELOR et al. 2006).

Laboratory Tests

- Laboratory tests should include a complete blood count, basic metabolic panel, and HIV test (Table 31.1). A 24-h urine creatinine clearance and liver function test should be drawn prior to initiation of methotrexate-based chemotherapy. Serum lactate dehydrogenase (LDH) should be performed, as it is a known prognostic factor (ABREY et al. 2005).

Imaging Studies

- Imaging of the central nervous system is essential and preferably performed with an MRI plus gadolinium. However, CT with contrast is acceptable when an MRI is contraindicated (ABREY et al. 2005).

- The location of the lesion should be noted, as deep lesions are a known adverse prognostic factor (Level IV) (FERRERI et al. 2003).

- Chest X-ray should be performed to rule out primary pulmonary disease.

- An extent of disease work-up includes a full body CT scan. Testicular ultrasound is recommended for elderly men to rule out testicular lymphoma (ABREY et al. 2005).

- FDG-PET or PET/CT scan can be considered and may be used in place of CT, bone marrow biopsy, and testicular ultrasound for non-Hodgkin's lymphoma; however, their utilization in PCNSL is still experimental.

Pathology

- Tissue diagnosis is required as multiple intracranial processes can mimic PCNSL on MRI, and therefore histological confirmation of the diagnosis is essential.

- The diagnostic procedure of choice is a stereotactic needle biopsy (Grade D) (ABREY et al. 2005). Surgical resection of the intracranial tumor is not recommended (Grade B). Results from a critical review of available publications revealed that no survival benefit is derived from a surgical resection (Level III) (RENI et al. 1997).

- If PCNSL is suspected, no corticosteroids should be administered prior to biopsy because its lymphocytic properties may make histological diagnosis difficult (Grade D) (BATCHELOR and LOEFFLER 2006; BATCHELOR et al. 2003).

- If the CSF fluid or a vitreous biopsy is positive, then a brain biopsy is not required, based on the consensus from the workshop on primary central nervous system lymphoma at the European Cancer Conference (Grade D) (BESSEL et al. 2007).

- Most cases of CNS lymphoma are B-cell, diffuse, high-grade lymphomas (Level IV) (JELLINGER et

Table 31.1. Imaging and laboratory work-ups for primary CNS non-Hodgkin's lymphoma

Imaging studies	Laboratory tests	Pathology
MRI + gadolinium	CBC	Stereotactic brain biopsy
CT with contrast (if MRI contraindicated)	Chemistries	CSF
CT of chest/abdomen/pelvis	LDH	Vitreous biopsy if slit-lamp positive
Testicular ultrasound	LFTs	Bone marrow biopsy
CXR	Renal function tests	
PET (experimental)		

al. 1995). Lymphoma of T-cell type is very rare and is usually supratentorial. Infratentorial primary T-cell lymphoma is exceedingly rare. In addition, there remains some debate on the prevalence of primary central nervous system lymphoma. Some studies have shown an increased in frequency in both immunocompromised and non-immunocompromised patients. A SEER analysis from 1973–1998, showed that the frequency was decreasing in all groups except for the highest risk group, those greater then 60 years (Level IV) (Miller et al. 1994; Kadan-Lottick et al 2001).

CSF and Bone Marrow Biopsy

- CSF sampling should be performed, if not medically contraindicated (Grade B). The CSF fluid should be tested for cell count, protein levels, cytology, flow cytometry, and immunoglobulin heavy chain gene rearrangement studies (Batchelor and Loeffler 2006).
  Positive leptomeningeal involvement may change management, and an elevated CSF protein is a poor prognostic factor (Level III) (Abrey et al. 2005).
- A bone marrow biopsy with aspirate is part of the recommended staging procedure (Grade D) (Level V) (O'Neil et al. 1995).

31.1.2 Staging

- PCNSL is staged as IE according to the Ann Arbor staging system, I denotes localized lymphoma, and E denotes extranodal disease (Batchelor and Loeffler 2006).
- The Ann Arbor staging system for non-Hodgkin's lymphoma is detailed in Table 27.3 (see Chap. 27).

31.1.3 Prognostic Factors

- PCNSL is viewed as multifocal disease that rarely has systemic involvement. Its main route of spread is along the craniospinal axis, which includes the eyes. When it recurs, it does so locally (RTOG 83-15, Level III) (Nelson et al. 1992).
- PCNSL prognosis is heavily dependent on a few factors, and survival can range from 1 month with

poor prognostic features and without treatment to a cure rate of over 30% with good prognostic features and with treatment (Level III) (Bessel et al. 2004).

- The International Extranodal Lymphoma Study Group (IELSG) developed a prognostic scoring system based on the following factors (Table 31.2): (1) age more than 60, (2) ECOG PS greater than 1, (3) elevated LDH, (4) elevated CSF protein, and (5) involvement of deep structures of the brain. The survival for these patients can be graded based on this system with one point for each factor (Level IV) (Ferreri et al. 2003).
- BCL-6 positives have been linked to an improved overall survival (Level IV) (Braaten et al. 2003).
- HIV status has been associated with a lower overall median survival (Level IV) (Jacomet et al. 1997).

31.2 Treatment of PCNSL

31.2.1 General Principles

- The data for treatment of this disease consist of phase II trials and retrospective analyses. The patient populations among these trials are heterogeneous, and comparison between studies is limited. As such, definitive evidence-based guidelines are limited (Fine 2001; Bessel et al. 2007).
- Primary treatment is a high-dose methotrexate (HD-MTX)-based chemotherapy regimen with or without radiation therapy (Grade B) (Level IV) (Reni et al. 2001).
- Radiation alone can be offered as treatment in patients with moderate or severe renal dysfunction (creatinine clearance <50 ml/min) and/or KPS less than 40.

Table 31.2. The International Extranodal Lymphoma Study Group (IELSG) prognostic scoring system

	Low (0–1)	Moderate (2–3)	High (4–5)
2-Year overall survival	85%	57%	8%

■ The role for surgical resection is reserved for relief of medically unresponsive increased intracranial pressure (Grade B). Results from a critical review of available publications revealed that no survival benefit is derived from a surgical resection (Level III) (Reni et al. 1997). Results of a retrospective series of 33 patients with PCNSL demonstrated that radiotherapy and chemotherapy improved survival, but no benefit could be demonstrated for the role of surgery. The author concluded that the role of surgery might be limited to a selected subset of patients presenting with large single space-occupying lesions and deteriorating neurological status (Level IV) (Bellinzona et al. 2005).

31.2.2 Chemotherapy

■ HD-MTX-based chemotherapy alone (>1.5 g/m^2) or in combination with other agents is recommended for definitive treatment of PCNSL (Grade B). Methotrexate crosses the blood-brain barrier and achieves therapeutic doses in the CNS. This treatment strategy has demonstrated good efficacy in a number of multicenter prospective trials achieving overall survival in excess of 30 months (Level III–IV) (Abrey et al. 1998; Blay et al. 1998; DeAngelis et al. 2002; Deangelis 2003; Bessel et al. 2001; Batchelor et al. 2003; Poortmans et al. 2003; Pels et al. 2003; Ferreri et al. 2006).

In a prospective phase II trial completed by the RTOG, 98 patients were treated with five cycles of multi-drug induction chemotherapy [methotrexate 2.5 g/m^2, vincristine, procarbazine, and intraventricular methotrexate (12 mg)]. Whole-brain radiotherapy was given to all patients. Initial radiation dose was 45 Gy delivered in 25 daily fractions, and then the study was amended to reduce the dose of irradiation for complete responders to induction chemotherapy to 36 Gy in 30 fractions in 3 weeks. All patients received high-dose cytarabine after RT. The results showed a complete response rate of 58%. The median progression-free survival and overall survival for the entire cohort were 24 months and 37 months, respectively. The study also demonstrated that the median survival for patients younger than 60 was 50.4 months, as compared to 21.8 months for those with more advanced age (RTOG 93-10, Level III) (DeAngelis

et al. 2002). A follow-up analysis revealed that for patients who received reduced doses of brain irradiation (to 36 Gy), the outcome in regard to progression-free survival and overall survival was not significantly affected. The lower dose irradiation delayed, but did not eliminate severe neurotoxicity from chemoradiation (RTOG 93-10, Level III) (Fisher et al. 2005).

In a more recently published retrospective series, 36 patients with PCNSL were treated using a multi-step schedule combining chemotherapy and deferred radiotherapy. The chemotherapy regimen was two modified M-BACOD cycles followed by further chemotherapy with a combination of HMTX, VCZ, PCB, and HD-Ara-C up to a total of nine cycles for patients achieving complete response, or in patients with partial response, stable and disease progression, chemotherapy was interrupted and radiotherapy initiated immediately (45 Gy whole-brain irradiation). The overall survival of the entire group was 42.1 months. In patients with a complete response, time to progression was 28.3 months. Salvage radiation was delivered at the time of recurrence, and 43.4% disease-free patients was observed at 2 years (Level IV) (Silvani et al. 2007).

■ Newer chemotherapeutic regimens including immunotherapy using rituximab in combination with methotrexate have been studied.

A prospective phase II trial studied the efficacy of two cycles of intrathecal (12 mg) and IV (1 g/m^2) methotrexate, thiotepa (30 mg/m^2), and procarbazine (75 mg/m^2) prior to whole-brain radiotherapy and found that complete response was achieved in approximately 40% of patients after chemotherapy, and 76% of patients achieved complete response after adjuvant radiation. The median disease-free survival and overall survival were 18 and 32 months, respectively. This regimen resulted in an efficacy and toxicity profile comparable to other combined modality treatments, despite the relatively low dose of methotrexate (Level III) (Omuro et al. 2005).

A more recently published prospective trial evaluated the safety and efficacy of adding rituximab to methotrexate-based chemotherapy (between five and seven cycles of R-MPV (rituximab, MTX, procarbazine, and vincristine). Patients who achieved complete response after induction chemotherapy were treated with whole-brain radiation up to 23.4 Gy, and those who had less than a CR received 45 Gy to the whole brain (two cycles of high-dose cytarabine were given with brain irradiation). The results revealed 44% of patients achieved a CR after five or fewer cycles, and 78% after seven cycles of R-MPV. Thus, additional cycles of R-MPV nearly doubled the CR rate. The 2-year overall and progression-free survival was 67% and 57%, respectively. Furthermore, reduced-dose radiation of 23.4 Gy was not associated with neurocognitive decline, and disease control at the time of analysis was optimal (Level III) (SHAH et al. 2007).

■ Methotrexate should be withheld for patients with moderate to severe renal dysfunction (creatinine clearance <50 ml/min) and KPS lower than 40.

■ Non-methotrexate-based chemotherapy is not recommended at this time outside of a clinical trial (Grade B). Results from a prospective phase II trial indicated that pre-radiation chemotherapy using a cyclophosphamide, doxorubicin, vincristine, and dexamethasone (CHOD) regimen did not significantly improve survival over RT alone for patients with PCNSL (RTOG 88-06, Level II) (SCHULTZ et al. 1996).

In addition, results from a phase III randomized trial (closed prematurely due to failure to accrue) revealed that when radiation therapy is used as the primary treatment, CHOP-based adjuvant chemotherapy has no clear role in the treatment of patients with PCNSL (MRC, Level II) (MEAD et al. 2000).

Imaging After Chemotherapy

■ An MRI and slit-lamp exam should be performed after completion of chemotherapy in order to assess response (Grade B). Tumor response after chemotherapy is prognostically significant and may direct consolidative treatment in patients younger than 60 (RTOG 93-10, Level II) (DEANGELIS et al. 2002).

■ The lesion should be graded based on response to treatment (Grade D) (ABREY et al. 2005) (CR, complete response; CRu, complete response unconfirmed; PR, partial response; POD, progression of disease) (Table 31.3).

31.2.3 Radiation Therapy

■ The use of radiation therapy in the definitive treatment of PCNSL is controversial.

■ For patients with poor performances status (KPS < 40) and/or who are not chemotherapy candidates, radiation alone to the whole brain is the treatment of choice (Grade B). When used, the whole brain should be treated, as a high rate of out-field recurrence can be observed if localized treatment is delivered without a generous margin (Level IV) (SHIBAMOTO et al. 2003).

PCNSL is a radiosensitive disease, and radiation alone can achieve a response rate of greater than 80% (RTOG 83-15, Level III) (NELSON et al. 1992). However, radiation alone has a short median survival of less than 12 months (RTOG 83-15, Level III) (NELSON et al. 1992) (Level IV) (SHIBAMOTO et al. 2004).

■ For patients with good performance status (KPS ≥ 40) and who are chemotherapy candidates, radiation alone is not routinely recommended as primary treatment (Grade B). Results from a number of prospective trials mentioned above have indicated methotrexate-based chemotherapy should be considered for definitive treatment and can provide a survival advantage over radiotherapy alone.

■ Radiation should begin after completion of chemotherapy (Grade B). Radiation may have the capacity to repair damage to the blood-brain barrier caused by bulky disease. As such, chemotherapy should be initiated prior to radiation in order to maximize this window of blood-brain barrier distribution (Level III) (RENI et al. 1997).

■ Concurrent chemoradiation should be used with caution as it has a high rate of neurocognitive toxicity in the elderly (Level III) (ABREY et al. 1998).

Immediate vs. Salvage Radiation

■ For chemotherapy candidates, some studies advocate immediate radiation treatment, and others have shown success with deferred radiation.

Table 31.3. Radiological response to treatment of PCNSL

	CR	CRu	PR	POD
Imaging	No contrast enhancement	Minimal abnormality	50% Decrease in enhancing tumor	25% Increase in lesion or any new disease

■ Results from a retrospective study have demonstrated that complete response has been associated with improved survival (Level IV) (Corn et al. 2000). A literature review of 19 prospective trials demonstrated no difference in survival between immediate and deferred radiation for patients who achieved a complete response after HD-MTX-based chemotherapy (Level III) (Reni et al. 2001). However, chemotherapy alone only provided a complete response rate of 50%, and radiation can elevate the response rate to greater than 80% (RTOG 93-10, Level III) (DeAngelis et al. 2002).

■ Salvage treatment causes radiation to be targeted against bulk disease, rather than at microscopic disease where it is more effective. A significant percentage of patients who defer radiation may die prior to receiving salvage radiation (Level III) (Pels et al. 2003).

Immediate Radiation

■ Patient's younger than 60 years of age who achieve a complete response with chemotherapy should receive ≤36 Gy of adjuvant radiation (Grade B). Radiation plus chemotherapy has shown improved disease control over chemotherapy alone (Level IV) (Gavrilovic et al. 2006). However, doses higher than 40 Gy showed no improvement in outcome for complete responders (Level IV) (Reni et al. 2001).

■ Decreased incidences of neurotoxicities are noted in patients who receive less than 36 Gy (Level IV) (Nguyen et al. 2005; Bessel et al. 2002).

■ Patients younger than 60 years of age who achieve a PR or who have stable disease after chemotherapy should receive 45 Gy.

Salvage Radiation

■ Radiation should be initially deferred for patients greater than 60 years of age and reserved for salvage (Grade B). Radiation showed no improvement in survival in patients 60 years or older (Level IV) (Gavrilovic et al. 2006). In addition, brain irradiation is associated with a high incidence of cognitive neurotoxicity and leukoencephalopathy (Level III) (Abrey et al. 1998).

■ Most relapses occur in the brain and intraocular region; therefore, local therapy is well suited after failure (Level IV) (Loeffler et al. 1985).

Radiation is an effective agent for local control of the recurrent disease. Studies have shown that recurrent disease maintains the same radiosensitivity (Level IV) (Nguyen et al. 2005). Furthermore, there may be decreased CNS toxicity from waiting more than 6 months between methotrexate and radiation (Level IV) (Hottinger et al. 2007).

Concurrent Dexamethasone

■ Concurrent dexamethasone should be started at 6 mg daily with radiation therapy, and the completion of the taper should coincide with the end of the course of treatment (Grade B). No corticosteroids are needed if minimal or no disease is noted prior to adjuvant radiotherapy (RTOG 93-10, Level III) (DeAngelis et al. 2002).

31.3 Treatment Technique of Radiation Therapy

31.3.1 Simulation

■ A head immobilization device should be used to ensure proper position during setup and treatment.

■ CT-based planning is usually not routinely required, and a clinical setup technique can be utilized according to the technique described in the RTOG 93-10 protocol (DeAngelis et al. 2002).

31.3.2 Physics and Treatment Planning

■ Treatment should be delivered with a megavoltage machine of energy ranging from 6 Mv to 10 Mv photons, with a source to skin distance that must be at least 80 cm.

■ The whole-brain treatment should be delivered by opposed lateral fields. The dose should be calculated at the mid-point of the two beams. The anterior, superior, and posterior borders of the treatment portal should include a 1-cm margin.

■ The caudal border should be the inferior aspect of C2 (Fig. 31.1). Custom-made blocks should

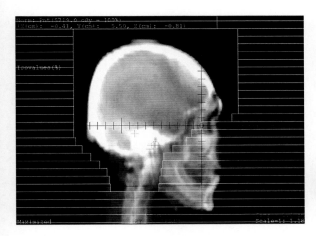

Fig. 31.1. A typical field arrangement (using opposed lateral fields) for whole brain irradiation of PCNSL. The inferior margin was set to the inferior border of the C2 vertebra. A minimum of 1 cm margins were given to the superior, anterior, and posterior borders. Caution was paid to include the frontal lobe in the treatment field

shield the lens with care to include the posterior one-third of the eyes and the frontal lobe. The block should also cover the nasopharynx-pharynx.

■ If ocular lymphoma is evident on initial slit-lamp examination prior to radiation, then both eyes should be included in the treatment field.

■ Spinal radiation is questionable for leptomeningeal involvement.

31.3.3 Dose and Fractionation

■ For patients less than 60 years of age who achieve a complete response after chemotherapy, a total dose of ≤ 36 Gy in 1.8 Gy fractions (Grade B) is required. As detailed above, a dose higher than 40 Gy delivered in conventional fractionation provided no survival advantage, and decreased incidences of neurotoxicities are noted in patients who receive ≤ 36 Gy.

■ For patients less than 60 years who have a partial response, stable disease, or progressive disease after chemotherapy, a total dose of 45 Gy in 1.8 Gy fractions is recommended.

31.3.4 Dose Constraints

■ The total dose to the cervical spinal cord should be limited to 45 Gy; the total dose to the brain stem should be limited to 50 Gy (Level IV) (EMAMI et al. 1991).

31.4 Treatment-Induced Side Effects and Complications

■ The most widely documented side effect of treatment for CNS lymphoma is the potential devastating neurotoxicity. With improvement in long-term survival, it is becoming of greater concern (PEREZ et al. 2004). Treatment-induced neurotoxicities can present in many ways, including cognitive impairment, ataxia, incontinence, and decline in quality of life (BATCHELOR and LOEFFLER 2006). There is no known treatment for this debilitating complication.

■ The most severe toxicity is seen in patients receiving combination therapy with radiation and chemotherapy, followed by radiation alone, and then chemotherapy alone (Level III) (CORREA et al. 2004).

■ Combined chemoradiotherapy is associated with cognitive impairment in patients of all age groups. In an evaluation of the cognitive status and quality of life in a cohort of 19 consecutive patients treated in a prospective European Organization for Research and Treatment of Cancer (EORTC) for PCNSL, cognitive impairment was found in more than 60% of patients despite a complete response. Close to 20% of patients experienced severe cognitive deficits. The study also demonstrated that impairment correlated with age (EORTC 20962, Level III) (HARDER et al. 2004). Other studies have also demonstrated that toxicity is significantly higher in patients older than 60 years of age, with some reports showing near 100% incidence (Level III) (ABREY et al. 1998).

■ Changes in white matter on MRI normally correspond to the neurocognitive changes (Level III) (BESSEL et al. 2001).

■ Retinopathy has been documented in 18.5% of 5-year survivors who received whole-brain irradiation (total dose 41–45 Gy) (Level IV) (GRIMM et al. 2006).

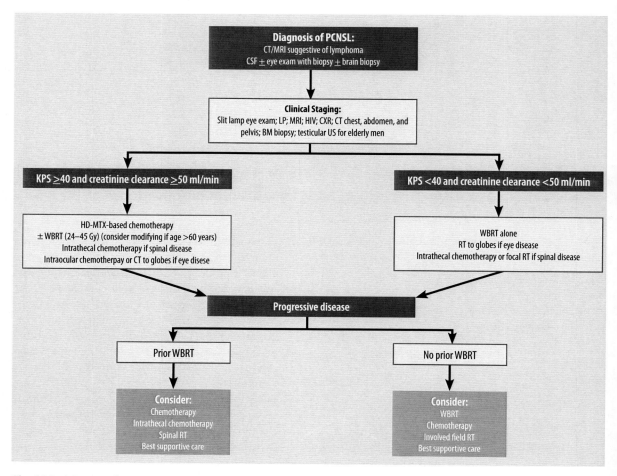

Fig. 31.2. A Proposed treatment algorithm for PCNSL

31.5 Follow-Up, Schedule, and Work-Up

- Long-term follow-up after treatment of PCNSL is indicated in all patients.
- Disease recurrence and neurotoxicities should be the two main points of concern in follow-up. It is important to note recurrence early in order to consider salvage treatment (with chemotherapy and/or radiation).

Schedule

- Patients should be evaluated every 3 months for the 1st year, every 4 months for the 2nd year, and every 6 months thereafter until they reach 5 years. After 5 years, patients should be evaluated annually (Grade D) (ABREY et al. 2005) (Table 31.4).

Table 31.4. Follow-up schedule after treatment for PCNSL

Interval	Frequency
First follow-up	2–4 weeks post-treatment
Year 1	Every 3 months
Year 2	Every 4 months
Year 3–5	Every 6 months
Over 5 years	Annually

Work-Up

- Each follow-up visit should include a history, physical, including MMSE, and an MRI scan with gadolinium.
- Patients with initial involvement of the CSF and eyes should undergo repeat lumbar puncture and ophthalmologic exam as needed (Grade D) (ABREY et al. 2005).

References

Abrey LE, Deangelis LM, Yahalom J (1998) Long-term survival in primary CNS lymphoma. J Clin Oncol 16:859–863

Abrey LE, Yahalom J, DeAngelis LM (2000) Treatment of primary CNS lymphoma: the next step. J Clin Oncol 18:3144–3150

Abrey LE, Batchelor TT, Ferreri MG et al (2005) Report of an international work shop to standardize baseline evaluation and response criteria for primary CNS lymphoma. J Clin Oncol 23:5034–5043

Braaten KM, Betensky RA, de Leval L et al (2003) BCL-6 expression predicts improved survival in patients with primary central nervous system lymphoma. Clin Cancer Res 9:1063–1069

Bataille B, Delwail V, Menet E et al (2000) Primary intracerebral malignant lymphoma: report of 248 cases. J Neurosurg 92:261–266

Batchelor T, Carson K, O'Neill A et al (2003) Treatment of primary CNS lymphoma with methotrexate and deferred radiotherapy: a report of NABTT 96-07. J Clin Oncol 21:1044–1049

Batchelor TT, Loeffler JS (2006) Primary CNS lymphoma. J Clin Oncol 24:1281–1288

Bellinzona M, Roser F, Ostertag H et al (2005) Surgical removal of primary central nervous system lymphomas (PCNSL) presenting as space occupying lesions: a series of 33 cases. Eur J Surg Oncol 31:100–105

Bessell EM, Graus F, López-Guillermo A et al (2001) CHOD/BVAM regimen plus radiotherapy in patients with primary CNS non-Hodgkin's lymphoma. Int J Radiat Oncol Biol Phys 50:457–464

Bessell EM, López-Guillermo A, Villá S et al (2002) Importance of radiotherapy in outcome of patients with primary CNS lymphoma: An analysis of the CHOD/BVAM regimen followed by two different radiotherapy treatments. J Clin Oncol 20:231–236

Bessell EM, Graus F, Lopez-Guillermo A et al (2004) Primary non-Hodgkin's lymphoma of the CNS treated with CHOD/BVAM or BVAM chemotherapy before radiotherapy: long-term survival and prognostic factors. Int J Radiat Oncol Biol Phys 59:501–508

Bessell EM, Hoang-Xuan K, Ferreri AJ et al (2007) Primary central nervous system lymphoma–Biological aspects and controversies in management. Eur J Cancer 43:1141–1152

Blay JY, Conroy T, Chevreau C et al (1998) High-dose methotrexate for the treatment of primary cerebral lymphomas: analysis of survival and late neurologic toxicity in a retrospective series. J Clin Oncol 16:864–871

Corn BW, Dolinskas C, Scott C et al (2000) Strong correlation between imaging response and survival among patients with primary central nervous system lymphoma: a secondary analysis of RTOG studies 83-15 and 88-06. Int J Radiat Oncol Biol Phys 47:299–303

Correa DD, DeAngelis LM, Shi W et al (2004) Cognitive functions in survivors of primary central nervous system lymphoma. Neurology 62:548–555

Deangelis LM, Seiferheld W, Schold SC et al. (2002) Combination chemotherapy and radiotherapy for primary central nervous system lymphoma: Radiation Therapy Oncology Group Study 9310. J Clin Oncol 20:4643–4648

DeAngelis LM (2003) Primary central nervous system lymphoma: a curable brain tumor. J Clin Oncol 21:4471–4473

Emami B, Lyman J, Brown A et al (1991) Tolerance of normal tissue to therapeutic irradiation. Int J Radiat Oncol Biol Phys 21:109–122

Ferreri AJ, Blay JY, Reni M et al (2003) Prognostic scoring system for primary CNS lymphomas: The International Extranodal Lymphoma Study Group experience. J Clin Oncol 21:266–272

Ferreri AJ, Dell'Oro S, Foppoli M et al (2006) MATILDE regimen followed by radiotherapy is an active strategy against CNS lymphoma. Neurology 66:1435–1438

Fine HA (2002) Primary central nervous system lymphoma: time to ask the question. J Clin Oncol 20:4615–4617

Fisher B, Seiferheld W, Schultz C et al (2005) Secondary analysis of RTOG 9310: an intergroup phase II combined modality treatment of primary CNS lymphoma. J Neurooncol 74:201–205

Gavrilovi IT, Hormigo A, Yahalom J et al (2006) Long-term follow-up of high-dose methotrexate-based therapy with and without whole brain irradiation for newly diagnosed primary CNS lymphoma. J Clin Oncol 24:4570–4574

Grimm SA, Yahalom J, Abrey LE et al (2006) Retinopathy in survivors of primary central nervous system lymphoma. Neurology:67:2060–2062

Harder H, Holtel H, Bromberg JE et al (2004) Cognitive status and quality of life after treatment for primary CNS lymphoma. Neurology 62:544–547

Hottinger AF, DeAngelis LM, Yahalom J et al (2007) Salvage whole brain radiotherapy for recurrent or refractory primary CNS lymphoma. Neurology 69:1178–1182

Jacomet C, Girard PM, Lebrette MG et al (1997) Intravenous methotrexate for primary central nervous system non-Hodgkin's lymphoma in AIDS. AIDS 11:1725–1730

Jellinger KA, Paulus W (1995) Primary central nervous system lymphomas – New pathological developments. J Neurooncol 24:33–36

Kadan-Lottick NS, Skluzacek MC, Gurney JG (2002) Decreasing incidence rates of primary central nervous system lymphoma. Cancer 95:193–202

Loeffler JS, Elvin TJ, Mauch P et al (1985) Primary lymphoma of the central nervous system: patterns of failure and factors that influence survival. J Clin Oncol 3:490–494

Mead GM, Bleehen NM, Gregor A et al (2000) A medical research council randomized trial in patients with primary cerebral non-Hodgkin lymphoma: cerebral radiotherapy with and without cyclophosphamide, doxorubicin, vincristine, and prednisone chemotherapy. Cancer 89:1359–1370

Miller DC, Hochberg FH, Harris NL et al (1994) Pathology with clinical correlations of primary central nervous system non-Hodgkin's lymphoma: The Massachusetts General Hospital experience in 1958–1989. Cancer 74:1383–1397

National Comprehensive Cancer Network (2008) Clinical practice guidelines in oncology: Central nervous system cancers. Version I/2008. Available at http://www.nccn.org/professionals/physician_gls/PDF/cns.pdf. Accessed on March 28, 2008

Nelson DF, Martz KL, Bonner H et al (1992) Non-Hodgkin's lymphoma of the brain: can high dose, large volume radiation therapy improve survival? Report on a prospective trial by the Radiation Therapy Oncology Group (RTOG): RTOG 8315. Int J Radiat Oncol Biol Phys 23:9–17

Nguyen PL, Chakravarti A, Finkelstein DM et al (2005) Results of whole brain radiation as salvage of methotrexate failure for immunocompetent patients with primary CNS lymphoma. J Clin Oncol 23:1507–1513

O'Neill BP, Dinapoli RP, Kurtin PJ et al (1995) Occult systemic non-Hodgkin's lymphoma (NHL) in patients initially diagnosed as primary central nervous system lymphoma (PCNSL): how much staging is enough? J Neurooncol 25:67–71

Omuro AM, DeAngelis LM, Yahalom J et al (2005) Chemoradiotherapy for primary CNS lymphoma: an intent-to-treat analysis with complete follow-up. Neurology 64:69–74

Pels H, Schmidt-Wolf I, Glasmacher A et al (2003) Primary central nervous system lymphoma: results of a pilot and phase II study of systemic and intraventricular chemotherapy with deferred radiotherapy. J Clin Oncol 21:4489–4495

Perez CA, Brady LW, Halperin EC, Schmidt-Ullrich RK (2004) Principles and practice of radiation oncology, 4th edn. Lippinicott, Williams, & Wilkins, Philadelphia, pp 2098–2100

Poortmans PMP, Kluin-Nelemans C, Haaxama-Reiche H et al (2003) High dose methotrexate-based chemotherapy followed by consolidating radiotherapy in non-AIDS related primary central nervous system lymphoma; European Organization for research and treatment of cancer lymphoma group phase II trial 20962. J Clin Oncol 21:4483–4488

Reni M, Ferreri AJ, Garancini MP et al (1997) Therapeutic management of primary central nervous system lymphoma in immunocompetent patients: results of a critical review of the literature. Ann Oncol 8:227–234

Reni M, Ferreri AJM, Guha-Thakurta N et al (2001) Clinical relevance of consolidation radiotherapy and other main therapeutic issues in primary central nervous system lymphomas treated with upfront high-dose methotrexate. Int J Radiat Oncol Biol Phys 51:419–425

Schultz C, Scott C, Sherman W et al (1996) Preirradiation chemotherapy with cyclophosphamide, doxorubicin, vincristine, and dexamethasone for primary CNS lymphomas: initial report of radiation therapy oncology group protocol 88-06. J Clin Oncol 14:556–564

Shah GD, Yahalom J, Correa DD et al (2007) Combined immunochemotherapy with reduced whole-brain radiotherapy for newly diagnosed primary CNS lymphoma. J Clin Oncol 25:4730–4735

Shibamoto Y, Hayabuchi N, Hiratsuka J et al (2003) Is whole brain irradiation necessary for primary central nervous system lymphoma? Cancer 97:128–133

Shibamoto Y, Ogino H, Hasegawa M et al (2004) Results of radiation monotherapy for primary central nervous system lymphoma in the 1990's. Int J Radiat Oncol Biol Phys 62:809–813

Silvani A, Salmaggi A, Eoli M et al (2007) Methotrexate based chemotherapy and deferred radiotherapy for primary central nervous system lymphoma (PCNSL): single institution. J Neurooncol 82:273–279

Section VIII:

Tumors of the Central Nervous System

Meningioma

32

Georges F. Hatoum and B-Chen Wen

Introduction and Objectives

Meningiomas are extra-axial central nervous system tumors that arise from the meninges which surround and protect the outer surface of the brain and the spinal cord (Fig. 32.1). Meningiomas account for 1%–30% of all primary intracranial tumors (Longstreth et al. 1993). Approximately 90% of all meningiomas occur in the supratentorial compartment (Bondy and Ligon 1996). Intracranial meningiomas are most common in adults in their fourth through sixth decades of life and are rare in children (2% of all meningiomas present in childhood). Meningiomas are more common in African-Americans and in females. There is a 2:1 female to male ratio in intracranial meningiomas.

The treatment of meningioma requires a multidisciplinary management, usually involving surgery and/or radiation therapy. This chapter examines:

● Diagnosis
● Treatment recommendations for meningiomas
● Systemic therapy
● Follow-up care and surveillance

32.1 Diagnosis, Staging, and Prognoses

32.1.1 Diagnosis

Initial Evaluation

■ Diagnosis and evaluation of intracranial meningioma start with a complete history and physical examination (H&P).

■ The clinical presentation of meningioma is dependent on tumor location, and symptoms are often insidious in nature. The commonly observed symptoms from intracranial meningiomas include headache, seizure, stroke, visual deficit, personality changes, frontal lobe syndrome, and contralat-

G. F. Hatoum, MD
Department of Radiation Oncology, Sylvester Comprehensive Cancer Center, 1475 NW 12th Avenue, D-31, Miami, FL 33136, USA
B-C. Wen, MD
Department of Radiation Oncology, Sylvester Comprehensive Cancer Center, 1475 NW 12th Avenue, D-31, Miami, FL 33136, USA

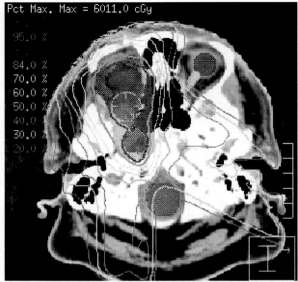

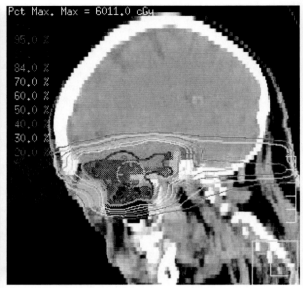

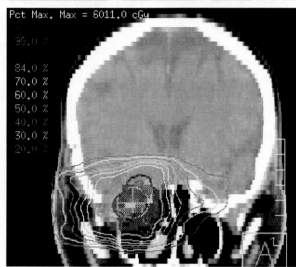

Fig. 32.1a–c. Intensity-modulated radiation therapy (IMRT) in a patient with optic meningioma and cavernous sinus extension (prescription: 1.8 Gy per fraction to a total dose of 50.4 Gy to 90% isodose line)

eral hemiparesis. For diseases located in cavernous sinus, ocular motor deficits, visual field deficits, trigeminal nerve dysfunction, ischemic deficits, and pituitary dysfunction are possible.
- History of ionizing radiation exposure is pertinent and should be recorded.

Imaging Studies

- MRI and CT scan of the brain with and without contrast are the imaging modalities of choice. Meningiomas have typical radiological findings and therefore a biopsy is generally not needed for the diagnosis.

- MRI is a preferred imaging study for the diagnosis of meningioma, although neither MRI nor CT of the brain demonstrated a universal superiority for the diagnosis of intracranial meningiomas. MRI commonly reveals a dural-based tumor, isointense with the gray matter with homogenous enhancement (in more than 95% of cases). MRI was better suited for identifying the extraaxial location of the tumor, the broad contact of the tumor to the meninges, the tumor capsule, and the meningeal contrast enhancement adjacent to the tumor (Level III) (SCHUBEUS et al. 1990).
CT scan proved to be superior in demonstrating calcifications and a typical tumor density, and

may demonstrate bone remodeling, intratumoral calcification (seen in 25%), and hyperostosis of the surrounding skull in base of skull tumors or peripherally located diseases.

Other findings on imaging studies include dilated middle meningeal artery groove, posterior clinoid erosion, and a secondary osteolytic lesion can occur. There is often an enhancing dural tail (60%). Between 10% and 15% of meningiomas are atypical in appearance showing a significant peritumoral edema.

- Positron emission tomography (PET) is not routinely indicated in the diagnosis and evaluation of meningioma, but may be used for meningiomas occuring in the base of skull meningiomas (Grade C) (Level IV) (RUTTEN et al. 2007).

- Frequent findings on plain X-ray are intratumoral calcifications and bone hyperostosis "sunray effect," although plain X-ray is not recommended routinely in the diagnosis and evaluation of meningioma.

- Octreotide brain scintigraphy is useful in differentiating post-surgical residual tumor from scarring in sub-totally resected or recurrent meningiomas, as meningiomas usually have a high somatostatin receptor density (Grade C) (Level IV) (REUBI et al. 1986).

- Cerebral angiography is important for patients requiring surgical resection. It may show sunburst effect and a prolonged vascular stain or so-called blushing as a result of intratumoral venous stasis.

- MRI spectroscopy is an important complementary study to MRI as it helps differentiate other tumors masquerading as meningiomas, and can differentiate typical from atypical meningiomas. Classically, there is an increase in the choline, creatine, and alanine peaks. A low inositol peak may distinguish a meningioma from a schwannoma. A lactate peak is seen in more than 60% of atypical meningiomas.

Pathology

- Meningioma can usually be diagnosed radiologically, and pathologic conformation is not required in most cases.

- Pathologic classification of meningioma (in resected specimen) is important in predicting the clinical behavior of the disease. The World Health Organization (WHO) classification is the most commonly used system for meningioma, classifying meningiomas into three categories:

Grade I or benign meningiomas: slow-growing tumors with well-defined borders, not invading the adjacent normal brain, and with low mitotic index (90% of all meningiomas).

Grade II or atypical meningiomas: higher mitotic index (>4 mitosis per 10 HPF) (5%–7% of all meningiomas). Variant of chordoid and clear cell are included.

Grade III or malignant meningiomas: highest mitotic index (>20 per 10 HPF) (1%–3% of all meningiomas). Variant types such as papillary and rhabdoid are considered malignant (Table 32.1).

Table 32.1. World Health Organization classification of tumors of meningothelial cell origin

Grade	Tumor types
I	Meningothelial (Syncytial), transitional, fibrous, psammomatous, angiomatous, microcystic, secretory, lymphoplasmocyte-rich, metaplastic variants (xanthomatous, myxoid, osseous, cartilaginous)
II	Atypical, chordoid, and clear cell
III	Anaplastic (malignant), papillary, and rhabdoid

32.1.2 Prognosis

- Differentiation of meningioma is of prognostic importance. More than 90% of meningiomas are WHO Grade I disease and are slow-growing in nature. The mean doubling time for WHO grade I, II, and III meningioma is 415, 178, and 205 days (Level IV) (JÄÄSKELÄINEN et al. 1985). The 5-year recurrence rates in benign, atypical, and anaplastic meningiomas were 3%, 38%, and 78%, respectively, after complete resection (Level IV) (JÄÄSKELÄINEN et al. 1986). Grade I meningioma does not metastasize. Although rare, grade II and III meningioma may metastasize outside of the central nervous system, especially in advanced or recurrent diseases.

- In patients requiring active treatment, completeness of surgery is associated with the probability of recurrence. MIRIMANOFF et al. (1985) reported a 10-year and a 15-year recurrence-free survival (RFS) of 80% and 68% after total resection. However, after partial resection, the 10-year and the 15-year RFS were 45% and 9%, respectively (Level IV).

- Other reported adverse factors associated with tumor growth include high mitotic index, younger age (age <40 is associated with higher incidence of recurrence), male gender, absence of calcification on CT scan, and infratentorial and petroclival location of the disease (Level IV) (Jääskeläinen et al. 1985; Nakamura et al. 2003; Van Havenbergh et al. 2003).

32.2 Treatment of Meningioma

32.2.1 General Principles

■ The primary management of intracranial meningiomas depends upon the presenting signs or symptoms, the location and size of the tumor, as well as patients' health condition and preference. Depending on characteristics of the disease and patient, long-term management may involve a combination of several modalities including

watchful waiting, surgery, and radiation therapy (Fig. 32.2).

■ Observation (watchful waiting) is only a valid option for patients with small and asymptomatic meningioma, especially in patients of advanced age (>65 years) or significant comorbidities (Grade A).

■ Surgical resection is the mainstay treatment for patients when treatment is indicated (Grade A).

■ Radiation therapy is usually recommended as adjuvant treatment for patients with WHO Grade II and III disease, or incompletely resected tumors (Grade A).

32.2.2 Watchful Waiting

■ The majority of asymptomatic meningiomas may be followed safely with serial brain imaging until either the tumor enlarges significantly or becomes symptomatic (Grade A). Watchful waiting is an option for patients with small and asymptomatic

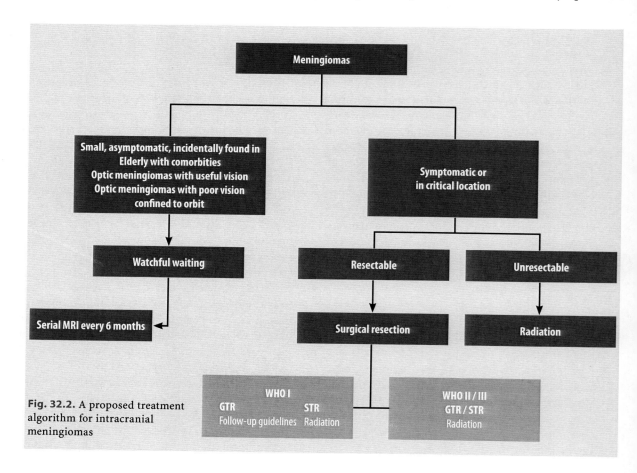

Fig. 32.2. A proposed treatment algorithm for intracranial meningiomas

intracranial meningiomas diagnosed incidentally, or optic sheath meningiomas with normal vision (asymptomatic). In patients with optic sheath meningiomas confined to the orbit without intact vision, active treatment can also be postponed.

The results from a number of retrospective studies have confirmed that watchful-waiting is a valid option for selected patients with meningioma: In an early retrospective review of 60 patients with asymptomatic meningioma, OLIVERO et al. (1995) reported that 35 patients had no evidence of tumor growth, and no patients in the entire group became symptomatic from an enlarging tumor during their follow-up period of 29 months (range 3–72 months) (Level IV).

In another retrospective study including 47 patients from Germany, 41 patients were managed conservatively with observation. The mean growth rate of tumors was 0.796 cm^3 per year, and approximately 66% of the tumors showed a growth rate of less than 1 cm^3 per year. The mean tumor doubling time was 22 years. Progression is less likely if the tumor had calcification; however, young age is associated with higher growth rates (Level IV) (NAKAMURA et al. 2003).

The retrospective study from the Mayo Clinic included 35 asymptomatic patients who were diagnosed with meningioma incidentally. Patients were followed-up for a median period of 6.2 years. The results showed that close to 90% of patients had stable disease without active treatment. In addition, progression is not likely if the tumor showed calcification on imaging studies (Level IV) (Go 1998).

The results of a smaller study of 12 incidentally diagnosed and asymptomatic patients who were followed-up for a median of 8.8 years revealed that disease progression is uncommon, in only one of the 12 cases (Level IV) (BRAUNSTEIN 1997).

32.2.3 Surgery

■ Surgical resection is the mainstay treatment for symptomatic meningioma. The goal of surgery for intracranial meningiomas is total resection whenever possible. Completeness of resection can be determined by early (<72 h) postoperative, contrast-enhanced CT scan or MRI of the brain.

■ The possibility of complete surgical resection depends on the location of meningiomas: Convexity and olfactory groove meningiomas have a high likelihood of complete resection; falx, parasagittal, sphenoid wing, suprasellar, and intraventricular meningiomas are usually subtotally resected; and clival, petroclival and cavernous sinus meningiomas are usually unresectable.

■ The probability of recurrence can be predicted by the Simpson grading system, which was developed based on the completeness of resection (Table 32.2) (Grade B). The 10-year recurrence rate is 9% for patients with a Simpson Grade of 1, compared to a 10-year recurrence rate of 29% for patients with a Simpson grade of 3 (Level IV) (SIMPSON 1957).

■ For symptomatic patients whose tumor is not completely resectable due to tumor location, decompression surgery followed by adjuvant radiotherapy is indicated in patients presenting with neurologic deficit caused by tumor compression (Grade B). Patients who underwent partial resection of their tumor followed by adjuvant radiotherapy had similar outcome as compared to those who received total resection, as described in the next section.

Table 32.2. Simpson grading system for meningiomas

Grade	Definition
1	Macroscopic GTR w/ excision of dura, sinus, and bone
2	Macroscopic GTR w/ coagulation of dural attachment
3	Macroscopic resection w/o resection or coagulation of dural attachment
4	STR
5	Biopsy

GTR, gross-total resection; STR, subtotal resection.

32.2.4 Radiation Therapy

■ Adjuvant radiation therapy is usually not recommended after complete resection for WHO Grade I meningioma (Grade B). The probability of recurrence after complete resection is less than 5% at 5 years after surgery for benign meningioma (Level IV) (JÄÄSKELÄINEN et al. 1986).

■ Adjuvant radiation therapy is indicated for WHO grade I meningioma after partial resection (Grade A). Patients underwent partial resection of their tumor followed by adjuvant radiotherapy had similar outcome as compared to those received total resection:

Results from a retrospective study reported by TAYLOR et al. (1988) revealed that the 10-year local control rates for 132 patients with WHO grade I meningioma were 77% and 82%, respectively, for those achieved gross total resection or received partial resection plus radiation therapy. However, the rate of patients who underwent partial resection only was 18% (Level IV). These findings were supported by the more recently published results of 92 patients with WHO grade I meningioma. The 5-year progression-free survival (PFS) rates for patients treated with partial resection followed by radiotherapy or partial resection alone were 91% versus 38%, respectively (p=0.0005). The PFS of patients achieved complete gross resection was 77% (Level IV) (SOYUER et al. 2004).

In a larger series including 262 patients with WHO Grade I, II, or III meningiomas, the cause-specific survival of patients receiving total resection or partial resection followed by adjuvant radiation approached 90% at 15 years, as compared to 50% in those who had partial resection only (p=0.0003) (Level IV) (CONDRA et al. 1997).

- Adjuvant therapy is indicated for patients with WHO Grade II or Grade III meningioma after surgery (Grade B). The 5-year recurrence rate of patients with atypical or anaplastic meningiomas were 38% and 78%, respectively, after complete resection (Level IV) (JÄÄSKELÄINEN et al. 1986; GOYAL et al. 2000). Adjuvant radiation therapy was found to be effective in reducing local recurrence for patients with atypical or malignant meningiomas after complete or partial resection in a number of retrospective studies with small sample sizes (Level IV) (COKE et al. 1998; MILOSEVIC et al. 1996).

- Definitive radiation therapy using external beam radiation therapy or stereotactic radiosurgery is the treatment of choice when surgery is contraindicated (e.g., meningioma of optic nerve sheath or cavernous sinus, or medically inoperable patients due to comorbidities). The purpose of radiation therapy is to retard the growth of the tumor and preserve the existing function. As most cases of meningioma are slow-growing, significant regression of the tumor after radiation therapy usually does not occur with a limited period of follow-up (Level IV) (DEBUS 2001).

Treatment Technique

- Radiation therapy can be delivered with conventional external beam radiation therapy or intensity-modulated radiation therapy. Newer radiation therapy modalities have also been explored.

3D Conformal Radiation Therapy or IMRT

- CT-based planning is highly recommended for radiation treatment of meningioma (Grade B). CT based simulation significantly improved the treatment outcome (overall survival) according to the results of a retrospective series of 140 patients treated between 1967 and 1990 for meningioma at the University of California, San Francisco (Level IV) (GOLDSMITH et al. 1994).

- The gross tumor volume (GTV) should be determined by fusion of the T1-weighted contrast-enhanced MRI with the planning CT (Grade B). The tumor volume is best determined by comparing preoperative and postoperative findings of a contrast-enhanced MRI of the brain. MRI defined meningioma volumes could be larger but not inclusive of CT-defined volumes, thus CT scan and MRI are complementary for the purpose of tumor delineation (Level III) (KHOO et al. 2000).

- The GTV for adjuvant radiation of WHO Grade I meningioma can include the postoperative residual tumor only. For atypical and malignant meningioma (i.e., WHO grade II and III), GTV should include the entire tumor bed on the preoperative MRI (Grade D).

- Radiation dose for the adjuvant treatment of WHO grade I meningioma ranges from 50 Gy to 54 Gy at 1.8–2.0 Gy per daily fraction (Grade B). Dose response of meningioma to radiation therapy has not been evaluated. Radiation dose of less than 50 Gy is associated with increased recurrence (Level IV) (MILOSEVIC et al. 1996). In a retrospective review reported by GOLDSMITH et al. (1994) the recurrence rate for patients treated with 54 Gy or lower was significantly higher (Level IV). However, doses of 54 Gy or higher using conventional radiotherapy is associated with increased long-term complications. For WHO Grade II or III diseases, higher dose (e.g., 59.4 Gy in 33 daily fractions at 1.8 Gy/fractions) is recommended.

- IMRT can be recommended for meningioma, and may produce improved outcome as compared to conventional radiotherapy, particularly for lesions located close to critical normal tissues (Grade B)

(Fig. 32.1). Results from dosimetric studies have demonstrated the benefit of IMRT on small intracranial tumors (Level IV) (CARDINALE et al. 1998). The clinical value of IMRT for meningioma was preliminarily demonstrated in a small retrospective series of 20 patients with recurrent, residual, or skull-base meningioma. Patients treated with IMRT experienced evident clinical and radiological regression of symptoms compared to those treated with 3D conformal radiotherapy, as the doses to the gross tumor volume were significantly higher in tumors treated with IMRT (Level IV) (PIRZKALL et al. 2003).

Stereotactic Radiosurgery or Radiotherapy

- Stereotactic radiosurgery may benefit meningioma patients with small residual tumors when the maximum tumor dimension does not exceed 3.5 cm and the separation between the tumor and critical structures, such as chiasm and brainstem, is sufficiently large (>3 mm) (Level III) (KONDZIOLKA et al. 2003).
- Single doses ranging from 10 Gy to 50 Gy have been utilized. For example, 10–50 Gy (mean dose of 29 Gy) has been applied at the German Cancer Research Center, and 10–25 Gy (mean dose of 17 Gy) has been utilized at the University of Pittsburgh. Dose to optic chiasm is limited to 8 Gy/single fraction (Level IV) (KONDZIOLKA et al. 2003). And dose to brainstem is limited to 12 Gy/single fraction (Level IV) (PERKS et al. 2003).
- With fractionated stereotactic conformal radiotherapy (50–55 Gy in 30–33 daily fractions), tumor control rates of more than 90% at 5 years have been reported (Level IV) (JALALI et al. 2002).

Intensity-Modulated Stereotactic Radiation Therapy

- Intensity-modulated stereotactic radiation therapy (IMSRT) using a micro multileaf collimator (μMLC) could be safely implemented for highly focused treatment of small skull-base meningiomas (Level IV) (BAUMERT et al. 2003). It remains to be observed whether the dosimetric improvements achievable with IMSRT will lead to significant clinical outcome improvements

Proton Therapy

- Proton therapy can be used in the treatment of meningioma as primary or adjuvant treatment;

however, facility of proton therapy is currently limited. Optimal control, PFS, and overall survival rates have been demonstrated with a median prescribed dose of 56–59 CGE (Level IV) (WEBER et al. 2004; WENKEL et al. 2000).

Radiation-Induced Side Effects and Dose Limiting Structures

Side Effects and Complications

- Acute toxicities include fatigue, skin erythema, alopecia, external otitis, and serous otitis media if the external and medial ear are in the field. Exacerbation of preradiation therapy deficits can occur, including sudden visual loss (Level IV) (CAPO and KUPERSMITH 1991). In patients presenting with visual disturbance, Decadron is strongly recommended.
- Late toxicities include retinopathy and optic neuropathy, memory deficit, cerebral necrosis, hearing deficit, and hypopituitarism depending on the area irradiated (Level IV) (GOLDSMITH et al. 1992; MIRALBELL et al. 1992; GLAHOLM et al. 1990).

Dose Limiting Structures

- Dose limiting structures of brain irradiation include brain, optic nerve and chiasm, pituitary gland, soft-tissue, and other tissues or organs in the radiation fields.
- Radiation dose to 1/3 of the brain should be limited to 60 Gy or less (Grade B) (Level IV) (EMAMI et al. 1991). The brain necrosis incidence was 18% with doses >64.8 Gy, compared to 0% with doses <57 Gy (Level IV) (MARKS and WONG 1985). Clinical/overt hypopituitarism was observed in 14% of patients who received a median dose of 62 Gy or more. The hypopituitarism was dependent on total dose more than fraction size (Level IV) (BHANDARE et al. 2007).
- Radiation dose to the optic pathway should be strictly limited to less than 60 Gy (Grade B). There was no optic neuropathy if the dose is <59 Gy. If the dose is more or equal to 60 Gy, the 15-year risk of optic neuropathy was 11% if the fraction size is less than 1.9 Gy and 47% if the fraction size is more or equal than 1.9 Gy (Level IV) (PARSONS et al. 1994).
- The estimated TD 5/5 and TD 50/5 for developing chronic otitis media is about 55 Gy and 65 Gy, respectively (Level IV) (EMAMI et al. 1991).

32.3　Systemic Therapy of Meningioma

32.3.1 Hormonal Therapy

- Although the growth of meningioma may be hormone dependent, systemic hormonal therapy should not be routinely used for the treatment, and should not be considered an alternative to adjuvant radiotherapy (Grade B). Meningiomas are more common in females and may increase in size during pregnancy. Approximately 70% of meningiomas are progesterone receptor positive and 30% are estrogen receptor positive (Sanson 2000). Several clinical findings support a link between female sex hormones and the risk of meningioma. In addition, there is also a well-known relationship between breast cancer and meningioma which could be explained by a hormonal effect or a shared chromosome 22 abnormality (Iida 1998).
- However, no evidence supports the use of hormonal therapy agents such as megestrol acetate, mifepristone and tamoxifen for the treatment of meningioma: Results from a small retrospective study showed that oral progesterone agonist megestrol acetate has no effect on tumor response in patients with unresectable meningioma. (Level IV) (Grunberg and Weiss 1990). The effect of tamoxifen in unresectable or refractory meningiomas was studied in a phase II trial of the Southwest Oncology Group, and the results showed that no objective improve was observed in patients treated with tamoxifen (SWOG, Level III) (Goodwin et al. 1993).

32.3.2 Biotherapy and Chemotherapy

- Systemic chemotherapy or biotherapy has a very limited role in the treatment of meningioma. Although recombinant interferon-α, oral temozolomide, and CPT-11 were studied, no clear benefit was demonstrated. Hydroxyurea has been shown with efficacy in three small trials (Level IV) (Shrell et al. 1997; Newton et al. 2000; Mason et al. 2002).
- Long-acting somatostatin showed a good efficacy in a small prospective trial. Somatostatin analogs may offer a novel relatively non-toxic alternative treatment for patients with surgical and radiotherapy refractory meningiomas (Level III) (Chamberlain et al. 2007). However, further investigation is needed before any conclusion can be made for the use of somatostatin in meningioma.

32.4　Follow-Ups

32.4.1 Post-Treatment Follow-Ups

- Long-term follow-up is indicated for patients with meningioma after definitive treatment or if observation is preferred. Tumors may require follow-up for more than 10 years regardless of tumor grade and completeness of resection.

Schedule

- The optimal imaging schedule is unknown and has not been addressed in any clinical trials. Initially, patients can be evaluated at 3 months after the completion of their treatment or diagnosis (if observation is chosen), then at 9 month, and annually thereafter for stable WHO grade I meningiomas (Table 32.3) (Grade D).
- For atypical and anaplastic meningiomas, follow-up every 6 months is indicated (Grade D).

Table 32.3. Follow-up schedule for WHO Grade I meningioma

Interval	Frequency
First follow-up	3 Months after treatment
Second follow-up	9 Months after treatment
Year 2 and after	Annually

Work-Ups

- Each follow-up should include neurological evaluations and appropriate history and physicals examinations.
- MRI of the brain with and without contrast can be performed initially within 72 h after surgery to access the residual disease. MRI can then be ordered at each follow-up session.

References

Bhandare N, Kennedy L, Malyapa RS et al. (2007) Primary and central hypothyroidism after radiotherapy for head-and-neck tumors. Int J Radiat Oncol Biol Phys 68:1131–1139

Baumert BG, Norton IA, Davis JB (2003) Intensity-modulated stereotactic radiotherapy vs. stereotactic conformal radiotherapy for the treatment of meningioma located predominantly in the skull base. Int J Radiat Oncol Biol Phys 57:580–592

Bondy M, Ligon BL (1996) Epidemiology and etiology of intracranial meningiomas: a review. J Neurooncol 29:197–205

Braunstein JB (1997) Meningiomas: the decision not to operate. Neurology 48:1459–1462

Capo H, Kupersmith MJ (1991) Efficacy and complications of radiotherapy of anterior visual pathway tumors. Neurol Clin 9:179–203

Cardinale RM, Benedict SH, Wu Q et al. (1998) A comparison of three stereotactic radiotherapy techniques; ARCS vs. noncoplanar fixed fields vs. intensity modulation. Int J Radiat Oncol Biol Phys 42:431–436

Chamberlain MC, Glantz MJ, Fadul CE (2007) Recurrent meningioma: salvage therapy with sandostatin. Neurology 69:969–973

Coke CC, Corn BW, Werner-Wasik M et al. (1998) Atypical and malignant meningiomas: an outcome report of seventeen cases. J Neurooncol 39:65–70

Condra KS, Buatti JM, Mendenhall WM et al. (1997) Benign meningiomas: primary treatment selection affects survival. Int J Radiat Oncol Biol Phys 39:427–436

Emami B, Lyman J, Brown A et al. (1991) Tolerance of normal tissue to therapeutic radiation. Int J Radiat Oncol Biol Phys 21:109–122

Glaholm J, Bloom HJ, Crow JH (1990) The role of radiotherapy in the management of intracranial meningiomas: the Royal Marsden Hospital experience with 186 patients. Int J Radiat Oncol Biol Phys 18:755–761

Go RS (1998) The natural history of asymptomatic meningiomas in Olmsted County, Minnesota. Neurology 51:1718–1720

Goldsmith BJ, Rosenthal SA, Wara WM et al. (1992) Optic neuropathy after irradiation of meningioma. Radiology 185:71–76

Goldsmith BJ, Wara WM, Wilson CB et al. (1994) Postoperative irradiation for subtotally resected meningiomas. A retrospective analysis of 140 patients treated from 1967 to 1990. J Neurosurg 80:195–201

Goodwin JW, Crowley J, Eyre HJ et al. (1993) A phase II evaluation of tamoxifen unresectable or refractory meningiomas: a Southwest Oncology Group Study. J Neurooncol 15:73–77

Goyal LK, Suh JH, Mohan DS et al. (2000) Local control and overall survival in atypical meningioma: a retrospective study. Int J Radiat Oncol Biol Phys 46:57–61

Grunberg SM, Weiss M (1990) Lack of efficacy of megestrol acetate in the treatment of unresectable meningioma. J Neurooncol 8:61–65

Jääskeläinen J, Haltia M, Laasonen E et al. (1985) The growth rate of intracranial meningiomas and its relation to histology. An analysis of 43 patients. Surg Neurol 24:165–172

Jääskeläinen J, Haltia M, Servo A (1986) Atypical and anaplastic meningiomas: radiology, surgery, radiotherapy, and outcome. Surg Neurol 25:233–242

Jalali R, Loughrey C, Baumert B et al. (2002) High precision focused irradiation in the form of fractionated stereotactic conformal radiotherapy (SCRT) for benign meningiomas predominantly in the skull base location. Clin Oncol (R Coll Radiol) 14:103–109

Khoo VS, Adams EJ, Saran F et al. (2000) A Comparison of clinical target volumes determined by CT and MRI for the radiotherapy planning of base of skull meningiomas. Int J Radiat Oncol Biol Phys 46:1309–1317

Kondziolka D, Nathoo N, Flickinger JC et al. (2003) Long-term results after radiosurgery for benign intracranial tumors. Neurosurgery 53:815–21; discussion 821–822

Marks JE, Wong J (1985) The risk of cerebral radionecrosis in relation to dose, time and fractionation. A follow-up study. Prog Exp Tumor Res 29:210–218

Mason WP, Gentili F, Macdonald DR et al. (2002) Stabilization of disease progression by hydroxyurea in patients with recurrent or unresectable meningioma. J Neurosurg 97:341–346

Milosevic MF, Frost PJ, Laperriere NJ et al. (1996) Radiotherapy for atypical or malignant intracranial meningioma. Int J Radiat Oncol Biol Phys 34:817–822

Miralbell R, Linggood RM, de la Monte S et al. (1992) The role of radiotherapy in the treatment of subtotally resected benign meningiomas. J Neurooncol 13:157–164

Mirimanoff RO, Dosoretz DE, Linggood RM et al. (1985) Meningiomas: analysis of recurrence following neurosurgical resection. J Neurosurg 62:18–24

Mirimanoff RO, Dosoretz DE, Linggood RM et al. (1985) Meningioma: analysis of recurrence and progression following neurosurgical resection. J Neurosurg 62:18–24

Nakamura M, Roser F, Michel J et al. (2003) The natural history of incidental meningiomas. Neurosurgery 53:62–70; discussion 70–71

Newton HB, Slivka MA, Stevens C (2000) Hydroxyurea chemotherapy for unresectable or residual meningioma. J Neurooncol 49:165–170

Olivero WC, Lister JR, Elwood PW (1995) The natural history and growth rate of asymptomatic meningiomas: a review of 60 patients. J Neurosurg 83:222–224

Parsons JT, Bova FJ, Fitzgerald CR et al. (1994) Radiation optic neuropathy after megavoltage external-beam irradiation. Int J Radiat Oncol Biol Phys 30:755–763

Perks JR, St George EJ, El Hamri K et al. (2003) Stereotactic radiosurgery XVI: isodosimetric comparison of photon stereotactic radiosurgery techniques (gamma knife vs. micromultileaf collimator linear accelerator) for acoustic neuroma – and potential clinical importance. Int J Radiat Oncol Biol Phys 57:1450–1459

Pirzkall A, Debus J, Haering P et al. (2003) Intensity modulated radiotherapy (IMRT) for recurrent, residual, or untreated skull-base meningiomas: preliminary clinical experience. Int J Radiat Oncol Biol Phys 55:362–372

Reubi JC, Maurer R, Klijn JG et al. (1986) High incidence of somatostatin receptors in human meningiomas: biochemical characterization. J Clin Endocrinol Metab 63:433–438

Rutten I, Cabay JE, Withofs N et al. (2007) PET/CT of skull base meningiomas using 2-18F-fluoro-L-tyrosine: initial report. J Nucl Med 48:720–725

Schrell UM, Rittig MG, Anders M et al. (1997) Hydroxyurea for treatment of unresectable and recurrent meningiomas. II. Decrease in the size of meningiomas in patients treated with hydroxyurea. J Neurosurg 86:840–844

Schubeus P, Schörner W, Rottacker C et al. (1990) Intracranial meningiomas: how frequent are indicative findings in CT and MRI? Neuroradiology 32:467–473

Simpson D (1957) The recurrence of intracranial meningiomas after surgical resection. J Neurol Neurosurg Psychiatry 201:22–39

Soyuer S, Chang EL, Selek U et al. (2004) Radiotherapy after surgery for benign cerebral meningioma. Radiother Oncol 71:85–90

Taylor BW Jr, Marcus RB Jr, Friedman WA et al. (1988) The meningioma controversy: postoperative radiation therapy. Int J Radiat Oncol Biol Phys 15:299–304

Van Havenbergh T, Carvalho G, Tatagiba M et al. (2003) Natural history of petroclival meningiomas. Neurosurgery 52:55–62; discussion 62–64

Weber DC, Lomax AJ, Rutz HP et al. (2004) Spot-scanning proton radiation therapy for recurrent, residual or untreated intracranial meningiomas. Radiother Oncol 71:251–258

Wenkel E, Thornton AF, Finkelstein D et al. (2000) Benign meningioma: partially resected, biopsied, and recurrent intracranial tumors treated with combined proton and photon radiotherapy. Int J Radiat Oncol Biol Phys 48:1363–1370

Adult Gliomas

33

Bernadine R. Donahue

CONTENTS

B. R. DONAHUE, MD
Department of Radiation Oncology, Maimonides Cancer
Center, 6300 Eighth Avenue, Brooklyn, NY 11220, USA

Introduction and Objectives

Malignant or high-grade gliomas account for approximately half of all primary brain tumors in adults. Malignant gliomas include anaplastic gliomas which are classified as WHO Grade III, and glioblastoma multiforme (GBM) which is classified as WHO Grade IV. GBM accounts for about 75% of high-grade gliomas in adults, and anaplastic gliomas account for the remaining 25% of high-grade gliomas. Surgery, radiation therapy, and chemotherapy are important therapeutic modalities in the curative treatment of high-grade gliomas.

Low-grade gliomas account for approximately 10% of all primary intracranial tumors in adults and are generally categorized as pilocytic astrocytoma (WHO Grade I) or diffusely infiltrating low-grade gliomas (WHO Grade II). Low-grade gliomas in adults are usually treated with surgery and/or radiation therapy, although the subtype of oligodendroglioma may be considered for treatment with chemotherapy.

This chapter includes:

● Recommendations for diagnosis and staging procedures

● The staging systems and prognostic factors

● Treatment recommendations as well as the supporting scientific evidence for surgery, radiation therapy, and chemotherapy for adult GBM

● Treatment recommendations as well as the supporting scientific evidence for surgery, radiation therapy, and chemotherapy for adult anaplastic gliomas (astrocytomas and oligodendrogliomas)

● Treatment recommendations as well as the supporting scientific evidence for surgery and/or radiation therapy for adult low-grade gliomas, as well as considerations for chemotherapy

● Follow-up care and surveillance of survivors

33.1 Diagnosis, Staging, and Prognoses

33.1.1 Diagnosis

Initial Evaluation

- Diagnosis and evaluation of any intracranial neoplasm starts with a complete history and physical examination, with particular attention to neurological signs and symptoms.
- Family history, screening for heritable disorders associated with CNS tumors (neurofibromatosis, Li-Fraumeni, von Hippel-Lindau, Turcot's, etc.), should be obtained.
- Thorough neurological examination should be performed including a baseline mini-mental status examination.
- Particular attention may need to be paid to ophthalmological findings and endocrine findings, depending on the location of the tumor.
- Additionally, patients with malignant gliomas have a high incidence of deep venous thrombosis and subsequent risk of pulmonary embolism, and thus attention should be paid to symptoms or physical findings associated with these.

Laboratory Tests

- Initial laboratory tests should include a complete blood count, comprehensive metabolic panel, and coagulation profile (the latter in anticipation of neurosurgical intervention).

Imaging Studies

- Magnetic resonance imaging (MRI) is the imaging modality of choice. Images should be obtained both with and without gadolinium. T1-weighted images are useful for defining anatomy and should be obtained pre- and post-contrast. FLAIR (fluid attenuation inversion recovery) and T2-weighted images aid in detecting edema or infiltration of brain parenchyma, including infiltration across the corpus callosum, a not infrequent finding in malignant gliomas. The pattern of enhancement is useful in the differential diagnosis of the lesion. In GBMs, MRI typically shows peripheral enhancement and a central necrotic region with surrounding FLAIR/T2 signal change indicative of vasogenic edema or tumor infiltration. Anaplastic gliomas, like GBMs, may have enhancement and necrosis; however, they frequently do not enhance. Pilocytic astrocytomas are usually well-circumscribed, vividly enhancing lesions, often with a cystic component. Low-grade infiltrating gliomas are hypointense and non-enhancing on T1-weighted images, and hyperintense on T2-weighted images.
- Computed tomography (CT) is utilized when patients cannot undergo MRI (implanted pacemaker/defibrillator or other non-MRI compatible implanted devices, surgical clips, or metals, etc.) or are unable to tolerate MRI. CT is useful for identifying calcifications, such as those seen in oligodendrogliomas.
- More advanced imaging such as MR spectroscopy, perfusion MRI, and PET can help provide further information regarding functional brain tissue or tumor (JENKINSON et al. 2007).

Pathology

- Tissue for pathologic diagnosis can be obtained during definitive surgical resection or biopsy.
- Pathologic confirmation of glioma is imperative prior to the initiation of any treatment (with the exception of "typical" infiltrating brainstem gliomas). Treatment and prognosis will vary depending upon the grade and subtype of glioma identified.
- The histopathologic features of GBM include nuclear atypia, mitotic activity, vascular proliferation, and necrosis. Anaplastic gliomas have nuclear atypia and mitotic activity, without necrosis or neovascularization. Oligodendrogliomas are frequently described as having cells with "fried egg" appearance. Pilocytic astrocytomas consist of astrocytes forming a glioma matrix with intermixed Rosenthal fibers. Infiltrating low-grade fibrillary gliomas are well differentiated and lack mitoses, nuclear pleomorphism, anaplasia, vascular proliferation, and necrosis.

33.1.2 Staging

- The American Joint Committee on Cancer Tumor Node Metastasis (TNM) staging system is not widely used in the staging of malignant gliomas. Tumor histology, location, and biology have proven to be more important in predicting outcome than a TNM system, and thus, in 1997 the CNS Tumor Task Force of the American Joint Committee on Cancer recommended that a formal classification and staging system not be included in the fifth edition of the staging manual (AMERICAN JOINT COMMITTEE ON CANCER 1997).

■ The RTOG recursive partitioning analysis (RPA) divides patients with GBM and anaplastic astrocytoma into classes, i.e., groups with similar outcomes (Table 33.1) (Level II) (CURRAN et al. 1993). There is not a widely recognized staging system for low-grade gliomas; however, in practical terms they can be thought of as disseminated or non-disseminated.

■ High-grade gliomas rarely metastasize to the spine, but neuroaxis imaging should be considered in symptomatic patients or in the presence of ventricular dissemination of tumor. MRI of the spine with and without gadolinium is the imaging of choice. Low-grade gliomas can disseminate to the neuroaxis and imaging should be obtained if clinically indicated (Level III) (MAMELAK et al. 1994; POLLACK et al. 1994; GAJJAR et al. 1995; HUKIN et al. 2003).

Table 33.1. Radiation Therapy Oncology Group recursive partitioning of malignant gliomas

Class	Patient characteristics	Median survival
I and II	Anaplastic astrocytomas with age ≤50 years and normal mental status or age >50 years and KPS >70 and symptom duration >3 months	40–60 months
III and IV	Anaplastic astrocytomas with age ≤50 years and abnormal mental status or age >50 years and symptom duration <3 months	11–18 months
	GBM with age <50 years or age >50 years and KPS ≥70	
V and VI	GBM with age >50 years, KPS <70 or abnormal mental status	5–9 months

33.1.3 Prognostic Factors

■ The prognosis of patients with GBM is poor with survival of only approximately 1 year. The survival of patients with anaplastic astrocytoma is longer, in the order of 3 years. The presence of an oligodendroglial component confers an improved survival with median survival of approximately 5 years (Level I and Level III) (DONAHUE et al. 1997; CAIRNCROSS et al. 2006). Prognostic factors for both GBM and anaplastic astrocytomas include age at diagnosis, Karnofsky performance status (KPS), histology, extent of resection, duration of symptoms, and neurologic functional/mental status (Level II) (CURRAN et al. 1993).

■ Prognostic factors for low-grade gliomas also have been identified. Factors influencing survival in adults with supratentorial low-grade glioma include histologic subtype, age, size of the tumor, presence of tumor across midline, and extent of surgical resection (Level II and III) (EYRE et al. 1993; PIGNATTI et al. 2002; KRETH et al. 1997). Age 40 is the most consistently used age cut-off for poor prognosis.

■ Molecular markers have also been identified as prognostic factors in GBM. MGMT gene promoter methylation status appears to have an impact on survival when patients are treated with temozolamide. In a landmark EORTC/NCIC study evaluating the impact of the addition of temozolamide to RT in the treatment of GBM, patients with methylated MGMT had improved median overall survival of 18.2 months as compared to those with unmethylated MGMT promoter regions whose median overall survival was 12.2 months ($p<.001$) (Level I) (HEGI et al. 2005).

■ Molecular markers have also been identified as prognostic factors in oligodendrogliomas. Allelic loss of 1 p and 19 q has been identified as a good prognostic factor in oligodendrogliomas. Both RTOG 94-02 and EORTC 26951 assessed 1 p and 19 q status in patients with anaplastic oligodendroglioma/oligoastrocytoma. Both of these trials evaluated RT alone versus RT and PCV chemotherapy. In the EORTC study, the presence of 1 p/19 q loss was found to be the most important factor to predict survival (HR = 0.27) (Level I) (VAN DEN BENT et al. 2006). In the RTOG study loss of both 1p and 19q resulted in a longer median survival time of >7 years versus 2.8 years ($p<.001$) (Level I) (CAIRNCROSS et al. 2006). 1 p/19 q status may also be predictive of outcome in low-grade oligodendrogliomas (Level III) (SMITH et al. 2000; FALLON et al. 2004; JEON et al. 2007).

33.2 Treatment of Glioblastoma Multiforme

33.2.1 General Principles

- For many years, the standard treatment of GBM was surgical resection followed by radiation therapy.
- Historically, nitrosoureas were added to surgery and RT.
- The RTOG conducted several Phase II trials during the past decade attempting to identify alternative agents which would be active with RT in the setting of high-grade glioma (Level III) (DELROWE et al. 2000; YUNG et al. 2001; LANGER et al. 2001; FISHER et al. 2002; COLMAN et al. 2006; ROBINS et al. 2006). Other treatments which have been explored include altered fractionation and dose escalation (MURRAY et al. 1995; WERNER-WASIK et al. 1996; CURRAN et al. 1996; SCOTT et al. 1998; WERNER-WASIK et al. 2004), SRS (SOUHAMI et al. 2004), FSRT (CARDINALE et al. 2006), brachytherapy (SELKER et al. 2002; WELSH et al. 2007), particle therapy (LARAMORE et al. 1988; PICKLES et al. 1997; CASTRO et al. 1985; BARTH and JOENSUU 2007), radiosensitizers (NELSON et al. 1986; MIRALBELL et al. 1999; FORD et al. 2007), and radioimmunotherapy (Levels I–IV) (QUANG and BRADY 2004). However, to date, none of these have shown a clinically meaningful improvement in survival and are not considered standard therapy.
- Recent experience has led to the widespread use of temozolamide in conjunction with RT as the standard of care.
- Currently, targeted agents are being explored in the treatment of GBM (Level III) (CHAKRAVARTI et al. 2006; KRISHNAN et al. 2006; SATHORNSUMETEE et al. 2006; NARAYANA et al. 2007b).

33.2.2 Surgery

- Surgery is considered as the initial treatment for GBM (Grade A). The intent of surgery may be biopsy for diagnosis, resection with definitive intent, palliative debulking for management of mass effect related symptoms, or shunting to relieve symptoms caused by increased intracranial pressure or hydrocephalus.

- When feasible, maximal surgical resection should be performed as resection appears related to outcome. The Glioma Outcomes Project was organized to generate a prospective database to track patients with malignant glioma (Level III) (LAWS et al. 2003). A total of 52 clinical sites across North America participated and enrolled patients from 1997 to 2001. This observational database was used to evaluate the influence of resection, as opposed to biopsy, on patient outcome with the primary outcome measure being length of survival. The median length of survival was 40.9 weeks for the 413 patients with GBM. In multivariate analysis, resection rather than biopsy was associated with a prolonged survival time for patients with GBM ($p<0.0001$). The prognostic value of resection compared with biopsy was maintained ($p<0.0001$), even after eliminating "poor risk" patients (those with age >60 years, KPS score <70, or presence of multifocal tumors).
- The current NCCN guidelines leave open the option to place a BCNU-impregnated biodegradable polymer (Gliadel wafer) intraoperatively if frozen section reveals high-grade glioma (Grade B). A Phase III randomized trial of the wafer compared to placebo showed an improvement in median survival from 11.6 months to 13.9 months ($p = .03$) (Level II) (WESTPHAL et al. 2003. It is important to note that for patients with GBM, the placebo arm of the trial did not allow systemic BCNU and thus the wafer was not measured against systemic chemotherapy, but rather radiation therapy alone. One potential problem with this approach is that conventional MRI may be difficult to interpret after wafer placement and MRSI may be a better tool for evaluating the presence of tumor (Level IV) (DYKE et al. 2007). Additionally, it should be remembered that the enthusiasm for wafers preceded the temozolamide experience, and thus their use in newly-diagnosed patients who will also get temozolamide is not clearly defined.

33.2.3 Chemoradiation

- Radiation therapy is indicated in the definitive treatment of GBM (Grade A) and most cooperative group trials have required that RT be started within 5 weeks of definitive resection.
- Randomized trials consistently have demonstrated a survival benefit to the use of radiotherapy after

surgery (Level I) (WALKER et al. 1978, 1980). It is clear that postoperative RT improves median survival from 14–22 weeks to 36–47 weeks; however, most patients still die within 2 years with local recurrence (although the pattern of failure remains to be defined in the era of temozolamide and targeted therapy). BTCG 6901 included 200 eligible patients (90% of patients had GBM) who had undergone surgery followed by randomization to supportive care, whole brain RT, BCNU, or whole brain RT and BCNU (Level II) (WALKER et al. 1978). The addition of WBRT improved median survival time from 14 weeks with supportive care alone (19 weeks with BCNU) to 36 weeks. In this study and a subsequent one evaluating methyl-CCNU (Level II) (WALKER et al. 1980), chemotherapy produced a modest benefit in survival, and the standard treatment for GBM in the United States became RT administered along with a nitrosourea, most commonly BCNU.

■ Standard treatment of GBM now includes postoperative chemoradiation with temozolamide followed by six cycles of adjuvant temozolamide (Grade A).

■ The results of the control arm of RTOG 9006, which employed the then-accepted standard of conventional RT and BCNU, serve as an excellent basis with which to compare more recent trials (Level I) (CURRAN et al. 1996). In that study, which was open from 1990–1994, 712 patients with high-grade glioma were randomized to partial brain RT at conventional fractionation of 2.0 Gy/fx daily to 60 Gy versus 1.2 Gy/fraction bid to a total of 72 Gy; patients in both arms received BCNU. The median survival time in the control arm was 13.2 months (it was 11.2 months in the hyperfractionated arm and there was no survival advantage for HFRT in any subgroup; in fact, the median survival time was statistically better for all patients under the age of 50 with conventional fractionation). However, despite multiple cooperative-group attempts, no randomized Phase III trial of nitrosourea-based adjuvant chemotherapy demonstrated a significant survival benefit as compared with radiotherapy alone (STEWART 2002) (although there were more long-term survivors in the chemotherapy groups in some studies) (Level I), and thus in many places, including Europe, RT alone remained the standard of care.

■ The role of chemotherapy in GBM has been redefined on the basis of a Phase III cooperative group trial conducted by the EORTC Brain and Radiotherapy Groups and National Cancer Institute of Canada (Level I) (STUPP et al. 2005). In this trial, 573 patients with GBM were randomized to receive either standard radiotherapy alone (total dose of 60 Gy given as 2 Gy fractions 5 days per week over 6 weeks) or concomitant daily temozolomide (75 mg/m^2 daily), an oral alkylating agent that is able to cross the BBB, with standard radiotherapy followed by six cycles of maintenance temozolomide (150–200 mg/m^2 daily on days 1–5 every 28 days). This trial showed a significant survival benefit in the temozolomide arm. In the original publication the median survival was 14.6 months with radiotherapy plus temozolomide and 12.1 months with radiotherapy alone. The 2-year survival rate was 26.5% with radiotherapy plus temozolomide and 10.4% with radiotherapy alone ($p<.0001$). A recent update reported the 4-year survival rate to be 12.1% in the combined arm and 3% in the RT alone arm (MIRIMANOFF et al. 2007). Toxicity with chemoradiotherapy was acceptable with 7% Grade 3 or 4 hematologic toxicity. Importantly, in the 45% of patients with MGMT methylation, the 2-year survival was 22.1% in the combined modality arm and 5.2% in the RT alone arm ($p=.04$). In the patients without methylation of the MGMT promoter, these numbers were 11.1% and 0% respectively ($p=.035$).

33.2.4 Radiation Therapy

Dose and Fractionation

■ External beam radiation therapy to a total dose of 60 Gy at 2 Gy/fraction (or 59.40 Gy at 1.8 Gy/fraction), in combination with concurrent temozolamide (75 mg/m^2 daily for 42 continuous days) is the standard regimen for definitive treatment (Grade A). A conedown is performed after 46 Gy (or 45 Gy).

■ Data from the original Brain Tumor Cooperative Group protocols showed a significant improvement in median survival from 28 to 42 weeks in the groups treated with doses of 50 to 60 Gy (Level III) (WALKER et al. 1979). A Medical Research Council study also showed a significant survival advantage in patients who received 60 Gy compared to those who received 45 Gy (12 vs. 9 months; $p=.007$) (Level II) (BLEEHEN and STENNING 1991). A benefit for doses >60 Gy using conventional treatment has not been demonstrated. The RTOG and

Eastern Cooperative Oncology Group (ECOG) randomized 253 patients to either whole brain irradiation conventionally fractionated to 60 Gy or 60 Gy plus a 10 Gy boost to a limited volume (Level II) (NELSON et al. 1988). Median survival was 9.3 months for patients receiving 60 Gy and 8.2 months for those receiving 70 Gy.

■ Radiation therapy is delivered in a conventional fractionation schedule as outlined above (Grade A).

■ Several groups have used hyperfractionated or accelerated regimens as a means to escalate dose. In a prospective, randomized Phase I/II trial, RTOG 83-02 examined dose escalation using twice daily fractionation and BCNU in patients with malignant gliomas (Level II) (WERNER-WASIK et al. 1996). Hyperfractionated regimens studied were 64.8, 72.0, 76.8, and 81.6 Gy given in 1.2-Gy fractions twice daily, and accelerated hyperfractionated regimens were 48 and 54.4 Gy given in 1.6-Gy twice-daily fractions. Patients also received chemotherapy with BCNU. Early results appeared to favor the 72-Gy arm which led to a Phase III trial comparing conventional radiotherapy of 60 Gy in 30 daily fractions to hyperfractionated radiotherapy to 72 Gy in fractions of 1.2 Gy given twice daily (BCNU was included in both arms) (Level I) (CURRAN et al. 1996). No difference in survival was found.

Volume

■ Partial brain RT is indicated in the treatment of GBM (Grade A). Historically, the entire cranial contents were irradiated, i.e., whole brain RT was the treatment of choice. However, a classic study by HOCHBERG and PRUITT (1980) (Level IV) showed that in 35 patients who had a CT scan within 2 months prior to autopsy, 78% of recurrences of GBM were within 2 cm of the margin of the initial tumor bed and 56% were within 1 cm or less of the volume visualized on the CT scan. As this type of information became available, and as the ability to image CNS tumors developed, partial brain RT was adopted. Subsequently, it was shown that the use of partial brain fields did not compromise outcome as the pattern of recurrence was predominantly still local (Level IV) (HESS et al. 1994), thus validating this approach. Even in patients treated with treated with 3D conformal radiotherapy with small margins to 90 Gy, CHAN et al. (2002) showed that 23/34 patients (68%) recurred in the high-dose region (Level IV).

Simulation and Planning

■ CT-based treatment planning with the utilization of MR fusion is highly recommended for defining GTV and PTV (Fig. 33.1).

■ Individualized immobilization device (e.g., headrest, aquaplast, tiltboards) should be used during planning and treatment.

■ Treatment planning CT should be obtained in treatment position. The head position depends upon the location of the tumor and the patient's ability to tolerate positioning. Slices, no more than 1.25 mm thick, should be obtained from the level of above the head (i.e., into air) through the shoulders. Thicker slices may not allow adequate visualization of structures such as optic nerves, chiasm, cochlea, etc.

■ The tumor volume should be defined using MRI fusion when possible (Fig. 33.2). In the future, there may be a role for incorporating more advanced imaging such as perfusion imaging, spectroscopy, or PET into RT planning (Level IV) (PIRZKALL et al. 2000; TSIEN et al. 2005; NARAYANA et al. 2007a), but to date these remain in the experimental stage. Additionally, the emerging knowledge that the neural stem cells reside in the subventricular zone adjacent to the lateral ventricles and the subgranular zone of the dentate gyrus (Level IV) (BARANI et al. 2007a,b) may affect RT planning in the future.

■ The gross target volume (GTV) for both the initial volume (GTV1) and the conedown volume (GTV2) is obtained from the MRI. GTV1 includes the contrast enhancing lesion, the surgical re-

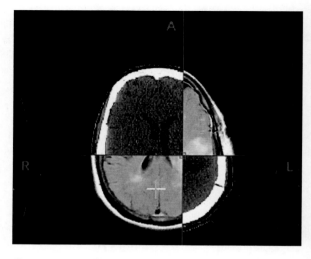

Fig. 33.1. Example of CT/MR fusion for treatment planning

Fig. 33.2. FLAIR abnormality outlined on MR and seen as color wash on treatment planning CT

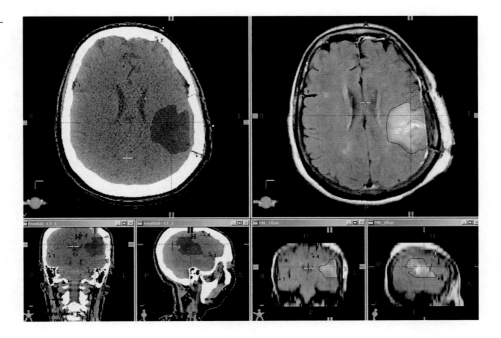

section cavity and surrounding edema; a 2.0-cm margin is added to form PTV1. GTV2 for the conedown treatment should include the contrast-enhancing lesion (without edema) plus a 2.5-cm margin to form PTV2. In anatomic regions in the brain where natural barriers would likely preclude microscopic tumor extension, such as the cerebellum, the contralateral hemisphere, the tentorium cerebri, and the ventricles, the margins may be modified. PTV1 is treated to 46 Gy in 23 fractions and after that there is a conedown to PTV2 which is treated for an additional 14 Gy in seven fractions.

■ Most cooperative group protocols originally specified volumes based on the preoperative imaging. However, recently there has been a trend to plan off postoperative images and to account for anatomic shifts which have occurred after surgery. The rationale for including surrounding T2 change with a margin is based on the knowledge that glioma cells migrate and infiltrate throughout brain parenchyma. Utilizing stereotactic guidance and serial biopsy technique, KELLY et al. (1987) showed that the region of contrast enhancement corresponds to tumor tissue without intervening parenchyma, and the regions of hypodensity and T2 changes correspond to parenchyma infiltrated by isolated tumor cells, to tumor in low-grade gliomas, or to edema (Level IV).

■ Critical structures such as the eyes, optic nerves, chiasm, hypothalamus, brainstem, cochlea, spinal cord, etc., should be outlined. Clinical judgment should be used to limit sensitive structures to within tolerance.

■ Isodose distributions for the PTV1 and PTV2 should be generated and evaluated for homogeneity and normal tissue tolerance. It may also be helpful to look at composite isodose lines in absolute dose when evaluating a plan. The inhomogeneity within the target volume should be kept to ≤10% and the minimum dose to the target volume should be kept within 10% of the dose at the center of the volume (Fig. 33.3).

Treatment Delivery

■ Treatment should be delivered with multiple fields in an attempt to achieve homogeneity throughout the volume and spare dose to uninvolved brain. This can be accomplished using 3D conformal techniques or intensity-modulated radiation therapy (IMRT). In general, parallel opposed portals are not used; however, in cases where tumor is infiltrating across midline through corpus callosum, this may be a very reasonable field arrangement for the initial PTV. Comparative dosimetric analyses suggest that IMRT may decrease dose to critical structures (Level IV) (NARAYANA et al. 2006; MACDONALD et al. 2007).

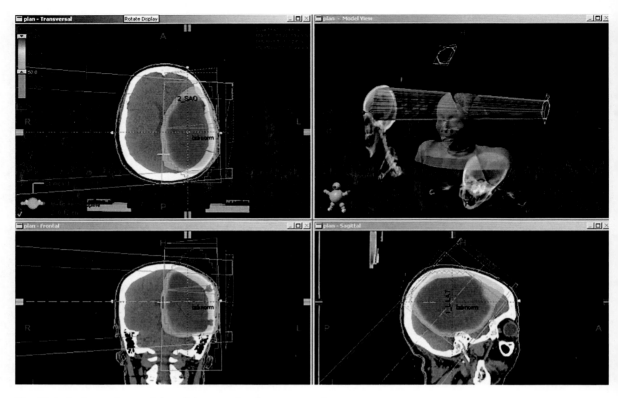

Fig. 33.3. Isodose color wash in axial, coronal and transverse planes

■ Portal imaging should be obtained for field and/ or isocentric verification. On-board imaging allows for daily inspection of accuracy of setup and if performed with kilovoltage probably contributes little to the overall dose; however, if frequent megavoltage imaging is done, care should be taken to evaluate what this will contribute to the total isodose plan, particularly in terms of critical structures.

Radiation Side Effects

■ Radiation-induced side effects and complications depend on the location of the primary tumor and volume of normal tissue treated.

■ Commonly observed acute effects associated with radiation include hair loss, fatigue, anorexia, and erythema or soreness of the scalp. Irritation of the external auditory canal and serous otitis may occur. Potential acute toxicities include nausea and vomiting as well as headaches, seizures, and exacerbation of focal neurologic deficits. Dry mouth or altered taste may be reported by patients.

■ Patients are usually maintained on decadron throughout treatment (a common dose is 2 mg po bid) along with appropriate proton-pump inhibitors or H2 agonists. However, there are some patients, particularly those with gross total resection and no residual edema, who complete RT without requiring steroids. Topical creams such as aquaphor may be required and otitis should be treated if observed. Nutritional counseling may be necessary for supportive care.

■ The radiation oncologist should be familiar with the dosing and side effects of temozolamide. In addition to anticipated side effects such as myelosupression, an increased incidence of PCP pneumonia has been noted in patients who are receiving temodar, and PCP prophylaxis is recommend by the manufacturer during the 42-day course of temozolamide.

■ Possible early delayed radiation effects include lethargy and transient worsening of existing neurological deficits occurring 1–3 months after radiotherapy treatment. Patients may experience somnolence syndrome and require a re-introduction of steroids. Possible late delayed effects of radiotherapy include radiation necrosis, endocrine dysfunction, and radiation-induced neoplasms. In addition, neurocognitive deficits, which could lead to mental slowing and behavioral change, are possible. Permanent hearing impairment and visual damage are rare. Cataracts may develop either associated with steroids or scattered dose to the lens.

with a median age of 75 years and a median KPS of 70 experienced a median overall survival of 6.4 months and a median progression-free survival of 5.0 months. Toxicity was comparable to other trials employing temozolamide.

33.2.5 Palliation

- Many patients with GBM present with a KPS that is poor and they are unable to tolerate a prolonged course of RT. Other patients, particularly the very elderly, may present with co-morbidities which preclude definitive chemoradiation. For these patients, short-course RT is considered. There may be a role for temozolamide alone in this setting.
- Although patients over age 60 were excluded from the EORTC study which established RT and temozolamide as the standard of care, there has not an been upper age limit in most North American glioma trials, and there is evidence that standard chemoradiation with RT and temozolamide is feasible in the "healthy" elderly (Level III) (MINNITI et al. 2008). Thus, age itself should not be the sole factor in determining the course of therapy.
- RT should be delivered to a partial brain field with a palliative regimen such as 30 Gy delivered in ten daily 3.0 Gy fractions delivered over 2 weeks (Grade B).
- No randomized controlled trials have compared 6 weeks of daily conventionally fractionated radiotherapy with short course hypofractionated radiotherapy in patients who are being treated with palliative intent. However, there is limited data for short-course RT comparing the outcome with well-matched cohorts or with historical controls (Level III) (BAUMAN et al. 1994; FORD et al. 1997). It appears that survival and palliative effect are similar as compared with conventional fractionation.
- Temozolamide alone may be a considered, although experience using this drug specifically for palliation is limited.
- There is data for the efficacy of temozolamide in the setting of recurrence (Level III) (CHANG et al. 2004). Additionally, temozolamide has been evaluated as a single agent in the de novo setting. CHINO et. al. (2004) conducted a Phase II study to evaluate the efficacy and safety of temozolamide without RT in elderly patients with newly diagnosed GBM (Level III). A total of 32 patients

33.2.6 Recurrence

- In patients with poor performance status or multiple medical co-morbidities precluding treatment, a palliative approach is warranted. This may include palliative debulking, but there is no data to show that this improves survival. Steroids and anticonvulsants may be employed as indicated, and referral to hospice is appropriate.
- Systemic chemotherapeutic agents have been tested mostly in the context of clinical trials and have not had a major impact on outcome (Level III) (HESS et al. 1999).
- Targeted therapies have been evaluated in the setting of recurrence as well. EGFR is amplified in approximately one half of malignant gliomas, and EGFR tyrosine kinase inhibitors have been evaluated in patients with recurrent GBM. Although retrospective analyses have highlighted co-expression of EGFRvIII and wild-type PTEN (phosphatase and tensin homologue deleted in chromosome 10) as a significant predictor of EGFR-tyrosine kinase inhibitor response in patients with GBM, to date, neither erlotinib or gefinitib has had a major impact on survival (VOELZKE et al. 2008) (review article). Neovascularization is a major feature of GBM, as is VEGF secretion, and hence strategies to inhibit angiogenesis are under active investigation. The agent that currently is receiving intense scrutiny is bevacizumab, an antibody to VEGF. Multiple reports have described marked radiographic responses with striking reductions in peritumoral edema, implying that bevacizumab has considerable effect on restoring the BBB (REARDON et al. 2008) (review article). Currently, bevacizumab is being evaluated by the RTOG in a randomized Phase II trial (with irinotecan versus temozolamide) for recurrent GBM.
- Repeat radiotherapy using one of several different methods (including radiosurgery, brachytherapy, GliaSite balloon brachytherapy, and even repeat external beam radiotherapy) may be considered for carefully selected patients (Grade C).

33.3 Treatment of Anaplastic Astrocytoma

33.3.1 General Principles

■ Anaplastic gliomas generally occur during young to middle adulthood.

■ Anaplastic gliomas include pure anaplastic astrocytomas, anaplastic oligodendrogliomas, and anaplastic mixed oligoastrocytomas.

■ Anaplastic astrocytomas display clinical and biologic heterogeneity. As previously mentioned, patients with anaplastic oligodendroglioma have a better prognosis, particularly those with tumor containing the chromosome changes characterized by loss of heterozygosity of 1 p and 19 q for whom median survival is approximately 5–7 years (Level I and Level III) (Van den Bent et al. 2006; Cairncross et al. 2006; Smith et al. 2000; Fallon et al. 2004; Jeon et al. 2007).

■ The current standard of care for patients with anaplastic gliomas is maximal surgical resection followed by postoperative radiotherapy (Grade A). The radiotherapy target volume and dose are the same as for GBM.

■ Unlike GBM, the survival benefit with chemotherapy is less dramatic, and given potential toxicity, its role in the treatment of anaplastic astrocytoma is more controversial.

33.3.2 RT and Chemotherapy for Pure Anaplastic Astrocytoma

■ The current standard of care is maximal surgical resection when feasible followed by postoperative RT (Grade A). This recommendation stems from the trials discussed in the section on GBMs, most of which included anaplastic astrocytomas.

■ The current NCCN guidelines currently leave chemotherapy as an option (Grade C). Many people have extrapolated the experience of temozolamide in GBM to the setting of anaplastic astrocytoma; however, this is somewhat controversial.

■ BCNU or PCV (procarbazine, CCNU, vincristine) used to be the most common drugs used in the treatment of anaplastic astrocytomas. In a Phase III randomized trial performed by the NCOG, the use of PCV was found to be associated with an improved outcome in patients with anaplastic glioma as compared with BCNU (Level II) (Levin et al. 1990). In contrast, a retrospective review of patients from the RTOG database with newly diagnosed anaplastic astrocytoma, showed no improvement in survival with PCV as compared with BCNU (Level III) (Prados et al. 1999).

■ Temozolomide has shown activity in patients with recurrent anaplastic astrocytoma with an objective response rate of 35% and an acceptable safety profile (Level III) (Yung et al. 1999). The Phase III portion of RTOG 98-13 evaluated RT and temozolamide versus RT and a nitrosourea for anaplastic astrocytomas (mixed anaplastic oligoastrocytoma was included if pathology showed a dominant astrocytic component). This study closed recently and results are pending. A new international study may help clarify the role of temozolamide in the setting of anaplastic astrocytoma. The EORTC is leading in a trial in which patients will be randomly assigned to concomitant RT and temozolamide versus RT alone, with a second random assignment for the administration of adjuvant temozolamide or observation. The trial end point is overall survival; enrollment of more than 800 patients is planned (Stupp et al. 2007) (review article).

33.3.3 RT and Chemotherapy for Anaplastic Oligodendrogliomas and Anaplastic Oligoastrocytomas

■ The current standard of care is maximal surgical resection when feasible followed by postoperative RT (Grade A).

■ The current NCCN guidelines leave chemotherapy as an option (Grade C).

■ Anaplastic oligodendroglioma and oligoastrocytoma are generally thought of as chemosensitive tumors based on their response to PCV (Level III) (Cairncross et al. 1992). Two randomized trials have now evaluated the efficacy of PCV and RT for these tumors. RTOG 94-02 randomized 289 patients with newly diagnosed anaplastic oligodendroglioma and oligoastrocytoma to either radiotherapy alone or neoadjuvant PCV (four cycles) followed by radiotherapy (Level I) (Cairncross et al. 2006). The median survival was 4.9 years in the combined arm, and 4.7 years in the RT alone arm radiotherapy alone ($p = 26$). Progression-free survival was better in the combined arm, 2.6 years versus 1.7 years with RT alone ($p = 008$). However, Grade 3 or 4 toxicity was observed much more frequently with PCV. It is important to note that 57% of patients treated with RT alone received salvage chemotherapy with PCV or temozolomide at the time of recurrence. The second study, EORTC 26951, assessed radiotherapy followed by adjuvant PCV chemotherapy (Level I) (VAN DEN BENT et al. 2006). In this trial 368 patients were randomized to receive either radiotherapy alone or radiotherapy followed by six cycles of adjuvant PCV. The difference in median survival, 40.3 months in the combined arm and 30.6 months in the RT alone arm was not statistically significant ($p = 23$); however, the median progression-free survival was 23 months in the group receiving RT plus PCV compared to 13.2 months in the group receiving radiotherapy alone ($p = 0018$). In this study, PCV was given at recurrence to 65% of patients in the RT alone arm. Thus, two large randomized trials investigating the use of sequential chemoradiotherapy in patients with anaplastic oligodendroglioma and oligoastrocytoma failed to show any overall survival advantage over radiotherapy alone. It is important to note the high number of patients who received chemotherapy at the time of progression: the lack of benefit observed in these trials may reflect the effect of salvage therapy in patients treated initially with RT alone.

- On the EORTC study, 25% of patient were identified as having both 1 p and 19 q loss; in the RTOG study, 1 p/19 q LOH was identified in 46% of the patients. In both studies, patients with loss of 1 p and 19 q survived significantly longer than patients without the chromosomal changes, despite which treatment they received.
- Temozolomide has produced high response rates in patients with anaplastic oligodendroglioma. Studies both in the setting of recurrence following PCV or in newly-diagnosed patients have showed objective responses in the range of 30%–40% (Level III) (CHINOT et al. 2001; VOGELBAUM et al. 2005). Most neuro-oncologists would now use temozolamide when choosing to use chemotherapy. In a survey of the Society of Neuro-oncology members, the majority of whom practiced at academic medical centers, the most common recommendation for the treatment of anaplastic oligodendroglioma, regardless of molecular status, was temozolamide with RT followed by adjuvant temozolamide (Level IV) (ABREY et al. 2007).

33.4 Treatment of Low-Grade Gliomas

33.4.1 General Principles

- Low-grade gliomas are relatively uncommon in adults accounting for approximately 10% of adult primary CNS tumors (www.cbtrus.org/2005-2006/tables/2006.table12.pdf)
- Pilocytic astrocytomas are generally considered a surgical disease and are not addressed in the NCCN guidelines.
- Low-grade gliomas comprise a heterogenous group of tumors including infiltrating fibrillary astrocytomas, pleomorphic xanthoastrocytoma, subependymal giant cell astrocytoma, and subependymoma. Comments will be limited to pilocytic astrocytoma and infiltrating fibrillary astrocytoma; optic tract gliomas will not be discussed.
- The timing of intervention for patients with low-grade tumors remains controversial. The clinical course is variable with some patients having long survival even without treatment and others suffering from progressive deterioration despite treatment. In RTOG 98-02 median time to progression in good risk patients (defined as <40 and gross total tumor resection) was 5 years (Level II) (SHAW et al. 2006). In general, early intervention is indicated for patients with increasing symptoms, radiographic progression, and high-risk features suggestive of transformation to a higher-grade tumor.

33.4.2 Pilocytic Astrocytoma

Surgery

- Pilocytic astrocytoma is a rare tumor in adults, and when it does occur it had been thought to have a relatively benign course. The median age at presentation is in the early 30s (Level III) (BROWN et al. 2004), and the most common symptom is headache (Level III) (BELL et al. 2004). Gross total resection should be performed when feasible, as this is the definitive treatment (Grade A).

Radiation Therapy

- Radiation therapy can be used in the setting of residual symptomatic or progressive, particularly when re-resection is not feasible (Grade B).

■ The use of RT for pilocytic astrocytoma in adults is not well-defined. BROWN et al. (2004) reported the results of a prospective NCCTG/RTOG trial in 20 adults with supratentorial PA treated between 1986 and 1994 (Level III). Patients who had subtotal or gross total resection were observed; patients with biopsy only were treated with postoperative RT with a dose of 50.4 Gy in 28 fractions delivered to the tumor volume and edema. Eleven patients underwent complete resection, six had incomplete resections, and three had biopsy only. At a median follow-up of 10 years, the 5-year progression-free and overall survival rates were 95%. One of the 17 patients who was observed experienced disease progression, but on retrospective review it appeared that only a "minimal" subtotal resection had been performed; this patient was salvaged with RT. One patient who had biopsy and postoperative RT died of unknown causes. Neurologic function remained high in the patients on this study.

■ In general, adults with pilocytic astrocytoma appear to have a favorable prognosis with regard to survival and neurologic function. A series from Germany described 45 patients over the age of 16 years who underwent surgery for primary or recurrent PA (Level III) (STUER et al. 2007). In this series, 18% of patients died from disease at a mean follow-up of greater than 6 years; however, slightly more than a quarter of the patients in this series had pathologic features of increased proliferation or anaplasia.

■ If RT is to be utilized, the dose and volumes treated are those described for pilocytic astrocytoma in children.

31.4.3 Infiltrating Fibrillary Astrocytoma

Surgery

■ Maximal safe surgical resection is the treatment of choice when possible (Grade A).

■ It is controversial as to when to proceed to surgery in a patient with a suspected low-grade glioma. Most patients undergo some type of surgery at presentation in order to establish the diagnosis and to determine histology, grade, and molecular characteristics that affect treatment. However, these tumors are often diffusely infiltrative and involve of eloquent regions making complete surgical resection difficult.

■ Many studies have found total or subtotal (>90%) resection to be associated with improved outcome (Level III) (BERGER et al. 1994; CLAUS et al. 2005; LEIGHTON et al. 1997) and aggressive resection may result in more accurate histopathologic diagnosis (Level IV) (JACKSON et al. 2001).

Radiation Therapy and Chemotherapy

■ The recommendation for a maximally resected tumor is observation for patients under the age of 45, and observation or RT for patients over the age of 45 (Grade B). Interestingly, the current NCCN guidelines use age 45 as a cut-off, whereas many of the cooperative group trials have identified 40 years of age as a cutoff.

■ Chemotherapy may be considered in oligodendrogliomas, particularly those with 1p or combined 1 p 19 q deletion (Grade C).

■ The recommendation for patients with subtotally resected or biopsy-only tumors with stable or controlled symptoms is observation or RT (Grade B). Again, chemotherapy may be considered in oligodendrogliomas, particularly those with 1p or combined 1 p 19 q deletion (Grade C).

■ Patients who have had less than gross total resection and who have uncontrolled or progressive symptoms should be treated with RT (Grade B), although for patients with oligodendrogliomas, particularly those with 1 p or combined 1 p 19 q deletion, chemotherapy may be considered (Grade C).

■ The most controversial issue in the management of the adult patient with a low-grade glioma is whether or not to administer immediate RT or at the time of progression. Many years ago, the Brain Tumor Study Group tried to randomize adults with low-grade glioma to immediate versus delayed postoperative radiation; however, the study was terminated because of poor accrual (likely based on physician bias). The RTOG completed a Phase II study of observation in favorable low-grade glioma (defined as <40 and gross total tumor resection) and a Phase III study of RT with or without PCV in unfavorable low-grade glioma (age >40 or subtotal resection/biopsy) (RTOG 9802) (Level II) (SHAW et al. 2006). Preliminary results were reported in 2006. For the 111 favorable patients who were observed, the

5-year progression-free survival was 50% and the 5-year overall survival was 94%. For the 251 unfavorable patients, there was no difference in overall survival at 5 years: 61% with RT alone and 70% with RT + PCV ($p = 0.72$), and the 5-year progression-free survival was only 39% and 61%, respectively. Analysis of outcome by 1 p 19 q status is pending.

- EORTC 22845 is the only randomized trial in low-grade glioma to compare immediate RT with deferred treatment (including radiotherapy) at the time of progression (Level I) (VAN DEN BENT et al. 2005). In that trial, 314 patients with low-grade gliomas were randomized to receive postoperative radiotherapy to 54 Gy in fractions of 1.8 Gy ($n = 157$) or radiotherapy at progression ($n = 157$). The median progression free survival was significantly better with immediate RT, 5.3 versus 3.4 years ($p < 0001$), but there was no difference in median survival, 7.4 versus 7.2 years ($p = .872$). Seizure control was reported as being better in the immediate RT group, but there was no in-depth quality of life adjusted analysis. Thus, it appears that immediate RT results in improved progression free survival, but withholding radiotherapy until tumor progression does not jeopardize overall survival.
- The RT dose that should be delivered is on the order of 50.4 Gy at 1.8 Gy/fraction daily (Grade A). Involved fields are treated and volumes should be outlined on MRI FLAIR images. Margins of 1–1.5 cm are added to create a PTV.
- This dose for the treatment of low-grade gliomas has been established in two Phase III trials. In EORTC 22844 379 patients were randomized to receive 45 Gy in 5 weeks or 59.4 Gy in 6.6 weeks (Level I) (KARIM et al. 1996). There was no difference in progression free survival or overall survival in either arm (50% and 60%, respectively). In a joint NCCTG/RTOG/ECOG study, 203 patients were randomized to 50.4 Gy in 28 fractions or 64.8 Gy in 36 fractions (Level I) (SHAW et al. 2002). This trial also showed no difference in progression-free survival or overall survival, and Grade 3–5 neurotoxicity occurred in 5% of patients in the high-dose arm as compared with 2.5% of patients in the low-dose arm.
- There is no clearly established role for chemotherapy in adult patients with low-grade gliomas.
- In the Phase III portion of RTOG 98-02, in which 251 patients age >40 or with subtotal resection or biopsy were randomized to receive radiotherapy alone to 54 Gy in 30 fractions or radiotherapy fol-

lowed by six cycles of PCV, the overall survival at 5 years was 61% in those treated with radiotherapy alone and 70 in those treated with radiotherapy plus PCV (Level II) (SHAW et al. 2006). Progression-free survival was not different between the two arms. There was more acute toxicity in the arm that included PCV. Currently, the EORTC is conducting a Phase III trial (EORTC 22033) comparing radiotherapy (50.4 Gy in 28 fractions) versus temozolomide in patients with supratentorial WHO Grade II gliomas who are ≥ 40 years of age or who have radiographic progression or new or worsening neurological symptoms (other than seizures only) or intractable seizures. Patients are stratified by 1 p and 19 q allele status. The RTOG is now testing concurrent temozolamide with RT (54 Gy) for high risk patients with supratentorial WHO Grade II astrocytoma, oligodendroglioma or oligoastrocytoma (RTOG 0424). Patients must have at least three of the following risk factors: age ≥40, largest preoperative diameter of tumor ≥6 cm, tumor crossing midline, tumor subtype of astrocytoma (astrocytoma dominant) or preoperative Neurological Function Status >1.

33.5 Follow-Ups

33.5.1 General Principles

- Follow-up after definitive treatment of brain tumors is imperative to monitor both for recurrence as well as treatment effects.
- The imaging schedule is dependent on the tumor type. Follow-up, however, must also include neurological evaluations and appropriate history and physicals with attention to late effects. Endocrine and neuropsychological screenings should be included based upon the volume and area treated. Screening for second malignancy may be appropriate in long-term survivors.

MRI Schedule

- MRI with and without gadolinium is the imaging of choice for follow-up examination.
- For high-grade gliomas, follow-up MRI should be scheduled 2–6 weeks after RT, then every

2–3 months for 2–3 years (Grade D) (NCCN 2007). In patients who survive longer than this, many clinicians would continue to follow with yearly or every other year MRI 5–10 years after treatment.

■ For low-grade gliomas, follow-up MRI should be scheduled every 3–6 months for 5 years and then at least annually (Grade D) (NCCN 2007).

■ Integration of metabolic scans into post-treatment follow-up may help distinguish between tumor recurrence and treatment-related changes (Grade C). Additional imaging may be warranted to help clarify changes on MRI. Spectroscopy, perfusion, or PET may help aid in the differential of tumor versus necrosis (HERHOLZ et al. 2007) (review article).

References

Abrey LE, Louis DN, Paleologos N et al. (2007) Survey of treatment recommendations for anaplastic oligodendroglioma. Neuro-Oncology 9:314–318

American Joint Committee on Cancer (AJCC) (1997) Cancer staging manual, 5th edn. Lippincott-Raven, Philadelphia, PA

Barani IG, Benedict SH, Peck-Sun L (2007a) Neural stem cells: implications for the conventional radiotherapy of central nervous system malignancies. Int J Radiat Oncol Biol Phys 68:324–333

Barani IG, Cuttino LW, Bendict SH et al. (2007b) Neural stem cell-preserving external-beam radiotherapy of central nervous system malignancies. Int J Radiat Oncol Biol Phys 68:978–985

Barth RF, Joensuu H (2007) Boron neutron capture therapy for the treatment of glioblastomas and extracranial tumours: as effective, more effective or less effective than photon irradiation? Radiother Oncol 82:119–122

Bauman GS, Gasper LE, Fischer BJ et al. (1994) A prospective study of short course radiotherapy in poor prognosis glioblastoma multiforme. Int J Radiat Oncol Biol Phys 29:835–839

Bell D, Chitnavis BP, Al-Sarraj S et al. (2004) Pilocytic astrocytoma of the adult – clinical features, radiological features and management. Br J Neurosurg 18:613–616

Berger MS, Deliganis AV, Dobbins J et al. (1994) The effect of extent of resection on recurrence in patients with low grade cerebral hemisphere gliomas. Cancer 74:1784–1791

Bleehen NM, Stenning SP (1991) A Medical Research Council trial of two radiotherapy doses in the treatment of Grades 3 and 4 astrocytoma. The Medical Research Council Brain Tumour Working Party. Br J Cancer 64:769–774

Brown PD, Buckner JC, O'Fallon JR et al. (2004) Adult patients with supratentorial pilocytic astrocytomas: a prospective multicenter clinical trial. Int J Radiat Oncol Biol Phys 58:1153–1160

Cairncross JG, Macdonald DR, Ramsay DA (1992) Aggressive oligodendroglioma: a chemosensitive tumor. Neurosurgery 31:78–82

Cairncross G, Berkey B, Shaw E et al. (2006) Phase III trial of chemotherapy plus radiotherapy compared with radiotherapy alone for pure and mixed anaplastic oligodendroglioma: Intergroup RadiationTherapy Oncology Group Trial 9402. J Clin Oncol 24:2707–2714

Cardinale R, Won M, Choucair A et al. (2006) A Phase II trial of accelerated radiotherapy using weekly stereotactic conformal boost for supratentorial glioblastoma multiforme: RTOG 0023. Int J Radiat Oncol Biol Phys 65:1422–1428

Castro JR, Saunders WM, Austin-Seymour MM et al. (1985) A Phase I–II trial of heavy charged particle irradiation of malignant glioma of the brain: a Northern California Oncology Group Study. Int J Radiat Oncol Biol Phys 11:1795–1800

Chakravarti A, Berkey B, Robins HI et al. (2006) An update of Phase II results from RTOG 0211: a Phase I/II study of gefitinib with radiotherapy in newly diagnosed glioblastoma. J Clin Oncol 24[Suppl]:1527

Chan JL, Lee SW, Fraass BA et al. (2002) Survival and failure patterns of high grade gliomas after three-dimensional conformal radiotherapy. J Clin Oncol 20:1635–1642

Chang SM, Theodosopoulos P, Lamborn K et al. (2004) Temozolamide in the treatment of recurrent malignant glioma. Cancer 100:605–611

Chinot OL, Honore S, Dufour H et al. (2001) Safety and efficacy of temozolomide in patients with recurrent anaplastic oligodendrogliomas after standard radiotherapy and chemotherapy. J Clin Oncol 19:2449–2455

Chinot OL, Barrie M, Frauger E et al. (2004) Phase II study of temozolomide without radiotherapy in newly diagnosed glioblastoma multiforme in an elderly populations. Cancer 100:2208–2214

Claus EB, Horlacher A, Hsu L et al. (2005) Survival rates in patients with low grade glioma after intraoperative magnetic resonance image guidance. Cancer 103:1227–1233

Colman H, Berkey BA, Moar MH et al. (2006) Phase II Radiation Therapy Oncology Group trial of conventional radiation therapy followed by treatment with recombinant interferon-beta for supratentorial glioblastoma: results of RTOG 9710. Int J Radiat Oncol Biol Phys 66:818–824

Curran WJ Jr, Scott CB, Horton J et al. (1993) Recursive partitioning analysis of prognostic factors in three Radiation Therapy Oncology Group malignant glioma trials. J Natl Cancer Inst 85:704–710

Curran W, Scott C, Yung W et al. (1996) No survival benefit of hyperfractionated radiotherapy (RT) to 72.0 Gy and carmustine versus standard RT and carmustine for malignant glioma patients: preliminary results of RTOG 90-06. J Clin Oncol 15[Suppl]:154, 280

DelRowe J, Scott C, Werner-Wasik M et al. (2000) A single-arm open label Phase II study of intravenously administered tirapazamine plus radiation therapy for glioblastoma multiforme. J Clin Oncol 18:1254–1259

Donahue B, Scott C, Nelson J et al. (1997) Influence of an oligodendroglial component on the survival of patients with anaplastic astrocytoma: a report of RTOG 83-02. Int J Radiat Oncol Biol Phys 38:911–914

Dyke JO, Sanelli PC, Voss HU et al. (2007) Monitoring the effects of BCNU chemotherapy wafers (Gliadel) in glioblastoma multiforme with proton magnetic resonance spectroscopic imaging at 3.0 Tesla. J Neurooncol 82:103–110

Eyre HJ, Crowley J, Townsend JJ et al. (1993) A randomized trial of radiotherapy versus radiotherapy plus CCNU for incompletely resected low-grade gliomas. A SWOG study. J Neurosurg 78:909–914

Fallon KB, Palmer CA, Roth KA et al. (2004) Prognostic value of 1 p, 19 q, 9 p, 10 q, and EGFR-FISH analyses in recurrent oligodendrogliomas. J Neuropathol Exp Neurol 63:314–322

Fisher B, Won M, Macdonald D et al. (2002) Phase II study of topotecan plus cranial radiation for glioblastoma multiforme: results of Radiation Therapy Oncology Group RTOG 95-13. Int J Radiat Onco Biol Phys 53:980–986

Ford JM, Stenning SP, Boote DJ et al. (1997) A short fractionation radiotherapy for poor prognosis patients with high-grade glioma. Clin Oncol 9:20–24

Ford JM, Seiferheld W, Alger JR et al. (2007) Results of the Phase I dose-escalating study of motexafin gadolinium with standard radiotherapy in patients with glioblastoma multiforme. Int J Radiat Oncol Biol Phys 69:831–838

Gajjar A, Bhargava R, Jenkins JJ et al. (1995) Low-grade astrocytoma with neuraxis dissemination at diagnosis. J Neurosurg 83:67–71

Hegi ME, Diserens AC, Gorlia T et al. (2005) MGMT gene silencing and benefit from temozolomide in glioblastoma. N Engl J Med 352:997–1003

Herholz K, Coope D, Jackson A (2007) Metabolic and molecular imaging in neuro-oncology. Lancet Neurol 6:711–724

Hess CF, Schaaf JC, Kortmann RD et al. (1994) Malignant glioma: patterns of failure following individually tailored limited volume irradiation. Radiother Oncol 30:146–149

Hess KR, Wong ET, Jaeckle KA et al. (1999) Response and progression in recurrent malignant glioma. Neuro Oncol 1:282–288

Hochberg FH, Pruitt A (1980) Assumptions in the radiotherapy of glioblastoma. Neurology 30:907–911

Hukin J, Siffert J, Cohen H et al. (2003) Leptomeningeal dissemination at diagnosis of pediatric low-grade neuroepithelial tumors. Neuro Oncol 5:188–196

Jackson RJ, Fuller GN, Abi-Said D et al. (2001)Limitations of stereotactic biopsy in the initial management of gliomas. Neuro Oncol 3:193–200

Jenkinson MD, Du Plessis DG, Walker C, Smith TS (2007) Advanced MRI in the management of adult gliomas. Br J Neurosurg 21:550–561

Jeon YK, Park K, Park CK et al. (2007) Chromosome 1 p and 19 q status and p 53 and p 16 expression patterns as prognostic indicators of oligodendroglial tumors: a clinicopathological study using fluorescence in situ hybridization. Neuropathology 27:10–20

Karim AB, Maat B, Hatlevoll R et al. (1996) A randomized trial on dose-response in radiation therapy of low-grade cerebral glioma: European Organization for Research and Treatment of Cancer (EORTC) Study 22844. Int J Radiat Oncol Biol Phys 36:549–556

Kelly PJ, Daumas-Duport C, Scheithauer BW et al. (1987) Stereotactic histologic correlations of computed tomography- and magnetic resonance imaging-defined abnormalities in patients with glial neoplasms. Mayo Clin Proc 62:450–459

Kreth FW, Faist M, Rossner R et al. (1997) Supratentorial World Health Organization Grade 2 astrocytomas and oligodendrogliomas. A new pattern of prognostic factors. Cancer 70:370–379

Krishnan S, Brown PD, Ballman KV et al. (2006) Phase I trial of erlotinib with radiation therapy in patients with glioblastoma multiforme: results of North Center Cancer Treatment Group protocol N0177. Int J Radiat Oncol Biol Phys 65:1192–1199

Langer C, Ruffer J, Rhodes H et al.(2001) Phase II Radiation Therapy Oncology Group Trial of weekly paclitaxel and conventional external beam radiation therapy for supratentorial glioblastoma multiforme. Int J Radiat Oncol Biol Phys 51:113–119

Laramore GE, Diener-West M, Griffin TW et al. (1988) Randomized neutron dose searching study for malignant gliomas of the brain: results of an RTOG study. Radiation Therapy Oncology Group. Int J Radiat Oncol Biol Phys 14:1093–1102

Laws ER, Parney IF, Huang W et al. (2003) Survival following surgery and prognostic factors for recently diagnosed malignant glioma: data from the Glioma Outcomes project. J Neurosurg 99:467–473

Leighton C, Fisher B, Bauman G et al. (1997) Supratentorial low-grade glioma in adults: an analysis of prognostic factors and timing of radiation. J Clin Oncol 15:1294–1301

Levin VA, Silver P, Hannigan J et al. (1990) Superiority of post-radiotherapy adjuvant chemotherapy with CCNU, procarbazine, and vincristine (PCV) over BCNU for anaplastic gliomas: NCOG 6G61 final report. Int J Radiat Oncol Biol Phys 18:321–324

MacDonald S, Ahmad S, Krachis S et al. (2007) Intensity modulated radiation therapy versus three-dimensional conformal radiation therapy for the treatment of high grade glioma: a dosimetric comparison. J Appl Clin Med Phys 8:47–60

Mamelak AN, Prados MD, Obana WG et al. (1994) Treatment options and prognosis for multicentric juvenile pilocytic astrocytoma. J Neurosurg 81:24–30

Minniti G, De Sanctis V, Muni R et al. (2008) Radiotherapy plus concomitant and adjuvant temozolomide for glioblastoma in elderly patients. J Neurooncol; published online Feb 5, 2008

Miralbell R, Mornex F, Greiner R et al. (1999) Accelerated radiotherapy, carbogen, and nicotinamide in glioblastoma multiforme: report of European Organization for Research and Treatment of Cancer trial 22933. J Clin Oncol 17:3143–3149

Mirimanoff R, Mason W, Van den Bent M et al. (2007) Is long-term survival in glioblastoma possible? Updated results of the EORTC/NCIC Phase III randomized trial on radiotherapy (RT) and concomitant and adjuvant temozolamide (TMZ) versus RT alone. Int J Radiat Oncol Biol Phys 69[Suppl]:S2

Murray KJ, Nelson DF, Scott C et al. (1995) Quality-adjusted survival analysis of malignant glioma. Patients treated with twice-daily radiation (RT) and carmustine: a report of Radiation Therapy Oncology Group (RTOG) 83-02. Int J Radiat Oncol Biol Phys 31:453–459

Narayana A, Yamada J, Berry S et al. (2006) Intensity-modulated radiotherapy in high-grade gliomas: clinical and dosimetric results. Int J Radiat Oncol Biol Phys 64:892–897

Narayana A, Chang J, Thakur S et al. (2007a) Use of MR spectroscopy and functional imaging in the treatment planning of gliomas. Br J Radiol 80:347–354

Narayana A, Golfinos J, Knopp E et al. (2007b) Feasibility of using bevacizumab with radiation therapy in high grade glioma. Int J Radiat Oncol Biol Phys 69[Suppl]:90,S51

Nelson DF, Diener-West M, Weinstein AS et al. (1986) A randomized comparison of misonidazole sensitized radiotherapy plus BCNU and radiotherapy plus BCNU for treatment of malignant glioma after surgery: final report of an RTOG study. Int J Radiat Oncol Biol Phys 12:1793–1800

Nelson DF, Diener-West M, Horton J et al. (1988) Combined modality approach to treatment of malignant gliomas – re-evaluation of RTOG 7401/ECOG 1374 with long-term follow-up: a joint study of the Radiation Therapy Oncology Group and the Eastern Cooperative Oncology Group. NCI Monogr (6):279–284

Pickles T, Goodman GB, Rheaume DE et al. (1997) Pion radiation for high grade astrocytoma: results of a randomized study. Int J Radiat Oncol Biol Phys 37:491–497

Pignatti F, van den Bent M, Curran D et al. (2002) Prognostic factors for survival in adult patients with cerebral low-grade glioma. J Clin Oncol 20:2076–2084

Pirzkall A, Larson DA, McKnight TR et al. (2000) MR-spectroscopy results in improved target delineation for high-grade gliomas. Int J Radiat Oncol Biol Phys 48[Suppl]:115

Pollack IF, Hurtt M, Pang D et al. (1994) Dissemination of low grade intracranial astrocytomas in children. Cancer 73:2671–2673

Prados MD, Scott C, Curran WJ Jr et al. (1999) Procarbazine, lomustine, and vincristine (PCV) chemotherapy for anaplastic astrocytoma: a retrospective review of Radiation Therapy Oncology Group protocols comparing survival with carmustine or PCV adjuvant chemotherapy. J Clin Oncol 17:3389–3395

Quang TS, Brady L (2004) Radioimmunotherapy as a novel treatment regimen: 125I-labeled monoclonal antibody 425 in the treatment of high-grade brain gliomas. Int J Radiat Onco Biol Phys 58:972–975

Reardon DA, Desjardins A, Rich JN, Vredenburgh JJ (2008) The emerging role of anti-angiogenic therapy for malignant glioma. Curr Treat Options Oncol; published online Feb 7, 2008

Robins HI, Won M, Seiferheld WF et al. (2006) Phase 2 trial of radiation plus high-dose tamoxifen for glioblastoma multiforme: RTOG protocol BR-0021. Neuro Oncol 8:47–52

Sathornsumetee S, Reardon DA, Quinn JA et al. (2006) An update on Phase I study of dose-escalating imatinib mesylate plus standard-dosed temozolomide for the treatment of patients with malignant glioma. J Clin Oncol 24[Suppl]:1560

Scott C, Curran W, Yung W et al. (1998) Long term results of RTOG 9006: a randomized trial of hyperfractionated radiotherapy (RT) to 72.0 Gy and carmustine vs. standard RT and carmustine for malignant glioma patients with emphasis on anaplastic astrocytoma (AA) patients. J Clin Oncol 16[Suppl]:384

Selker RG, Shapiro WR, Burger P et al. (2002) The Brain Tumor Cooperative Group NIH Trial 87-01: a randomized comparison of surgery, external radiotherapy, and carmustine versus surgery, interstitial radiotherapy boost, external radiation therapy, and carmustine. Neurosurgery 51:343–355

Shaw E, Arusell R, Scheithauer B et al. (2002) Prospective randomized trial of low-versus high-dose radiation therapy in adults with supratentorial low-grade glioma: initial report of a North Central Cancer Treatment Group/

Radiation Therapy Oncology Group/Eastern Cooperative Oncology Group study. J Clin Oncol 20:2267–2276

Shaw EG, Berkey BA, Coons SW et al. (2006) Initial report of Radiation Therapy Oncology Group (RTOG) 9802: prospective studies in adult low-grade glioma (LGG). J Clin Oncol 24[Suppl]:1500

Smith JS, Perry A, Borell TJ et al. (2000) Alterations of chromosome arms 1 p and 19 q as predictors of survival in oligodendrogliomas, astrocytomas, and mixed oligoastrocytomas. J Clin Oncol 18:636–645

Souhami L, SeiferheldW, Brachman D et al. (2004) Randomized comparison of stereotactic radiosurgery followed by conventional radiotherapy with carmustine to conventional radiotherapy with carmustine for patients with glioblastoma multiforme: report of Radiation Therapy Oncology Group 93-05 protocol. Int J Radiat Oncol Biol Phys 60:853–860

Stewart LA (2002) Chemotherapy in adult high grade glioma: a systematic review and metaanalysis of individual patient data from 12 randomised trials. Lancet 359:1011–1018

Stuer C, Vilz B, Majores M et al. (2007) Frequent recurrence and progression in pilocytic astrocytoma in adults. Cancer 110:2799–2808

Stupp R, Mason WP, Van den Bent MJ et al. (2005) Radiotherapy plus Concomitant and Adjuvant Temozolomide for Glioblastoma. N Engl J Med 352:987–996

Stupp R, Hegi ME, Gilbert MR and Chakravarti A (2007) Chemoradiotherapy in malignant glioma: standard of care and future directions. J Clin Oncol 25:4127–4136

Tsien C, Piert M, Junck D et al. (2005) The impact of 11C methionine (11C MET) positron emission tomography (PET) imaging in target volume delineation of glioblastoma multiforme. Int J Radiat Oncol Biol Phys 63[Suppl]:S63–S64

Van den Bent MJ, Afra D, de Witte O et al. (2005) Long-term efficacy of early versus delayed radiotherapy for low-grade astrocytoma and oligodendroglioma in adults: the EORTC 22845 randomised trial. Lancet 366:985–990

Van den Bent MJ, Carpentier AF, Brandes AA et al. (2006) Adjuvant procarbazine, lomustine, and vincristine improves progression-free survival but not overall survival in newly diagnosed anaplastic oligodendrogliomas and oligoastrocytomas: a randomized European Organization for Research and Treatment of Cancer Phase III trial. J Clin Oncol 24:2715–2722

Voelzke WR, Petty WJ, Lesser GJ (2008) Targeting the epidermal growth factor receptor in high-grade astrocytomas. Curr Treat Options Oncol; published online Feb 5, 2008

Vogelbaum MA, Berkey B, Peereboom D et al. (2005) RTOG 0131: Phase II trial of pre-irradiation and concurrent temozolomide in patients with newly diagnosed anaplastic oligodendrogliomas and mixed anaplastic oligodendrogliomas. J Clin Oncol 23[Suppl]:1520

Walker MD, Alexander E, Jr, Hunt WE et al. (1978) Evaluation of BCNU and/or radiotherapy in the treatment of anaplastic gliomas. A cooperative clinical trial. J Neurosurg 49:333–343

Walker MD, Strike TA, Sheline GE (1979) An analysis of dose-effect relationship in the radiotherapy of malignant gliomas. Int J Radiat Oncol Biol Phys 5:1725–1731

Walker MD, Green SB, Byar DP et al. (1980) Randomized comparisons of radiotherapy and nitrosoureas for the treatment of malignant glioma after surgery. N Engl J Med 303:1323–1329

Welsh J, Sanan A, Gabayan AJ et al. (2007) GliaSite brachytherapy boost as part of initial treatment of glioblastoma multiforme: a retrospective multi-institutional pilot study. Int J Radiat Oncol Biol Phys 68:159–165

Werner-Wasik M, Scott CB, Nelson DF et al. (1996) Final report of a Phase I/II trial of hyperfractionated and accelerated hyperfractionated radiation therapy with carmustine for adults with supratentorial malignant gliomas. Radiation Therapy Oncology Group Study 83-02. Cancer 77:1535–1543

Werner-Wasik M, Seiferheld W, Michalski J et al. (2004) Phase I/II conformal three-dimensional radiation therapy dose escalation study in patients with supratentorial glioblastoma multiforme: report of the Radiation Therapy Oncology Group 98-03 Protocol. Int J Radiat Oncol Biol Phys 60[Suppl]:S163–164, 58

Westphal M, Hilt DC, Bortey E et al. (2003) A Phase 3 trial of local chemotherapy with biodegradable carmustine (BCNU) wafers (Gliadel wafers) in patients with primary malignant glioma. Neuro Oncol 5:79–88

Yung WK, Prados MD, Yaya-Tur R et al. (1999) Multicenter Phase II trial of temozolomide in patients with anaplastic astrocytoma or anaplastic oligoastrocytoma at first relapse. Temodal Brain Tumor Group. J Clin Oncol 17:2762–2771

Yung WA, Seiferheld W, Donahue B et al. (2001) A RTOG (Radiation Therapy Oncology Group) Phase II study of conventional radiation therapy plus thalidomide followed by thalidomide post XRT for supratentorial glioblastoma. J Clin Oncol 20[Suppl]:206, 52a

Pituitary Tumors

34

Walter H. Choi and Matthew C. Biagioli

W. H. Choi, MD
Department of Radiation Oncology, Beth Israel Medical Center, 10 Union Square East, Suite 4G, New York, NY 10003, USA
M. C. Biagioli, MD, MS
Division of Radiation Oncology, Department of Interdisciplinary Oncology, University of South Florida, 12902 Magnolia Drive, Tampa, FL 33612-9416, USA

Introduction and Objectives

Pituitary adenoma is a relatively common disease entity of the CNS, and accounts for 10%–15% of all diagnosed primary intracranial tumors. Results of autopsy series demonstrated that pituitary adenomas are detected in 3%–25% of pituitary glands. Approximately 70% of all pituitary cases are endocrinologically functional. Localized tumors may have both local and systemic signs and symptoms, and a multidisciplinary approach to evaluation and management is necessary. Randomized studies of different treatment modalities in the management of pituitary adenomas do not exist.

This chapter examines:

● **Recommendations for diagnosis and work-up**

● **Treatment recommendations for various tumor types as well as the supporting scientific evidence**

● **The use of medical, surgical, and radiotherapeutic intervention for management of pituitary tumors**

● **Radiation therapy techniques for the treatment of pituitary tumors**

● **Follow-up care and surveillance after treatment**

34.1 Diagnosis, Staging, and Prognoses

34.1.1 Diagnosis

Initial Evaluation

■ Diagnosis and initial evaluation of pituitary tumor should include a detailed history and physical examination, with particular emphasis on neurologic and cranial nerve examination, especially the optic nerves and cranial nerves III, IV, V_1, V_2 and VI, which travel through the cavernous sinus.

■ Approximately 70% of pituitary adenomas are functional. Among functional tumors, prolactin-secreting adenomas are the most common, followed by GH- and ACTH-secreting tumors.

- Ophthalmologic evaluation and visual field testing should be performed. The most common visual field deficit is a bitemporal hemianopsia, although other deficits, including superior temporal deficits, homonymous hemianopsias may occur.
- In patients with known diagnosis of malignancies, metastasis should be considered in the differential diagnosis.

Laboratory Tests

- Laboratory tests including a complete blood count and serum chemistries should be performed, as well as baseline measurements of endocrine hormones. The majority of pituitary tumors arise from the anterior pituitary, which is derived from Rathke's pouch (ectodermal origin) and produces ACTH, FSH, LH, GH, TSH and prolactin. The posterior pituitary and infundibulum arise from an outgrowth of the diencephalon, and stores and releases ADH and oxytocin, which are produced by the hypothalamus.
- Patients with prolactinomas will demonstrate an elevated serum prolactin level. Although moderately elevated levels can have several causes, a level >200 ng/ml is usually diagnostic. Prolactinomas are more common in women. Premenopausal women may present with galactorrhea, and oligomenorrhea or amenorrhea. Men may present with impotence and decreased libido secondary to low testosterone levels. Alterations in mood may also be present.
- ACTH-secreting tumors can cause Cushing's disease, with symptoms secondary to adrenal hyperplasia and elevated cortisol levels. Symptoms include thin, brittle skin, hypertension, glucose intolerance, osteoporosis, easy bruisability, central obesity, buffalo hump, moon facies, abdominal striations, proximal muscle weakness, acne, hirsutism, and psychological disturbances.
- Laboratory tests should include a 24-h urine free cortisol level and a dexamethasone suppression test. Patients are given 1 mg of dexamethasone in the evening; normally, ACTH is suppressed and cortisol levels decrease by 50%. Elevated levels suggest Cushing's syndrome. Petrosal sinus venous sampling can also be performed when the diagnosis is difficult.
- Growth hormone secreting adenomas can cause gigantism in children and acromegaly in adults. Laboratory tests should include a fasting growth hormone level, which is usually greater than 10 ng/mL, and a glucose suppression test, where after 100 g bolus of oral glucose, GH levels are measured. Normally, GH levels will be suppressed to <5 ng/mL.

Imaging Studies

- Contrast enhanced MRI is the imaging study of choice for evaluating pituitary tumors (Fig. 34.1) (Grade B). When contraindicated, a high-resolution CT scan is recommended. Results from a prospective comparison between MRI and CT for the diagnosis and evaluation of pituitary tumor revealed that MRI is more sensitive for certain types of pituitary adenoma, such as ACTH secreting tumors (Level III) (ESCOUROLLE et al. 1993).
- Patients with acromegaly should also undergo skeletal surveys.

34.1.2 Staging

- Pituitary tumors can be classified by size into microadenomas (≤1 cm) and macroadenomas (>1 cm). Other considerations include tumor invasion and vision defects requiring decompression.
- Hardy's classification for pituitary adenomas and grading for suprasellar extension is listed in Table 34.1. The classification utilized information from radiographic studies as well as intraoperative findings of sellar destruction and extrasellar invasion.
- Functionally, they are separated into functioning (secretory) and nonfunctioning (nonsecretory) tumors.

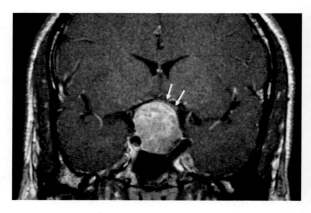

Fig. 34.1. Coronal T1 post-contrast MR image of a pituitary macroadenoma. Note the displacement of the optic nerve (*arrows*)

Table 34.1. Hardy's radiographic classification for pituitary adenomas and grading schema for suprasellar extensions

Hardy's radiographic classification for pituitary adenomas	
0:	Normal pituitary appearance
I:	Enclosed within the sella, microadenoma, <10 mm
II:	Enclosed within the sella, macroadenoma, ≥10 mm
III:	Invasive, locally, into the sella
IV:	Invasive, diffusely, into the sella
Hardy's grading schema for suprasellar extensions	
A:	0–10 mm suprasellar extension occupying the suprasellar cistern
B:	10–20 mm extension, elevation of the third ventricle
C:	20–30 mm extension, occupying the anterior third ventricle
D:	Greater than 30 mm extension, beyond the foramen of Monro, or Grade C with lateral extensions.

34.2 Treatment of Pituitary Tumors

34.2.1 General Principles

- The management of pituitary tumors is by nature multimodal. Surgery, medical management and radiation therapy are all therapeutic options, each with advantages and disadvantages (Fig. 34.2).
- The goal of management is the normalization and alleviation of symptoms from excessive pituitary secretion, shrinkage of tumors and decompression of contiguous structures, maintaining normal pituitary function, as well as preventing recurrence.
- Secretory tumors must further be classified by the hormones they secrete. The primary approach is dependent on the classification of a given diagnosed adenoma. What follows is an integrated approaches based on tumor classification.

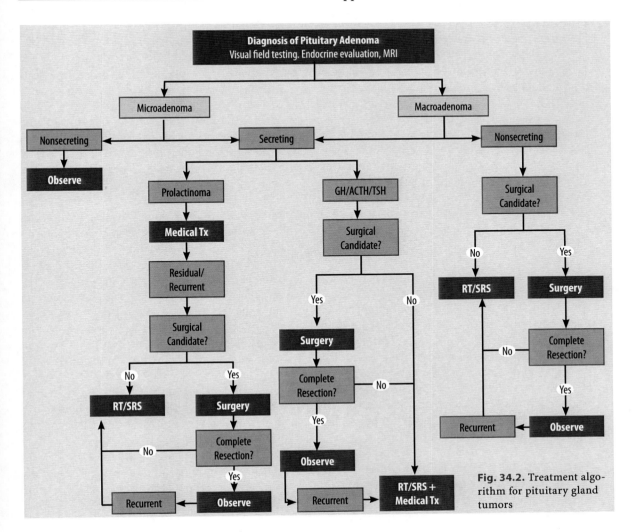

Fig. 34.2. Treatment algorithm for pituitary gland tumors

Nonfunctioning Tumors

■ Nonfunctioning tumors comprise one third of pituitary adenomas. Because they are non-secreting, they usually present as macroadenomas with neurological symptoms associated with compression.

■ Nonfunctioning microadenomas that are incidentally detected (i.e., asymptomatic) can be observed with serial MRIs.

■ Surgical resection from a transsphenoidal approach with a sellar fat graft is the preferred primary treatment (Grade B). However, due to frequent supra- and parasellar extension, surgery is infrequently curative, leaving tumor remnant to regrow with long-term follow-up (Level IV) (TURNER et al. 1999). Close to 20% of patients with macroadenomas who achieved radiographic complete resection will recur as opposed to 58% of those with residual disease (Level IV) (FERRANTE et al. 2006).

■ Patients with adenoma remnant after surgery can be radiographically followed or undergo re-resection or radiotherapy (Grade B). In a group of 122 patients with clinically nonfunctioning pituitary adenomas followed using a prospective protocol, no patient received immediate adjuvant radiation. Periodical MRI scans were performed. The researchers found that disease progression that necessitated radiotherapy occurred in 14 patients (Level III) (GREENMAN et al. 2003). Most retrospective series using either fractionated irradiation (BRADA et al. 1993; BREEN et al. 1998; PARK et al. 2004) or stereotactic radiosurgery (SRS) (FEIGL et al. 2002; PETROVICH et al. 2003; LISCAK et al. 2007) report a tumor control rate of >90% (Level IV).

Prolactinomas

■ Prolactinomas are the most common type of hyper-secreting pituitary adenomas accounting for 60% (MELMED 1995). They generally present in women as microadenomas with lower prolactin levels and symptoms of amenorrhea, galactorrhea, and infertility as compared with men who predominately present with macroadenomas with higher prolactin levels and symptoms of impotence, loss of libido, and infertility.

■ Medical management is the preferred approach for prolactinomas (Grade B). Primary surgical approaches alone only cure about 70% of microadenomas and 30% of macroadenomas (MELMED 1995).

■ Bromocriptine in the management of prolactinomas was first introduced in the 1970s. Its mechanism of action inhibits prolactin secretion by binding D2 dopamine receptors in the anterior pituitary. It is indicated as initial therapy for both microadenomas and macroadenomas in both men and women. Bromocriptine is successful in 80%–90% of patients with microadenomas, normalizing prolactin levels, decreasing tumor size, and normalizing sexual function (VANCE et al. 1984). In patients with macroadenomas normalized prolactin levels and decreasing tumors size by > 50% occurred in 75% of patients treated with bromocriptine (Level III) (LIUZZI et al. 1985; MOLITCH et al. 1985; BEREZIN et al. 1995). Though resistance to bromocriptine is rare, the drug is not curative, and discontinuation usually results in recurrence (Level III) (JOHNSTON et al. 1984; VAN'T VERLAAT and CROUGHS 1991). Maintenance therapy is usually indicated with the exception of rare small microadenoma in which the drug can be withdrawn (Level III) (JOHNSTON et al. 1984).

■ Cabergoline is a long-acting D2 receptor agonist which can be used to suppress prolactin levels for 14 days with single oral administration (Grade A). A double-blind comparison of bromocriptine with cabergoline involving 459 women with amenorrheic prolactinomas demonstrated that cabergoline better normalized prolactin levels (83% vs. 59%), resumed normal gonadal function (72% vs. 52%), and resolved galactorrhea (90% vs. 78%) than bromocriptine (Level I) (WEBSTER et al. 1994). Cabergoline has also been reported to shrink 75% of macroadenomas and may be effective in bromocriptine resistant patients (Level III) (BILLER et al. 1996; COLAO et al. 1997).

■ Surgery is indicated in hyperprolactinemic patients intolerant or resistant to dopamine agonists and in patients with invasive macroadenomas and compromised vision with no immediate response to medical treatment (Grade B). Surgical debulking alone is rarely curative and dopamine agonist therapy is usually required after surgery. Primary surgical approaches alone only cure about 70% of microadenomas and 30% of macroadenomas (MELMED 1995).

■ Radiation therapy is typically reserved for patients in whom medical and surgical treatments have failed, or if patients are not surgical candidates (Grade B). Biochemical cure rates are typically slow to achieve, with variable long-term hormonal control rates reported in single-institution series, ranging from approximately 20% to 50%. These levels can be achieved with either fractionated radiation therapy (Level IV) (GRIGSBY et al. 1989; TSAGARAKIS et al. 1991) or SRS (Level IV) (PAN et al. 2000). Continued medical treatment after radiation therapy is required. As with other secreting adenomas, tumor control is more successful than hormonal control.

ACTH Secreting Tumors

- Adrenocorticotropin hormone (ACTH)-producing tumors make up 15% of functioning pituitary adenomas of which 90% are microadenomas.

- The primary management of Cushing's disease is transsphenoidal surgery (Grade B) (MELBY 1988). The cure rate of this procedure is about 80%–90% for microadenomas but only up to 50% for macroadenomas (Level IV) (MAMPALAM et al. 1988). Hypopituitarism associated with permanent hypocortisolism may occur. In most cured patients, a postoperative period of adrenal insufficiency lasts as long as 6 months. Hypocortisolism recurs in approximately 5% of patients who have had successful surgery.

- Mitotane or ketoconazole therapy in combination with irradiation is the preferred treatment after surgical failure. It is usually used for several months until the delayed biochemical effects of the irradiation occur. Combined treatment results in biochemical remission in 80%–100% of patients after 8–16 months.

- Other less frequently used drugs include etomidate, metyrapone, and aminoglutethimide. Bromocriptine and octreotide have no role in the treatment of Cushing's disease.

- In rare circumstances bilateral adrenalectomy is indicated to treat Cushing's disease that has failed other treatments.

- Radiation is offered in patients in whom surgery is contraindicated, or for patients in whom ACTH secretion persists or recurs (Grade B). Compared with other functional adenomas, ACTH-secreting tumors seem to have an overall better hormonal control rate after irradiation, with results ranging around 50% for either fractionated RT (HOWLETT et al. 1989; LITTLEY et al. 1990) or SRS (SHEEHAN et al. 2000; DEVIN et al. 2004) (Level IV).

GH Secreting Tumors

- Somatotroph adenomas account for 20% of functional pituitary adenomas, with 75% being macroadenomas. Diagnosis may be delayed by up to 10 years because the symptoms of acromegaly are slow to develop.

- The primary management of GH-secreting micro- and macroadenomas is transsphenoidal surgery (Grade B). The cure rates are approximately 70% and 50%, respectively (FAHLBUSCH et al. 1992; MELMED et al. 1995).

- Growth hormone levels usually return to normal within 1 h, and IGF-I levels become normal after 1 week. Residual pituitary function is usually preserved after resection of well-encapsulated tumors, and signs of preoperative tumor compression are often restored by surgery. However, acromegaly may recur several years after surgery in 5%–10% of patients who have had the operation, and pituitary failure is found in up to 15% of patients.

- Somatostatin analogues may be used as adjuvant therapy or as primary treatment in selected cases. Octreotide is the most commonly used analogue and its indication includes presurgical therapy in patients with large invasive macroadenomas, immediate relief of symptoms, and reduction of growth hormone hypersecretion in patients awaiting surgery or those with recurrent disease, morbidity in elderly patients, and a patient's decision not to undergo surgery. Treatment with somatostatin analogues or bromocriptine should also be initiated when previous surgical therapy has not achieved biochemical remission. Pegvisomant, a new GH-receptor antagonist, is indicated in case of resistance to somatostatin analogs. Patients who are resistant to medical management should be referred for sellar irradiation or additional surgery.

- As in other functional adenomas, radiation is reserved for patients with residual or recurrent disease (Grade B). Either fractionated radiation therapy or SRS can be offered, with slow improvement in growth hormone levels over several years. Hormonal cure rates vary in reported series, and may depend on length of follow-up, but generally are in the range of 20%–40% after RT (LUDECKE et al. 1989; MACLEOD et al. 1989) or stereotactic radiosurgery (Level IV) (ZHANG et al. 2000; CASTINETTI et al. 2005).

Thyroid-Stimulating Hormone-Secreting Adenomas

- Thyroid-stimulating hormone (TSH)-secreting adenomas are very rare, accounting for <1% of adenomas, of which 70% are macroadenomas.
- Transsphenoidal adenoma resection is the primary treatment of choice. Patients with continued TSH hypersecretion after surgery or who are inoperable should be treated with octreotide with or without radiotherapy (Grade B). Preoperative treatment with octreotide has been shown to produce euthyroid (BECK-PECCOZ and PERSANI 2002). However, there is currently only limited data to suggest that it may improve the success of or obviate total resection (Level IV) (SOCIN et al. 2003).
- As in other functional tumors, radiation is reserved for patients who have incomplete resections or recurrence of disease (Grade B). Radiotherapy is successful in controlling hormone secretion in approximately two thirds of patients (Level IV) (BECK-PECCOZ et al. 1996).

34.3 Surgical Intervention

- A transsphenoidal approach is the preferred management and can be performed microscopically or endoscopically. The endoscopic approach offers advantages of a wider close-up view of the surgical field and the possibility of "looking around the corners" by using differently angled lenses. These gains can be clinically expressed by minimization of surgical trauma, obviation of the nose speculum and nasal packing, as well as easier treatment of recurrences. In select invasive cases an intracranial approach is necessitated.
- After surgical decompression, 79% of patients with preoperative diminished visual acuity have improvement in their symptoms (BLACK et al. 1988).
- Surgical complications occur in 6.5%–29% of patients. Commonly observed surgical complications include CSF leaks, paranasal sinusitis, septal perforation, meningitis, empty sella syndrome, and intracranial bleeding. Operative mortality rates are between 1%–3% (Level IV) (CIRIC et al. 1983; MOHR et al. 1990; COMTOIS et al. 1991; ORUCKAPTAN et al. 2000).

34.4 Radiation Therapy

- There are no randomized studies comparing the various techniques of irradiation for pituitary adenomas. Selection of modality is often influenced by the clinical presentation, availability of resources, and physician and patient preference.

External-Beam Radiation Therapy

- External-beam radiation therapy is the most common radiation technique in the treatment of pituitary tumors.
- Positioning and immobilization of patients is critical to minimize morbidity of normal structures. An Aquaplast mask is used to reproduce the patient's head position during daily setup.
- With two-dimensional planning techniques, patients were typically treated with a three-field approach, using two lateral opposed fields and an anterior/superior field. Patients are typically positioned with maximal head flexion; this allows the orbital structures to be avoided in the anterior/superior field. Treatment with two opposed lateral fields alone should be avoided, in order to decrease the temporal lobe dose.
- 3D planning techniques are recommended for patients undergoing radiation therapy. Patients should undergo contrast-enhanced CT-based simulation and treatment planning. MRI aids in delineating the GTV for pituitary adenomas, and should be coregistered with the simulation CT.
- Additional margin expansion from GTV to CTV is unnecessary in pituitary adenomas. With conventional external RT planning techniques, an expansion of approximately 1 cm is required for the PTV.
- Doses of 45–54 Gy are recommended with a daily dose of 1.8 Gy, with nonsecreting tumors typically receiving 45–50.4 Gy and secreting tumors receiving 50.4–54 Gy (Grade B). Doses of <45 Gy are associated with higher relapse rates (Level III) (GRIGSBY et al. 1989; MCCOLLOUGH et al. 1991; ZIERHUT et al. 1995).

Stereotactic Radiosurgery (SRS)

- Stereotactic radiosurgery is an alternative to external-beam radiation therapy for pituitary adenomas (Grade B). Prescribed doses range widely, from 10–30 Gy, but mean doses of approximately 16 Gy to the margin have been demonstrated to be effective, with higher doses often delivered for functional tumors (Level III) (SHEEHAN et al. 2002). Although some reports have suggested a more rapid decline of hormone levels with SRS compared with fractionated RT, this has not consistently proven to be the case (BRADA et al. 2004).

- The dose to the optic chiasm should be kept below 8 Gy in order to minimize the risk of radiation-induced optic neuropathy (Level III) (TISHLER et al. 1993; GIRKIN et al. 1997). If the optic chiasm is prohibitively close to the tumor, fractionated radiation should be recommended.

Fractionated Stereotactic Radiation Therapy (FSRT)

- Fractionated stereotactic radiation therapy (FSRT) utilizes stereotactic guidance to maximize precision of radiation delivery and minimize the PTV expansion required for setup variability, thereby minimizing the risk of damage to normal structures (Fig. 34.3).
- FSRT can be offered in patients with larger tumors and those that are close to the optic apparatus.
- Various immobilization techniques are available, including noninvasive headframes, masks with bite-blocks/radiocamera systems, and standard thermoplastic masks. Image-guidance techniques are often utilized as well, in order to maximize treatment accuracy.

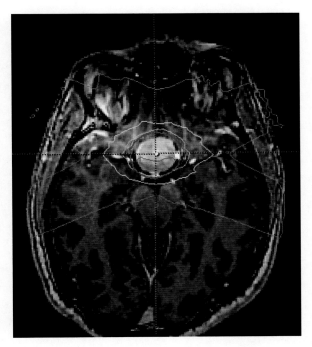

Fig. 34.3. Fractionated stereotactic radiation therapy plan for treatment of a pituitary macroadenoma

- The optimal imaging schedule is unknown and has not been addressed in any clinical trials. MRI of the brain with contrast should be performed annually.
- Hormone levels should also be performed. In patients undergoing surgery or radiation, panhypopituitarism may be a sequela of treatment, and close follow-up with an endocrinologist is necessary.
- In patients undergoing radiation, regular visual field testing is also recommended.

34.5 Follow-Up

34.5.1 Post-Treatment Follow-Ups

- Long-term follow-up is indicated for patients with pituitary adenoma after definitive treatment or if observation is usually required.

Schedule and Work-Ups

- Each follow-up should include neurological evaluations and appropriate history and physical examinations.

References

Beck-Peccoz P, Persani L (2002) Medical management of thyrotropin-secreting pituitary adenomas. Pituitary 5:83–88

Beck-Peccoz P, Brucker-Davis F et al. (1996) Thyrotropin-secreting pituitary tumors. Endocr Rev 17:610–638

Berezin M, Shimon I et al. (1995) Prolactinoma in 53 men: clinical characteristics and modes of treatment (male prolactinoma). J Endocrinol Invest 18:436–441

Biller BM, Molitch ME et al. (1996) Treatment of prolactin-secreting macroadenomas with the once-weekly dopamine agonist cabergoline. J Clin Endocrinol Metab 81:2338–2343

Black PM, Zervas NT et al. (1988) Management of large pituitary adenomas by transsphenoidal surgery. Surg Neurol 29:443–447

Brada M, Rajan B et al. (1993) The long-term efficacy of conservative surgery and radiotherapy in the control of pituitary adenomas. Clin Endocrinol (Oxf) 38:571–578

Brada M, Ajithkumar TV, Minniti G (2004) Radiosurgery for pituitary adenomas. Clin Endocrinol (Oxf) 61:531–543

Breen P, Flickinger JC et al. (1998) Radiotherapy for nonfunctional pituitary adenoma: analysis of long-term tumor control. J Neurosurg 89:933–938

Castinetti F, Taieb D et al. (2005) Outcome of gamma knife radiosurgery in 82 patients with acromegaly: correlation with initial hypersecretion. J Clin Endocrinol Metab 90:4483–4488

Ciric I, Mikhael M et al. (1983) Transsphenoidal microsurgery of pituitary macroadenomas with long-term follow-up results. J Neurosurg 59:395–401

Colao A, Di Sarno A, Sarnacchiaro F et al. (1997) Prolactinomas resistant to standard dopamine agonists respond to chronic cabergoline treatment. J Clin Endocrinol Metab 82:876–883

Comtois R, Beauregard H et al. (1991) The clinical and endocrine outcome to trans-sphenoidal microsurgery of non-secreting pituitary adenomas. Cancer 68:860–866

Devin JK, Allen GS et al. (2004) The efficacy of linear accelerator radiosurgery in the management of patients with Cushing's disease. Stereotact Funct Neurosurg 82:254–262

Escourolle H, Abecassis JP et al. (1993) Comparison of computerized tomography and magnetic resonance imaging for the examination of the pituitary gland in patients with Cushing's disease. Clin Endocrinol (Oxf) 39:307–313

Fahlbusch R, Honegger J et al. (1992) Surgical management of acromegaly. Endocrinol Metab Clin North Am 21:669–692

Feigl GC, Bonelli CM et al. (2002) Effects of gamma knife radiosurgery of pituitary adenomas on pituitary function. J Neurosurg 97[5 Suppl]:415–421

Ferrante E, Ferraroni M, Castrignanò T et al. (2006) Nonfunctioning pituitary adenoma database: a useful resource to improve the clinical management of pituitary tumors. Eur J Endocrinol 155:823–829

Girkin CA, Comey CH et al. (1997) Radiation optic neuropathy after stereotactic radiosurgery. Ophthalmology 104:1634–1643

Greenman Y, Ouaknine G, Veshchev I et al. (2003) Postoperative surveillance of clinically nonfunctioning pituitary macroadenomas: markers of tumour quiescence and regrowth. Clin Endocrinol (Oxf) 58:763–769

Grigsby PW, Simpson JR et al. (1989) Prognostic factors and results of surgery and postoperative irradiation in the management of pituitary adenomas. Int J Radiat Oncol Biol Phys 16:1411–1417

Howlett TA, Plowman PN et al. (1989) Megavoltage pituitary irradiation in the management of Cushing's disease and Nelson's syndrome: long-term follow-up. Clin Endocrinol (Oxf) 31:309–323

Johnston DG, Hall K et al. (1984) Effect of dopamine agonist withdrawal after long-term therapy in prolactinomas. Studies with high-definition computerised tomography. Lancet 2:187–192

Liscak R, Vladyka V, Marek J, Simonová G, Vymazal J (2007) Gamma knife radiosurgery for endocrine-inactive pituitary adenomas. Acta Neurochir (Wien) 149:999–1006; discussion 1006

Littley MD, Shalet SM et al. (1990) Long-term follow-up of low-dose external pituitary irradiation for Cushing's disease. Clin Endocrinol (Oxf) 33:445–455

Liuzzi A, Dallabonzana D et al. (1985) Low doses of dopamine agonists in the long-term treatment of macroprolactinomas. N Engl J Med 313:656–659

Ludecke DK, Lutz BS et al. (1989) The choice of treatment after incomplete adenomectomy in acromegaly: proton-versus high voltage radiation. Acta Neurochir (Wien) 96:32–38

Macleod AF, Clarke DG et al. (1989) Treatment of acromegaly by external irradiation. Clin Endocrinol (Oxf) 30:303–314

Mampalam TJ, Tyrrell JB et al. (1988) Transsphenoidal microsurgery for Cushing disease. A report of 216 cases. Ann Intern Med 109:487–493

McCollough WM, Marcus RB Jr et al. (1991) Long-term follow-up of radiotherapy for pituitary adenoma: the absence of late recurrence after greater than or equal to 4500 cGy. Int J Radiat Oncol Biol Phys 21:607–614

Melby JC (1988) Therapy of Cushing disease: a consensus for pituitary microsurgery. Ann Intern Med 109:445–446

Melmed S (1995) The pituitary. Blackwell Science, Cambridge, Mass.

Melmed S, Ho K, Klibanski A, Reichlin S, Thorner M (1995) Clinical review 75: recent advances in pathogenesis, diagnosis, and management of acromegaly. J Clin Endocrinol Metab 80:3395–3402

Mohr G, Hardy J et al. (1990) Surgical management of giant pituitary adenomas. Can J Neurol Sci 17:62–66

Molitch ME, Elton RL et al. (1985) Bromocriptine as primary therapy for prolactin-secreting macroadenomas: results of a prospective multicenter study. J Clin Endocrinol Metab 60:698–705

Oruckaptan HH, Senmevsim O et al. (2000) Pituitary adenomas: results of 684 surgically treated patients and review of the literature. Surg Neurol 53:211–219

Pan L, Zhang N et al. (2000) Gamma knife radiosurgery as a primary treatment for prolactinomas. J Neurosurg 93[Suppl 3]:10–13

Park P, Chandler WF et al. (2004) The role of radiation therapy after surgical resection of nonfunctional pituitary macroadenomas. Neurosurgery 55:100–106; discussion 106–107

Petrovich Z, Yu C et al. (2003) Gamma knife radiosurgery for pituitary adenoma: early results. Neurosurgery 53:51–59; discussion 59–61

Sheehan JM, Vance ML et al. (2000) Radiosurgery for Cushing's disease after failed transsphenoidal surgery. J Neurosurg 93:738–742

Sheehan JP, Kondziolka D et al. (2002) Radiosurgery for residual or recurrent nonfunctioning pituitary adenoma. J Neurosurg 97[5 Suppl]:408–414

Socin HV, Chanson P et al. (2003) The changing spectrum of TSH-secreting pituitary adenomas: diagnosis and management in 43 patients. Eur J Endocrinol 148:433–442

Tishler RB, Loeffler JS et al. (1993) Tolerance of cranial nerves of the cavernous sinus to radiosurgery. Int J Radiat Oncol Biol Phys 27:215–221

Tsagarakis S, Grossman A et al. (1991) Megavoltage pituitary irradiation in the management of prolactinomas: long-term follow-up. Clin Endocrinol (Oxf) 34:399–406

Turner HE, Stratton IM et al. (1999) Audit of selected patients with nonfunctioning pituitary adenomas treated without irradiation – a follow-up study. Clin Endocrinol (Oxf) 51:281–284

Vance ML, Evans WS et al. (1984) Drugs five years later. Bromocriptine. Ann Intern Med 100:78–91

van't Verlaat JW, Croughs RJ (1991) Withdrawal of bromocriptine after long-term therapy for macroprolactinomas; effect on plasma prolactin and tumour size. Clin Endocrinol (Oxf) 34:175–178

Webster J, Piscitelli G et al. (1994) A comparison of cabergoline and bromocriptine in the treatment of hyperprolactinemic amenorrhea. Cabergoline Comparative Study Group. N Engl J Med 331:904–909

Zhang N, Pan L et al. (2000) Radiosurgery for growth hormone-producing pituitary adenomas. J Neurosurg 93[Suppl 3]:6–9

Zierhut D, Flentje M et al. (1995) External radiotherapy of pituitary adenomas. Int J Radiat Oncol Biol Phys 33:307–314

Section IX:

Skin Cancers and Soft Tissue Sarcoma

Cutaneous Malignant Melanoma

Michael F. Back

CONTENTS

M. F. Back, MD
Department of Radiation Oncology, Northern Sydney Cancer Centre, Royal North Shore Hospital, St Leonards NSW 2065, Australia

Introduction and Objectives

Cutaneous melanoma is a significant oncological condition in countries with large Caucasian populations. Not only is there a rising incidence rate, but mortality rates have also increased in many countries (Jemal et al. 2008). As demonstrated from Cancer Registry Data in NSW Australia, the age standardized incidence has risen by 16% in males and 24% in females over the 10 years from 1996 to 2005. It accounts for almost 10% of malignancies, with an incidence of 59.8 new cases per 100,000 in males. One in 24 males and one in 33 females will develop a melanoma by age 75. Melanoma ranks as the 7th most common cause for cancer related mortality in males (Tracey et al. 2006).

Cutaneous malignant melanoma is a cancer that has a poor prognosis despite the early presentation of relatively small bulk primary tumors. Initial surgical therapy involves a structured management for achieving adequacy of resection and pathological staging. Multidisciplinary management is beneficial for decision-making regarding the optimal adjuvant therapies, including clinical trial involvement. Radiation oncology has an evolving role for selected patients with high risk locoregional disease and palliation.

This chapter examines:
- Approaches to clinical and pathological diagnosis, prognostic factors, and staging
- Initial surgical management of primary and nodal sites
- Selection of patients for adjuvant radiation therapy at primary and nodal sites
- Radiobiological issues and dose/fractionation for adjuvant radiation therapy
- Techniques for adjuvant regional radiation therapy post nodal dissection
- Issues regarding adjuvant systemic therapy and interferon-α-2b therapy
- Approaches to palliative interventions in advanced disease

35.1 Diagnosis, Staging, and Prognosis

35.1.1 Diagnosis

Initial Diagnosis

- Diagnosis and evaluation of malignant melanoma starts with a complete history and physical examination. Given its relatively high incidence, awareness of melanoma is an important aspect of initial evaluation of skin lesions. Risk factors for melanoma predominantly relate to individuals at high risk with history of sun exposure. Individuals with fair skin complexion or hair, blue eyes, poor ability to tan, or with a prior history of pigmented skin lesions have a greater risk of developing melanoma (BLISS et al. 1995).
- A thorough skin examination is usually required.
- Melanoma may be differentiated from benign pigmented lesions by demonstrating features that are changing, display variation in pigmentation, border, or shape, or are symptomatic such as with ulceration.
- Clinico-pathological subtypes of melanoma and related clinical importance to radiation oncologists are listed in Table 35.1.
- Lesion sites are generally in sun exposed regions of the trunk and limbs. Acral lentiginous melanoma is less frequent and may occur in subungal sites, mucosal surface, or soles of feet.

- Amelanotic melanoma demonstrating minimal or absent pigmentation are unusual but may occur with nodular melanoma or naevoid melanoma.
- Lentigo maligna refers to the in situ variant of melanoma and generally presents as a large macular pigmented lesion, often located in the face of elderly patients. Transformation to invasive melanoma (lentigo maligna melanoma) occurs over a long natural history and the rate of concurrent clinically occult invasive melanoma at time of excision is 5%–15% (HAZAN et al. 2008).
- Metastatic spread is generally to regional lymph nodes and then to distant sites. Most common systemic sites of spread are skin, lung, and brain.

Imaging Studies

- There is a minimal role for imaging modalities in asymptomatic patients with localized lesions or nodal metastases detected on sentinel lymph node biopsy (SLNB) (Grade B). A recent retrospective study on 183 patients with SLNB-positive melanoma undertaking thorough CT demonstrated only one patient with detectable metastatic disease (Level IV) (MIRANDA 2006).
- Similarly, patients with palpable nodal disease or clinically advanced melanoma can undertake baseline staging investigations with CT of chest, abdomen, and brain, although there is no evidence to confirm cost-effectiveness of these procedures (Grade D). The rate of positive detection is reported at 5%–20% (Level IV) (BUZAID et al. 1995).

Table 35.1. Clinico-pathological subtypes of malignant melanoma

Pathological subtype	Proportion	Relevant clinical features
Superficial spreading	60%	Radial growth and may have single cell or pagetoid spread throughout epidermis, thus risk for satellite metastases
Nodular	15%–30%	Early deep invasion. Well defined as no lateral growth phase. May be amelanotic
Acral lentiginous	5%	Palmar, plantar, subungual, and mucosal surfaces
Lentigo maligna melanoma	5%	Invasive lesion of lentigo maligna (LM). Long history of radial growth as LM before vertical growth phase
Desmoplastic	2%–3%	May resemble scar tissue and prone for neurotropic spread. Risk for local recurrence
Nevoid	<2%	Misdiagnosed as benign nevus

- Positron emission tomography (FDG-PET) scan has utility in the detection of metastatic melanoma and as a marker of response in advanced disease (Level III). In one retrospective study of 250 patients at various stages of management, accuracy of PET/CT was significantly higher than either PET alone or CT in the detection of metastatic disease (0.98 vs. 0.93 and 0.84) (Level IV) (REINHARDT et al. 2006). However, it has low specificity or sensitivity as an initial staging investigation (Level IV) (CONSTANTINIDOU et al. 2008).

Biopsy and Pathology

- Lesions with any of the above clinical features in individuals at risk should be managed promptly with an incisional biopsy or, if cosmetically feasible, excisional biopsy with narrow (2-mm) margins (TSAO et al. 2004).
- All excised pigmented or atypical lesions in an at-risk population should undergo pathological review. Surveillance photography and clinical mapping of atypical lesions or dysplastic naevi can be utilized to detect early malignant change (Grade D).
- Malignant melanoma is confirmed on microscopic appearance of mitoses, invasion, and immunohistochemical staining to S100 protein and HMB-45 antibody. The pathological report should include description of size, presence of ulceration, maximum thickness, and level of invasion and microscopic margins of resection. Other immunohistochemical markers include MART-1 and MAGE-1 (BLESSING et al. 1998).
- Maximum thickness to be reported as per Breslow thickness (mm); level of invasion should be reported as per the Clark's level (Levels I–V) (Table 35.2). It is important to note that Level I in the Clark's level is technically non-existent (in situ melanoma has other names), and if there is involvement of lymph nodes or distant metastases, another staging system must be used.

Table 35.2. Clark's level of invasion

Level I:	Confined to epidermis (in situ); never metastasizes; 100% cure rate
Level II:	Invasion into papillary dermis; invasion past basement membrane (localized)
Level III:	Tumor filling papillary dermis (localized), and compressing the reticular dermis
Level IV:	Invasion of reticular dermis (localized)
Level V:	Invasion of subcutaneous tissue (regionalized by direct extension)

- A potential genetic link is suggested as family history and history of prior melanoma are associated with risk of melanoma. A hereditary melanoma condition is proposed with mutations in CDK4, CDKN2a genes (GOLDSTEIN et al. 2007).

35.1.2 Staging

- The American Joint Committee on Cancer (AJCC) Tumor Node Metastasis (TNM) staging system incorporates lesion thickness, ulceration, and nodal involvement for non-metastatic melanoma. Level of invasion is utilized only for lesions <1.0 mm thick (Table 35.3) (GREENE et al. 2002).

35.1.3 Prognostic Factors

- Stage at presentation is the most important prognostic factor for malignant melanoma. Prognosis is related to stage of melanoma as demonstrated in Figure 35.1.
- Tumor thickness, ulceration, and level of invasion are the major factors associated with survival in localized melanoma. Long-term results from a prospective surgical trial aimed to compare various surgical margins for resection showed that depth of invasion is a significant factor for outcome in lesions measuring 1–4 mm in depth (Intergroup Melanoma Surgical Trial, Level III) (BALCH 2001a). Mitotic rate and presence of vessel invasion are also associated with poor survival.
- Desmoplastic and neurotropic melanoma are associated with increased local relapse (Level IV) (QUINN et al. 1998).

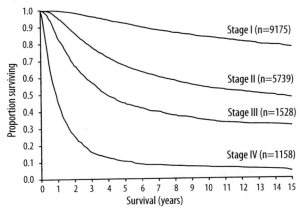

Fig. 35.1. 15-Year survival curves for AJCC stage [From GREENE et al. (2002) with permission]

Table 35.3. American Joint Committee on Cancer (AJCC) TNM classification of carcinoma cancer of melanoma of the skin. [From GREENE et al. (2002) with permission]

Primary tumor (T)	
TX	Primary tumor cannot be assessed (e.g., shave biopsy or regressed melanoma)
T0	No evidence of primary tumor
Tis	Melanoma in situ
T1	Melanoma ≤ 1.0 mm in thickness with or without ulceration
T1a	Melanoma ≤ 1.0 mm in thickness and level II or III, no ulceration
T1b	Melanoma ≤ 1.0 mm in thickness and level IV or V or with ulceration
T2	Melanoma 1.01–2 mm in thickness with or without ulceration
T2a	Melanoma 1.01–2 mm in thickness, no ulceration
T2b	Melanoma 1.01–2 mm in thickness, with ulceration
T3	Melanoma 2.01-4 mm in thickness with or without ulceration
T3a	Melanoma 2.01-4 mm in thickness, no ulceration
T3b	Melanoma 2.01–4 mm in thickness, with ulceration
T4	Melanoma greater than 4.0 mm in thickness with or without ulceration
T4a	Melanoma >4.0 mm in thickness, no ulceration
T4b	Melanoma >4.0 mm in thickness, with ulceration
Regional lymph nodes (N)	
NX	Regional lymph nodes cannot be assessed
N0	No regional lymph node metastasis
N1	Metastasis in one lymph node
N1a	Clinically occult (microscopic) metastasis
N1b	Clinically apparent (macroscopic) metastasis
N2c	Satellite or in-transit metastasis without nodal metastasis
N3	Metastasis in four or more regional nodes, or matted metastatic nodes, or in-transit metastasis or satellite(s) with metastasis in regional node(s)
Distant metastasis (M)	
MX	Distant metastasis cannot be assessed
M0	No distant metastasis
M1	Distant metastasis
M1a	Metastasis to skin, subcutaneous tissues or distant lymph nodes
M1b	Metastasis to lung
M1c	Metastasis to all other visceral sites or distant metastasis at any site associated with an elevated serum lactic dehydrogenase (LDH)
STAGE GROUPING	
0:	Tis N0 M0
IA:	T1a N0 M0
IB:	T1b N0 M0, T2a N0 M0
IIA:	T2b N0 M0, T3a N0 M0
IIB:	T3b N0 M0, T4a N0 M0
IIC:	T4b N0 M0
III:	Any T N1 M0, Any T N2 M0, Any T N3 M0
IV:	Any T Any N M1

35.2 Treatment for Localized Melanoma

35.2.1 General Principles

- Management of malignant melanoma is recommended to be undertaken in specialist units with access to surgical staging and multidisciplinary care (Grade D). Although no study has demonstrated improved outcome, there is evidence for cost-effectiveness (Level IV) (FADER et al. 1998).
- Definitive surgery with wide surgical excision and appropriate nodal management is the principal modality of care in localized melanoma (Grade A).
- Adjuvant locoregional and systemic therapies could be considered (Grade C). However, adjuvant treatment remains controversial with minimal or conflicting evidence as the improvement in outcome.
- The high risk of occult metastatic disease in the presence of a generally young, good performance status patient promotes the participation of patients with high risk lesions into clinical trial protocols.

35.2.2 Definitive Surgery

Primary Surgery Margin Width

- Wide local excision (minimum 1 cm to maximum 3 cm) is the definitive treatment for melanoma with the macroscopic margin width determined on thickness of the lesion from prior biopsy (Grade A). Recommendations for margin width interpreted from randomized clinical trials are listed in Table 35.4.

  Margin width for lesions 2–4 mm remains controversial with the UK Melanoma Study Group Trial of 1 cm versus 3 cm for lesions greater than 2 mm thickness demonstrating a greater risk of locoregional recurrence for the 1 cm margin, but no impact on overall survival (THOMAS and CLARK 2004). Interpreting all studies, there is no evidence to support a margin greater than 2 cm for this subgroup (TSAO et al. 2004).

Table 35.4. Interpretations for margin width extrapolated from randomised clinical trials

Melanoma tumor stage/thickness	Optimal surgical margin	Local recurrence	Reference
T1: <1.0 mm	10 mm	1.6% at 12 years	WHO Study; Cascinelli et al. (1998)
T2: 1.01–2.0 mm	20 mm	<1% at 16 years	French Cooperative Trial; Khayat et al. (2003)
T3: 2.01–4.0 mm	20 mm	3% at 10 years	US Intergroup; Balch et al. (2001b)
T4: >4.0 mm	30 mm	Not specified	UK Melanoma Study Group; Thomas and Clark (2004)

Nodal Management

- Pathological staging of regional lymph nodes is recommended with the use of sentinel-lymph-node biopsy for patients with melanoma greater than 1.0 mm (Grade A).
  The Multicenter Selective Lymphadenectomy Trial (MSLT) Group confirmed the role of SLNB in a large randomized controlled trial published in 2006. Patients with melanoma of intermediate thickness of 1.2–3.5 mm were randomized to SLNB or observation. The incidence of sentinel-node micrometastases was 16.0% (122 of 764 patients), and the rate of nodal relapse in the observation group was 15.6% (78 of 500 patients). Patients with positive SLNB proceeded to formal axillary dissection. There was an improvement in overall survival in patients with nodal disease managed with SLNB (MSLT, Level I) (Morton et al. 2006).
- Both blue dye and radiocolloid should be used to detect the sentinel lymph node during surgery (Grade B). The chance of detecting sentinel lymph node reached 96% using lymphoscintigraphy, intraoperative gamma probe, and isosulfan blue dye in a prospective clinical trial (Level III) (Schmalbach et al. 2003). The MSLT Group used both blue dye and radiocolloid to detect the sentinel lymph node, and examined nodes with both H+E and immunohistochemical analysis (Morton et al. 2006).
- Patients with melanoma <1.0 mm have a low rate of nodal metastases and in the absence of other adverse pathological features there is no role for SLNB.

35.2.3 Adjuvant Radiation Therapy

- The natural history in melanoma suggests that after definitive surgical therapy for localized disease, the most significant risk for the patient is systemic rather than locoregional relapse. Even patients with advanced melanoma who are at higher risk for locoregional failure, have a competing higher risk for distant metastatic disease. The low rate of locoregional relapse in patients with localized melanoma demonstrates that the indications for adjuvant radiation therapy are potentially limited to a poorly defined subgroup of patients, principally with lesions at sites where surgical resection is limited, or demonstrate less common pathological subtypes (Grade B).
  The outcome from randomized clinical trials investigating margin width in localized melanoma demonstrates a local relapse rate of <3% at 10 years after definitive surgical therapy with optimal margin (Tsao et al. 2004). Similarly, in patients managed with SLNB, the MSLT Group demonstrated only a 4.2% risk of regional lymph nodes being site of initial relapse (Level I) (Morton et al. 2006).
- The most significant impact for adjuvant radiation therapy is with patients who have high risk regional disease, where data is evolving as to the role of RT after positive lymph node dissection or in lieu of nodal dissection after a positive SLNB in patients with clinically negative regional nodes.

Radiobiologic Issues

- Melanoma has been presumed to be a relatively radioresistant tumour based on cell survival models showing an enhanced capacity for sublethal damage repair. To overcome the repair capacity hypofractionated regimens were recommended, though total dose was limited by the paralleled reduced capacity for normal tissue repair (Stevens and McKay 2006).

- It is postulated that there is a wide range of radiation sensitivities for melanoma and that a high biological total dose for both conventional and hypofractionated regimens is important to deliver for effective tumour response.

Clinical data on optimal radiation therapy dose/fractionation is conflicting and generally limited to assessing response in metastatic skin nodules. Retrospective data showed an improved response rate for large fraction size (Level IV) (OVERGAARD et al. 1986). However, the only small randomized trial (RTOG 83–05) showed no difference in response rate in 137 patients for a hypofractionated (32 Gy in four fractions delivered weekly) versus conventional schedule (50 Gy in 25 fractions over 5 weeks) (Level II) (SAUSE et al. 1991).

Indications of Local Primary Site Radiation

Melanoma with Limited Surgical Margins

- For most sites re-excision with wide margins is the recommended procedure if initial margins are suboptimal (Grade B). The local control for melanoma excised with 2-cm margins is generally >95%–97%, then adjuvant radiation therapy to the primary site is not appropriate, as detailed above.

- In some local sites, especially in the head and neck region, wide surgical margins may be difficult to achieve without major cosmetic deficit. Radiation therapy can be recommended in these cases (Grade B). Clinical data utilizing adjuvant radiation therapy to high risk local sites are suggestive of an equivalent or acceptable rate of local control. Local control rate of 88% after combined surgery and hypofractionated radiation therapy (30 Gy in five fractions) was reported in a non-randomized series (Level III) (ANG 1994).

Lentigo Maligna Melanoma

- Lentigo maligna melanoma (LMM) and lentigo maligna (LM) refer to the melanoma-in-situ lesions with or without invasive melanoma, respectively. Often situated in the head and neck region the lesions occur in an elderly population, can be more extensive or poorly defined. Thus the ability to remove with wide margins may be limited due to tumour or patient related factors.

- The surgical margins required for LMM and LM are not well defined. Review of the literature utilizing staged excision or Moh's serial mapping procedures confirmed local control rates at 5-year follow-up of >95% (BUB et al. 2004). However, margins of >5 mm for LM and >10 mm for LMM may be required (Level III) (HUILGOL et al. 2004). This may limit patient selection for resection. A benefit of surgical excision may also upstage patients with LM to LMM in 5%–15% of patients (Level IV) (HAZAN et al. 2008).

- Radiation therapy is recommended in the treatment of LM where surgery is not feasible or resection margins will be limited (Grade B). Results from retrospective trials have demonstrated that radiotherapy provided durable local control in patients with LM in retrospective series (Level IV) (FARSHAD et al. 2002).

- The invasive (often nodular) component of LMM is recommended to be excised prior to radiation therapy.

Desmoplastic-Neurotropic Melanoma

- Desmoplastic-neurotropic melanoma is a rare, atypical form of melanoma with a reported incidence of 2%–4%. Characteristically there are dominant spindle cell features with dense fibrosis, and association with neural involvement.

- Radiation has a potential role in the treatment of desmoplastic melanoma (Grade B). Initial reports described high rates of local relapse after complete resection and thus potential benefit from RT (Level IV) (POSTHER et al. 2006).

- In the presence of adequately wide surgical margins (>2 cm) more recent data suggests local relapse rates equivalent to similar thickness melanoma; however, with a greater requirement for re-excision to achieve the margin width (Level IV) (QUINN et al. 1998).

RT may be considered in patients with inadequate margin width of <2 cm (Grade D) (STEVENS et al. 2000).

Presence of Satellite Lesions

- The presence of satellite lesions or adjacent in-transit metastases is a potential indication for adjuvant RT. This may imply more extensive occult disease locally with skip lesions or result in an inability to achieve wide surgical margins.

- The beneficial impact of improved local control by radiation therapy in this clinical scenario is likely to be outweighed by the competing risks of distant metastatic disease in this poor prognostic local factor.

Thick Ulcerated Lesions

- T4b lesions (>4 mm and ulcerated) have a local relapse rate after surgery alone of 10%–15%. Margins of >3 cm are recommended.
- Radiation therapy may potentially improve local control; however, as with the presence of satellite nodules, the competing risks of distant metastatic disease minimizes the benefit of improved local control.

Regional Nodal Irradiation for High Risk Pathological Features After Nodal Dissection

- Regional relapse after nodal dissection has been described to occur at rates of 10%–80% and be associated with potential reduced survival, as well as significant morbidity (Calabro et al. 1989). Risk factors for subsequent regional relapse post nodal dissection include:
  - Residual disease or positive margin
  - Extracapsular extension
  - Multiple nodal involvement
  - Nodal size >3 cm
- The number of nodes to define multiple nodal involvement has been poorly described in clinical series, and it is likely to vary between regional sites.
- In the current Australasian Trans-Tasman Radiation Oncology Group (TROG) Phase III study the eligibility criteria defines the high-risk number of nodes as one or more parotid node, two or more cervical or axillary nodes, and three or more inguino-femoral nodes (Level III) (Burmeister et al. 2002).
- The use of adjuvant radiation therapy in patients with high risk features post dissection has been demonstrated to reduce subsequent regional relapse to less <15% and thus less than historical controls (Grade B). However, aggressive adjuvant regional therapy may be associated with increased treatment related morbidity with lymphedema, without the improved regional control impacting on survival.

Adjuvant radiation therapy delivered after nodal excision without formal lymph node dissection produced an actuarial 5-year regional control and distant metastasis-free survival rates of 93% and 59%, respectively (Level IV) (Ballo et al. 2003). A recent Australasian Phase II multicentre study in 234 high risk patients described a 9.3% regional relapse at 5 years after adjuvant high dose regional RT with acceptable morbidity (Burmeister et al.

2006). This is now being assessed in the TROG phase III study to determine the magnitude of improved regional control and the impact of subsequent regional control on overall survival.

Prophylactic Nodal Irradiation

- The acceptance of pathological staging of regional lymph nodes with SLNB has reduced the requirement for prophylactic nodal management. However, in the absence of SLNB or a decision to avoid nodal dissection after positive SLNB, there is a role for elective RT as nodal management (Grade B). A literature review showed that the likelihood of a positive SLNB exceeds 20% for melanomas >2 mm thick and approximately ≥20% of those patients with positive SLNB will be found to have residual positive lymph nodes on completion of lymph node dissection. Furthermore, patients with positive regional lymph nodes have an approximately ≥20% risk of regional recurrence after surgery alone, particularly if multiple lymph nodes are involved and/or extracapsular extension is present. Postoperative adjuvant radiation therapy results in locoregional control rates of more than 85% in high-risk patients (Mendenhall et al. 2008).

In the head and neck region the single centre experience from Houston demonstrates the effectiveness of elective nodal RT. A hypofractionated regimen of 30 Gy in five fractions using electrons was delivered in 157 patients with clinically node negative disease and 35 patients with positive nodal disease post simple nodal excision. The 10-year actuarial regional control rate was 89%. Treatment related morbidity was acceptable with 6% of patients experiencing a symptomatic treatment related complication, including one patient with temporal lobe necrosis (Level IV) (Bonnen et al. 2004).

35.2.4 Radiation Therapy Regimens

Irradiation of Local Primary Site

- Depending on the site of lesion, conventional or hypofractionated RT regimens may be considered because of the low volume of tissue within portals at primary sites. Cosmetic appearance may be inferior with large dose per fraction.

- The RT field arrangement will depend on the site, surgical scar, and patient contour. Generally, it would involve either an electron field with bolus or kilovoltage superficial RT. The clinical tumor volume (CTV) encompasses the primary tumor surgical bed and a margin of 3 cm. The planned tumor volume (PTV) covers the CTV plus 0.5 cm margin (Grade D).
- 45–50 Gy in 20–25 fractions over 5 weeks or 30 Gy in five fractions over 3 weeks can be recommended for adjuvant treatment after complete resection.
- The acute and delayed side effects and complications induced by radiotherapy is generally dependent on the site and volume irradiated. Acute side effects are usually limited to radiation dermatitis. Late subcutaneous tissue fibrosis or epidermal atrophy and telangiectasia, especially with hypofractionated regimens, may lead to a late cosmetic deficit.

Irradiation of Regional Lymph Nodes

- Although the larger tissue volume to treat the entire nodal surgical bed and proximity to major neural structures potentially increases the risk of late morbidity with hypofractionation regimens, the most recent prospective data has utilized these regimens (Level III) (BURMEISTER et al. 2006).
- Toxicity from nodal irradiation is usually acceptable; however it is important to consider the dosimetry policies utilized in these studies to achieve consistent results.

Target Volume

- Three major nodal sites are treated after regional nodal dissection. For head and neck region, ipsilateral parotid bed, posterior auricular region, levels I–V nodal regions, and the surgical scar should be included. For axilla region, ipsilateral levels I–III axillary nodal regions, adjacent supraclavicular fossa, and the surgical scar should be encompassed. For inguino-femoral regions, ipsilateral femoral, inguinal and external inguinal nodal regions, and the surgical scar should be included.

Dose and Fractionation

- Brief hypofractionation used in the M. D. Anderson Cancer Center (30 Gy in five fractions over 2.5 weeks) can be considered (Grade B). The major experience with this regimen has been in the head

and neck region with the use of direct 9- to 12-MeV electron fields, though inguinal and axillary sites have also been studied (Level III) (BALLO et al. 2003). Radiation therapy is delivered twice weekly with 2–3 days' break. The dose is specified at the dose maximum. For matched electron fields junctions are moved after the second and fourth fractions to avoid dose inhomogeneity. In the head and neck fields, individualized bolus is used to minimize the dose to underlying temporal lobe to less than 24 Gy.

- Prolonged hypofractionation, as used in the TROG protocols (48 Gy in 20 fractions over 4 weeks), can also be utilized (BURMEISTER et al. 2006). Radiotherapy is delivered daily over a period of 4 weeks, dosed at 100%. For matched electron fields the junction should be moved 10 mm for half of the treatment course. As the radiation dose per fraction is higher (2.4 Gy), the brain and spinal cord should be limited to 40 Gy; larynx and brachial plexus less than 45 Gy; and neck of femur less than 35 Gy.

Radiation Techniques

- Irradiation to the head and neck region can generally utilize a direct electron field or 3D conformal photon fields. In the direct electron field technique, the patient is immobilized supine in an individualized vacuum bag or equivalent stabilization device. The head is rotated to the opposite side to expose and flatten the contour over the ipsilateral parotid and cervical nodes. The fields are marked with clinically non-anatomical boundaries and then confirmed on CT simula-

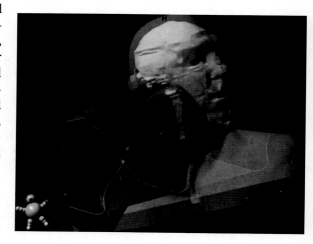

Fig. 35.2. The field borders for direct electron treatment of surgical bed post right cervical lymph nodal dissection

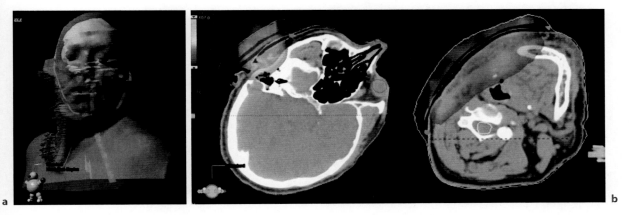

Fig. 35.3a,b. Individualized bolus is used to optimize the dose to surgical bed target volume and reduce the dose at depth at the temporal lobe

tion. Wire is used to mark the surgical scar and subsequent bolus. The field borders are demonstrated in Figure 35.2. Wax is placed in the external ear canal, and an intraoral shield should be placed on the ipsilateral buccal mucosa. Electron energy is determined by patient anatomy, but generally 9–12 MeV is used. Individualized bolus is used to optimize the dose to surgical bed target volume, and reduce the dose at depth over sites such as the temporal lobe, spinal cord, and larynx (Fig. 35.3).

■ In the 3D conformal technique for the head and neck region, the patient is immobilized in a rigid cast system with the neck extended. CT simulation is performed with wire over surgical scars to guide bolus placement. Between 4 and 6 MV photons with wedged pairs for a superior aspect of the field and AP/PA for the lower neck are used. Surgical bed and residual nodal sites are contoured for CTV with a field uncertainty margin added for PTV.

■ Irradiation to the axilla region can generally utilize an AP/PA field to cover the supraclavicular fossa to the lower axilla. Immobilization in an individualized stabilization device with the arm abducted at 30°–45°. CT simulation with wire over surgical scars to guide bolus placement. 4–18 MV photons often with combination energies to reduce the dose to the posterior compartment. Surgical bed and residual nodal sites contoured for CTV with field uncertainty margin added for PTV.

■ Irradiation to the inguino-femoral region can utilize a 3D conformal photon approach to cover the surgical bed and residual nodal sites, as well as to limit dose to the underlying femoral neck and surrounding small bowel. Immobilization in an individualized stabilization device with hips abducted. CT simulation with wire over surgical scars to guide bolus placement. CTV contoured and uncertainty margin (approximately 10 mm) added for PTV depending upon individual center's immobilization. The PTV generally would correspond to the lower sacroiliac joint level superiorly and extend to the proximal third of the femur inferiorly. 3D conformal fields cover PTV but minimize dose to small bowel and neck of femur.

Radiation-Induced Mobility

■ Acute and late toxicity will be influenced by treatment site, post surgical complications, patient performance status, and volume irradiated. Hypofractionation schedules reported have acceptable morbidity, but have to be administered with care so as to avoid potential effects of the increased dose per fraction (STEVENS and McKAY 2006).

■ Concurrent interferon-α therapy should be avoided given anecdotal reports of enhanced radiosensitization on normal tissues, resulting in increased acute and late radiation-induced toxicity (Level IV) (HAZARD et al. 2002).

■ Lymphedema: This is the major concern of delivery of adjuvant RT following nodal dissection in the axillary and inguinal regions. The Australasian TROG study has produced prospective toxicity data on lymphedema to aid decision-making (BURMEISTER et al. 2006). Grade 3 lymphedema was recorded in 9% of 109 patients who received

RT to the axilla and 19% of 48 patients received RT to the inguinal region

- Neural injury: The high dose per fraction of the MDAH regimen (30 Gy in five fractions) may predispose to late neural injury. However, the reported toxicity data from accumulated series describes acceptable neural toxicity with rates <5% (MENDENHALL et al. 2008).
- Bone/joint injury: Bone and joint injuries are unusual with Grade 3 or 4 effects such as severe limitation of movement occurring in less than 2% in the TROG study patients (BURMEISTER et al. 2006).

35.2.5 Adjuvant Systemic Therapies

- The high rate of subsequent distant metastatic failure in patients with high risk locoregionally confined melanoma indicates a potential role for adjuvant systemic therapy.
- The response rate to systemic cytotoxic chemotherapy in advanced melanoma is only 10%–25% (TSAO et al. 2004), thus limiting its effectiveness in an adjuvant therapy role.
- Historically it has been known that host immunological responses influence melanoma response (MORTON et al. 1970); thus systemic therapies have been utilized to augment host defenses or induce immune responses against melanoma antigens. Single agent or combination immunotherapy using interferon-α and interleukin-2 have demonstrated potential effectiveness in advanced disease with response rates of 15%–30% including complete responses (TSAO et al. 2004). However, acute toxicity is significant and provides a challenge to their use in newly diagnosed patients as an adjuvant therapy.
- Clinical trials are an important aspect of management to define a patient population and systemic agents that may improve survival with acceptable toxicity. Novel immune therapies are being investigated including melanoma specific cell and antigen defined vaccines. Biochemotherapy or combined cytotoxic chemotherapy and immunotherapy are being investigated to enhance potential response.

Interferon-α 2b

- Only interferon-α 2b has consistently demonstrated a clinical benefit as an adjuvant therapy with improvement in relapse free survival (Grade A); however, uncertainty regarding overall survival benefit and issues of toxicity remain.
- Patients with melanoma >4 mm thick or with nodal disease were the patient subgroup enrolled in the interferon-α randomized clinical trials. This correlates with AJCC 2002 Stages IIB–III and predicts for a greater than 40% risk of distant metastatic disease (Level I) (KIRKWOOD et al. 1996).
- High dose interferon-α has been extensively studied in multicenter randomized clinical trials and all studies demonstrated improvement in relapse free survival compared to observation or vaccine therapy (Level I) (WHEATLEY et al. 2003). The 5-year overall survival was improved in two major trials, but pooled analysis of long-term data suggested no benefit at 10 years.
- The recommended regimen is a 12-month course with initial induction therapy at a dose of 20×10^6 IU/m² daily for 5 days a week intravenously over a 4-week period. This is followed by maintenance treatment at a dose of 10×10^6 IU/m² subcutaneously 3 days a week for 48 weeks (Grade A). The ECOG 1690 study comparing high to low dose interferon-α and observation demonstrated a significant benefit in relapse free survival with high dose that was not achieved with low dose (Level I) (KIRKWOOD et al. 2000).
- Interferon-α toxicity is significant with constitutional symptoms of fatigue, fever, myalgia, and nausea, as well as myelosuppression and autoimmune responses. Treatment delay is seen in 35%–50% of patients due to toxicity (Level IV) (KIRKWOOD et al. 2002).

Other Adjuvant Systemic Regimens

- Single or multiagent chemotherapy is currently not recommended routinely in the adjuvant treatment of malignant melanoma (Grade B). There is no evidence to support the use of systemic cytotoxic chemotherapy as adjuvant therapy. The agent most studied has been dacarbazine, either as a single agent or in combination with cisplatin, tamoxifen, or with high dose stem cell transplant (MEISENBERG et al. 1993). Current study protocols are investigating cytotoxic chemotherapy as biochemotherapy in combination with immunotherapies.
- Vaccines may be cellular (whole melanoma cells) or antigen based (gangliosides or peptide anti-

gen presenting cells). Although phase II studies are promising, there is no evidence to support vaccine therapy as adjuvant therapy (Grade B) (CHAPMAN 2007).

<h2>35.3 Treatment of Advanced Melanoma</h2>

35.3.1 General Principles

■ Palliative interventions for metastatic melanoma should follow rules of palliation for other tumour pathologies, with treatment designed to improve quality of life by reducing symptoms or limiting progression of disease (Grade B).
■ There is a poorly defined subgroup of patients with oligometastases which have a potentially long natural history disease and would be suitable for more aggressive treatment that includes surgical resection. This may include patients with lung or limited cutaneous metastatic disease who have an improved 12-month survival compared with patients with visceral metastases.
■ Most patients with stage IV metastatic disease will have a median survival of 9–12 months. Patients with lung or limited cutaneous metastatic disease have an improved 12-month survival compared with patients with visceral metastases.

35.3.2 Palliative Surgical Therapy

Resection of Oligometastases

■ There is a poorly defined subgroup of patients with oligometastases which have a potential long natural history disease and would be suitable for more aggressive treatment that includes surgical resection (Grade C). However, results from a limited number of publications have not been conclusive. This may include resection of limited cutaneous, lung, cerebral, and liver metastases (MOSCA et al. 2008).
Decision making should be individualized and based on the number of metastases and number of sites involved. Survival after resection was also influenced by earlier primary tumor stage and

a long (>36 months) disease-free interval before metastatic disease (ESSNER et al. 2004).

Isolated Limb Perfusion (ILP) and Limb Infusion (ILI)

■ Regionally infused drug therapy is an appropriate option for patients with multiple, rapidly progressive satellite in-transit lesions on limbs. ILP using melphalan in combination with hyperthermia may achieve response rates of 60%–90% (Level II) (CORNETT et al. 2006).
■ The procedure requires a specialized unit with experience in regional drug delivery.

35.3.3 Palliative Radiation Therapy

■ The radiobiological principles in adjuvant radiation therapy of melanoma should also be considered in palliation. The improved response to high total dose or high dose per fraction will need to be balanced against potential morbidity and inconvenience of treatment in the palliative setting.

Major Sites for Palliation

Cerebral Metastases

■ The median survival of patients is 3–6 months, though dependent upon disease natural history, number of cerebral metastases, and presence of extracranial disease (FIFE et al. 2004).
■ The standard of care for the majority of patients with multiple brain metastases is whole brain radiation therapy (WBRT). However, the optimal dose regimen has not been established for melanoma.
■ Patients with oligometastases and good performance status (between one and three cerebral lesions) should be assessed for more aggressive intervention which would include surgical resection or stereotactic radiosurgery (SRS) (Grade B).
RTOG 95-08 demonstrated a benefit of SRS and WBRT over WBRT alone for patients with oligometastases and excellent performance status. However, only 4% of patients had melanoma (ANDREWS 2004).
The role of WBRT after local cerebral therapy such as surgery or SRS is controversial because of concerns over neurotoxicity from radiation. However, ECOG E6397 Phase II study in relatively

radioresistant pathologies provides evidence for the use of WBRT. In this study patients were managed with SRS alone for oligometastases and demonstrated a 48.3% intracranial relapse rate at 6 months. A total of 45% of patients had melanoma pathology. A total of 38% of patients died from neurological causes (Level III) (Manon et al. 2005). Retrospective studies have provided more evidence to confirm a role for more aggressive interventions in selected patients (Level IV) (Buchsbaum et al. 2002).

Cutaneous and Nodal Metastases

■ Palliative radiation is indicated for symptomatic cutaneous and nodal metastases (Grade B). Radiation therapy can provide effective local palliation with response rates of >75% (Level IV) (Seegenschmiedt et al. 1999).

■ Higher dose of radiation therapy (doses >30 Gy and a BED >39.0 Gy) should be considered for palliation (Grade C). A higher total dose is associated with improved response rate and more durable palliation was demonstrated in a retrospective study (Level IV) (Olivier et al. 2007). However, dose was not a significant factor predicting treatment outcome in the above-mentioned study reported by Seegenschmiedt et al. (1999).

Skeletal Metastases

■ Extrapolated from bone metastases in other pathologies external beam radiation can provide clinical response and palliation in 70%–75% (Grade A) (Wu et al. 2003).

■ Single fraction radiotherapy is as effective as multi-fraction radiotherapy in relieving metastatic bone pain. However, the re-treatment rate and pathological fracture rates were higher after single fraction radiotherapy (Grade A) (Sze et al. 2004).

■ Palliative radiation therapy for bone metastases is detailed in Chapter 43.

35.3.4 Palliative Systemic Therapy

■ Single agent dacarbazine is the agent of choice for patients with stage IV melanoma when considering response rate (10%–25%) and an acceptable toxicity profile (nausea) (Grade B). The median duration of response is only 4 months (Tsao et al. 2004).

■ Other systemic cytotoxic agents such as fotemustine, temozolomide, and platinum compounds can be suggested (Grade C). These agents have demonstrated activities, but no improvement in median survival over dacarbazine in clinical trials (Level II) (Middleton et al. 2000). There is less morbidity with temozolomide compared to dacarbazine (Level II) (Kiebert et al. 2003).

■ Multi-agent chemotherapy is not recommended currently for palliation of metastatic melanoma (Grade A). According to the results of a systemic review of 41 randomized clinical trials, there is no benefit of combination over single agent therapy in palliation of metastatic disease (Level I) (Eigentler et al. 2003).

■ Interferon-α and interleukin-2 are active with response rates of 10%–30%, and can be recommended in a selective group of patients (Grade A). Results of a meta-analysis indicated that high-dose interleukin-2 is a reasonable treatment option for patients with good performance status (ECOG 0-1), a normal lactate dehydrogenase level, fewer than three organs involved, or have cutaneous and/or subcutaneous metastases only, and no evidence of central nervous system metastases. However, there is associated toxicity that limits efficacy in palliation, especially with interleukin-2 (Level I) (Petrella et al. 2007).

■ Combination cytotoxic chemotherapy and immunotherapy cannot be routinely recommended in the palliative treatment of melanoma (Grade A). The combination treatment may potentially enhance response rates. However, the results of a meta-analysis failed to demonstrate an improved survival even in the presence of improved response rate (Level I) (Sasse et al. 2007).

35.4 Follow-Up

35.4.1 Post-Treatment Follow-Up

■ Long-term follow-up for melanoma patients after treatment for detection of disease recurrence and new skin cancer is recommended (Grade B). Results of the Surveillance, Epidemiology and End Results (SEER) database analysis indicates the risk of developing a subsequent melanoma to be ten times the rate of a first melanoma among the general SEER population. The lifetime risk of a second melanoma is approximately 5% (TSAO et al. 2004).

■ There is no clinical evidence to guide clinicians on a follow-up regimen for patients managed with localized or metastatic melanoma. Guidelines based on expert opinion have been developed (Grade D) (FRANCKEN et al. 2005, 2007).

■ A follow-up regimen should be based on tumor thickness with local examination, surveillance for new lesions, and education as to self-detection

of melanoma and non-melanomatous skin cancer (Grade C) (MCCARTHY et al. 1988).

■ For patients with high risk localized melanoma, a potential follow-up schedule would be history, physical examination including regional lymph nodes, skin inspection, and palpation of primary tumor location every 3 months for 2 years and every 6–12 months thereafter for 10 years (Grade D) (JOST et al. 2005).

■ There is no role for laboratory and imaging investigations for asymptomatic surveillance.

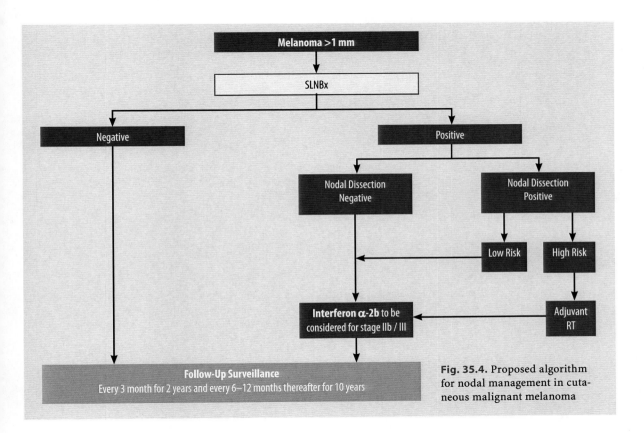

Fig. 35.4. Proposed algorithm for nodal management in cutaneous malignant melanoma

References

Andrews DW, Scott CB, Sperduto PW (2004) Whole brain radiation therapy with or without stereotactic radiosurgery boost for patients with one to three brain metastases: phase III results of the RTOG 9508 randomised trial. Lancet 363:1665–1672

Ang KK, Peters LJ, Weber RS et al. (1994) Postoperative radiotherapy for cutaneous melanoma of the head and neck region. Int J Radiat Oncol Biol Phys 30:795–798

Balch CM, Soong SJ, Smith T et al. (2001a) Long-term results of a prospective surgical trial comparing 2 cm vs. 4 cm excision margins for 740 patients with 1–4 mm melanomas. Ann Surg Oncol 8:101–108

Balch CM, Soong SJ, Gershenwald JE et al. (2001b) Prognostic factors analysis of 17,600 melanoma patients: validation of the American Joint Committee on Cancer melanoma staging system. J Clin Oncol 19:3622–3634

Ballo MT, Bonnen MD, Garden AS et al. (2003) Adjuvant irradiation for cervical lymph node metastases from melanoma. Cancer 97:1789–1796

Blessing K, Sanders DS, Grant JJ (1998) Comparison of immunohistochemical staining of the novel antibody melan-A with S100 protein and HMB-45 in malignant melanoma and melanoma variants. Histopathology 32:139–146

Bliss JM, Ford D, Swerdlow AJ et al. (1995) Risk of cutaneous melanoma associated with pigmentation characteristics and freckling: systematic overview of 10 case-control studies. The International Melanoma Analysis Group (IMAGE). Int J Cancer 62:367–376

Bonnen MD, Ballo MT, Myers JN et al. (2004) Elective radiotherapy provides regional control for patients with cutaneous melanoma of the head and neck. Cancer 100:383–389

Bub JL, Berg D, Slee A, Odland PB (2004) Management of lentigo maligna and lentigo maligna melanoma with staged excision: a 5-year follow-up. Arch Dermatol. May 140:552–558

Buchsbaum JC, Suh JH, Lee SY et al. (2002) Survival by radiation therapy oncology group recursive partitioning analysis class and treatment modality in patients with brain metastases from malignant melanoma: a retrospective study. Cancer 94:2265–2272

Burmeister BH, Smithers BM, Davis S et al. (2002) Radiation therapy following nodal surgery for melanoma: an analysis of late toxicity. ANZ J Surg 72:344–348

Burmeister BH, Mark Smithers B, Burmeister E et al. (2006) A prospective phase II study of adjuvant postoperative radiation therapy following nodal surgery in malignant melanoma-Trans Tasman Radiation Oncology Group (TROG) Study 96.06. Radiother Oncol 81:136–142

Buzaid AC, Tinoco L, Ross MI, Legha SS, Benjamin RS (1995) Role of computed tomography in the staging of patients with local-regional metastases of melanoma. J Clin Oncol13:2104–2108.

Calabro A, Singletary SE, Balch CM (1989) Patterns of relapse in 1001 consecutive patients with melanoma nodal metastases. Arch Surg 124:1051–1055

Cascinelli N, Belli F, Santinami M et al. (2000) Sentinel lymph node biopsy in cutaneous melanoma: the WHO Melanoma Program experience. Ann Surg Oncol 7:469–474

Chapman PB (2007) Melanoma vaccines. Semin Oncol 34:516–523

Constantinidou A, Hofman M, O'Doherty M et al. (2008) Routine positron emission tomography and positron emission tomography/computed tomography in melanoma staging with positive sentinel node biopsy is of limited benefit. Melanoma Res 18:56–60

Cornett WR, McCall LM, Petersen RP et al. (2006) Randomized multicenter trial of hyperthermic isolated limb perfusion with melphalan alone compared with melphalan plus tumor necrosis factor: American College of Surgeons Oncology Group Trial Z0020. J Clin Oncol 24:4196–4201

Eigentler TK, Caroli UM, Radny P, Garbe C (2003) Palliative therapy of disseminated malignant melanoma: a systematic review of 41 randomised clinical trials. Lancet Oncol 4:748–759

Essner R, Lee JH, Wanek LA et al. (2004) Contemporary surgical treatment of advanced-stage melanoma. Arch Surg 139:961–966

Fader DJ, Wise CG, Normolle DP, Johnson TM (1998) The multidisciplinary melanoma clinic: a cost outcomes analysis of specialty care. J Am Acad Dermatol 38(5 Pt 1):742–751

Farshad A, Burg G, Panizzon R, Dummer R (2002) A retrospective study of 150 patients with lentigo maligna and lentigo maligna melanoma and the efficacy of ra-

diotherapy using Grenz or soft X-rays. Br J Dermatol 146:1042–1046

Fife KM, Colman MH, Stevens GN et al. (2004) Determinants of outcome in melanoma patients with cerebral metastases. J Clin Oncol 22:1293–300

Fife KM, Colman MH, Stevens GN et al. (2004) Determinants of outcome in melanoma patients with cerebral metastases. J Clin Oncol 22:1293–1300

Francken AB, Bastiaannet E, Hoekstra HJ (2005) Follow-up in patients with localised primary cutaneous melanoma. Lancet Oncol 6:608–621

Francken AB, Shaw HM, Accortt NA et al. (2007) Detection of first relapse in cutaneous melanoma patients: implications for the formulation of evidence-based follow-up guidelines. Ann Surg Oncol 14:1924–1933

Goldstein A, Chan M, Harland M et al. (2007) Features associated with germline CDKN2A mutations: a GenoMEL study of melanoma-prone families from three continents. J Med Genet 44:99–106

Greene F, Page D, Fleming I et al. (2002) AJCC Cancer Staging Manual, 6th edn. Springer, Berlin Heidelberg New York

Hazan C, Dusza SW, Delgado R et al. (2008) Staged excision for lentigo maligna and lentigo maligna melanoma: a retrospective analysis of 117 cases. J Am Acad Dermatol 58:142–148

Hazard LJ, Sause WT, Noyes RD (2002) Combined adjuvant radiation and interferon-alpha 2B therapy in high-risk melanoma patients: the potential for increased radiation toxicity. Int J Radiat Oncol Biol Phys 52:796–800

Huilgol SC, Selva D, Chen C et al. (2004) Surgical margins for lentigo maligna and lentigo maligna melanoma: the technique of mapped serial excision. Arch Dermatol 140:1087–1092

Jemal A, Siegel R, Ward E et al. (2008) Cancer Statistics 2008. CA Cancer J Clin 58:71–96

Jost LM, Jelic S, Purkalne G (2005) ESMO Minimum Clinical Recommendations for diagnosis, treatment and follow-up of cutaneous malignant melanoma. Ann Oncol 16[Suppl 1]:i66–i68

Khayat D, Rixe O, Martin G et al. (2003) Surgical margins in cutaneous melanoma (2 cm versus 5 cm for lesions measuring less than 2.1-mm thick). Cancer 97:1941–1946

Kiebert GM, Jonas DL, Middleton MR (2003) Health-related quality of life in patients with advanced metastatic melanoma: results of a randomized phase III study comparing temozolomide with dacarbazine. Cancer Invest 21:821–829

Kirkwood JM, Strawderman MH, Ernstoff MS et al. (1996) Interferon alfa-2b adjuvant therapy of high-risk resected cutaneous melanoma: the Eastern Cooperative Oncology Group Trial EST 1684. J Clin Oncol 14:7–17

Kirkwood JM, Ibrahim JG, Sondak VK et al. (2000) High- and low-dose interferon alfa-2b in high-risk melanoma: first analysis of intergroup trial E1690/S9111/C9190. J Clin Oncol 18:2444–2458

Kirkwood JM, Bender C, Agarwala S et al. (2002) Mechanisms and management of toxicities associated with high-dose interferon alfa-2b therapy. J Clin Oncol 20:3703–3718

Manon R, O'Neill A, Knisely J et al. (2005) Phase II trial of radiosurgery for one to three newly diagnosed brain metastases from renal cell carcinoma, melanoma, and sarcoma: an Eastern Cooperative Oncology Group study (E 6397). J Clin Oncol 23:8870–8876

McCarthy WH, Shaw HM, Thompson JF et al (1988) Time and frequency of recurrence of cutaneous stage I malignant melanoma with guidelines for follow up study. Surg Gynecol Obstet 166:497–502

Meisenberg BR, Ross M, Vredenburgh JJ et al. (1993) Randomized trial of high-dose chemotherapy with autologous bone marrow support as adjuvant therapy for high-risk, multi-node-positive malignant melanoma. J Natl Cancer Inst 85:1080–1085

Mendenhall WM, Amdur RJ, Grobmyer SR et al. (2008) Adjuvant radiotherapy for cutaneous melanoma. Cancer 112:1189–1196

Middleton MR, Grob JJ, Aaronson N et al. (2000) Randomized phase III study of temozolomide versus dacarbazine in the treatment of patients with advanced metastatic malignant melanoma. J Clin Oncol 18:158–166

Miranda EP (2006) Utility of computed tomography and magnetic resonance imaging staging before completion lymphadenectomy in sentinel lymph node-positive melanoma. J Clin Oncol 24:5178

Morton D, Eilber FR, Malmgren RA, Wood WC (1970) Immunological factors which influence response to immunotherapy in malignant melanoma. Surgery 68:158–163

Morton DL, Thompson JF, Cochran AJ et al. (2006) Sentinel-node biopsy or nodal observation in melanoma. N Engl J Med 355:1307–1317

Mosca PJ, Teicher E, Nair SP, Pockaj BA (2008) Can surgeons improve survival in stage IV melanoma? J Surg Oncol [Epub ahead of print]

Olivier KR, Schild SE, Morris CG et al. (2007) A higher radiotherapy dose is associated with more durable palliation and longer survival in patients with metastatic melanoma. Cancer 110:1791–1795

Overgaard J, Overgaard M, Hansen PV, von der Maase H (1986) Some factors of importance in the radiation treatment of malignant melanoma. Radiother Oncol 5:183–192

Petrella T, Quirt I, Verma S et al. (2007) Single-agent interleukin-2 in the treatment of metastatic melanoma. Curr Oncol 14:21–26

Posther KE, Selim MA, Mosca PJ et al. (2006) Histopathologic characteristics, recurrence patterns, and survival of 129 patients with desmoplastic melanoma. Ann Surg Oncol 13:728–739

Quinn MJ, Crotty KA, Thompson JF et al. (1998) Desmoplastic and desmoplastic neurotropic melanoma: experience with 280 patients. Cancer 83:1128–1135

Reinhardt MJ, Joe AY, Jaeger U et al. (2006) Diagnostic performance of whole body dual modality 18F-FDG PET/CT imaging for N- and M-staging of malignant melanoma: experience with 250 consecutive patients. J Clin Oncol 24:1178–1187

Sasse AD, Sasse EC, Clark LG et al. (2007) Chemoimmunotherapy versus chemotherapy for metastatic malignant melanoma. Cochrane Database Syst Rev. Jan 24; (1):CD005413

Sause WT, Cooper JS, Rush S et al. (1991) Fraction size in external beam radiation therapy in the treatment of melanoma. Int J Radiat Oncol Biol Phys 20:429–32

Seegenschmiedt MH, Keilholz L, Altendorf-Hofmann A et al. (1999) Palliative radiotherapy for recurrent and metastatic malignant melanoma: prognostic factors for tumor response and long-term outcome: a 20-year experience. Int J Radiat Oncol Biol Phys 44:607–618

Schmalbach CE, Nussenbaum B, Rees RS et al. (2003) Reliability of sentinel lymph node mapping with biopsy for head and neck cutaneous melanoma. Arch Otolaryngol Head Neck Surg 129:61–65

Stevens G, Thompson JF, Firth I, O'Brien CJ, McCarthy WH, Quinn MJ (2000) Locally advanced melanoma: results of postoperative hypofractionated radiation therapy. Cancer 88:88–94

Stevens G, McKay M (2006) Dispelling the myths surrounding radiotherapy for treatment of cutaneous melanoma. Lancet Oncol 7:575–583

Sze WM, Shelley M, Held I, Mason M (2004) Palliation of metastatic bone pain: single fraction versus multifraction radiotherapy – a systematic review of the randomised trials. Cochrane Database Syst Rev. (2):CD004721

Thomas JM, Clark MA (2004) Selective lymphadenectomy in sentinel node-positive patients may increase the risk of local/in-transit recurrence in malignant melanoma. Eur J Surg Oncol 30:686–691

Tracey EA, Chen S, Baker D, Bishop J, Jelfs P (2006) Cancer in New South Wales: incidence and mortality 2004. Cancer Institute NSW, Sydney, November

Tsao H, Atkins M, Sober A (2004) Management of cutaneous melanoma. N Engl J Med 351:998–1012

Wheatley K, Ives N, Hancock B et al. (2003) Does adjuvant interferon-alpha for high-risk melanoma provide a worthwhile benefit? A meta-analysis of the randomised trials. Cancer Treat Rev 29:241–252

Wu JS, Wong R, Johnston M et al. (2003) Meta-analysis of dose-fractionation radiotherapy trials for the palliation of painful bone metastases. Int J Radiat Oncol Biol Phys 55:594–605

Squamous and Basal Cell Carcinoma of the Skin

36

José A. Peñagarícano and Vaneerat Ratanatharathorn

J. A. PEÑAGARÍCANO, MD
University of Arkansas for Medical Sciences, Department of
Radiation Oncology, 4301 W. Markham Street #771, Little
Rock, AR 72205, USA
V. RATANATHARATHORN, MD
Winthrop P. Rockefeller Cancer Institute, 4301 W. Markham
Street #623, Little Rock, AR 72205, USA

Introduction and Objectives

Basal and squamous cell carcinomas of the skin are the most common histologic types of skin cancer and the most common malignancies. They are significantly associated with ultraviolet light exposure, exposure to ionizing radiation, exposure to chemical carcinogens such as arsenic, chronic irritation, and gene mutations. Squamous cell carcinoma is also related to alterations in immune system. The incidence of non-melanoma skin cancer in the United States in 2007 was more than 1 million cases with an annual mortality of less than 2000. Approximately 20% of the American population will develop basal cell carcinoma and/or squamous cell carcinoma during their lifetime.

This chapter examines:

● Recommendations for diagnosis and staging procedures for both basal and squamous cell carcinomas
● Prognostic factors
● Definitive and adjuvant treatment recommendations for both diseases
● Radiation therapy techniques for definitive and adjuvant treatment
● Follow-up care and surveillance after treatment

36.1 Diagnosis, Staging, and Prognoses

36.1.1 Diagnosis

■ Definitive diagnosis can only be made by biopsy.
■ Types of skin biopsies include:
– Shave: adequate for raised lesions.
– Punch: adequate for flat lesions.
– Excisional: used to sample deep dermal and subcutaneous tissue with post-operative margin assessment.

- Patients with poor prognostic factors or clinically evident metastasis should undergo work-up for systemic disease.

Laboratory Tests and Imaging Studies

- Laboratory tests are usually not required for diagnosis and evaluation of basal and squamous cell carcinomas, except for those required for screening prior to surgery and anesthesia.
- Imaging studies are usually not required for diagnosis and evaluation of basal and squamous cell carcinomas. However, for locally advanced diseases, CT scan or MRI for evaluating the depth of invasion and regional lymph node is indicated.

Pathology

Basal Cell Carcinoma

- Basal cell carcinoma of the skin is the most common histological type of skin cancer. It is a non-keratinizing neoplasm arising from the basal layer of the epidermis.
- Basal cell carcinoma has a low metastatic potential with predilection for local invasion (BERTI and SHARATA 1999).
- Perineural invasion from basal cell carcinoma is uncommon but occurs in recurrent and aggressive lesions (McCORD et al. 1999).
- Histological sub-types of basal cell carcinoma include:
- Nodular: raised nodule with telangiectasia in sun-exposed areas
- Superficial: erythematous or eroded macule, which mimic eczema or psoriasis
- Morpheaform: flat, firm lesion without well-defined margins

Squamous Cell Carcinoma

- Squamous cell carcinoma of the skin is the second most common histological type of skin cancer.
- Squamous cell carcinoma is a neoplasm of keratinizing malignant cells, and arises from keratinocytes of the epidermis, and actinic keratosis is a precancerous condition of squamous cell carcinoma of the skin.
- Pathologic grading of squamous sell carcinoma of the skin depends on the magnitude of polymorphism, mitosis, and keratinization, and classifies the disease to poorly, moderately, or well differentiated categories.

Staging

- Carcinoma of the skin is staged clinically, and the American Joint Committee on Cancer (AJCC) TNM Staging System is the most commonly utilized classification for both basal cell carcinoma and squamous cell carcinoma (Table 36.1) (GREENE et al. 2002).
- For patients with multiple skin lesions, the tumor with highest T-classification should be staged and used as the primary reporting lesion, and the number of lesions should be presented in parentheses (GREENE et al. 2002).

Table 36.1. American Joint Committee on Cancer staging system for carcinoma of the skin (excluding eyelid, vulva, and penis). [From GREENE et al. (2002) with permission]

Primary tumor (T)	
TX	Primary tumor cannot be assessed
T0	No evidence of primary tumor
Tis	Carcinoma in situ
T1	Tumor 2 cm or less in greater dimension
T2	Tumor more than 2 cm, but not more than 5 cm, in greatest dimension
T3	Tumor more than 5 cm in greatest dimension
T4	Tumor invades deep extradermal structures (i.e., cartilage, skeletal muscle, or bone)
Regional lymph nodes (N)	
NX	Regional lymph nodes cannot be assessed
N0	No regional lymph node metastasis
N1	Regional lymph node metastasis
Distant metastasis (M)	
MX	Distant metastasis cannot be assessed
M0	No distant metastasis
M1	Distant metastasis
STAGE GROUPING	
0:	Tis N0 M0
1:	T1 N0 M0
II:	T2-T3 N0 M0
III:	T4 N0 M0 or Any T N1 M0
IV:	Any T Any N M0

36.1.2 Prognostic Factors

- Overall basal and squamous cell carcinoma of the skin has good prognosis. The presenting staging of the disease, including regional nodal involvement status, is the most important prognostic factor.
- The size of the primary tumor (i.e., T-classification) is a major determinant for local recurrence after definitive radiation. The local control rates were more than 95%, 80%, and 53% for lesions of T1, T2, and T3 classifications, respectively, according to a number of large retrospective series (Level IV) (FITZPATRICK et al. 1984; MAZERON et al. 1988).

Basal Cell Carcinoma

- Recurrences are seen most commonly with morpheaform and nodular (when micronodules are present) histological sub-types when margins of resection are small (ROWE et al. 1989).
- Location and size is a known factor for basal cell carcinoma recurrence. Tumors in the head and neck area are more likely to recur and carry a worse prognosis (Level IV) (BOETA-ANGELIS and BENNETT 1998; MENDENHALL et al. 1989).

Squamous Cell Carcinoma

- Squamous cell carcinoma is usually more aggressive than the basal cell carcinoma of the skin. The probability of regional lymph node involvement and distant metastasis is higher than that of basal cell carcinoma and occurs in approximately 10% of all cases.
- The presenting staging of the disease, including overall invasiveness and depth of the primary disease, as well as regional nodal involvement status, is the most important prognostic factor for squamous cell carcinoma of the skin (IMMERMAN et al. 1983; FRIEDMAN 1985). Tumors of at least 4 mm deep or invading the reticular dermis and subcutis have a high recurrence rate or nodal involvement. Tumor size of larger than 2 cm in diameter carries an increased risk or local recurrence (ROWE et al. 1992).
- Degree of cellular differentiation is of prognostic significance. Poorly differentiated tumors are more likely to metastasize (ROWE et al. 1992).
- Location is a known factor for squamous cell carcinoma recurrence. Tumors in the head and neck area, genitalia, mucosal surfaces, and ear are at higher risk of metastasizing (HAAS 1998).

- Perineural invasion is an indicator for local and/or regional recurrence or distant metastasis (TERASHI et al. 1997).
- Locally recurrent squamous cell carcinoma of the skin has an overall metastatic rate of 30% (ROWE et al. 1992).
- Immunosuppression as seen in organ transplantation is a risk for development of squamous cell carcinoma of the skin (GUPTA et al. 1986).

36.2 Treatment of Basal and Squamous Cell Carcinomas of the Skin

36.2.1 General Principles

- Treatment of basal and squamous cell carcinomas is similar. Both diseases are most commonly treated with surgery (Mohs or post-operative margin assessment), radiation therapy, or a combination of both.
- Selection of therapy is based on preservation of function and cosmesis, location of the lesion(s), patient preference and general health status. Surgery is preferred over radiation therapy for small sized (<4 cm) and resectable basal cell carcinoma of the face (Grade C). Results from a randomized trial from France showed that the 4-year actuarial failure rate was 0.7% after surgery and 7.5% after radiation ($p=0.003$) However, more than 50% of the patients in this study received interstitial radiation therapy and only 12% received conventional radiation. (Level II) (AVRIL et al. 1997).
- In patients with no poor prognostic factors (such as morpheaform histology), negative histo-pathological margins can be followed-up after surgery; Patients with no poor prognostic factors and positive margins should be re-excised in order to achieve negative margins or receive adjuvant radiation therapy.
- Patients with poor prognostic factors, negative histo-pathological margins, and no evidence of perineural invasion can be followed-up. Patients with poor prognostic factors and positive histo-pathological margins should be re-excised in order to achieve negative margins or receive adjuvant radiation therapy.

- Adjuvant radiotherapy is recommended for diseases with perineural invasion (including large named nerves), regional lymph node involvement, and large primary disease for prevention of local recurrences.
- For squamous cell carcinoma patients with regional disease (clinically or radiographically abnormal adenopathy) and after diagnosis is establish via biopsy of primary and regional disease, a regional lymph node dissection followed by adjuvant radiation therapy is recommended.

36.2.2 Radiation Therapy

- Radiation therapy can be used in patients who are not surgical candidates in both diseases, and is commonly used in treating lesions on the face for better cosmetic and functional results (Grade A). The local control rate after definitive radiation therapy was approximately 90% for all sizes of basal cell carcinoma, comparable to that after surgical excision (Level IV) (KOPF 1979; FREEMAN et al. 1964). Similar results after radiation for both basal and squamous cell carcinoma were reported in a retrospective study, in which patients were treated with radiation for initial treatment or after failing initial surgical excision. The local control rates were 97% versus 91%, respectively, for basal or squamous cell carcinoma smaller than 1 cm, and 87% versus 76% for those measuring between 1 and 5 cm (Level IV) (LOVETT et al. 1990). The local control rates were more than 95%, 80%, and 53% for lesions of T1, T2, and T3 classifications, respectively, according to a number of large retrospective series which studied the prognostic effect of tumor size after radiation (Level IV) (FITZPATRICK et al. 1984; MAZERON et al. 1988).
- The radiation therapy volumes and definitive doses depend on the size and extent of disease, the need to irradiate any high risk areas, and the expected cosmetic result. Typically, the treatment field should encompass the gross tumor and 1–2 cm margin. A smaller margin of 1 cm or less is recommended for lesions close to critical organs or tissues such as eye, or for tumors less than 1 cm in largest diameter.
- For lesions in the eyelid, protection of the ocular structures can be achieved with a led eye shield placed into the conjunctival sac daily.

- Orthovoltage X-rays (75–150 kVp depending on the depth of tumor) or more commonly electron-beams (6–12 MeV depending on the depth of tumor) can be used for the treatment of cutaneous tumors. The 90% isodose line of the electron-beam should cover the entire depth of the tumor (including bolus) with a few millimeters deeper than the base of the tumor. The size of the electron beams should be at least 4 × 4 cm for reliable dosimetry.
- Elective radiation to the lymph node is not recommended for both basal and squamous cell carcinoma of the skin, except in patients with large infiltrative squamous cell carcinoma (Grade A). Recurrences in the regional lymph nodes after definitive surgery or radiation is exceedingly rare in the above-mentioned studies (Levels II and IV) (AVRIL et al. 1997; KOPF 1979; LOVETT et al. 1990; FITZPATRICK et al. 1984; MAZERON et al. 1988).
- The use of standard fractionation (1.8–2 Gy per fraction) is expected to show an improved cosmetic result as a higher dose per fraction is associated with increased late effects of normal tissue (Grade B) (Level III) (TURESSON and NOTTER 1984a,b, 1986).
- When cosmetic result is not important or other patient related issues (transportation, performance status, etc.) preclude a protracted course of treatment, shorter courses may be used (i.e. 50 Gy in 15 fractions over 3 weeks).
- Definitive radiation therapy doses for basal and squamous cell carcinoma can be recommended as follows according to the size and pathology of the primary disease (Grade B), based on a large retrospective analysis of 531 lesions at the Washington University (Level IV) (LOCKE et al. 2001).
  - For basal cell carcinoma lesions <1 cm, 40 Gy
  - For basal cell carcinoma lesions ≤3 cm or squamous cell carcinoma <1 cm, 45–50 Gy
  - For basal cell carcinoma >3 cm and squamous cell carcinoma >1 cm, 60 Gy
  - All treatment is given in 2.5-Gy fractions per day, 4 days per week.
- Alternatively, when a conventional fraction (i.e., 2.0 Gy) is used, a total dose of 60–64 Gy in 30–32 fractions and 66 Gy in 33 fractions can be recommended to tumors ≤2 cm or >2 cm in diameter, respectively.
- A local control rate of approximately 90% was reported, in line with those rates reported by the retrospective studies mentioned above.
- In the postoperative adjuvant setting for basal and squamous cell carcinomas with adverse

prognostic factors, the recommended radiation therapy dose is 60 Gy at 2 Gy per fraction. Higher doses are required for positive histo-pathological margins (66–70 Gy per fraction at 2 Gy per fraction). The course of radiation may be modified for small volumes or when cosmesis is not an issue (i.e., 50 Gy in 15 fractions over 3 weeks).

■ Radiation therapy can be used as a salvage therapy for patients in whom initial radiation failed for their disease (Grade C). Retrospective experience of 17 patients with recurrent skin cancer from Washington University demonstrated that a local control rate of more than 50% can be expected in patients who received a second course of radiation after local recurrence. Squamous cell carcinoma was more resistant to reirradiation as compared to basal cell carcinoma, and six of seven patients with resistant disease had squamous cell carcinoma (Level IV) (CHAO et al. 1995).

36.3   Post-Treatment Follow-Ups

■ Follow-up after definitive treatment of basal or squamous cell carcinomas of the skin is recommended (Grade A) (NATIONAL COMPREHENSIVE CANCER NETWORK 2008). Approximately 30%–50% of patients develop another non-melanoma skin cancer (Level III) (ROBINSON 1998). Most recurrences of squamous cell carcinoma of the skin occur within the initial 2 years after the completion of treatment (Level III) (SHIN et al. 1998). MENDENHALL et al. (1987) reported that close to 85% of recurrences were noted within 2 years of radiation therapy, and almost all cases within 5 years of treatment (Level IV).

Schedule

■ In general, patients can be followed-up every 3–6 months for the first 2 years and every 6–12 months thereafter with their surgeon, radiation oncologist, or dermatologist (Grade D).

Work-Ups

■ Each follow-up should include complete physical examination. Imaging studies and laboratory tests are usually not indicated for follow-up on

basal or squamous cell carcinomas of the skin after treatment.

■ Patients should be educated about self-skin examination and sun protection.

References

Avril MF, Auperin A, Margulis A et al. (1997) Basal cell carcinoma of the face: surgery or radiotherapy? Results of a randomized study. Br J Cancer 76:100–106

Boeta-Angeles L, Bennett RG (1998) Features associated with recurrence (basal cell carcinoma). In Miller SJ, Maloney ME (eds) Cutaneous oncology. Pathophysiology, diagnosis, and management. Blackwell Science, Malden, MA, p 646

Berti JJ, Sharata HH (1999) Metastatic basal cell carcinoma to the lung. Cutis 63:165–166

Chao CK, Gerber RM, Perez CA (1995) Reirradiation of recurrent skin cancer of the face: a successful salvage modality. Cancer 75:2351–2355

Fitzpatrick PJ, Thompson GA, Easterbrook WM et al. (1984) Basal and squamous cell carcinoma of the eyelids and their treatment by radiotherapy. Int J Radiat Oncol Biol Phys 10:449–454

Freeman RG, Knox JM, Heaton CL (1964) The treatment of skin cancer: a statistical study of 1,314 skin tumors comparing results obtained with irradiation, surgery, and curettage followed by electrodesiccation. Cancer 17:535–538

Friedman HI, Cooper PH, Wanebo HJ (1985) Prognostic and therapeutic use of microstaging of cutaneous squamous cell carcinoma of the trunk and extremities. Cancer 56:1099–1105

Greene F, Page D, Fleming I et al. (2002) AJCC Cancer Staging Manual, 6th edn. Springer, Berlin Heidelberg New York

Gupta AK, Cardella CJ, Haberman HF (1986) Cutaneous malignant neoplasms in patients with renal transplants. Arch Dermatol 122:1288–1293

Haas AF (1998) Features associated with metastasis (squamous cell carcinoma). In Miller SJ, Maloney ME (eds) Cutaneous oncology. Pathophysiology, diagnosis, and management. Blackwell Science, Malden, MA, p 500

Immerman SC, Scanlon EF, Christ M et al. (1983) Recurrent squamous cell carcinoma of the skin. Cancer 51:1537–1540

Kopf AW (1979) Computer analysis of 3531 basal cell carcinoma of the skin. J Dermatol 6:267–281

Locke J, Karimpour S, Young G et al. (2001) Radiotherapy for epithelial skin cancer. Int J Radiat Oncol Biol Phys 51:748–755

Lovett RD, Perez CA, Shapiro SJ et al. (1990) External irradiation of epithelial skin cancer. Int J Radiat Oncol Biol Phys 19:235–242

Mazeron JJ, Chassagne D, Crook J et al. (1988) Radiation therapy of carcinomas of the skin of the nose and nasal vestibule. A report of 1676 cases by the Groupe Europeen de Curietherapie. Radiother Oncol 13:165–173

Mendenhall WM, Parsons JT, Mendenhall NP et al. (1987) T2–T4 carcinoma of the skin of the head and neck treated with radical irradiation. Int J Radiat Oncol Biol Phys 13:975–981

Mendenhall WM, Parsons JT, Mendenhall NP et al. (1989) Carcinoma of the skin of the head and neck with perineural invasion. Head Neck 11: 301–308

McCord MW, Mendenhall WM, Parsons JT et al. (1999) Skin cancer of the head and neck with incidental microscopic perineural invasion. Int J Radiat Oncol Biol Phys 43:591–595

National Comprehensive Cancer Network (2008) Clinical practice guidelines in oncology: esophageal cancer. Version 2.2007. Available at http://www.nccn.org/professionals/physician_gls/PDF/esophageal.pdf.

Robinson JK (1998) Follow-up and prevention. Follow-up and prevention (basal cell carcinoma). In Miller SJ, Maloney ME (eds) Cutaneous oncology. Pathophysiology, diagnosis, and management. Blackwell Science, Malden, MA, pp 695–698

Rowe DE, Carroll RJ, Day CL (1989) Long-term recurrence rates in previously untreated basal cell carcinoma: implications for patient follow-up. J Dermatol Surg Ocol 15:315–328

Rowe DE, Carroll RJ, Day CL (1992) Prognostic factors for local recurrence metastasis and survival rates in squamous cell carcinoma of the skin, ear and lip. Implications for treatment modality selection. J Am Acad Dermatol 26:976–990

Shin DM, Maloney ME, Lippman SM (1998) Follow-up and prevention (squamous cell carcinoma). In Miller SJ, Maloney ME (eds) Cutaneous oncology. Pathophysiology, diagnosis, and management. Blackwell Science, Malden, MA, pp 565–570

Terashi H, Kurata S, Tadokoro T et al. (1997) Perineural and neural involvement in skin cancers. Dermatol Surg 23:259–264

Turesson I, Notter G (1984) The influence of fraction size in radiotherapy on the late normal tissue reaction-I: comparison of the effects of daily and once-a-week fractionation on human skin. Int J Radiat Oncol Biol Phys 10:593–598

Turesson I, Notter G (1984) The influence of fraction size in radiotherapy on the late normal tissue reaction-II: comparison of the effects of daily and twice-a-week fractionation on human skin. Int J Radiat Oncol Biol Phys 10:599–606

Turesson I, Notter G (1986) The predictive value of skin telangiectasia for late radiation effects in different normal tissues. Int J Radiat Oncol Biol Phys 12:603–609

Soft Tissue Tumors

Atif J. Khan

CONTENTS

Introduction and Objectives

Soft tissue sarcomas are uncommon tumors that can arise from any of a number of mesenchymal cell types. A little over half of these tumors arise from extremities, a little over a third arise from within the abdomen/pelvis (retroperitoneal and visceral), and 10% or so arise from the head and neck.

Radiation therapy plays a critical role in the local management of sarcomas, and is an intrinsic component of limb-preserving combined modality therapy for extremity lesions. Radiation therapy can be delivered preoperatively or postoperatively. Both external beam radiation therapy and brachytherapy can play roles in the adjuvant setting. The benefit of chemotherapy has been difficult to demonstrate, but may be indicated in certain high-risk patient cohorts.

This chapter focuses on the management of extremity/girdle and retroperitoneal soft tissue sarcomas.

- Recommendations for diagnoses and staging procedures
- The staging systems and prognostic factors
- Treatment recommendations for extremity and girdle sarcomas and the supporting peer-reviewed scientific evidence
- Treatment recommendations for retroperitoneal sarcoma and the supporting peer-reviewed scientific evidence
- Follow-up care and surveillance of survivors

The management of bone malignancies are not discussed. The management of rhabdomyosarcoma and extraskeletal Ewing's are discussed elsewhere.

37.1 Diagnosis, Staging, and Prognoses

37.1.1 Diagnosis

Initial Evaluation

- Diagnosis and evaluation of soft tissue sarcomas (STS) usually starts with a complete history and

A. J. Khan, MD
Robert Wood Johnson Medical School-UMDNJ, Cancer Institute of New Jersey, 195 Little Albany St, New Brunswick, NJ 08901, USA

physical examination. An antecedent history of trauma may bring a previously unnoticed lesion to attention, although a causal relationship between trauma and STS is unlikely. A painless mass is the usual presentation, although additional associated signs and symptoms can be attributable to the location of the lesion: obstructive GI or head/neck symptoms, neuropathies, pain, or uterine bleeding.

- A history of radiation exposure should be recorded.
- A thorough physical examination with special attention directed towards externally palpable lesions should be performed. The exam should focus on assessing fixation to overlying skin or underlying bone. Although uncommonly involved, regional lymph nodes should be examined.
- The examination of the abdomen in patients with retroperitoneal lesions should attempt to palpate the primary lesion and assess for metastatic hepatomegaly.

Laboratory Tests

- Initial laboratory tests should include a complete blood count, basic blood chemistry, liver and renal function tests. Renal function tests are relevant for retroperitoneal lesions that may be in the vicinity of a kidney or ureter.

Imaging Studies

- CT scans of the chest, abdomen, and pelvis are required to appropriately evaluate and stage STS.
- CT scan and MRI scans are necessary to adequately evaluate the primary lesion. CT will typically provide better bony detail while MRI is the definitive imaging modality for STS. MRI provides excellent contrast resolution within soft tissues, allows discernment of peritumoral edema, and acquires images in multiple viewing planes.
- CT scan of the chest should always be performed. Abdomen and pelvis scans are indicated in retroperitoneal lesions and myxoid liposarcomas of the extremity which can involve the abdomen.
- Renal perfusion scans should be ordered for retroperitoneal lesions that will require irradiation.
- PET scans should not be used routinely for the primary lesion (Grade D). The National Comprehensive Cancer Network (NCCN) modified its recommendation for PET scan to "it may be useful in prognostication, grading and determining

response to chemotherapy" (Level V) (NATIONAL COMPREHENSIVE CANCER NETWORK 2007).

- In the absence of neurologic symptoms, a CT or MRI of the brain is not routinely recommended.

Pathology

- Core needle biopsy is preferred over fine-needle aspiration (FNA) as the diagnostic tool of choice because the tissue specimen retrieved by core needle is usually adequate for characterization.
- Occasional situations will require an open biopsy, in which case an incisional biopsy should be performed. Diagnostic excisional biopsies are non-oncological and can lead to tumor contamination and spillage into the relevant body compartment.
- Pathological subtypes of soft tissues sarcomas can behave differently.
- Malignant fibrous histiocytoma is the most common subtype although this is largely attributable to its status as a diagnosis of exclusion for undifferentiated spindle cell neoplasms. More recent evidence indicates that as many as 80% of these can exhibit features suggestive of differentiation along other subtypes using immunohistochemistry and ultrastructural features (FLETCHER et al. 2001).
- Liposarcomas display an unusual pattern of multifocal, soft tissue recurrences with a predilection for the abdomen/retroperitoneum. Myxoid liposarcomas show radiosensitivity.
- Synovial sarcomas have biphasic, epithelial, and spindle-cell components and tend to arise in the tendons and articular areas around the distal extremities.

Table 37.1. Imaging and laboratory work-ups for soft tissue sarcoma

Imaging studies	Laboratory tests
– CT of primary lesion	– Complete blood count
– MRI of primary lesion	
– CT of thorax	– Serum chemistry
– CT/MRI abdomen/pelvis (in certain situations)	– Liver function tests
– FDG-PET (Optional)	– Renal function tests
– CT/MRI of the brain (if symptomatically indicated)	
– Renal perfusion scan (if indicated)	

- Gastrointestinal stromal tumors (GISTs) are rare tumors that arise in the abdominal viscera or in the retroperitoneum and can have activating mutations in the c-kit or platelet derived growth factor receptor A gene, making these tumors potentially responsive to molecular targeted therapy.
- Clear cell sarcomas (malignant melanoma of soft parts) has intracellular melanin and stains for S100; recent genomic analysis indicates this tumor may be a subtype of melanoma.
- ■ Regional nodal disease is uncommon in STS with the important exceptions of epithelioid, clear cell, angiosarcoma, and rhabdomyosarcoma, which can show nodal involvement in approximately 10%–30% of cases.
- ■ Translocations (selected)
  - t(12;16)   Liposarcoma, myxoid type
  - t(12;22)   Clear cell sarcoma
  - t(17;22)   Dermatofibrosarcoma protuberans
  - t(x;17)   Alveolar sarcoma of soft parts
  - t(x;18)   Synovial sarcoma

- ■ Tumor differentiation
- Grade is an important prognostic feature and can be based on mitoses, necrosis, differentiation, cellularity, and nuclear pleomorphism.
- In TNM classification, grade is assigned as either high or low in a two-tiered system.
- A four grade system (Grades 1–4) is used by the AJCC and the UICC. This system can be collapsed such that grades 1–2 are "low grade" and grades 3–4 are "high grade".
- The three-tier system used by the French Federation may provide better correlation with overall survival (OS) (GUILLOU et al. 1997); grade 1 is considered low grade while grades 2 and 3 are high grade.

Table 37.2. American Joint Committee on Cancer (AJCC) TNM Classification of soft tissue sarcomas. [From GREENE et al. (2002) with permission]

Primary tumor (T)	
TX	Primary tumor cannot be assessed
T0	No evidence of primary tumor
T1	Tumor ≤5 cm in greatest dimension
T1a	Superficial tumor*
T1b	Deep tumor*
T2	Tumor >5 cm in greatest dimension
T2a	Superficial tumor*
T2b	Deep tumor*
Regional lymph nodes (N)	
NX	Regional lymph nodes cannot be assessed
N0	No regional lymph node metastasis
N1	Regional lymph node metastasis
Distant metastasis (M)	
MX	Distant metastasis cannot be assessed
M0	No distant metastasis
M1	Distant metastasis
STAGE GROUPING	
I:	G1–2 T1a/T1b/T2a/T2b N0 M0
II:	G3–4 T1a/T1b/T2a N0 M0
III:	G3–4 T2b N0 M0
IV:	G1–4 T1–2 N1 or M1

*Superficial tumor is located exclusively above the superficial fascia without invasion of the fascia; deep tumor is located either exclusively beneath the superficial fascia, superficial to the fascia with invasion of or through the fascia, or both superficial yet beneath the fascia

37.1.2 Staging

- ■ Soft tissue sarcomas are staged clinically based on results of physical examination, laboratory tests, imaging studies, and relevant biopsies.

37.1.3 Prognostic Factors

- ■ The most important prognostic factors for disease-free survival (DFS) and distant metastases are tumor size, tumor grade, and location deep to the superficial investing fascia (PISTERS et al. 1996b; COINDRE et al. 2001).
- ■ Prognostic factors for local control include prior recurrence, microscopically positive margins, age >50, and certain histologies (fibrosarcoma, peripheral nerve sheath tumors) (PISTERS et al. 1996b). Other potential factors for local control may include non-extremity location and non-use of radiation. Tumor size, grade, and location (deep versus superficial) do not seem to impact local control.

37.2 Treatment of Extremity Soft Tissue Sarcomas

37.2.1 General Principles

- Surgery is the mainstay therapy for sarcoma of the extremities, and limb-preservation therapy has largely replaced amputation for the majority of extremity soft tissue sarcomas (Grade A).
- Radiation therapy is usually indicated after local resection (Grade A).
- Local control rates with current local therapies is favorable – typically greater than 80% at 5 years, and OS of 50%–60% at 5 years can be expected.

37.2.2 Surgery

- Surgery is the mainstay of local therapy for sarcoma (Grade A). The extent of surgery can vary widely from marginal excisions on the least aggressive end and continuing through to radical amputations. Amputations have historically been associated with high local control rates – 75%–85% at 5 years.
- Local control rates have not been shown to impact OS due to micrometastatic disease and inactive systemic agents.
- Conservative, limb-preserving resections coupled with adjuvant radiation therapy can produce equivalent OS and DFS as amputation (Level II) (Rosenberg et al. 1982), and also result in high local control rates. The NCI trial reported by Rosenberg randomized 43 adult patients (2:1) with high-grade soft tissue sarcoma to either amputation ($n=16$) or limb-sparing resection and external beam radiation therapy (EBRT) ($n=27$) to a dose of 60–70 Gy. Both arms received chemotherapy. There were four local recurrences on the limb-preservation arm and 0 on the amputation arm ($p=0.06$), while actuarial 5-year rates of DFS and OS were equal (71% vs. 78% and 83% vs. 88%, respectively).
- Conservative, limb-preserving resections without adjuvant radiation therapy result in suboptimal local control rates (Level II) (Pisters et al. 1996b); (Level I) (Yang et al. 1998).

37.2.3 Radiation Therapy

Radiation Modality

- EBRT delivered adjuvantly after limb-preserving surgery is indicated (Grade A). Adjuvant therapy improves local control over surgery alone for both high-grade and low-grade sarcomas: Yang et al. (1998) randomized 141 patients with extremity sarcomas after limb-preserving resection to EBRT 63 Gy (45 Gy to compartment then 18 Gy cone-down) or observation. Statistically significant benefits in local control were shown for both high-grade and low-grade ($n=50$) lesions. No differences in OS were seen (Level I) (Yang et al. 1998).
- Post-operative brachytherapy after limb-preserving resection is indicated. The American Brachytherapy Society also recommends brachytherapy as monotherapy be used only in patients with high-grade tumors and negative margins (Grade B). Adjuvant radiotherapy improves local control compared to surgery alone. However, this benefit may be restricted to high-grade lesions.
- Pisters et al. (1996a) randomized 164 patients to a prospective institutional trial of limb-preserving surgery alone or with adjuvant brachytherapy. Brachytherapy catheters were placed to include the tumor bed with 2 cm sup-inf margin and 1.5–2 cm lateral margin, in a single plane, with dose of 42–45 Gy delivered over 4–6 days. With a median follow-up of 76 months, there were 13/78 recurrences on the radiation arm and 25/86 recurrences on the observation arm ($p=0.04$). There was no difference in DFS or OS. There was no significant benefit in local control for patients with low-grade lesions ($n=45$). Patients with positive margins did not seem to benefit from the brachytherapy, although numbers were small (Level II).
- Brachytherapy with additional comprehensive EBRT may be considered in the treatment of soft tissue sarcoma (Grade C). Combined external beam radiation and brachytherapy may improve local control for patients with positive margins (Level IV) (Alekhteyar et al. 1996).

Sequence/Timing

- Radiation therapy can be delivered in the adjuvant setting or preoperatively. The decision for preoperative versus postoperative radiation needs to be made on a case-by-case basis: Adjuvant radiation therapy allows for full pathological review prior to irradiation and allows earlier definitive surgical therapy.

■ Preoperative radiation therapy allows smaller treatment volumes and lower treatment doses (by virtue of treating an oxygenated treatment volume), and may increase resectability by downstaging disease. Hypothetically, preoperative radiation therapy may limit dissemination of viable tumor cells at the time of surgery.

■ The Canadian SR.2 study was a direct, randomized comparison (n=190) of preoperative (50 Gy) versus postoperative (66–70 Gy) external beam radiation and revealed no differences in local control. Higher wound complications occurred in the preoperative arm (35% vs. 17%, p=0.01). This difference was attributable mostly to wound complications resulting in treatment of the proximal lower extremity (thigh). Higher late complications occurred in the postoperative arm. Surprisingly, patients who had preoperative radiotherapy had better OS than those who had postoperative treatment (p=0.0481), although this finding was likely due to statistical chance (Level I) (O'SULLIVAN et al. 2002).

■ In a subsequent report on the late effects of pre- versus postoperative radiotherapy on the SR.2 trial (DAVIS et al. 2005), non-significant increases in late toxicity were shown for postoperative RT, translating into statistically significant impairment of limb function. Field size was predictive of fibrosis and joint stiffness.

Patient Selection

■ Taken together, results from the randomized trials of PISTERS et al. (1996b) and YANG et al. (1998) would seem to indicate that all patients undergoing limb-preserving surgery should receive adjuvant radiation therapy. Investigators have attempted to define subgroups in whom radiation may be safely omitted.

■ Certain patients with small, high-grade lesions may not require adjuvant radiation therapy (Grade B). At present, radiation can probably be omitted for small (<5 cm) low grade lesions. Large low-grade lesions and small superficial high-grade lesions can potentially omit radiation if surgical margins are widely negative, the patient is a good candidate for follow-up, and a potential local recurrence would not be limb-threatening. Large and/or deep high-grade lesions should continue to be offered adjuvant radiation routinely (Grade B).

– In a single institution report of 204 patients with stage IIB sarcomas of the extremity, ALEKTIAR et al. (2002) reported high 5-year local control rates in patients who did (n=88) and did not receive RT (n=116) in addition to surgery (84% vs. 80%). The only independent correlates of local failure were age >50 and central tumor location. All patients in this report had microscopically negative margins (Level IV).

– The group at Dana Farber/Brigham and Women's reported on 74 patients with sarcoma of the extremity or trunk who were treated with function-sparing surgery alone without radiation. Of these, 40 were low grade while 34 were grade 2–3. The 10-year actuarial local control rate was 93%. Multivariate analysis was not performed due to the small number of events. Margin status <1 cm predicted for worse local control on univariate analysis (crude rates 4/38 vs. 0/36, 10-year actuarial 87% local control vs 100%, p=0.04). No other associations for local control were found (Level IV) (BALDINI et al. 1999).

– The MD Anderson group conducted a prospective trial of observation alone for sarcomas less than 5 cm resected with microscopically negative margins. A total of 74 patients were enrolled, cumulative rates of local recurrence at 5 and 10 years were 8% and 11%, respectively. Approximately 60% of lesions were high-grade and two thirds were superficial. In total, 11/12 recurrences were high-grade and 8/12 recurrences were deep tumors (T1b) (Level II) (PISTERS et al. 2007).

■ The issue of accurate patient selection for radiation versus observation after conservative surgical resection is the subject of ongoing study.

Dose

■ Radiation dose of 50 Gy delivered preoperatively is sufficient if subsequent R0 resections are achieved (Grade B). Postoperative boosts (external beam, IORT or brachytherapy) for close or positive margins (R1 resections) should bring the total dose to 60–66 Gy (10–16 Gy boosts). An additional 20–24 Gy should be delivered for R2 resections (total dose 70–76 Gy). In the adjuvant setting, 60–76 Gy should be delivered with EBRT with or without brachytherapy for R0–R2 disease (Grade A) (NATIONAL COMPREHENSIVE CANCER NETWORK 2007).

- When brachytherapy is used as monotherapy after resection for high-grade, margin-negative cases, a dose of 45 Gy prescribed at a depth of 1 cm from the plane of the implant is used (Grade A).

Simulation and Field Arrangement

- The relevant extremity or girdle should be immobilized using thermoplastic or other molds. The relevant extremity should be positioned to maximize access of potential beam arrangements while minimizing incidental dose to normal tissues. Between 5- and 7-cm cranio-caudad expansions on the resection bed (postoperative) or gross tumor (preoperative) coupled with a 1.5- to 2-cm radial expansion, all confined within the relevant fascial compartment and limited by natural barriers (bone), but inclusive of the scar and drains sites, is the volume treated to 50 Gy with EBRT. Areas of peritumoral edema on T2 MRI should be considered CTV (White et al. 2005). Subsequent conedowns to the final dose are limited to 2- to 3-cm cranio-caudad expansions.
- In contrast, the brachytherapy target volume for adjuvant monotherapy is limited to 2-cm expansion beyond the resection cavity without any attempt to include the entire scar or drain sites, and results in excellent local control rates (Grade A) (Pisters et al. 1996a).

37.2.4 Chemotherapy

- The benefit of adjuvant cytotoxic chemotherapy remains uncertain and should not be offered routinely. Certain chemosensitive subtypes (synovial sarcoma), and high-risk stage III disease can be considered for chemotherapy (Grade C). The Sarcoma Meta-analysis Collaboration pooled data on over 1500 patients treated on 14 randomized trials with or without adriamycin-based chemotherapy. In all, 5% of cases were low-grade and 18% were less than 5 cm. Adjuvant chemotherapy produced statistically significant improvements in distant metastases, local control, relapse-free survival, but not OS (non-significant 4% benefit). In the subgroup of patients with extremity lesions, an OS advantage was reported (HR 0.80, $p=0.029$, 7% overall benefit). However, the analysis has been criticized for lack of central pathology review and inclusion of visceral soft tissue sarcomas (17% were uterine) (Level I) (Sarcoma Meta-analysis Collaboration 1997).

The Italian Sarcoma group randomized 104 patients with high-grade and large (>5 cm) tumors to observation or epirubicin/ifosfamide after definitive local therapy. At the most recently reported follow-up (90 months median for alive patients), the improvement in OS and DFS previously reported was no longer statistically significant (Level I) (Frustaci et al. 2003). However, this small and underpowered trial did show a clear improvement in interval to disease progression.
- Neoadjuvant chemotherapy remains less studied and should be considered investigational at present.

37.3 Treatment of Abdominal/Retroperitoneal Sarcomas

37.3.1 General Principles

- Retroperitoneal tumors are rare tumors; approximately 80% of retroperitoneal tumors are STS. Retroperitoneal tumors can grow insidiously and are often of substantial size before they cause symptoms that lead to detection.
- Pain or compressive symptoms attributable to the location of these tumors are the usual clinical presentation.
- CT-guided biopsies are the initial diagnostic procedure of choice in most cases.
- Surgical resection is required for treatment that is curative in intent; however, resectability may be limited by invasion of major vasculature or vertebral column structures. Macroscopically positive margins decrease the likelihood of local control and limit OS. Even with R0 or R1 resections, local control and OS at 5 years is typically 40%–60%.
- Radiation therapy is indicated as adjuvant or neoadjuvant therapy (Grade B).

37.3.2 Radiation Therapy

- Adjuvant radiation therapy is indicated as adjuvant or neoadjuvant therapy (Grade B). Retrospective data have demonstrated lower local failure rates with adjuvant radiation therapy (Level IV) (CATTON et al. 1994; STOECKLE et al. 2001).

Timing/Sequence

- Radiation therapy can be delivered adjuvantly or preoperatively. As with extremity lesions, postoperative therapy requires irradiation of the entire operative field.
- Preoperative radiation should be considered unless the patient requires palliation that can only be achieved by initial surgical resection (Grade C). Preoperative irradiation is particularly advantageous for retroperitoneal lesions due to the more limited treatment volume (tumor vs. entire operative field) and displacement of the small bowel and other organs by the mass.

Dose

- Radiation dose is 45–50 Gy delivered in conventional fractionation in both the preoperative and adjuvant setting.
- In the postoperative setting, an external beam boost of 5.4–9 Gy can be considered if organs at risk can be spared (Level III) (FEIN et al. 1995).
- An intraoperative boost may increase local control over EBRT alone (Grade B). Intraoperative boosts of 10–15 Gy can be delivered using electron-beam therapy (Level III) (GEISCHEN et al. 2001; PETERSEN et al. 2002) or brachytherapy techniques (Level III) (ALEKTIAR et al. 2000; JONES et al. 2002).

Simulation and Field Arrangement

- 3D-conformal therapy or other highly conformal technologies (IMRT, helical tomotherapy, and proton therapy) should be used.
- The gross tumor volume (GTV) equals the imaging defined tumor, the clinical tumor volume (CTV) is a 1- to 2-cm margin on GTV, and the planned tumor volume (PTV) expansions are specific to institutional and patient set-up parameters.

37.3.3 Chemotherapy

- The role of cytotoxic chemotherapy in retroperitoneal sarcomas is currently undefined.
- Imatinib can be considered for the treatment of GISTs (Grade A). It has proven efficacy in GISTs in the adjuvant setting (DEMATTEO et al. 2007), as well as in advanced or metastatic settings (Level I) (DEMETRI et al. 2002; VERWEIJ et al. 2004).

37.4 Follow-Ups

37.4.1 Post-Treatment Follow-Ups

- Life-long follow-up after definitive treatment of extremity and abdominal soft tissue sarcomas is recommended for detecting recurrence, secondary tumors, or other long-term complications of radiation therapy or chemotherapy.

Schedule

- Follow-ups could be scheduled every 3 months for 3 years, then every 6 months for two additional years, then annually thereafter (Grade D) (NATIONAL COMPREHENSIVE CANCER NETWORK 2007) (Table 37.3).

Work-Ups

- Each follow-up should include a complete history and physical examination.
- Follow-up imaging of the primary site (MRI and/or CT) should be based on the locoregional recurrence risk and should not be excessive in low-risk subsets (NATIONAL COMPREHENSIVE CANCER NETWORK 2007). Every 3–6 months for the first

Table 37.3. Follow-up schedule after treatment of soft tissue sarcoma

Interval	Frequency
First 3 years	Every 3 months
Year 4–5	Every 6 months
Over 5 years	Annually

5 years and then annually is reasonable for high-risk lesions.

▪ For stage IIB–III disease, chest imaging (either CT or chest X-ray) should be performed every 3–6 months for 5 years, then annually thereafter. Chest imaging every 6–12 months should be considered for stage I–IIA disease.

▪ Patients with low-grade abdominal lesions should have follow-up history and physicals every 3–6 months for 2–3 years and then annually thereafter. In contrast, patients with high-grade lesions should have scans every 6 months for years 4–5, then annually. Chest imaging should also be considered (Grade D) (NATIONAL COMPREHENSIVE CANCER NETWORK 2007).

References

Alekhteyar KM, Leung DH, Brennan MF et al. (1996) The effect of combined external beam radiotherapy and brachytherapy on local control and wound complications in patients with high-grade soft tissue sarcomas of the extremity with positive microscopic margin. Int J Radiat Oncol Biol Phys 36:321–324

Alektiar KM, Hu K, Anderson L et al. (2000) High-dose rate intraoperative radiation therapy (HDR-IORT) for retroperitoneal sarcomas. Int J Radiat Oncol Biol Phys 47:157–163

Alektiar KM, Leung D, Zelefsky MJ et al. (2002) Adjuvant radiation for stage IIB soft tissue sarcoma of the extremity. J Clin Oncol 20:1643–1650

Baldini EH, Goldberg J, Jenner C et al. (1999) Long-term outcomes after function-sparing surgery without radiotherapy for soft-tissue sarcoma of the extremities and trunk. J Clin Oncol 17:3252–3259

Catton CN, O'Sullivan B, Kotwall C et al. (1994) Outcome and prognosis in retroperitoneal soft tissue sarcoma. Int J Radiat Oncol Biol Phys 29:1005–1010

Coindre JM, Terrier P, Guillou L et al. (2001) Predictive value of grade for metastasis development in the main histologic types of adult soft tissue sarcomas: a study of 1240 patients from the French Federation of Cancer Centers Sarcoma Group. Cancer 91:1914–1926

Davis AM, O'Sullivan B, Turcotte R et al. (2005) Late radiation morbidity following randomization to preoperative versus postoperative radiotherapy in extremity soft tissue sarcoma. Radiother Oncol 75:48–53

DeMatteo R, Owzar K, Maki R et al. (2007) Adjuvant imatinib mesylate increases recurrence free survival (RFS) in patients with completely resected localized primary gastrointestinal stromal tumor (GIST): North American Intergroup Phase III trial ACOSOG Z9001. 2007 ASCO annual meeting. Abstract 10079

Demetri GD, Von Mehren M, Blancke CD et al. (2002) Effi-

cacy and safety of imatinib mesylate in advanced gastrointestinal stromal tumors. N Engl J Med 347:472–480

Fein DA, Corn BW, Lanciano RM et al. (1995) Management of retroperitoneal sarcomas: does dose escalation impact locoregional control. Int J Radiat Oncol Biol Phys 31:129–134

Fletcher CD, Gustafson P, Rydholm A et al. (2001) Clinicopathological re-evaluation of 100 malignant fibrous histiocytomas: prognostic relevance of subclassification. J Clin Oncol 19:3045–3050

Frustaci S, DiPaoli A, Bidoli E et al. (2003) Ifosfamide in the adjuvant therapy of soft tissue sarcomas. Oncology 65[Suppl 2]:80–84

Gieschen HL, Spiro IJ, Suit HD et al. (2001) Long-term results of intraoperative electron beam radiotherapy for primary and recurrent retroperitoneal soft tissue sarcoma. Int J Radiat Oncol Biol Phys 50:127–131

Greene F, Page D, Fleming I et al. (2002) AJCC Cancer Staging Manual, 6th edn. Springer, Berlin Heidelberg New York

Guillou L, Coindre JM, Bonichon F et al. (1997) Comparative study of the National Cancer Institute and French Federation of Cancer Centers Sarcoma Group grading systems in a population of 410 adult patients with soft tissue sarcoma. J Clin Oncol 15:350–362

Jones JJ, Catton CN, O'Sullivan B et al. (2002) Initial results of a trial of preoperative external-beam radiation therapy and postoperative brachytherapy for retroperitoneal sarcoma. Ann Surg Oncol 9:346–354

Nag S, Shasha D, Janjan N et al. (2001) The American Brachytherapy Society Recommendations for brachytherapy of soft tissue sarcomas. Int J Radiat Oncol Biol Phys 49:1033–1043

National Comprehensive Cancer Network (2007) Practice Guidelines in Oncology-V.1.2007, www.nccn.org./professionals/physicians_gls/PDF/sarcoma.pdf. Accessed March 2008.

O'Sullivan B, Davis AM, Turcotte R et al. (2002) Preoperative versus postoperative radiotherapy in soft-tissue sarcoma of the limbs: a randomized trial. Lancet 359:2235–2241

Petersen IA, Haddock MG, Donohue JH et al. (2002) Use of intraoperative electron beam radiotherapy in the management of retroperitoneal soft tissue sarcoma. Int J Radiat Oncol Biol Phys 52:469–475

Pisters PW, Harrison LB, Leung DH et al. (1996a) Long-term results of prospective randomized trial of adjuvant brachytherapy in soft tissue sarcoma. J Clin Oncol 14:859–868

Pisters PW, Leung DH, Woodruff JM et al. (1996b) Analysis of prognostic factors in 1041 patients with localized soft tissue sarcomas of the extremities. J Clin Oncol 14:1679–1689

Pisters PW, Ballo MT, Fenstermacher MJ et al. (2003) Phase I trial of preoperative concurrent doxorubicin and radiation therapy, surgical resection, and intraoperative electron-beam radiation therapy for patients with localized retroperitoneal sarcoma. J Clin Oncol 21:3092–2097

Pisters PW, Pollock RE, Lewis VO et al. (2007) Long-term results of prospective trial of surgery alone with selective use of radiation for patients with T1 extremity and trunk soft tissue sarcomas. Ann Surg 246:675–682

Rosenberg SA, Tepper JE, Glatstein EJ et al. (1982) The treatment of soft-tissue sarcomas of the extremities: prospective randomized evaluations of (1) limb-sparing surgery plus radiation therapy compared with amputation and (2) the role of adjuvant chemotherapy. Ann Surg 196:305–315

Sarcoma Meta-analysis Collaboration (1997) Adjuvant chemotherapy for localized resectable soft-tissue sarcoma of adults: meta-analysis of individual data. Lancet 350:1647–1654

Stoeckle E, Coindre JM, Bonvalot S et al. (2001) Prognostic factors in retroperitoneal sarcoma: a multivariate analysis of a series of 165 patients of the French Cancer Center Federation Sarcoma Group. Cancer 92:359–368

Verweij J, Casali PG, Zalcberg J et al. (2004) Progression-free survival in gastrointestinal stromal tumors with high-dose imatinib: randomized trial. Lancet 364:1127–1134

White LM, Wunder JS, Bell RS et al. (2005) Histologic assessment of peritumoral edema in soft tissue sarcoma. Int J Radiat Oncol Biol Phys 61:1439–1445

Yang JC, Chang AE, Baker AR et al. (1998) Randomized prospective study of the benefit of adjuvant radiation therapy in the treatment of soft tissue sarcomas of the extremity. J Clin Oncol 16:197–203

Section X:
Pediatric Tumors

CNS Tumors in Children

38

CRISTIANE TAKITA and GEORGES F. HATOUM

CONTENTS

Introduction and Objectives

Pediatric CNS malignancies represent 20% of all pediatric malignancies, and approximately 3,000 cases occur in the United States annually. CNS malignancies are the most frequent tumors in childhood after hematological malignancies and require a multidisciplinary management. Surgery, chemotherapy, and radiation therapy play a prominent role in the management of nearly all pediatric CNS malignancies; however, the selection of treatment is based on the pathology as well as the extent of the disease.

This chapter examines:

● Recommendations for diagnosis and work-up of most common pediatric CNS malignancies

● The prognostic factors of various types of pediatric CNS malignancies

● Treatment recommendations as well as supporting scientific evidence

● Radiation treatment techniques

● Follow-up care of survivors

C. TAKITA, MD
Department of Radiation Oncology, Sylvester Comprehensive Cancer Center, University of Miami Miller School of Medicine, 1475 NW 12th Avenue, D-31, Suite 1500, Miami, FL 33136, USA
G. F. HATOUM, MD
Department of Radiation Oncology, Sylvester Comprehensive Cancer Center, University of Miami Miller School of Medicine, 1475 NW 12th Avenue, D-31, Suite 1500, Miami, FL 33136, USA

Diagnosis, Staging, and Prognoses

38.1.1 Diagnosis

Initial Evaluation

- Diagnosis and evaluation of pediatric CNS tumors start with a complete history and physical examination (H&P).
- Presenting signs and symptoms depend on the location and extent of the tumor. Attention should be paid to specific neurological symptoms and signs such as:
  - Increased intracranial pressure leading to vomiting, morning headache, ataxia, nausea, and papilledema.
  - Parinaud's syndrome associated with pineal tumors (diminished upward gaze, diminished convergence, and diminished pupillary constriction to light).
  - Precocious or delayed puberty, diabetes insipidus, and visual field defects in suprasellar tumors (pineal tumors, craniopharyngioma).
  - Cranial nerve palsies mainly seen in brainstem gliomas.
- Thorough neurological and visual exam including a funduscopic examination should be performed.

Laboratory Tests

- Initial laboratory tests should include a complete blood count, basic blood chemistry, serum markers (β-HCG and AFP elevated in germinomas).
- CSF cytology for all embryonal tumors, including CSF serum markers in case of pineal tumors, and ependymomas.

Imaging Studies

- MRI of the CNS (brain) with and without contrast is the gold standard imaging study for pediatric CNS tumors.
- CT scan of the brain can be useful for calcified tumors such as craniopharyngiomas and germ cell tumors.
- Spinal axis MRI is mandatory for PNET and ependymomas.

Table 38.1. Imaging and laboratory work-ups for pediatric CNS tumors

Imaging studies	Laboratory tests
– MRI of the brain – CT of the brain (optional) – Spinal axis MRI for PNET, ependymomas	– Complete blood count – Serum chemistry – APF, β-HCG, LDH – CSF cytology – CSF serum markers

38.1.2 Staging

- Clinical or pathological staging is generally not applicable to pediatric CNS tumors.
- The Chang staging system for medulloblastoma is presented in Table 38.2.

Table 38.2. Chang-Harisiadis tumor classification system

Tumor stage	Size/extension	Metastasis stage	Invasiveness
T1	Tumor < 3 cm in diameter	M0	No evidence of subarachnoid or hematogenous metastasis
T2	Tumor ≥ 3 cm	M1	Tumor cells found in cerebrospinal fluid
T3a	Tumor > 3 cm with extension	M2	Intracranial tumor beyond primary site
T3b	Tumor > 3 cm with unequivocal extension into the brain stem	M3	Gross nodular seeding in spinal subarachnoid space
T4	Tumor > 3 cm with extension beyond the Sylvian aqueduct and/or beyond the foramen magnum	M4	Metastasis outside the cerebrospinal axis

38.1.3 Prognostic Factors

■ The prognosis of patients with pediatric CNS tumors depends on the type of the tumor.

■ Metastases stage, adjuvant treatment, and residual tumor are important adverse prognostic factors in medulloblastoma (CCG 921, Level II) (ZELTZER et al. 1999).

■ Histology is the most important prognostic factor for pineal tumors. Non-germinomatous tumors are aggressive, relatively less radiosensitive, and have a poor outcome compared to germinoma.

■ Diffuse infiltrating pattern, WHO high grade histology, lack of enhancement on MRI, and duration of symptoms to diagnosis of less than 6 months are adverse prognostic factors for brainstem gliomas (Level IV) (MAUFFREY 2006).

■ Extent of resection and amount of residual tumor on postoperative imaging are important prognostic factors for ependymomas, according to a retrospective cohort study reported by Children's Cancer Group (CCG) (Level IV) (ROBERTSON et al. 1998).

38.2 Treatment of Medulloblastoma

38.2.1 Surgery

■ Complete surgical resection remains the primary treatment modality of medulloblastoma (Grade B). Gross total resection and near total resection (> 90% resection estimated by the surgeon and < 1.5 cm2 residual on postoperative imaging) are associated with superior outcome compared to subtotal resection (defined as 51%–90% of tumor removal), partial resection (11%–50%), or biopsy (≤ 10%) (Level IV) (ALBRIGHT et al. 1996).

■ Invasion of the brainstem or cerebellopontine peduncle is often the limiting factor for complete resection.

■ A ventriculoperitoneal (VP) shunt may be performed in cases of increased intracranial pressure before or after resection (Grade B). Seeding of malignant cells into the peritoneal cavity through the shunt is rare (Level IV) (BERGER et al. 1991).

38.2.2 Adjuvant Chemotherapy

■ Chemotherapy is indicated in the treatment of high risk (T3/T4, residual tumor, M+) medulloblastoma, and low risk (T1/T2, complete resection, M0) medulloblastoma in the hope of decreasing the dose of CSI (craniospinal irradiation) (Grade B). All current trials use chemotherapy for low and high risk patients.
The most common regimen used is Vincristine (VCR) weekly with radiation followed by maintenance therapy with CCNU/VCR/CDDP (Grade B). The efficacy of the VCR based chemotherapy followed by radiation has been demonstrated in a prospective trial from CCG. A total of 65 patients with nondisseminated medulloblastoma were treated with postoperative, reduced-dose craniospinal radiation therapy (23.4 Gy) and 55.8 Gy of local radiation therapy. Adjuvant vincristine based chemotherapy was concurrently given with radiation, and lomustine, vincristine, and cisplatin chemotherapy was administered during and after radiation. Progression-free survival was approaching 80% at 5 years (Level III) (PACKER et al. 1999).

■ Adjuvant chemotherapy delivered prior to irradiation (i.e., sequential chemotherapy followed by radiation) is not recommended in the treatment of non-metastatic medulloblastoma (Grade A). Preradiation chemotherapy was compared with radiation therapy alone in a prospective randomized trial from the United Kingdom. Although event-free survival was significantly improved for sequential chemotherapy and radiotherapy, there was no statistically significant difference in 3- and 5-year overall survival between patients treated with combined treatment or radiation only (SIOP/UKCCSG, Level I) (TAYLOR et al. 2003).

■ As concurrent chemoradiation therapy provides improved treatment outcome and can reduce the required irradiation dose, surgery followed by concurrent chemoradiotherapy is the current standard of treatment of non-metastatic medulloblastoma.

38.2.3 Adjuvant Radiation Therapy

■ Adjuvant radiation therapy is indicated in the treatment of medulloblastoma (Grade B). The volume to be treated in medulloblastoma is the entire neuraxis (craniospinal irradiation) in all patients ≥ 3 years of age. It consists of the cranial field, spinal field, and the posterior fossa boost field.

- Recommended total dose to the craniospinal axis is 36 Gy for high risk patients and 23.4 Gy along with chemotherapy for low risk patients (Grade B). In a prospective randomized trial reported by POG/CCG, reduced dose neuraxis irradiation was associated with reduced rate of event-free survival, although the difference did not reach statistical significance at 8 years after treatment (Level II) (Thomas et al. 2000). As detailed above, the results of a prospective trial conduced by CCG demonstrated that combined reduced-dose radiation and multi-drug chemotherapy provided similar outcome as the standard dose irradiation (Level III) (Packer et al. 1999).
  Lower dose irradiation dose is associated with less severe neuropsychological toxicity (Level IV) (Mulhern et al. 1998). Current trials are evaluating 18 Gy to spinal field for low risk patients along with chemotherapy.
- An overt meningeal seeding should receive a total dose of 39.6 Gy. Nodular leptomeningeal disease should receive a dose of 45–50 Gy.
- The posterior fossa needs to be boosted to a total dose of 54–55.8 Gy (Grade B). A dose below 50 Gy to the posterior fossa was associated with increased risk of local failure (Level IV) (Berry et al. 1981).

Treatment Technique

- The patient is simulated in a prone position with an aquaplast for the cranial field and the spinal fields. The posterior fossa field can be treated prone or supine.
- The cranial field (whole brain) is treated with bilateral parallel opposed fields, whereas the spinal volume is treated with a direct posterior field.
- At the discretion of the treating physician, an asymmetric collimation technique (single isocentric technique) or symmetric collimation technique can be used.
- If a symmetric collimation technique is used, there might be a skin gap of no more than 0.5 cm between the whole brain field and the spinal field. The collimator angle of the lateral cranial field should be adjusted so that the inferior border of the cranial field is parallel to the superior border of the divergent spinal field in the sagittal plane. A couch rotation may also be used to align the infe-

rior edge of the cranial field with the superior edge of the spinal field. The junction may be "feathered" (moved by 1–2 cm) every five to six fractions or at least twice during the treatment course.
- The cranial field should extend anteriorly to cover the entire frontal sinus and the cribriform plate region.
- The spinal field should cover the recesses of the entire vertebral bodies with at least a 1-cm margin on either side. The inferior border should be placed after review of the termination of the subdural space on MRI. The inferior border should be 2 cm below the termination of the subdural space (at least bottom of S2), but may be as low as bottom of S4. If there is a need for two spinal fields, then a skin gap between the two fields is calculated so that the 50% decrement lines of each field meet at the posterior margin of the vertebral body.
- In the case of spinal metastases, a portal field to include all visible disease with a margin of one vertebral body on each side of the lesions is to be used.
- The posterior fossa boost field has an inferior border at C1–C2 interspace, a superior border at least 1 cm superior to the midpoint distance between the foramen magnum and the vertex, an anterior border encompassing the posterior clinoids, and a margin fall off posteriorly. Posterior oblique fields to reduce the dose to the inner ear are used, which is an important consideration in children who also will receive chemotherapy with cisplatin. The optimal clinical target volume (CTV) remains to be defined; reduction of the target volume combined with 3D conformal planning is currently being evaluated, as this offers a potentially significant benefit in greater sparing not only of the cochlea but also the pituitary gland, the hypothalamus, and the temporal lobes.

38.3 Brainstem Gliomas

38.3.1 Surgery

- Surgery can be recommended for the treatment of brainstem gliomas; however, its role is determined by the location of the lesion. Surgery is the treatment of choice for dorsal exophytic tumors, focal non-tectal lesions surgically accessible, and for cervicomedullary tumors. However, surgery has no role in the management of patients with diffuse intrinsic lesions and biopsies are no longer considered necessary.

38.3.2 Radiation Therapy

■ Radiotherapy is the mainstay treatment for pediatric brainstem glioma, as surgical resection often has limited usage in the treatment of diffuse disease (Grade A). Neurological improvement can be expected in close to 80% of patients after radiation; however, overall survival is usually disappointing and ranges below 10% at 2 years after treatment.

■ Total dose of 54–55.8 Gy in standard fractionation is recommended when radiation therapy is used (Grade A). Results from prospective randomized trials reported by POG have confirmed that hyperfractionation has no benefit on treatment outcome (POG 9293, Level I) (Mandell et al. 1999). In addition, higher dose of irradiation to a total dose of 75.6 Gy (at 1.26 Gy twice a day in 60 fractions) provided no survival or local control benefits (POG 8495, Level III) (Freeman et al. 1993, 1996).

■ The target volume consists of gross tumor volume (GTV) (determined best by T2 weighted/FLAIR MRI). The clinical tumor volume consists of GTV and a margin of 1.5–2 cm.

38.3.3 Chemotherapy

■ High dose cyclophosphamide, cisplatinum/cyclophosphamide, and oral VP-16 have been tested without a durable response. At the present time, there is no evidence that intervening chemotherapy will enable the delay of radiation.

38.4 Germinomas

38.4.1 Surgery

■ Surgery plays an important role in the diagnosis of germinomas. However, radical resection of germinoma has shown no benefit.

38.4.2 Radiation Therapy

■ Radiotherapy is the mainstay treatment of germinomas (Grade B). If radiation is used alone, a craniospinal irradiation dose of 24–36 Gy, followed by a boost to the primary site to a total dose of 45–50 Gy, can be recommended. The results from a multi-institutional prospective nonrandomized trial from Germany demonstrated that complete response can be expected in all patients treated in such regimens, and the 5-year relapse-free survival rate was over 90% (Level III) (Bamberg et al. 1999).

■ The treatment volume is controversial (craniospinal irradiation versus involved field). Craniospinal irradiation is recommended if no chemotherapy is used. Most recent trials use chemotherapy followed by involved field radiation.

38.4.3 Chemotherapy

■ Chemotherapy is recommended in the treatment of pediatric CNS germinomas (Grade B). CNS germinomas are highly sensitive to chemotherapy. Medications such as cyclophosphamide, ifosfamide, etoposide, cisplatin, and carboplatin are highly active and have been studied in prospective trials. The current COG trial is using neoadjuvant chemotherapy followed by localized radiation. The dose and volume of the radiation treatment fields depend on the response to chemotherapy.

38.5 Treatment of Low-Grade Astrocytomas

38.5.1 Surgery

■ For some asymptomatic children with neurofibromatosis type 1 (NF-1) diagnosed with low-grade astrocytoma (LGA), close follow-up is an appropriate initial management. Treatment is reserved for progression of disease.

■ Surgery is the mainstay treatment of low-grade astrocytoma (Grade B). Complete resection can be achieved in approximately 80% of cerebral and cerebellar tumors and 40% of the diencephalic tumors. Complete surgical resection for children with cerebellar and hemispheric tumors results in disease-free and overall survival rates of 80%–100% (Level IV) (Gajjar et al. 1997).

- After subtotal resection in neurologically stable patients, the recommendation is to follow-up patients closely. At the time of progression, a second surgical resection should be considered if possible.

38.5.2 Radiation Therapy

- Radiotherapy is not indicated after complete resection, but is recommended after incomplete resection for patients who may develop loss of vision or impaired neurological function, if disease progresses.
- Radiotherapy is recommended for patients ≥ 3 years of age with unresectable tumors that have progressed or cause symptoms.

Radiation Therapy Techniques

- In pilocytic tumors, the CTV is GTV (tumor bed and residual gross tumor, best seen in T1 MRI) with a 0.5-cm margin. Planning target volume (PTV) is CTV plus 0.3–0.5 cm margin. Studies are currently evaluating the treatment of the residual postoperative tumor only with margins.
- In infiltrative diffuse fibrillary tumors, margins of 1.5–2 cm around the tumor using T2-weighted or FLAIR MRI are more appropriate.
- In children ≥ 3 years of age, doses of 54–55 Gy, in 150–180 cGy/fraction, are used. For children < 3 years of age, if radiation can not be delayed, doses of about 45–50 Gy to small volumes are appropriate.
- 3D treatment planning using MRI/CT image fusion increases target volume conformality and better assessment of normal tissue doses with evaluation of dose-volume histograms (DVH).
- For small tumors (< 3.5 cm), stereotactic fractionated radiotherapy or stereotactic radiosurgery techniques are promising. In a prospective trial reported by Marcus et al. (2005), 50 patients with low-grade astrocytoma were treated with stereotactic fractionated radiation therapy when progression occurred during or after chemotherapy or after surgery. The progression-free survival rate was 82.5% at 5 years and 65% at 8 years, and the overall survival was 97.8% at 5 years and 82%

at 8 years after treatment. No marginal failure was observed, and only one patient developed a presumed radiation-induced primitive neuroectodermal tumor 6 years after initial treatment (Level III).

38.5.3 Chemotherapy

- Chemotherapy can be used, particularly for infants and young children (< 3 years of age), to delay radiotherapy (Grade B). Complete responses are low with chemotherapy, but partial responses or stable disease can be up to 70%–100% (Level III) (Walker et al. 1999).

38.6 Treatment of High-Grade Astrocytomas

38.6.1 Surgery

- Surgery is the most important treatment for high-grade astrocytomas (HGA) (Grade B). Results from the analysis of patients treated in a randomized study demonstrated a clear survival benefit for patients undergoing complete resection (CCG 945, Level IV) (Wisoff et al. 1998).
- A second surgical procedure should be considered if there is significant residual disease after the initial surgery.

38.6.2 Radiation Therapy

- Postoperative radiotherapy is always recommended in the treatment of high-grade astrocytoma (Grade B). The most common site of failure is local, despite the incidence of leptomeningeal seeding of about 10%–30%.
- Target treatment volume is CTV-1 which includes GTV (tumor bed, residual macroscopic disease best seen on gadolinium enhanced T1 MRI), peritumoral edema (T2 MRI) with a 2-cm margin. PTV-1 is CTV-1 with 0.3–0.5 cm margin. After 45–50 Gy, a field reduction is done to include the tumor bed and residual macroscopic disease with 1-cm margin (CTV-2), adding a 0.3- to 0.5-cm margin for the PTV-2.

- Dose to the CTV-1 should be around 45–50 Gy with final boost to the tumor bed/residual disease to about 60 Gy.
- There is no data to support that higher doses of radiation, use of radiosurgery, stereotatic boost, or hyperfractionated radiotherapy improve outcome of these patients.

38.6.3 Chemotherapy

- Chemotherapy is currently not recommended for the treatment of high-grade astrocytoma in children (Grade A). Results from two randomized phase III trials have been disappointing. Both studies failed to show a definite benefit for high-grade astrocytoma patients (CHILDREN'S CANCER STUDY GROUP 943 and 945, Level I) (SPOSTO et al. 1989; FINLAY et al. 1995). Chemotherapy agents most commonly used in clinical trials are vincristine, lomustine (CCNU), and prednisone.
- Chemotherapy should be considered in infants to delay radiation after 3 years of age (Grade B). Partial response to chemotherapy was demonstrated according to the Pediatric Oncology Group experience (Level III) (DUFFNER et al. 1996).

38.7 Craniopharyngiomas

38.7.1 Surgery

- For small, localized tumors, treatment of choice is an attempt at complete resection with preservation of visual, hypothalamic, and pituitary function (Grade B). Disease-free survival of about 75%–80% at 10 years can be expected after complete resection (Level IV) (DE VILE et al. 1996; SANFORD 1994).
- In larger tumors, a planned limited resection (biopsy/partial/subtotal resection) followed by radiation is associated with less morbidity than attempting radical surgery alone. After subtotal resection, residual tumor progression is seen in about 71%–90% of the patients collectively according to one literature review (HOFFMAN 1990).

38.7.2 Radiation Therapy

- Radiotherapy is not indicated after gross total resection of craniopharyngiomas. However, adjuvant radiation therapy is indicated after incomplete surgical resection (Grade B). A subtotal resection (biopsy/partial/subtotal resection) followed by postoperative radiation gives local control in approximately 80%–95% (Level IV) (HETELEKIDIS et al. 1993; WEN et al. 1989).
- Immediate postoperative radiation provides better outcome than radiation therapy delivered at the time of recurrence. The 20-year overall survival for patients irradiated for primary disease was 78% versus 25% for those irradiated for recurrence (Level IV) (REGINE et al. 1992, 1993).
- 3D conformal RT with multiple fields and IMRT can be used to decrease normal tissue irradiation and late sequelae.
  The PTV includes GTV (solid and cystic components of the tumor) plus a 1-cm margin. If cyst aspiration or partial resection is performed, attention should be made to cover the cystic wall.
- The recommended doses are 54–55.8 Gy at 1.8-Gy daily fraction (Level IV) (BLOOM et al. 1990; RAJAN et al. 1993; REGINE et al. 1992). Doses above 60 Gy were associated with late complications such as brain necrosis and optic neuropathy.
- In primary or recurrent large cystic tumors, implantation of intracystic catheter allows decompression of the cyst and instillation of radioactive material into the cystic area (^{90}Y or ^{32}P) (JULOW et al. 2007; POLLOCK et al. 1995).
- Stereotatic radiosurgery can be considered for residual or recurrent tumors after surgery (Grade B). A retrospective study of 98 consecutive cases of craniopharyngioma treated with stereotactic radiosurgery (maximal dose was 21.8 Gy and tumor margin dose was 11.5 Gy) for residual or recurrent disease demonstrated complete and partial response rates of 19.4% and 67.4%, respectively. The actuarial 5- and 10-year progression-free survival rates were 60.8 and 53.8%, respectively (Level IV) (KOBAYASHI et al. 2005).

38.8 Ependymoma

38.8.1 Surgery

- Complete resection of ependymoma is the initial treatment of choice (Grade A). Extent of surgical resection is the most important prognostic factor for ependymomas (Level IV) (Robertson et al. 1998). The rate of gross total resection has been increased to 85% of ependymomas in the newer series.
- The rate of complete resection is lower for infratentorial ependymomas, especially for tumors extending through the Foramen of Magendie and Luschka, or large tumors at presentation. Second-look surgery should be considered in these patients.

38.8.2 Radiation Therapy

- Postoperative radiotherapy is considered the standard of care for children older than 3 years of age with ependymomas (Grade A). The most effective treatment for localized ependymoma (no evidence of neuraxis dissemination) is gross total resection followed by postoperative radiation, with progression-free survival of 50%–60% at 5 years, for children above 3 years of age (Level IV) (Merchant and Fouladi 2005).
- Standard volume for patients with localized ependymoma is local radiation field (Grade B). Based on results of a number of retrospective studies, craniospinal irradiation (CSI) does not improve outcome in adequately staged patients (Level IV) (Merchant et al. 1997; Paulino et al. 2002).
  Frequency of neuraxis dissemination at diagnosis is less than 7% with the use of MR spinal imaging and CSF cytologic evaluation (Level IV) (Perilongo et al. 1997).
- The target volume for infratentorial ependymoma should include the tumor bed, based on the preoperative images, considering changes from surgery, including residual macroscopic disease, plus a margin for the CTV of 1–1.5 cm around the GTV. For PTV, add a margin of 0.3–0.5 cm around the CTV.

For anaplastic ependymomas, the target volume consists of tumor bed and macroscopic residual disease with a 1.5- to 2-cm margin.
- CSI is recommended only for patients with leptomeningeal seeding at presentation and ependymoblastomas.
- The current standard doses for brain lesions are 54–55 Gy. If there is gross residual disease, boost doses might be given to about 60 Gy to GTV (Grade B). Results of a retrospective review of 51 cases of pediatric ependymoma demonstrated a dose-response relationship showing better local control with doses ≥ 45 Gy (32%) as compared to those received lower dose (0%) (Level IV) (Goldwein 1990).
  CSI doses are 36 Gy in 1.8-Gy fractions; patients with overt meningeal seeding at diagnosis typically receive CSI higher dose of about 38–40 Gy, and a boost to areas of focal spinal involvement of about 45–50 Gy.
- Use of 3D conformal radiotherapy is encouraged to decrease late side effects.
- Intensity-modulated radiation therapy (IMRT) might be an option to decrease long-term side effects in childhood ependymoma (Grade C). All failures were within the high-dose region according to a clinical study from the University of New Mexico, suggesting that IMRT does not diminish local control (Level III) (Schroeder et al. 2008).
- The use of stereotactic radiosurgery (SRS) in the treatment of ependymoma awaits further investigation. SRS has been used in small intracranial tumors or spinal target, as boost treatment or at time of recurrence, with limited success (Level V) (Mansur et al. 2004).

38.8.3 Chemotherapy

- Chemotherapy is usually not recommended in the treatment of ependymoma (Grade B). Combination chemotherapy in older patients has failed to improve results after surgery and radiation, despite sensitivity for chemotherapy agents such as platinum compounds and alkylating agents (Evans et al. 1996).
- Chemotherapy can be used in patients ≤ 3 years of age after surgical resection (Grade B). The efficacy of chemotherapy in this group of patients aimed to delay radiotherapy was demonstrated in a prospective trial (SIOP/ UKCCSG, Level III) (Grundy et al. 2007).

38.9 Radiation-Induced Side Effects and Complications

38.9.1 Cranial Radiotherapy

- Acute side effects associated with cranial irradiation include hair loss, skin reactions, headache, nausea, and vomiting. A potential subacute toxicity associated with cranial irradiation is the somnolence syndrome.
- Late side effects are mainly neuropsychological and endocrine.
  Neuropsychological sequelae are mainly lower levels of IQ with deficits in verbal coding and memory. Lower levels of IQ after radiation therapy are associated with younger age at treatment (Level IV) (Hirsh et al. 1979). Behavioral disturbances such as attention deficits, negative attitudes, emotional regression, defective spatial orientation, and dysgraphia can also occur.
  Endocrine sequelae may be secondary to tumor location in addition to the effects of radiation on the hypothalamic-pituitary axis. Between 70% and 100% of children show abnormal GH tests on provocation, and decreased growth rate is described in 30%–100%.

38.9.2 Spinal Radiotherapy

- The most pronounced acute side effect is the hematologic suppression. Other acute side effects include nausea with or without vomiting or acute effects related to the exit dose through the mouth such as mucositis, sore throat, dry mouth, thickened saliva, altered taste, and esophagitis.
- Late side effects might include growth retardation, short stature, and secondary thyroid carcinoma.

38.10 Follow-Ups

38.10.1 Post-Treatment Follow-Ups

- Life-long follow-up is required for all children after treatment.

- Patients should be followed-up according to the treatment protocol.
- Follow up with clinical exam, neurological evaluation, and neuroimaging is recommended approximately every 6–12 months for several years.
- Patients with neuroendocrine abnormalities are likely to need lifelong care in association with an endocrinologist.
- Careful neuropsychological testing, educational interaction, and vocational rehabilitation are necessary to improve the quality of life for survivors of pediatric CNS tumors.

References

Albright AL, Wisoff JH, Zeltzer PM (1996) Effects of medulloblastoma resections on outcome in children: a report from the Children's Cancer Group. Neurosurgery 38:265–271

Bamberg M, Kortmann RD, Calaminus G et al. (1999) Radiation therapy for intracranial germinoma: results of the German cooperative prospective trials MAKEI 83/86/89. J Clin Oncol 8:2585–2592

Berger MS, Baumeister B, Geyer JR et al. (1991) The risks of metastases from shunting in children with primary central nervous system tumors. J Neurosurg 74:872–877

Berry MP, Jenkin RDT, Keen CW et al. (1981) Radiation treatment for medulloblastoma: a 21-year review. J Neurosurg 55:43–51

Bloom HJG, Glees J, Bell J (1990) The treatment of long-term prognosis of children with intracranial tumors: a study of 610 cases, 1951–1981. Int J Radiat Oncol Biol Phys 18:723–745

De Vile CJ, Grant DB, Kendall BE et al. (1996) Management of childhood craniopharyngioma: can the morbidity of radical surgery be predicted? J Neurosurg 85:73–81

Duffner PK, Krischer JP, Burger PC et al. (1996) Treatment of infants with malignant gliomas: the Pediatric Oncology Group experience. J Neurooncol 28:215–222

Evans AE, Anderson JR, Lefbowitz-Boudreaux IB et al. (1996) Adjuvant chemotherapy of childhood posterior fossa ependymoma: cranio-spinal irradiation with or without adjuvant CCNU, vincristine, and prednisone: a Children's Cancer Group study. Med Pediatr Oncol 27:8–14

Finlay JL, Boyett JM, Yates JA et al. (1995) Randomized phase III trial in childhood high-grade astrocytoma comparing vincristine, lomustine, and prednisone with eight-drugs-1-day regimen. J Clin Oncol 13:112–123

Freeman CR, Krischer JP, Sanford RA et al. (1993) Final results of a study of escalating doses of hyperfractionated radiotherapy in brain stem tumors in children: a Pediatric Oncology Group study. Int J Radiat Oncol Biol Phys 27:197–206

Freeman CR, Bourgouin PM, Sanford RA et al. (1996) Long term survivors of childhood brain stem gliomas treated with hyperfractionated radiotherapy. Clinical characteristics and treatment related toxicities. The Pediatric Oncology Group. Cancer 77:555–562

Gajjar A, Sanford RA, Heideman R et al. (1997) Low-grade astrocytoma: a decade of experience at St. Jude Children's Research Hospital. J Clin Oncol 15:2792–2799

Goldwein JW, Leahy JM, Packer RJ, Sutton LN, Curran WJ, Rorke LB, Schut L, Littman PS, D'Angio GJ (1990) Intracranial ependymomas in children. Int J Radiat Oncol Biol Phys 19:1497–1502

Grundy RG, Wilne SA, Weston CL et al. (2007) Primary postoperative chemotherapy without radiotherapy for intracranial ependymoma in children: the UKCCSG/SIOP prospective study. Lancet Oncol 8:696–705

Hetelekidis S, Barnes PD, Tao ML et al. (1993) 20-year experience in childhood craniopharyngioma. Int J Radiat Oncol Biol Phys 27:189–195

Hirsch JF, Renier D, Czernichow P et al. (1979) Medulloblastoma in childhood: survival and functional results. Acta Neurochir 48:1–15

Hoffman HJ (1990) Craniopharyngiomas. The role for resection. Neurosurg Clin N Am 1:173–180

Julow J, Backlund EO, Lanyi F et al. (2007) Long-term results and late complications after intracavitary Yttrium-90 colloid irradiation of recurrent cystic craniopharyngioma. Neuros 61:288–295

Kobayashi T, Kida Y, Mori Y et al. (2005) Long-term results of gamma knife surgery for treatment of craniopharyngioma in 98 consecutive cases. J Neuros 103[6 Suppl]:482–488

Mandell LR, Kadota R, Freeman C et al. (1999) There is no role for hyperfractionated radiotherapy in the management of children with newly diagnosed diffuse intrinsic brainstem tumors: results of a Pediatric Oncology Group phase III trial comparing conventional vs. hyperfractionated radiotherapy. Int J Radiat Oncol Biol Phys 43:959–964

Mansur DB, Drzymala RE, Rich KM et al. (2004) The efficacy of stereotatic radiosurgery in the management of intracranial ependymoma. J Neurooncol 66:187–190

Marcus KJ, Goumnerova L, Billett AL et al. (2005) Stereotactic radiotherapy for localized low-grade gliomas in children: final results of a prospective trial. Int J Radiat Oncol Biol Phys 61:374–379

Mauffrey C (2006) Pediatric brainstem gliomas: prognostic factors and management. J Clin Neurosci 13:431–437

Merchant TE, Fouladi M (2005) Ependymomas: new therapeutic approaches including radiation and chemotherapy. J Neurooncol 75:287–299

Merchant TE, Haida T, Wang MH et al. (1997) Anaplastic ependymoma: treatment of pediatric patients with or without craniospinal radiation therapy. J Neurosurg 86:943–949

Mulhern RK, Kepner JL, Thomas PR et al. (1998) Neuropsychologic functioning of survivors of childhood medulloblastoma randomized to receive conventional or reduced-dose craniospinal irradiation: A Pediatric Oncology Group study. J Clini Oncol 16:1723–1728

Packer RJ, Goldwein J, Nicholson HS et al. (1999) Treatment of children with medulloblastomas with reduced-dose craniospinal radiation therapy and adjuvant chemotherapy: A Children's Cancer Group Study. J Clin Oncol 17:2127–2136

Paulino AC, Wen BC, Buatti JM et al. (2002) Intracranial ependymomas: an analysis of prognostic factors and patterns of failure. Am J Clin Oncol 25:117–122

Perilongo G, Massimino M, Sotti G et al. (1997) Analyses of prognostic factors in a retrospective review of 92 children with ependymoma: Italian Pediatric Neuro-Oncology Group. Med Pediatr Oncol 29:79–85

Pollock BE, Lunsford LD, Kondziolka D et al. (1995) Phosphorus-32 intracavitary irradiation of cystic craniopharyngioma: current technique and long-term results. Int J Radiat Oncol Biol Phys 33:437–446

Rajan B, Ashley S, Gorman C et al. (1993) Craniopharyngioma – long term results following surgery and radiotherapy. Radiother Oncol 26:1–10

Regine WF, Kramer S (1992) Pediatric craniopharyngiomas: long-term results of combined treatment with surgery and radiation. Int J Radiat Oncol Biol Phys 24:611–617

Regine WF, Mohiuddin M, Kramer S (1993) Long-term results of pediatric and adult craniopharyngiomas treated with combined surgery and radiation. Radiother Oncol 27:13–21

Robertson PL, Zelter PM, Boyett JM et al. (1998) Survival and prognostic factors following radiation therapy and chemotherapy for ependymomas in children: a report of the Children's Cancer Group. J Neurosurg 88:695–703

Sanford RA. (1994) Craniopharyngioma: results of survey of the American Society of Pediatric Neurosurgery. Pediatr Neurosurg 21[Suppl 1]:39–43

Schroeder TM, Chintagumpala M, Okcu MF et al. (2008) Intensity modulated radiation therapy in childhood ependymoma. Int J Radiat Oncol Biol Phys 71:987–993

Sposto R, Ertel IJ, Jenkin RDT et al. (1989) The effectiveness of chemotherapy for treatment of high-grade astrocytoma in children: results of a randomized trial. A report from the Children's Cancer Study Group. J Neurooncol 7:165–177

Taylor RE, Bailey CC, Robinson K et al. (2003) Results of a randomized study of preradiation chemotherapy versus radiotherapy alone for nonmetastatic medulloblastoma: the International Society of Paediatric Oncology/United Kingdom Children's Cancer Study Group PNET-3 Study. J Clin Oncol 21:1581–1591

Thomas PR, Deutsch M, Kepner JL et al. (2000) Low-stage medulloblastoma: final analysis of trial comparing standard-dose with reduced-dose neuraxis irradiation. J Clin Oncol 18:3004–3011

Walker DA, Perilongo G, Zanetti I, Gnekow A, Taylor R (1999) Vincristine carboplatin in low grade glioma: an interim report of the international consortium on low grade glioma. Med Ped Onc 33:178

Wen BC, Hussey DH, Staples J et al. (1989) A comparison of the roles of surgery and radiation therapy in the management of craniopharyngiomas. Int J Radiat Oncol Biol Phys 16:17–24

Wisoff JH, Boyett JM, Berger MS et al. (1998) Current neurosurgical management and the impact of the extent of resection in the treatment of malignant gliomas in childhood: a report of the Children's Cancer Group Trial No CCG-945. J Neurosurg 89:52–59

Zeltzer PM, Boyett JM, Finlay JL et al. (1999) Metastasis stage, adjuvant treatment, and residual tumor are prognostic factors for medulloblastoma in children: conclusions from the Children's Cancer Group 921 randomized phase III study. J Clin Oncol 17:832–845

Pediatric Lymphomas

B-Chen Wen and Kelly LaFave

CONTENTS

Introduction and Objectives

Malignancies of the lymphoid system (including Hodgkin's and non-Hodgkin's lymphoma, and acute leukemias) account for approximately 40% of pediatric malignancies.

Hodgkin's lymphoma (HL) in the pediatric population has distinct characteristics, and is associated with Epstein-Barr virus (EBV) infection. It is uncommon before age 5 and most patients are 11 years of age and older (Cleary et al. 1994), and has a predominance in male. The incidence of this malignancy is highest in North America and Europe, being relatively rare in Asian countries.

Approximately 500 cases of non-Hodgkin's lymphoma (NHL) are diagnosed in the United States in patients younger than 15 years, and the median age at diagnosis is 11. It is rare for children <3 to develop NHL. NHL is the third most commonly diagnosed malignancy in childhood. The majority of cases of pediatric NHL are of Burkitt's, lymphoblastic, and large-cell lymphomas, and their clinical characteristics and management differ significantly from those commonly diagnosed in adults.

Contemporary treatment regimens for both HL and NHL have evolved to limit the potential related toxicities.

Chemotherapy plays a major role in the treatment of pediatric HL and NHL. However, radiation therapy remains an important treatment modality for consolidation treatment in selected patients presenting with bulky disease.

This chapter examines:

● Recommendations for initial evaluation, laboratory studies, and imaging studies for both HL and NHL

● Staging system, pathology, and prognostic factors

● Treatment recommendations for both disease entities accompanied by supporting literature

● Indications for radiation therapy and radiation technique

● Treatment-related toxicities

As the characteristics and treatment of acute leukemias differ significantly from those of HL and NHL, the management of ALL and AML are not included in this chapter.

B-C. Wen, MD
Kelly LaFave, MD
Department of Radiation Oncology, Sylvester Comprehensive Cancer Center, University of Miami, 1475 NW 12th Avenue, D-31, Miami, FL 33136, USA

39.1 Diagnosis, Staging, and Prognoses in Pediatric Hodgkin's Lymphoma

39.1.1 Diagnosis

Initial Evaluation

- Diagnosis and evaluation of HL in children starts with a complete history and physical examination; presenting signs and symptoms depend on the location and extent of the tumor. Full history and physical examination allow for evaluation of the involved lymph node chains.
- Patients may present with mediastinal and cervical lymphadenopathy and "B" symptoms (unexplained fever >38°C for 3 days, drenching night sweats, weight loss of 10% in previous 6 months).
- The majority of affected children up to age 10 are male (80%), while in adolescents the male and female ratio is 1:1 (CLEARLY et al. 1994; NACHMAN et al. 2002).
- In a developed country, HL is commonly associated with higher socioeconomic status, small family size, and early birth order in siblings; in developing countries, HL is more likely in children under age 10 and associated with EBV (KANDIL et al. 2001).
- HIV, inherited immunodeficiency disorders, environmental and familial causes may predispose children to HL.

Laboratory Tests

- Laboratory studies performed at diagnosis include complete blood count with differential, ESR, liver function tests, and renal function tests.
- Patients presenting with "B" symptoms or advanced disease (i.e., stage III or IV) should undergo bone marrow aspiration and biopsy.

Imaging Studies

- Imaging studies essential in the staging workup include chest X-ray (posteroanterior and lateral) and CT of neck, chest, abdomen, and pelvis (HANNA et al. 1993). Oral and IV contrast assist in defining lymphadenopathy in the infradiaphragmatic region.

- Bulky disease of the mediastinum is classified as the ratio of the mediastinal mass to the largest intrathoracic diameter ≥1/3 on a PA chest X-ray. Greater than or equal to 6 cm in peripheral nodal disease is also considered bulky (Level III) (SMITH et al. 2003).
- MRI may assist in distinguishing infradiaphragmatic lymph nodes in children as there is less fat, making CT more difficult to differentiate retroperitoneal lymph nodes.
- FDG-PET scan or PET/CT should be considered in the initial evaluation (Grade B). FDG-PET scan, PET/CT, and high dose gallium studies in children are most helpful in determining the response to treatment, but may also provide more information on initial staging. FDG-PET is superior to gallium in the infradiaphragmatic region (Level IV) (HUELTENSCHMIDT et al. 2001; RHODES et al. 2006).
- Lymphangiography and staging laparotomy were routinely used for staging purposes in the past. Lymphangiography is not considered part of the standard work-up in the modern age.

Pathology

- Pathologic confirmation of a diagnosis of HL is required prior to any treatment.
- Excisional lymph node biopsy should be performed to determine the histological subtype. Fine needle aspiration or core biopsies are generally not adequate for making a diagnosis.
- A staging laparotomy could be considered for patients to be treated without chemotherapy.
- HL is classified into five subtypes by the World Health Organization (HARRIS et al. 1999; CLEARLY et al. 1994).
- Classical HL (CHL) includes: nodular sclerosis (NSHL), mixed cellularity (MCHL), lymphocyte depleted (LDHL), lymphocyte-rich classical (LRCHL).
  - NSHL: Most common HL in all child age groups and is more frequently seen in adolescents as compared to children under age 10. NSHL commonly presents with mediastinal, cervical, and supraclavicular lymphadenopathy and also with bulky disease.
  - MCHL: Second most common HL and is relatively more common in children under age 10. MCHL usually presents with more advanced stage.
  - LDHL: Rare in children but more common in HIV+ patients.

Table 39.1. CHL and NLPHL group characteristics. [Adapted from HERBST et al. (1991) and HALUSKA et al. (1994) with permission]

	Classical HL	NLPHL
Characteristic cell	Reed-Sternberg cell	Lymphocytic and histiocytic cell "Popcorn cells"
Surface antigens	CD15+, CD30+, CD20+/−, CD45−, EMA−	CD15−, CD30−, CD20+, CD45+, EMA+
EBV	EBV+ in 50%	EBV−

– LRCHL: Uncommon type of HL in children. May present with localized peripheral lymphadenopathy.
■ Nodular lymphocyte predominant HL (NLPHL): Relatively more common in children under age 10, NLPHL most often presents with early stage disease (Table 39.1).
■ In the group under age 10, NSHL is most common (44%), followed by MCHL (33%), and NLPHL (13%).

39.1.2 Staging

■ Pediatric HL is usually staged clinically. Staging of patients requires evaluation of disease extent.

Table 39.2. Modified Ann Arbor Staging System. [From CARBONE et al. (1971) with permission]

Stage I	Involvement of single lymph node (I) or extralymphatic site (IE)
Stage II	Involvement of two or more involved lymph node sites on the same side of the diaphragm (II) or localized involvement of one extralymphatic organ or site plus one or more lymph node regions on the same side of diaphragm (IIE)
Stage III	Involvement of lymph node regions on both sides of the diaphragm (III) which can include involvement of the spleen (IIIS) or localized extralymphatic site or organ extension (IIIE) or both (IIISE)
Stage IV	Diffuse (multifocal) involvement of one or more extralymphatic organs or sites
Descriptors	A= "B" symptoms "B" Unexplained fever >38°C, weight loss >10% in previous 6 months, drenching night sweats X=Bulky disease (The Ann Arbor Staging System does not include descriptors of bulk of disease)

The Ann Arbor staging system for HL is presented in Table 39.2.

39.1.3 Prognosis

■ Overall the prognosis of pediatric HL is superior to that of adults. The presenting stage at diagnosis is the most important prognostic factor. The 10-year overall survival rates is >90% for early stage and is 75%–80% for patients with stage IV disease.
■ "B" symptoms are present in 25% of patients and are of prognostic significance (Level IV) (NACHMAN et al. 2002).
■ A retrospective review of a large series from Stanford University (including 328 patients with lymphoma from 1990–2000) revealed that male gender, stage IIB/IIIB/IV, bulky mediastinal disease, WBC >13.5×10³/mm³ and hemoglobin <11 g/dl are prognostic factors on multivariate analysis (Level IV) (SMITH et al. 2003).

39.2 Treatment of Pediatric Hodgkin's Lymphoma

39.2.1 General Principles

■ Children with HL should be treated on clinical protocol whenever possible. The goal is to use non-cross resistant chemotherapy regimens with the least amount of toxicity as possible.
■ In order to minimize the treatment-related toxicities, risk adapted combined-modality therapy and response-based involved field radiotherapy is commonly utilized in treatment regimens for pediatric HL, especially in the United States.

■ It is essential that the side-effect profile and treatment complications are avoided and reduced as much as possible since these patients enjoy an excellent prognosis. VAMP is an example of a toxicity reduced chemotherapy regimen, without alkylating agents, bleomycin, or etoposide, designed to retain normal fertility and organ function while reducing the risk of developing a second malignancy (DONALDSON 2004).

■ Commonly used chemotherapy regimens in pediatric HL include MOPP, ABVD, COPP, OEPA (boys), OPPA (girls), and VAMP:
 - MOPP   Nitrogen mustard, Oncovin (vincristine), procarbazine, prednisone
 - ABVD   Adriamycin (doxorubicin), bleomycin, vinblastine, dacarbazine
 - COPP   Cyclophosphamide, Oncovin, procarbazine, prednisone
 - OEPA (boys) Oncovin, etoposide, prednisone, adriamycin
 - OPPA (girls) Oncovin, procarbazine, prednisone, adriamycin
 - VAMP   Vinblastine, adriamycin, methotrexate, prednisone

■ Low-dose involved-field radiation therapy (IFRT) can be considered in the treatment of bulky disease.

39.2.2 Treatment of Early-Stage Favorable Classical Hodgkin's Lymphoma

■ Favorable early-stage patients include those with stage IA and IIA classical HL with less than four involved nodal regions, without bulky adenopathy, extranodal extension, or "B" symptoms.

■ Standard treatment for early-stage favorable classical HL include between two and four cycles of chemotherapy without alkylating agents followed by IFRT. A total dose of 15–21 Gy can be considered for patients who achieve complete response; 25.5–35 Gy can be considered for patients with partial response (Grade C). Alternatively, patients can be treated with between four and six cycles of chemotherapy alone without radiation therapy (Grade B).
 The POG 8625 study evaluated 159 pathologically staged IA, IIA, and IIIA patients who received

four cycles of alternating MOPP/ABVD. Patients who had complete response were randomized to two more cycles of alternating MOPP/ABVD or IFRT to a total of 25.5 Gy. Overall survival rates at 8 years were 96.8% with radiation as compared to 93.6% without radiation. The event-free survival (EFS) rates were 91.1% versus 82.6%, respectively, for those with or without radiation (POG 8625, Level II) (KUNG et al. 2006).

The GPOH-HD 95 study evaluated early stage I and IIA patients treated with two cycles of OPPA chemotherapy for girls and two cycles of OEPA chemotherapy for boys. Patients who achieved complete response did not receive adjuvant radiotherapy. Patients who achieved partial response of more than 75% of the tumor bulk received 20 Gy IFRT, and those less responsive to chemotherapy (i.e., partial response <75%) received 30 Gy of irradiation. A higher radiation dose (35 Gy) was delivered to residual masses of more than 50 ml. The results revealed that no difference could be observed in the 5-year disease-free survival rates in favorable early-stage patients treated with or without radiation (HR 0.97 vs 0.94) (CPOH-HD 95, Level III) (DÖRFFEL et al. 2003).

A prospective trial from CCG 5942 evaluated early-stage favorable patients with four cycles of COPP/ABV followed by IFRT (21 Gy) or no irradiation. Patients with early-stage unfavorable disease received six cycles of COPP/ABV followed by the IFRT (21 Gy) or no further irradiation. Stage IV patients received two courses of intensive chemotherapy followed by the same radiation arrangements. The 3-year event-free survival rates were statistically improved with the addition of IFRT in the as-treated analysis (93% vs. 85%). However, there was no difference in the 3-year overall survival rates (98 vs. 99%) (CCG 5942, Level II) (NACHMAN et al. 2002).

39.2.3 Treatment of Early-Stage Unfavorable Classical Hodgkin's Lymphoma

■ Unfavorable early-stage patients include patients with stage IB, IIB, and IIIA disease with bulky mediastinal disease, peripheral lymph nodes larger than 6 cm, or with three involved lymph node groups.

■ Standard treatment for this group of patients includes between four and six cycles of chemotherapy plus IFRT to a total of 15–25 Gy. Radiation doses up to 35 Gy may be considered for patients with residual disease (Grade C).

Alternatively, patients can be treated with between six and eight cycles of chemotherapy alone (Grade B).

■ Results from clinical trials have been mixed as to whether radiation therapy is required for complete responders. However, radiation should be considered in patients with partial response after chemotherapy: The GPOH-HD 95 detailed above evaluated intermediate staged patients given two cycles of OPEA (boys)/OPPA (girls) plus two cycles of COPP, followed by radiation therapy to a total dose of 20–35 Gy depending on extent of disease for partial responders, and no radiation for complete responders. Radiation therapy provided an improved 5-year disease-free survival (HR 0.92 vs. 0.78); however, no difference in overall survival was observed (Level III) (DÖRFFEL et al. 2003).

39.2.4 Treatment of Advanced-Stage Classical Hodgkin's Lymphoma

■ Advanced-stage patients include those with stage IIIB and IV disease. Some research groups include stage IIB in the advanced stage category when fever and weight loss are present.

■ Standard treatment for this group of patients includes between six and eight cycles of chemotherapy, with or without IFRT to a total dose of 15–25 Gy (Grade C). Radiation doses up to 35 Gy may be considered for patients with residual disease.

Alternatively, patients can be treated with eight cycles of chemotherapy alone (Grade B).

A trial reported by the Pediatric Oncology Group studied patients with clinical stage IIB, IIIA2, IIIB, and IV treated with eight cycles of MOPP/ABVD, followed by total nodal irradiation (TNI) or no further treatment. The results showed that the 5-year event free survival and overall survival rates have no differences between the two groups (Level II) (WEINER et al. 1997).

The above-mentioned GPOH-HD 95 treated advanced-stage HL patients with OEPA/OPPA × 2 + COPP × 4. Patients with partial response received adjuvant radiation to 20–35 Gy, and those who achieved complete response received no further irradiation. The 5-year disease-free survival was significantly improved in irradiated patients (HR 0.91 vs. 0.79); however, no difference in overall survival was observed (Level III) (DÖRFFEL et al. 2003).

39.2.5 Treatment of Nodular Lymphocyte Predominant Hodgkin's Lymphoma

■ Stage IA nodular lymphocyte predominant HL may be treated with complete nodal excision followed by observation. IFRT is recommended in a fully mature adolescent.

■ Chemotherapy alone is not recommended for NLPHL IA patients (Grade C). Results from a retrospective review revealed a 67% progression-free survival and a 100% overall survival at 3.5 years follow-up (Level IV) (MAUZ-KARHOLZ et al. 2007). However, a local relapse rate of more than 50% was reported with chemotherapy alone (Level IV) (VAN GROTEL 2006).

A COG trial is currently ongoing to assess the efficacy of chemotherapy alone in stage IA patients.

■ Treatment of stage II-IV NLPHL should follow the strategy used in classical HL management.

39.2.6 Treatment of Recurrent or Refractory Disease

■ Treatment of recurrent pediatric HL depends on prior treatment regimens. Chemotherapy or combined chemoradiotherapy can be considered in patients previously treated with radiation alone, and salvage rates between 50% and 80% can be expected.

■ If recurrence occurs after more than 1 year of disease-free interval, combined chemoradiation therapy or radiation therapy alone could result in a salvage rate of 40%–50% (Level III) (WIMMER et al. 2006; SCHELLONG et al. 2005).

■ Patients who relapsed less than 1 year after completion of treatment, or those who failed to respond to initial therapy, have a poor prognosis. High-dose chemotherapy followed by hematopoietic stem cell transplantation (HSCT) is the best option with salvage rates of approximately 50%

(Level III)–(Majhail et al. 2006; Baker et al. 1999).

■ IFRT before or after the HSCT may be helpful in reducing disease (Grade D).

39.2.7 Techniques of Radiation Therapy

■ Most patients who will receive radiation therapy should receive low-dose IFRT as part of a combined treatment regimen.

■ The field arrangement of radiation therapy is similar to that used in adult HL detailed in Chapter 28. When planning the radiation dose and field set-up, careful attention is needed to reduce the potential long-term complications in pediatric patients.

■ For unilateral cervical lesion(s), the medial border should be placed at the contralateral transverse process to cover the entire vertebral body to avoid asymmetric bone growth.

■ Mediastinal field width is determined by postchemotherapy residual disease while the craniocaudad height is determined by pre-chemotherapy extent of disease.

39.2.8 Treatment Complications

Radiation-Induced Side Effects and Complications

■ Most data from the literature regarding complications comes from the treatment technique with extended fields and higher radiation dose. With lower dose and smaller volume of radiation (e.g., in IFRT), the likelihood of the various organs being exposed to radiation and the risk of radiation-induced organ toxicity is significantly reduced.

■ *Musculoskeletal asymmetry.* With lower dose and smaller volume of radiation, the risk of skeletal abnormalities is minimized. Height reduction is most severe in prepubertal children treated with full-dose radiation. However, dose reduction to less than 33 Gy in a restricted volume showed no clinically significant height impairment (Willman 1994). Asymmetric mantle fields with doses as low as 15 Gy could impact the growth of the clavicle. In addition, the patient age and volume of clavicle irradiated increase the risk of clavicle asymmetry (Merchant et al. 2004).

■ *Pulmonary toxicity.* The incidence is lower with less RT dose, smaller RT volumes, and by omitting bleomycin in combined modality. The data from CCSG reported that 9% of children treated with ABVD followed by 21 Gy to mantle field developed clinically significant pulmonary damage.

■ *Infertility.* Oophoropexy in girls may allow preservation of ovarian function. Risk factors for premature menopause include exposure to increasing doses of ovarian radiation and increasing alkylating agent score (Sklar et al. 2006). In boys, fertility is affected by alkylators and the dose of radiation to the testicles. Reversible oligospermia (usually within 18–24 months) is common if testicular shield is applied.

■ *Cardiac toxicity.* The incidence and severity of cardiac toxicity is related to the radiation dose, irradiated volume, and the use of anthracyclines. With a modern treatment approach, cardiac sequelae, including pericarditis/effusion, valvular thickening, biventricular dysfunction, and coronary artery disease is expected to be reduced.

■ *Hypothyroidism.* Constine et al. (2004) reported elevation of TSH in 17% of those who received mantle radiation of ≤ 26 Gy , and in 78% of those who received greater than 26 Gy.

■ *Secondary malignancies.* The reported risk of secondary malignancy is based on older treatment studies and does not reflect contemporary therapy which has reduced the radiation dose and treatment volume. HL patients have an increased risk of second malignancies including solid tumors such as thyroid, breast, sarcomas, and lung cancers. A review of 930 children from 1960–1990 from five institutions with median follow up 16.7 years showed that 11% of patients developed a secondary malignancy with actuarial rate of 19% at 25 years. On multivariate analysis, female and mantle radiation dose were associated with increased risk of secondary malignancy. Increased radiation dose showed increased risk of secondary malignancy (Constine et al. 2004).

Chemotherapy-Induced Complications

■ Chemotherapy-induced long-term complications are drug specific: Procarbazine: Infertility in boys

■ Nitrogen mustard, six cycles: Irreversible azoospermia. Limiting to three or less cycles may maintain fertility.

- Nitrogen mustard: Increased risk of secondary acute myeloid leukemia and myelodysplastic syndrome.
- Adriamycin: Cardiac toxicity especially greater than cumulative 500 mg/m^2 (STEINHERZ et al. 1991).
- Bleomycin: Pulmonary fibrosis.

39.3 Follow-Up

39.3.1 Post-Treatment Follow-Ups

- Life-long follow-up after definitive treatment of HL in the pediatric population is recommended for detecting recurrence, secondary tumors, or other long-term complications of radiation therapy or chemotherapy.

Schedule

- Follow-ups should be scheduled according to the treatment protocol. Alternatively, follow-up could be scheduled every 3–4 months for 2 years, then every 6 months for 3 additional years, then annually thereafter (Grade D) (Table 39.3).

Work-Ups

- Each follow-up should include a complete history and physical examination.
- Laboratory tests and imaging studies at each follow-up should follow the requirement of treatment protocol.
- Alternatively, complete blood count, ESR, and alkaline phosphatase can be ordered every 3–4 months for 2 years, every 6 months for an addition 3 years, then annually thereafter (Grade D). Chest X-ray or CT of thorax every 3–6 months for first 2–3 years, then annually up to 5 years can be recommended (Grade D).

Table 39.3. Follow-up schedule after treatment for pediatric Hodgkin's lymphoma

Interval	Frequency
First 2 years	Every 3-4 months
Year 3-5	Every 6 months
Over 5 years	Annually

39.4 Diagnosis, Staging, and Prognoses in Pediatric Non-Hodkin's Lymphoma

39.4.1 Diagnosis

Initial Evaluation

- The diagnosis and evaluation of pediatric NHL start with a complete history and physical examination, with particular attention to all lymph node regions.
- History of inherited immunodeficiencies and acquired immunodeficiency disorders should be recorded, as they predispose patients to NHL.
- Compared to adults, children with NHL tend to have higher grade and more diffuse disease.
- Special characteristics at presentations of the different histological subtypes of NHL:
  - Endemic Burkitt's lymphoma: Child presents with rapidly growing abdominal mass, commonly in ileocecal region, which can lead to intussusception; can also present with cervical lymphadenopathy or enlarged tonsils.
  - Lymphoblastic: Adolescent male with rapidly growing large anterior mediastinal mass. The patient may present with shortness of breath or superior vena cava syndrome (SVC).
  - Anaplastic Large Cell Lymphoma (ALCL): ALCL commonly presents with extranodal disease in skin, lung, bone, and/or soft tissues.

Laboratory Tests

- Laboratory studies should include complete blood count, basic serum chemistry, calcium, lactate dehydrogenase (LDH), liver function tests, renal function tests, uric acid, bilirubin, and alkaline phosphatase.
- CSF analysis and bilateral bone marrow aspirate and biopsy can be performed for staging.
- Endemic Burkitt's, mostly in Africa, are mostly EBV-positive, while only 15% of sporadic cases in the US are positive.

Imaging Studies

- Imaging studies should include CT scan of the neck, thorax, abdomen, and pelvis. Chest X-ray (posteroanterior and lateral) should also be performed.

■ Gallium scan and FDG-PET scan can be used in pediatric patients to assess response to treatment, but their value is limited in lymphoblastic and Burkitt's lymphoma.

■ Bone scan is indicated for patients with elevated alkaline phosphatase or bone pain.

Pathology

■ Pathologic diagnosis of NHL is required prior to determining treatment recommendations. The treatment strategies of various types of NHL differ significantly from each other and from those used for HL.

■ Tissue obtained by core needle biopsy or open biopsy is recommended to evaluate histological, cytogenetic, and immunophenotyping features. Cytology of any fluid, i.e., pleural or ascites, should be obtained.

■ Most pediatric NHL fall into four categories, in decreasing order of frequency: small noncleaved cell (Burkitt's and Burkitt-like) lymphoma, lymphoblastic lymphoma, diffuse large B cell lymphoma, and anaplastic large lymphoma (Table 39.4).

■ Patients with a history of transplant are at risk for a post-transplant lymphoproliferative disease.

■ Immuno-phenotyping and cytogenetic analysis are routinely obtained for more precise subclassification of NHL and to better understand its prognostic implications.

39.4.2 Staging

■ Pediatric NHL is usually staged clinically using information from history and physical examination, laboratory tests (including bone marrow aspiration and biopsy), and imaging tests.

■ The most commonly used staging system for pediatric NHL is the St. Jude staging system (Table 39.5).

39.4.3 Prognostic Factors

■ Stage at diagnosis is of prognostic significance for pediatric NHL (MURPHY 1980) (Table 39.5).

■ C-myc is associated with favorable prognosis in Burkitt's lymphoma; ALK in anaplastic large-cell lymphoma is associated with favorable prognosis.

39.5   Treatment of Pediatric Non-Hodgkin's Lymphoma

39.5.1 General Principles

■ Patients with pediatric NHL should be treated on research protocol whenever possible.

Table 39.4. Major histology types and characteristics. [Modified from WEINSTEIN and TARBELL (2004) and HEEREMA et al. (2005) with permission]

Histology	Frequency	Location	Immunophenotype	Cytogenetics
Burkitt's and Burkitt-like lymphoma	45%	Waldeyer's ring, neck, abdomen, Ileocecal, ovary, kidney, CNS, bone, bone marrow	IgM, κ or λ light chains	cmyc t(8;14), t(8;22), t(2;8), t(14;18)
Lymphoblastic B cell	5%	Neck, skin, Waldeyer's ring	CD10, CD19	Hyperdiploid
Lymphoblastic T cell	25%	Mediastinum, bone, bone marrow, CNS, peripheral LN	CD 2, CD5, CD7	t(1;14), t(5;14), t(8;14), t(10;14), t(11;14), t(11;19)
Diffuse large B cell lymphoma	15%	Mediastinum, abdomen, bone, peripheral LN	CD 19, CD20, CD22, sIg+/–	cmyc t(8;14)
Anaplastic large cell lymphoma	10%	Mediastinum, abdomen, skin, soft tissues, lung, bone	CD30+	ALK t(2;5)

Table 39.5. St. Jude staging system for pediatric non-Hodgkin's lymphoma. [From Murphy (1980) with permission]

Stage I	Single tumor (extranodal) or single anatomic area (nodal) excluding the mediastinum or abdomen
Stage II	Single tumor (extranodal) with regional node involvement Two or more nodal areas on the same side of diaphragm Two tumors (extranodal) on the same side of diaphragm with or without regional nodal involvement Primary GI tumor with or without associated mesenteric LN, gross total resection
Stage III	Two single tumors extranodal on both sides of diaphragm Two or more nodal areas on both sides of diaphragm Primary intrathoracic tumors (mediastinal, pleural, thymic) Extensive intraabdominal disease, unresectable Primary paraspinal or epidural tumors
Stage IV	Any of the above with CNS or bone marrow involvement (<25% blasts)

- Chemotherapy plays a major role in the treatment of pediatric NHL.
- Radiation therapy is only indicated in patients with CNS involvement, airway compromise, or spinal cord compression for palliation (Grade B). In contrast to HL, IFRT has not shown any benefit in patients with lymphoblastic lymphomas or diffuse large cell-lymphomas.
- In patients with CNS involvement, craniospinal axis irradiation should be considered (Grade B). The dose to the whole brain is 18 Gy in ten fractions and the dose to spinal cord is 6–12 Gy in four to eight fractions.
- Low-dose radiation to alleviate the compression from tumor bulk can be considered in symptomatic cases when proper diagnosis cannot be urgently established (Grade D). Doses as low as 4–4.5 Gy in two to three fractions is usually adequate. Additional RT should be considered if there is no improvement. Chemotherapy should start promptly once the compression symptoms are relieved.
- CNS prophylaxis was often recommended in the past for patients with Burkitt's, non-Burkitt's, or lymphoblastic lymphoma. With the progress of chemotherapy in preventing CNS recurrence,

whole brain irradiation is no longer utilized, except in advanced lymphoblastic lymphoma.
- Bone marrow transplant may be considered for relapsed or refractory disease.

Treatment Complications

- Tumor lysis syndrome can occur within 48–72 h after initiation of treatment and is more likely in Burkitt's lymphoma. The syndrome consists of elevated uric acid, potassium, phosphate levels, and hypocalcemia. It is essential to monitor electrolytes, provide vigorous hydration, alkalinize the urine and administer allopurinol to prevent tumor lysis syndrome.

References

Baker KS, Gordon BG, Gross TG et al. (1999) Autologous hematopoietic stem-cell transplantation for relapsed or refractory Hodgkin's disease in children and adolescents. J Clin Oncol 17:825–831

Carbone PP, Kaplan HS, Musshoff K, Smithers DW, Tubiana M (1971) Report of the Committee on Hodgkin's Disease Staging Classification. Cancer Res 31:1860–1861

Cleary SF, Link MP, Donaldson SS (1994) Hodgkin's disease in the very young. Int J Radiat Oncol Biol Phys 28:77–83

Constine LS, Tarbell N, Hudson M et al. (2004) Second malignancies after pediatric Hodgkin lymphoma: Associations with radiation dose and volume. Proceedings of the American Society for Therapeutic Radiology and Oncology 46th annual meeting

Donaldson SS, Link MP, Weinstein HJ et al. (2007) Final results of a prospective clinical trial with VAMP and low-dose involved-field radiation for children with low-risk Hodgkin's disease. J Clin Oncol 25:332–337

Dörffel W, Lüders H, Rühl U et al. (2003) Preliminary results of the multicenter trial GPOH-HD 95 for the treatment of Hodgkin's disease in children and adolescents: analysis and outlook. Klin Padiatr 215:139–145

Haluska FG, Brufsky AM, Canellos GP (1994) The cellular biology of the Reed-Sternberg cell. Blood 84:1005–1019

Hanna SL, Fletcher BD, Boulden TF et al. (1993) MR imaging of infradiaphragmatic lymphadenopathy in children and adolescents with Hodgkin disease: comparison with lymphography and CT. J Magn Reson Imaging 3:461–470

Harris NL, Jaffe ES, Diebold J et al. (1999) The World Health Organization classification of neoplastic diseases of the hematopoietic and lymphoid tissues: report of the Clinical Advisory Committee meeting, Airlie House, Virginia, November. J Clin Oncol 17:3835–3849

Heerema NA, Bernheim A, Lim MS et al. (2005) State of the art and future needs in cytogenetic/molecular genetics/arrays in childhood lymphoma: summary report of workshop at the First International Symposium on childhood and adolescent non-Hodgkin lymphoma, April 9, 2003, New York City, NY. Pediatr Blood Cancer 45:616–622

Herbst H, Dallenbach F, Hummel M et al. (1991) Epstein-Barr virus latent membrane protein expression in Hodgkin and Reed-Sternberg cells. Proc Natl Acad Sci USA 88:4766–4770

Hueltenschmidt B, Sautter-Bihl ML, Lang O et al. (2001) Whole body positron emission tomography in the treatment of Hodgkin disease. Cancer 91:302–310

Kandil A, Bazarbashi S, Mourad WA et al. (2001) The correlation of Epstein-Barr virus expression and lymphocyte subsets with the clinical presentation of nodular sclerosing Hodgkin disease. Cancer 91:1957–1963

Kung FH, Schwartz CL, Ferree CR et al. (2006) POG 8625: a randomized trial comparing chemotherapy with chemoradiotherapy for children and adolescents with stages I, IIA, IIIA1 Hodgkin disease: a report from the Children's Oncology Group. J Pediatr Hematol Oncol 28:362–368

Majhail NS, Weisdorf DJ, Defor TE et al. (2006) Long-term results of autologous stem cell transplantation for primary refractory or relapsed Hodgkin's lymphoma. Biol Blood Marrow Transplant 12:1065–1072

Mauz-Körholz C, Gorde-Grosjean S, Hasenclever D et al. (2007) Resection alone in 58 children with limited stage, lymphocyte-predominant Hodgkin lymphoma – experience from the European network group on pediatric Hodgkin lymphoma. Cancer 110:179–185

Merchant TE, Nguyen I, Nguyen D et al. (2004) Differential attenuation of clavicle growth after asymmetric mantle radiotherapy. Int J Radiat Oncol Biol Phys 59:556–561

Murphy SB (1980) Classification, staging and end results of treatment of childhood non-Hodgkin's lymphomas: dissimilarities from lymphomas in adults. Semin Oncol 7:332–339

Nachman JB, Sposto R, Herzog P et al. (2002) Randomized comparison of low-dose involved-field radiotherapy and no radiotherapy for children with Hodgkin's disease who achieve a complete response to chemotherapy. J Clin Oncol 20:3765–3771

Rhodes MM, Delbeke D, Whitlock JA et al. (2006) Utility of FDG-PET/CT in follow-up of children treated for Hodgkin and non-Hodgkin lymphoma. J Pediatr Hematol Oncol 28:300–306

Schellong G, Dörffel W, Claviez A et al. (2005) Salvage therapy of progressive and recurrent Hodgkin's disease: results from a multicenter study of the pediatric DAL/GPOH-HD study group. J Clin Oncol 23:6181–6189

Sklar CA, Mertens AC, Mitby P et al. (2006) Premature menopause in survivors of childhood cancer: a report from the childhood cancer survivor study. J Natl Cancer Inst 98:890–896

Smith RS, Chen Q, Hudson MM et al. (2003) Prognostic factors for children with Hodgkin's disease treated with combined-modality therapy. J Clin Oncol 21:2026–2033

Steinherz LJ, Steinherz PG, Tan CT et al. (1991) Cardiac toxicity 4 to 20 years after completing anthracycline therapy. JAMA 266:1672–1677

van Grotel M, Lam KH, de Man R et al. (2006) High relapse rate in children with non-advanced nodular lymphocyte predominant Hodgkin's lymphoma (NLPHL or nodular paragranuloma) treated with chemotherapy only. Leuk Lymphoma 47:1504–1510

Weiner MA, Leventhal B, Brecher ML et al. (1997) Randomized study of intensive MOPP-ABVD with or without low-dose total-nodal radiation therapy in the treatment of stages IIB, IIIA2, IIIB, and IV Hodgkin's disease in pediatric patients: a Pediatric Oncology Group study. J Clin Oncol 15:2769–2779

Weinstein HJ, Tarbell NJ (2004) Leukemias and lymphomas of childhood. In: Devita VT, Hellman S, Rosenberg SA (eds) Cancer: principles and practice of ncology (1939–1957). Lippincott Williams & Wilkins, Philadelphia

William KY, Cox RS, Donaldson SS (1994) Radiation induced height impairment in pediatric Hodgkin's disease. Int J Radiat Oncol Biol Phys 28:85–92

Wimmer RS, Chauvenet AR, London WB et al. (2006) APE chemotherapy for children with relapsed Hodgkin disease: a Pediatric Oncology Group trial. Pediatr Blood Cancer 46:320–324

Retinoblastoma

40

Beatriz E. Amendola

B. E. AMENDOLA, MD FACR
Innovative Cancer Institute, 6141 Sunset Drive, Miami, FL
33143, USA

Introduction and Objectives

The estimated number of new cases of retinoblastoma occurring each year in USA is about 250 (ABRAMSON et al. 2003). Retinoblastoma is usually confined to the eye, as a result, more than 90% of children with intraocular retinoblastoma will be cured. The present challenge for those who are specialized in retinoblastoma treatment is to prevent loss of an eye, blindness, and other serious effects of treatment that reduce life span or quality of life.

This capter examines:

● Recommendations for diagnosis and staging procedures

● Staging systems and prognostic factors

● Treatment recommendations for both

● Techniques of radiation

● Follow-up care and surveillance of survivors

40.1 Diagnosis, Staging, and Prognosis

40.1.1 Diagnosis

Initial Evaluation

■ Diagnosis and evaluation of retinoblastoma starts with a complete patient history and physical examination. Attention should be paid to history, signs, and symptoms specific to the ocular tumor.

■ Retinoblastoma commonly presents with a white papillary light reflex (namely, leukocoria). Parents may notice this abnormal appearance in flash photography (Fig. 40.1).

■ Leukocoria can also be seen with a handheld ophthalmoscope during a routine examination by a pediatrician with a positive family history or during the course of a follow-up examination.

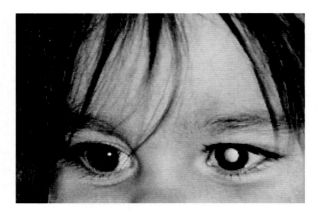

Fig. 40.1. Child with white pupillary reflex (Leukocoria). Courtesy of Paul T. Finger MD, http://eyecancer.com

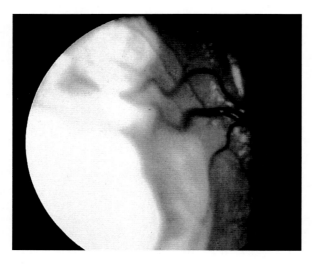

Fig. 40.2. Opthalmoscopic evaluation demonstrating a raised white mass consistent with retinoblastoma

- On ophthalmoscopic examination one notes a raised white, white-yellow, or white-pink mass (Fig. 40.2). Tortuous vessels may be seen feeding the tumor. Cells may break off from the main tumor mass and grow as small vitreous seeds (Fig. 40.3). Retinoblastoma may be multifocal, it is necessary to examine the entire retinal surface, generally with the patient under anesthesia.

Differential Diagnosis

- When retinoblastoma presents as a mass, the differential diagnosis includes astrocytic hamartoma, *Toxocara canis* granuloma, the infected emboli of subacute bacterial endocarditis or toxoplasmosis, and other severe uveitis. When retinoblastoma causes retinal detachment, the differential diagnosis includes Coat's disease, retrolental fibroplasias, and persistent hyperplastic vitreous (Abramson and Ellsworth 1980).
- Retinal drawings and photographs, along with a written description, are used to record whether single or multifocal tumors are present. Ultrasound is also useful for documenting tumor location and size (Fig. 40.4) The distance from the cornea to the back of the lens can also be measured with ultrasound to aid in lateral field radiotherapy planning.

Laboratory Tests

- Among the tests used to detect metastatic disease are a lumbar puncture with cerebrospinal fluid

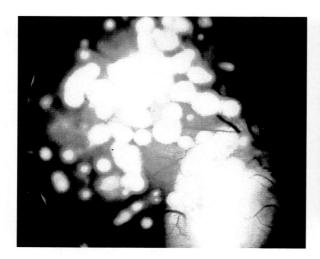

Fig. 40.3. Vitreus Seeding (Snow storm effect)

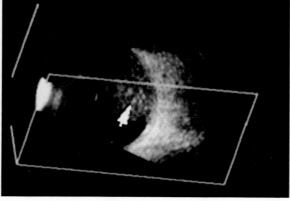

Fig. 40.4. A 3D ultrasound image of a large retinoblastoma with spots of calcification within the tumor. Courtesy of Paul T. Finger MD, http://eyecancer.com

(CSF) cytology and a bone marrow biopsy, when extensive disease is suspected.

Lumbar puncture with cerebrospinal fluid (CSF) cytology and bone marrow biopsy aspirate is needed for patients with symptoms suggestive of metastasis (Grade B). The results of a retrospective series of 23 patients showed that useful tests for determining the extent of disease were bone marrow aspiration, lumbar puncture, skull films, EEG, and brain scan (Level IV) (MACKAY et al. 1984).

In modern practice, routine lumbar puncture and bone marrow aspiration are not justified for retinoblastoma confined to the retina without optic nerve involvement or other suggestion of extraocular extension.

Imaging Studies

■ MRI of the orbits and brain is the imaging study of choice (Grade A). Computed tomography (CT) scan is effective in demonstrating tumor calcification (Fig. 40.5). DE GRAAF et al. (2005) evaluated the value of MRI in the evaluation of disease extent in 58 cases of retinoblastoma, and found that the sensitivity and specificity of choroidal invasion were 73% and 72%, respectively. Those for postlaminar optic nerve invasion were 50% for sensitivity, and 100% for specificity. Scleral and extrascleral tumor invasion were correctly excluded in all eyes using MRI (Level IV). In a more recently published retrospective series of 150 patients, the sensitivity and specificity of detecting of postlaminar invasion were 60% and 95% for MRI, as compared to 0% and 100% for CT scan, respectively (Level IV).

■ In the presence of symptoms suggestive of metastatic disease, a bone scan is indicated.

Pathology

■ Retinoblastoma is a poorly differentiated malignant neuroectodermal tumor. The tumor is composed mainly of undifferentiated anaplastic cells that arise from the nuclear layers of the retina. Histology shows similarity to neuroblastoma and medulloblastoma, including aggregation around blood vessels, necrosis, calcification, and Flexner-Wintersteiner rosettes. Retinoblastomas are characterized by marked cell proliferation as

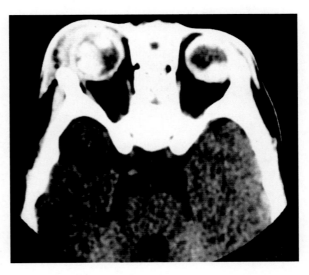

Fig. 40.5. CT images of a child with bilateral Retinoblastoma. Calcifications are easily seen

evidenced by high mitosis counts and extremely high MIB-1 labeling indices (SCHWIMER and PRAYSON 2001).

■ Classically, four growth patterns are recognized in retinoblastoma:

■ Endophytic RB, which grows from the retina toward the vitreous, appears to be a mass protruding into the vitreous chamber. These often friable and necrotic tumors may produce small clusters of tumor cells that are detached from the main mass and form satellite tumor nodules. These can range from localized tumor nodules within the vitreous, known as vitreous seeding, up to diffuse involvement, which some call the *snowstorm effect*.

■ Exophytic retinoblastoma typically grows from the outer retinal layers and extends beneath the detached retina toward the choroid. Dislodged masses may implant on the retinal pigment epithelium and erode through Bruch's membrane into the choroid.

■ Diffuse plaque-like retinoblastoma defies common morphologic patterns. It grows diffusely without forming a detectable mass. Such a growth pattern can present a confusing clinical picture.

■ Biopsy of a suspected retinoblastoma or vitreous aspiration for enzyme studies is generally felt to be contraindicated because of the risk of choroidal seeding (Grade B) (REESE 1976).

40.1.2 Staging and Prognosis

■ Prognostic factors depend on the ocular status. The staging system for retinoblastoma must fulfill at least two requirements. First, it must predict likelihood of cure, a requirement of all malignancy staging systems. However, an important goal of retinoblastoma treatment is preservation of sight in the affected eye (i.e., ocular survival).

■ The most widely used grouping system for retinoblastoma was proposed by REESE (1976) and ELLSWORTH (1969) (Table 40.1). This system does not predict survival probability. However, it predicts the chance of visual preservation with conservative therapy.

■ At least two staging systems have attempted to predict prognosis for survival and include information on disease extension beyond the globe (SCHVARTZMAN et al. 1996). One of these systems, the St. Jude Children's Research Hospital (SJCRH) system has been used more frequently. The most recent clinical protocols for combined-modality retinoblastoma therapy use a new system based on the work of the Children's Oncology Group and MURPHEE et al. (2007) of the Children's Hospital of Los Angeles. This staging system is gaining increasing popularity.

■ The Reese-Ellsworth system for intraocular retinoblastoma has been shown to have prognostic significance for maintenance of sight and control of local disease at a time when surgery and external-beam radiation therapy were the only treatment options. The Reese-Ellsworth system is relevant to decisions regarding the use of local treatment modalities and chemoreduction (Table 40.1).

■ The other classification systems for retinoblastoma include the SJCRH. This classification assists in predicting those who are likely to be cured without the need for enucleation or external-beam radiotherapy (SCHVARTZMAN et al. 1996) (Table 40.2.).

■ The International Classification for Intraocular Retinoblastoma currently used is another staging system that offers greater precision to predict prognosis for survival and include information on disease extension beyond the globe, as well as stratifying risk for newer therapies (SHIELDS et al. 2006) (Table 40.3).

Table 40.1. Reese-Ellsworth classification for intraocular tumors

Group I: Very favorable for maintenance of sight	
1	Solitary tumor, smaller than 4 DD, at or behind the equator
2	Multiple tumors, none larger than 4 DD, all at or behind the equator
Group II: Favorable for maintenance of sight	
1	Solitary tumor, 4–10 DD at or behind the equator
2	Multiple tumors, 4–10 DD behind the equator
Group III: Possible for maintenance of sight	
1	Any lesion anterior to the equator
2	Solitary tumor, larger than 10 DD behind the equator
Group IV: Unfavorable for maintenance of sight	
1	Multiple tumors, some larger than 10 DD
2	Any lesion extending anteriorly to the ora serrata
Group V: Very unfavorable for maintenance of sight	
1	Massive tumors involving more than one half of the retina
2	Vitreous seeding. DD, disc diameter.

Table 40.2. The St. Jude Children's Research Hospital staging system of retinoblastoma

Intraocular disease
● Retinal tumor, single or multiple
● Extension to lamina cribrosa
● Uveal extension
Orbital disease
● Orbital tumor
Scattered episcleral cells
Orbital invasion
● Optic nerve
Invasion of optic nerve to cut end
Invasion of optic nerve beyond cut nerve
Intracranial metastases
● Positive cerebrospinal fluid
● Mass lesion in the central nervous system
Hematogenous metastasis
● Positive bone marrow
● Facial bone lesions with or without positive marrow
● Other organ involvement

Table 40.3. International classification system for intraocular retinoblastoma

Group A: Small intraretinal tumors away from foveola and disc
All tumors are 3 mm or smaller in greatest dimension, confined to the retina and
All tumors are located further than 3 mm from the foveola and 1.5 mm from the optic disc
Group B: All remaining discrete tumors confined to the retina
All other tumors confined to the retina not in Group A
Tumor-associated subretinal fluid less than 3 mm from the tumor with no subretinal seeding
Group C: Discrete local disease with minimal subretinal or vitreous seeding
Tumor(s) are discrete
Subretinal fluid, present or past, without seeding involving up to ¼ retina
Local fine vitreous seeding may be present close to discrete tumor
Local subretinal seeding less than 3 mm (2 DD) from the tumor
Group D: Diffuse disease with significant vitreous or subretinal seeding
Tumor(s) may be massive or diffuse
Subretinal fluid present or past without seeding, involving up to total retinal detachment
Diffuse or massive vitreous disease may include "greasy" seeds or avascular tumor masses
Diffuse subretinal seeding may include subretinal plaques or tumor nodules
Group E: Presence of any one or more of these poor prognostic features
Tumor touching the lens
Tumor anterior to anterior vitreous face involving ciliary body or anterior segment
Diffuse infiltrating retinoblastoma
Neovascular glaucoma
Opaque media from hemorrhage
Tumor necrosis with aseptic orbital cellulites
Phthisis bulbi

40.1.3 Prognostic Factors

- Staging classifications detailed above are of prognostic significance.
- Other reported poor prognostic factors include: optic nerve invasion, uveal invasion, orbital invasion, and choroidal involvement.

40.2 Treatment of Retinoblastoma

40.2.1 General Principles on Selection of Therapy

- The primary goal of retinoblastoma therapy is cure (Grade A). Retinoblastoma rarely metastasizes, and the chance of cure remains excellent. The actuarial overall 5-year survival rate for 731 children with retinoblastoma seen at St. Bartholomew's Hospital and Moorfield's Eye Hospital from 1960 to 1988 was 87% (Level IV) (KINGSTON and HUNGERFORD 1992). The 50-month actuarial overall survival of 52 SJCRH patients with initial intraocular disease was 97% (Level IV) (PRADHAN et al. 1997).

40.2.2 Surgery

Enucleation

- The majority of the children present with a large tumor in one eye that requires an aggressive approach. In 25%–40% of cases both eyes are affected.
- Enucleation is indicated in unilateral retinoblastoma, where the eye is blind. In bilateral retinoblastoma when both eyes are blind, a bilateral enucleation is done.
- In an enucleation for retinoblastoma, the rectus muscles are severed. The optic nerve is then cut near its exit from the socket. Obtaining a long segment of nerve is important if the tumor is within the nerve. In young children, orbital growth slows after enucleation. As the child grows, the orbit appears small. This is overcome by using properly fitting orbital prosthesis.

Exenteration

- An exenteration is the removal of the globe, extraocular muscles, lids, nerves, and orbital fat. Blood loss may be significant. In the opinion of some ophthalmologists, the indications for exenteration in retinoblastoma include extensive local tumor breaching the globe (orbital exenteration generally is followed by postoperative irradiation and chemotherapy). Prognosis is poor.

40.2.3 Other Local Therapies

Cryotherapy

- Cryotherapy is based on the same principles as photocoagulation. The tumor is localized, transsclerally, with a nitrous oxide cryoprobe. The freeze (–80°C) is then applied until the tumor is completely covered with a frozen vitreous. The freeze-thaw cycle is repeated at least three times. Cryotherapy is indicated for the primary treatment of retinoblastoma in small tumors anterior to the equator, without vitreous seeding, which can be reached with the cryoprobe (posterior tumors are difficult to reach and the risks of freezing the macula or nerve are high). Cryotherapy can be used for treatment of local recurrence and/or tumor persistence after irradiation, and in conjunction with chemotherapy (ABRAMSON et al. 1994a).
- Cryotherapy can induce acute retinal edema and accumulation of subretinal fluid. To avoid retinal detachment, some ophthalmologists use the laser to create a retinal barrier to fluid leakage. Disruption of the retina by cryotherapy may increase intravitreal penetration of systemic Carboplatin (WILSON et al. 1994).

Photocoagulation

- The technique of photocoagulation is based on obliteration of the retinal vessels. The procedure produces a white retinal burn surrounding the tumor. Approximately 1 mm area is painted with the laser beam. Special attention is directed to closing feeding vessels. The tumor is encircled by the burn, and regression depends on interruption of blood supply (SHIELDS et al. 1995). Direct photocoagulation of retinoblastoma should be avoided because small explosions can release viable tumor cells into the vitreous and lead to tumor recurrence (KINGSTON and HUNGERFORD 1992). Vitreous seeding is a contraindication for the procedure (CASSADY et al. 1969; ABRAMSON and ELLSWORTH 1980). With proper case selection, photocoagulation has a local tumor control probability of about 70% (SHIELDS et al. 1995).

40.2.4 Radioactive Plaque Application

- Radioactive plaques are used for solitary 2- to 16-mm basal diameter unilateral lesions located more then 3 mm from the optic disk or fovea, generally less then 10 mm thick, for two lesions that are small enough or close enough to be covered by one plaque, and for local failure after other therapy (Grade B). Plaques can be used if there is a small amount of vitreous seeding over the tumor apex (Level IV) (AMENDOLA et al. 1989, 1990; SHIELDS et al. 1993, 2001).

Techniques

- Before the operative procedure, the tumor's maximum base diameter and maximum height are ascertained by physical examination and ultrasonography. In treatment planning, it is customary to allow 1 mm for sclera thickness, although there is some normal variation in this measurement. The operative procedure begins with a careful eye examination using magnifying lenses. After confirming the tumor anatomy, the surgeon opens the conjunctiva around the periphery of the limbus (a peritomy). Muscle hooks are used to snare rectus muscles and rotate the eye. Traction sutures are sometimes used. It may be necessary to disinsert a muscle in order to visualize the tumor. With the room darkened, a transilluminator is placed over the pupil. The shadow cast by the tumor is marked on the sclera with a marking pen or with electrocautery. Tumors that cannot be transilluminated are located by ultrasound. A clear dummy plaque is then brought into the operative field. Allow 2 mm of margin on either side of the basal diameter; that is, an 8-mm tumor is plaqued with a 12-mm device. The dummy is used to place the two sutures through the lug holes and into the sclera. The dummy is then replaced with the radioactive plaque. The retention sutures are tied and the eye is rotated back into place. The conjunctiva is then closed. The patient generally remains hospitalized for the duration of the application. The plaque is then removed (FREIRE et al. 1997).

■ Several plaque types are available. The ^{60}Co plaque (1.17 and 1.33 MeV, half-life of 5.2 years) may be purchased in a circular or crescentic configuration to fit around the optic nerve. The ^{60}Co ball applicator is a platinum-coated 6-mm sphere attached to a ring. The ^{125}I plaque (27–35 keV, half-life of 60 days) with lip consists of ^{125}I seeds glued in a carrier within a gold shield. These plaques can be custom made in a circular or notched configuration (Fig. 40.6). ^{192}Ir (295–612 keV, half-life of 74.5 days) and ^{109}Ru (beta emitter) plaques are also available. Each of the four available plaques (^{60}Co, ^{125}I, ^{192}Ir, and ^{109}Ru) has advantages and disadvantages (Fig. 40.7)

■ Using ^{60}Co plaques, STALLARD (1966) (Fig. 40.8) administered 35 Gy to the tumor apex in 7 days. Of 69 children with tumor involving one-fourth of the retinal area or less, 63 were successfully treated with a plaque. When the tumor involved one-fourth to one-half of the retinal area, success was achieved in eight of ten instances (Level IV).

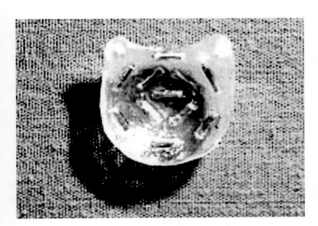

Fig. 40.6. Custom made Iodine 125 Episcleral plaque

40.2.5 External-Beam Radiotherapy

■ If retinoblastoma is multifocal, close to the macula or optic nerve, and vision is well preserved, cryotherapy, photocoagulation, or plaque therapy as a monotherapy is inadequate, while enucleation is too aggressive. In these circumstances,

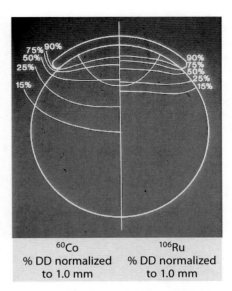

^{60}Co	^{106}Ru
% DD normalized to 1.0 mm	% DD normalized to 1.0 mm

Fig. 40.7. Comparison of dose distribution from a ^{60}Co versus ^{106}Ru plaques

external-beam irradiation or chemotherapy with focal therapy is recommended (Grade A). External-beam radiation therapy and chemotherapy are also indicated for large tumors and vitreous seeding. HILGARTNER (1910) reported treatment of a case of bilateral retinoblastoma with X-rays in 1910. Verhoeff cured a case of retinoblastoma with X-ray treatment in 1918. The patient died in 1972 with tumor controlled (Level V) (MARCUS et al. 1990). The efficacy of external-beam radiation therapy has been confirmed in a number of retrospective studies as detailed below. Historically, the Reese-Ellsworth grouping system has been used to predict the probability of success for external-beam irradiation.

Technique of External-Beam Radiotherapy

■ The goals of conventional external-beam radiotherapy are to provide a homogenous and tumoricidal dose to the entire retina and vitreous while maintaining tolerance of normal tissue structures. The rational to cover the entire volume is based on the following facts:
– In many cases retinoblastoma represents a field change in which all retinal cells have a genetic neoplastic potential; therefore, the entire retina must be treated.
– Presence of vitreous seeding.
– Multiple tumors may arise from a primary retinoblastoma.

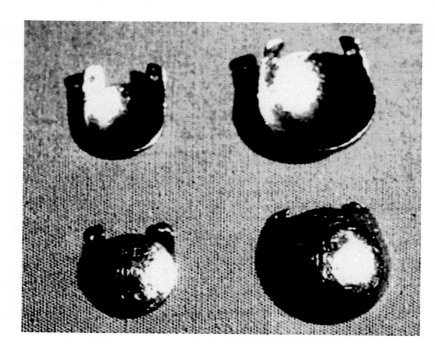

Fig. 40.8. Examples of ^{60}Co plaques

- The tumor could spread via the subretinal space.
- Retinal differentiation progress from posterior to anterior and from superior to inferior. Subclinical disease may exist in the immature retina and must be included in the treatment (Level IV) (FOOTE et al. 1989).
■ One of the earliest techniques for the external-beam irradiation of retinoblastoma was developed by Algernon Reese in the 1930s. Using an orthovoltage unit, treatment was delivered through temporal and nasal portals. The technique attempted to avoid the lens (ABRAMSON 1982).

Immobilization

■ Patient immobilization is crucial to delivering the designated treatment volume precisely while minimizing radiation to normal tissue. Sedation is usually necessary.
■ Either a whole body device or a thermoplastic head holder can be used for treatment.

Beam Arrangement

■ Any external-beam irradiation technique for retinoblastoma treatment should encompass the entire retina, avoiding the contralateral eye, and limit the dosage to normal tissue.
■ The most commonly used techniques are lateral-beam megavoltage technique with the anterior field border set at the lateral bony orbit, and a direct lateral field is utilized. A half-beam blocked lateral field has been used to sharpen the beam edge. Field sizes ranging from 3×6 cm to 5×10 cm are typically used for a 3×3-cm to 5×5-cm treatment area.
■ Lateral-beam technique with the beam edge set 2–3 mm behind the limbus is preferred to a technique using a more posteriorly set lateral beam and an anterior electron field with lens-sparing block (Grade B).
BLACH et al. (1996) updated a retrospective series previously reported by MCCORMICK et al. (1988, 1989) (Level IV). The more posterior field arrangement was associated with anterior failures. Many other series confirm anterior failures with anterior segment-sparing techniques are used (MCCORMICK et al. 1988). In all, 20 patients with large macular retinoblastoma were treated at Duke with a lateral 4-MV photon half-blocked beam set halfway between the limbus and bony orbit and an anterior field.
■ A two-field technique using a lateral field and an anterior field with a hanging lens block can also be used in an attempt to achieve a homogeneous retinal dosage.

Dosage of Radiation Therapy

■ Total dose of 36–46 Gy delivered in conventional fractionation can be prescribed for external-bean radiotherapy for retinoblastoma, depending on the extent of the disease (Grade B). Results from retrospective studies showed that 32–35 Gy was no less effective then 40–45 Gy and the observation that late ill effects of irradiation on the retina (i.e., chorioretinitis) are uncommon at dosages of <50 Gy or less (CASSADY et al. 1969; McCORMICK et al. 1988, 1989). The dose response analysis reported by FOOTE et al. (1989) revealed that a dose of 45 Gy in 1.8-Gy fractions was adequate for local control of tumors smaller than 10 disc diameters, and no differences could be observed for doses higher than 45 Gy at 1.8 Gy per fraction (Level IV).

■ MERCHANT et al. (2004) demonstrated a difference in the ocular preservation rates for patients with advanced disease (Reese-Ellsworth group III–V) compared with early disease when treated with lower doses of radiation. Patients treated with en face electrons experienced a lower 5-year estimate of ocular preservation than those treated with photons. In his experience the use of low-dose external-beam radiation therapy (36 Gy) results in ocular preservation rates that are comparable to those of high-dose external-beam radiation therapy. The use of electrons requires careful treatment planning and computerized dosimetry. The author suggested 36 Gy for newly diagnosed patients with Reese-Ellsworth group I and II, and 44–46 Gy for Reese-Ellsworth group III–V.

■ Two recent studies have evaluated the radiosensitivity for retinoblastoma grown in culture, and 35 Gy was the appropriate dosage delivered in 7 days. A large number of dosage and fraction schemes have been proposed for external-beam treatment, ranging from 2 to 3.8 Gy per fraction.

■ The risk of side-effects and late complications is higher if hypofractionation or doses higher than 50 Gy is used (Grade B). Data from Lausanne, Switzerland, demonstrated an increase in retinopathy at 2.5 Gy or more per fraction (PRADHAN et al. 1997). Patients with retinoblastoma should be treated 5 days per week at 2 Gy or less per fraction. Daily dosages of 1.8–2.0 Gy, 5 days per week, are used.

After reviewing 44 eyes in 38 children with retinoblastoma treated with external-beam radiotherapy, COUCKE et al. (1993) found that the only significant factor associated with retinopathy were total dose multiplied by dose per fraction, or total dose normalized to the equivalent total dose in 2-Gy fractions as estimated from the LQ model (Level IV).

■ Although hypofractionation seemed to be associated with high complications radiation to a total of 35–36 Gy in 9–12 fractions has been used to avoid sedation.

40.2.6 Chemotherapy for Intraocular Disease

■ Cooperative group trials are in preparation to optimize chemotherapy regimens. Several protocols have been drafted to test the benefits of carboplatin, etoposide, and vincristine regimens. These protocols generally address and combine more advanced cases of disease (CHAN et al. 2005; KIM et al. 2007).

■ Given the absence of mature trials, it will be critical to monitor the long-term side effects of multiagent chemotherapy, especially as regards the development of secondary malignancies (HALPERIN et al. 2005).

40.3 Special Situations

Trilateral Disease

■ Trilateral retinoblastoma is a rare but well-recognized entity consisting of bilateral retinoblastoma associated with ectopic retinoblastoma of the pineal or suprasellar region. The intracranial lesion can cause signs of raised intracranial pressure: anorexia, ataxia, lethargy, and vomiting (Level V) (AMOAKU et al. 1996).

Retreatment

■ Among the most difficult problems confronting the pediatric radiation oncologist is therapy selection in a child who has suffered recurrent retinoblastoma in an eye previously treated with external-beam radiation to full dosage. If the recurrent lesion is small and favorably located, it may be treated with photocoagulation, cryotherapy, or a radioactive plaque, often with success.

■ In a series reported by AMENDOLA et al. (1989, 1990), 29 eyes (in which 28 had group V diseases) were treated with plaque for recurrent tumor.

Tumor progression in 14 eyes was observed which ultimately necessitated enucleation. The remaining 15 eyes (52%) had preservation of vision (Level IV).

■ There appears to be no increase in secondary nonocular tumors in children receiving two courses of radiotherapy (Level IV) (ABRAMSON et al. 1982).

Palliation of Metastases

■ For bony metastases causing pain, palliative radiotherapy is appropriate. A dosage of 25–30 Gy is usually given.

40.4 Treatment-Induced Complications

Secondary Nonocular Tumors

■ The evidence is persuasive that the 13q–14q deletion of heritable retinoblastoma produces a malignant diathesis. The relative risk (RR) for death from a second tumor is much higher among patients with bilateral retinoblastoma (RR=60) than among those with unilateral disease (R=60 vs. 3.8). This first manifests itself in the development of the index case of retinoblastoma. In long-term survivors of heritable retinoblastoma, there is an extremely high incidence of secondary nonocular tumors.
The most common secondary malignant neoplasms (SMNs) occurring in the radiation field in survivors of heritable retinoblastoma are osteosarcoma, fibrosarcoma, and other spindle cell sarcomas.

Cataracts

■ Radiation-induced cataracts are common after external-beam radiotherapy. Clinically significant posterior pole cataracts developed in 23 of 27 cases (85%), according to a retrospective series (Level IV) (FONTANESI et al. 1996). A series from the Mayo Clinic reported four of 14 (28%) posterior cataracts using a lens-sparing technique (Level IV) (FOOTE et al. 1989). In seven eyes treated with lateral and anterior fields and followed-up for more then 36 months, HERNANDEZ et al.

(1996) observed lens changes in all cases, with three necessitating lens extraction (Level IV). Radiation-induced cataracts after radiotherapy of retinoblastoma can be removed successfully (Level IV) (BROOKS et al. 1990).

Orbital Development

■ Children treated with radiotherapy or enucleations for retinoblastoma are at significant risk for orbital and facial growth retardation.

Lacrimal Gland

■ Irradiated eyes had significantly less tear production and significantly less tear protein production than a control group.

40.5 Follow-Up

■ The familial form of retinoblastoma may manifest as unilateral or bilateral disease. In familial retinoblastoma, tumors tend to occur at a younger age. Children with the familial form who have a normal examination in at least one eye on initial presentation need to be examined frequently for the development of new retinoblastoma tumors.

■ It is recommended that they be examined every 2–4 months for at least 28 months. Following treatment, patients require careful surveillance until age 5 years (ABRAMSON and FRANK 1998).

■ Patients with the familial type of retinoblastoma have an increased frequency of SMN. The cumulative incidence is about 26% (± 10%) in nonirradiated patients and 58% (± 10%) in irradiated patients by 50 years after diagnosis of retinoblastoma – a rate of about 1% per year (Level IV) (WONG et al. 1997). Most SMNs are osteosarcomas, soft tissue sarcomas, or melanomas.

Future Directions

■ Studies are planned for a variety of patient groups. The International Classification system is being utilized for these trials. This classification schema is based on the extent and location of intraocular retinoblastoma and is being used in the upcoming series of protocols from the COG. The preliminary version of this system was verified to be reproducible with preliminary data from five centers that staged their patients on an Internet site in August 2000 (SHIELDS et al. 2004). Experience with a closely related grouping system has been published. Data have been published using this system in a study of chemotherapy for intraocular retinoblastoma, where stage appeared to assist in prognosis for successful treatment without enucleation or external-beam radiotherapy (SHIELDS et al. 2001).

■ For patients with Group B disease, the COG is investigating the use of vincristine and carboplatin chemoreduction combined with local ophthalmic therapies, without the use of etoposide. For patients with Group C or D disease, the COG is investigating use of higher doses of systemic carboplatin, combined with subconjunctival carboplatin and lower doses of external-beam radiation therapy, using intensity-modulated approaches. Also under investigation is the use of adenovirus-mediated gene therapy for treatment of vitreous tumor seeding (CHÉVEZ-BARRIOS et al. 2005; KIM et al. 2007).

References

Abramson DH (1982) Retinoblastoma: diagnosis and management. CA Cancer J Clin 32:130–140

Abramson DH, Ellsworth RM (1980) The surgical management of retinoblastoma. Ophthalmic Surg Lasers 11:596–598

Abramson DH, Frank CM (1998) Second nonocular tumors in survivors of bilateral retinoblastoma: a possible age effect on radiation-related risk. Ophthalmology 105:573–579; discussion 579–580

Abramson DH, Ellsworth RM, Rosenblatt M et al. (1982) Retreatment of retinoblastoma with external beam irradiation. Arch Opthalmol 100:1257–1260

Abramson DH, Niksarli K, Ellsworth RM et al. (1994a) Changing trends in the management of retinoblastoma: 1951–1965 vs. 1966–1980. J Pediatr Ophthalmol Strabismus 31:32–37

Abramson DH, Beaverson K, Sangani P et al. (2003) Screening for retinoblastoma: presenting signs as prognosticators of patient and ocular survival. Pediatrics 112(6 Pt 1):1248–1255

Amendola BE, Markoe AM, Augsburger JJ et al. (1989) Analysis of treatment results in 36 children with retinoblastoma treated by sclera plaque irradiation. Int J Radiat Oncol Biol Phys 17:63–70

Amendola BE, Lamm FR, Markae AM et al. (1990) Radiotherapy of retinoblastoma: a review of 63 children treated with different irradiation techniques. Cancer 66:21–26

Amoako WMK, Willshaw HE, Parkes SE et al. (1996) Trilateral retinoblastoma: a report of five patients. Cancer 78:858–863

Blach LE, McCormic B, Abramson DH (1996) External beam radiation therapy and retinoblastoma: long-term results in the comparison of two techniques. Int J Radiat Oncol Biol Phys 35:45–51

Brooks HL Jr, Meyer D, Shields JA et al. (1990) Removal of radiation-induced cataracts in patients treated for retinoblastoma. Arch Ophthalmol 108:1701–1708

Cassady JR, Sagerman RH, Tretter P et al. (1969) Radiation therapy in retinoblastoma. Radiology 93:405–409

Chan HS, Gallie BL, Munier FL et al. (2005) Chemotherapy for retinoblastoma. Ophthalmol Clin North Am 18:55–63, viii

Chévez-Barrios P, Chintagumpala M, Mieler W et al.(2005) Response of retinoblastoma with vitreous tumor seeding to adenovirus-mediated delivery of thymidine kinase followed by ganciclovir. J Clin Oncol 23:7927–7935

Coucke PA, Schmid C, Balmer A et al. (1993) Hypofractionation in retinoblastoma: an increased risk of retinopathy. Radiother Oncol 28:157–161

de Graaf P, Barkhof F, Moll AC et al. (2005) Retinoblastoma: MR imaging parameters in detection of tumor extent. Radiology 235:197–207

Ellsworth RM (1969) The practical management of retinoblastoma. Trans Am Ophthalmol Soc 67:462–534

Fontanesi J Pratt CB, Kun LE et al. (1996) Treatment outcome and dose-response relationship in infants younger than 1 year treated for retinoblastoma with primary irradiation. Med Pediatr Oncol 26:297–304

Foote RL, Garretson BR, Schamberg PJ et al. (1989) External beam irradiation for retinoblastoma: patterns of failure and dose-response analysis. Int J Radiat Oncol Biol Phys 116:823–830

Freire JE, DePotter P, Brady LW et al. (1997) Brachytherapy in primary ocular tumors. Semi Surg Oncol 13:167–176

Halperin EC et al. (2005) Pediatric radiation oncology, 4th edn. Lippincott Williams & Wilkins, Philadelphia, pp 135–177

Hernandez JC, Brady LW, Shields JA et al. (1996) External beam radiation for retinoblastoma: results, patterns of failure, and a proposal for treatment guidelines. Int J Radiat Oncol Biol Phys 35:125–132

Hilgartner HL (1910) Report of a case of double glioma treated by X-rays. Tex Med J 18:322

Kim JW, Abramson DH, Dunkel IJ et al. (2007) Current management strategies for intraocular retinoblastoma. Oncol 67:2173–2185

Kingston JE, Hungerford JL (1992) Retinoblastoma. In: Plowman PN, Pinkerton CR (eds) Paediatric oncology: clinical practice and controversies. Chapman & Hall, London, pp 268–290

MacKay CJ, Abramson DH, Ellsworth RM (1984) Metastatic patterns of retinoblastoma. Arch Ophthalmol 102:391–396

Marcus DM, Craft JL, Albert DM (1990) Histopathology verification of Verhoeff's 1918 irradiation cure of retinoblastoma. Ophthalmol 97:221–224

McCormick B, Ellsworth R, Abramson D et al. (1988) Radiation therapy for retinoblastoma: comparison of results with lens-sparing versus lateral beam techniques. Int J Radiat Oncol Biol Phys 15:567–574

McCormick B, Ellsworth R, Abramson D et al. (1989) Results of external beam radiation for children with retinoblastoma: a comparison of two techniques. J Pediatr Ophthalmol Strabismus 26:239–243

Merchant TE, Gould CJ, Wilson MW et al. (2004) Episcleral plaque brachytherapy for retinoblastoma. Pediatr Blood Cancer 43:134–139

Murphree L (2007) Staging and grouping of retinoblastoma. In: Singh A, Damato B (eds) Clinical ophthalmic oncology. Saunders Elsevier, Philadelphia, p 422

Pradhan DG, Sandridge AL, Mullaney P et al. (1997) Radiation therapy for retinoblastoma: a retrospective review of 120 patients. Int J Radiat Oncol Biol Phys 39:3–13

Reese AB (1976) Tumors of the eye, 3rd ed. Harper & Row, Hagerstown, MD, pp 90–122

Schvartzman E, Chantado G, Fandino A, et al. (1996) Results of a stage-based protocol for the treatment of retinoblastoma. J Clin Oncol 14:1532–1536

Schwimer CJ, Prayson RA (2001) Clinicopathologic study of retinoblastoma including MIB-1, p53, and CD99 immunohistochemistry. Ann Diagn Pathol 5:148–154

Shields CL, Shields JA, DePotter P et al. (1993) Plaque radiotherapy for retinoblastoma. Int Ophthalmol Clin 33:107–118

Shields CL, Shields JA, Kiratli H et al. (1995) Treatment of retinoblastoma with indirect ophthalmoscope laser photocoagulation. J Pediatr Ophthalmol Strabismus 114:1348–1356

Shields CL, Meadows AT, Shields JA et al. (2001) Chemoreduction for retinoblastoma may prevent intracranial neuroblastic malignancy (trilateral retinoblastoma). Arch Ophthalmol 119:1269–1272

Shields CL, Mashayekhi A, Demirci H et al. (2004) Practical approach to management of retinoblastoma. Arch Ophthalmol 122:729–735

Shields CL, Mashayekhi A, Au AK et al. (2006) The International Classification of Retinoblastoma predicts chemoreduction success. Ophthalmology 113:2276–2280

Stallard HB (1966) The treatment of retinoblastoma. Ophthalmologica 51:214–230

Wilson AH, Karr DJ, Kalina RE et al. (1994) Visual outcomes of macular retinoblastoma after external beam radiation therapy. Opthalmology 101:1244–1249

Wong FL, Boice JD Jr, Abramson DH et al. (1997) Cancer incidence after retinoblastoma. Radiation dose and sarcoma risk. JAMA 278:1262–1267

Ewing's Sarcoma Family of Tumors

Hiram A. Gay and Ron R. Allison

CONTENTS

H. A. Gay, MD
Department of Radiation Oncology, The Brody School of
Medicine at ECU, 600 Moye Blvd., Greenville, NC 27834,
USA
R. R. Allison, MD
Department of Radiation Oncology, The Brody School of
Medicine at ECU, 600 Moye Blvd., Greenville, NC 27834,
USA

Introduction and Objectives

Ewing's sarcoma (ES) is second only to osteosarcoma as the most common primary bone tumor in children. The Ewing's sarcoma family of tumors (EFT) includes extraosseous Ewing sarcoma (ES), peripheral primitive neuroectodermal tumor (pPNET), and malignant small cell tumor of the thoracopulmonary region (Askin tumor). All these are considered manifestations of a single neoplastic entity with characteristic phenotypic and molecular features.

This chapter focuses on the rapidly evolving management of the EFT:

- Recommendations for diagnostic and staging procedures
- The staging systems and prognostic factors
- Treatment recommendations and the supporting peer-reviewed scientific evidence
- Follow-up care and surveillance of survivors

41.1 Diagnosis, Staging, and Prognoses

41.1.1 Diagnosis

Initial Evaluation

- Diagnosis and evaluation of EFT starts with a complete history and physical examination. EFT can develop in almost any bone or soft tissue. Patients typically present with localized pain or swelling of a few weeks or months duration; a distinct soft tissue mass can sometimes be appreciated; rib lesions usually present as a palpable mass with pleural effusion on CXR; spine or sacrum involvement may have associated neurologic symptoms.

■ A multidisciplinary approach with participation of the pediatric oncologist, surgeon, radiation oncologist, radiologist, and pathologist is essential.

Imaging Studies

■ Imaging studies are essential for staging and include evaluation of the: primary tumor, skeletal system, and lung/pleura.

Primary Tumor

■ A current review article on EFT imaging recommends MRI as the study of choice for local tumor staging due to its excellent contrast, usefulness for evaluating tumor extension, and delineation of the neurovascular bundle and other critical structures when planning surgery. The lesions usually have a mildly heterogeneous hypointense signal on T1 weighted images, heterogeneous increased signal on the fluid sensitive sequences, and heterogeneous variable enhancement on the postcontrast sequences (MAR et al. 2008).

■ CT was found to be helpful for identifying subtle pathological fractures or cortical breakthrough, determining the extent of extraosseous tumor extension, and evaluating primary extraosseous tumors (Fig. 41.1) (MAR et al. 2008).

■ CT, MRI, and FDG-PET (Sect. 41.1.3) may be useful for assessing tumor response to treatment.

Skeletal System

■ FDG-PET is more sensitive than bone scintigraphy (bone scan) for the evaluation of skeletal me-

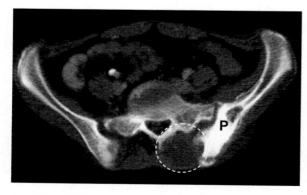

Fig. 41.1. Axial post-contrast CT scan of the pelvis demonstrating a left sacroiliac joint Ewing's sarcoma. The left sacrum and ilium demonstrate a permeative lesion with cortical destruction and periosteal reaction (*P*). There is tumor extension into the adjacent parapelvic and paraspinous musculature (*dashed circle*)

tastases in ES (Grade A). A prospective study of children and young adults who underwent whole-body spin-echo MR imaging, bone scintigraphy, and FDG-PET for the initial staging of bone marrow metastases included 20 patients with ES. The sensitivity for MRI imaging and bone scan for ES was 80% (20/25 lesions), and 88% (22/25 lesions) for FDG-PET (Level III) (DALDRUP-LINK et al. 2001). In addition, the results of a retrospective study of 24 ES patients who underwent FDG-PET studies included 14 patients who also underwent bone scintigraphy for evaluation of bone metastases. Although bone scintigraphies detected all 11 primary bone lesions present at the time of investigation, these only detected eight of 70 bone metastases revealed by PET and MRI. Moreover, 62 metastases in four patients remained undetected by bone scintigraphy (Level IV) (GYORKE et al. 2006). A retrospective study comparing FDG-PET with bone scintigraphy included 38 patients with ES. The sensitivity, specificity and accuracy for ES were 100%, 96%, and 97% for FDG-PET versus 68%, 87%, and 82% for bone scan on an examination-based analysis (Level IV) (FRANZIUS et al. 2000).

■ Recent Children's Oncology Group protocols such as AEWS07P1 (COG 2007a) and AEWS0621 (COG 2007b) include FDG-PET as a recommended, but not mandatory, imaging study.

■ One problem with FDG-PET is the identification of skull metastases which may be obscured by the high glucose metabolism in the normal brain.

■ There is insufficient evidence in ES to determine how whole-body MRI compares to FDG-PET or bone scintigraphy for skeletal staging. Figure 41.2 shows an MRI of a patient with thoracolumbar metastases. MRI may be very useful when evaluating cord compression (Fig. 41.3) and skull metastases (Fig. 41.4).

Lung/Pleura

■ CT is more sensitive than chest X-ray for detecting pulmonary metastases (Fig. 41.5).

■ Spiral CT is superior to FDG-PET for detecting pulmonary metastases, and FDG-PET is not recommended for excluding lung metastases (Grade B). A retrospective study comparing FDG-PET with spiral CT which included 61 ES examinations, showed that FDG-PET had a sensitivity of 56%, specificity of 91%, positive predictive value of 69%, and negative predictive value of 85%. The study also analyzed an additional

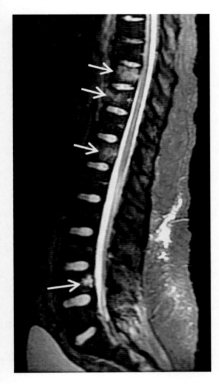

Fig. 41.2. Sagittal STIR MRI sequence of the thoracolumbar spine demonstrating abnormal T2 signal hyperintensity in the T9, T10, T12, and L4 vertebral bodies (*arrows*) with loss of height of the T10 vertebral body representing pathologic fracture

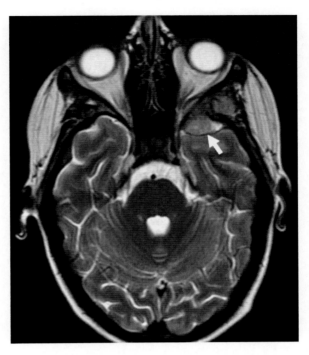

Fig. 41.4. Axial post-contrast T2 MRI image of the brain demonstrating a metastatic Ewing's sarcoma enhancing soft tissue mass centered in the greater wing of the sphenoid bone on the left (*arrow*), extending into orbital apex, temporal fossa, and middle cranial fossa. There is mild mass effect on the ventral left temporal lobe. The patient had left facial numbness

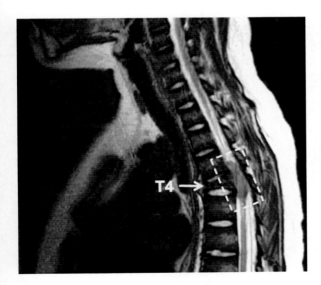

Fig. 41.3. Sagittal T2 weighted MRI image of the cervicothoracic spine. There is a pathologic compression fracture (*arrow*) of the T4 vertebral body with anterior wedge deformity. A metastatic Ewing's sarcoma soft tissue mass with paraspinous and epidural extension is compressing the spinal cord (*box*) which resulted in lower extremity weakness. No cord signal abnormality was identified

49 osteosarcoma examinations. Analyzing both groups together, the authors observed that spiral CT was superior to FDG-PET for detecting pulmonary metastases. Nevertheless, since the specificity of FDG-PET was high, FDG-PET could be used to confirm abnormalities seen on a thoracic CT scan.

Emerging Role of Hybrid PET/CT

■ Hybrid PET/CT is significantly more accurate than FDG-PET for the detection and localization of lesions and improves staging for patients with ES (Grade B). A retrospective study of 53 patients with ES who had a total of 91 hybrid PET/CT imaging studies from the base of skull to feet observed that, as determined by a lesion-based analysis, the sensitivity, specificity, and accuracy of FDG-PET were 71%, 95%, and 88%, respectively, while the corresponding values for the hybrid PET/CT technique were 87%, 97%, and 94% ($p<0.0001$). The advantage of hybrid PET/CT is mainly due to the detection of new lesions (Level IV) (GERTH et al. 2007). The authors used a special weight-adapted

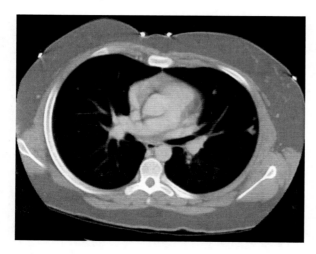

Fig. 41.5. Axial post-contrast CT scan of the chest demonstrating multiple pulmonary metastatic lesions

protocol to minimize FDG-PET radiation exposure to approximately 5 mSv, as well as a low-dose CT scan contributing an estimated 0.7 mSv. Care should be taken so that the lower extremities are completely visualized, which is not routinely the case with hybrid PET/CT.

■ Whether hybrid PET/CT improves on the low sensitivity of FDG-PET in detecting pulmonary metastases remains to be evaluated.

Laboratory Tests

■ Initial laboratory tests should include an LDH which, if elevated, is of negative prognostic value. Complete blood count, liver, and renal function tests are often necessary when evaluating chemotherapy suitability and protocol eligibility (Table 41.1).

Biopsy

■ The surgeon should be consulted after the imaging studies are obtained and prior to tumor biopsy to avoid compromising future surgery. Some surgical principles for the biopsy include:
- Longitudinal incisions to avoid spread to additional compartments
- Planning so that the biopsy tract is removed with the lesion at the time of surgery due to the risk of tumor seeding the scar
- Avoiding neurovascular structures which may result in the need for amputation rather than a limb-sparing procedure due to contamination
- Following a direct route to the tumor through muscles without retracting the muscles
- Careful hemostasis since a hematoma may permit tumor spread to other compartments
- Open, incisional biopsy of the primary is recommended to obtain enough tissue for all biologic studies, which are becoming increasingly important. Fresh tissue is needed for molecular studies. Often the diagnosis can be made from the surrounding involved soft tissues without having to obtain bone. Bone biopsy may increase the risk of a pathologic fracture. Bone biopsy also prevents the possibility of performing a frozen section to determine if the material is satisfactory for diagnosis.

■ Biopsy specimen analysis should include:
- Gross and hematoxylin and eosin staining microscopic examinations
- Immunohistochemical evaluation to exclude other entities (Table 41.2)

Table 41.2. Immunohistochemistry panel frequently employed when working-up EFT. [Adapted with permission from KHOURY (2008)]

Marker	EFT	ALL	Neuro-blastoma	Rahabdomyo-sarcoma
CD99	+	+/--	+/-	+/-
TdT	-	+	-	-
Synaptophysin	-/+	-	+	-
NB84	-	-	+	-
Myogenin	-	-	-	+
MyoD1	-	-	-	+

EFT, Ewing family of tumors; ALL, acute lymphoblastic leukemia/lymphoma; CD99, cluster of differentiation 99; TdT, terminal deoxynucleotidyl transferase; NB84, neuroblastoma 84

Table 41.1. Imaging and laboratory work-ups for EFT

Imaging studies	Laboratory tests
- MRI ± CT of primary	- LDH
- FDG-PET for detecting bone metastases	- Complete blood count
- Spiral chest CT to rule out lung metastases	- Liver function tests
- MRI for suspected skull metastases or cord compression	- Renal function tests

- Molecular (RT-PCR or FISH) or cytogenetic studies demonstrating an EFT chromosomal translocation
- Bone marrow biopsy and aspirate from at least two sites distant from the primary tumor or known metastases. There is some variability among ES protocols on the recommended number and location for bone marrow biopsies and aspirates.

Pathology

- The EFT is generally included in the loosely defined "small round cell tumors" group. Whether the EFT have a neuroectodermal or mesenchymal origin is a matter of debate.
- The defining feature of the EFT is the presence of non-random chromosomal translocations leading to the fusion of the *EWS* gene on chromosome 22p12 with one of several members of the ETS family of transcription factors (KHOURY 2008). The two most common translocations are t(11;22)(q24;q12) and t(21;22)(q22;q12) with an approximate prevalence of 90% and 10%, respectively.
- A variety of molecular techniques may be used to detect EFT-specific translocations including reverse transcriptase (RT)-PCR and fluorescence in situ hybridization (FISH). Currently, FISH is regarded as the technique of choice for confirming *EWS/ETS* translocations, in part due to its higher sensitivity and specificity than RT-PCR (KHOURY 2008). The main limitation of FISH is its inability to define the type of t(11;22) translocation if present.
- The immunophenotypic hallmark of EFT is the expression of CD99. However, CD99 is not a specific feature of the EFT and is insufficient for diagnosis.

41.1.2 Staging

- No widely accepted staging system exists for EFT.
- The AJCC bone and soft tissue sarcoma staging may be used for staging EFT (GREENE et al. 2002a,b). ES of the bone had more influence on the bone staging system. For example, T1 is defined as a tumor 8 cm or less in greatest dimension and T2 as more than 8 cm. The 8 cm cutoff for T1 and T2 was primarily based on the ES literature. The distinction of lung metastases (M1a) from distant sites of metastases (M1b) which carry a worse prognosis is also supported by the EFT literature. Unfortunately, the AJCC staging system currently does not address other important prognostic factors mentioned in the next section.

41.1.3 Prognostic Factors

- In the absence of an accepted staging system, prognostic factors are essential for patient risk stratification. There are two major types of prognostic factors for patients with EFT: pretreatment factors and treatment response factors.

Pretreatment Factors

- *Metastases:* The presence of metastases is the main adverse prognostic factor and is associated with a significantly worse relapse-free survival. For patients with metastases, patients with lung metastases only have a better survival than those with bone metastases or both (Level II) (COTTERILL et al. 2000).
- *Site:* For patients with non-metastatic EFT, axial sites (pelvis, rib, spine, scapula, skull, clavicle, sternum) have a worse survival than extremities (Level II) (COTTERILL et al. 2000; BACCI et al. 2006a). Distal extremity tumors have the highest event-free survival (EFS), followed by proximal extremity tumors and finally pelvic tumors which have the lowest EFS (Level II) (GRIER et al. 2003).
- *Size and volume:* Tumors with a maximal diameter of at least 8 cm have a poorer outcome than those with smaller tumors (Level II) (GRIER et al. 2003). Tumor volume has been shown to be an important prognostic factor in most studies. Cutoffs of either 100 ml (COTTERILL et al. 2000), 150 ml (BACCI et al. 2006a) or 200 ml (PAULUSSEN et al. 2001) have been found prognostic.
- *Serum lactate dehydrogenase (LDH):* For patients with non-metastatic EFT, elevated LDH is associated with a worse disease-free survival (Level II) (BACCI et al. 2006a).
- *Age:* Younger patients have better outcome than older patients (Level II) (COTTERILL et al. 2000; BACCI et al. 2006a; GRIER et al. 2003).
- *Gender:* For patients with non-metastatic EFT, girls with have a better disease-free survival than boys (Level II) (BACCI et al. 2006a). Gender did

not reach statistical significance in the INT-0091 study (Level II) (Grier et al. 2003).

- *Molecular findings:* Type 1 *EWS-FLI1* fusion is a positive predictor of overall survival (Level IV) (de Alava et al. 1998). More than 90% of ES contain a fusion of the *EWS* and *FLI1* genes, due to the t(11;22)(q24;q12) translocation. At the molecular level, the *EWS-FLI1* rearrangements show great diversity. In the most common fusion type (type 1), *EWS* exon 7 is linked in frame with exon 6 of *FLI1*. The prognostic significance of *EWS-Fli1* transcript type is being prospectively evaluated in the EURO-E.W.I.N.G. 99 protocol (EURO-E.W.I.N.G.99 2006).

Treatment Response Factors to Preoperative Therapy

- *Response to chemotherapy:* The higher the grade of tumor necrosis after preoperative chemotherapy, the better the disease-free-survival (Level III) (Picci et al. 1997; Lin et al. 2007). Females and younger patients are more likely to achieve complete tumor necrosis or only scattered foci of viable tumor cells (Level III) (Ferrari et al. 2007).
- *FDG-PET response to chemotherapy:* FDG-PET imaging of EFT correlates with histologic response to neoadjuvant chemotherapy. A retrospective study of 36 patients with EFT were evaluated by FDG-PET before and after neoadjuvant chemotherapy. The positive predictive value of an SUV less than 2.5 after neoadjuvant chemotherapy for a favorable response (≤10% viable tumor) was 79%, whereas the negative predictive value for an unfavorable response (>10% viable tumor) was 40%. An SUV less than 2.5 after neoadjuvant chemotherapy was predictive of progression-free survival (PFS) independent of initial disease stage (Level IV) (Hawkins et al. 2005).
- *Relapse:* Patients who relapse within 2 years of diagnosis have a less favorable prognosis than those who relapse later (Level II) (Cotterill et al. 2000: Bacci et al. 2006b). Patients who relapse 2 or more years after primary treatment, patients who relapse with only lung metastases, and patients whose recurrences can be surgically treated may still be cured even after two or three relapses (Level III) (Bacci et al. 2006b).

41.2 Treatment of EFT

41.2.1 General Principles

- EFT should be regarded as a systemic disease.
- To improve EFS for patients with ES, most of the European cooperative groups [including UKCCSG, SFOP, EORTC, GPOH (Germany and Austria), and SIAK] initiated EURO-E.W.I.N.G. 99, a phase III three arm trial based on risk stratification for treatment selection. In the United States, the Children's Oncology Group (COG) has opened the treatment arm for patients with isolated pulmonary metastases (R2pulm).
- For more information on open clinical trials for EFT visit:
- *http://www.kinderkrebsinfo.de/studien* (Germany, Austria)
- *http://www.e-cancer.fr/ (France)*
- *http://www.sakk.ch/ (Switzerland)*
- *http://www.cancerhelp.org.uk/trials/trials/ (UK)*
- *http://www.cancer.gov/clinicaltrials/search (USA)*

Pelvic Primary

- VACA-IE seems to confer a local failure benefit over VACA for pelvic primaries irrespective of local control modality (11% vs. 30%; $p=0.06$) (Grade B). As previously mentioned in Section 41.1.3, compared to other locations, pelvic primaries are associated with the worst EFS. A subset analysis of 75 patients with nonmetastatic pelvic ES treated on INT-0091 showed no significant difference in EFS or local failure (LF) by tumor size (<8 cm, ≥8 cm), local control (LC) modality, or chemotherapy. Although not statistically significant, surgery and radiotherapy seemed to have comparable LF rates at 5 years of 25% each, in contrast to an 11% LF rate at 5 years for patients treated with both (Level IV) (Yock et al. 2006).

Chest Wall/Rib Primary

- The likelihood of complete tumor resection with a negative microscopic margin and consequent avoidance of external-beam radiation is increased with neoadjuvant chemotherapy and delayed resection of chest wall EFT (Grade D). A restrospective study of 98 EFT patients with chest wall primaries observed that 10 of 20 (50%) initial resections resulted in negative margins compared with 41 of 53 (77%) negative margins with delayed resections after chemotherapy (*p*=0.043). EFS did not differ by timing of surgery or type of local control. Of 24 patients with initial surgery, 17 (70.8%) received radiotherapy compared with 25 of 62 patients (40.3%) who had delayed operations (*p*=0.016) (Level IV) (SHAMBERGER et al. 2003).

Lower Extremity

■ There is an increased risk of relapse and local failure in patients treated with radiotherapy alone (Grade D). A retrospective study of 53 patients with ES of the lower extremity with median follow-up of 19.2 years, noted that although overall survival was not statistically compromised, there was an increased risk of relapse and local failure in patients treated with radiotherapy alone. The 15-year actuarial local control rate was 100% for the surgery ± radiotherapy group and 68% for the definitive radiotherapy group (*p*=0.03) (Level IV) (INDELICATO et al. 2008). Using the Toronto Extremity Salvage Score (TESS), the study suggested that patients believe their lower extremitiy function after definitive radiotherapy is excellent and at least equivalent to patients treated with surgery.

41.2.2 Chemotherapy

■ Systemic chemotherapy has a central role in EFT treatment. Without systemic treatment, more than 90% of patients die from secondary metastases (PATRICIO et al. 1991). The use of chemotherapy impacts local control (LC) (Level IV) (PAULINO et al. 2007a).

■ The following chemotherapy combinations have proven to be effective: VAC (vincristine, actinomycin-D, cyclophosphamide), VACA (VAC plus doxorubicin alternating with actinomycin-D), the IESS II schedule (alternating the combination of ifosfamide plus etoposide and VACA), VAIA and EVAIA (ifosfamide replacing cyclophosphamide in VACA, either without or with additional etoposide), and the INT-0091 VACA-IE (vincristine, actinomycin-D which is substituted for doxorubicin when a total doxorubicin dose of 375 mg/m^2 is reached, cyclophosphamide, and doxorubicin, alternating with ifosfamide plus etoposide).

■ In the United States, the standard chemotherapy regimen for patients with nonmetastatic EFST is the INT-0091 VACA-IE (Grade B). Among 398 patients with non-metastatic disease, the mean 5-year EFS for the 198 patients in the VACA-IE group was 69%, as compared with 54% among the 200 patients in the VACA group (*p*=0.005). Overall survival was also significantly better among patients in the VACA-IE group than in the VACA group, 72% vs. 61%, respectively (*p*=0.01) (Level II) (GRIER et al. 2003). The addition of IE to VACA did not affect the outcome for patients with metastatic disease.

■ In Europe, based on the experience from the ET-1, ET-2, EW88, EW93, CESS81, CESS 86, EICESS92, and other clinical trials, the standard arm of EURO-E.W.I.N.G. 99 for localized disease includes induction VIDE (vincristine, ifosfamide, doxorubicin and etoposide) for six cycles and consolidation VAI (vincristine, actinomycin-D, and ifosfamide) for eight cycles.

■ Current chemotherapeutic strategies being explored to improve outcome involve increasing the intensity of chemotherapy and incorporating promising chemotherapeutic agents. The reader is advised to look for the results of COG AEWS0031 and EURO E.W.I.N.G. 99 once they are published. Protocol AEWS0031 was presented at ASCO in 2008 and showed promising results which will likely change the standard of care in the USA.

41.2.3 Surgery

■ The trend for local management of ES has changed recently toward surgical resection whenever feasible based on retrospective reports (Grade C) (Level IV) (INDELICATO et al. 2008; SCHUCK et al. 2003; BACCI et al. 2006c). Nevertheless, whether surgery followed by adjuvant radiation, surgery alone, or definitive radiation is superior for local control has yet to be evaluated in a prospective randomized trial.

■ Surgical highlights from EURO-E.W.I.N.G. 99 COG section:

– In patients with a poor radiographic and clinical response to preoperative chemotherapy, one should consider preoperative radiotherapy.

– If radiation is to be followed by posterior consideration of surgery, the delayed surgery should be done after the end of chemotherapy.

- Surgical resection of primary lesions arising in the vertebrae is seldom indicated, due to involvement of epidural and adjacent structures.
- Initial resection is not encouraged for a rib primary, and most patients should receive induction chemotherapy prior to resection (see Chest Wall/ Rib Primary heading on Section 41.2.1).
- Additional practical surgical advice is given for specific tumor locations in the COG protocol section which may be accessed on *http://www.childrensoncologygroup.org/* (EURO-E.W.I.N.G.99 2006).
- Note that the EURO-E.W.I.N.G. 99 protocol's European section bases the need for adjuvant radiotherapy on the extent of surgical margins, while the COG section of the protocol takes a somewhat different approach based on defining the extent of resection and tumor volume.

41.2.4 Radiation Therapy

General Principles

- For patients receiving busulfan:
- Large irradiation portals including bowel or lung need to be avoided. Whole-lung radiotherapy prior to or after busulfan may result in severe lung fibrosis.
- Radiation doses planned or administered involving spinal cord or brain must not exceed 30 Gy in the EURO-E.W.I.N.G. 99 protocol (EURO-E.W.I.N.G.99 2006).

Primary Tumor

Field Coverage and Arrangement

- Involved-field (IF) radiation is currently recommended over whole-bone radiation for local tumor control in EFT (Grade D). POG 8346 attempted to answer whether involved field radiation is equivalent to whole bone radiation in terms of local control. As DONALDSON et al. (1998) have pointed out, there were several problems with the study which hindered confidently answering the question (Level II). Nevertheless, INT-0091 successfully applied the IF approach with a promising LF rate of 11 % for the VACA-IE arm.
- Gross tumor volume (GTV) definitions in the COG section of the EURO-E.W.I.N.G. 99 protocol (see Table 41.3):

- GTV_1 for primary tumors is defined as the visible and/or palpable bony or soft tissue disease prior to treatment defined by physical examination or imaging (MRI optimal).
- GTV_2 for unresected tumors is defined as the pretreatment bony abnormalities and residual soft tissue following induction chemotherapy.
- GTV_2 for inadequately resected tumors is defined as the site of microscopic residual disease or the site of the less than minimal margin (for patients with intra-operative spill, $GTV_2 = GTV_1$).
- GTV_2 for partially resected tumors is defined as the residual soft tissue and bony abnormalities following induction chemotherapy and surgical debulking.
- Clinical tumor volume (CTV):
- $CTV_1 = GTV_1 + 1.5$ cm
- $CTV_2 = GTV_2 + 1$ cm
- Radiotherapy technique highlights from EURO-E.W.I.N.G. 99:
- Areas of scars after biopsy or tumor resection are to be included in the radiation fields.
- If the patient has a diaphyseal lesion, every attempt should be made to exclude at least one epiphysis (or both, if possible) of the affected bone.
- If any of the recommended treatment margins necessitates irradiating the epiphysis of an adjacent bone and there is no extension across the joint space, a smaller margin should be used, so that the adjacent epiphysis can be excluded.
- The epiphyseal plates should be spared if possible.
- An adequate strip of skin and subcutaneous tissues should be spared to avoid constrictive extremity fibrosis and/or lymphatic obstruction.
- In postoperative irradiation following implantation of prosthetic material, the prosthetic material should be included with a safety margin of 2 cm.
- The radiation field should not extend across a joint unless absolutely necessary for tumor coverage in which case the dose to the joint should not exceed 45 Gy.
- In some instances, 3D-conformal radiotherapy (3D-CRT) which satisfies the recommended tumor primary coverage and dose guidelines and at the same time minimizes the irradiation of grossly uninvolved bone marrow, could potentially reduce the risk of compromising the essential adjuvant chemotherapy. In addition, 3D-CRT may minimize the volume receiving 48 Gy and above

which has been associated with an increased risk of secondary sarcoma (see Sect. 41.2.5).

- EFT protocols usually specify additional tumor volume and dose constraints for special situations such as pathologically involved lymph nodes, chest wall tumors, pathologically involved pleural fluid, pleural nodules, residual lesions after whole lung radiotherapy, vertebral body primaries, and others.

Dose and Fractionation

- Table 41.3 lists the EURO-E.W.I.N.G. 99 COG section partial list of recommended doses. The doses are in agreement with the review article on radiation dose and target volume by DONALDSON (2004). Of note, in the EURO-E.W.I.N.G. 99 European section radiotherapy is deemed essential for a tumor volume ≥200 ml.

- Patients who receive definitive radiotherapy doses ≥49 Gy for tumor size ≤8 cm, or ≥54 Gy for tumor size >8 cm have improved local control (Grade C). A retrospective study of 40 patients with localized ES treated at a single institution observed that for tumors ≤8 cm, the 5- and 10-year local control rate was 94.1% for a dose ≥49 Gy and 50.0% for a dose <49 Gy ($p=0.01$). For tumors >8 cm, the 5- and 10-year local control rate was 85.7% for a dose ≥54 Gy and 26.7% for a dose <54 Gy ($p=0.006$) (Level IV) (PAULINO et al. 2007b).

Table 41.3. Doses for EFT. [Based on COG section of EURO-E.W.I.N.G. 99 protocol (EURO-E.W.I.N.G.99 2006)]

	Clinical scenario	GTV[a]	Dose
Primary	– Unresected – Inadequately resected – Partial resection, PR	GTV1 GTV2	45 Gy 10.8 Gy (1.8 Gy fx.)
	– Partial resection, GR – GTR with adequate margins, PR	GTV1	45 Gy (1.8 Gy fx.)
	– GTR with adequate margins, GR		
Lung	– Lung metastases on presentation, no busulfan	GTV1	15 Gy (< 14 yo) 18 Gy (> 14 yo) (1.5 Gy fx.)

[a] See Section 41.2.4 for GTV and CTV descriptions for the primary and lung. GTV, gross tumor volume; CTV, clinical tumor volume; GTR, gross total resection; PR, poor histological response (≥10% residual tumor cells); GR, good histological response (<10% residual tumor cells); fx., fractions; yo, years old.

Whole-Lung Radiotherapy

Patients Presenting with Lung Metastases

- Whole-lung radiotherapy (WLR) (see Fig. 41.6) is recommended in EFT patients presenting with lung metastases unless treatment includes busulfan chemotherapy (Grade B). A retrospective study of 114 patients with ES presenting with synchronous pulmonary and/or pleural metastases treated in protocol CESS81, CESS86, or EICESS92 observed that 40% of patients who did not receive WLR had first relapses confined to the lungs or pleural space only, while following WLR, isolated pulmonary/pleural relapses occurred in 20% ($p=0.046$). The 5-year EFS rate was 38% with WLR versus 27% without WLR ($p=0.0022$) (Level IV) (PAULUSSEN et al. 1998).

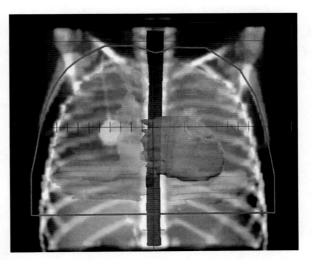

Fig. 41.6. Whole-lung radiotherapy anterior treatment field. Margins should take into account lung motion and potential setup errors

- EURO-E.W.I.N.G. 99 highlights:
- GTV$_1$ for lung is defined as the entire thoracic contents from the attachments of the diaphragm to the apices.
- The whole-lung CTV$_1$ = GTV$_1$ + 1 cm.
- Not that the COG section allows boosts to residual lung lesions.

Prophylactic Lung Radiotherapy

- Prophylactic WLR is currently not recommended outside of a clinical trial based on the results of the IESS I study (Grade C). The first Intergroup Ewing's Sarcoma Study (IESS I) randomized a total of 342 ES patients according to institution group. In group I institutions, patients were randomized between treatment 1 [radiotherapy to primary lesion plus vincristine, actinomycin-D, cyclophosphamide, and doxorubicin (VACA)] or treatment 2 (VAC), and group II institutions randomized patients between treatment 2 or treatment 3 (VAC plus bilateral pulmonary radiotherapy). The RFS at 5 years for treatments 1, 2, and 3 were 60%, 24%, and 44%, respectively. The occurrence of lung metastases was 15% (22 of 148) for treatment 1, 30 of 74 (40%) for treatment 2, and 20% (22 of 109) for treatment 3. Since the VACA treatment was superior to the other two groups in terms of RFS, prophylactic radiation therapy to the lung was not studied in subsequent trials (Level II) (NESBIT et al. 1990).

Total Body Irradiation

■ Total body irradiation is currently not recommended outside a clinical trial (Grade B). As a component of systemic treatment, it has been investigated in a limited fashion usually with disappointing results (MEYERS et al. 2001; HOROWITZ et al. 1993; BURDACH et al. 2003) .

Palliation

■ Metastases from EFT can result in pain, neurologic symptoms, and painful lymphadenopathy (KOONTZ et al. 2006).
■ Palliative radiotherapy without a protracted treatment course is appropriate for providing symptom relief in patients with metastatic ES (Grade B). A retrospective study of 21 patients with metastatic ES who received palliative radiotherapy (median dose, 30 Gy; range, 4.5–68.5 Gy) to a total of 63 metastatic sites (median three sites per patient; range, 1–16), observed that of all sites 55% had a complete clinical response of symptoms, and 29% had a partial response. The median response duration was 4.0 months (range, 10 days–4.8 years). The only long-term survivor was noted to have a treatment complication consisting of growth hormone insufficiency (Level IV) (KOONTZ et al. 2006).

41.2.5 Multimodality Treatment Late Side Effects and Complications

■ The most common late effects in patients receiving radiotherapy are: muscular atrophy, limb length growth delay, and development of secondary malignancy (Level IV) (PAULINO et al. 2007a).
■ Both radiotherapy and surgery may cause scoliosis and decrease the range of movement of an extremity (Level IV) (PAULINO et al. 2007a).
■ The overall risk of second malignancies after Ewing's sarcomas is similar to that associated with treatment for other childhood cancers. The estimated cumulative incidence rates at 20 years for any second malignancy and for secondary sarcoma were 9.2% and 6.5%, respectively. The cumulative incidence rate of secondary sarcoma was radiation dose-dependent ($p=.002$), and no secondary sarcomas developed among patients who had received less than 48 Gy (Level IV) (KUTTESCH et al. 1996). Nevertheless, PAULINO et al. (2007b) reported a radiation-induced osteosarcoma after a dose of 45 Gy in a retrospective review of 40 cases treated with definitive radiotherapy.
■ A retrospective study noted that five of eight patients with ES developed a pathologic fracture. One patient with a pathologic fracture was found to have a malignant fibrous histiocytoma in the irradiated bone, while two others were found to have osteogenic sarcoma 2.3–4 years later. The authors noted that a pathologic fracture in an irradiated field is important to consider as it may be a sign of a radiation-induced malignancy, or an early warning of someone at risk for a second malignant neoplasm in the bone (Level IV) (PAULINO 2004).
■ Among the various potential late effects from chemotherapy, doxorubicin may result in cardiomyopathy and cyclophosphamide in infertility.

41.3   Follow-Ups

41.3.1 Post-Treatment Follow-Ups

■ Life-long follow-up after definitive treatment of EFT is recommended for detecting recurrence, secondary tumors, or other long-term complications of treatment.

Schedule

- EFT may relapse as late as 5–10 years after initial diagnosis.
- There is no consensus on the optimal follow-up schedule or imaging studies for EFT. Table 41.4 is based on the EURO-E.W.I.N.G. 99 protocol (EURO-E.W.I.N.G.99 2006) follow-up schedule (Grade D).
- A baseline MRI or CT scan of the primary at the end of treatment is advisable if the patient has been treated with radiotherapy only or incomplete surgery for local control of the primary (EURO-E.W.I.N.G.99 2006) (Grade D).

Table 41.4. Follow-up schedule after treatment for EFT

Interval	Frequency
1st year	2-monthly examination and chest X-ray
2nd year	3-monthly examination and chest X-ray
3rd year	4-monthly examination and chest X-ray
4th and 5th years	6-monthly examination and chest X-ray
Over 5 years	Annual examination and chest X-ray

Work-Ups

- Each follow-up should include a complete history and physical examination.
- Chest X-ray examinations as in Table 41.4.

Acknowledgments

Thanks to Ron Sayers, MD, Department of Radiology, Pitt County Memorial Hospital, for his review of the diagnostic images and image capture, Leo Mascarenhas, MD, MS, for his valuable help in clarifying the European and United States standard of care for EFT, and Darin Noble, medical dosimetrist, for his assistance with capturing and editing Figure 41.6.

References

Bacci G, Longhi A, Ferrari S, Mercuri M, Versari M, Bertoni F (2006a) Prognostic factors in non-metastatic Ewing's sarcoma tumor of bone: an analysis of 579 patients treated at a single institution with adjuvant or neoadjuvant chemotherapy between 1972 and 1998. Acta Oncol 45:469–475

Bacci G, Longhi A, Ferrari S et al. (2006b) Pattern of relapse in 290 patients with nonmetastatic Ewing's sarcoma family tumors treated at a single institution with adjuvant and neoadjuvant chemotherapy between 1972 and 1999. Eur J Surg Oncol 32:974–979

Bacci G, Longhi A, Briccoli A, Bertoni F, Versari M, Picci P (2006c) The role of surgical margins in treatment of Ewing's sarcoma family tumors: experience of a single institution with 512 patients treated with adjuvant and neoadjuvant chemotherapy. Int J Radiat Oncol Biol Phys 65:766–772

Burdach S, Meyer-Bahlburg A, Laws HJ et al. (2003) High-dose therapy for patients with primary multifocal and early relapsed Ewing's tumors: results of two consecutive regimens assessing the role of total-body irradiation. J Clin Oncol 21:3072–3078

COG (2007a) AEWS07P1, A Pilot Study of Chemotherapy Intensification by Adding Vincristine, Topotecan and Cyclophosphamide to Standard Chemotherapy Agents with an Interval Compression Schedule in Newly Diagnosed Patients with Localized Ewing Sarcoma Family of Tumors https://members.childrensoncologygroup.org/Prot/AEWS07P1/AEWS07P1DOC.pdf

COG (2007b) AEWS0621, Phase II Trial of Intermediate-Dose Cytarabine to Modulate EWS/FLI for Children and Young Adults with Recurrent or Refractory Ewing Sarcoma https://members.childrensoncologygroup.org/Prot/AEWS0621/aews0621doc.pdf

Cotterill SJ, Ahrens S, Paulussen M et al. (2000) Prognostic factors in Ewing's tumor of bone: analysis of 975 patients from the European Intergroup Cooperative Ewing's Sarcoma Study Group. J Clin Oncol 18:3108–3114

Daldrup-Link HE, Franzius C, Link TM et al. (2001) Whole-body MR imaging for detection of bone metastases in children and young adults: comparison with skeletal scintigraphy and FDG PET. AJR Am J Roentgenol 177:229–236

de Alava E, Kawai A, Healey JH et al. (1998) EWS-FLI1 fusion transcript structure is an independent determinant of prognosis in Ewing's sarcoma. J Clin Oncol 16:1248–1255

Donaldson SS (2004) Ewing sarcoma: radiation dose and target volume. Pediatr Blood Cancer 42:471–476

Donaldson SS, Torrey M, Link MP et al. (1998) A multidisciplinary study investigating radiotherapy in Ewing's sarcoma: end results of POG #8346. Pediatric Oncology Group. Int J Radiat Oncol Biol Phys 42:125–135

EURO-E.W.I.N.G.99 (2006) AEWS0331, European Ewing Tumor Working Initiative of National Groups Ewing Tumour Studies 1999(EURO-E.W.I.N.G. 99) https://members.childrensoncologygroup.org/Prot/AEWS0621/aews0621doc.pdf

Ferrari S, Bertoni F, Palmerini E et al. (2007) Predictive factors of histologic response to primary chemotherapy in patients with Ewing sarcoma. J Pediatr Hematol Oncol 29:364–368

Franzius C, Sciuk J, Daldrup-Link HE, Jurgens H, Schober O (2000) FDG-PET for detection of osseous metastases from malignant primary bone tumours: comparison with bone scintigraphy. Eur J Nucl Med 27:1305–1311

Gerth HU, Juergens KU, Dirksen U, Gerss J, Schober O, Franzius C (2007) Significant benefit of multimodal imaging: PET/CT compared with PET alone in staging and follow-up of patients with Ewing tumors. J Nucl Med 48:1932–1939

Greene F, Page D, Fleming I et al. (eds) (2002a) Bone. In: AJCC Cancer Staging Manual, 6th edn. Springer, Berlin Heidelberg New York, pp 187–192

Greene F, Page D, Fleming I et al. (eds) (2002b) Soft tissue sarcoma: In: AJCC Cancer Staging Manual, 6th edn. Springer, Berlin Heidelberg New York, pp 193–200

Grier HE, Krailo MD, Tarbell NJ et al. (2003) Addition of ifosfamide and etoposide to standard chemotherapy for Ewing's sarcoma and primitive neuroectodermal tumor of bone. N Engl J Med 348:694–701

Gyorke T, Zajic T, Lange A et al. (2006) Impact of FDG PET for staging of Ewing sarcomas and primitive neuroectodermal tumours. Nucl Med Commun 27:17–24

Hawkins DS, Schuetze SM, Butrynski JE et al. (2005) [18F] Fluorodeoxyglucose positron emission tomography predicts outcome for Ewing sarcoma family of tumors. J Clin Oncol 23:8828–8834

Horowitz ME, Kinsella TJ, Wexler LH et al. (1993) Total-body irradiation and autologous bone marrow transplant in the treatment of high-risk Ewing's sarcoma and rhabdomyosarcoma. J Clin Oncol 11:1911–1918

Indelicato DJ, Keole SR, Shahlaee AH et al. (2008) Long-term clinical and functional outcomes after treatment for localized Ewing's tumor of the lower extremity. Int J Radiat Oncol Biol Phys 70:501–509

Khoury JD (2008) Ewing sarcoma family of tumors: a model for the new era of integrated laboratory diagnostics. Expert Rev Mol Diagn 8:97–105

Koontz BF, Clough RW, Halperin EC (2006) Palliative radiation therapy for metastatic Ewing sarcoma. Cancer 106:1790–1793

Kuttesch JF Jr, Wexler LH, Marcus RB et al. (1996) Second malignancies after Ewing's sarcoma: radiation dose-dependency of secondary sarcomas. J Clin Oncol 14:2818–2825

Lin PP, Jaffe N, Herzog CE et al. (2007) Chemotherapy response is an important predictor of local recurrence in Ewing sarcoma. Cancer 109:603–611

Mar WA, Taljanovic MS, Bagatell R et al. (2008) Update on imaging and treatment of Ewing sarcoma family tumors: what the radiologist needs to know. J Comput Assist Tomogr 32:108–118

Meyers PA, Krailo MD, Ladanyi M et al. (2001) High-dose melphalan, etoposide, total-body irradiation, and autologous stem-cell reconstitution as consolidation therapy for high-risk Ewing's sarcoma does not improve prognosis. J Clin Oncol 19:2812–2820

Nesbit ME, Jr., Gehan EA, Burgert EO, Jr. et al. (1990) Multimodal therapy for the management of primary, nonmetastatic Ewing's sarcoma of bone: a long-term follow-up of the First Intergroup study. J Clin Oncol 8:1664–1674

Patricio MB, Vilhena M, Neves M et al. (1991) Ewing's sarcoma in children: twenty-five years of experience at the Instituto Portuges de Oncologia de Francisco Gentil (I.P.O.F.G.). J Surg Oncol 47:37–40

Paulino AC (2004) Late effects of radiotherapy for pediatric extremity sarcomas. Int J Radiat Oncol Biol Phys 60:265–274

Paulino AC, Nguyen TX, Mai WY (2007a) An analysis of primary site control and late effects according to local control modality in non-metastatic Ewing sarcoma. Pediatr Blood Cancer 48:423–429

Paulino AC, Nguyen TX, Mai WY, Teh BS, Wen BC (2007b) Dose response and local control using radiotherapy in non-metastatic Ewing sarcoma. Pediatr Blood Cancer 49:145–148

Paulussen M, Ahrens S, Craft AW et al. (1998) Ewing's tumors with primary lung metastases: survival analysis of 114 (European Intergroup) Cooperative Ewing's Sarcoma Studies patients. J Clin Oncol 16:3044–3052

Paulussen M, Ahrens S, Dunst J et al. (2001) Localized Ewing tumor of bone: final results of the cooperative Ewing's Sarcoma Study CESS 86. J Clin Oncol 19:1818–1829

Picci P, Bohling T, Bacci G et al. (1997) Chemotherapy-induced tumor necrosis as a prognostic factor in localized Ewing's sarcoma of the extremities. J Clin Oncol 15:1553–1559

Schuck A, Ahrens S, Paulussen M et al. (2003) Local therapy in localized Ewing tumors: results of 1058 patients treated in the CESS 81, CESS 86, and EICESS 92 trials. Int J Radiat Oncol Biol Phys 55:168–177

Shamberger RC, LaQuaglia MP, Gebhardt MC et al. (2003) Ewing sarcoma/primitive neuroectodermal tumor of the chest wall: impact of initial versus delayed resection on tumor margins, survival, and use of radiation therapy. Ann Surg 238:563–567; discussion 7–8

Yock TI, Krailo M, Fryer CJ et al. (2006) Local control in pelvic Ewing sarcoma: analysis from INT-0091 – a report from the Children's Oncology Group. J Clin Oncol 24:3838–3843

Wilms' Tumor

42

Arnold C. Paulino and Bin S. Teh

CONTENTS

A. C. PAULINO, MD
Department of Radiation Oncology, The Methodist Hospital/
Weill Medical College, 6565 Fannin Street, DB1-077, Houston,
TX 77030, USA
B. S. TEH, MD
Department of Radiation Oncology, The Methodist Hospital/
Weill Medical College, 6565 Fannin Street, DB1-077, Houston,
TX 77030, USA

Introduction and Objectives

Wilms' tumor or nephroblastoma is the most common abdominal tumor of childhood, and accounts for 6%–7% of childhood cancer in North America. It is comparatively more common in African Americans and least common in the East Asian population. The male-to-female ratio is 0.92:1. The median age at initial diagnosis is 36.1 months. For patients with bilateral disease, it is 25.5 months.

Recent trials have focused on limiting treatment-related toxicity from chemotherapy and radiotherapy. Dramatic improvement in the outcome of patients with Wilms' tumor has been a result of cooperative group studies utilizing a multidisciplinary approach. At present, approximately 90% of children will survive Wilms' tumor.

This chapter examines:
- Recommendations for work-up of a child with Wilms' tumor
- Staging system and prognostic factors
- Treatment recommendations for favorable histology and anaplastic Wilms' tumor
- Treatment recommendations for rhabdoid tumor and clear cell sarcoma of the kidney
- Radiotherapy guidelines for management of Wilms' tumor
- Follow-up recommendations

42.1 Clinical Presentation, Diagnosis, and Staging

42.1.1 Clinical Presentation

- The most common presentation is a painless abdominal mass in an otherwise healthy child.
- Abdominal pain or hematuria are seen in about 25% of cases. Several syndromes are associated with Wilms' tumor including the WAGR syndrome (Wilms' tumor, aniridia, genitourinary

anomalies, mental retardation) and the Beckwith-Wiedemann syndrome (overgrowth syndrome characterized by visceromegaly, macroglossia, and hypoglycemia).

■ The most common congenital anomalies seen are genitourinary (cryptorchidism, hypospadias, double collecting system, uterine abnormalities, horseshoe kidney).

■ Approximately 2% of Wilms' tumor patients have hemihypertrophy and 1% has aniridia.

Diagnosis

■ Work-up is shown in Table 42.1. This includes history and physical examination with special attention to possible congenital anomalies.

■ CT scan of the abdomen is performed if ultrasound shows an abdominal mass. The CT scan helps identify the origin of tumor (kidney vs. non-kidney, lymph node involvement, invasion into major vessels, liver metastases, and bilateral kidney involvement).

■ In North America, patients with suspected Wilms' tumor undergo nephrectomy. Biopsy of renal mass violates the renal capsule and upstages the patient to at least a Stage II. The exception is bilateral Wilms' tumor where renal preservation is paramount.

■ In contrast, most European centers make a presumptive diagnosis of Wilms' tumor based on imaging studies and give preoperative chemotherapy.

Pathology

■ The most common type of kidney cancer in children is a favorable histology Wilms' tumor. In the National Wilms Tumor Study (NWTS) publications, approximately 90% have favorable histology and 4% have anaplastic (focal or diffuse) Wilms' tumor.

■ Other types of kidney cancer which have been enrolled on NWTS protocols include clear cell sarcoma and rhabdoid tumor of the kidney. Clear cell sarcoma has a higher incidence of spread to the bone compared to other renal tumor types, while rhabdoid tumor has a predisposition to the brain. The most common site of distant metastases is pulmonary, similar to favorable and anaplastic histology Wilms' tumor.

■ Approximately 20% of renal tumors in those ≤6 months of age have congenital mesoblastic nephroma.

42.1.2 Staging

■ The staging system currently used in North America was devised by the NWTS and is shown in Table 42.2.

■ Most patients present with Stage I or II disease. Only about 5% of patients present with bilateral kidney involvement or Stage V disease.

42.1.3 Prognostic Factors

■ The most important prognostic factor is histology. Anaplastic tumors have a worse prognosis compared to favorable histology (FH) Wilms' tumor.

Table 42.1. Work-up for Wilms' tumor

Imaging studies	Laboratory tests
– Abdominal ultrasound	– Complete blood count
– CT scan of the abdomen	– Chemistry profile including BUN, creatinine, and calcium
– CT scan of the chest	– Urine analysis including catecholamines

Table 42.2. National Wilms' Tumor Study staging system

Stage I	Tumor confined to kidney and completely resected. No penetration of the renal capsule or involvement of renal sinus vessels
Stage II	Tumor extends beyond kidney but completely resected. (a) Penetration of renal capsule; (b) invasion of renal sinus vessels; (c) biopsy of tumor before removal
Stage III	Gross or microscopic residual disease remains postoperatively (inoperable tumor, positive surgical margins, tumor spillage involving peritoneal surfaces, regional lymph node involvement, transected tumor thrombus)
Stage IV	Hematogenous or lymph node metastases outside the abdomen
Stage V	Bilateral Wilms' tumor at onset

- The 4-year overall survival rates for the different histologies according to stage are as follows: Stage I FH, 97%; Stage II FH, 92%; Stage III FH, 87%; Stage IV FH, 82%; Stage I anaplastic, 89%; Stage II–IV anaplastic, 68%; Stage I–IV clear cell sarcoma, 75%; Stage I–IV rhabdoid tumor, 25%.
- The 5-year overall survival rates for synchronous and metachronous bilateral Wilms tumor are 73% and 49%, respectively.
- Children with both loss of heterozygosity (LOH) at 1p and 16q have worse survival than those with no LOH or only 1p or 16q LOH.
- Stage I and II FH patients with LOH at 1p **and** 16q have a 4-year relapse-free survival (RFS) of 74.9% and overall survival rate of 90.5%.
- Stage III and IV FH patients with LOH 1p and 16q have a 4-year RFS of 65.9% and overall survival rate of 77.5%.

42.2   Treatment of Wilms' Tumor

- Treatment of Wilms' tumor is determined by the risk of the disease (Fig. 42.1).

42.2.1 Very Low Risk

- Children <2 years of age with Stage I tumor and kidney weight of <550 grams undergo nephrectomy and are observed on the current Children's Oncology Group (COG) AREN0532 study.
- For these children, it is expected that 85% will be cured with surgery alone. Chemotherapy will be offered to <15% of these patients, and an overall survival of 95% is predicted for those undergoing this approach.

42.2.2 Low Risk

- Stage I and II FH children without LOH 1p and 16q undergo nephrectomy followed by chemotherapy consisting of vincristine and actinomycin-D. They are treated according to COG AREN03B2 protocol.

42.2.3 Standard Risk

- Stage I and II FH children with LOH at 1p and 16q are treated with nephrectomy followed by vin-

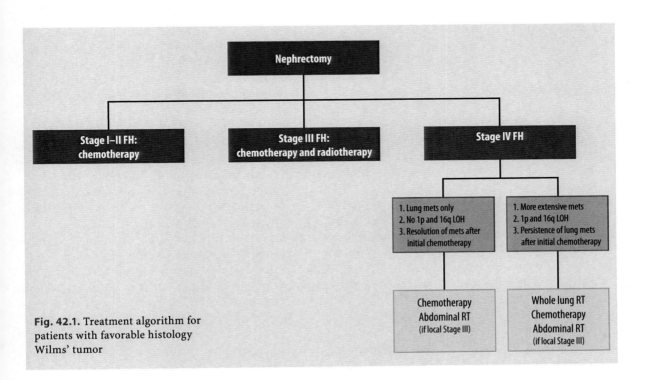

Fig. 42.1. Treatment algorithm for patients with favorable histology Wilms' tumor

cristine, actinomycin-D, and doxorubicin and are treated on the COG AREN0532 study.

■ Stage III FH children with no LOH at 1p and 16q are treated with nephrectomy, followed by vincristine, actinomycin-D, and doxorubicin and postoperative radiotherapy (RT) and are treated on the COG AREN0532 study.

42.2.4 Higher Risk

■ Stage III FH children with LOH 1p and 16q are treated with nephrectomy, followed by vincristine, actinomycin D, doxorubicin, cyclophosphamide, etoposide and postoperative RT on the COG AREN0533 protocol.

■ For patients with Stage IV FH tumors, all receive 6 weeks of vincristine, actinomycin D, and doxorubicin following nephrectomy. If the tumor has no LOH, is Stage IV because of pulmonary lesions only, and the pulmonary lesions disappear at week 6, patients continue with the same chemotherapy and are treated with abdominal RT based on local stage; they do not receive pulmonary RT. For all other Stage IV FH patients, pulmonary RT is given and the chemotherapy is changed to include cyclophosphamide and etoposide with local RT, given if needed as well as RT, to nonpulmonary metastatic sites. These children are treated on the COG AREN533 protocol.

42.2.5 High Risk

■ Patients with focal anaplastic Stage I–III and diffuse anaplastic Wilms' tumor undergo nephrectomy, vincristine, actinomycin-D, doxorubicin, and local RT on the COG AREN0321 protocol.

■ Patients with clear cell sarcoma Stage I–III tumors undergo nephrectomy, vincristine, actinomycin-D, doxorubicin, cyclophosphamide, etoposide, and local RT on COG AREN0321 protocol. Stage I patients do not require local RT.

■ Patients with focal anaplastic Stage IV, diffuse anaplastic Stage II–III, Stage I–III rhabdoid tumor, and Stage IV clear cell sarcoma undergo nephrectomy, vincristine, actinomycin-D, doxorubicin, cyclophosphamide, etoposide, carboplatin, and RT on the COG AREN0321 protocol.

■ Patients with Stage IV diffuse anaplastic Wilms' or rhabdoid tumor undergo nephrectomy and undergo therapy with irinotecan and vincristine followed by more extensive chemotherapy which also includes actinomycin-D, doxorubicin, cyclophosphamide, carboplatin, etoposide, and RT. These patients are treated on the COG AREN0321 protocol.

42.3 Radiotherapy Guidelines

42.3.1 Irradiation to the Primary Site

■ Successive studies have shown that adjuvant RT is not indicated for Stage I and II FH Wilms' tumor provided that vincristine and actinomycin-D are given (Grade A) (NWTS-3, Level I) (D'Angio et al. 1989), (NWTS-2, Level II) (D'Angio et al. 1981).

■ An adjuvant RT dose of approximately 1000 cGy is sufficient to control the primary site in Stage III FH Wilms' tumor provided triple drug chemotherapy (vincristine, actinomycin-D, and doxorubicin) is delivered (Grade A) (NWTS-3, Level I) (D'Angio et al. 1989). A boost dose of another 1000 cGy in 150- to 180-cGy fractions can be delivered to areas of gross disease.

■ For patients who need local RT, the preoperative tumor and kidney with a 2 cm margin is the treatment volume. The medial border of the RT field is extended medially encompassing the entire vertebral width to minimize development of scoliosis.

■ For patients with diffuse peritoneal implants or diffuse spillage of tumor, the whole abdomen is treated to approximately 1000 cGy given in 150- to 180 cGy fractions. When there are gross peritoneal deposits, a dose of approximately 2000 cGy is recommended with the remaining kidney receiving not more than 1400 cGy.

■ Patients with local spillage of tumor used to be classified as Stage II and did not receive postoperative RT; they were found to have a higher risk of local relapse compared to Stage III patients receiving RT. These patients now require RT to the primary site (Grade B) (NWTS-4, Level III) (Shamberger et al. 1999).

■ For patients with anaplastic Wilms' tumor, there is no evidence of a dose response; hence, the recommended dose is similar to FH Wilms' tumor (Grade B) (NWTS, Level III) (GREEN et al. 1994a). For Stage III, diffuse anaplastic Wilms' tumor, the recommended dose, however, is 2000 cGy because of the poorer outcome of these patients. Previously, Stage I anaplastic tumors did not require RT, but now they do secondary to inferior EFS and overall survival rates when compared to FH tumors of the same stage (Grade B) (NWTS-5, Level III) (DOME et al. 2006).

■ For patients with clear cell sarcoma, the current recommended dose is approximately 1000 cGy in 150- to 180-cGy fractions based on the absence of a dose response (Grade B) (NWTS, Level III) (GREEN et al. 1994b). Stage I patients are now recommended not to receive postoperative RT based on their excellent survival and local control rates (Grade B) (NWTS-4, Level III) (SEIBEL et al. 2004).

■ On the current COG AREN0321 study, patients with rhabdoid tumor receive local RT regardless of stage. The recommended dose is approximately 2000 cGy for children >1 year old and 1000 cGy for those <1 year old (Grade D).

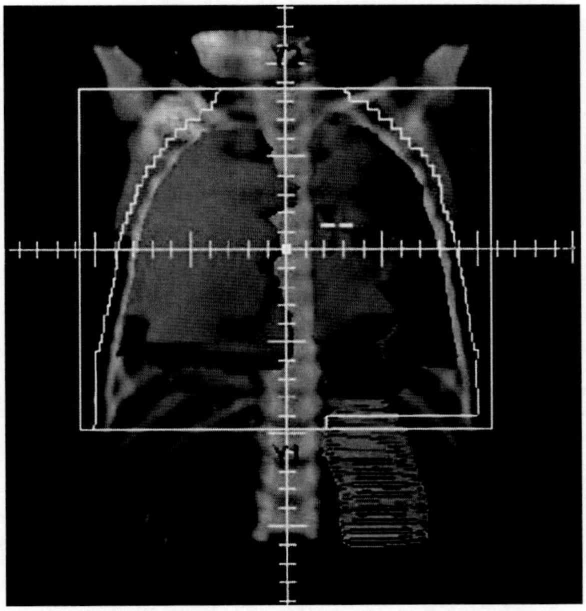

Fig. 42.2. Pulmonary irradiation in patient with Wilms' tumor and lung metastases

42.3.2 Pulmonary Irradiation

■ In previous NWTS protocols, patients with pulmonary metastases have received pulmonary RT to a dose of 1200 cGy in eight fractions (Grade B). There is controversy as to whether pulmonary irradiation is needed in children with CT positive, chest X-ray negative pulmonary metastases with the idea being that chemotherapy can control these lesions well without RT (Grade C). The NWTS and International Society of Pediatric Oncology (SIOP) trials have not shown an EFS or overall survival benefit with pulmonary irradiation (Level III) (GREEN et al. 1991; MEISEL et al. 1999; DEKRAKER et al. 1990); however, a recent trial from the United Kingdom shows a worse EFS without improvement in overall survival in those not receiving pulmonary RT (Level III) (NICOLIN et al. 2008) (Fig. 42.2).

■ Currently, patients enrolled on COG studies who have Stage IV FH, no LOH 1p and 16q, and who achieve a complete response in the lungs after the initial 6 weeks of chemotherapy are not given pulmonary RT.

42.4 Follow-Up

■ Post-treatment follow-up should include studies to detect recurrence and late effects of treatment including radiotherapy.

Schedule

■ Children are generally followed every 3 months for 5 years with a history and physical exam.

Post-Treatment Studies

■ Chest X-ray and abdominal ultrasound are performed every 6 months. These studies alternate with a CT scan of the chest, abdomen, and pelvis every 6 months, beginning 3 months after the first follow-up chest X-ray and abdominal ultrasound.

■ Patients with anaplastic histology may need more aggressive imaging (CT scan of the chest, abdomen, and pelvis) every 3 months for the first 2 years followed by less aggressive imaging, similar to FH tumors, for the next 3 years.

- Both clear cell sarcoma and rhabdoid tumor need bone scan for 2 years (every 3 months for the first year then every 6 months for the second year) and MRI of the brain for 3 years (every 6 months).
- For tests involving diagnosis of late effects, the "Long-Term Follow-Up Guideline for Survivors of Childhood, Adolescent, and Young Adult" from the Children's Oncology Group should be followed (Grade D) (CHILDREN'S ONCOLOGY GROUP 2006).

References

Children's Oncology Group (2006) Long-term follow-up guideline for survivors of childhood, adolescent, and young adult. http://www.survivorshipguidelines.org/pdf/LTFUGuidelines.pdf. Accessed on March 31, 2008

D'Angio GJ, Evans A, Breslow N et al. (1981) The treatment of Wilms' tumor: results of the Second National Wilms' Tumor Study. Cancer 47:2302–2311

D'Angio GJ, Breslow N, Beckwith JB et al. (1989) Treatment of Wilms' tumor: results of the Third National Wilms' Tumor Study. Cancer 64:349–360

DeKraker J, Lemerle J, Voute PA et al. (1990) Wilms tumor with pulmonary metastases at diagnosis: the significance of primary chemotherapy. International Society of Pediatric Oncology Nephroblastoma Trial and Study Committee. J Clin Oncol 8:1187–1190

Dome JS, Cotton CA, Perlman EJ et al. (2006) Treatment of anaplastic histology Wilms' tumor: results of the fifth National Wilms' Tumor Study. J Clin Oncol 24:2352–2358

Green DM, Fernbach DJ, Norkool P et al. (1991) The treatment of Wilms' tumor patients with pulmonary metastases detected only with computed tomography: a report from the National Wilms' Tumor Study. J Clin Oncol 9:1776–1781

Green DM, Beckwith JB, Breslow NE et al. (1994a) Treatment of children with stages II to IV anaplastic Wilms' tumor: a report from the National Wilms' Tumor Study Group. J Clin Oncol 12:2136–2131

Green DM, Breslow NE, Beckwith JB et al. (1994b) Treatment of children with clear cell sarcoma of the kidney: a report from the National Wilms' Tumor Study Group. J Clin Oncol 12:2132–2137

Meisel JA, Guthrie KA, Breslow NE et al. (1999) Significance and management of computed tomography detected pulmonary nodules: a report from the National Wilms Tumor Study Group. Int J Radiat Oncol Biol Phys 44:579–585

Nicolin G, Taylor R, Baughan C et al. (2008) Outcome after pulmonary radiotherapy in Wilms' tumor patients with pulmonary metastases at diagnosis: a UK Children's Cancer Study Group, Wilms' Tumour Working Group Study. Int J Radiat Oncol Biol Phys 70:175–180

Seibel NL, Li S, Breslow NE et al. (2004) Effect of duration of treatment on treatment outcome for patients with clear cell sarcoma of the kidney: a report from the National Wilms Tumor Study Group. J Clin Oncol 22:468–473

Shamberger RC, Guthrie KA, Ritchey ML et al. (1999) Surgery-related factors and local recurrence of Wilms tumor in the National Wilms Tumor Study-4. Ann Surg 229:292–297

Section XI:
Metastatic Diseases

Management of Bone Metastases

Vaneerat Ratanatharathorn and José A. Peñagarícano

CONTENTS

Introduction and Objectives

Bone is the most common organ affected by metastatic cancers (Coleman 2006). Bone metastases are the most common condition referred for palliative radiation therapy and the most common cause of cancer-related pain. Patients with bone metastases also have a more prolonged duration of survival compared to patients with visceral metastases. There is no reliable prevalence figure for bone metastases, but estimates can be made that approximately 350,000 people in the United States who die each year from cancer had bone metastases. The numbers of patients living with bone metastases increase when we consider patients who are living with the condition, since some patients with bone metastases, especially from breast and prostate cancer, generally live longer than 1 year (Mundy 2002). Treatment must be selected based on the predicted duration of patients' survival and any need to prevent catastrophic complications from bone metastases. Thus treatments are multi-disciplinary. The appropriate selection and sequencing of therapeutic modalities is crucial in maximizing the extent and duration of the benefits with the least toxicities.

This chapter examines:

- Recommendations for diagnosis and staging procedures
- Prognostic factors
- Complications of bone metastases
- Treatment recommendations including multi-disciplinary management plans
- Radiation therapy dose-fractionation and techniques for delivery including external beam and radionuclides
- Follow-up care and surveillance of survivors

V. Ratanatharathorn, MD
Winthrop P. Rockefeller Cancer Institute, 4301 W. Markham Street, #623, Little Rock, AR 72205, USA
J. A. Peñagarícano, MD
University of Arkansas for Medical Sciences, Department of Radiation Oncology, 4301 W. Markham Street, #771, Little Rock, AR 72205, USA

Diagnosis, Staging, and Prognosis

43.1.1 Diagnosis

Initial Evaluation

- Patients referred to the radiation therapy clinic for consideration of palliative radiation therapy for bone metastases usually have obvious other metastases or multiple bone metastases. Solitary bone metastases occur in <10% of patients (FALKMER et al. 2003).
- Primary sites with high propensity for bone metastases include prostate, breast (70% of these two primaries had bone metastases at autopsy), lung, kidney, and thyroid (30%–40% of these three primaries had bone metastases at autopsy) (COLEMAN 2006). Most bone metastases seen in the clinic come from prostate, breast, and lung primaries due to their high incidence in addition to the great propensity for bone involvement. Some malignancies, such as gastrointestinal, rarely go to bone (<10%). If clinical evidence is inconsistent with the diagnosis of bone metastasis, or if this is the first metastasis, then biopsy is warranted. (RATANATHARATHORN et al. 2004).
- Assess patients' performance status, pain sites, and severity using visual analog scale, analgesic usage, mobility, urinary and fecal continence, weight loss, and mental status.
- Obtain the history of prior and on-going treatments and patients' responses to treatments.

Laboratory Tests

- Initial laboratory tests should include a complete blood count, biochemical profile including kidney and liver function tests, alkaline phosphatase, serum LDH, and serum calcium (total, ionized, and adjusted for albumin level).
- Initial and then monthly measurements of the bone resorption marker, n-telopeptide of type 1 collagen are recommended in patients with bone metastases from breast and prostate cancers (Grade C). The test is useful for monitoring patients and for predicting the risks of skeletal complications (COLEMAN 2006).

Imaging Studies

- Whole-body bone scintigraphy or FDG-PET/CT is required to evaluate the extent and distribution of bone metastases, as well as other metastases (Grade B). The information of the entire metastatic burden in the body is important for assessing patients' prognoses. CT portion of PET/CT allows clinicians to more accurately assess patients for risks of fractures of weight-bearing long bone than bone X-ray. Any potential concerns for neurologic complications from bone metastases may also be assessed (Level III) (ANTOCH et al. 2004; RATANATHARATHORN et al. 2004)
- Although PET/CT is widely used to assess whole-body tumor extent, bone scintigraphy will need to be performed in patients considered for radionuclide therapy such as Sr^{89} or SM^{153} (Grade A). These radionuclides mimic pathways of calcium metabolism in the body and the information is needed to determined the patient's candidacy for radionuclide therapy (Level I) (HOLMES 1993; RESCHE et al. 1997; SERAFINI et al. 1998).
- Magnetic resonance imaging studies are crucial in assessing any potential neurologic complications indicated by patients' symptoms or concerns discerned from other studies such as CT scans. The entire spine must be examined for precise management plans to be formulated (RATANATHARATHORN et al. 2004).

Pathology

- First metastasis should be biopsied. Any clinical evidence or cancer natural history inconsistent with bone metastases may also necessitate biopsy. At times, tissue diagnosis may be established through surgical procedures such as laminectomy or open reduction and internal fixation done for therapeutic purposes.
- Breast, prostate, and lung primaries account for 80% of bone metastases. Two-thirds of bone metastases produce symptoms such as pain, fractures, hypercalcemia, nerve root or cord compression. Solitary bone metastases occur in <10% of patients. Greater than 80% of bone metastases are in axial skeletons. Primary sites generally do not correlate with localization patterns of bone metastases, except that pelvic primaries such as prostate, bladder, etc., tend to involve pelvic bones (FALKMER et al. 2003).

43.1.2 Complications of Bone Metastases

■ The risks of developing skeletal morbidity depends on the primary sites, the pattern of bone metastases, and the presence of other co-existing distant metastases. More than 50% of breast cancer patients with bone metastases develop skeletal complications. In breast cancer patients with bone-only metastases at the first relapse, 81% develop skeletal morbidity with 83% of patients needing palliative radiation therapy and 60% needing more than one course of treatment. In breast cancer with no bone metastases at the first relapse, only 21% of patients develop skeletal morbidities and the median time to the first skeletal complication is 56 months versus 11 months for the first group (COLEMAN 2006).

■ Complications of bone metastases include:
- *Pain* – 75% of patients will have pain and, in general, pain symptoms are severe. The mechanisms of pain are not completely understood. Pain is usually worse at night, which is opposite to the pattern of pain from degenerative diseases (COLEMAN 2006).
- *Fractures* – Pathologic fractures occur in 8%–30% of patients and usually involve femurs (FALKMER et al. 2003). Fractures actually occur most frequently in ribs and vertebrae (COLEMAN 2006). But it is the fractures of the weight-bearing long bones, such as femurs, or the epidural extension of tumors into the spine that cause the most disability. MIRELS (1989) proposed a scoring system to assess the fracture risks based on the site, nature, size, and symptoms from the metastatic lesions. Based on this system, lesions that score >7 generally require surgical intervention; scores ≥10 had an estimated risk of fracture of >50%. Again, CT may provide a more accurate assessment of fracture risks than planar X-ray since, depending on the location and extent of the bone lesions and cortical erosion, such risks may not be obvious on planar X-ray (COLEMAN 2006).
- *Compression of nerve roots and/or spinal cord* – Neurologic complications from cord/nerve root compression occur in 5% of patients with bone metastases. Pain is common and is usually localized to the area overlying the tumor. Local pain usually precedes radicular pain. Other symptoms include motor weakness (96%), pain (94%), sensory disturbances (79%), and sphincteric disturbances (61%) (COLEMAN 2006). Frequently, spinal instability is also present and surgery is required

to relieve the pain. When the compression is from bone fragments, surgery is needed. Early treatment offers the best chance of reversing neurologic deficits. When treatment is delayed, results depend more on the radiosensitivity of the tumors than other factors (FALKMER et al. 2003).
- *Hypercalcemia* – Hypercalcemia most often occurs in patients with squamous cell lung cancer, breast cancer, kidney cancers, and certain hematologic malignancies such as myeloma and lymphoma and it is seen in approximately 10% of patients (MUNDY 2002). Osteolysis accounts for about 80% of patients with hypercalcemia. It is rare in certain cancers such as small cell lung cancer and prostate cancer even in the presence of extensive bone metastases. Parathyroid hormone-related peptide (PTHrP) seems to play an important role in hypercalcemia of malignancies. Its level is elevated in two-thirds of patients with hypercalcemia and bone metastases and in almost all patients with humoral hypercalcemia. In breast cancer, there is also an association between hypercalcemia and liver metastases, which may reflect the relationship between liver involvement and production or reduced metabolism of PTHrP or RANKL (receptor activator of nuclear factor-κβ ligand). Patients' volume depletion with the action of PTHrP on renal tubular reabsorption of calcium further increases serum calcium level. Death generally results from renal failure and cardiac arrhythmias (COLEMAN 2006).
- *Leuko-erythroblastic anemia* – This is associated with marrow replacement by cancer cells resulting in production of young white blood cells. Thus it is seen in patients with extensive bone metastases (MUNDY 2002).

43.1.3 Prognostic Factors

■ There is no established staging system for bone metastases. It is important to understand the prognostic and predictive factors for more individualized treatments to achieve more cost-effective use of health care resources, as well as the best use of patients' remaining time.

■ Many factors have been shown to be predictive of patients' duration of survival and/or risks of developing complications of bone metastases The parameters for the assessment of patients' prognosis include: primary sites (median survival from the time of diagnosis of bone metastasis from breast and prostate cancers is measurable in years; from lung cancer, typically in months), the distribution of bone metastases, the extent and volume of bone metastases (imaging, bone resorption markers, serum LDH), presence or absence of visceral metastases (lung, liver, and brain), cachexia, and performance status (COLEMAN 2006; MUNDY 2002; FALKMER et al. 2003; RATANATHARATHORN et al. 2004; CHOW et al. 2002).

- The ability to predict the risks of skeletal complications is important since patients may acutely decompensate should such complications develop, such as fracture of weight-bearing long bones in elderly patients.

43.2 Treatment of Bone Metastases

43.2.1 General Principles

- Any management plan of bone metastases must take into account predicted duration of patients' survival. Prognostic factors predicting survival duration of <6 months include low performance status such as ECOG ≥3 or Karnofsky performance status of ≤50, visceral organ involvement, the extent and tempo of bone metastases, and cachexia (FALKMER et al. 2003).
- There are generally two phases in the management of bone metastases: Initially, when the metastatic burden is low, anti-neoplastic therapy may be given in an aggressive manner with the intent of prolonging patient's survival. However, the majority of patients with bone metastases are treated with the intent to relieve distressing symptoms or to prevent catastrophic complications such as spinal cord compression or fracture of weight-bearing long bones. The risk:benefit ratio must be carefully weighed for each patient.
- Management of the complications of bone metastases is a crucial and integral part of cancer management. Commonly observed complications of bone metastases include pain, potential fractures, and compression of nerve roots and/or spinal cord, as well as hypercalcemia.

- Therapy of bone metastases is multi-disciplinary. Judicious use of these disciplines in combination and in the appropriate sequence maximizes the benefits for patients. Different treatment modalities will be mentioned herein.

43.2.2 Management of Hypercalcemia

- The truly effective long-term management in controlling hypercalcemia of malignancies is to treat the underlying tumor.
- Symptomatic therapy is indicated in the acute phase, including the administration of volume and sodium repletion with saline until serum calcium values are below 3.0 mM and/or adequate oral fluid intake has been established.
- Loop diuretics should be avoided because of the risk of causing extra-cellular fluid volume contraction. An exception is in elderly patients, in whom extra fluid may cause heart failure in the presence of limited cardiac reserve.
- Bone resorption must be inhibited using intravenous bisphosphonates in the acute phase due to the general presence of gastrointestinal (GI) symptoms with relatively poor GI absorption. The newer generation and more potent preparations of bisphosphonates, such as pamidronate and zoledronic acid, are not yet available as an oral preparation (RALSTON 2000).
- Patients with humoral hypercalcemia may remain mildly hypercalcemic even after adequate volume and sodium repletion and administration of bisphosphonates. This is due to the effect of PTHrP on the distal renal tubules with increased renal tubular reabsorption of calcium (RALSTON 2000). Many patients will die within a month of the development of hypercalcemia of malignancies, so the mildly persistent hypercalcemia may not be relevant or observed due to the terminal condition of patients. Neutralizing antibodies to PTHrP was shown in preclinical studies to be effective in the treatment of hypercalcemia of malignancies.
- Nearly all patients show a beneficial response to bisphosphonates in the acute phase management of bone metastasis-related hypercalcemia (Grade A). Bisphosphonates block bone resorption but may also block tumor cell mitosis and stimulate tumor cell apoptosis. Bisphosphonates also help alleviate bone pain in certain subset of patients (Level I) (KOHNO et al. 2005).

43.2.3 Current Use of Bisphosphonates

■ It is reasonable to begin bisphosphonates when there are lytic or mixed lytic/blastic bone metastases, when painful sites correspond to areas of bone destruction on bone imaging studies, when bone metastases appear to progress rapidly, after failure of a first-line anti-neoplastic therapy, and following the first skeletal-related events.

■ Bisphosphonates should probably be recommended for all patients with bone metastases from hormone refractory prostate cancer (Grade C). Although bone metastases from prostate cancer are typically osteoblastic, osteolytic components are frequently present and there is enough evidence to show that they are effective in reducing skeletal-related morbidity in bone metastases from prostate cancer as well (Level III) (Heidenreich et al. 2002; Michaelson and Smith 2005).

■ Standard doses of bisphosphonates such as pamidronate 90 mg IV over 2 h every 3–4 weeks, or zoledronic acid 4 mg IV over 15 min every 3–4 weeks are typically associated with moderate bone pain relief benefits.

In patients with compromised renal function such as creatinine clearance of <30 ml/min or patients receiving other nephrotoxic drugs, ibandronate should be used instead of zoledronic acid, according to the American Society of Clinical Oncology Update (Grade A) (Hillner et al. 2003). Loading dose of IV ibandronate 6 mg IV over 3 consecutive days or 4 mg IV over 4 consecutive days have been shown in open trials to rapidly relieve severe or refractory metastatic bone pain from urologic cancers, breast cancer, and other tumor types (Grade B) (Level III) (Heidenreich et al. 2002, 2003; Mancini et al. 2004).

■ The role of bisphosphonates in the adjuvant setting to inhibit the appearance of bone metastases is under study for patients at high risk of developing bone metastases from different tumors.

■ Bisphosphonates can also be used to prevent treatment-induced bone loss from chemotherapy, castration, steroidal or non-steroidal aromatase inhibitors, and complete androgen blockade (Grade B). The efficacy of ibandronate on the prevention of treatment-induced bone loss has been demonstrated in a number of prospective non-randomized trials (Level III) (Hillner et al. 2003; Michaelson and Smith 2005; Ralston 2000).

43.2.4 Orthopedic Management

■ Bone metastases alter two basic and inter-related elements of bone: the material properties of bone tissues (determined by osteoid and the hard mineralized matrices) and the structural properties of the entire bone (Rubert et al. 2000). The restoration of the material properties of the bone is achieved by anti-neoplastic therapy such as local radiation therapy, systemic therapy, which allows normal bone mechanisms to replace the areas of tumor-induced lysis with new bone. It can also be assisted by the use of bisphosphonates. The process may be slow but complete restoration of bone properties may be achieved provided that local tumor control is maintained and the host status is healthy enough to allow healing to take place (nutritional status and calcium homeostasis).

■ The goal of orthopedic management is to restore the normal structural integrity of the bone and to achieve local control of tumor, thereby preventing further deterioration of the remaining bone. Mirels (1989) proposed a scoring system for prediction of pathologic fractures based on a score of 1–3 and four variables of site (upper limb, lower limb, and peritrochanter with a progressive score from 1–3), pain (mild, moderate and functional pain with progressive scores from 1–3), lesion characteristics (blastic, mixed, and lytic with progressive scores from 1–3), and size (bone diameter divided into a third with score of 1 for <1/3 and score of 2 for 1/3–2/3, and score of 3 for >2/3). For weight-bearing long bones, patients with pathologic fractures had a mean summed score of 1. Pain that is aggravated by function appears to be an important predictor of fracture, presumably because functional pain signifies diminution in the mechanical strengths of the bone and Mirels (1989) found that this is invariably followed by fractures.

Harrington (1972) recommends complete removal of tumor and replacement with bone cement with internal fixation, and classifies acetabular bone destruction into three categories based on the location and extent of the disease and the technical requirement necessary for stable reconstruction:

Class I: Disease has sufficient lateral cortices and medial and superior wall and may be reconstructed with the conventional total hip acetabular component.

Class II: Has deficient medial wall and requires transfer of weight-bearing to intact acetabular rim using devices such as antiprotrusio cup or shell.

Class III: Diseases are large and there is extensive destruction of all walls requiring reconstruction with transfer of weight-bearing to the upper ilium and adjacent SI joint using multiple Steinman pin-reinforced bone cement with saddle prosthesis (HARRINGTON 1981, 1995; RUBERT et al. 2000)

■ CT remains the standard for the evaluation of cortical bone involvement and must be performed in lesions of the pelvis, shoulder girdle, and spine prior to reconstructions. MRI is useful in evaluating the soft tissue extent of the tumor and may detect intramedullary lesions (intertrabecular involvement without lytic or blastic response of the involved bone) (RUBERT et al. 2000). For difficult reconstructions of vertebral lesions and large pelvic lesions, both CT and MRI should be preformed. Preoperative embolization of suspected vascular lesions is useful in reducing blood loss and makes the procedures safer for patients. The standard surgical approach may need to be modified in patients with prior radiation therapy and surgeons must ensure adequate soft tissue coverage and closure. Gross disease should be curetted. Internal rigid fixation or prosthetic replacement with bone cement must be used to provide immediate structural strength to the compromised bone. Adjuvant radiation therapy should be given if this has not yet been done to reduce the chance of tumor progression and loss of the surgical fixation (RUBERT et al. 2000).

■ HARRINGTON (1988a) set up criteria for surgical stabilization of spinal metastases from class I–V based on the extent of the vertebral destruction, presence or absence of fractures/instability/spinal canal compromise/pain/neurologic deficits, and the extent of such deficits. Patients in Harrington's class III–V are candidates for surgical management, based on the results of their retrospective series (Level IV). In the management of spinal metastases, one must also determine the stabilization of the spine using the 6 column classification system of KOSTUIK et al. (1988). The spine is divided into six columns: anterior, middle, and posterior with each subdivided into the right and the left sides. The destruction of ≤2 columns is considered stable provided that any angulation, if present, is <20%. The destruction of 2–4 columns destabilizes the spine. The destruction of 5–6 columns makes the spine markedly unstable. MCLAIN and WEINSTEIN (1990) proposed a classification system of the zone for the surgical approach for spinal surgery depending upon the location of the instability and/or epidural compression.

43.2.5 External-Beam Radiation Therapy

■ External-beam radiation therapy can be offered for local fields to target painful or involved sites, or half-body irradiation to target the symptomatic half of the body, or sequential half-body irradiation to treat symptoms, as well as adjuvant treatment to reduce subsequent development of painful sites (Grade A). However, the optimal dose level and fractionation has not been established.

■ Duration of survival of patients with bone metastases is usually 3–12 months (FALKMER et al. 2003). However, some patients may survive several years. Most studies aim at bone pain palliation, fracture prevention and treatment, as well as spinal cord compression. The role of radiation therapy in preventing or healing fractures has not been fully evaluated.

■ The vast majority of patients were treated with palliative goals with RR >80% in pain relief with at least 50% of patients having relief for >6 months. The reported controlled clinical trials showed no correlation between treatment results and RT dose/fractionation schemes. Dose fractionation schemes were reported to have no impact on complications of bone metastases such as spinal cord compression, fractures, etc. Such complications within the index fields are low. Early diagnoses and treatments of potential complications of bone metastases hold the best promise for favorable outcomes. Otherwise, radioresponsiveness of cancers comes into play more (FALKMER et al. 2003).

Dose and Fractionation

■ Various doses and fractionations have been tested in randomized trials, and results from most trials demonstrated that a large single dose (e.g., 8 Gy) and more fractionated radiation (e.g., 30 Gy in 10 fractions) provided similar symptomatic control (Level I) (HARTSELL et al. 2005; KOSWIG and BUDACH 1999; NIELSEN et al. 1998; STEENLAND et al. 1999; BONE PAIN TRIAL WORKING PARTY 1999). However, the authors of various clinical trials of palliative radiation therapy for bone metastases recommend that the dose-fractionation scheme recommended to patients take into account the predicted duration of patients' survival and the treatment goals.

For patients with survival duration of <3–6 months in non-weight-bearing bones, a single fraction of 8 Gy encompassing the entire targets including the extra-osseous component is reasonable.

In weight-bearing long bones in patients with indolent bone metastases (e.g., bone metastases from differentiated thyroid carcinoma, adenoid cystic carcinoma, etc.) or predicted prolonged survival in the order of years (first and only metastasis to bone from breast cancer), dose fractionation in the order of 40–50 Gy with conventional fractionation is appropriate.

For "radioresistant" tumors such as renal cell carcinoma with large expansile mass and otherwise low distant metastatic burden, higher dose per fraction and higher total dose is appropriate. Patients with metastases to weight-bearing long bones should receive higher total dose such as 40 Gy or its biologically equivalent doses to effectuate tumor cell kill and bone healing in order to circumvent pathologic fracture. In other words, cases and their treatment must be highly individualized. Most cases, however, are appropriately treated with 20–24 Gy in between four and six fractions for pain relief (FALKMER et al. 2003; RATANATHARATHORN et al. 1999).

■ Doses less than 8 Gy delivered as a single-dose radiation treatment is usually not recommended (Grade B). The results of a prospective randomized trial showed that the actual response rates were 69% for 8 Gy and 44% for 4 Gy at 4 weeks after treatment ($p<0.001$) (Level II) (HOSKIN et al. 1992). However, lower dose is indicated in patients unable to tolerate higher dose irradiation.

■ For palliation with half-body irradiation, a total dose of 15 Gy delivered in five daily fraction at 3 Gy/fraction is recommended (Grade A). A randomized trial reported by SALAZAR et al. (1996, 2001) using 3 Gy/Fx, 5 Fx, 15 Gy/week; 4 Gy/Fx, 2 Fx/d, 8 Gy/1 d; 3 Gy/Fx, 1 Fx/d, 6 Gy/2 d, had the same overall pain relief, side effects, and quality of life with all three dose-fractionation regimens, but had significantly longer duration of pain re-

lief with 15-Gy total dose in 1 week (155 days vs. 101 days vs. 112 days, respectively) (Level I)

Issues of Clinical Trials on Radiotherapy for Bone Metastases

■ There are several barriers to conducting meaningful trials on bone metastases: (1) Patients are generally in advanced stage of disease and large randomized trials with follow-up of at least 1 year is difficult to conduct. (2) Results of trials may lack clarity due to a lack of adequate methods for the assessment of pain. (3) Dose levels and fractionation schemes used for RT for pain relief often turned out to be based on empirical knowledge of both the patients' individual characteristics and the local institution practice (FALKMER et al. 2003).

■ There are several problems about studying dose-response in bone metastases trials as follow:

– Dose-response is not well known. At least three large controlled trials did not prescribe dose appropriately (Dmax, 5 cm depth to all spine fields) or did not describe the technique at all. There is no description of: prescribed isodose or minimal dose to targets, single vs. multiple port arrangements, beam energy and beam geometry, imaging used to delineate target, technique to daily localized targets. So the actual delivered doses to targets are not documented or known. The extent of the geographic misses due to factors other than technique, such as missing extra-osseous components, is also unknown.

– Studies look mainly at pain relief and mostly quite short term, with few having at least 1 year of follow-up.

– Studies did not formulate radiation dose regimens based on, or taking into account, the biology of bone metastases, bone healing mechanism, predictive model of patients' survival duration, and development of skeletal complications and morbidity.

– All dose fractionation regimens studied [single (8 Gy) vs. multi-fraction regimens (20–24 Gy in 5–6 fractions)] used relatively low doses, which may all be biologically equivalent once we look at the actual dose applied or delivered to the targets.

■ It is also crucial to evaluate the management strategy in the era of rapid advancement both in systemic therapy (patients with metastatic diseases living longer than in previous eras) and radiation therapy delivery technology. Only a few of the 13 controlled clinical trials meet the criteria for high weight of evidence (Level I) (BONE PAIN TRIAL WORKING PARTY 1999; NIELSEN et al. 1998; STEENLAND et al. 1999). Nine of the 13 controlled clinical trials reported the duration of pain relief. Seven of the 13 trials reported retreatment rates, which varied from 2%–44%, with single fraction regimens (23%–25% re-treatment) having 2.5–3 times more retreatment compared with multi-fraction regimens (7%–10% re-treatment). Six of the 13 trials reported pathologic fracture rates after local RT, varying from 1%–10% with single-fraction regimens having between two- and three-fold greater fracture rates compared with multi-fraction regimens. This is remarkable in that the multi-fraction regimens used in these clinical trials used low doses of only 20–24 Gy total doses. It is not known if using a higher total dose than 24 Gy will further improve these results (FALKMER et al. 2003). KOSWIG and BUDACH (1999) also reported a significantly higher rate of remineralization of the index lesions with 30 Gy in 10 fractions than with 8 Gy in a single fraction at 6 months. Remineralization of osteolytic lesions appears to be dose-dependent and a more fractionated schedule appears to be obviously more advantageous (Level I). This finding is supported by the work of MATSUBAYASHI et al. (1981), looking at remineralization of vertebral lesions, which appears only at higher dose levels of 40 Gy. It appears that adequate local tumor cell kill must take place for bone healing to occur (Level III). This is a good point to bear in mind when treating weight-bearing bone to prevent fractures.

■ It is difficult to obtain complete response rates of bone pain relief due to the lack of set criteria or common end points. Overall pain relief varies from 59%–90% (FALKMER et al. 2003). The lowest single-dose regimen for pain relief was 6 Gy (Level III) (UPPELSCHOTEN et al. 1995). Half a year after local RT, at least 50% of the patients with overall pain relief are still pain-free. Complications of bone metastases such as pathologic fractures and spinal cord compression at the index field are rare.

■ Another problem in interpreting the trial results came from the lack of descriptions of radiation therapy techniques in most trials and the use of inadequate techniques in some trials. The Bone Pain Trial Working Party prescribed all spine field doses to a depth of 5 cm regardless of the depths of the index lesions and the patients' body habitus (Level I) (BONE PAIN TRIAL WORKING PARTY 1999). The Dutch Bone Metastases Trial provided no description of techniques (Level I) (STEENLAND et al. 1999). NIELSEN et al. (1998) prescribed the dose to Dmax in their randomized trial (Level I). It is easy to glean that the actual dose delivered to the index lesions would be different from the prescribed dose, thus making the report of the existence of dose-response or lack thereof unreliable.

■ Different trials also had different patient selection criteria. BREMER et al. (1999) excluded patients with vertebral lesions or lesions in weight-bearing bones in their prospective trials (nonrandomized) (Level III). In contrast, HUGUENIN et al. (1998) included only patients with malignant melanoma and renal cell carcinoma, both of which were more "radioresistant," in their non-randomized trial (Level III).

43.2.6 Bone Healing After External-Beam Radiation Therapy

■ External-beam irradiation produces some healing and re-ossification in 65%–85% of lytic lesions in bone (BODY 1992; FORD and YARNOLD 1983; GARMATIS and CHU 1978); in most cases, there is formation of mature organized bone in the healed lesions, seemingly by direct osteogenesis. GAINOR and BUCHERT (1992) reported that radiation doses of more than 30 Gy are detrimental to bone healing in fractured long bones (Level IV). However, MATSUBAYASHI and colleagues (1981) reported that bone healing of spinal lesions was achieved with doses higher than 40 Gy and with patient survival of 6 months for bone healing to take place (Level III). These are not conflicting reports since fractured long bone heals by endochondral bone formation and vertebra heals by intra-membranous bone formation. Endochondral bone formation involves the radiosensitive chondrogenic phase, whereas the intra-membranous bone formation occurs by direct osteogenesis, which is more radioresistant.

■ If external-beam irradiation is given after fracture has occurred in a long bone, the chondrogenic phase of fracture healing can be impaired by doses usually used for treatment of bone metastases, such as 30 Gy in 10 fractions (GAINOR and BUCHERT 1992; HARRINGTON 1988b; PROBERT and

PARKER 1975). This is one of the major arguments for performing prophylactic internal fixation of impending fractures, so that the non-fractured long bone will heal by direct osteogenesis and will not be impaired by irradiation. For actual fractures of long bones, rigid immobilization with internal fixation is required for healing.

■ Duration of survival of 6 months or longer and performance of internal fixation are the important predictors of fracture healing HARRINGTON (1988c). Postoperative local irradiation is necessary, because local tumor progression has been reported to cause higher failure rates of internal fixation devices SIM et al. (1992).

43.2.7 Systemic Radionuclide Therapy

■ Radionuclide (such as Sr^{89} or Sm^{153}) therapy can be offered to patients with multiple painful bone metastases for symptomatic control (Grade A). Bone metastases treated with radionuclides generally come from breast and prostate primaries with a small number from lung primaries. The efficacy of radionuclide therapy has been demonstrated in prospective randomized trials (Level I) (HOLMES 1993; RESCHE et al. 1997; SERAFINI et al. 1998). However, studies of palliative therapy for patients with bone metastases usually suffer from high attrition rates. In the above-mentioned randomized study from SERAFINI et al. (1998), only 30% of patients completed the 16-week follow-up. The majority discontinued due to disease progression. This high attrition rate of patients in clinical trials occurred frequently in other trials as well, such as in the external-beam radiation therapy trials reported from the Royal Marsden (Level I, Level III) (PRICE et al. 1986, 1988).

■ The criteria for treatment generally require predicted duration of survival of 3 if not 6 months, adequate blood count, adequate renal function, good urinary control, and uptake of radionuclide at the index lesions. The dose of Sr^{89} and Sm^{153} suitable for bone pain now seems to be agreed upon (Grade A): 150–200 MBq for Sr^{89} and 1.0 mCi/kg for Sm^{153} (Level I) (HOLMES 1993; RESCHE et al. 1997; SERAFINI et al. 1998).

■ The onset of pain relief for radionuclide therapy varies with the half-life of the radionuclides: Sr^{89} 15 days, Sm^{153} 2–7 days, and Re^{186} 7–20 days, with duration of relief of 2–4 months (FALKMER et al.

2003). In almost all studies, a mild and transient myelosuppression was reported 3–6 weeks after the treatment depending on the radionuclide used.

■ Adequate pain medication must be administered to prevent pain flare after the radionuclide injection (Grade B). Pain flare may occur in a significant number of patients. In the series reported by KRAEBER-BODÉRÉ et al. (2003) using Sr^{89}, pain flare was observed in 23% of cases (Level IV).

■ Repeated administration of radionuclide can be offered for pain control (Grade B). However, response to repeated treatment varies, and in a phase I/II trial, ALBERTS et al. (1997) reported that only 38% of patients treated with Sm^{153} qualified for multiple treatments and toxicities increase with dosage (Level III).

 ## 43.3 Special Therapeutic Considerations for Patients with Solitary Bone Metastasis

■ Less than 10% of patients with bone metastases present with solitary bone metastases. These patients may warrant special consideration for aggressive therapy with "curative intent."

■ Selected groups of patients with a long disease-free interval with solitary bone metastasis from breast, renal, or thyroid cancer may be considered for surgical resection (Grade B). If the resection is complete, there is no need for adjuvant radiation therapy. There are reports that some patients are rendered disease-free (Level IV) (GOKASLAN et al. 1998): Patients with bone metastases from thyroid carcinoma have been reported to have 13% survival rate at 10 years (Level IV) (McLAIN and WEINSTEIN 1990). Studies of patients with bone metastases repeatedly showed that patients with lung primary fare much worse than patients with breast, prostate, and thyroid primaries (Level IV) (COLEMAN and RUBENS 1987; KOENDERS et al. 1992; LEONE et al. 1988; PITTAS et al. 2000; SCHEID et al. 1986; SHERRY et al. 1986). Patients with renal primary have an intermediate prognosis (Level IV) (HARRINGTON 1981). However, patients with solitary metastases from renal primaries have been reported to have survival rate as high as 16% at 10 years when aggressive treatments were pursued (Level IV) (KJAER 1987).

43.4   Follow-Ups and Surveillance of Survivors

■ Follow-up schedule and work-ups of patients with bone metastasis depend on the primary malignancy as well as the status of metastatic diseases.

■ Patient education regarding physical activities may help minimize the chance of fractures. Patients with spine involvement should be instructed to avoid bending positions, especially bending at the waist to pick up objects from the floor since this posture will acutely increase the load on the lumbar spine (BULLOUGH 1992). The use of a long handle grasper may help with daily routines such as putting on socks or picking up objects without bending. Twisting motion of any involved long bone should be avoided, such as twisting the legs while getting out of an automobile (Grade D) (RUBERT et al. 2000).

■ No conclusive recommendation can be provided for patient selection for an aggressive rehabilitation program. Patients who are considered for such intensive rehabilitation are usually those operated on for impending or actual fractures with remaining functional deficits. BUNTING et al. (1985) reported that 23 of 58 such patients could ambulate independently after intensive rehabilitation. Fractures rarely occur as a result of rehabilitation (Level IV).

■ Monitoring response to therapy is usually done radiographically. Radiographic studies during the follow-up phase are usually done as indicated by clinical history and/or problems (COOK and FOGELMAN 2000; PECHERSTORFER and VESELY 2000). Sclerotic healing of an initially osteolytic lesion extends from the periphery of the lesion to gradually fill in the center. Sclerosis may also appear in areas of previously normal appearing bone when healing of clinically occult lesions take place. Ultimately, areas of sclerosis from healing will diminish leaving normal looking bone. Any "flare" response to treatment is also confined to the first several months after therapy and should subside by 6 months after therapy. Radiographic monitoring of osteoblastic metastases is more challenging since an increase in size and number of lesions may be the result of response to therapy. When it presents as a diagnostic dilemma, correlation with clinical picture and laboratory evidence may be helpful.

References

Alberts AS, Smit BJ, Louw WK et al (1997) Dose response relationship and multiple dose efficacy and toxicity of samarium-153-EDTMP in metastatic cancer to bone. Radiother Oncol 43:175–179

Antoch G, Saoudi N, Kuehl H et al (2004) Accuracy of whole-body dual-modality fluorine-18-2-fluoro-2-deoxy-D-glucose positron emission tomography and computed tomography (FDG-PET/CT) for tumor staging in solid tumors: comparison with CT and PET. J Clin Oncol 22:4357–4368

Body JJ (1992) Metastatic bone disease: clinical and therapeutic aspects. Bone 13[Suppl]:557–562

Bone Pain Trial Working Party (1999) 8 Gy single fraction radiotherapy for the treatment of metastatic skeletal pain: randomised comparison with a multifraction schedule over 12 months of patient follow-up. Radiother Oncol 52:111–121

Bremer M, Rades D, Blach M (1999) Effectiveness of hypofractionated radiotherapy in painful bone metastases. Two prospective studies with 1×4 Gy and 4×4 Gy. Strahlenther Onkol 175:382–386

Bullough PG (1992) Atlas of orthopaedic pathology with clinical and radiologic correlations, 2nd ed. Gower Medical Publishing, New York, pp 6, 17–29

Bunting R, Lamont-Havers W, Schweon D et al (1985) Pathologic fracture risk in rehabilitation of patients with bony metastases. Clin Orthop Relat Res 192:222–227

Chow E, Fung K, Panzarella T et al. (2002) A predictive model for survival in metastatic cancer patients attending an outpatient palliative radiotherapy clinic. Int J Radiat Oncol Biol Phys 53:1291–1302

Coleman RE (2006) Clinical features of metastatic bone disease and risk of skeletal morbidity. Clin Cancer Res 12(20 Pt 2):6243s–6249s

Coleman RE, Rubens RD (1987) The clinical course of bone metastases from breast cancer. Br J Cancer 55:61–66

Cook GJR, Fogelman I (2000) Diagnosis and monitoring of bone metastases: scintigraphy. In: Body JJ (ed) Tumor bone disease and osteoporosis in cancer patients. Marcel Dekker, Inc., New York, pp 131–154

Falkmer U, Järhult J, Wersäll P et al (2003) A systematic overview of radiation therapy effects in skeletal metastases. Acta Oncol 42:620–633

Ford HT, Yarnold JR (1983) Radiation therapy: pain relief and medication. In: Stoll BA, Parbhoo S (eds) Bone metastases: monitoring and treatment. Raven Press, New York, p 343

Gainor BJ, Buchert P (1992) Fracture healing in metastatic bone disease. Clin Orthop Relat Res 178:297–302

Garmatis CJ, Chu FC (1978) The effectiveness of radiation therapy in the treatment of bone metastases from breast cancer. Radiology 126:235–237

Gokaslan ZL, York JE, Walsh GL et al. (1998) Transthoracic vertebrectomy for metastatic spinal tumors. J Neurosurg 89:599–609

Harrington KD (1972) The use of methacrylate as an adjunct in the internal fixation of malignant neoplastic fractures. J Bone and Joint Surg 54:1665–1676

Harrington KD (1981) The management of acetabular insufficiency secondary to metastatic malignant disease. J Bone Joint Surg Am 63:653–664

Harrington KD (1988a) Anterior decompression and stabilization of the spine as a treatment for vertebral collapse and spinal cord compression from metastatic malignancy. Clin Orthop Relat Res 233:177–197

Harrington KD (1988b) Irradiation for bone metastases. In: Harrington KD (ed) Orthopaedic management of metastatic bone disease. CV Mosby, St Louis, pp 83–94

Harrington KD (1988c) Prophylactic management of impending fractures. In: Harrington KD (ed) Orthopaedic management of metastatic bone disease. CV Mosby, St Louis, pp 283–307

Harrington KD (1995) Orthopaedic management of pelvic and extremity lesions. Clin Orthop 312:136–147

Hartsell WF, Scott CB, Bruner DW et al. (2005) Randomized trial of short- versus long-course radiotherapy for palliation of painful bone metastases. J Natl Cancer Inst 97:798–804

Heidenreich A, Elert A, Hofmann R (2002) Ibandronate in the treatment of prostate cancer associated with painful osseous metastases. Prostate Cancer Prostatic Dis 5:231–235

Heidenreich A, Ohlmann C, Olbert P et al (2003) High dose ibandronate is effective and well tolerated in the treatment of pain and hypercalcemia due to metastatic urologic cancer. Eur J Cancer 1[Suppl 5]:S270

Hillner BE, Ingle JN, Chlebowski RT et al (2003) American Society of Clinical Oncology 2003 update on the role of bisphosphonates and bone health issues in women with breast cancer. J Clin Oncol 21:4042–4057

Holmes RA (1993) Radiopharmaceuticals in clinical trials. Semin Oncol 20[Suppl 2]:22–26

Hoskin PJ, Price P, Easton D et al. (1992) A prospective randomised trial of 4 Gy or 8 Gy single doses in the treatment of metastatic bone pain. Radiother Oncol 23:74–78

Huguenin PU, Kieser S, Glanzmann C et al. (1998) Radiotherapy for metastatic carcinomas of the kidney or melanomas: an analysis using palliative end points. Int J Radiat Oncol Biol Phys 41:401–405

Kjaer M (1987) The treatment and prognosis of patients with renal adenocarcinoma with solitary metastasis. 10 Years survival results. Int J Radiat Oncol Biol Phys 13:619–621

Koenders PG, Beex LV, Kloppenborg PW et al. (1992) Human breast cancer: survival from first metastasis. Breast Cancer Study Group. Breast Cancer Res Treat 21:173–180

Kohno N, Aogi K, Minami H et al. (2005) Zoledronic acid significantly reduces skeletal complications compared with placebo in Japanese women with bone metastases from breast cancer: a randomized, placebo-controlled trial. J Clin Oncol 23:3314–3321

Kostuik JP, Errico TJ, Gleason TF et al. (1988) Spinal stabilization of vertebral column tumors. Spine 13:250–256

Koswig S, Budach V (1999) Remineralization and pain relief in bone metastases after different radiotherapy fractions (10 times 3 Gy vs. 1 time 8 Gy). A prospective study. Strahlenther Onkol 175:500–508

Kraeber-Bodéré F, Campion L, Rousseau C et al. (2000) Treatment of bone metastases of prostate cancer with strontium-89 chloride: efficacy in relation to the degree of bone involvement. Eur J Nucl Med 27:1487–1493

Leone BA, Romero A, Rabinovich MG et al. (1988) Stage IV breast cancer: clinical course and survival of patients with osseous versus extraosseous metastases at initial diagnosis. The GOCS (Grupo Oncológico Cooperativo del Sur) experience. Am J Clin Oncol 11:618–622

Mancini I, Dumon JC, Body JJ (2004) Efficacy and safety of ibandronate in the treatment of opioid-resistant bone pain associated with metastatic bone disease: a pilot study. J Clin Oncol 22:3587–3592

Matsubayashi T, Koga H, Nishyama Y et al (1981) The reparative process of metastatic bone lesions after radiotherapy. Jpn J Clin Oncol 11[Suppl]:253–264

McLain RF, Weinstein JN (1990) Tumors of the spine. Sem Spine Surg 2:157–180

Michaelson MD, Smith MR (2005) Bisphosphonates for treatment and prevention of bone metastases. J Clin Oncol 23:8219–8224

Mirels H (1989) Metastatic disease in long bones: a proposed scoring system for diagnosing impending pathologic fractures. Clin Orthop 249:256–264

Mundy GR (2002) Metastasis to bone: causes, consequences and therapeutic opportunities. Nat Rev 2:584–593

Nielsen OS, Bentzen SM, Sandberg E et al. (1998) Randomized trial of single dose versus fractionated palliative radiotherapy of bone metastases. Radiother Oncol 47:233–240

Pecherstorfer M, Vesely M (2000) Diagnosis and monitoring of bone metastases: clinical means. In: Body JJ (ed) Tumor bone disease and osteoporosis in cancer patients. Marcel Dekker, Inc., New York, pp 97–129

Pittas AG, Adler M, Fazzari M et al. (2000) Bone metastases from thyroid carcinoma: clinical characteristics and prognostic variables in one hundred forty-six patients. Thyroid 10:261–268

Price P, Hoskin PJ, Easton D et al. (1986) Prospective randomised trial of single and multifraction radiotherapy schedules in the treatment of painful bony metastases. Radiother Oncol 6:247–255

Price P, Hoskin PJ, Easton D et al. (1988) Low dose single fraction radiotherapy in the treatment of metastatic bone pain: a pilot study. Radiother Oncol 12:297–300

Probert JC, Parker BR (1975) The effects of radiation therapy on bone growth. Radiology 114:155–162

Ralston SH (2000) Treatment of tumor-induced hypercalcemia. In: Body JJ (ed) Tumor bone disease and osteoporosis in cancer patients. Marcel Dekker, Inc., New York, pp 131–154

Ratanatharathorn V, Powers WE, Moss WT et al (1999) Bone metastasis: review and critical analysis of random allocation trials of local field treatment. Int J Radiat Oncol Biol Phys 44:1–18

Ratanatharathorn V, Powers, WE, Temple HT (2004) Palliation of bone metastases. In: Perez CA, Brady LW (eds) Principles and practice of radiation oncology, 4th ed. JB Lippincott Co, Philadelphia, pp 2385–2404

Resche I, Chatal JF, Pecking A et al. (1997) A dose-controlled study of 153Sm-ethylenediaminetetramethylenephosphonate (EDTMP) in the treatment of patients with painful bone metastases. Eur J Cancer 33:1583–1591

Rubens RD (1991) The nature of metastatic bone disease. In: Rubens RD, Fogelman I (eds) Bone metastses: diagnosis and treatment. Springer-Verlag, London, pp 1–10

Rubert CK, Henshaw RM, Malawer MM (2000) Orthopedic management of skeletal metastases. In Body JJ (ed) Tumor bone disease and osteoporosis in cancer patients. Marcel Dekker, Inc., New York, pp 305–356

Salazar OM, DaMotta NW, Bridgman SM et al. (1996) Fractionated half-body irradiation (HBI) for pain palliation in widely metastatic cancer: comparison with single dose. Int J Radiat Oncol Biol Phys 36:49–60

Salazar OM, Sandhu T, da Motta NW et al. (2001) Fractionated half-body irradiation (HBI) for the rapid palliation of widespread, symptomatic, metastatic bone disease: a randomized Phase III trial of the International Atomic Energy Agency (IAEA). Int J Radiat Oncol Biol Phys 50:765–775

Scheid V, Buzdar AU, Smith TL et al. (1986) Clinical course of breast cancer patients with osseous metastasis treated with combination chemotherapy. Cancer 58:2589–2593

Serafini AN, Houston SJ, Resche I et al. (1998) Palliation of pain associated with metastatic bone cancer using samarium-153 lexidronam: a double-blind placebo-controlled clinical trial. J Clin Oncol 16:1574–1581

Sherry MM, Greco FA, Johnson DH et al. (1986) Metastatic breast cancer confined to the skeletal system. An indolent disease. Am J Med 81:381–386

Sim FH, Frassica FJ, Frassica DA (1992) Metastatic bone disease: current concepts of clinicopathophysiology and modern surgical treatment. Ann Acad Med Singapore 21:274–279

Steenland E, Leer JW, van Houwelingen H et al. (1999) The effect of a single fraction compared to multiple fractions on painful bone metastases: a global analysis of the Dutch Bone Metastasis Study. Radiother Oncol 52:101–109

Uppelschoten JM, Wanders SL, de Jong JM (1995) Single-dose radiotherapy (6 Gy): Palliation in painful bone metastases, Radiother Oncol 36:198–202

Central Nervous System Metastases

Iris C. Gibbs and Scott G. Soltys

CONTENTS

Introduction and Objectives

The central nervous system is one of the most common sites of cancer metastases; up to 40% of cancer patients develop brain metastasis in the course of their disease. Radiation plays an important role in the palliative treatment of brain metastasis. Whole brain irradiation following surgical resection (or stereotactic radiosurgery) is considered the mainstay treatment for solitary brain metastasis. Whole-brain irradiation with or without stereotactic radiosurgery is the choice of treatment for palliation in patients with more than one intracranial metastatic lesions. Stereotactic radiosurgery alone for 4 or fewer brain metastases is also a reasonable option in selected patients.

Malignant spinal cord compression is a common complication in cancer management. More than 20,000 cancer patients suffer from cord compression annually in the United States. Many commonly diagnosed malignancies, including prostate cancer, breast cancer, and lung cancer, have the propensity to cause spinal cord compression. Management of malignant spinal cord compression is challenging. Early detection and treatment of spinal cord compression is crucial for neurologic function preservation and quality of life. Treatment of malignant spinal cord requires multidisciplinary approach which often includes medication (steroids), surgery, and radiotherapy.

This chapter examines:

- Recommendations for diagnosis and evaluation for metastases to brain and malignant spinal cord compression

- Prognostic factors in patients with brain metastases and spinal cord compression

- Treatment recommendations including multi-disciplinary management plans and supporting scientific evidence

- Radiation therapy dose-fractionation and techniques for delivery including external-beam and stereotactic radiosurgery

- Follow-up care and surveillance of survivors

I. C. Gibbs, MD
S. G. Soltys, MD
Department of Radiation Oncology, Stanford University Medical Center, 875 Blake Wilbur Drive, MC 5847, Stanford, CA 94305-5847, USA

44.1 Diagnosis, Staging, and Prognoses

44.1.1 Diagnosis

Initial Evaluation

■ The diagnosis and evaluation of potential brain metastases begins with a thorough history and physical examination (H&P). Brain metastases should be suspected in patients with a known history of cancer who present with headache (40%–50%), seizure (15%–25%), impaired cognitive function (up to 65%), or neurologic symptoms (40%) such as hemiparesis, aphasia, or hemianopsia.
Although initial physical examination and neurologic exam are commonly negative, they may reveal papilledema or focal neurologic deficits.

■ The spine is the most common site of osseous tumor spread of cancer comprising 40% of skeletal metastases (Level IV) (HARRINGTON 1988; KLIMO and SCHMIDT 2004; WISE et al. 1999; WONG et al. 1990). Spinal metastases may be asymptomatic or associated with pain. More than 80% of patients with metastatic epidural spinal cord compression (MESCC) present with back pain, and symptoms progress to weakness and inability to ambulate in 60%–85% of cases. Incontinence or urinary retention may occur in up to half of patients (PRASAD and SCHIFF 2005).

Laboratory Tests

■ There are no specific laboratory tests required for the evaluation of brain metastases.
■ Basic blood chemistries including liver and renal function tests may be helpful to assess possible systemic metastases and the patient's suitability for contrast administration.

Imaging Studies

■ Contrast-enhanced magnetic resonance imaging (MRI) is the gold standard imaging modality for brain metastases. Contrast-enhanced computed tomography (CT) may be used in patients with implantable metallic devices who are unable to undergo MRI.

■ Approximately 80%, 15%, and 5% of brain metastases occurs in cerebral hemisphere, cerebellum, and brain stem, respectively. Approximately 70% of patients presenting with brain metastases have more than one intracranial lesion (DEVITA et al. 2001).
■ MRI scanning is the definitive modality for diagnosing MESCC (Grade A). Results of a systemic review supported the use of MRI as a preferred imaging technique for detecting and evaluating malignant spinal cord compression (Level I) (LOBLAW et al. 2005).
■ CT imaging of the chest, abdomen, and pelvis may be indicated in patients who present with no prior known cancer.

Pathology

■ Tissue biopsy or resection is warranted when there is uncertainty about the etiology of the brain mass(es) or when no other extracranial tumor is readily accessible for biopsy.
■ Tissue diagnosis may also be warranted for single, dural-based tumor in the setting of breast cancer as benign meningioma may co-exist.

44.1.2 Staging

■ Brain metastases generally represent distant spread and therefore, Stage IV for staging of the primary tumor.

44.1.3 Prognosis

Brain Metastasis

■ The most important prognostic factors for patients with brain metastases are age, performance status, and the status of extracranial disease.
■ Recursive partitioning analysis (RPA) of multiple trials has identified three prognostic groups based on these three factors. An analysis of the 432 patients studied in a RTOG randomized trial (RTOG 9104) was performed, and validated the three prognostic classes (Level IV) (GASPAR et al. 2000) (Table 44.1).

Table 44.1. Recursive partitioning analysis classification for brain metastases. [Adapted from GASPAR et al. (2000) and LUTTERBACH et al. (2002)]

	Median survival (months)
RPA class 1	
KPS ≥70, age <65, controlled primary, no extracranial disease	7.1
Single metastasis	13.5
Multiple metastases	6.0
RPA class 2	
KPS ≥70, and one or more of the following: age ≥65, uncontrolled primary tumor, presence of extracranial metastases	4.2
Single metastasis	8.1
Multiple metastases	4.1
RPA class 3	
KPS <70	2.3

■ The number of metastatic brain lesions may also be prognostic. A retrospective study from Germany reviewed the outcome of 916 patients with brain metastasis, and found that survival was significantly better for patients with a single brain metastasis compared with those patients having multiple metastases. The overall survival was 5.6%, 2.9%, 1.8%, and <1%, respectively, at 2, 3, 5, and 10 years (Level IV) (LUTTERBACH et al. 2002).

■ Based on patients treated with radiosurgery, another prognostic system has been devised using additional factors including age, Karnofsky performance status (KPS), systemic disease status, number of metastatic brain lesions, and volume of the largest brain lesion (Level IV) (WELTMAN et al. 2000).

■ Using these factors, each of five prognostic factors is classified into three categories and a numeric value of 0, 1, or 2 is assigned. The score index for radiosurgery (SIR) is generated by summing the values of each factor yielding a sum ranging from 0 to 10.

■ SIR sum scores of 1–3 yield median survival of 2.9 months; scores of 4–7 yield median survival of 7 months, and 8–10 yield median survival of 31.4 months (Level IV) (WELTMAN et al. 2000) (Table 44.2).

Spinal Metastasis

■ Survival of patients with MESCC varies from 0%–89%, based on the following prognostic factors:
- Tumor histology
- Time to diagnosis of MESCC
- Presence other metastatic sites
- Ambulatory status
- Duration of motor deficits

■ A scoring system using the above-listed factors was developed based on a multivariate survival analysis of 1852 patients who were treated with radiotherapy, and can be used to predict the overall survival of patients presented with MESCC (Level IV) (RADES et al. 2008). However, the scoring system awaits validation.

■ The speed of symptomatic onset is of prognostic value. Postradiation ambulatory rates are higher (86% vs. 35%) in patients with a slower onset of neurologic symptoms (>14 days) than those with acute neurologic deterioration (<7 day) (Level IV) (RADES et al. 2002).

Table 44.2. Score index for radiosurgery. [Adapted from WELTMAN et al. (2000)]

	Score Index for Radiosurgery		
	0	**1**	**2**
Age (years)	≥60	51–59	≤50
KPS	<50	60–70	>70
Systemic disease status	Progressive disease	Partial remission or stable disease	Complete clinical remission or no evidence of disease
Largest brain lesion volume (cm³)	>13	5–13	<5
Number of brain lesions	≥3	2	1

44.2 Treatment of Brain Metastases

44.2.1 General Principles

- Brain metastases are often associated with peritumoral edema; corticosteroids play an important role in initial management of symptomatic tumors and should be considered (Grade B) (Level II) (HORTON et al. 1971).
- Routine use of prophylactic anti-convulsants is not recommended for most patients with brain metastases (Grade A). The report of the Quality Standards Subcommittee of the American Academy of Neurology revealed that the lack of efficacy and potential side effects prevented the recommendation of routine use of prophylactic anti-convulsants (Level I) (GLANTZ et al. 2000).
- Traditionally, whole-brain radiotherapy (WBRT) is the mainstay of treatment of brain metastases (Grade A).
- Treatment options for brain metastases include: WBRT with or without surgery; WBRT with or without radiosurgery; or radiosurgery alone.

44.2.2 Surgical Resection of Intracranial Lesion(s)

- The role of surgery in brain metastases is generally limited to one of the following situations:
- To establish a tissue diagnosis when there is uncertainty
- To resect a single accessible brain metastasis in patients with limited or absent systemic disease
- To relieve acute mass effect in symptomatic patients (particularly tumors >3 cm in the posterior fossa)
- Surgery for multiple brain metastases remains controversial and currently is not routinely recommended (Grade C). Results from a case controlled retrospective studies demonstrated that intracranial control rates and median survival rates were similar after resection of one or more than one brain metastasis (Level IV) (BINDAL et al. 1993). A similar conclusion was found in a more recently published retrospective series of 208 patients treated with surgery in addition to WBRT from Korea (Level IV) (PAEK et al. 2005). However, conclusions from other retrospective

reviews indicated that surgery should be used with caution in patients with more than one intracranial metastasis (Level IV) (HAZUKA et al. 1993; MARTIN and KONDZIOLKA 2005).

44.2.3 Whole-Brain Radiation Therapy

- WBRT is the mainstay of treatment of brain metastases (Grade A). Radiation fields should aim to gain adequate coverage of all intracranial contents by ensuring that the blocked edges sufficiently cover the anterior cranial fossa, middle cranial fossa, and skull base (Fig 44.1)
- Results from two randomized trials from RTOG revealed that WBRT improves survival over supportive care and is associated with improved neurologic function in about half of patients (Level I) (BORGELT et al. 1980).
- Multiple dose schedules can be recommended for WBRT. A standard dose of 30 Gy delivered in 10 daily fractions or 20 Gy in five fractions can be considered (Grade A). Results from multiple retrospective series have indicated that dose escalation beyond 30 Gy in 10 daily fractions for WBRT

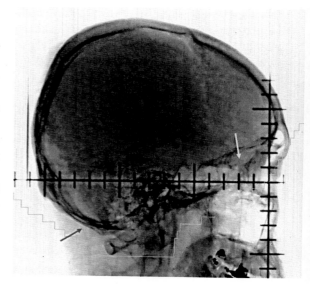

Fig. 44.1. Whole-brain radiotherapy treatment field. The field is blocked by a multi-leaf collimator and the field edge is indicated by the *cyan-colored line*. The blocked field ensures coverage of the inferior extent of the anterior cranial fossa (*yellow arrow*), middle fossa (*magenta arrow*), and the posterior fossa (*red arrow*)

was not associated with improved outcome in patients with brain metastasis.

WBRT using accelerated hyperfractionated regimen to 54.4 Gy or similar doses (using twice daily treatment at 1.6–1.8 Gy per fraction) is not recommended (Grade A). Results of a phase III randomized trial from RTOG revealed that the median survival time was 4.5 months in patients treated with accelerated hyperfractionated regimen or standard dose schedule at 30 Gy in 10 fractions, and the 1-year survival rates were 19% and 16%, respectively, without significant difference (RTOG 9104, Level I) (Murray et al. 1997).

The results from a Cochrane review demonstrated that none of the randomized clinical trials with altered dose-fractionation schemes as compared to standard delivery (30 Gy in 10 fractions) found a benefit in terms of overall survival, neurologic function, or symptom control (Level I) (Tsao et al. 2006). These findings supported the recommendation from an evidence-based clinical practice guideline on the optimal radiotherapeutic management of single and multiple brain metastases was developed and published in 2005: 30 Gy delivered in 10 daily fractions or 20 Gy in five fractions are considered standard dose for WBRT for brain metastasis (Tsao et al. 2005).

■ Acute effects of WBRT include hair loss, scalp erythema or pigmentation, somnolence, and fatigue. Late effects induced by WBRT include: dementia (2%–5%), reduced memory, radiation necrosis, leukoencephalopathy, and cerebral atrophy. Symptoms observed may include sluggishness, distractibility, personality change, memory impairment, and motor weakness (Level IV) (Conill et al. 2007; DeAngelis et al. 1989; Nieder et al. 1999).

44.2.4 Stereotactic Radiosurgery

■ Stereotactic radiosurgery is defined by highly precise beams of radiation delivered with rapid dose fall-off at the periphery of discrete, well-demarcated targets.

■ Stereotactic radiosurgery can be recommended to patients with between one and three brain metastatic lesions in combination with WBRT (Grade A). The American Society for Therapeutic Radiology and Oncology (ASTRO)'s evidence-based review of the role of radiosurgery for brain metastases re-

vealed three randomized clinical trials and seven retrospective series which compared the efficacy of WBRT alone versus WBRT plus radiosurgery boost. For patients with up to three newly diagnosed brain metastases (and in one study up to four brain metastases), the use of radiosurgery boost in addition to WBRT significantly improves intracranial control rates as compared with WBRT alone. However, no survival benefits could be observed for patients with multiple brain metastases (Level I) (Mehta et al. 2005).

■ Radiosurgery alone, deferring WBRT for salvage in patients with newly diagnosed brain metastases likely yields comparable overall survival compared to up-front WBRT alone (Level II–IV) (Chougule et al. 2000; Pirzkall et al. 1998; Rades et al. 2007a,b; Sneed et al. 1999, 2002).

The comprehensive review mentioned above from ASTRO also compared the effect of stereotactic radiosurgery alone versus radiosurgery plus WBRT and found that overall survival was not compromised in patients who did not receive WBRT; however, intracranial control was reduced if WBRT was omitted (Level I) (Mehta et al. 2005).

■ Radiation dosing for radiosurgery should be based on the size, location, and histology of the lesion. Radiation dose guidelines have been developed based on minimizing the risk of radiation necrosis.

■ General radiation dose guidelines are 15–24 Gy depending on the diameter of the lesion. These guidelines have evolved from the integrated logistic formula and an RTOG dose escalation trial (Level III–IV) (Flickinger 1989; Shaw et al. 2000; Shehata et al. 2004). The following guidelines are based on the maximum tolerated dose determined by the RTOG trial in patients with recurrent brain tumors: 24 Gy for tumors <20 mm in diameter; 18 Gy for tumors 21–30 mm; and 15 Gy for tumors 31–40 mm (Level III) (Shaw et al. 2000).

■ Radiation necrosis is the most important risk of radiosurgery.

44.2.5 Treatment of Single Brain Metastasis

■ **Combined surgical resection or stereotactic radiosurgery with WBRT should be recommended to patients with a single intracranial metastatic** lesion (Grade A). However, reasonable treatment options for single, resectable brain metastasis also include: stereotactic radiosurgery alone for tumors <3.5 cm in largest dimension; stereotactic radiosurgery plus WBRT; surgical resection followed by local therapy (e.g. GliaSite®, or postoperative radiosurgery to the resection cavity).

■ Surgical resection followed by WBRT is considered the mainstay treatment for single brain metastasis (Grade A). Several randomized trials have addressed the role of radiation and surgery for single brain metastases, and most trials demonstrated that combined surgery and radiation therapy provided improvement in neurologic functions and/or survival over either surgery or WBRT alone:

A small trial from the Netherlands randomized patients with single brain metastasis to neurosurgical excision plus radiotherapy as compared with radiotherapy alone. The results found that survival and functionally independent survival (FIS) were significantly prolonged in the group of patients treated with combined therapy. The improvement was most pronounced in patients with stable extracranial disease: the median survival and FIS were 17 months and 9 months, respectively. Patients with progressive extracranial cancer had a median overall survival of 5 months and an FIS of 2.5 months irrespective of treatment administered (Level II) (VECHT et al. 1993).

A randomized trial reported by PATCHELL et al. (1990) studied patients with single brain metastasis who were treated with WBRT alone or surgery followed by whole WBRT. The results showed that recurrence at the site of the original metastasis was less frequent in the surgery plus radiation group than in the radiation only group. The median survival times were 40 weeks versus 15 weeks, in favor of combined surgery and radiation therapy. In addition, patients treated with surgery and WBRT remained functionally independent longer as compared to those received radiation only. All differences were statistically significant (Level II).

In a second randomized trial reported by PATCHELL et al. (1998), patients with single brain metastasis were treated with surgery alone or surgery followed by WBRT. The results showed that although survival was not different between the groups, the patients treated by surgery plus WBRT experienced fewer local relapses at the original tumor site (10% vs. 46%), fewer relapses elsewhere in the brain (14% vs. 37%), and were less likely to die of neurologic causes than patients treated by surgery alone (Level II).

■ Radiosurgery can be used in combination with WBRT for the treatment of single brain metastasis (Grade A). For lesions <3.5 cm in largest dimension, results from retrospective studies have confirmed that stereotactic radiosurgery is comparable to surgery when used in combination with WBRT in terms of local control (Level IV) (MUACEVIC et al. 1999; O'NEILL et al. 2003; SCHÖGGL et al. 2000).

Furthermore, a systemic review and meta-analysis showed that although among patients with multiple metastases, no difference in survival between those treated with WBRT and stereotactice radiosurgery and those treated with WBRT was found, a significant survival benefit was observed in patients with single metastasis favoring those treated with WBRT + stereotactic radiosurgery. Intracranial tumor control at 2 years was improved with the addition of SRS to WBRT, regardless of the number of brain lesions (Level I) (STAFINSKI et al. 2006).

■ Surgical resection followed by local therapy [e.g. GliaSite (Proxima Therapeutics Inc., Alpharetta, Ga.) or postoperative radiosurgery to the resection cavity] can be recommended in selected patients with single brain metastasis (Grade B). The efficacy of GaliaSite brachytherapy prescribed to 60 Gy to 1 cm depth after resection of a single brain metastasis was studied in a multi-institutional prospective phase II trial. The local control rate, median patient survival time, and duration of functional independence were similar to those achieved with resection plus WBRT (Level III) (ROGERS et al. 2006). The effect of local treatment to the resection cavity using stereotactic radiosurgery was demonstrated in a retrospective series from Stanford University. The results of the series showed that radiosurgery administered to the resection cavity of brain metastases resulted in a 79% local control rate at 12 months, which compares favorably with historic results with observation alone (54%) and postoperative WBI (80%–90%) (Level IV) (SOLTYS et al. 2008).

■ As detailed in Section 44.2.4, other acceptable treatment options for single but unresectable brain metastasis include WBRT plus stereotactic radiosurgery (Grade A). Alternatively, radiosurgery alone can be considered (Grade C). WBRT plus stereotactic radiosurgery (Level II) (STAFINSKI et al. 2006; KONDZIOLKA et al. 1999).

44.2.6 Treatment of Oligometastases (1–3 Intracranial Lesions)

■ The management of multiple brain metastases has historically been WBRT alone. Currently, treatment options for patients with oligometastases in the brain include: (1) WBRT, (2) WBRT in combination with stereotactic radiotherapy, and (3) stereotactic radiotherapy alone.

■ Recently published evidence supports the use of stereotactic radiosurgery in combination with WBRT (Grade A). The efficacy of combined stereotactic radiosurgery and WBRT was reported in a prospective randomized study from the University of Pittsburgh. Patients with between two and four brain metastases of ≤2.5 cm in diameter were randomized to WBRT alone or WBRT plus stereotactic radiosurgery. The total dose of WBRT was 30 Gy delivered in 12 daily fractions. The results showed that there was no neurologic or systemic morbidity related to stereotactic radiosurgery. Local tumor control was significantly improved with the use of SRS: The median time to local failure was 6 months and 36 months after WBRT or WBRT plus radiosurgery, respectively; the median time to any brain failure was improved in the radiosurgery group. No significant difference was detected in median survival time in both groups (7.5 vs. 11 months, $p=0.22$) (Level II) (KONDZIOLKA et al. 1999). Randomizing patients with between one and three brain metastases between WBRT and stereotactic radiosurgery versus WBRT alone, RTOG 9508 showed that patients treated by the combined therapy experienced improved functional autonomy compared to those treated by WBRT alone. Patients with a single brain metastasis also experienced improved survival with the combined treatment (RTOG 9508, Level I) (ANDREWS et al. 2004).

■ Stereotactic radiosurgery alone can be considered for patients with up to four intracranial lesions (Grade B). Omission of WBRT in patients with between one and three metastatic intracranial lesion(s) did not appear to adversely affect survival, according to the results of a number of retrospective series (Level IV) (SNEED et al. 1999, 2002). A study randomizing patients with 1–4 brain metastases between radiosurgery alone versus WBRT plus radiosurgery, there was no survival difference observed. However, the intracranial relapse rate was more frequent when WBRT was not given (Level I) (AOYAMA et al. 2006).

44.2.7 Treatment of Multiple Brain Metastases (≥4 Intracranial Lesions)

■ Currently, WBRT therapy is the treatment of choice for patients with multiple brain metastases. Results from currently available publications do not support the routine use of surgery or stereotactic radiosurgery for treating patients with four or more intracranial metastatic lesions.

44.3 Management of Spinal Metastases

44.3.1 Treatment of Spinal Metastases Without Cord Compression

■ Orthopedic consultation is recommended for patients who may present with spinal instability, i.e., pathologic fracture, significant kyphosis, deformity, and significantly retropulsed bone fragments. Surgery followed by adjuvant radiotherapy or radiotherapy alone are traditional options for palliation of spinal metastases.

■ Radiotherapy without surgery is recommended for the following clinical presentations:

– Painful spinal metastases without epidural spinal compression
– Epidural spinal cord compression caused by radioresponsive tumors (e.g., lymphoma, multiple myeloma, leukemia, germ cell tumors)
– Medically inoperable patients
– Multiple levels of disease (POSNER 1995; SPINAZZE et al. 2005)

■ Radiotherapy can achieve greater than 80% overall pain relief for skeletal metastases including spinal metastases (FALKMER et al. 2003).

■ The treatment strategy for spinal metastasis without cord compression assimilates that of bone metastasis: Total dose of radiation dose to 30–40 Gy in 10–20 fractions is generally the preferred palliative course of treatment when a patient has a favorable life expectancy; those patients with a limited survival may be treated with 8 Gy in a single fraction (Grade A).

Multiple randomized trials and retrospective reviews have confirmed that short and long schedules of radiotherapy have similar effectiveness in early pain relief (70%–75% pain relief); however, re-treatment is required more frequently after the shorter courses (Level I and IV) (Bone Pain Trial Working Party 1999; Blitzer 1985; Hartsell et al. 2005; Niewald et al. 1996; Rasmusson et al. 1995; Tong et al. 1982). Re-irradiation rates are 20%–25% for short course (8 Gy×1) compared to 10%–15% for longer courses (20–30 Gy in 5–10 fractions) (Level I) (Wu et al. 2003).

The details of palliative radiation therapy for bone metastasis are detailed in Chapter 43.

44.3.2 Treatment of Metastatic Epidural Spinal Cord Compression (MESCC)

■ Spinal metastases may evolve to cause epidural compression of the spinal cord or cauda equine. High-dose dexamethasone should be given as an adjunct treatment in patients with metastatic epidural spinal cord compression prior to palliative radiotherapy (Grade B). A minimum dose of dexamethasone of 4 mg every 6 h can be recommended.

Treatment with dexamethasone and radiotherapy improves the gait preservation rate compared to radiotherapy alone in patients with MESCC: higher ambulation rates in patients with MSCC who received high-dose dexamethasone before radiotherapy compared with patients who did not receive corticosteroids before radiation therapy (81% vs. 63% at 3 months, respectively; $p=.046$). (Level II) (Sørensen et al. 1994).

The preservation of neurologic function is associated with the severity of neurologic symptoms and the onset of the treatment. Treatment should be initiated as soon as possible without delay.

■ Currently, combined surgery and radiation therapy is the recommended strategy for the treatment of MESCC (Grade A). Results from a retrospective study reported by Sundaresan et al. (1995) revealed that more than 80% of the patients with symptomatic malignant spinal cord compression were improved in terms of pain relief and ambulatory status after surgery. The overall median survival duration was 16 months and, apart from primary tumor, the presence of preoperative paraparesis had the most significant impact on survival (Level IV). Based on these

results and results from other retrospective data, an evidence-based guideline supported the use of surgery in combination with radiation as the emergent treatment for patients with malignant spinal cord compression (Loblaw and Laperriere 1998).

The results from a randomized phase III study confirmed that direct decompressive surgery given prior to palliative radiotherapy (30 Gy given in 10 daily fractions) improved prognosis: Approximately 84% of patients were able to ambulate after combined surgery and radiotherapy, as compared to 57% among patients received radiation only. In addition, patients treated with surgery also retained the ability to walk significantly longer, and more patients in the surgery group regained the ability to walk than patients in the radiation group (62% vs. 19%) (Level I) (Patchell et al. 2005).

Radiation Therapy

■ Similar to bone metastases, the rate of pain and neurologic symptom relief are the same for short- or long-course radiotherapy schedules, with approximately 25%–30% of patients with improved motor function.

■ A total dose of 30 Gy in 10 fractions is considered the standard for radiation therapy for MESCC (Grade B). When radiation therapy is used alone, the failure rate at 2 years is 24%–26% for short-course (8 Gy×1, 5 Gy×4) vs. 7%–14% for long-course (3 Gy×10, 2.5 Gy×15, 2 Gy×20) radiotherapy (Level IV) (Rades et al. 2005). In addition, there is no apparent benefit to treatment schedules escalated beyond 30 Gy in 10 fractions (Level IV) (Rades et al. 2007c, 2008).

■ Results from prospective trials show that approximately three-quarters of patients are ambulatory post-treatment and 54%–59% show complete relief of back pain (Maranzano and Latini 1995; Maranzano et al. 1997, 2005).

Surgery and Radiotherapy

■ Patients with neurologic symptoms due to a single level of MESCC due to a non-radiosensitive histology, who have <48 h of paraplegic symptoms, >3-month life expectancy, and are medically operable, should be treated with direct decompressive surgery (not a simple laminectomy) followed by 30 Gy radiotherapy rather than radiotherapy alone (Grade A). As detailed above, patients with these characteristics treated with surgery followed by palliative radiation in the randomized trial reported by PATCHELL et al. (2005) had significantly improved outcome as compared to those received radiation only: overall post-treatment ambulatory rates were 84% in surgical patients compared to only 57% with radiation alone. In non-ambulatory patients, 62% vs. 19% regained the ability to walk with surgery compared to radiotherapy alone (Level I).

Spinal Stereotactic Radiosurgery

■ With advances in linear accelerator technology, the application of stereotactic radiosurgical principles for the treatment of spinal lesions is an emerging option (Fig. 44.2).
■ Spinal stereotactic radiosurgery, given in one to five days, may be used in the primary setting or in those who have already received prior radiotherapy (Grade B). Pain relief and local control from a short course of SRS appear comparable to a long course of radiotherapy; with better local control than short course schedules (Level IV) (Table 44.3).
■ Dose guidelines are evolving for stereotactic radiosurgery. Typical doses are 16–30 Gy in between one and five fractions. Dose prescriptions also take into account the dose delivered to the spinal cord and cauda equina.
■ Although the tolerance of neural structures in stereotactic radiosurgery is unknown, care is taken to avoid complications by limiting the partial volume of the neural contents in the high-dose region.
■ Typical dose constraints are:
– Limit the volume of cord/cauda that receives the single-dose equivalent of 8–12 Gy to <1 cm^3 or
– Limit no more than 10% of the volume of the cord/cauda to receive 10 Gy or higher (GERSZTEN et al. 2007; CHANG 2007; GIBBS et al. 2007)

44.4 Follow-Ups

44.4.1 Post-Treatment Follow-Ups

■ Life-long follow-up after treatment of malignant CNS metastasis is recommended (Grade D) (NATIONAL COMPREHENSIVE CANCER NETWORK 2008). However, no conclusive recommendation can be provided for patient selection for an aggressive rehabilitation program.

Schedule and Work-Ups

■ Follow-ups could be scheduled every 3 months.
■ Each follow-up after treatment of brain metastasis should include a complete history and physical examination, including a neurologic examination. MRI of the brain every 3 months for 1 year and then as clinically indicated can be recommended (Grade D) (NATIONAL COMPREHENSIVE CANCER NETWORK 2008). Further treatment after

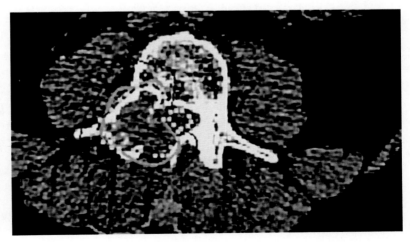

Fig. 44.2. Stereotactic radiosurgery isodose plan for a spinal metastasis involving the right L4 lamina and transverse process. The target tumor is outlined in *red* with *yellow points* while the prescription isodose line is indicated by the *green curve*. The spinal neural contents are shown centrally. The 50% isodose surface (*purple curve*) shows the rapid dose fall-off and the selective dose gradient to spare the neural structure

Table 44.3. Results from initial studies of spinal stereotactic radiosurgery

Reference	No. of targets	Median follow-up (months)	Prior radiation (%)	Local control (%)	Pain relief (%)
RYU et al. (2008)	61	13	0	NR	84
DEGEN et al. (2005)	58	12	53	88	97
GIBBS et al. (2007)	102	9	74	NR	84
GERSZTEN et al. (2007)	500	21	87	92	86
CHANG et al. (2007)	74	21	56	84	NR
YAMADA et al. (2008)	103	15	0	90	NR

NR, not reported

intracranial recurrence depends on the status of patients' general condition, systemic disease, and previous treatment.

■ Each follow-up after treatment of spinal cord compression should include a complete history and physical examination, including a neurologic examination. Laboratory tests and imaging studies can be ordered as clinically indicated.

References

Aoyama H, Shirato H, Tago M et al. (2006) Stereotactic radiosurgery plus whole-brain radiotherapy vs. stereotactic radiosurgery alone for treatment of brain metastases: a randomized controlled trial. JAMA 295:2483–2491

Andrews DW, Scott CB, Sperduto PW et al. (2004) Whole brain radiation therapy with or without stereotactic radiosurgery boost for patients with one to three brain metastases: phase III results of the RTOG 9508 randomised trial. Lancet 363:1665–1672

Bindal RK, Sawaya R, Leavens ME et al. (1993) Surgical treatment of multiple brain metastases. J Neurosurg 79:210–216

Blitzer PH (1985) Reanalysis of the RTOG study of the palliation of symptomatic osseous metastasis. Cancer 55:1468–1472

Bone Pain Trial Working Party (1999) 8 Gy single fraction radiotherapy for the treatment of metastatic skeletal pain: randomised comparison with a multifraction schedule over 12 months of patient follow-up. Bone Pain Trial Working Party. Radiother Oncol 52:111–121

Borgelt B, Gelber R, Kramer S et al. (1980) The palliation of brain metastases: final results of the first two studies by the Radiation Therapy Oncology Group. Int J Radiat Oncol Biol Phys 6:1–9

Chang EL, Shiu AS, Mendel E, et al. (2007) Phase I/II study of stereotactic body radiotherapy for spinal metastasis and its pattern of failure. J Neurosurg Spine 7:151–160

Chougule P, Burton-Williams M, Saris S, Zheng Z (2000) Randomized treatment of brain metastases with gamma knife radiosurgery, whole brain radiotherapy or both. Int J Radiat Oncol Biol Phys 48[Suppl 3]:114

Conill C, Berenguer J, Vargas M et al. (2007) Incidence of radiation-induced leukoencephalopathy after whole brain radiotherapy in patients with brain metastases. Clin Transl Oncol 9:590–595

DeAngelis LM, Delattre JY, Posner JB (1989) Radiation-induced dementia in patients cured of brain metastases. Neurology 39:789–796

Degen JW, Gagnon GJ, Voyadzis JM et al. (2005) CyberKnife stereotactic radiosurgical treatment of spinal tumors for pain control and quality of life. J Neurosurg Spine 2:540–549

DeVita VT Jr, Hellman S, Rosenberg SA (2001) Principle and practice of oncology, 6th ed. Lippincott Williams & Wilkins, Philadelphia

Falkmer U, Jarhult J, Wersall P, Cavallin-Stahl E (2003) A systematic overview of radiation therapy effects in skeletal metastases. Acta Oncol 42:620–633

Flickinger JC (1989) An integrated logistic formula for prediction of complications from radiosurgery. Int J Radiat Oncol Biol Phys 17:879–885

Gaspar LE, Scott C, Murray K et al. (2000) Validation of the RTOG recursive partitioning analysis (RPA) classification for brain metastases. Int J Radiat Oncol Biol Phys 47:1001–1006

Gerszten PC, Burton SA, Ozhasoglu C, Welch WC (2007) Radiosurgery for spinal metastases: clinical experience in 500 cases from a single institution. Spine 32:193–199

Gibbs IC, Kamnerdsupaphon P, Ryu MR et al. (2007) Image-guided robotic radiosurgery for spinal metastases. Radiother Oncol 82:185–190

Glantz MJ, Cole BF, Forsyth PA et al. (2000) Practice parameter: anticonvulsant prophylaxis in patients with newly diagnosed brain tumors. Report of the Quality Standards Subcommittee of the American Academy of Neurology. Neurology 54:1886–1893

Harrington KD (1988) Anterior decompression and stabilization of the spine as a treatment for vertebral collapse and spinal cord compression from metastatic malignancy. Clin Orthop (233):177–197

Hartsell WF, Scott CB, Bruner DW et al. (2005) Randomized trial of short- versus long-course radiotherapy for palliation of painful bone metastases. J Natl Cancer Inst 97:798–804

Hazuka MB, Burleson WD, Stroud DN et al. (1993) Multiple brain metastases are associated with poor survival in patients with surgery and radiotherapy. J Clin Oncol 11:369–373

Horton J, Baxter DH, Olson KB (1971) The management of metastases to the brain by irradiation and corticosteroids. Am J Roentgenol Radium Ther Nucl Med 111:334–336

Klimo P Jr, Schmidt MH (2004) Surgical management of spinal metastases. Oncologist 9:188–196

Kondziolka D, Patel A, Lunsford LD, Kassam A, Flickinger JC (1999) Stereotactic radiosurgery plus whole brain radiotherapy versus radiotherapy alone for patients with multiple brain metastases. Int J Radiat Oncol Biol Phys 45:427–434

Loblaw DA, Laperriere NJ (1998) Emergency treatment of malignant extradural spinal cord compression: an evidence-based guideline. J Clin Oncol 16:1613–1624

Loblaw DA, Perry J, Chambers A et al. (2005) Systematic review of the diagnosis and management of malignant extradural spinal cord compression: the Cancer Care Ontario Practice Guidelines Initiative's Neuro-Oncology Disease Site Group. J Clin Oncol 23:2028–2037

Lutterbach J, Bartelt S, Ostertag C (2002) Long-term survival in patients with brain metastases. J Cancer Res Clin Oncol 128:417–425

Maranzano E, Latini P (1995) Effectiveness of radiation therapy without surgery in metastatic spinal cord compression: final results from a prospective trial. Int J Radiat Oncol Biol Phys 32:959–967

Maranzano E, Latini P, Perrucci E, Beneventi S, Lupattelli M, Corgna E (1997) Short-course radiotherapy (8 Gy × 2) in metastatic spinal cord compression: an effective and feasible treatment. Int J Radiat Oncol Biol Phys 38:1037–1044

Maranzano E, Bellavita R, Rossi R et al. (2005) Short-course versus split-course radiotherapy in metastatic spinal cord compression: results of a phase III, randomized, multicenter trial. J Clin Oncol 23:3358–3365

Martin JJ, Kondziolka D (2005) Indications for resection and radiosurgery for brain metastases. Curr Opin Oncol 17:584–587

Mehta MP, Tsao MN, Whelan TJ et al. (2005) The American Society for Therapeutic Radiology and Oncology (ASTRO) evidence-based review of the role of radiosurgery for brain metastases. Int J Radiat Oncol Biol Phys 63:37–46

Muacevic A, Kreth FW, Horstmann GA et al. (1999) Surgery and radiotherapy compared with gamma knife radiosurgery in the treatment of solitary cerebral metastases of small diameter. J Neurosurg 91:35–43

Murray KJ, Scott C, Greenberg HM et al. (1997) A randomized phase III study of accelerated hyperfractionation versus standard in patients with unresected brain metastases: a report of the Radiation Therapy Oncology Group (RTOG) 9104. Int J Radiat Oncol Biol Phys 39:571–574

National Comprehensive Cancer Network (2008) Clinical practice guidelines in oncology: central nervous system cancers. Version I.2008. Available at http://www.nccn.org/professionals/physician_gls/PDF/cns.pdf. Accessed on March 28, 2008

Nieder C, Leicht A, Motaref B, Nestle U, Niewald M, Schnabel K (1999) Late radiation toxicity after whole brain radiotherapy: the influence of antiepileptic drugs. Am J Clin Oncol 22:573–579

Niewald M, Tkocz HJ, Abel U et al. (1996) Rapid course radiation therapy vs. more standard treatment: a randomized trial for bone metastases. Int J Radiat Oncol Biol Phys 36:1085–1089

O'Neill BP, Iturria NJ, Link MJ, Pollock BE, Ballman KV, O'Fallon JR (2003) A comparison of surgical resection and stereotactic radiosurgery in the treatment of solitary brain metastases. Int J Radiat Oncol Biol Phys 55:1169–1176

Paek SH, Audu PB, Sperling MR, Cho J, Andrews DW (2005) Reevaluation of surgery for the treatment of brain metastases: review of 208 patients with single or multiple brain metastases treated at one institution with modern neurosurgical techniques. Neurosurgery 56:1021–1034; discussion 1021–1034

Patchell RA, Tibbs PA, Walsh JW et al. (1990) A randomized trial of surgery in the treatment of single metastases to the brain. N Engl J Med 322:494–500

Patchell RA, Tibbs PA, Regine WF et al. (1998) Postoperative radiotherapy in the treatment of single metastases to the brain: a randomized trial. JAMA 280:1485–1489

Patchell RA, Tibbs PA, Regine WF et al. (2005) Direct decompressive surgical resection in the treatment of spinal cord compression caused by metastatic cancer: a randomised trial. Lancet 366:643–648

Pirzkall A, Debus J, Lohr F et al. (1998) Radiosurgery alone or in combination with whole-brain radiotherapy for brain metastases. J Clin Oncol 16:3563–3569

Posner JB (1995) Spinal metastases. In: Neurologic complications of cancer. FA Davis Company, Philadelphia, pp 111–142

Prasad D, Schiff D (2005) Malignant spinal-cord compression. Lancet Oncol 6:15–24

Rades D, Heidenreich F, Karstens JH (2002) Final results of a prospective study of the prognostic value of the time to develop motor deficits before irradiation in metastatic spinal cord compression. Int J Radiat Oncol Biol Phys 53:975–979

Rades D, Stalpers LJ, Veninga T et al. (2005) Evaluation of five radiation schedules and prognostic factors for metastatic spinal cord compression. J Clin Oncol 23:3366–3375

Rades D, Bohlen G, Pluemer A et al. (2007a) Stereotactic radiosurgery alone versus resection plus whole-brain radiotherapy for 1 or 2 brain metastases in recursive partitioning analysis class 1 and 2 patients. Cancer 109:2515–2521

Rades D, Pluemer A, Veninga T et al. (2007b) Whole-brain radiotherapy versus stereotactic radiosurgery for patients in recursive partitioning analysis classes 1 and 2 with 1 to 3 brain metastases. Cancer 110:2285–2292

Rades D, Karstens JH, Hoskin PJ et al. (2007c) Escalation of radiation dose beyond 30 Gy in 10 fractions for metastatic spinal cord compression. Int J Radiat Oncol Biol Phys 67:525–531

Rades D, Dunst J, Schild SE (2008) The first score predicting overall survival in patients with metastatic spinal cord compression. Cancer 112:157–161

Rasmusson B, Vejborg I, Jensen AB et al. (1995) Irradiation of bone metastases in breast cancer patients: a randomized study with 1 year follow-up. Radiother Oncol 34:179–184

Rogers LR, Rock JP, Sills AK et al. (2006) Results of a phase II trial of the GliaSite radiation therapy system for the treatment of newly diagnosed, resected single brain metastases. J Neurosurg 105:375–384

Ryu S, Jin R, Jin JY et al. (2008) Pain control by image-guided radiosurgery for solitary spinal metastasis. J Pain Symptom Manage 35:292–298

Schöggl A, Kitz K, Reddy M et al. (2000) Defining the role of stereotactic radiosurgery versus microsurgery in the treatment of single brain metastases. Acta Neurochir (Wien) 142:621–626

Shaw E, Scott C, Souhami L et al. (2000) Single dose radiosurgical treatment of recurrent previously irradiated primary brain tumors and brain metastases: final report of RTOG protocol 90-05. Int J Radiat Oncol Biol Phys 47:291–298

Shehata MK, Young B, Reid B et al. (2004) Stereotactic radiosurgery of 468 brain metastases < or =2 cm: implications for SRS dose and whole brain radiation therapy. Int J Radiat Oncol Biol Phys 59:87–93

Sneed PK, Lamborn KR, Forstner JM et al. (1999) Radiosurgery for brain metastases: is whole brain radiotherapy necessary? Int J Radiat Oncol Biol Phys 43:549–558

Sneed PK, Suh JH, Goetsch SJ et al. (2002) A multi-institutional review of radiosurgery alone vs. radiosurgery with whole brain radiotherapy as the initial management of brain metastases. Int J Radiat Oncol Biol Phys 53:519–526

Soltys SG, Adler JR, Lipani JD et al. (2008) Stereotactic radiosurgery of the postoperative resection cavity for brain metastases. Int J Radiat Oncol Biol Phys 70:187–193

Sørensen S, Helweg-Larsen S, Mouridsen H et al. (1994) Effect of high-dose dexamethasone in carcinomatous metastatic spinal cord compression treated with radiotherapy: a randomised trial. Eur J Cancer 30A:22–27

Spinazze S, Caraceni A, Schrijvers D (2005) Epidural spinal cord compression. Crit Rev Oncol Hematol 56:397–406

Sundaresan N, Sachdev VP, Holland JF et al. (1995) Surgical treatment of spinal cord compression from epidural metastasis. J Clin Oncol 13:2330–2335

Stafinski T, Jhangri GS, Yan E, Menon D (2006) Effectiveness of stereotactic radiosurgery alone or in combination with whole brain radiotherapy compared to conventional surgery and/or whole brain radiotherapy for the treatment of one or more brain metastases: a systematic review and meta-analysis. Cancer Treat Rev 32:203–213

Tong D, Gillick L, Hendrickson FR (1982) The palliation of symptomatic osseous metastases: final results of the Study by the Radiation Therapy Oncology Group. Cancer 50:893–899

Tsao MN, Lloyd NS, Wong RK et al. (2005) BMC Clinical practice guideline on the optimal radiotherapeutic management of brain metastases. BMC Cancer 5:34

Tsao MN, Lloyd NS, Wong RK et al. (2006) Cochrane Database Syst Rev. 2006 Jul 19;3:CD003869

Vecht CJ, Haaxma-Reiche H, Noordijk EM et al. (1993) Treatment of single brain metastasis: radiotherapy alone or combined with neurosurgery? Ann Neurol 33:583–590

Weltman E, Salvajoli JV, Brandt RA et al. (2000) Radiosurgery for brain metastases: a score index for predicting prognosis. Int J Radiat Oncol Biol Phys 46:1155–1161

Wise JJ, Fischgrund JS, Herkowitz HN, Montgomery D, Kurz LT (1999) Complication, survival rates, and risk factors of surgery for metastatic disease of the spine. Spine 24:1943–1951

Wong DA, Fornasier VL, MacNab I (1990) Spinal metastases: the obvious, the occult, and the impostors. Spine 15:1–4

Wu JS, Wong R, Johnston M, Bezjak A, Whelan T (2003) Meta-analysis of dose-fractionation radiotherapy trials for the palliation of painful bone metastases. Int J Radiat Oncol Biol Phys 55:594–605

Yamada Y, Bilsky MH, Lovelock DM et al. (2008) High-dose, single-fraction image-guided intensity-modulated radiotherapy for metastatic spinal lesions. Int J Radiat Oncol Biol Phys, Epub ahead of print

Section XII:
Radiation Biology and Physics

Medical Imaging Modalities in Radiotherapy

45

Dimitre Hristov and Lei Xing

CONTENTS

Introduction and Objectives

Therapeutic ratio improvement by exploiting the highly conformal distributions that are enabled by current image-guided radiation delivery systems depends on the accurate identification and localization of both treatment targets and healthy structures. While imaging is indispensable in accomplishing this task, the reflection of disease-related morphological and functional features in 3D and 4D medical image datasets is determined by: physical contrast generation mechanisms; imaging system design, performance, and capabilities; and clinical acquisition protocols. The intent of this chapter is to provide an overview of the above factors for the most widely used medical imaging modalities in radiotherapy. Thus this chapter examines, to varying degrees of detail:

● Computed tomography (CT)
● Positron emission tomography-computed tomography (PET/CT)
● Magnetic resonance imaging (MRI)

45.1 Computed Tomography

45.1.1 Imaging Principles and Information Content

Image Acquisition and Reconstruction

■ A modern multi-slice CT scanner and its major components are illustrated in Figure 45.1. A gantry-mounted fan pair comprising an X-ray source and detector array (Fig. 45.1) rotates continuously around a subject at between one and three revolutions per second as the subject is advanced through the scanner bore in continuous (spiral or helical scanning) or incremental (axial scanning)

D. Hristov, PhD; L. Xing, PhD
Department of Radiation Oncology, Stanford University School of Medicine, 875 Blake Wilbur Drive, Stanford, CA 94305-5847, USA

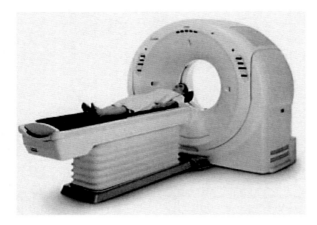

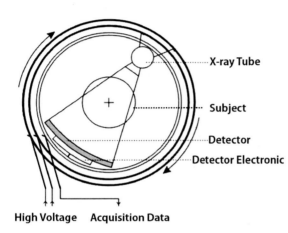

Fig. 45.1. A modern multi-slice CT scanner and its major component

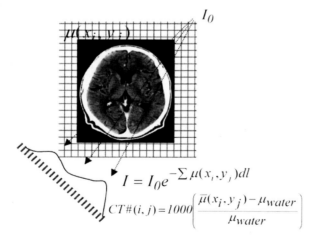

$$I = I_0 e^{-\sum \mu(x_i, y_j) dl}$$

$$CT\#(i, j) = 1000 \left(\frac{\bar{\mu}(x_i, y_j) - \mu_{water}}{\mu_{water}} \right)$$

Fig. 45.2. The physical principles of CT acquisition. The CT detector array registers projections comprising the subject integral attenuation along rays between individual detectors and the X-ray source

fashion. Projection data containing the integral X-ray attenuation along paths connecting the X-ray source and the individual detectors within the array is measured (Fig. 45.2). These projections are filtered with various convolution kernels depending on the selected clinical reconstruction protocol and then backprojected to reconstruct a CT image or slice (Oppelt 2006).

- Current multi-slice CT scanners use many (16–320) detector rows allowing a number of slices to be measured simultaneously. This leads to reduction in scan time and better utilization of the X-ray source output. However, depending on the clinical protocol only a subset of the detector rows may be used (Oppelt 2006).

Acquisition Parameters

- Scan type: spiral (or helical) and axial.
- X-ray tube high voltage measured in kVs. It controls the X-ray source radiation exposure rate (for fixed tube current) as well as the spectrum of the X-ray beam. The latter influences the radiographic contrast of the CT images. Typical high voltage values range between 80 and 140 kV.
- X-ray tube current measured in mA. It controls the radiation exposure rate and thus the signal-to-noise ratio in the CT images. The latter directly affect the detection of low-contrast objects (Sprawls 1992). While CT systems allow a large range from ~10 mA to ~500 mA, for given scan parameters the maximum value of the X-ray tube current is most often limited automatically by the finite X-ray tube heat load capacity. The product of the X-ray tube current and the scan exposure time (measured in mAs) is the major dose determining parameter. Typical effective dose values range between 1–15 mSv depending on the acquisition technique and the body site (McCollough et al. 2008a).
- Pitch defined as the ratio of table travel per rotation in millimeters divided by the beam collimation. Typical pitch values range between 0.1 and 2. While small pitch values improve the image resolution along the scan axis, larger pitch values result in smaller imaging doses.

Information Content

- A CT image is a discrete 2D matrix representation of the spatial distribution of the X-ray attenuation coefficient within a scanned object. For a particular matrix element or pixel (i, j), the corresponding CT number $CT\#(i, j)$ measures the relative value of the average attenuation coefficient $\mu(x_i, y_j)$ in Hounsfield units (HU), thus

$$CT\#(i, j) = 1000 \left(\frac{\bar{\mu}(x_i, y_j) - \mu_{water}}{\mu_{water}} \right)$$

- where μ_{water} is adjusted so as to give water a pixel value of zero independent of the X-ray spectrum. A normal CT scale ranges from −1024 HU to 3071 HU. Extended CT scales are available as an off-line post-processing option for patients with metallic implants (COOLENS and CHILDS 2003).
- The CT value of human tissues depends on the kV setting for the CT scan. Representative CT values for some human tissues are given in Figure 45.3.
- A typical patient's 3D CT data set comprises more than 100 2D images (or slices), each of which contains 512×512 pixels. With 16 bits per pixel, the size of such dataset exceeds 50 megabytes.
- CT imaging is characterized by high spatial integrity, excellent reproducibility, high cross sectional spatial resolution (<1 mm) and low contrast sensitivity (<0.5%) for typical imaging doses.

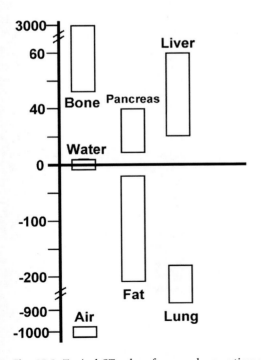

Fig. 45.3. Typical CT values for some human tissues

45.1.2 CT Simulators

Specifications for Hardware and Software Components

- A CT simulator is a CT system with additional hardware and software components to enable radiation therapy simulation and planning based on CT-generated model of the patient anatomy.
- A flat table top is necessary to reproduce the treatment position intended for radiation delivery.
- Large bore size (~80 cm) is required to provide maximum flexibility for patient setup. For instance, such a bore facilitates the CT simulation of breast patients on inclined breast boards.
- Extended field-of-view (FOV) reconstruction is necessary to capture the anatomy of large patients and provide skin contours for evaluation of the delivered dose. Since extended FOV reconstruction requires projection extrapolation beyond the acquisition FOV (~50 cm), the fidelity of the CT numbers in the periphery of the FOV needs to be examined.
- Localizing (movable) lasers are to be included for facilitating the radiation therapist with the patient setup and skin marks.
- Large X-ray tube heat capacity exceeding 6 Mega Heat Units (MHU) is necessary to enable four-dimensional respiratory correlated CT scans (4D CT) with clinically useful scan range as well thin slice CT scans.
- Large detector array (>16 rows) is necessary to allow large scan coverage at high resolution. This is beneficial for single breath-hold imaging as well as 4D imaging.
- Extended HU scale is beneficial in scanning patients with metal implants.
- Respiratory gating option is to be included for retrospective 4D CT or prospective gated CT acquisition.

CT Scanning and Image Interpretation Principles

- Scan limits need to encompass all relevant anatomy for accurate calculation of dose and dose derived indices such as dose-volume histograms (DVHs).
- Thin slice imaging is important for treatment sites such as head and neck (H&N), prostate, and lung since the CT volume or digitally reconstructed radiographs (DRRs) derived from the CT are subsequently used as reference data in image-guided radiation delivery.

- Extended HU scale with proper HU-to-electron density calibration can reduce dose calculation uncertainty for patients with metal implants. However, an extended scale does not necessarily eliminate image artifacts.
- Clinical scanning protocols need to be created and used consistently since HU, depending on the kV settings and reconstruction algorithms, are converted to electron density for accurate dose calculation.
- Visualization and interpretation of CT images depend on the acquisition and the reconstruction parameters as well as the display setting used for viewing the data. The apparent size of a structure depends on the window-level settings. These need to be standardized and followed consistently.

45.1.3 4D CT Imaging

Description and Clinical Applications

- 4D CT imaging refers to CT imaging techniques that allow the acquisition of respiratory-correlated scans (VEDAM et al. 2003; RIETZEL et al. 2005b; PAN et al. 2004; KEALL et al. 2004; LI et al. 2005). Such scans can be acquired by prospective gating whereby imaging is performed only during a predetermined respiratory state or by retrospective respiratory correlated sorting of CT images that capture several states of the breathing cycle. The latter approach is referred to as retrospective 4D CT.
- A retrospective 4D CT allows: (i) mitigation of image artifacts caused by respiratory-correlated internal anatomy motion; (ii) evaluation of the pattern and magnitude of the internal motion; and (iii) design of strategies for its management in the course of radiotherapy. These strategies include generation of patient-specific margins for target volumes (UNDERBERG et al. 2004, 2005; RIETZEL et al. 2005a), breath-hold radiation delivery (WONG et al. 1999), or gated delivery (VEDAM et al. 2001, KUBO and HILL 1996, OHARA et al. 1989, WINK et al. 2008). 4D CT forms the basis for respiratory motion management in radiation therapy (KEALL et al. 2006; WINK et al. 2008).

Acquisition and Reconstruction

- The retrospective 4D CT scanning process includes three relatively independent steps: record-

ing of respiratory signal(s), acquisition of time-dependent CT projection data, and construction of a 4D image from these data.
- 4D CT patient setup proceeds along the same lines as a standard 3D CT exam. The patient is immobilized on the scanner bed and aligned using room and scanner lasers. Sagittal and coronal scout images are used to verify patient positioning, and the setup is adjusted as necessary. At this stage of the setup, the 4D procedure begins to diverge from the 3D exam.
- Respiratory signal is recorded by tracking a surrogate of respiration-related organ and tumor motion, such as chest expansion monitored by pneumatic bellows (KLESHNEVA et al. 2006) or displacements of a reflecting external marker placed on the abdomen and tracked with a camera (PAN et al. 2004) (Fig. 45.4).
- Once a sufficiently regular breathing pattern is established, time-stamped CT data is acquired in either over-sampled helical (pitch ~0.1) or "cine" mode. The latter is a step-and-shoot technique, whereby the gantry completes several rotations at each bed position in order to acquire data over the full respiratory cycle. With either mode, several CT slices are generated that capture the anatomy over the full respiratory cycle at each axial location. Because several respiratory points are sampled at each bed position, a 4D CT scan can take several times as long as a corresponding 3D CT. A 4D CT scan typically results in 1500–3000 CT slices for a 20- to 40-cm axial FOV.
- Upon scan completion, phase or amplitude at each point of the respiratory trace is calculated. In the

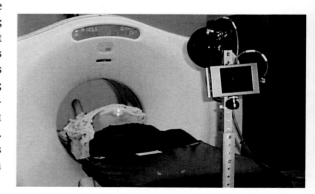

Fig. 45.4. 4D CT acquisition with an infrared camera tracking system consisting of an infrared source, CCD camera, and a reflecting block. The block is attached to the patient's abdomen, typically just inferior to the xiphoid process, and the motion of the block is captured by the camera

case of phase calculation, the location of the peaks at end-inspiration is determined, and percentages to inter-peak points are assigned by a linear interpolation of the peak-to-peak distance. For example, under this scheme, end-inspiration occurs at 0%, while end-expiration typically appears near 50%–60%. The peak-to-peak distance can vary between respiratory cycles, as can the position of end-expiration with respect to end-inspiration.

■ The respiratory and scan data are combined by sorting the over-sampled time-stamped CT slices according to their phase. Thus different CT series labeled in accordance with the respiratory state are generated (Fig. 45.5). These form the basis for 4D treatment planning.

■ 4D CT effective doses are about a factor of 5–10 larger than those for standard thorax exams (LI et al. 2005).

45.1.4 Linac Integrated CT and Cone-Beam CT

■ Cone-beam CT (CBCT) is an imaging modality which employs a large area (cone) X-ray beam and a flat panel detector technology for the reconstruction of 3D dataset from a number of 2D projections acquired from a subject (XING et al. 2006).

■ While analogous to CT, CBCT differs in two main aspects: detector technology and collimation of the imaging beam impinging on the subject. For comparable imaging doses, these factors result in CBCT image quality somewhat inferior to that of CT.

■ Linac-integrated kV CBCT refers to a combination a kV range X-ray source and a flat-panel detector mounted on the drum of a medical accelerator with the kV imaging axis orthogonal to that of MV therapy beam (JAFFRAY and SIEWERDSEN 2000).

■ Linac-integrated megavoltage CBCT refers to an imaging mode of the linac delivery system that employs the megavoltage treatment beam as an imaging source in combination with a flat-panel detector mounted opposing to the treatment source (POULIOT et al. 2005). The physics of radiation-matter interaction at megavoltage energies affects the MV CBCT image quality.

■ Linac-integrated CT refers to a dedicated delivery system that integrates a 6 MV MV treatment source and an array of CT detectors on a CT gantry (MEEKS et al. 2005; LANGEN et al. 2005a,b; KUPELIAN et al. 2005).

■ 3D CBCT (or CT) images are used for on-line verification and correction of patient setup. The images are registered with the planning CT data through the use of either manual or automated 3D image registration software that calculates shifts in x-, y- and z-directions (depending on the manufacturer, rotations can also be included). The movements determined during the registration represent the required setup corrections that are applied by displacing the treatment couch (WHITE et al. 2007; MOSELEY et al. 2007; LETOURNEAU et al. 2005; GAYOU and MIFTEN 2007; XING et al. 2006).

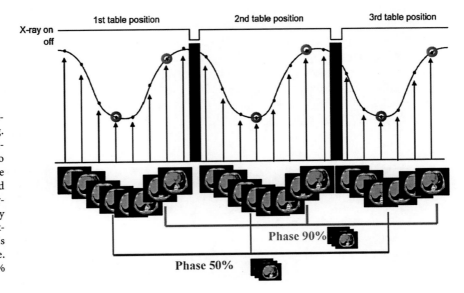

Fig. 45.5. 4D CT reconstruction by retrospective sorting. At each table position time-stamped images belonging to a particular respiratory state are selected and combined in a separate 3D dataset corresponding to the respiratory state. (In this particular example the respiratory state is labeled by a respiratory phase. The 50% phase and the 90% phase are reconstructed)

45.1.5 Quality Assurance

- CT scanner quality assurance programs need to target the minimum standards for dose and image quality established by the American College of Radiology (ACR) Computed Tomography Accreditation Program.
- Quality assurance guidelines for CT simulators covering radiation and patient safety, electromechanical components, as well as imaging performance are provided in an American Association of Physicists in Medicine (AAPM) report by Task Group 66 (MUTIC et al. 2003).
- CBCT quality assurance, methods, and guidelines are described in (LETOURNEAU et al. 2007; MAO et al. 2008; YOO et al. 2006).

45.2   Positron Emission Tomography–Computed Tomography (PET/CT)

45.2.1 PET Principles and Information Content

PET Physical Basis and Data Acquisition

- A radioactive isotope (Table 45.1) typically conjugated to some molecule of biological interest, decays via positron emission (Fig. 45.6a). The emitted positron travels some distance based on its energy (<1 mm–4 mm) before it encounters an electron and annihilates. The annihilation produces two 511 keV photons at approximately 180°, minus some small angle (~0.5°) due to the energy of the positron (Fig. 45.6b).
- The 511 keV photons are stopped by scintillation detectors coupled to photomultiplier tubes (Fig. 45.6b). The light signal produced in the

scintillation detectors decays with characteristic times ranging from 40–300 ns depending on the detector scintillation material.

- After energy discrimination (between ~370 keV and ~650 keV, depending on the scintillating material), a detected photon (single) that qualifies as an annihilation γ-ray is time stamped. A coincidence event is registered by identifying detectors that count a single energy-qualifying photon within a "coincidence window" of 10–20 ns. Thus each coincidence event is assigned to a particular line of response (LOR) which is the volume spanned by a pair of coincidence detectors (Fig. 45.6d).

PET Data Corrections and Image Reconstruction

- The finite processing time (dead time) associated with the detection of a γ-ray results in loss of coincidence events. Known relationships between measured and true events are used to estimate true count rates from the detected ones (TOWNSEND 2004, 2006; STEVEN and BADAWI 2004; CHERRY et al. 2003).
- Accidental ("randoms") coincidences result from separate electron-positron annihilation events when the photons originating in such events are registered in the coincidence window (Fig. 45.7). Since these events are temporarily uncorrelated, their number is estimated in a delayed coincidence window in which there are no true coincidence events. The random coincidence correction is a subtraction of the delayed-window counts from the coincidence window counts corrects for each LOR (TOWNSEND 2004, 2006; STEVEN and BADAWI 2004; CHERRY et al. 2003).
- Non-uniform response of the detector elements results in different LOR count rates for the same activity. For each LOR, the raw count rates are corrected by normalization factors estimated by scanning a positron-emitting source that exposes the detector pairs to uniform photon flux.
- When an annihilation γ-ray is scattered, a coincidence event is registered in a misplaced LOR (Fig. 45.7) if the γ-ray falls within the energy discrimination window. Such scatter events result in image quality deterioration manifested in diffuse background counts. Scatter correction is build via scatter models into the reconstruction process (STEVEN and BADAWI 2004).

Table 45.1. Some radioisotopes for PET imaging

Isotope	Half life (h)	Decay mode abundance (%)	Maximum β + energy (keV)	Mean β + energy (keV)
^{11}C	0.34	β + (99.8%)	960.2	385.6
^{13}N	0.17	β + (99.8%)	1198.4	491.8
^{15}O	0.03	β + (99.9%)	1731.9	735.3
^{18}F	1.83	β + (96.7%)	633.5	249.8

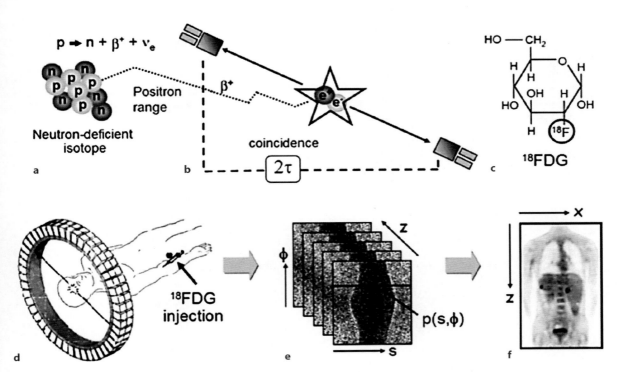

Fig. 45.6a–f. The principles of PET imaging shown schematically: (**a**) the decay of a neutron-deficient, positron emitting isotope; (**b**) the detection in coincidence of the annihilation photons within a time window of 2 (10–20 ns); (**c**) the glucose analogue deoxyglucose labeled with the positron emitter ^{18}F to form the radiopharmaceutical FDG; (**d**) the injection of the labeled pharmaceutical and the detection of a pair of annihilation photons in coincidence by a multi-ring PET camera. A line of response is shown; (**e**) the collection of the positron annihilation events into sinograms wherein each element of the sinogram contains the number of annihilations in a specific projection direction; and (**f**) a coronal section of the final, reconstructed whole-body image mapping the utilization of glucose throughout the patient. [Reproduced from TOWNSEND (2006) with permission]

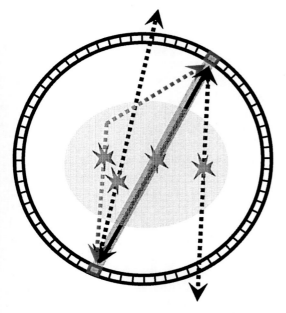

Fig. 45.7. True coincidence (*solid black*), random coincidence (*dotted black*), and scatter coincidence (*dotted red*) events assigned to one and the same line of response (*thick red line*)

- Annihilation events in a particular spatial location result in different coincidence counts along different LORs because the photon flux attenuation varies from LOR to LOR. The attenuation factor is given by $\exp(-\int_{0}^{L} \mu(x, y)dl)$ which measures the total attenuation at 511 keV along a LOR of length L. The attenuation corrections are derived either from transmission scans employing a single radioactive source (Cs-137 or Ge-68) or from attenuation maps reconstructed from the 3D dataset provided by the CT scanner in a PET/CT system (STEVEN and BADAWI 2004).

- PET image reconstruction is based on iterative algorithms that refine estimates of the activity distribution by optimizing a target function which incorporates models of the data acquisition process, statistical noise models and prior constraints such as the non-negativity of the count values (BOELLAARD et al. 2001; HUDSON and LARKIN 1994; RIDDELL et al. 2001; CHERRY et al. 1992; YAO et al. 2000).

PET Image Content and Quantitation

- Reconstructed PET images represent count rate (counts per second, or cps) per voxel provided that PET raw data is corrected for deadtime, randoms, detector response, scatter, and attenuation.
- With the application of a measured system calibration factor given in (Bq/cc)/(cps/voxel), the PET images yield activity concentration $A(i,j,k)$ ($[A(i,j,k)]$=Bq/cc) for each voxel (i,j,k). The system calibration factor is determined by a PET scan of water-filled volume source with uniform activity concentration.
- Another clinically widely used representation of the activity concentration is the standard uptake value (SUV) which, under specific conditions, can approximate the net rate of radiotracer flux into the tissue (WEBER 2005). SUV is defined as:

$$SUV = \frac{decay\ corrected\ activity/tissue\ volume}{injected\ activity/body\ mass}$$

and measured in g/cc.

45.2.2 PET Performance Parameters

Spatial Resolution

- Positrons are emitted over a spectrum of kinetic energies with maximum energies ranging from 0.58 MeV to 1.73 MeV depending on the radioisotope. The finite travel range of positrons prior to annihilation degrades the spatial resolution by ~0.1 mm for F-18 and 0.5 mm for O-15 (LEVIN and HOFFMAN 1999, 2000).
- Non-colinearity of the annihilation photons results in blurring that depends on the PET scanner bore diameter. This spatial resolution degradation is about ~2 mm for an 80-cm bore scanner (ZANZONICO 2004; CHERRY et al. 2003).
- Finite detector size (~4–6×4–6×20–30 mm^3) and depth-of-interaction effects directly affect spatial resolution in radially dependent manner (CHERRY et al. 2003).
- The overall spatial resolution of last generation commercial whole-body PET scanners as measured by full width half maximum (FWHM) of the line spread function is in the range of 4 mm–8 mm (TERAS et al. 2007; SURTI et al. 2007; BETTINARDI et al. 2004).

Sensitivity

- System sensitivity is defined by the measured count rate per unit activity. It depends on two parameters. The first one is the scanner geometric efficiency as determined by the fraction of emitted photons striking the detector. The second one is the detector quantum detection efficiency as determined by the fraction of photons striking a detector that are stopped and counted by the detector. System sensitivity is a measure of the utilization of the injected activity for imaging.
- Representative value for last generation commercial whole-body PET scanners range between 3–7 cps/kBq (TERAS et al. 2007; SURTI et al. 2007; BETTINARDI et al. 2004).

Noise-Equivalent Count Rate (NECR)

- The noise-equivalent count rate (NECR) (NU2-2001, 2001) is defined as

$$NECR = \frac{T^2}{T + S + R}, \text{ where } T, S, \text{ and } R \text{ are True,}$$

scatter and random count rates.
- NECR provides a metrics for comparing different PET systems and acquisition modes by equating count rates to the count rate that would have resulted in the same signal-to-noise ratio in the data in the absence of randoms and scatter.

45.2.3 PET/CT Integration

System Description

- A PET/CT system integrates a CT scanner and a PET scanner via a common which transfers a subject between the imaging bores of axially aligned CT and PET scanners by simple linear motion (TOWNSEND and CHERRY 2001; TOWNSEND et al. 2003). The known couch positions during the CT and the PET scan form the basis for the hardware fusion between the PET and CT datasets (Fig. 45.8).
- Additional software integration incorporates CT data in the calculation of attenuation maps and other radiological properties necessary for the attenuation and scatter correction of the PET raw data (Fig. 45.9d).

Fig. 45.8. A hybrid PET/CT scanner. [Adapted from TOWNSEND (2006) with permission]

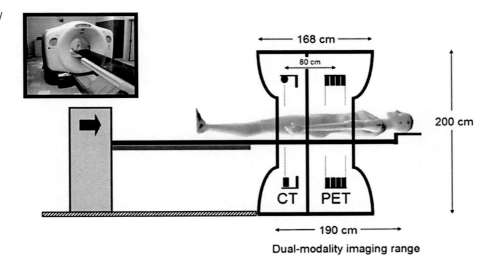

Fig. 45.9a–f. A typical imaging protocol for a combined PET/CT study that comprises (**a**) a topogram, or scout scan, for positioning; (**b**) a spiral CT scan; (**c**) a PET scan over the same axial range as the CT scan; (**d**) the generation of CT-based attenuation correction factors; (**e**) reconstruction of the attenuation-corrected PET emission data; and (**f**) display of the final fused images. [Reproduced from TOWNSEND (2006) with permission]

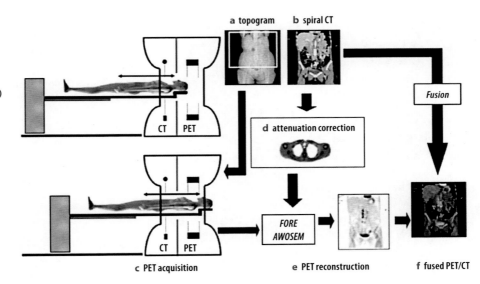

Clinical Advantages Over Independent PET and CT Scans

- PET/CT is a hardware-based image-fusion technology that virtually eliminates the uncertainty and inconvenience of the software fusion of separate PET and CT images, which are often acquired with the patients in different positions during the two exams. Thus the PET/CT improves the accuracy of the anatomical localization of the metabolic signal and therefore the physician confidence in making diagnostic and treatment decisions.
- Incorporation of CT attenuation maps reduces whole-body scan times by about 40% (TOWNSEND 2004).

- PET/CT is more convenient for the patient and the physician in comparison to a combination of separate PET and CT exams.

PET/CT Radiotherapy Simulator

- A PET/CT simulator is a PET/CT system with additional hardware and software components to enable radiation therapy simulation and planning based on CT-generated model of the patient anatomy and PET-generated models of biological processes.
- Hardware and software requirements with respect to the CT subsystem are equivalent to these for a CT simulator.

- A flat table top is necessary to reproduce the intended treatment position during radiation delivery.
- Depending on the design, the extended range of the patient support system (couch) can lead to couch flex between the PET and CT exams. This effect results in some uncertainty of the hardware fusion process.
- Localizing (movable) lasers are to be included for facilitating the radiation therapist with the patient setup and skin marks.
- Additional facilities such as injection/patient waiting room in the vicinity of the PET/CT room need to be available.

45.2.4 FDG Imaging

Underlying Mechanism

- By far the most commonly used radiotracer for diagnosis, staging, detection of recurrent disease and monitoring of cancer therapy is the fluorine-labeled glucose analog [^{18}F]2-fluoro-2-deoxy-D-glucose (FDG, shown in Fig. 45.6c) (FLETCHER et al. 2008; KRAUSE et al. 2007).
- Once inside a cell, FDG is phosphorylated to FDG-6-phosphate but it is not metabolized beyond this step because of the fluorine substitution in the molecule (REIVICH et al. 1979).
- Compared to normal tissues many tumors are characterized by glucose avidity (WARBURG 1956) which results in preferential uptake of FDG and therefore in elevated accumulation of the emitter activity imaged by PET.

Imaging Protocol

- Patients are instructed to have no caloric intake for at least 4 h before imaging.
- FDG activity of about 5 MBq per kilogram of body weight is administered, with typical values ranging between 370 MBq and 740 MBq.
- During a tracer uptake phase lasting between 45–120 min the patient sits in a quiet resting room.
- After the uptake phase, the patient is placed on the PET/CT table in a comfortable position that allows the entire anatomy of interest to be captured in the CT reconstruction field-of-view. This minimizes errors in CT-based PET attenuation correction (NESTLE et al. 2006). A topogram

(scout)view is acquired to determine the extent of the PET/CT scan (Fig. 45.9a–f.a).
- The patient is instructed to hold their breath at end tidal volume or breathe shallowly to minimize the mismatch between the PET and the CT data.
- A spiral CT dataset is acquired followed by a PET scan (Fig. 45.9a–f.a,b). PET images are reconstructed with and without CT attenuation correction. The latter set of images facilitate interpreting and resolving ambiguities resulting from CT attenuation corrections in the presence of CT contrast, CT truncation artifacts, and metal implants (NESTLE et al. 2006).

Image Interpretation Principles

- Increased blood glucose level prior to scanning results in lower FDG uptake.
- Increased tracer uptake time results in increased FDG uptake.
- Imaged maximum activity concentration is markedly underestimated when significantly different uptake occurs across spatial scales smaller than twice the PET resolution. Examples are small lesions and large tumors with necrotic centers and thin viable rims.
- Visualization interpretation of lesion size depends on the display window-level settings.

45.2.5 4D PET

Description and Clinical Application

- 4D PET imaging refers to PET imaging techniques that allow the acquisition of respiratory-correlated scans (NEHMEH et al. 2002, 2003; KLEIN et al. 1998; HUESMAN et al. 1997, 1998; LI et al. 2006b; THORNDYKE et al. 2006).
- The most common solutions gated PET acquisition and list mode acquisition with retrospective reconstruction (NEHMEH et al. 2002, 2003; KLEIN et al. 1998; HUESMAN et al. 1997, 1998).
- A 4D PET scan allows: (i) evaluation of the pattern and magnitude of the internal motion, and (ii) better estimation of the maximum activity uptake because of the elimination of motion blurring.

Acquisition and Reconstruction

- For gated PET acquisition mode, patient setup proceeds in the same manner as an un-gated PET one.

- For systems with an optical respiratory trace monitor, an infrared camera tracks a reflecting block placed on the patient abdomen (Fig. 45.4.).
- An acquisition trigger is set by the user to occur at some given point (e.g., end inspiration) in the respiratory cycle. When this point is detected by the optical tracking system, a trigger is sent to the scanner and data accumulation is initiated.
- In gated mode, the user selects both the width of the acquisition window and the number of sequential bins to be recorded within each respiratory cycle. The bin width directly affects image quality, since the signal-to-noise ratio within an image asymptotically approaches the square root of the signal level. Multiple bin acquisition allows capture of the full respiratory cycle in several bins, offering the possibility of retrospectively sorting into two or more respiratory phases.
- Each time a trigger is received, data is directed to the initial bin, and then to the remaining bins sequentially until the next trigger. This process continues for the duration of the scan.

45.2.6 Quality Assurance and Radiation Safety

- The quality assurance program for the CT subsystem of a PET/CT scanner needs to target the minimum standards for dose and image quality established by the ACR Computed Tomography Accreditation Program.
- Quality assurance guidelines covering radiation and patient safety, electromechanical components, as well as imaging performance provided in an AAPM report by Task Group 66 (MUTIC et al. 2003) for CT simulators are applicable to PET/CT simulators as well.
- The quality assurance program for the PET subsystem of a PET/CT scanner needs to target the minimum standards established by the ACCR Accreditation of Nuclear Medicine and PET Imaging Departments Program with respect to performance testing and quality control (MACFARLANE 2006).
- Compliance with radiation safety standards needs to be observed including adequate shielding of PET/CT facilities. Guidelines for shielding of PET/CT facilities are discussed in an AAPM report by Task Group 108 (MADSEN et al. 2006).

45.3 Magnetic Resonance Imaging

45.3.1 Physical Basis and Instrumentation

- Most MRI techniques involve generation and manipulation of bulk magnetization of soft tissue water protons within a given voxel through use of radio-frequency (RF) radiation and magnetic fields (MCROBBIE 2007). Magnitude, relaxation, and resonance properties of this bulk magnetization can be interrogated by MR to serve as contrast generating mechanism. RF signal generated by temporally changing bulk magnetization is detected, digitized, and processed in order to reconstruct the MR images.
- The major components of an MRI system include: (1) magnetically shielded main magnet with a static field strength between 0.2–3 Tesla (T) in order to generate bulk net magnetization along the magnetic field direction; (2) gradient-coils creating linear variations of the main magnetic field with maximum gradient values between 10–50 mT/m in order to spatially encode the bulk magnetization; (3) a radiofrequency system with a transmitting coil to tip the bulk magnetization away from the static magnetic field direction and receiving coils to detect the radiofrequency signal resulting from the temporal variations of the bulk magnetization (OPPELT 2006; MCROBBIE 2007).
- With a patient positioned within the main magnetic field, a typical MR acquisition protocol involves a sequence of gradient coil and transmitter coil activations along with RF signal detection by the receiving coils. In addition to the magnitude, relaxation, and resonance properties of the bulk magnetization, timing and order of coil activations and readout significantly influence the MR signal (WESTBROOK et al. 2005).

45.3.2 MRI Radiotherapy Applications

- Typical MR protocols include several sequences to generate images that are weighted with respect to proton density and tissue (magnetization) spin-lattice (T_1) and spin–spin (T_2) relaxation times (VILLEIRS and DE MEERLEER 2007; JENKINSON et al. 2007).

- MRI provides superior soft tissue discrimination, especially for CNS structures (JENKINSON et al. 2007; HENSON et al. 2005) and within the abdomen and pelvis (VILLEIRS and DE MEERLEER 2007; KHOO and JOON 2006).
- Fast MRI can be used for imaging temporal variations of the anatomy to design appropriate motion management strategies in the course of radiotherapy (CHAN et al. 2008; PLATHOW et al. 2006; KAUCZOR and PLATHOW 2006).
- MRI is typically employed together with CT images with the help of image fusion software to delineate the extent of the malignancy. Incorporation of MR for the delineation of target volumes requires proper accounting for MR system and object-induced distortions, as well as anatomy variations resulting from differences between the MR and CT imaging setups.

45.4 Outlook

45.4.1 CT and CBCT

- CT scanners with very large numbers of detector rows (256 or more) are becoming available that may enable 4D CT imaging of adequate anatomical extents without external respiratory signal. With proper imaging dose management, true anatomy motion evaluation even in the presence of irregular breathing patterns may be possible.
- Dual X-ray source scanners are being commercialized (ENGEL et al. 2008; FLOHR et al. 2006; McCOLLOUGH et al. 2008b; YAN et al. 2006). These may offer the opportunity for radiotherapy relevant tissue characterization by dual-energy volumetric imaging.
- 4D CBCT is being developed to obtain phase resolved volumetric images that eliminate motion artifacts. This can improve image interpretation and localization accuracy prior to treatment delivery (DIETRICH et al. 2006; HARSOLIA et al. 2008; LI et al. 2006a,c, 2007, 2008; LI and XING 2007; LU et al. 2007; PURDIE et al. 2006; RIT et al. 2005; SONKE et al. 2005, 2008).

45.4.2 PET/CT

- A number of radiotracers are being investigated as agents for imaging biological processes and microenvironment parameters of interest to radiotherapy: proliferation, hypoxia, apoptosis, and angiogenesis [NIMMAGADDA et al. (2008) and references therein].
- Fast scintillation detectors and new reconstruction algorithms are being pursued to enable time-of-flight PET imaging that will potentially improve image quality and PET quantification (KARP et al. 2008; SURTI et al. 2006, 2007).

45.4.3 MRI

- Dynamic contrast enhanced MRI (DCE-MRI) is being actively explored as a predictor of tumor response to radiotherapy [ZAHRA et al. (2007) and references therein].
- Magnetic resonance spectroscopy (MRS) is a focus of investigations as a potential tool for treatment planning and treatment response evaluation in brain tumors and prostate cancer [PAYNE and LEACH (2006) and references therein].
- Available open-bore (>70 cm) MR systems outfitted with MR compatible flat table tops and laser systems may be adopted as dedicated MR simulators.

References

Bettinardi V, Danna M, Savi A et al. (2004) Performance evaluation of the new whole-body PET/CT scanner: discovery ST. Eur J Nucl Med Mol Imaging 31:867–881

Boellaard R, Van Lingen A, Lammertsma AA (2001) Experimental and clinical evaluation of iterative reconstruction (OSEM) in dynamic PET: quantitative characteristics and effects on kinetic modeling. J Nucl Med 42:808–817

Chan P, Dinniwell R, Haider MA et al. (2008) Inter- and intrafractional tumor and organ movement in patients with cervical cancer undergoing radiotherapy: a cinematic-MRI point-of-interest study. Int J Radiat Oncol Biol Phys 70:1507–1515

Cherry SR, Dahlbom M, Hoffman EJ (1992) Evaluation of a 3D reconstruction algorithm for multi-slice PET scanners. Phys Med Biol 37:779–790

Cherry SR, Phelps ME, Sorenson JA (2003) Physics in nuclear medicine. Saunders, Philadelphia

Coolens C, Childs PJ (2003) Calibration of CT Hounsfield units for radiotherapy treatment planning of patients with metallic hip prostheses: the use of the extended CT-scale. Phys Med Biol 48:1591–1603

Dietrich L, Jetter S, Tucking T, Nill S, Oelfke U (2006) Linac-integrated 4D cone beam CT: first experimental results. Phys Med Biol 51:2939–2952

Engel KJ, Herrmann C, Zeitler G (2008) X-ray scattering in single- and dual-source CT. Med Phys 35:318–332

Fletcher JW, Djulbegovic B, Soares HP et al. (2008) Recommendations on the use of 18F-FDG PET in oncology. J Nucl Med 49:480–508

Flohr TG, Mccollough CH, Bruder H et al. (2006) First performance evaluation of a dual-source CT (DSCT) system. Eur Radiol 16:256–268

Gayou O, Miften M (2007) Commissioning and clinical implementation of a mega-voltage cone beam CT system for treatment localization. Med Phys 34:3183–192

Harsolia A, Hugo GD, Kestin LL et al. (2008) Dosimetric advantages of four-dimensional adaptive image-guided radiotherapy for lung tumors using online cone-beam computed tomography. Int J Radiat Oncol Biol Phys 70:582–589

Henson JW, Gaviani P, Gonzalez RG (2005) MRI in treatment of adult gliomas. Lancet Oncol 6:167–175

Hudson HM, Larkin RS (1994) Accelerated image reconstruction using ordered subsets of projection data. IEEE Trans Med Imaging 13:601–609

Huesman RH, Klein GJ, Reutter BW (1997) Respiratory compensation in cardiac PET using doubly-gated acquisitions. J Nucl Med 38:426–426

Huesman RH, Klein GJ, Reutter BW et al. (1998) List mode data acquisition for retrospective respiratory-cardiac gated PET. J Nucl Med 39:93p–93p

Jaffray DA, Siewerdsen JH (2000) Cone-beam computed tomography with a flat-panel imager: initial performance characterization. Med Phys 27:1311–1323

Jenkinson MD, Du Plessis DG, Walker C, Smith TS (2007) Advanced MRI in the management of adult gliomas. Br J Neurosurg 21:550–561

Karp JS, Surti S, Daube-Witherspoon ME, Muehllehner G (2008) Benefit of time-of-flight in PET: experimental and clinical results J Nucl Med 49:462–470

Kauczor HU, Plathow C (2006) Imaging tumour motion for radiotherapy planning using MRI. Cancer Imaging 6:S140–144

Keall PJ, Starkschall G, Shukla H et el. (2004) Acquiring 4D thoracic CT scans using a multislice helical method. Phys Med Biol 49:2053–2067

Keall PJ, Mageras GS, Balter JM et al. (2006) The management of respiratory motion in radiation oncology report of AAPM Task Group 76. Med Phys 33:3874–3900

Khoo VS, Joon DL (2006) New developments in MRI for target volume delineation in radiotherapy. Br J Radiol 79 Spec No 1: S2–15

Klein GJ, Reutter BW, Ho MH, Reed JH, Huesman RH (1998) Real-time system for respiratory-cardiac gating in positron tomography. IEEE Transactions on Nuclear Science 45:2139–2143

Kleshneva T, Muzik J, Alber M (2006) An algorithm for automatic determination of the respiratory phases in four-dimensional computed tomography Phys Med Biol 51:N269–276

Krause BJ, Beyer T, Bockisch A et al. (2007) [FDG-PET/CT in oncology. German Guideline]. Nuklearmedizin 46:291–301

Kubo HD, Hill BC (1996) Respiration gated radiotherapy treatment: a technical study. Phys Med Biol 41:83–91

Kupelian PA, Ramsey C, Meeks SL et al. (2005) Serial megavoltage CT imaging during external beam radiotherapy for non-small-cell lung cancer: observations on tumor regression during treatment. Int J Radiat Oncol Biol Phys 63:1024–108

Langen KM, Meeks SL, Poole DO et al. (2005a) The use of megavoltage CT (MVCT) images for dose recomputations. Phys Med Biol 50:4259–4276

Langen KM, Zhang Y, Andrews RD et al. (2005b) Initial experience with megavoltage (MV) CT guidance for daily prostate alignments. Int J Radiat Oncol Biol Phys 62:1517–1524

Letourneau D, Martinez AA, Lockman D et al. (2005) Assessment of residual error for online cone-beam CT-guided treatment of prostate cancer patients. Int J Radiat Oncol Biol Phys 62:1239–1246

Letourneau D, Keller H, Sharpe MB, Jaffray DA (2007) Integral test phantom for dosimetric quality assurance of image guided and intensity modulated stereotactic radiotherapy. Med Phys 34:1842–1849

Levin CS, Hoffman EJ (1999) Calculation of positron range and its effect on the fundamental limit of positron emission tomography system spatial resolution. Phys Med Biol 44:781–799

Levin CS, Hoffman EJ (2000) Calculation of positron range and its effect on the fundamental limit of positron emission tomography system spatial resolution (vol 44, p 781, 1999). Phys Med Biol 45:559–559

Li T, Xing L (2007) Optimizing 4D cone-beam CT acquisition protocol for external beam radiotherapy. Int J Radiat Oncol Biol Phys 67:1211–1219

Li T, Schreibmann E, Thorndyke B, Tillman G, Boyer A, Koong A, Goodman K, Xing L (2005) Radiation dose reduction in 4D computed tomography. Med Phys 32:3650–3660

Li T, Schreibmann E, Yang Y, Xing L (2006a) Motion correction for improved target localization with on-board cone-beam computed tomography. Phys Med Biol 51:253–267

Li T, Thorndyke B, Schreibmann E, Yang Y, Xing L (2006b) Model-based image reconstruction for four-dimensional PET. Med Phys 33:1288–1298

Li T, Xing L, Munro P, Mcguinness C, Chao M, Yang Y, Loo B, Koong A (2006c) Four-dimensional cone-beam computed tomography using an on-board imager. Med Phys 33:3825–3833

Li T, Koong A, Xing L (2007) Enhanced 4D cone-beam CT with inter-phase motion model. Med Phys 34:3688–3695

Li G, Citrin D, Camphausen K, Mueller B et al. (2008) Advances in 4D medical imaging and 4D radiation therapy. Technol Cancer Res Treat 7:67–81

Lu J, Guerrero TM, Munro P et al. (2007) Four-dimensional cone beam CT with adaptive gantry rotation and adaptive data sampling. Med Phys 34:3520–3529

Macfarlane CR (2006) ACR accreditation of nuclear medicine and PET imaging departments. J Nucl Med Technol 34:18–24

Madsen MT, Anderson JA, Halama JR et al. (2006) AAPM Task Group 108: PET and PET/CT shielding requirements. Med Phys 33:4–15

Mao W, Lee L, Xing L (2008) Design of multi-purpose phantom and automated software analysis tool for quality assurance of onboard kV/MV imaging system. Med Phys 35:1497–1506

Mccollough C, Cody D, Edyvean S, Geise R, Gould G (2008a) The measurement, reporting, and management of radiation dose in CT. American Association of Physicists in Medicine, College Park, MD

Mccollough CH, Schmidt B, Yu L et al. (2008b) Measurement of temporal resolution in dual source CT. Med Phys 35:764–768

McRobbie DW (2007) MRI from picture to proton. Cambridge University Press, Cambridge, UK, New York

Meeks SL, Harmon JF Jr, Langen KM et al. (2005) Performance characterization of megavoltage computed tomography imaging on a helical tomotherapy unit. Med Phys 32:2673–2681

Moseley DJ, White EA, Wiltshire KL et al. (2007) Comparison of localization performance with implanted fiducial markers and cone-beam computed tomography for online image-guided radiotherapy of the prostate. Int J Radiat Oncol Biol Phys 67:942–953

Mutic S, Palta JR, Butker EK et al. (2003) Quality assurance for computed-tomography simulators and the computed-tomography-simulation process: report of the AAPM Radiation Therapy Committee Task Group No. 66. Med Phys 30:2762–2792

Nehmeh SA, Erdi YE, Ling CC et al. (2002) Effect of respiratory gating on quantifying PET images of lung cancer. J Nucl Med 43:876–881

Nehmeh SA, Erdi YE, Rosenzweig KE et al. (2003) Reduction of respiratory motion artifacts in PET imaging of lung cancer by respiratory correlated dynamic PET: methodology and comparison with respiratory gated PET. J Nucl Med 44:1644–1648

Nestle U, Kremp S, Grosu AL (2006) Practical integration of [18F]-FDG-PET and PET-CT in the planning of radiotherapy for non-small cell lung cancer (NSCLC): the technical basis, ICRU-target volumes, problems, perspectives. Radiother Oncol 81:209–225

Nimmagadda S, Ford EC, Wong JW, Pomper MG (2008) Targeted molecular imaging in oncology: focus on radiation therapy. Semin Radiat Oncol 18:136–148

Nu2-2001 NSP (2001) Performance measurement of positron emission tomographs. National Electrical Manufacturers' Association (NEMA), Washington, DC

Ohara K, Okumura T, Akisada M, Inada T, Mori T, Yokota H, Calaguas MJ (1989) Irradiation synchronized with respiration gate. Int J Radiat Oncol Biol Phys 17:853–857

Oppelt A (2006) Imaging systems for medical diagnostics: fundamentals, technical solutions and applications for systems applying ionizing radiation, nuclear magnetic resonance and ultrasound. Publicis Corporate Publishing, Erlangen

Pan T, Lee TY, Rietzel E, Chen GT (2004) 4D-CT imaging of a volume influenced by respiratory motion on multi-slice CT. Med Phys 31:333–340

Payne GS, Leach MO (2006) Applications of magnetic resonance spectroscopy in radiotherapy treatment planning. Br J Radiol 79 Spec No 1:S16–26

Plathow C, Hof H, Kuhn S et al. (2006) Therapy monitoring using dynamic MRI: analysis of lung motion and intrathoracic tumor mobility before and after radiotherapy. Eur Radiol 16:1942–1950

Pouliot J, Bani-Hashemi A, Chen J et al. (2005) Low-dose megavoltage cone-beam CT for radiation therapy. Int J Radiat Oncol Biol Phys 61:552–560

Purdie TG, Moseley DJ, Bissonnette JP et al. (2006) Respiration correlated cone-beam computed tomography and 4DCT for evaluating target motion in stereotactic lung radiation therapy. Acta Oncol 45:915–922

Reivich M, Kuhl D, Wolf A et al. (1979) The [18F]fluorodeoxyglucose method for the measurement of local cerebral glucose utilization in man. Circ Res 44:127–137

Riddell C, Carson RE, Carrasquillo JA et al. (2001) Noise reduction in oncology FDG PET images by iterative reconstruction: a quantitative assessment. J Nucl Med 42:1316–1323

Rietzel E, Chen GT, Choi NC, Willet CG (2005a) Four-dimensional image-based treatment planning: target volume segmentation and dose calculation in the presence of respiratory motion. Int J Radiat Oncol Biol Phys 61:1535–1550

Rietzel E, Pan T, Chen GT (2005b) Four-dimensional computed tomography: image formation and clinical protocol. Med Phys 32:874–889

Rit S, Sarrut D, Ginestet C (2005) Respiratory signal extraction for 4D CT imaging of the thorax from cone-beam CT projections. Med Image Comput Comput Assist Interv Int Conf Med Image Comput Comput Assist Interv 8:556–563

Sonke JJ, Zijp L, Remeijer P, Van Herk M (2005) Respiratory correlated cone beam CT. Med Phys 32:1176–1186

Sonke JJ, Lebesque J, Van Herk M (2008) Variability of four-dimensional computed tomography patient models. Int J Radiat Oncol Biol Phys 70:590–598

Sprawls P (1992) AAPM tutorial. CT image detail and noise. Radiographics 12:1041–1046

Steven RM, Badawi RD (2004) Quantitative techniques in PET. In: Valk P, Bailey D, Townsend DW, Michael M (eds) Positron emission tomography: basic science and clinical applications. Springer, London

Surti S, Karp JS, Popescu LM et al. (2006) Investigation of time-of-flight benefit for fully 3-D PET. IEEE Trans Med Imaging 25:529–538

Surti S, Kuhn A, Werner ME et al. (2007) Performance of Philips Gemini TF PET/CT scanner with special consideration for its time-of-flight imaging capabilities. J Nucl Med 48:471–840

Teras M, Tolvanen T, Johansson JJ et al. (2007) Performance of the new generation of whole-body PET/CT scanners: discovery STE and Discovery VCT. Eur J Nucl Med Mol Imaging 34:1683–1692

Thorndyke B, Schreibmann E, Koong A et al. (2006) Reducing respiratory motion artifacts in positron emission tomography through retrospective stacking. Med Phys 33:2632–2641

Townsend DW (2004) Physical principles and technology of clinical PET imaging. Ann Acad Med Singapore 33:133–145

Townsend D (2006) Basic science of PET and PET/CT. Positron emission tomography. Springer, London

Townsend DW, Cherry SR (2001) Combining anatomy and function: the path to true image fusion. Eur Radiol 11:1968–1974

Townsend DW, Beyer T, Blodgett TM (2003) PET/CT scanners: a hardware approach to image fusion. Semin Nucl Med 33:193–204

Underberg RW, Lagerwaard FJ, Cuijpers JP et al. (2004) Four-dimensional CT scans for treatment planning in stereotactic radiotherapy for stage I lung cancer. Int J Radiat Oncol Biol Phys 60:1283–1290

Underberg RW, Lagerwaard FJ, Slotman BJ et al. (2005) Use of maximum intensity projections (MIP) for target volume generation in 4DCT scans for lung cancer. Int J Radiat Oncol Biol Phys 63:253–260

Vedam SS, Keall PJ, Kini VR, Mohan R (2001) Determining parameters for respiration-gated radiotherapy. Med Phys 28:2139–2146

Vedam SS, Keall PJ, Kini VR et al. (2003) Acquiring a four-dimensional computed tomography dataset using an external respiratory signal. Phys Med Biol 48:45–62

Villeirs GM, De Meerleer GO (2007) Magnetic resonance imaging (MRI) anatomy of the prostate and application of MRI in radiotherapy planning. Eur J Radiol 63:361–368

Warburg O (1956) On the origin of cancer cells. Science 123:309–314

Weber WA (2005) Use of PET for monitoring cancer therapy and for predicting outcome. J Nucl Med 46:983–995

Westbrook C, Kaut-Roth C, Talbot J (2005) MRI in practice. Blackwell Pub, Oxford, Malden, MA

White EA, Cho J, Vallis KA et al. (2007) Cone beam computed tomography guidance for setup of patients receiving accelerated partial breast irradiation. Int J Radiat Oncol Biol Phys 68:547–554

Wink NM, Chao M, Antony J, Xing L (2008) Individualized gating windows based on four-dimensional CT information for respiration-gated radiotherapy. Phys Med Biol 53:165–175

Wong JW, Sharpe MB, Jaffray DA et al. (1999) The use of active breathing control (ABC) to reduce margin for breathing motion. Int J Radiat Oncol Biol Phys 44:911–919

Xing L, Thorndyke B, Schreibmann E, Yang Y, Li TF, Kim GY, Luxton G, Koong A (2006): Overview of image-guided radiation therapy. Med Dosim 31:91–112

Yan M, Zhang C, Liang H (2006) A new scheme and reconstruction algorithm for dual source circular CT. Conf Proc IEEE Eng Med Biol Soc 1:3783–3786

Yao R, Seidel J, Johnson CA et al. (2000) Performance characteristics of the 3-D OSEM algorithm in the reconstruction of small animal PET images. Ordered-subsets expectation-maximization. IEEE Trans Med Imaging 19:798–804

Yoo S, Kim GY, Hammoud R et al. (2006) A quality assurance program for the on-board imagers. Med Phys 33:4431–4447

Zahra MA, Hollingsworth KG, Sala E et al. (2007) Dynamic contrast-enhanced MRI as a predictor of tumour response to radiotherapy. Lancet Oncol 8:63–74

Zanzonico P (2004) Positron emission tomography: a review of basic principles, scanner design and performance, and current systems. Semin Nucl Med 34:87–111

The Technical Infrastructure of a
Modern Radiation Oncology Department

Xiaodong Wu

Introduction and Objectives

The style of radiation therapy practice has evolved drastically since the early days when the field was first established. The technical advancement has played a decisive role in this evolution. Whatever the changes might have been, the objective remains the same: to eradicate tumors and to eliminate all cells in the regions at risk with minimized normal tissue toxicity. All along, this objective has been the guiding principle in the progress of radiation therapy. The clinical and technical aspects of radiation oncology equally govern the structure of its operation. In this chapter, we briefly update our readers on the current technical status in a rather general form and then postulate in some detail the configuration of a typical radiation therapy center – albeit small in size, the principles demonstrated throughout can be easily generalized.

The objective of the chapter was conceived with the intention to help the readers gain a wider perspective of the radiation therapy practice and therefore examines:

● The current available imaging technologies in radiation therapy
● Treatment planning, delivery, and informatics systems
● Configuration of a modern radiation therapy facility
● Issues of staffing and clinical operation

46.1 A Brief Overview of the Current Technical Status

46.1.1 Imaging Technologies in Radiation Therapy

Images for Treatment Planning

■ CT scanners are now considered part of the essential components in a modern radiation therapy department. CT images are generally the primary imaging modality for delineating treatment tar-

X. Wu, PhD
Department of Radiation Oncology, University of Miami,
1475 N.W. 12th Avenue, Miami, FL 33136, USA

gets, defining critical structures, and for dose computation, while other imaging modalities (MRI, PET, ultrasound, MRSI, etc.) have been used (through fusions) in most of the treatment-planning systems to further enhance the accuracy in targets and critical structure delineation. There is good indication that multiple-slice 4D CT would soon become standard, as the 4D radiation therapy may soon take center stage.

Image-Guided Treatment Delivery

■ Following the rapid adoption of advanced imaging technologies for treatment planning, the technologies of image guidance for treatment delivery (IGRT) quickly emerged, with electronic portal imagers (EPID), ultrasound-based systems, kV X-ray- based radiographic setup systems (CyberKnife by Accuray Inc., ExacTrac by BrainLab), CT-based IGRT systems (in-room CT configuration, Tomotherapy unit, on-board kV cone-beam CT and MV cone-beam CT) sequentially coming into prime application (DAWSON and JAFFRAY 2007). The implementation of the volumetric image acquisition during treatment makes it possible for the adaptive radiation therapy (modifying dose plan based on daily acquired volumetric images) with desirable frequency.

Target Motion Management

■ Tumor motion management has been part of the IGRT effort (KEALL et al. 2006). The first generation of tumor motion management utilizes passive methods, which include respiratory gating and active breathing control (breath-hold). Neither technique involves directly quantitative acquisition of target position or active radiation beam tracking to follow the target motion in real-time. Active or dynamic motion management (real-time or near real-time targeting) involves both direct tumor-motion monitoring and active beam targeting. The current commercially available active-targeting system is the Accuray's CyberKnife, an image-guided robotic radiosurgery system, which has both static, periodic beam correction and continuous respiratory tracking (Synchrony, Accuray Inc., Sunnyvale, CA). Synchrony provides real-time radiation beam targeting for tumors that move in relation to respiration. In Synchrony the target position is periodically localized by radiographic images and correlated to the respiratory motion moni-

tored by an optical system comprising a camera and light beacons affixed to the patient's chest wall. This correlation is represented by a mathematical model to proactively project the target location and instruct the robot-mounted linac to follow the tumor motion during beam-on time. Active or real-time beam tracking is markedly more difficult for gantry-mounted linacs. The general approaches are dynamic MLC-based beam tracking, or treatment couch-based motion compensation. Real-time tumor motion monitoring can now be achieved by the Calypso 4D Localization System (Calypso Medical, Inc., Seattle, WA) using non-ionizing electromagnetic guidance. Active motion management capabilities for gantry-mounted linacs are expected to be commercially available in the near future. The final solution for the tumor motion management will include both geometric and dosimetric corrections for the tumor deformation. 4D-CT acquisition with information synchronization during treatment delivery will be indispensable in this endeavor.

46.1.2 Radiation Delivery Systems

External Beam Radiation Therapy System

■ From its early commercial introduction in the late 1960s, linear accelerators (linac) providing MV X-rays and electron beams with a sufficiently wide range of energy selections have undergone remarkable improvement. All linacs manufactured are now providing a fully computer-controlled user interface, built-in beam shaping systems (MLC), built-in image-guided setup systems of different kinds (EPID and on-board imager, or OBI), and respiratory gating systems of different kinds. At the present time, the treatment using MV X-rays and electron beams is still the primary modality of external-beam radiation therapy. The successful introduction and implementation of intensity-modulated radiation therapy (IMRT) marked the quantum leap in photon-based radiation treatment. As the crowning technical achievement, IMRT provides flexibility of achieving the most complex dose distribution ever imagined (BOYER et al. 2001). It should be commemorated that the "Peacock" of the binary IMRT system by NOMOS was the first deliverable IMRT system. The binary configuration of the IMRT system underwent immediate development into a dedicated IMRT/IGRT machine known as the Tomotherapy unit (MACKIE et al. 1999). All modern linacs are now capable of delivering IMRT using either binary MLC or conventional dynamic MLC. The present ongoing development of the IMRT has been focused on both a better optimization algorithm and the faster treatment-delivery mechanism with a minimal amount of MUs. Some recent developments show promise of an aperture-modulated dynamic arc (or volumetric-modulated arc known as VMAT) as the solution to deliver a complex IMRT plan at high speed (CROOKS et al. 2003). Both Varian and Elekta have announced the availability of such a product.

Intra-operative Radiotherapy (IORT)

■ IORT with high-energy electron beam has proven to be beneficial for a number of clinical indications. Traditionally, IORT was performed using a conventional linac with special IORT cone applicators. The patient was transported from the operating room to the linac treatment room, which was sterilized prior to receiving the patient. A large fractional dose (15–20 Gy) was then delivered to the treatment site with the direct interface through the IORT cone applicator. Many centers are now using a dedicated portable IORT linac, which can be transported to the OR and administers the dose on-site (Mobetron by IntraOp Medical). A more recent development involves the use of low energy (up to 50 kV) X-ray source (Intrabeam by Carl Zeiss Meditec). The introduction of mobile IORT systems significantly improves the practicality and efficiency of IORT (BEDDAR et al. 2006; VAIDYA et al. 2002).

Radiosurgery Systems

■ Contrary to most people's perception of being a modern development, radiosurgery indeed bears its unique path of history as long and glorious as conventional radiation therapy. The first full-scale successful radiosurgery system is the Leksell GammaKnife, which took its final shape in the late 1960s. Its successful clinical utilization had established the concrete notion and foundation for intracranial radiosurgery and radiosurgery in general. Following its success, a number of modified linac-based systems have been developed since the 1980s. Although the latest models of a conventional linac from the three major vendors (Varian, Elekta, and Siemens) all claim their abilities to deliver radiosurgery, there are a number of systems that are considered specialized for radiosurgery. They are Elekta's GammaKnife, Accuray's CyberKnife, BrainLab's Novalis and OUR's Rotating Gamma Unit (and its modified models). A parallel development using proton beams, although small in number, has demonstrated equal clinical efficacy with greater dose sparing capability.

■ The goal of radiosurgery is to administer an ablative dose without damaging the surrounding normal tissue and thus achieve complete or much higher local control compared with conventional radiotherapy. The unique physical characteristics of radiosurgery are: high precision (sub-millimeter), highly-focused dose distribution (about a 10% dose fall-off per millimeter outside the treatment margin), and high dose (10 Gy and higher) (PHILLIPS et al. 1994). It should be noted that the term "stereotactic" has always been attached to radiosurgery. The modern IGRT treatments are in fact all stereotactic (3D) in nature. The differences are in the implication of accuracy.

■ The concept of intracranial radiosurgery was first applied to other body sites in the early 1990s using modified conventional linacs. The introduction of the dedicated radiosurgery systems (such as Accuray's CyberKnife and BrainLab's Novalis) has widened the application in this avenue, most noticeably from the early 2000s. Clinical efficacy has been well demonstrated (KAVANAGH and TIMMERMAN 2004). Due to the fact that most of these treatments were carried out in more than one fraction, the term SBRT (stereotactic body radiotherapy) was introduced, despite the fact that the fractional dose is comparable to that of the traditional intracranial radiosurgery. While the term SBRT has gained wide adoption, it should be remembered that the essential difference between radiotherapy and radiosurgery lies in the fractional-dose size which leads to their different therapeutic effects – as a result of different radiobiological effects. The term stereotactic only indicates the method of target localization.

■ The stereotactic localization methods vary among different delivery systems. For intracranial indications, both frame-based and image-guided, frameless approaches are equally effective, with the frameless approach being more patient-friendly and easier for a fractionated scheme. For body radiosurgery, image-guidance, with or without radio-opaque fiducial markers, is essential.

■ It has been recognized from the outset that tumor motion in body radiosurgery presents a serious challenge. Different approaches have been employed to minimize the motion-related errors. For tumors that move with a respiratory cycle, gating, shallow breathing, breath-hold, or real-time active beam tracking by robotic linac are used in different settings. A proper treatment margin should be used based on the tumor geometric uncertainties anticipated with different motion-management techniques.

■ Due to its nature of having highly-focused dose distribution, radiosurgery can be a good alternative for brachytherapy in certain indicated areas. As an example, clinical trials have been established to administer hypofractionated treatment (for example 725 cGy × 5) for early-stage prostate cancer, as a similar approach to the HDR monotherapy.

Brachytherapy Systems

■ Both LDR and HDR, permanent or temporary implants are still active parts in the field of radiation therapy. Image-based planning has become standard for brachytherapy, replacing the rather historical dose template methods. Brachytherapy delivery also enjoys the advances of image-guided technology. The technical advancements of brachytherapy are reflected in both general instrumental innovations and site-specific development. The following are some observations of the current status of brachytherapy:

■ Remote after-loading systems (HDR or LDR) have a strong tendency of replacing the manual-loading applications. Even the systems for prostate permanent-seed implants are evolving with increasing automation.

■ The brachytherapy approach of partial breast irradiation (PBI) has matured on both forms of the MammoSite balloon technique and multi-catheter technique with an HDR-delivery method.

■ Brachy-embolization for treatment of hepatic tumors using yttrium-90 beta microspheres has been introduced clinically (www.nordion.com; www.sirtex.com).

■ The multiple-source HDR unit is commercially available, which can potentially achieve more flexible and complex isodose distributions (www.isodosecontrol.com).

■ An electronic brachytherapy system has been developed for clinical use that utilizes a miniature X-ray source (50 kV) instead of radioactive material. The system can potentially offer greater flexibility in carrying out brachytherapy procedures due to the simplified requirement for protection (www.xoftinc.com).

Particle Beam Therapy

■ As IMRT marks the crowning achievement of photon-based external-beam radiation therapy, the next step of improving physical-dose distribution naturally points to the heavy-charged particle beams, of which Robert Wilson foresaw the application of Bragg peak in radiation therapy in 1946 (WILSON 1946).

■ The first hospital-based proton therapy facility, Loma Linda Proton Treatment Center, was operational in 1990. At the present time there are six operational proton facilities in the US and about 25 worldwide. There are a dozen more centers currently in planning or under construction. Despite its unique advantage of physical dose distribution, proton beam treatment is not considered as the ultimate, all-inclusive radiation treatment modality. Clinical indications are often focused on well-localized tumors or benign conditions that are more radioresistant for conventional photon treatment. The noted particle therapy vendors are IBA, Varian, Siemens, Hitachi, and Optivus.

■ There had been none to few clinical trials performed prior to the full clinical implementation of proton beam therapy, due to the fact that the therapeutic proton beam has similar RBE as photons. Most of the proton treatment regimens follow the data established from photon beam clinical trials. Similar to IMRT, proton beam therapy is taken as an advance in pure physical dose distribution. The implication of a higher RBE with heavier ion beams has stimulated intense international interest in heavier ion beam. There are currently four carbon-12 ion beam therapy facilities operational worldwide (two in Japan, two in Germany). There has been interesting and encouraging clinical data indicating the potential clinical advantages of using carbon-12 and other heavy ion beams (SCHULZ-ERTNER and TSUJII 2007). However, unlike the situation for proton beam therapy, more systemic clinical trials are called for to arrive at conclusive evidence and guidelines for heavier ion beam therapy due to the insufficiently-known radiobiological complexity to date.

46.1.3 Treatment Planning Systems

- Full 3D dose computation capability is now a common standard for major treatment-planning systems. Convolution-superposition has been the most widely used 3D dose computation algorithm with heterogeneity correction using the 3D CT data set. One can optimistically expect that a full Monte Carlo dose computation engine will soon become the gold standard which will offer the platform for dose computation with ultimate accuracy. The current commercially-available systems using the Monte Carlo method include the Peregrine from NOMOS (Sewickley, PA), the Multiplan from Accuray (Sunnyvale, CA), and the Eclipse from Varian (Palo Alto, CA).

- Algorithms for IMRT inverse planning have been constantly investigated by researchers for better efficiency. Combined with rapidly improved computer hardware, the inversed planning time for IMRT has been significantly shortened. It should be understood that the delivery system would ultimately dictate the limit in the advancement of the IMRT planning algorithm. The current efforts from gantry-mounted linac vendors of delivering TOMO-like IMRT seem to point to the aperture-modulated arc therapy (AMAT) or volumetric-modulated arc therapy (VMAT) as mentioned earlier. VMAT in theory could deliver very complex IMRTs in a very short time (less than 4 min following the treatment setup for an H&N case). This places demands, higher than ever before, on the mechanical performance and the accelerator output control.

46.1.4 Guidance of Radiobiology in Radiation Therapy

- Radiation therapy was initiated shortly after the discovery of X-ray and radioactive radium, with intuitive perception of the biological effects. Quantitative studies quickly followed and the field of radiobiology was established. The principles derived primarily from laboratory research and the biological insights, such as the "Four Rs", combined with carefully developed mathematical models (FOWLER 1992) have served as a guiding light for establishing clinical trials that have led to most of the quantitative treatment protocols – forming evidence-based clinical practice.

- Extensive efforts have been put forth for quantitative analysis to guide treatment planning. Although provisional in essence, they provide indispensable margins and fences protecting one from wandering too far into danger.

- Radiobiology also leads the field to explore new types of radiation that would give better therapeutic gain. The early attempts of neutron therapy and the more recent efforts of heavier (compared with proton) ion beam therapy have all been results inspired by the radiobiology initiative.

- One can envision that modern radiobiology would ultimately integrate with imaging technologies, providing heterogeneous information on cancer cells and direct more efficient dose-targeting that would lead to markedly improved clinical outcomes.

46.1.5 Informatics in Radiation Therapy

- The practice of radiation oncology has also benefited greatly from the advancement of computer hardware and the software industry. Electronic record and verification systems have become standard components in all modern linacs. A complete electronic management system for a radiation oncology department, integrating complete medical records, image management, scheduling, and billing has become readily available and has been adopted in ever more centers. The high-speed connectivity between image acquisition, treatment planning, plan transfer (to linac), and final treatment delivery not only improves the efficiency of the whole process, it also eliminates much of the potential operator-related errors. The easily available internet services allow efficient intra- and inter-institutional medical record and image transfer. Remote planning and plan review/ evaluation can also be easily done. This leads to the recently merged practice of centralized treatment planning. Caution, however, should be exercised in order to maintain close interaction between physician, physicist, and dosimetrist, thereby ensuring that quality patient care is not compromised. In general, the development and implementation of modern informatics have profoundly changed the management and practice of radiation therapy.

46.2 Configuration of a Radiation Therapy Facility

- The practice of radiation oncology defined itself and developed into a distinct discipline in the 1980s. A radiation therapy program can be configured in many different ways based on the operational objectives. A comprehensive radiation therapy department could include all treatment modalities. However, only a well-developed academic department would have an integrated radiobiology program.

- Currently, external-beam radiation therapy with high-energy photon and electron beams makes up the major portion of all radiation therapy patients. Indications for brachytherapy are selective and site-specific, such as a GYN implant with LDR or HDR, partial breast irradiation (PBI) with HDR, prostate seed implant, Y-90 microsphere liver implant, etc. The treatment modalities that are considered less conventional include radiosurgery, intra-operative radiation therapy (IORT), proton or heavier ion beam therapy, neutron therapy, hyperthermia, photodynamic therapy, radiofrequency ablation, and high-intensity focused ultrasound ablation, etc., which make up approximately 10%–15% of all the radiation therapy population. Notice that some of these "nonconventional" treatment modalities fall into the category of non-ionizing radiation, and ultrasound is naturally not radiation. Nevertheless, they all involve the process of energy deposition as the therapeutic mechanisms. Therefore they are natural extensions of the domain in which radiation oncologists and medical physicists are practicing.

- Although some radiation therapy procedures would always require hospital services, the majority of radiation treatments are done as outpatient procedures. The nature of outpatient services has resulted in the merging of many free-standing radiation therapy centers with one or two linacs and sometimes with a remote after-loading HDR brachytherapy unit. The "non-conventional" treatment modalities are mostly available in hospital-based radiation therapy departments or free-standing specialty centers such as particle therapy centers or radiosurgery centers.

- Planning a comprehensive radiation therapy program involves extensive work. The general principles are commonly derived from the Blue Book (ISCRO 1991) and the ACR standards (AMERICAN COLLEGE OF RADIOLOGY 1995). One must bear in mind that the modern technical developments had not been fully anticipated in the earlier writings. One should always orient his/her judgment according to the latest developments. However complicated it might be, an example of constructing a small-scale modern radiation therapy center could offer much insight that may well be suited to an "evidence-based" discussion. For many radiation oncologists, such an approach might be more informative for grasping the infrastructure of a functional radiation therapy program. In light of this, the following describes the making of: *A typical functional radiation therapy department with a single linac and an HDR brachytherapy unit.*

46.2.1 Operation Objectives

- Single linac to accommodate up to 40 external-beam treatments/day, with an occasional stereotactic hypo-fractionation treatment.
- A remote after-loading HDR unit to perform outpatient oriented brachytherapy procedures (between one and five procedures/day). It should be noted that such an HDR addition would not necessarily alter much of the manpower structure.
- Complete electronic operation with a comprehensive network platform to facilitate: (1) an all-inclusive treatment management connectivity between CT scanner, treatment-planning system, treatment delivery systems (linac and HDR unit), and on-board imaging system for setup and verification; (2) integrated electronic charting system including medical record management, treatment parameters management, patient scheduling, and electronic billing; (3) office management, and (4) high-speed internet connection.

46.2.2 Staffing

- Radiation oncologist: 2
- Medical physicist: 1 FTE + locum availability
- Dosimetrist: 1 FTE + locum availability
- Radiation therapist: 3 (including the chief therapist)

- Nurse/PA: 2
- Receptionist: 1
- Billing manager: 1
- Operation manager: 1
- IT support: Outsourced
- Equipment support: Outsourced
- Cleaning service: Outsourced

46.2.3 Equipment

- Linac:
- Dual photon energies, multiple electron energies, Dynamic MLC (0.5/1.0 cm resolution), IMRT, EPID, kV-OBI/CBCT, stereotactic (tight spec) option.
- HDR:
- Single Ir-192, or multiple-source after-loader.
- The device can be housed in the linac vault (cost effective). However, a dedicated vault is desirable for optimal throughput (exchange for additional cost). Since the CT room has lower occupancy, it is an ideal location to house the HDR unit.
- Electronic brachytherapy system with a soft X-ray source can be considered, since the procedures can be performed in a regular exam room. However, the X-ray energy of the current system may not be suited for the cases in which deeper penetration is desired.
- CT Scanner:
- A multiple-slice CT simulator with gating interface.
- Treatment planning system:
- Full-capacity external-beam/brachytherapy RT planning system.
- DICOM connections to receive images from the in-house CT, linac's CBCT, and from outside imaging centers, to directly transfer planning parameters to the record/verification electronic charting system.
- Remote planning capability, allowing physicians, physicists and dosimetrists to review and participate in the planning process remotely.
- Physics equipment:
- Water-phantom scanner.
- Calibration ion chambers, electrometer.
- Machine periodic QA devices (for linac, HDR and imaging systems).
- Safety survey meter.
- Patient-specific QA device (in-vivo dosimetry; IMRT QA device).

- Treatment aids:
- Fixation device/system.
- Mold room equipment (additional ventilation is usually required for a mold room).
- Additional aids, such as eye shield, bolus material, etc.
- Exam room:
- Standard medical exam room equipment.
- Electronic charting:
- Patient database management.
- Medical records management.
- Prescription/clinical treatment plans.
- Record/verification-linac interface.
- Image application/archiving management system.
- Departmental computer network:
- Network equipment.
- Computer servers.
- Office management software.
- Billing system.
- Internet/phone service.

46.2.4 Space Program

- In most cases, un-limited space is not a likely scenario. An economic space design is generally called for. Figure 46.1 demonstrates a practical space program designed for this operation, with typical dimensions. It shows that a 5000 sq. ft. footage can serve the operation well.
- For a radiation oncology department, the treatment vault occupies a significant portion of the space. High-density concrete or special shielding blocks with a direct-entry door is a good option to minimize the space required for shielding, and is adopted in this example. The linac size should be part of the initial consideration (without compromising functionalities), as different linac models have different space requirements. In this example, the vault is designed for a Varian Trilogy Silhouette linac. It should be stressed that the shielding design forms a subspecialty in medical physics. There are, in reality, very limited opportunities for every qualified physicist to become well-versed in shielding design. Contracting a reputable shielding expert is highly recommended.
- Additional space would certainly make way for a more luxurious layout. Less footage would require further optimization of space usage so that a normal operational work-flow is still attainable.

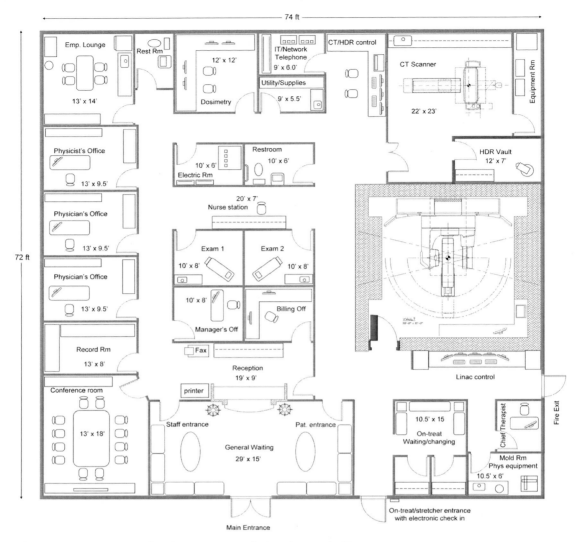

Fig. 46.1. Space program of a 1-linac, 1-HDR radiation therapy facility

- A conventional simulator is not included in the operational planning. The simulation and initial setup will be performed with linac's EPID and OBI.
- Notice that there is no dark room for film development as all image modalities are handled electronically. In case of the need for film dosimetry, GAFChromic films can be used.
- In this design, all environment-control equipment (air-conditioning units, etc.) are suspended above the ceiling finishes.
- The design shows that the operational traffic is well-differentiated. The clinical area and the office area are optimally partitioned without affecting easy access to both sides. A separate entrance allows daily entry for on-treat patients with personalized electronic check-in cards.

46.2.5 Essential Elements of the Initiative Team

- Just like every other established discipline, the advancement of radiation therapy practice also leads to internal differentiation into subspecialties: clinical, technical, and administrative. To warrant the successful development of an operation, resources must be placed effectively. The following are considered essential, although different in the level of involvement, for the initiation of the program:
- Radiation oncologist (medical director)
- Medical physicist
- Financial consultant
- Legal consultant

IT services: For any modern radiation oncology department, an efficient IT configuration is indispensable, professional IT services should be contracted to work with the initiators to design the network layout. A realistic network diagram for this demonstrative project is shown in Figure 46.2.

Project manager: A person who is experienced in the construction of a radiation therapy center. To contract such a person to oversee the project development is desirable if the initiators are not experienced in building such a center or are too busy to be involved in the ongoing progress of the project.

Architect: A qualified architectural firm or engineer with experience in radiation therapy installation is crucial and is the central element of the project, one who will integrate all necessary sources to direct the construction. Based on the preliminary space program with specific equipment installation information, including the shielding calculation (needs to be reiterated several times between the physicist and the architect to work out all details), a final architect plan is generated. After being reviewed by the physician and the physicist to ensure correct functionality of all areas, the plan is submitted for the approval by the proper regulatory body.

General contractor: The entity responsible for building the facility is contracted to work under the direction of the architect. A construction time-line is drawn and the work underway.

46.2.6 Clinical Operation

Prior to operation, a proper radiation machine license and radioactive material license must be obtained.

A radiation safety program must be developed by the physicist.

A comprehensive policy and procedure manual should be formulated.

Typical length for physicist(s) to commission such a center is 3–4 weeks. Due to the rapid merging and implementation of new technologies, in order to maximally and optimally utilize the lat-

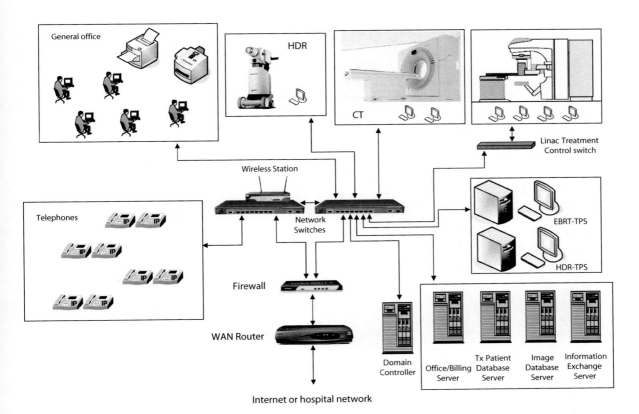

Fig. 46.2. Network scheme

est technologies, a rigorous training program for technical staff should be carefully planned and given prior to the operation.

■ An ongoing educational/training program is also essential, as many new technologies will take time to mature. It should be noted that many skills we are now comfortable with have been as the result of many people's cumulative experience over many years. We are now exposed to an increasing number of new procedures associated with the new technologies. The things for which we have now been trained or taught do not necessarily bear the same benefit as the long and cumulative experience. For many new procedures, we have not yet arrived at their optimal protocols. For example, opinion is still split regarding the optimal ratio between the cone-beam CT setup and orthogonal kV radiographic setup. Likewise, the definitions of 4D treatment also vary – they differ not because of the disagreement, but because of varying perspective and focus.

■ Standard clinical flow can be found in many good reference sources. The flow chart presented in Figure 46.3 reflects the influence of the new technologies. A modern radiation therapy center could follow this chart with different efficiency levels at different stages of the process/cycle, depending on the hardware in use, the clinical decisions, and the technical operation philosophy.

46.3 Final Remarks

■ It is worth noting that most of the decisive steps in the progress of modern radiation oncology were not met without skepticism, from the early implementation of dedicated CT simulators, 3D-CRT, MLC, IMRT, robotic radiosurgery, IGRT to the more-recent efforts in 4D-RT and particle beam therapy. The field of radiation oncology has been blessed and is indebted to those who have pioneered and ventured with conviction into new and better technologies. And the efforts of advancing the field will be continued, again, in three major directions: better accuracy

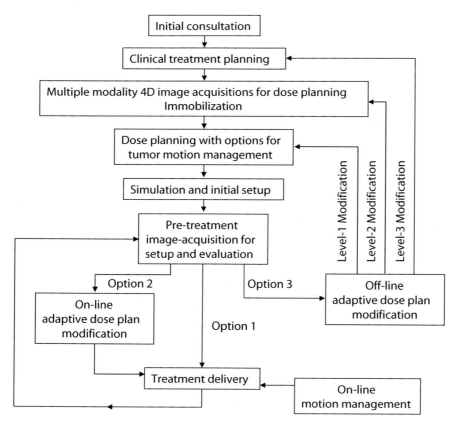

Fig. 46.3. A modern radiation therapy process

of dose targeting (in both target delineation and dose delivery), better physical-dose distribution using either a better algorithm or new radiation sources, and an enhanced radiobiological gain through cellular/genetic pathways or different radiation sources.

■ There is seemingly an underlying desire to create a super radiation machine that would cover all aspects of radiation therapy. This vision, however, has not yet been made reality. The statement made by Gilbert Fletcher in 1976, *"There is no alternative to electron beam therapy,"* still seems to hold true, not only for electron beam but also for other sub-branches in radiation therapy (FLETCHER 1976). Whether a stand-alone radiation therapy center or a full-scale institutional radiation therapy department, an objective evaluation of the equipment acquisition will determine its operational style and ultimately its success. The idea of a unifying super machine might be conceptually attractive; however, the optimal way of approaching it might not lie in the hope of a single machine, but rather a unified operational structure in which machineries are optimally specialized for individual treatment modalities and are effectively shared by a globally-integrated healthcare system. This might hold the key to the future technical advancement in our field.

■ The rate of technical advancement in our field has accelerated, which puts a growing demand on all of us to stay alert and informed, not only on what is new in our field but also on what is new out there that could impact the advancement of our field.

References

American College of Radiology (1995) ACR standards for radiation oncology. American College of Radiology, Reston, VA

Beddar A, Biggs P, Chang S et al. (2006) Intraoperative radiation therapy using mobile electron linear accelerators: report of AAPM Radiation Therapy Committee Task Group No. 72. Med Phys 33:1476–1489

Boyer A, Butler E, DiPetrillo A et al. (2001) Intensity-modulated radiotherapy: current status and issues of interest. Int J Radiat Oncol Biol Phys 51:880–914

Crooks S, Wu X, Takita C et al. (2003) Aperture modulated arc therapy. Phys Med Bio 48:1–12

Dawson L, Jaffray D (2007) Advances in image-guided radiation therapy. J Clin Oncol 25:938–946

Fletcher G (1976) Introduction. Clinical application of the electron beam. Wiley, New York

Fowler J (1992) Brief summary of radiobiological principles in fractionated radiotherapy. Semin Radiat 2:16–21

ISCRO (1991) Radiation oncology in integrated cancer management: report of the Inter-Society Council for Radiation Oncology (Blue book). American College of Radiology, Reston, VA

Kavanagh B, Timmerman R (2004) Stereotactic body radiation therapy. Lippincott Williams & Wilkins, Philadelphia

Keall P, Mageras G, Balter J et al. (2006) The management of respiratory motion in radiation oncology report of AAPM Task Group 76. Med Phys 33:3874–3900

Mackie T, Balog J, Ruchala K et al. (1999) Tomotherapy. Semin Radiat Oncol 9:108–117

Phillips M, Stelzer K, Griffin T et al. (1994) Stereotactic radiosurgery: a review and comparison of methods. J Clin Oncol 12:1085–1099

Schulz-Ertner D, Tsujii H (2007) Particle therapy using proton and heavier ion beams. J Clin Oncol 25:953–964

Vaidya J, Baum M, Tobias J, D'Suoza D (2002) The novel technique of delivering targeted intraoperative radiotherapy (Targit) for early breast cancer. Eur J Surg Oncol 28:447–454

Wilson R (1946) Radiological use of fast protons. Radiology 47:498–491

Appendix I: Performance Status Scales

ECOG Performance Status[a]

Grade	ECOG
0	Fully active, able to carry on all pre-disease performance without restriction
1	Restricted in physically strenuous activity but ambulatory and able to carry out work of a light or sedentary nature, e.g., light housework, office work
2	Ambulatory and capable of all self-care but unable to carry out any work activities. Up and about more than 50% of waking hours
3	Capable of only limited self-care, confined to bed or chair more than 50% of waking hours
4	Completely disabled. Cannot carry on any self-care. Totally confined to bed or chair
5	Dead

[a]As published in OKEN et al. (1982)

The Karnofsky Performance Scale Index allows patients to be classified according to their functional impairment. This can be used to compare effectiveness of different therapies and to assess the prognosis in individual patients. The lower the Karnofsky score, the worse the survival for most serious illnesses.

Karnofsky Performance Status Scale Definitions Rating (%) Criteria

Able to carry on normal activity and to work; no special care needed	100	Normal no complaints; no evidence of disease
	90	Able to carry on normal activity; minor signs or symptoms of disease
	80	Normal activity with effort; some signs or symptoms of disease
Unable to work; able to live at home and care for most personal needs; varying amount of assistance needed	70	Cares for self; unable to carry on normal activity or to do active work
	60	Requires occasional assistance, but is able to care for most of his personal needs
	50	Requires considerable assistance and frequent medical care
Unable to care for self; requires equivalent of institutional or hospital care; disease may be progressing rapidly	40	Disabled; requires special care and assistance
	30	Severely disabled; hospital admission is indicated although death not imminent
	20	Very sick; hospital admission necessary; active supportive treatment necessary
	10	Moribund; fatal processes progressing rapidly
	0	Dead

References

Brezinski D, Stone PH et al. (1991) Prognostic significance of the Karnofsky performance status score in patients with acute myocardial infarction: comparison of the left ventricular ejection fraction and the exercise treadmill test performance. Am Heart J 121:1374–1381

Crooks, V, Waller S et al. (1991) The use of the Karnofsky Performance Scale in determining outcomes and risk in geriatric outpatients. J Gerontol 46:M139–M144

de Haan R, Aaronson A et al. (1993) Measuring quality of life in stroke. Stroke 24:320–327

Hollen PJ, Gralla RJ et al. (1994) Measurement of quality of life in patients with lung cancer in multicenter trials of new therapies. Cancer 73:2087–2098

Oken MM, Creech RH, Tormey DC, Horton J, Davis TE, McFadden ET, Carbone PP (1982) Toxicity and response criteria of the Eastern Cooperative Oncology Group. Am J Clin Oncol 5:649–655

O'Toole DM, Golden AM (1991) Evaluating cancer patients for rehabilitation potential. West J Med 155:384–387

Schag CC, Heinrich RL, Ganz PA (1984) Karnofsky performance status revisited: reliability, validity, and guidelines. J Clin Oncology 2:187–193

Appendix II: Estimated Normal Tissue

Tolerance Dose to Conventionally Fractionated Radiation Oncology

Organ	TD5/5 (Gy) Volume of organ/tissue			TD50/5 (Gy) Volume of organ/tissue			Clinical end point
	3/3	2/3	1/3	3/3	2/3	1/3	
Bladder	65	80	N/A	80	85	N/A	Symptomatic bladder contracture and volume loss
Brachial plexus	60	61	62	75	76	77	Clinically apparent nerve damage
Brain	45	50	60	60	65	75	Necrosis/infraction
Brainstem	50	53	60	65	–	–	Necrosis/infraction
Cauda equina	60	–	–	75	–	–	Clinically apparent nerve damage
Colon	45	–	55	55	–	65	Obstruction, perforation, ulceration
Ear	30	30	30	40	40	40	Acute serous otitis
Ear	55	55	55	65	65	65	Chronic serous otitis
Esophagus (stricture, perforation)	55	58	60	68	70	72	Clinical stricture/perforation
Femoral head	52	–	–	65	–	–	Necrosis
Heart (pericarditis)	40	45	60	50	55	70	Pericarditis
Kidney	23	30	50	28	40	–	Clinical nephritis
Larynx	70	70	79	80	80	90	Cartilage necrosis
Larynx	45	45	–	80	–	–	Laryngeal edema
Lens	10	–	–	18	–	–	Cataract requiring intervention
Liver	30	35	50	40	45	55	Liver failure
Lung	17.5	30	45	24.5	40	65	Pneumonitis
Optic chiasm	50	–	–	65	–	–	Blindness
Optic nerve	50	50	50	65	–	–	Blindness
Parotid gland	32	32	–	46	46	–	Xerostomia
Rectum	60	–	–	80	–	–	Severe proctitis/necrosis/stenosis/fistula
Retina	45	–	–	65	–	–	Blindness
Rib cage	–	–	50	–	–	65	Pathologic fracture
Skin	(100cm^2) 5000	(30cm^2) 6000	(10cm^2) 7000	(100cm^2) 6500	–	–	Necrosis/ulceration
Spinal cord	(20 cm) 47	(10 cm) 50	(5 cm) 50	–	(10cm) 70	(5cm) 70	Myelitis/necrosis
Small intestine	40	–	50	55	–	60	Obstruction/perforation
Stomach	50	55	60	65	67	70	Ulceration/perforation
Temporomandibular joint and mandible	60	60	65	72	72	77	Marked limitation of the joint function
Thyroid	45	–	–	80	–	–	Clinical thyroiditis

Reference

Emami B, Lyman J, Brown A et al. (1991) Tolerance of normal tissue to therapeutic irradiation. Int J Radiat Oncol Biol Phys 21:109–122

Subject Index

List of Contributors

Andre A. Abitbol, MD
Department of Radiation Oncology
Baptist Hospital
8900 North Kendall Drive
Miami, FL 33176
USA
Email: AndreA@baptisthealth.net

Ron R. Allison, MD
Professor and Chairman
Department of Radiation Oncology
The Brody School of Medicine at ECU
600 Moye Blvd.
Greenville, NC 27834
USA
Email: allisonr@ecu.edu

Beatriz Amendola, MD, FACR
Innovative Cancer Institute
6141 Sunset Drive
Miami, FL 33143
USA
Email: dramendola@bellsouth.net

Michael F. Back, MD
Associate Professor of Radiation Oncology
Director and Senior Specialist
Department of Radiation Oncology
Northern Sydney Cancer Centre
Royal North Shore Hospital
St Leonards, NSW 2065
Australia
Email: mback@nsccahs.health.nsw.gov.au

Jonathan J. Beitler, MD, MBA, FACR
Professor of Radiation Oncology
Professor of Otolaryngology
Departments of Radiation Oncology
and Otolaryngology
Emory University School of Medicine
1365 Clifton Road NE
Atlanta, GA 30322-1013
USA
Email: jjbeitler@radonc.emory.org

Matthew Biagioli, MD, MS
Assistant Member, Chief of Brachytherapy
Division of Radiation Oncology
Department of Interdisciplinary Oncology
University of South Florida
12902 Magnolia Drive
Tampa, FL 33612-9416
USA

E. Brian Butler, MD
Department of Radiation Oncology
The Methodist Hospital
Cornell University/Weill Medical College
6565 Fannin St., DB1-077
Houston, TX 77030
USA

James S. Butler, MD
Department of Radiation Oncology
Maimonides Cancer Center
6300 Eighth Avenue
Brooklyn, NY 11020
USA
Email: jabutler@maimonidesmed.org

Luther W. Brady, MD
Professor, Hylda Cohn/American Cancer Society
Professor of Clinical Oncology, and
Professor, Department of Radiation Oncology
Drexel University College of Medicine
Broad & Vine Streets, Mail Stop 200
Philadelphia, PA 19102-1192
USA
Email: Luther.Brady@drexelmed.edu

Manjeet Chadha, MD
Associate Professor
Department of Radiation Oncology
Beth Israel Medical Center
10 Union Square East, Suite 4G
New York, NY 10003
USA
Email: mchadha@chpnet.org

Amy Y. Chen, MD, MPH
Associate Professor of Otolaryngology
Emory University School of Medicine
1365 Clifton Road NE
Atlanta, GA 30322-1013
USA
Email: achen@emory.edu

Wee Joo Chng, MD
Associate Professor and Consultant
Department of Hematology Oncology
National University Cancer Institute of Singapore
National University Health System
National University of Singapore
5 Lower Kent Ridge Road
Singapore 119074
Singapore
Email: mdccwj@nus.edu.sg

Walter H. Choi, MD
Department of Radiation Oncology
Beth Israel Medical Center
10 Union Square East, Suite 4G
New York, NY 10003
USA
Email: wachoi@chpnet.org

Hans T. Chung, MD, FRCPC
Consultant and Director of Postgraduate Research
Department of Radiation Oncology
National University Cancer Institute of Singapore
National University Health System
National University of Singapore
5 Lower Kent Ridge Road
Singapore 119074
Singapore
Email: Tse-Kan_Hans_Chung@nuh.com.sg

Jay S. Cooper, MD
Professor and Chairman
Department of Radiation Oncology
Maimonides Cancer Center
6300 Eighth Avenue
Brooklyn, NY 11220
USA
Email: jcooper@maimonidesmed.org

Bernadine R. Donahue, MD
Clinical Director, Department of Radiation Oncology
Maimonides Cancer Center
6300 Eighth Avenue
Brooklyn, NY 11220
USA
Email: bdonahue@maimonidesmed.org

Shen Fu, MD
Professor and Chairman
Department of Radiation Oncology
The 6th Hospital of Jiao Tong University
600 Yi Shan Road
Shanghai 200233
P.R. China
Email: shen_fu@hotmail.com

Hiram A. Gay, MD
Clinical Assistant Professor
Department of Radiation Oncology
The Brody School of Medicine at ECU
600 Moye Blvd.
Greenville, NC 27834
USA
Email: GAYH@ecu.edu

Iris C. Gibbs, MD
Associate Professor
Department of Radiation Oncology
Stanford University Medicine Center
875 Blake Wilbur Drive, MC 5847
Stanford, CA 94305-5847
USA
Email: iris.gibbs@stanford.edu

Stephanie C. Han, MD
Department of Radiation Oncology
Maimonides Cancer Center
6300 Eighth Avenue
Brooklyn, NY 11220
USA
Email: shan@maimonidesmed.org

Louis B. Harrison, MD
Professor and Chairman
Department of Radiation Oncology
Beth Israel Medical Center
10 Union Square East, Suite 4G
New York, NY 10003
USA

Georges F. Hatoum, MD
Assistant Professor
Department of Radiation Oncology
Sylvester Comprehensive Cancer Center
1475 NW 12th Avenue, D-31, Suite 1500
Miami, FL 33136
USA
Email: GHatoum1@med.miami.edu

JOSEPH M. HERMAN, MD, MSc
Assistant Professor of Radiation Oncology and
Molecular Sciences
Department of Radiation Oncology and
Molecular Radiation Sciences
Sidney Kimmel Comprehensive Cancer Center at
Johns Hopkins
401 N. Broadway Suite 1440
Baltimore, MD 21224
USA

Email: jherma15@jhmi.edu

DIMITRE HRISTOV, PhD
Assistant Professor
Department of Radiation Oncology
Stanford University School of Medicine
875 Blake Wilbur Drive
Stanford, CA 94305-5847
USA

Email:dimitre.hristov@stanford.edu

KENNETH HU, MD
Assistant Professor
Department of Radiation Oncology
Beth Israel Medical Center
10 Union Square East, Suite 4G
New York, NY 10003
USA

Email: khu@chpnet.org

BRADLEY J. HUTH, MD
Department of Radiation Oncology
Drexel University College of Medicine
216 N. Broad St.
1st Floor Feinstein Building
Mail Stop 200
Philadelphia, PA 19102-1192
USA

Email: bradley.huth@drexelmed.edu

ATIF J. KHAN, MD
Assistant Professor
Robert Wood Johnson Medical School-UMDNJ
Cancer Institute of New Jersey
195 Little Albany St.
New Brunswick, NJ 08901
USA

Email: atif.j.khan@gmail.com

FENG-MING (SPRING) KONG, MD, PhD, MPH
Chief, Radiation Oncology
Veteran Administration Health Center and University
Hospital Department of Radiation Oncology
University of Michigan
1500 E. Medical Center Drive
Ann Arbor, MI 48109
USA

Email: fengkong@med.umich.edu

LIN KONG, MD
Associate Professor
Department of Radiation Oncology
Cancer Hospital of Fudan University
270 Dong An Road
Shanghai 200032
P.R. China
E-mail: konglinj@gmail.com

KELLY LaFAVE, MD
Department of Radiation Oncology
Sylvester Comprehensive Cancer Center
University of Miami
1475 N.W. 12th Avenue, D-31
Miami, FL 33136
USA

EVAN M. LANDAU, MD
Department of Radiation Oncology
Montefiore Medical Center
111 East 210th Street
Bronx, NY 10467
USA

KHAI MUN LEE, MD
Senior Consultant and Chief
Department of Radiation Oncology
National University Cancer Institute of Singapore
National University Health System
National University of Singapore
5 Lower Kent Ridge Road
Singapore 119074
Singapore
Email: khai_mun_lee@nuh.com.sg

NANCY LEE, MD
Associate Attending
Department of Radiation Oncology
Memorial Sloan Kettering Cancer Center
1275 York Avenue, Box 22
New York, NY 10021
USA
Email: leen2@mskcc.org

Yexiong Li, MD
Professor and Chairman
Department of Radiation Oncology
Cancer Hospital, Chinese Academy of
Medical Sciences and Peking Union Medical College
P.O. Box 2258, Beijing 100021
P.R. China
Email: yexiong@yahoo.com

Jiade J. Lu, MD, MBA
Associate Professor and Consultant
Department of Radiation Oncology
National University Cancer Institute of Singapore
National University Health System
National University of Singapore
5 Lower Kent Ridge Road
Singapore 119074
Singapore
Email: jiade.lu.2005@anderson.ucla.edu
and
Distinguished Clinical Professor
Department of Radiation Oncology
Cancer Hospital of Fudan University
270 Dong An Road
Shanghai 200232
P.R. China

Arnold M. Markoe, MD
Professor and Chairman
Department of Radiation Oncology
Sylvester Comprehensive Cancer Center
University of Miami/Miller School of Medicine
1475 N.W. 12th Avenue, D-31
Miami, FL 33136
USA
Email: amarkoe@med.miami.edu

Vivek K. Mehta, MD
Swedish Cancer Institute
1221 Madison Street
Seattle, WA 98104
USA
Email: Vivek.Mehta@swedish.org

Subhakar Mutyala, MD
Director of Brachytherapy, Assistant Professor
Department of Radiation Oncology
Montefiore Medical Center
1665 Poplar St.
Bronx, NY 10461
USA
Email: smutyala@montefiore.org

Roger Ove, MD, PhD
Associate Professor
Department of Radiation Oncology
Leo Jenkins Cancer Center
The Brody School of Medicine at ECU
600 Moye Blvd.
Greenville NC, 27834
USA
Email: OVER@ecu.edu

Arnold C. Paulino, MD
Associate Professor
Department of Radiation Oncology
The Methodist Hospital
Cornell University/Weill Medical College
6565 Fannin St., DB1-077
Houston, TX 77030
USA
E-mail: apaulino@tmhs.org

Timothy M. Pawlik, MD, MPH
Assistant Professor, Surgery and Oncology
Division of Surgical Oncology at Johns Hopkins
600 N. Wolfe Street
Halsted 614
Baltimore, MD 21287
USA

José A. Peñagarícano, MD
Associate Professor
University of Arkansas for Medical Sciences
Department of Radiation Oncology
4301 W. Markham St. #771
Little Rock, AR 72205
USA
Email: PenagaricanoJoseA@uams.edu

Charles L. Perkins, MD, PhD
Assistant Professor
Department of Radiation Oncology
Emory University School of Medicine
1365 Clifton Road NE
Atlanta, GA 30322-1013
USA
Email: trey@radonc.emory.org

Vaneerat Ratanatharathorn, MD
Professor and Chairman
Winthrop P. Rockefeller Cancer Institute
4301 W. Markham St. #623
Little Rock, AR 72205
USA
Email: ratanatharathornvan@uams.edu

SCOTT G. SOLTYS, MD
Associate Professor
Department of Radiation Oncology
Stanford University Medicine Center
875 Blake Wilbur Drive, MC 5847
Stanford, CA 94305-5847
USA

MARNEE M. SPIERER, MD
Assistant Professor
Department of Radiation Oncology
Montefiore Medical Center
111 East 210th Street
Bronx, NY 10467
USA
Email: mspierer@montefiore.org

CRISTIANE TAKITA, MD
Assistant Professor
Department of Radiation Oncology
Sylvester Comprehensive Cancer Center
University of Miami Miller School of Medicine
1475 NW 12 Avenue, D-31, Suite 1500
Miami, FL 33136
USA

BIN S. TEH, MD
Professor
Department of Radiation Oncology
The Methodist Hospital
Cornell University/Weill Medical College
6565 Fannin St., DB1-077
Houston, TX 77030
USA
Email: BTeh@tmhs.org

B-CHEN WEN, MD
Professor, Department of Radiation Oncology
Sylvester Comprehensive Cancer Center
University of Miami
1475 NW 12th Avenue, D-31
Miami, FL 33136
USA
Email: bwen@med.miami.edu

AARON H. WOLFSON, MD
Professor and Vice Chair
Department of Radiation Oncology
University of Miami Miller School of Medicine
1475 NW 12th Avenue
Miami, FL 33136
USA
Email: awolfson@med.miami.edu

XIAODONG WU, PhD
Associate Professor and Chief
Division of Medical Physics
Department of Radiation Oncology
University of Miami
1475 N.W. 12th Avenue
Miami, FL 33136
USA
Email: XWu@med.miami.edu

LEI XING, PhD
Associate Professor
Department of Radiation Oncology
Stanford University School of Medicine
875 Blake Wilbur Drive
Stanford, CA 94305-5847
USA
Email: lei@reyes.stanford.edu

THEODORE E. YAEGER, MD
Associate Professor of Radiation Oncology
Director, Caldwell Memorial Hospital
321 Mulberry Street, SW
P.O. Box 1890
Lenoir, NC 28645
USA
Email: ted.yaeger@caldwell-mem.org

QING ZHANG, MD
Associated Professor
Department of Radiation Oncology
The 6th Hospital of Jiao Tong University
600 Yi Shan Road
Shanghai 200233
P.R. China
Email: zhangqingcyw@hotmail.com

ZHEN ZHANG, MD
Professor and Chairman
Department of Radiation Oncology
Cancer Hospital of Fudan University
270 Dong An Road
Shanghai 200232
P.R. China
Email: zhenzhang6@yahoo.com

MEDICAL RADIOLOGY Diagnostic Imaging and Radiation Oncology
Titles in the series already published

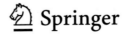

MEDICAL RADIOLOGY Diagnostic Imaging and Radiation Oncology

Titles in the series already published

Focal Liver Lesions
Detection, Characterization, Ablation
Edited by R. Lencioni, D. Cioni,
C. Bartolozzi

**Imaging in Treatment Planning
for Sinonasal Diseases**
Edited by R. Maroldi, P. Nicolai

Clinical Cardiac MRI
With Interactive CD-ROM
Edited by J. Bogaert, S. Dymarkowski,
A. M. Taylor

**Dynamic Contrast-Enhanced Magnetic
Resonance Imaging in Oncology**
Edited by A. Jackson, D. L. Buckley,
G. J. M. Parker

Contrast Media in Ultrasonography
Basic Principles and Clinical Applications
Edited by Emilio Quaia

Paediatric Musculoskeletal Disease
With an Emphasis on Ultrasound
Edited by D. Wilson

**MR Imaging in White Matter Diseases of the
Brain and Spinal Cord**
Edited by M. Filippi, N. De Stefano,
V. Dousset, J. C. McGowan

Imaging of the Hip & Bony Pelvis
Techniques and Applications
Edited by A. M. Davies, K. Johnson,
R. W. Whitehouse

Imaging of Kidney Cancer
Edited by Ali Guermazi

**Magnetic Resonance Imaging in
Ischemic Stroke**
Edited by R. von Kummer, T. Back

Diagnostic Nuclear Medicine
2nd Revised Edition
Edited by Christiaan Schiepers

**Imaging of Occupational and
Environmental Disorders of the Chest**
Edited by P. A. Gevenois, P. De Vuyst

Virtual Colonoscopy
A Practical Guide
Edited by P. Lefere, S. Gryspeerdt

Contrast Media
Safety Issues and ESUR Guidelines
Edited by H. S. Thomsen

Head and Neck Cancer Imaging
Edited by R. Hermans

Vascular Embolotherapy
A Comprehensive Approach
Volume 1: *General Principles, Chest,
Abdomen, and Great Vessels*
Edited by J. Golzarian. Co-edited by
S. Sun, M. J. Sharafuddin

Vascular Embolotherapy
A Comprehensive Approach
Volume 2: *Oncology, Trauma, Gene
Therapy, Vascular Malformations,
and Neck*
Edited by J. Golzarian. Co-edited by
S. Sun, M. J. Sharafuddin

Vascular Interventional Radiology
Current Evidence in Endovascular Surgery
Edited by M. G. Cowling

Ultrasound of the Gastrointestinal Tract
Edited by G. Maconi, G. Bianchi Porro

Parallel Imaging in Clinical MR Applications
Edited by S. O. Schoenberg, O. Dietrich,
M. F. Reiser

MRI and CT of the Female Pelvis
Edited by B. Hamm, R. Forstner

Imaging of Orthopedic Sports Injuries
Edited by F. M. Vanhoenacker,
M. Maas, J. L. Gielen

Ultrasound of the Musculoskeletal System
Edited by S. Bianchi, C. Martinoli

Clinical Functional MRI
Presurgical Functional Neuroimaging
Edited bei C. Stippich

**Radiation Dose from Adult and Pediatric
Multidetector Computed Tomography**
Edited by D. Tack, P. A. Gevenois

Spinal Imaging
*Diagnostic Imaging of the Spine and
Spinal Cord*
Edited by J. Van Goethem,
L. van den Hauwe, P. M. Parizel

Computed Tomography of the Lung
A Pattern Approach
Edited by J. A. Verschakelen,
W. De Wever

Imaging in Transplantation
Edited by A. Bankier

Radiological Imaging of the Neonatal Chest
2nd Revised Edition
Edited by V. Donoghue

**Radiological Imaging of the Digestive Tract
in Infants and Children**
Edited by A. S. Devos, J. G. Blickman

Pediatric Chest Imaging
Chest Imaging in Infants and Children
2nd Revised Edition
Edited by J. Lucaya, J. L. Strife

Color Doppler US of the Penis
Edited by M. Bertolotto

Radiology of the Stomach and Duodenum
Edited by A. H. Freeman, E. Sala

Imaging in Pediatric Skeletal Trauma
Techniques and Applications
Edited by K. J. Johnson, E. Bache

Image Processing in Radiology
Current Applications
Edited by E. Neri, D. Caramella,
C. Bartolozzi

**Screening and Preventive Diagnosis with
Radiological Imaging**
Edited by M. F. Reiser, G. van Kaick,
C. Fink, S. O. Schoenberg

**Percutaneous Tumor Ablation in
Medical Radiology**
Edited by T. J. Vogl, T. K. Helmberger,
M. G. Mack, M. F. Reiser

**Liver Radioembolization
with ⁹⁰Y Microspheres**
Edited by J. I. Bilbao, M. F. Reiser

Pediatric Uroradiology
2nd Revised Edition
Edited by R. Fotter

Radiology of Osteoporosis
2nd Revised Edition
Edited by S. Grampp

**Gastrointestinal Tract Sonography
in Fetuses and Children**
Edited by A. Couture, C. Baud,
J. L. Ferran, M. Saguintaah, C. Veyrac

**Intracranial Vascular Malformations and
Aneurysms**
2nd Revised Edition
Edited by M. Forsting, I. Wanke

**High-Resolution Sonography of the
Peripheral Nervous System**
2nd Revised Edition
Edited by S. Peer, G. Bodner

Imaging Pelvic Floor Disorders
2nd Revised Edition
Edited by J. Stoker, S. A. Taylor,
J. O. L. DeLancey

Coronary Radiology
2nd Revised Edition
Edited by M. Oudkerk, M. F. Reiser

Cardiothoracic Imaging with MDCT
Edited by M. Rémy-Jardin, J. Rémy

Multislice CT
3rd Revised Edition
Edited by M. F. Reiser, M. Takahashi,
M. Modic, C. R. Becker

MRI of the Lung
Edited by H.-U. Kauczor

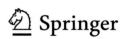

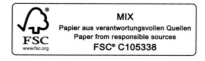
Printed by Books on Demand, Germany